Questions, Tricks, and Tips for the
ECHOCARDIOGRAPHY BOARDS

Second Edition

Questions, Tricks, and Tips for the
ECHOCARDIOGRAPHY BOARDS

Second Edition

Vincent L. Sorrell, MD, FACC, FACP, FASE

The Anthony N. DeMaria Chair in Cardiovascular Imaging
Professor of Medicine
Assistant Chief for the Division of Cardiovascular Medicine
Director of Cardiovascular Imaging
The Linda and Jack Gill Heart Institute
University of Kentucky
Lexington, Kentucky

Sasanka Jayasuriya, MBBS, FACC, FASE, FSCAI

Assistant Professor of Medicine
Section of Cardiovascular Medicine
Division of Medicine
Yale University School of Medicine
New Haven, Connecticut

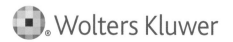

Philadelphia • Baltimore • New York • London
Buenos Aires • Hong Kong • Sydney • Tokyo

Acquisitions Editor: Sharon Zinner
Editorial Coordinator: Anne Seitz/Annette Ferran
Senior Production Project Manager: Alicia Jackson
Team Lead, Design: Stephen Druding
Senior Manufacturing Coordinator: Beth Welsh
Marketing Manager: Rachel Mante Leung
Production Service: SPi Global

Second Edition

Library of Congress Cataloging-in-Publication Data

Names: Sorrell, Vincent L., editor. | Jayasuriya, Sasanka, editor.
Title: Questions, tricks, and tips for the echocardiography boards / [edited by] Vincent L. Sorrell, Sasanka Jayasuriya.
Description: Second edition. | Philadelphia : Wolters Kluwer, [2019] | Includes bibliographical references and index.
Identifiers: LCCN 2018023919 | ISBN 9781496370297 (paperback)
Subjects: | MESH: Heart Diseases—diagnostic imaging | Ultrasonography | Echocardiography | Examination Questions
Classification: LCC RC683.5.U5 | NLM WG 18.2 | DDC 616.1/207543076—dc23 LC record available at
    https://lccn.loc.gov/2018023919

With this second edition, I am grateful for the many readers who have provided much feedback and support. Each and every one of you motivate me to continue to improve on this product. With the passing of time, some material becomes stale while much remains relevant. I am fortunate to work with so many outstanding University of Kentucky Imaging Specialists that were tasked with deciphering what material to replace. I am also grateful for the friendship, intelligence, and drive of my co-editor, Sasanka. She has become such a gifted cardiologist with many skills beyond echocardiography. Most important, I remain forever grateful to my family—my lovely wife, Amanda (Staffordshire Born & Bred); my beautiful daughter, Zoe (a musician through & through); and my son, Jack (making tomorrow a better place). Their love and support, encouragement, and subtle reminders of what's really important in life help me keep one eye on a career goal while fixing the other always on a life goal. I love you all! This edition is a culmination of many individual's dedication to education leaving me forever indebted to them. I hope that you find this material valuable to your education and use it to better care for your patients.

—VLS

Dedicated to my parents, Jayantha and Janes, who raised me with love, affection, and correct values in a beautiful rural Sri Lankan village; my husband, Aravinda, whose constant unwavering support, encouragement, and devotion to our children, Aneesha and Isha, that enabled me to commit long hours to complete this book; and to all the teachers, family, and friends who through the years wholeheartedly supported me in every step.

—SJ

Contributors to the First Edition

Aiden Abidov, MD, PhD, FACC, FAHA, FASE
Associate Professor, Medicine and Radiology
Division of Cardiology
Department of Medicine
The University of Arizona College of Medicine
Medical Director
Echocardiography/Cardiovascular Imaging
The University of Arizona Medical Center
Tucson, Arizona

Masood Ahmad, MD, FRCP(C), FACP, FACC, FAHA, FASE
Professor of Medicine, Director of Echocardiography Laboratory
Division of Cardiology
Department of Internal Medicine
University of Texas
Galveston, Texas

Mohamed Ahmed, MD
Postdoctoral Associate
University of Pittsburgh Medical Center
Heart and Vascular Institute
University of Pittsburgh
Pittsburgh, Pennsylvania

Andre Babak Akhondi, MD
Interventional Cardiology Fellow
Division of Cardiology
University of California
Los Angeles
Los Angeles, California

Edgar Argulian, MD, MPH
Attending Physician
Division of Cardiology
Department of Medicine
St. Luke's Roosevelt Hospital Center,
Mount Sinai Health Network
New York, New York

Reza Arsanjani, MD
Staff Physician
Department of Cardiology
Cedars Sinai Medical Center
Los Angeles, California

Ayman Haj Asaad, MD
Instructor Fellow
Division of Cardiovascular Disease
University of Alabama at Birmingham
Instructor Fellow
Division of Cardiovascular Disease
University of Alabama Hospital
Birmingham, Alabama

Robert Attaran, MD, FACC, FSCAI, FASE
Attending Cardiologist
Department of Cardiology
Aventura Hospital
Aventura, Florida

Alison L. Bailey, MD
Assistant Professor of Medicine
Gill Heart Institute
University of Kentucky
Lexington, Kentucky

Brent J. Barber, MD
Associate Professor
Section of Pediatric Cardiology
College of Medicine
University of Arizona
Tucson, Arizona

Daniel Berman, MD, FACC
Chief of Cardiac Imaging and Nuclear Cardiology
Medical Director, Artificial Intelligence in Medicine Program
Medical Director, Biomedical Research Institute
Cedars-Sinai Medical Center
West Hollywood, California
Professor of Imaging and Medicine
David Geffen School of Medicine
University of California, Los Angeles
Los Angeles, California

Louis I. Bezold, MD
Associate Professor and Vice-Chair
Department of Pediatrics
University of Kentucky College of Medicine
Enterprise Quality Director
Kentucky Children's Hospital
Lexington, Kentucky

Kunal Bodiwala, MD, FACC
Staff Cardiologist, Director of Cardiac Imaging
Advocate Medical Group
Illinois Heart and Lung
Normal, Illinois

Charles L. Campbell, MD
Associate Professor of Medicine
Division of Cardiovascular Disease
Department of Medicine
University of Kentucky Lexington
Veterans Administration Hospital
Lexington, Kentucky

Farooq A. Chaudhry, MD, FACP, FACC, FASE, FAHA
Professor of Medicine, Cardiology
Director, Echocardiography Laboratories
Associate Director, Mount Sinai Heart Network
Icahn School of Medicine at Mount Sinai
Zena and Michael A. Wiener Cardiovascular Institute
Marie-Josée and Henry R. Kravis Center for Cardiovascular Health
New York, New York

Andrew Cheng, MD
Acting Instructor/Senior Fellow
Department of Medicine
Division of Cardiology
University of Washington
Seattle, Washington

Patrick Collier, MD, PhD, FASE
Associate Staff Cardiologist
Robert and Suzanne Tomsich
Department of Cardiovascular Medicine
Cleveland Clinic Foundation
Cleveland, Ohio

Dennis M. Enomoto, MD, FACC
Staff Cardiologist
Division of Cardiology
Department of Medicine
St. Luke's Magic Valley Medical Center
Twin Falls, Idaho

Francesco F. Faletra, MD
Staff Cardiologist
Cardiocentro Ticino
University of Zurich
Lugano, Switzerland

Paul E. Fenster, MD, FACC
Associate Professor of Medicine
The University of Arizona College of
    Medicine
Tucson, Arizona

John Gorcsan III, MD
Professor of Medicine
University of Pittsburgh
Pittsburgh, Pennsylvania

Jeffrey K. Gregoire, RDCS, RRT
Technical Director, Outpatient
Echocardiography Lab
Department of Medicine
University of Arizona Medical Center
Tucson, Arizona

Brian Griffin, MD, FACC
Head, Imaging Section
Cardiovascular Medicine
Cleveland Clinic
Cleveland, Ohio

M. Reza Habibzadeh, MD
Staff Cardiologist
Carondelet Heart and Vascular Institute
St Mary's Hospital
Tucson, Arizona

Kamran Haleem, MD
Non-Invasive Cardiologist
Cardiovascular Medicine
Hudson Valley Heart Center
Poughkeepsie, New York

Arzu Ilercil, MD
Associate Professor of Medicine
Cardiovascular Sciences
University of South Florida
Staff Physician
Cardiovascular Disease
Tampa General Hospital
Tampa, Florida

Jooby John, MD, MPH, FACC, FSCAI
Staff Cardiologist
Cardiovascular Associates Inc.
Kissimmee, Florida

Elizabeth B. Juneman, MD
Associate Professor
Department of Medicine
University of Arizona
Director of Echocardiography
Department of Medicine
Southern Arizona VA Health Care
    System
Tucson, Arizona

Nishant Kalra, MD
Interventional Fellow
Cardiovascular Diseases
Gill Heart Institute
University of Kentucky
Lexington, Kentucky

Divya Kapoor, MD, FACC
Assistant Professor
Sarver Heart Center
University of Arizona
Director Tele-Cardiology Program
Cardiology Division
Southern Arizona VA Health Care
    System
Tucson, Arizona

Dalane W. Kitzman, MD
Professor of Internal Medicine
Section on Cardiology
Kermit G. Phillips, II Chair in
    Cardiology
Wake Forest School of Medicine
Winston-Salem, North Carolina

Scott Klewer, MD, FAAC
Professor
Chief, Division of Pediatric
    Cardiology
Peggy M. Barrett Endowed Chair for
    Congenital Heart Disease in
    Adults
Department of Pediatrics
The University of Arizona College of
    Medicine
Tucson, Arizona

Konstantinos P. Koulogiannis, MD
Associate Director, Cardiovascular Core
    Lab
Department of Cardiovascular
    Medicine
Morristown Medical Center
Gagnon Cardiovascular Institute
Morristown, New Jersey

**Itzhak Kronzon, MD, FASE, FACC,
FACP, FESC, FAHA**
Professor of Cardiology
Hofstra University
Chief
Non-Invasive Cardiac Imaging
North Shore-Long Island Jewish/
    Lenox
Hill Hospital
New York, New York

Daniela Lax, MD
Associate Professor
Department of Pediatrics (Section of
    Pediatric Cardiology)
University of Arizona
University of Arizona Medical Center
Tucson, Arizona

Kwan S. Lee, MD
Assistant Professor
Department of Cardiology
University of Arizona
Medical Director of Cardiology
Department of Cardiology
University of Arizona Medical Center
South Campus
Tucson, Arizona

**Steven J. Lester, MD, FACC,
FRCP(C), FASE**
Associate Professor of Medicine
Mayo Clinic College of Medicine
Scottsdale, Arizona

Rekha Mankad, MD, FACC
Instructor of Medicine
Division of Cardiovascular
Diseases
Mayo Clinic School of Medicine
Rochester, Minnesota

Sunil Mankad, MD, FACC, FASE
Associate Professor of Medicine
Director of Transesophageal
    Echocardiography
Associate Director, Cardiology
    Fellowship
Division of Cardiovascular Diseases
Mayo Clinic College of Medicine
Rochester, Minnesota

**Marti L. McCulloch, BS, MBA,
RDCS, FASE**
Director of Cardiovascular Imaging
Cardiovascular Imaging Section
Department of Cardiology
Houston Methodist DeBakey Heart and
    Vascular Center
Houston, Texas

**Mohamed Morsy, MD, FACC,
FASE, FACP**
Assistant Professor
Division of Cardiology
Department of Medicine
University of Texas Medical Branch
Galveston, Texas

Steven D. Mottl, BS, DO
Director of Non-Invasive Cardiology
The Heart Hospital
Baylor Denton
Denton, Texas

Navin C. Nanda, MD
Distinguished Professor of Medicine
    and Cardiovascular Disease
Director
Heart Station/Echocardiography
    Laboratories
University of Alabama at Birmingham
Birmingham, Alabama

Jacqueline A. Noonan, MD
Pediatric Cardiologist
UK Healthcare's Kentucky Children's
    Hospital
Professor Emeritus
Department of Pediatrics
University of Kentucky College of
    Medicine
Lexington, Kentucky

Natesa G. Pandian, MD, FACC
Professor, Tufts University School of
    Medicine
Director, Heart Valve Center
Co-Director, Cardiovascular Imaging
    Center
Director, Cardiovascular Ultrasound
    Research
Boston, Massachusetts

John P. Panidis, MD, FACC, FASE
Professor of Medicine
Department of Medicine
Temple School of Medicine
Attending
Department of Cardiology
Temple University Hospital
Philadelphia, Pennsylvania

Ayan R. Patel, MD
Professor
Department of Medicine
Tufts University School of Medicine
Director
Cardiovascular Imaging Center
The Cardiovascular Center
Tufts Medical Center
Boston, Massachusetts

Pravin Patil, MD
Assistant Professor of Medicine
Division of Cardiology
Temple University Hospital
Philadelphia, Pennsylvania

Dermot Phelan, MD, PhD
Cardiologist
Cardiovascular Imaging
Cleveland Clinic Foundation
Cleveland, Ohio

Min Pu, MD, PhD
Professor of Internal Medicine
Department of Cardiology
Wake Forest University
Director of Echocardiography and
    Stress Laboratory
Department of Cardiology
Wake Health Baptist Medical
    Center
Winston-Salem, North Carolina

Amit Pursnani, MD
Assistant Professor of Medicine
Division of Cardiology
Temple University Hospital
Philadelphia, Pennsylvania

Peter S. Rahko, MD
Professor of Medicine
Department of Medicine
University of Wisconsin School of
    Medicine and Public Health
Director
Adult Echocardiography Laboratory
Cardiovascular Medicine
University of Wisconsin Hospital and
    Clinics
Madison, Wisconsin

Louai Razzouk, MD, MPH
Cardiovascular Fellow
Division of Cardiology
Department of Medicine
New York University School of
    Medicine
New York, New York

Vera H. Rigolin, MD
Professor of Medicine
Division of Cardiology
Department of Medicine
Northwestern University Feinberg
    School of Medicine
Medical Director
Echocardiography Laboratory
Northwestern Memorial Hospital
Chicago, Illinois

Benjamin Sanchez, MD
Associate Professor of Medicine
Division of Cardiology
Temple University Hospital
Philadelphia, Pennsylvania

Muhamed Saric, MD, PhD
Associate Professor
Leon H. Charney Division of
    Cardiology
Director
Echocardiography Lab
New York University Langone Medical
    Center
New York, New York

Chetan Shenoy, MBBS
Fellow
Division of Cardiology
Department of Medicine
Tufts Medical Center
Boston, Massachusetts

William Stewart, AB, MD
Professor
Cleveland Clinic Lerner College of
    Medicine
Staff Physician
Cardiovascular Medicine
Cleveland Clinic
Cleveland, Ohio

Lissa Sugeng, MD, MPH
Associate Professor of Medicine
Cardiovascular Medicine
Yale Cardiovascular Clinical
Research
Yale School of Medicine
New Haven, Connecticut

**Prakash Suryanarayana,
MBBS, MD**
Assistant Professor
Division of Cardiology
University of Arizona Medical
    Center
Assistant Professor
Division of Cardiology
University of Arizona Medical
    Center,
South Campus
Tucson, Arizona

Gabriel Vorobiof, MD, FACC, FASE
Assistant Clinical Professor of
    Medicine (Cardiology) and
    Molecular & Medical Pharmacology
Division of Cardiology
Department of Medicine
David Geffen School of Medicine
University of California, Los Angeles
Director
Non-Invasive Cardiology Laboratories
University of California, Los Angeles
    Cardiovascular Center
Ronal Reagan University of California,
    Los Angeles Medical Center
Los Angeles, California

R. Parker Ward, MD
Professor of Medicine Director
Cardiovascular Fellowship Program
Non-Invasive Imaging Laboratories
Section of Cardiology
University of Chicago Medicine
Chicago, Illinois

Russell Witte, PhD
Associate Professor
Medical Imaging, Optical Sciences,
Biomedical Engineering
University of Arizona
Tucson, Arizona

Contributors

Niti Aggarwal, MD, FACC, FASNC
Associate Director of Cardiac MRI
Associate Professor of Medicine and
   Radiology
University of Wisconsin
Madison, Wisconsin

Paul Anaya, MD, PhD
Associate Professor of Medicine
Medical Director of Inpatient Cardiology
   Service
Gill Heart Institute
University of Kentucky
Lexington, Kentucky

Kristopher M. Cumbermack, MD
Associate Professor, Pediatrics
Medical Director of Congenital Echo
   Lab and Fetal Cardiac Program
University of Kentucky
Lexington, Kentucky

**Edward A. Gill, MD, FASE, FAHA,
FACC, FACP, FNLA**
Professor of Medicine
Division of Cardiology
Department of Medicine
Adjunct Professor of Radiology
Director of Harborview Medical Center
   Echocardiography
University of Washington School of
   Medicine
Clinical Professor of Diagnostic
   Ultrasound
Seattle University
Seattle, Washington

Maya E. Guglin, MD, PhD
Professor of Medicine
Director, Mechanical Assisted
   Circulation Gill Heart Institute
University of Kentucky
Lexington, Kentucky

Vedant A. Gupta, MD
Assistant Professor of Internal
   Medicine
Gill Heart and Vascular Institute
University of Kentucky
Lexington, Kentucky

**Sasanka Jayasuriya, MBBS,
FACC, FASE, FSCAI**
Assistant Professor of Medicine
Section of Cardiovascular Medicine
Division of Medicine
Yale University School of Medicine
New Haven, Connecticut

John R. Kotter, MD
Assistant Professor of Medicine
University of Kentucky
Lexington, Kentucky

Steve Leung, MD, FACC, FASE
Assistant Professor in Medicine and
   Radiology
Division of Cardiovascular Medicine
University of Kentucky
Lexington, Kentucky

Majd Makhoul, MD
Assistant Professor of Pediatrics
University of Kentucky
Kentucky Children's Hospital
Lexington, Kentucky

**Vidya Nadig, MBBS,
MRCP, FACC**
Associate Professor of Medicine
Department of Medicine
University of Connecticut
Heart and Vascular Institute
Hartford Hospital
Glastonbury, Connecticut

Mikel D. Smith, MD, FASE
Alberto Massoleni Professor
Internal Medicine
CV Imaging Research Team
Cardiovascular Research Center
Gill Heart and Vascular Institute
University of Kentucky
Lexington, Kentucky

**Vincent L. Sorrell, MD, FACC,
FACP, FASE**
The Anthony N. DeMaria Chair in
   Cardiovascular Imaging
Professor of Medicine
Assistant Chief for the Division of
   Cardiovascular Medicine
Director of Cardiovascular Imaging
The Linda and Jack Gill Heart Institute
University of Kentucky
Lexington, Kentucky

Each year, I am impressed by the dedication of the Cardiology Fellows as they prepare to sit for the Certifying Examination in Echocardiography. The depth of echocardiographic knowledge gained during this preparation period is indeed impressive. It serves as a reminder to me of my preparation for the initial ASE exam more than 20 years ago. At that time, there were only a limited number of available questions to review and a proportionate degree of anxiety. Since no previous exams had been given, there was no one to speak with regarding their preparation, successful or otherwise.

In the past decade, however, I have witnessed many fellows become expert in echocardiography through a committed process of dedicated reading, small group review sessions, and, importantly, liberal use of question and answer practice exams. Importantly, in addition to gained textbook knowledge, fellows demonstrated improved daily clinical echo lab interpretations and were better prepared during their daily patient management activities. Echocardiography is universal. Interventionalists, electrophysiologists, heart failure specialists, and general cardiologists alike are each better prepared for their daily practice if their echocardiography knowledge base is strong.

I am so pleased to be able to bring *Questions, Tricks, and Tips for the Echocardiography Boards, Second Edition*, to you. This book permits readers to evaluate their knowledge about a broad range of cardiovascular conditions and diagnostic techniques commonly encountered during the certifying examination in echocardiography. This second edition maintains many of the high-quality teaching points and individual expert teaching styles that contributed to the success of the first edition, all in an effort to maximize your learning.

There are more than 725 questions in this edition. There are new chapters on recent Echo Guidelines and Position Papers, expanded congenital heart disease questions, and questions aimed at addressing imaging acquisition skills: *"From Here to There."* There are more than 70 new figures and more than 70 new videos. Like the first edition, all Questions and Answers, including figures, tables, and movies, will be available on your personal devices providing access wherever you want. Also, new to this edition, there will be a Practice Exam with a potpourri of questions randomly provided to separate your material from a subject-specific chapter. This should be an excellent tool during your exam preparation.

This book is not intended to be a comprehensive textbook of echocardiography. However, unlike other Q & A books, it is purposefully designed to provide the reader with more than a simple one-line answer. Each wrong answer is described in detail with additional information for the reader to build on. Feedback from the first edition suggests that this book contains many difficult questions—more difficult than other Q & A books—but, once mastered, is an excellent barometer for exam preparedness. If you have difficulty in a particular chapter, please take the time to focus your studies in that area and read the additional recommended reading on those topics.

This book would not have been possible without the immense efforts of the contributing authors of the first and second editions. Through their insight and expertise in question writing, the readers must use second and third derivative reasoning that requires higher-level thinking than rote memory. Since the contributing authors come from a vast array of subspecialty backgrounds, no aspect of echocardiography is excluded.

Through feedback from exam takers, I have provided insights into successful study practices. A specific chapter on general preparation techniques and insights for standardized examinations is once again included in this second edition. This chapter provides the reader with successful test-taking techniques and published evidence from experts on other general test-taking skills.

This material should be valuable to the cardiology fellow trainee, recent fellow graduate, cardiac sonographer, junior faculty maintaining their echocardiography skills, and senior cardiology faculty considering sitting for the recertification ASCexam. Since echocardiography has evolved beyond the sole practice of the cardiologist, this book may be of value to anesthesiologists, hospitalists and internists, intensivists and surgeons, as well as pediatric cardiologists.

Many important images, figures, and tables are reproduced from *Feigenbaum's Echocardiography* and other key echocardiography resources and are included to specifically address critical topics. With Wolters Kluwer's willingness to include movies as well as still images, readers are able to understand dynamic principles. "A picture is worth a thousand words" is apropos and relevant in this book.

Every effort has been taken to ensure that the questions and answers are accurate and reflect the recommended standard guidelines at the time of publication, but errors may have occurred. Please notify us in those circumstances.

It is with the greatest of sincere appreciation that I personally thank each of contributing authors to the first edition as well as the Section Editors and contributing authors on this second edition project. Many are great friends and colleagues that I have admired or worked with over my career. Some I have only recently met, but I have already learned a great deal from. All are prodigious teachers in echocardiography and cardiovascular imaging.

My deepest appreciation is given to my coeditor, Sasanka Jayasuriya. She is one of the best cardiovascular fellows I have had the distinct pleasure to work with and has now distinguished herself as an outstanding Junior Faculty member at Yale. It was her initial idea to create a Q & A textbook on echo since she found this was missing from her own ASCexam preparation.

I wish you the best on an improved understanding of echocardiographic principles and applications. Good luck on your exam!

Vincent L. Sorrell

Contents

Contributors to the First Edition   vi
Contributors   x
Preface   xi

SECTION I   INTRODUCTION   1

Vincent L. Sorrell and Sasanka Jayasuriya

1   Tricks and Tips for Optimal Standardized
    Test-Taking   1
    Vincent L. Sorrell and Sasanka Jayasuriya

2   Statistics for the Echo Boards   7
    Sasanka Jayasuriya

SECTION II   PHYSICS   11

Vedant A. Gupta and Vincent L. Sorrell

3   Basic Principles of 2D Ultrasound   11
    Vedant A. Gupta and Vincent L. Sorrell

4   Basic Principles of Doppler Ultrasound   23
    Vincent L. Sorrell

5   Instrumentation and Knobology   29
    Vedant A. Gupta

6   Understanding Spatial and Temporal Resolution   39
    Vedant A. Gupta and Vincent L. Sorrell

7   Microbubbles   45
    Vincent L. Sorrell

8   Common and Uncommon 2D Artifacts   54
    Vedant A. Gupta and Vincent L. Sorrell

9   Artifact with Doppler Echo   68
    Vedant A. Gupta and Vincent L. Sorrell

10   Biologic Effects of Ultrasound   72
     Vedant A. Gupta

SECTION III   THE ECHO EXAMINATION   75

Vincent L. Sorrell and Sasanka Jayasuriya

11   Understanding the AUC Guidelines   75
     Sasanka Jayasuriya

12   Common TTE Anatomy   85
     Sasanka Jayasuriya

13   Normal TEE Anatomy   94
     Vincent L. Sorrell

14   Abnormal TEE Anatomy   103
     Sasanka Jayasuriya

15   Noncardiac Findings on Echocardiograms   106
     Vincent L. Sorrell

16   Image Acquisition (from Here to There)   112
     Vincent L. Sorrell

SECTION IV   VALVULAR HEART DISEASE   115

John R. Kotter

17   Aortic Stenosis   115
     John R. Kotter

18   Aortic Regurgitation   128
     John R. Kotter

19   Mitral Stenosis   137
     John R. Kotter

20   Mitral Regurgitation   145
     John R. Kotter

21   Tricuspid and Pulmonic Pathology   155
     John R. Kotter

22   Normal and Abnormal Prosthetic
     Valve Features   163
     Vincent L. Sorrell

**SECTION V   VENTRICULAR
     MEASUREMENTS**   179

Vidya Nadig

23   2D Measures   179
     Sasanka Jayasuriya

24   Doppler Measurements   188
     Vidya Nadig

25   M-Mode Findings   202
     Sasanka Jayasuriya

26   Diastolic Physiology   208
     Vidya Nadig

27   Right Ventricular Physiology   222
     Vidya Nadig

**SECTION VI   CORONARY ARTERY
     DISEASE**   229

Vincent L. Sorrell

28   Acute Coronary Syndromes and Infarct
     Complications   229
     Vincent L. Sorrell

29   Echo Features of Chronic CAD   239
     Vincent L. Sorrell

30   Stress Echocardiography   248
     Vincent L. Sorrell

SECTION VII **CARDIOMYOPATHIES** 259

Maya E. Guglin

31 Dilated Cardiomyopathy 259
Maya E. Guglin

32 Hypertrophic Cardiomyopathy 268
Maya E. Guglin

33 Echo Features of Restrictive Cardiomyopathy 276
Vincent L. Sorrell

34 Echo Features of Other Cardiomyopathies 286
Maya E. Guglin

35 Normal and Abnormal Appearance of Cardiac Devices 295
Maya E. Guglin

36 LV Dyssynchrony and Resynchronization Therapy 302
Vincent L. Sorrell

SECTION VIII **CONGENITAL HEART DISEASES** 309

Kristopher M. Cumbermack

37 Echo in Cardiac Shunt Lesions 309
Majd Makhoul

38 Congenital Valve Lesions 318
Kristopher M. Cumbermack

39 Arterial Anomalies 326
Majd Makhoul

40 Venous Malformations 335
Kristopher M. Cumbermack

41 Heart Diseases in Congenital Syndromes 341
Majd Makhoul

42 Fetal Echocardiography for the Boards 349
Kristopher M. Cumbermack

SECTION IX **MASSES AND TUMORS** 355

Mikel D. Smith

43 Pathologic Masses in the Atria 355
Mikel D. Smith

44 Masses and Tumors of the Ventricles 359
Vincent L. Sorrell

45 Pathologic Masses on the Valves 367
Mikel D. Smith

SECTION X **PERICARDIUM** 391

Steve Leung

46 Normal and Abnormal Pericardial Findings 391
Steve Leung

47 Pericardial Effusions 396
Steve Leung

48 Pericardial Constraint 405
Vincent L. Sorrell

SECTION XI **AORTA** 423

Steve Leung

49 Echo of the Normal and Diseased Aorta 423
Steve Leung

50 Acute Aortic Syndromes 429
Steve Leung

SECTION XII **THE GUIDELINES** 439

Vincent L. Sorrell

51 59 Case Examples Using Recent Echo-Relevant Guidelines and Consensus Documents 439
Vincent L. Sorrell

SECTION XIII **NEWER APPLICATIONS** 471

Paul Anaya

52 3-Dimensional Echocardiography 471
Paul Anaya

53 Echo Strain for the Boards 486
Paul Anaya

54 Echocardiography during Interventional Procedures 499
Paul Anaya

55 Intraoperative Echocardiography for the Boards 515
Vincent L. Sorrell

56 Invasive Echo for the Boards 523
Vincent L. Sorrell

SECTION XIV **MULTIMODAL CONCEPTS** 531

Vincent L. Sorrell

57 Echo as It Relates to Multimodal Imaging 531
Vincent L. Sorrell

SECTION XV **PRACTICE EXAM** 545

Vincent L. Sorrell and Niti Aggarwal

58 Practice Exam 545
Vincent L. Sorrell and Niti Aggarwal

Index 575

Chapter 1

Tricks and Tips for Optimal Standardized Test-Taking

Vincent L. Sorrell and Sasanka Jayasuriya

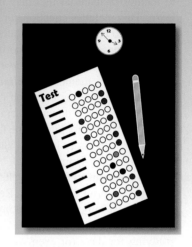

Many physicians believe that the use of standardized testing to obtain board certification is more a test of "test-taking skills" rather than knowledge. In fact, this has been studied. Published in the Journal of the American Board of Family Medicine (1), these authors attempted to study the relative impact of these "nonclinical skills" compared with the perceived necessary background of residency training knowledge. In this study, the nonphysicians managed to succeed beyond chance alone confirming their ability to perform well on standardized tests. However, they were not even close to the minimum value required to pass the board examination.

It is our belief that the most well-prepared candidate will be both knowledgeable in the examination material as well as having an advanced understanding of some of these test-taking "tips and tricks." The following suggestions were obtained after discussion with many past students, reviewing the available literature, and our own proven strategies from past successes as well as failures. These are provided as additional guides and should never persuade the reader from selecting a best answer from his or her knowledge. However, when stumped or befuddled, these strategies may be of value.

General Concepts

It has been demonstrated that there are three primary types of guessing: *random, cued, and informed* (2). *Random* guessing occurs when examinees respond in a completely blind manner with no insight whatsoever to the best answer. *Cued* guessing occurs when a response is based on a stimulus in the prompt. *Informed* guessing is often referred to as an "educated guess" and occurs when the response is based on partial knowledge.

Medical examinees rarely result to *random* guessing but often make decisions based on *cued* or *informed* guesses (3). An important test-taking strategy is to remove responses that are thought to be incorrect. By simply removing these wrong

options, the examinee increases one's chances of answering an item correctly. However, if one is able to eliminate all but two response options, one still has, at best, a 50% random chance of answering correctly.

ABIM officials have been reported as stating that nearly 85% of the test questions are presented as clinical scenarios rather than remote knowledge-based facts. Twenty-two percent of the questions recite material from previous exams, and most questions emphasize general knowledge. It is rare for a highly up-to-date material to be tested since these questions are compiled more than a year prior to the examination date. Certainly, late-breaking clinical studies will not be tested.

The ASCeXAM is now provided at computer testing centers. Multiple-choice and case-based questions are included. At the time this review book was written, the content outline stated that the ASCeXAM will consist of a total of four testing blocks: three multiple-choice blocks (60 minutes) and one case-oriented block (90 minutes). The questions will be categorized as being obtained from one of the following categories:

1. Physical principles of ultrasound
2. Valvular heart disease
3. Ventricular size and function, coronary artery disease, cardiomyopathies
4. Congenital heart disease and fetal echocardiography
5. Cardiac masses, pericardial disease, myocardial contract, and new applications of echocardiography

Examinees will be tested on knowledge of M-mode, 2D and Doppler echocardiography, TEE, contrast, and stress echocardiography.

"Cramming" data in for a couple days prior to the ASCeXAM may cause *retroactive inhibition*. This is the phenomenon in which longer-term "knowledge" is replaced by short-term "memory." Since it is unlikely that one can add enough short-term facts to offset the loss of long-term knowledge, this becomes a poor trade-off. Despite that fact, however, some successful examinees have used the few days before an exam to memorize material that they have found to be difficult to learn. This includes equations or quantitative parameters that are likely to be needed. For example, some test takers may be weak in physics and will memorize equations for *wavelength, bandwidth, attenuation coefficient, Doppler shift*, etc.

Others may memorize the *mild* and *severe* categories of quantitative valve regurgitation (all else is moderate) and be able to write these down on scrap paper once the test starts. Doing so prior to looking at the first question will provide the examinee with his or her own table to use when these values are called upon. Doing a quick "mind dump" of information you do not want to forget is valuable and should be practiced for accuracy prior to the exam. Repetition is important.

The most important test-taking strategy we can offer is to "anticram." If cramming is the art of spending hours nonstop studying for days (or even weeks) prior to the examination, then *anticramming* is practicing test taking in the first year of your fellowship. Adult cardiovascular fellowship programs that incorporate practice questions on a weekly basis are more likely to have well-prepared graduates that will succeed in passing their certifying exams on the first attempt. Creating a culture of practice exams and having trainees actively answer board-type questions fulfill one of the most important tenets of test-taking skills: practice, practice, practice! Although "practice may *not* make perfect," it will create a level of confidence that reduces the memory-taxing anxiety component for many examinees. Importantly, this practice helps to provide a structured format to identify weak areas requiring additional study. Take notes during your conferences and practice sessions.

Some past ASCeXAM diplomats have found that "small study groups" were highly rewarding. Even though this practice may have been new to the examinee, the highly specialized knowledge required for this exam tended to benefit from small group discussions. According to the individuals who benefited from this practice, it seems that regular consistent meetings (usually weekly) were most valuable. Limiting the groups to only those three to six fellows actually taking the next echo boards kept the discussion focused. If other fellows wanted to "get a leg up" and attend, they were asked to take notes and learn, but not interfere by talking or asking many questions. In 4 to 6 months, a small group setting can cover an entire textbook. At each 45- to 90-minute review session, some of the time should be dedicated for practice questions. Keep notes during your review sessions and record frequently poorly understood concepts and disease or technical categories for additional focused study.

Most of the fellows and faculty we spoke with highly recommend the ASE review and Mayo Review courses as a means to review material, to add confidence to current knowledge, and to fill in the remaining gaps of knowledge. In our opinion, these review courses are useful toward the end of the study period, but would not make up for 4 to 6 months of paced study.

When using this review book and other sample questions, it is most important to study the incorrect choices as well as understanding why an answer was correct. Simply answering a question correct is not nearly as valuable as carefully understanding why the other options were incorrect. At times, you may answer a question correct without sufficiently understanding the material. Moving on in this circumstance would subject the examinee to missing this same (or similar) question in the future. However, taking the time to study the other options and moving on only after truly understanding the educational teaching point(s) will go a long way to adding to your knowledge base and preparing you for a future similar question. For this reason, our book was designed to have extensive discussion after each question to provide the necessary material for knowledge growth.

Board-type questions contain initial prompts or stems. These are often clinical based. The examinee who performs well is often able to "pick out" pertinent details and create his or her own answer prior to looking at the options offered. Although there are no trick questions, it is important to remember that just like patients, partially correct answers are common, and therefore the *entire sentence* in *each of the answers* should be read prior to selecting your final answer.

In answering long questions, especially when extensive clinical details are provided (occasionally as red herrings), it is always *worthwhile to review the last sentence of the stem and selected options initially* so as to assist you in picking out important facts when reading through the lengthy prompt. This focuses your attention on the critical portions of the written material. This "tip" is equivalent to hearing a lengthy case history on consultation rounds and at the end of the presentation, learning the reason for the consult. You are better off knowing the reason for the consultation request at the beginning of the presentation, which allows the expert consultant the opportunity to "filter" the relevant from the unnecessary information being presented. With this approach, the best answer may be obvious prior to reading the entire prompt. Over the course of a multihour examination, this practice reduces the common ailments of mental and eye fatigue. See example.

An 82-year-old male with aortic stenosis and mitral regurgitation (MR) presents for follow-up. The patient was diagnosed with severe aortic stenosis 5 years ago and has continued to be physically active walking up to 3 miles a day on a track around the lake. A routine surveillance echocardiogram was performed 2 weeks ago. The aortic valve was noted to be calcified and stenotic with a valve area of 0.9 cm^2 and mean and peak gradients of 41 and 62 mm Hg, respectively. This was not significantly changed from before. The mitral valve was reported to be thickened with some degenerative changes. Moderate MAC was present. Moderate MR was qualitatively reported. You are being asked to reevaluate the MR and apply quantitative criteria.

Question 1. Which of the following criteria is LEAST consistent with moderate mitral regurgitation?

A. ERO 0.30 cm^2
B. Vena contracta 0.6 cm
C. Regurgitant fraction 55%
D. Regurgitant volume of 42 mL
E. Regurgitant jet area 6 cm^2

Answer C is correct. A, B, D, and E are quantitative values indicative of moderate MR. Option C is consistent with severe MR (>50%). To answer this question correctly, all that was required was the last sentence of the question stem and a quick glance at the answers. Although it is refreshing to read about the daily walk around the lake of an 82-year-old male with severe aortic stenosis, a time-sensitive exam would not be the best venue for enjoying short stories!

Always eat before your exam. Avoid heavy foods, which may make you groggy. Apples enhance memory recall more than coffee, but consistency is most important. If your practice study sessions involved coffee, then coffee it is. However, you should neither start drinking nor stop drinking coffee (or eating apples) just for the exam.

Specific Concepts

It is always important to *look for the central idea of each question*. What is the main point? Most question writers have a single teaching point they want to emphasize, and if you are able to identify this, then the answer may become more visible. Avoid the temptation to read too much into the question and make it harder than it was intended to be.

Example: "Which one of the following echo findings is *most predictive of cardiac events* in patients with this cardiac pathology?" may have a very different answer than "Which one of the following is *the best indication that this patient could benefit from repair* of this cardiac pathology?" Knowing this while reading through the prompt is valuable.

Consider ethnicity, race, gender, geography, and occupation when you read case studies. For example, African Americans are at higher risk for sarcoid; young women have a higher incidence of lupus erythematosus compared to men; and many congenital lesions are gender specific.

Do not agonize and get "hung up" over a question you do not know the answer to. Skip it and come back to the question later. Sometimes, later questions can provide hints to the answer or simply jog your memory to increase your chance of a correct answer.

The following "test-taking" tricks have been shown to assist examinees when they are truly stumped. How valuable these will be regarding the ASCeXAM in particular is not known.

1. **Grammatical cues**—one or more distracters do not follow grammatically from the stem.

Question 1. Example: What is the next best step for making a diagnosis in the patient scenario provided above?

A. Immediate CT surgery consultation.
B. Schedule elective outpatient clinic follow-up.
C. Perform emergent bedside TEE.
D. Give aminophylline ASAP.
E. Ask ID consulting physician to see patient.

Answer C is correct. The informed test taker will recognize that ONLY option C is a "diagnostic" option, and options A, B, D, and E are not "steps for making a diagnosis." Therefore, even though the "patient scenario" was not provided, the only diagnostic option as requested in the prompt was this choice. This is a grammatical clue.

2. **Logical cues**—a subset of the options is collectively exhaustive.

Question 1. Example: Which statement is most correct?

A. Raising the transducer frequency will increase depth resolution.
B. Raising the transducer frequency does not alter the depth resolution.
C. Raising the transducer frequency will lower the depth resolution.
D. Transducer frequency cannot be changed.
E. Depth resolution cannot be changed.

Answer C is correct. The informed test taker realizes that all three possibilities are offered in A, B, and C, making one of these the logical answer and only briefly considers D or E as possibilities.

3. **Absolute/closed terms versus open terms**—terms such as "always, never, all, and none" are often (not "always") indicators of an incorrect option since they are "closed" and restricting. These limit the actual possibilities, but in medicine, this phenomenon is rare. Open terms such as "usually, frequently, mostly, may, and generally" are often (but again not "always") found in correct options since they are less confining and open to various clinical possibilities.

Example: Contrast echocardiography will:

A. Always improve endocardial definition.
B. Never enhance the LV myocardium.
C. Commonly improve the visualization of the LV apex.
D. Frequently (>20%) cause minor adverse events such as back pain.
E. Always result in a higher LV volume compared to noncontrast echo.

Answer C is correct. Although contrast echo will very commonly (A) improve endocardial definition and (E) result in a higher LV volume compared to noncontrast echo, there are a number of circumstances (mostly technical) where these do not apply. The informed test taker is aware of this and eliminates these options due to the use of the term "always." Similarly, "never" is used in option B, but at times, contrast will definitely enhance the LV myocardium (especially with the use of perfusion imaging sequences). That leaves only options C and D for the informed test taker to select from.

4. Long correct answer—the correct answer is longer, more specific, or more complete than other options.

Question 1. Example: Which statement best describes the differences between M-mode and 2D echocardiography?

A. M-mode has superior spatial resolution compared with 2D.
B. Both 2D and M-mode require adherence to optimal scanning techniques to obtain the highest-quality temporal and spatial resolution.
C. M-mode temporal resolution may be 100× greater than 2D.
D. 2D temporal resolution will equal M-mode temporal resolution by narrowing the image sector.
E. Altering probe frequency will alter the 2D, but not the M-mode appearance.

Answer B is correct. It is unlikely that this practice will outweigh the other "tips and tricks" listed. It is but one of the many tried and true techniques voiced by the skilled test taker. These editors recommend using this with caution and as a last resort when you are thoroughly stumped.

---

5. All-of-the-above and **none-of-the-above** choices—although this is not one of the commonly reported "tricks," these editors have learned that this option is frequently the correct choice. When "all of the above" is an option, once you identify two answers as correct, then the answer would be "all of the above." For this reason, this was rarely allowed in our review book and was frequently included as an incorrect option to de-emphasize this practice. How this plays out in the ASCeXAM is not entirely known.

Remember, if any part of an option is false, then the entire statement is false! However, having part of the option true does not make that option the single best answer.

6. Opposite options—if two answers are opposite, then one of these may be the correct answer.

Question 1. Example:

A. The color flow Doppler signal will be increased.
B. The color flow Doppler signal will be decreased.

---

7. The never before heard of option—if it sounds "crazy," it may be "crazy." Do not select an answer by assuming that since you never heard of this before, it must be correct. It often is "crazy."

Question 1. Example:

A. The visible width of the modal velocity from the transmitral spectral Doppler flow signal is falsely narrowed when contrast microbubble enhancement has washed out of the arterial circulation.
 This is an entirely fictitious statement created for your enjoyment!

---

8. I saw my answer, so it must be correct—when selecting the correct answer on a mathematical question, be careful *not* to select your choice simply because it is one of the available options. Many question writers have learned that exam takers look for their "answer," and when it is not there, they reassess if they chose the correct formula or made a mathematical error. To address this, exam writers now commonly provide you options based upon incorrect formulas or incorrect numbers filled in correct formulas.

Note: Choice C is an alternative method when the LVOT data are not available or inaccurate (outflow gradient, etc.) and there is no cardiac-level shunt.

Note: Choice D is the dimensionless index. This value, when <0.25, is another marker of severity and a good technique when the LVOT diameter is not accurate (prosthetic valves, etc.).

When solving a mathematical question, carry your number values with you to assist in selecting the correct choice. TIP: Keep all values as cm (move the decimal point as needed; for example, 1.2 m/s = 120 cm/s; 12 mm = 1.2 cm).

---

1. Example: What is the AV area given the following parameters?

LVOT 2.0 cm	RVOT 2.2 cm	RVOT vti 17 cm
LVOT vti 20 cm	AR pht 400 m	
AV vti 100 cm	AV mean gradient 60 mm Hg	AV peak V = 5.0 m/s

A. $0.63 \text{ cm}^2 = ([2.0 \times 2.0 \times 0.785 \text{ or } 1.0 \times 1.0 \times 3.14] \times 20 \text{ cm}/100 \text{ cm})$
B. $0.13 \text{ cm}^2 = (2.0 \times 2.0 \times 0.785 \text{ or } 1.0 \times 1.0 \times 3.14/500)$
C. $0.65 \text{ cm}^2 = (2.2 \times 2.2 \times 0.785 \text{ or } 1.1 \times 1.1 \times 3.14/100 \text{ cm})$
D. $0.2 \text{ cm}^2 = 20 \text{ cm}/100 \text{ cm}$

Answer A is the correct answer based upon the correct formula. All other choices use incorrect formulas to obtain the listed choices B to D.

---

9. Stick with your initial answer—Think about the advice you received to improve your score on standardized multiple-choice exams? Some have been advised to trust their instincts and never go back and change an answer. Others have been instructed to go back and reconsider the questions they were not sure about. In looking for the best advice to give our readers, we reviewed the available literature and have created the following overview (TABLE 1.1) for your consideration (4). Based upon this, *it may be worthwhile to save time to reconsider changing answers* on questions where you are uncertain.

Dealing with Stress and Anxiety

Finally, any discussion on test-taking practices should at least mention the importance of the negative effects of stress and anxiety. The above tips and tricks are offered in the hopes of

Table 1.1	Strategy of Changing Your Initial Answer			
AUTHOR	**TOTAL QUESTIONS**	**% CHANGED**	**RIGHT TO WRONG**	**WRONG TO RIGHT**
Davis (1929)	22,000	2.50%	21%	53%
Shahabudin (1929)	21,903	2.90%	34%	66%
Bath (1967)	7,700	4.30%	20%	60%
Mathews (1975)	11,630	5.40%	20%	58%
Lowe and Crawford (1983)	39,380	4.60%	22%	46%
Fabry and Case (1985)	123,175	3.80%	23%	48%
Totals	**225,788**	**3.9%**	**23%**	**55%**

Adapted from Croskerry P. The importance of cognitive errors in diagnosis and strategies to minimize them. *Acad Med* 2003;78:775–780. Ref. (4)

reducing these aspects. Unfortunately, some examinees remain "stressed out" despite careful study and practice. In these circumstances, and knowing that adrenergic stimulation is partly responsible, the question sometimes arises: *should I take a beta blocker (BB) to minimize anxiety and enhance my performance?* Some individuals use BBs to enhance "high-stress" performances. Two recent Olympic athletes were banned from testing positive for PEDs. The drug: propranolol. In the music world, Inderal is considered the "underground musician's drug." Thus, certain individuals rely on the "performance-enhancing" capabilities of BB. But, does this apply to test takers?

Although the final answer is not known to these editors, the following study attempted to address this issue.

In one of the few published studies to address this issue, these authors gave students 5 or 10 mg mepindolol prior to their examination to study the impact of beta-adrenergic blockade on test-taking proficiency (5). In two placebo-controlled trials of $N = 55$ and $N = 49$ students, a reduction in self-rated anxiety could not be confirmed despite lower pulse rates. No improvement (nor worsening) in exam performance could be confirmed. To conclude, the anxiolytic effect of beta blocker and associated enhanced test-taking performance could not be confirmed. On a side note, 10 examinees suffered dizziness, fatigue, and/or headaches.

Nearly four decades ago, a team of British researchers tested the effects of BBs on the performances of skilled musicians (6). Under the most stressful settings, musicians were asked to perform four times each, twice on placebo and twice on BBs, in a double-blind, crossover clinical trial. Their performances were scored by two professional judges. The results demonstrated that the musicians trembled less on the BB but also performed better. The improvement was minimal, greatest for the first performance (highest anxiety), and most dramatic for those suffering the greatest from nervousness.

In our review, it seems that BBs reduce the outward expression of anxiety but do not modify the damaging "memory recall" impact of stress. Since it is the outward expression of anxiety that negatively impacts athletes (e.g., pistol shooters and archers) and musicians, a benefit from BB "doping" may be more predictable—at least in the most anxious individuals likely to demonstrate these physiologic expressions (e.g., tremors).

Unfortunately, stress and anxiety are two of the worst mental enemies as well as physical. When test takers suffer from stress or anxiety, they lose synchronization and focus. This is a bad combination for examinees, leads to unclear thinking

and poor memory recall, and lowers the likelihood for optimal exam performance.

To reduce the adverse mental component of stress and anxiety, it is our recommendation to practice *rhythmic breathing* and *muscle relaxation* and *improve your cardiovascular fitness*. There are definite mental (as well as physiologic) effects of these activities.

Rhythmic breathing helps bring about calmness of the mind, increase your level of self-confidence, and improve concentration ability. Many believe it restores your body's natural rhythms. Although not well studied in the test taker, these benefits should help improve your performance in an examination setting. Retention and recall of important learned information are the specific goal of practicing this particular yoga breathing technique.

Deep breathing consists of full breaths known to effectively reduce stress. Use your nose for breathing in and use your mouth for exhalation. Do this in a sudden and forceful manner to empty out your lungs.

Progressive muscle relaxation is another proven strategy to relieve stress. This relaxation technique is particularly useful if you suffer from muscular tension in a specific area. This practice may be effective to perform a few minutes before starting your examination. If neck pain or frontal headaches are common, try tensing the particular muscles that ache (e.g., lift shoulders, extreme head turn for neck pain; tightly close eyes for frontal headaches) for 10 seconds and then relaxing these same muscles for the same amount of time. Creating and releasing tension are a great stress reducer.

One of the most important activities for reducing stress and anxiety that should result in improved test-taking capabilities is enhancing your *cardiovascular fitness*. Importantly, even if it fails at giving you an improved exam score, it will help you to live longer.

Some very up-to-date tips to reduce anxiety specifically related to the ASCeXAM are to carefully plan ahead for the necessary details of that day. Locating the test center and parking options prior to the day of the exam is warranted. Identifying the required documents for the day and having these set aside and easy to find is important. Familiarize yourself with the computer software (online practice modules are available and should be utilized). Last, but certainly not least, be certain you understand the rules and regulations of the test. Do not assume that every test has the same rules. While mobile phones might be allowed to be used during break time of some tests, they are not allowed in others. We are aware of one recent test taker's entire test being invalidated (and no refund) due to a phone call made to the spouse during the final break. As they tell the story, that turned out to be an expensive phone call to make dinner plans.

Study Tips

Creating a study plan and sticking to are important to make sure you cover the necessary material. Making assumptions that certain categories of the exam may be skipped over due to perceived strengths may result in a suboptimal performance. Remember that only *10% of driver's rate themselves as "below average" drivers.*

In our opinion, preparing to sit for a multihour exam takes similar training to athletics. You do not just decide to run a 4-hour race a week before; instead you have to build up to it. This concept applies to sitting for long exams such as the ASCeXAM. *Build up your endurance for Q & A* over weeks to months prior to the exam. Get normal amounts of sleep. Wake up at the same time. Eat the same breakfast that "works for you" without causing GI symptoms or grogginess. Start answering questions at the same time you will be taking the exam. Complete full practice tests, answering more question blocks than the test to minimize mental fatigue on the day of the exam. Practicing each of these activities will make the actual exam seem commonplace and secondary to your routine.

We strongly encourage our fellows in training and course attendees to review all published images used in societal guidelines and consensus documents, as well as major cardiac imaging textbooks. *A fantastic practice review session is to "mask" the figure legend(s)* and have the video or figure projected on the screen using an overhead projector (or similar). Describing the image and highlighting the pertinent details and characteristics on the blinded figure initially and then having the figure legend unmasked for immediate recall may be *the single most important "test-taking tip."*

Some examinees have found value in *creating flash cards* with common formulas and other facts. The act of writing the flash card stores the material deeper in your long-term memory. Also, they can be rapidly called upon to practice throughout the working day.

Others have successfully used *audio recordings* of facts to play during car travel such as morning commutes or evenings after study completion such as preparing to sleep.

The use of *mnemonics* to remember certain facts or key points is also a common tool that has demonstrated success

with many (e.g., RIPCHAT = etiology of AF, R = rheumatic heart disease, I = ischemia, P = pericardial disease and pulmonary disease, C = CAD or congenital heart disease, H = HBP, A = alcohol, T = thyroid).

In our opinion, learning concepts is more valuable than mnemonics, both for test-taking preparation as well as patient care. For this purpose, it is valuable to *create diagrams and graphs* to illustrate and fully understand difficult concepts.

Rapid revision of all material in the days prior to the exam enhances recall during the test. It is less productive to attempt to grasp new concepts in the final few days leading up to the test.

During the actual exam, some examinees have found it productive to *underline keywords* in the question prompt and answer options that help distinguish the basis of the question and the relevant variables that separate one answer from another.

Summary

Eat right, sleep well, and be prepared. Learn a few test-taking skills to assist those rare situations where you are stumped. "Anticram" and reduce stress and anxiety by whatever means you have found useful. Find a small group of similar-focused colleagues and regularly cover the vast curriculum. Practice answering board-type questions. Review all answers—correct and incorrect. Get into a routine of waking, eating right, and answering questions, weeks before your exam date. Increase your cardiovascular fitness. Review figures from textbooks and guidelines in a blinded fashion. Understand the meaning of the question prior to answering. Do not be afraid of changing your answer when rechecking an answer you were initially unsure of Good luck!

References

1. O'Neill TR, et al. Performance on the American Board of Family Medicine (ABFM) certification examination: are superior test-taking skills alone sufficient to pass? *J Am Board Fam Med* 2011;24:175–180.
2. Rogers HJ. Guessing in multiple-choice tests. In: Masters GN, Keeves JP, eds. *Advances in Measurement in Educational Research and Assessment.* Oxford, UK: Pergamon, 1999:235–243.
3. Downing SM. Guessing on selected-response examinations. *Med Educ* 2003;37:670–671.
4. Croskerry P. The importance of cognitive errors in diagnosis and strategies to minimize them. *Acad Med* 2003;78:775–780.
5. Krope P, et al. Evaluating mepindolol in a test model of examination anxiety in students. *Pharmacopsychiatria* 1982;15(2):41–47.
6. James IM, et al. Effect of oxprenolol on stage-fright in musicians. *Lancet* 1977;2:952–954.

Chapter 2

Statistics for the Echo Boards

Sasanka Jayasuriya

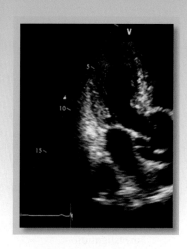

1. A 64-year-old male with a history of chronic obstructive pulmonary disease (COPD) and diabetes mellitus was admitted with sepsis due to gram-positive cocci and no definite focus of infection. The transthoracic echocardiogram (TTE) did not demonstrate a definite vegetation. Therefore, he was referred for a transesophageal echocardiogram (TEE). Which of the following is correct?

   A. Transesophageal echo is not indicated in native valve endocarditis in a patient with a normal transthoracic echocardiogram.
   B. In diagnosing native valve endocarditis, the specificity of TEE is significantly higher than TTE.
   C. Increased accuracy in the diagnosis of a paravalvular abscess is a proven benefit of TEE in comparison to TTE.
   D. TEE has a higher sensitivity for the diagnosis of endocarditis in right-sided cardiac valves in drug addicts.
   E. Two of the statements are true.

2. A 65-year-old male presented with syncope and substernal chest pain. A stat transthoracic echocardiogram was ordered, and the images in FIGURE 2.1 and VIDEO 2.1 are obtained.

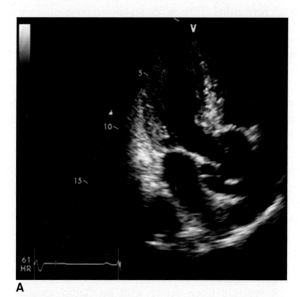

A

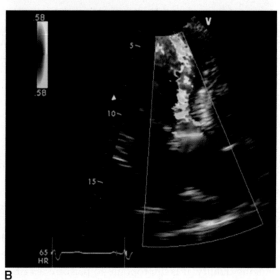

B

FIGURE 2.1 Reprinted from Brunson JM, Fine RL, Schussler JM. Acute ascending aortic dissection diagnosed with transthoracic echocardiography. *J Am Soc Echocardiogr* 2009;22(9):1086.e5–1086.e7. Copyright © 2009 American Society of Echocardiography. With permission.

Table 2.1	Sensitivity and Specificity of TTE and TEE in Different Pathologic Conditions		
		SENSITIVITY	SPECIFICITY
Endocarditis of native valves	TTE	40%–60%	90%–100%
	TEE	90%–100%	90%–100%
Prosthetic valve endocarditis	TTE	20%–40%	90%–100%
	TEE	80%–100%	90%–100%
Aortic type A dissection	TTE	80%–94%	60%–90%
	TEE	97%–100%	94%
Patent foramen ovale	TTE	50%–60%	100%
	TEE	100%	100%
Thrombus of left atrial appendage	TTE	60%	—
	TEE	100%	95%–100%

The most accurate diagnosis is:

A. Acute valvular lesion
B. Acute coronary syndrome
C. Acute aortic syndrome
D. Acute pulmonary embolism
E. Acute valvular lesion and acute aortic syndrome

3. In diagnosing the condition in Question 2, which of the following is true?

A. Echocardiography is the commonly used first line of investigation.
B. Sensitivity of transthoracic echocardiography is superior to computed tomography.
C. Microbubble contrast imaging may aid in echocardiographic diagnosis.
D. Sensitivity of transthoracic echocardiography is <50% when related valvular lesions are present.
E. A pericardial effusion has no known prognostic value in this setting.

4. A 56-year-old male with hypertension and dyslipidemia complained of left shoulder pain when walking the dog. An exercise stress echocardiogram (ESE) was performed (VIDEO 2.2). The patient exercised to reach 8.4 metabolic equivalents and target heart rate. Which of the following is correct considering the given information?

A. The peak wall motion score index (WMSI) is 1.0.
B. Ischemia in the left anterior descending artery (LAD) territory is present.
C. Ischemia in the circumflex territory is present.
D. A dobutamine stress echocardiogram (DSE) would have been the appropriate test.
E. An exercise stress echocardiogram is the most sensitive noninvasive cardiac stress test.

5. A 54-year-old truck driver with no cardiovascular risk factors is admitted due to a transient ischemic attack. A paradoxical embolus is suspected, and a transesophageal echocardiogram (TEE) with a bubble study is ordered. What are the sensitivity and specificity, respectively, of this test to detect a patent foramen ovale (PFO)?

A. 60% and 80%
B. 100% and 60%
C. 80% and 100%
D. 60% and 100%
E. 100% and 100%

Answer 1: *C.* The clinical scenario describes a patient who may well have endocarditis. Depending on the severity of COPD, the image quality may significantly deteriorate due to emphysematous lungs. Therefore, in a patient with a high clinical suspicion of endocarditis or in the setting of suboptimal imaging quality, it is appropriate to perform a TEE when the TTE did not reveal a vegetation. Therefore, answer A is incorrect.

The specificity of diagnosing endocarditis is similar in TTE and TEE and ranges from 90% to 100%. This means that in patients who do not have endocarditis, the false-positive diagnosis of endocarditis is very low and is similar between the two imaging modalities. Therefore, answer B is incorrect.

TEE is capable of diagnosing more paravalvular abscesses and abscesses of the intervalvular fibrosa than TTE. Therefore, a patient diagnosed with endocarditis who is not clinically improving on appropriate therapy should receive TEE to evaluate for abscesses as the management may require cardiac surgery. Hence, answer C is correct.

TEE is not known to have an increased sensitivity compared to TTE in diagnosing right-sided endocarditis in studies with a limited number of patients. However, in overall diagnosis of endocarditis, TEE has a much higher sensitivity of 90% to 100% compared to TTE, which has a sensitivity of 40% to 60%. Therefore, answer D is incorrect as it refers to only right-sided valves.

Only one of the options is correct. Hence, answer E is wrong.

Suggested Readings

Baddour LM, Wilson WR, Bayer AS, et al. Infective Endocarditis in Adults: Diagnosis, Antimicrobial Therapy, and Management of Complication: a Scientific Statement for Healthcare Professionals From the American Heart Association. *Circulation* 2015;132(15):1435–1486.
Evangelista A, Gonzalez-Alujas MT. Echocardiography in infective endocarditis. *Heart* 2004;90(6):614–617.

Answer 2: *E.* The image shows a dissection flap of the ascending aorta with severe aortic regurgitation, likely caused due to dissection disrupting the anatomy of the aortic annulus. Therefore, the correct answer is acute aortic valvular lesion and acute aortic syndrome. Acute aortic syndrome includes aortic dissection, intramural hematoma, penetrating aortic ulcer, and aortic transection. There are no definite regional wall motion abnormalities suggestive of acute coronary syndrome. Hence, answer B is incorrect. A pulmonary embolism large enough to cause syncope would likely cause the right ventricle to be dilated and akinetic, which are not seen in the given image. Hence, D is incorrect. While A and C are both correct, the most accurate diagnosis is E.

According to the Stanford classification, the aortic dissection shown in FIGURE 2.1 is a type A dissection, as the ascending aorta is involved. This condition requires emergency cardiothoracic surgery, as the mortality rate is 1% to 2% per hour. Type B dissections are dissections distal to the left subclavian artery and are usually managed conservatively unless further vascular compromise is present.

Answer 3: *C.* The above image shows a type A dissection. According to the IRAD registry that is the largest worldwide registry of aortic dissection, the commonest first-line diagnostic test was a CT. CT has a higher sensitivity of approximately 87% to 100% compared to TTE in the diagnosis of aortic dissection. Therefore, answers A and B are incorrect. However, TTE has a higher sensitivity of approximately 80% to 94% for type A dissections in comparison to type B dissections for which the sensitivity is low at 30% to 50%. Answer D implies a type A dissection and not a type B dissection by stating, "when related valvular lesions are present," referring to aortic regurgitation.

Therefore, answer D is incorrect. However, it is important to appreciate the utility of transthoracic echocardiography in diagnosing type A dissections, as this could be a valuable, rapid, bedside test performed in patients who are unstable. TEE has a very high sensitivity of 97% to 100% in diagnosing type A dissections. Therefore, TEE and CT have the highest sensitivity in diagnosing aortic dissection.

Microbubble contrast administration may help to identify the true lumen and the false lumen when the dissection flap is inconspicuous by administering contrast, which would opacify the true lumen and less of the false lumen (FIG. 2.2). Further, following dissipation of contrast, the dissection flap would be more obvious.

It is important to evaluate the pericardial space for an effusion, which would likely be a hemopericardium as this is a poor prognostic sign and may rapidly progress to tamponade. Hence, answer E is incorrect.

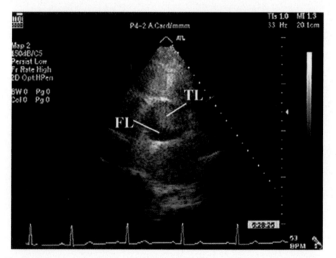

FIGURE 2.2 Reprinted from McRee D. Transthoracic contrast echocardiographic detection of ascending aortic dissection. *J Am Soc Echocardiogr* 1999;12(12):1122–1124. Copyright © 1999 American Society of Echocardiography. With permission.

Suggested Readings

Meredith EL, Masani ND. Echocardiography in the emergency assessment of acute aortic syndromes. *Eur J Echocardiogr* 2009;10(1):i31–i39.
Nienaber CA, Eagle KA. Aortic dissection: new frontiers in diagnosis and management: part I: from etiology to diagnostic strategies. *Circulation* 2003;108(5):628–635.

Answer 4: *A.* The images given (which are only of the apical four-chamber view) show normal regional wall motion abnormalities following stress. The wall motion score index is a score used to evaluate the severity of wall motion abnormalities. In stress echocardiography, a normal peak WMSI of 1.0 represents normal wall motion. Hence, answer A is correct.

There are no wall motion abnormalities suggestive of LAD or circumflex territory. Therefore, answers B and C are incorrect.

When a patient has reasonable exercise capacity and is able to reach target heart rate, ESE is more appropriate in comparison to DSE. The added benefit of an ESE is the ability of evaluating exercise capacity, symptoms, ECG changes, and hemodynamic response, all of which are of prognostic value during ESE but not as beneficial during DSE. Hence, answer D is incorrect.

Considering noninvasive stress testing, stress myocardial perfusion imaging is more sensitive than exercise stress echocardiography. Hence, answer E is incorrect. Studies have shown ESE and DSE to have a sensitivity of approximately 80%, although there is a wide range reported. Myocardial perfusion stress testing has a higher sensitivity of 85% to 90%.

Suggested Readings

American College of Cardiology Foundation Appropriate Use Criteria Task Force, et al. ACCF/ASE/AHA/ASNC/HFSA/HRS/SCAI/SCCM/SCCT/SCMR 2011 Appropriate Use Criteria for Echocardiography. A Report of the American College of Cardiology Foundation Appropriate Use Criteria Task Force, American Society of Echocardiography, American Heart Association, American Society of Nuclear Cardiology, Heart Failure Society of America, Heart Rhythm Society, Society for Cardiovascular Angiography and Interventions, Society of Critical Care Medicine, Society of Cardiovascular Computed Tomography, Society for Cardiovascular Magnetic Resonance American College of Chest Physicians. *J Am Soc Echocardiogr* 2011;24(3):229–267.
Armstrong WF, Zoghbi WA. Stress echocardiography: current methodology and clinical applications. *J Am Coll Cardiol* 2005;45(11):1739–1747.
Klocke FJ, et al. ACC/AHA/ASNC guidelines for the clinical use of cardiac radionuclide imaging—executive summary. *Circulation* 2003;108:1404–1418.
Yao S, Chaudhry FA, et al. Practical applications in stress echocardiography: risk stratification and prognosis in patients with known or suspected ischemic heart disease. *J Am Coll Cardiol* 2003;42(6):1084–1090.

Answer 5: *E.* TEE with a bubble study during a Valsalva maneuver and color Doppler is considered the gold standard in diagnosing PFOs. The sensitivity and specificity were nearly 100% and 100% when correlated with autopsy studies.

The current-generation transthoracic echocardiographic evaluation is also considered to be quite accurate when multiple bubble studies are performed with the Valsalva maneuver. However, the sensitivity and specificity are lower than that of TEE.

Suggested Readings

Di Tullio MR. Patent foramen ovale: echocardiographic detection and clinical relevance in stroke. *J Am Soc Echocardiogr* 2010;23(2):144–155.
Schneider B, Zienkiewicz T, Jansen V, et al. Diagnosis of patent foramen ovale by transesophageal echocardiography and correlation with autopsy findings. *Am J Cardiol* 1996;77:1202–1209.

Chapter 3

Basic Principles of 2D Ultrasound

Vedant A. Gupta and Vincent L. Sorrell

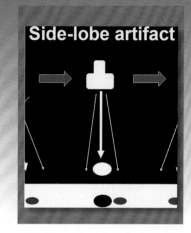
Side-lobe artifact

1. Which of the following statements is most accurate?

A. Ultrasound consists of waves of compression and decompression, traveling at a variable speed through a specific medium (such as fat or blood).

B. Ultrasound is considered too high for human hearing (generally >2,000 Hz), and infrasound is too low for human hearing (generally <200 Hz).

C. Ultrasound travels in a "longitudinal" (not sinusoidal) wave oscillating back and forth within the direction the sound was transmitted.

D. Most 2D ultrasound probes used in cardiac imaging consist of a range of 2.5 to 5.0 Hz.

E. Unlike audible frequencies, which are difficult to "hear" around objects, ultrasound is more likely to travel around tissue planes, become distorted, and create artifacts.

2. Which of the following is considered a disadvantage of ultrasound?

A. Ultrasound is poorly transmitted through a gaseous medium, and attenuation is marked.

B. As ultrasound passes through a medium, particles within this path vibrate parallel to the line of propagation.

C. Sound waves can be characterized by regions of closely related particles within the medium (compression) and regions of loosely related particles (rarefaction).

D. Reflection, refraction, and attenuation are each dependent on the acoustic properties of the medium.

E. As ultrasound moves through the medium, particle oscillations may become marked, and this particle motion may result in tissue heating and injury.

3. Which of the following is the correct order of the velocity of sound within the medium, from fastest to slowest tissue?

A. Blood, bone, and air

B. Air, bone, and blood

C. Air, blood, and bone

D. Bone, blood, and air

E. Bone, air, and blood

4. Match the following terms with the most accurate definition:

A. Gain	1. The transfer of ultrasound energy to the tissue during propagation
B. Intensity	2. The net loss of ultrasound energy during propagation
C. Acoustic impedance	3. The degree of amplification of the returning ultrasound signal
D. Absorption	4. Product of tissue density and the velocity of sound
E. Attenuation	5. Distribution of power within an area, analogous to *loudness*

5. Which of the following statements regarding the interaction between ultrasound and tissue is the least accurate?

A. The shorter the wavelength, the smaller the structures that can be accurately resolved.

B. The higher the frequency of ultrasound, the higher the axial spatial resolution.

C. The lower the frequency of ultrasound, the higher the tissue penetration.

D. Attenuation is independent of the frequency or tissue type.

E. The ratio of energy reflection versus transmission is directly related to the degree of acoustic mismatch.

6. Which of the following statements regarding the use of ultrasound gel is most accurate?

A. Acoustic coupling gels must always be used because the transducer footprint might otherwise create friction on the skin with resultant tissue injury from heating.

B. Acoustic coupling gels are required to form an image because otherwise 99% of the ultrasound energy is reflected prior to being transmitted into the skin.

C. The use of gel between the transducer and skin surface lowers the percentage of energy transmitted into the body.

D. Acoustic coupling gel is not mandatory to create an ultrasound image but helps to enhance the signal-to-noise ratio.

E. The use of gel alters the ultrasound frequency, increasing the penetration of the energy.

7. Which of the following tissues is not an example of a specular reflector?

A. Left ventricular endocardium
B. Left ventricular myocardial texture or speckles
C. Pericardium
D. Mitral valve
E. Right ventricular epicardium

8. Based upon the 2D short-axis images shown in FIGURE 3.1, which of the following statements is most accurate?

A. The image on the left was obtained using much higher gain than the image on the right.

B. The image on the right has the focus much closer to the near field than does the image on the left.

C. The image on the left was obtained with fundamental frequency, and the image on the right was obtained using a harmonic multiband imaging probe.

D. The image on the left used a lower-frequency imaging probe compared with the image on the right.

E. The image on the left has higher spatial resolution than does the image on the right.

9. Which of the following statements regarding 2D image acquisition is most accurate?

A. Bursts, or pulses, of ultrasound are transmitted after a brief excitation of the piezoelectric elements to create a pulsed-wave Doppler image, but continuous transmission is necessary for 2D imaging.

B. Pulse repetition rates (or frequencies) between 1,000 and 2,000 per second are used for M-mode scanning but higher in 2D scanning and usually between 3,000 and 5,000 per second.

C. Since M-mode scanning has a higher pulse repetition rate than 2D scanning, M-mode has a higher temporal resolution compared to 2D echocardiography.

D. Conventional 2D ultrasound requires very sensitive receivers since up to 50% of the emitted ultrasound energy may be lost (attenuated) prior to reflecting back to the transducer.

E. Pulse repetition frequencies are indeed lower for 2D scanning since the pulses are transmitted across a 90-degree sector scan.

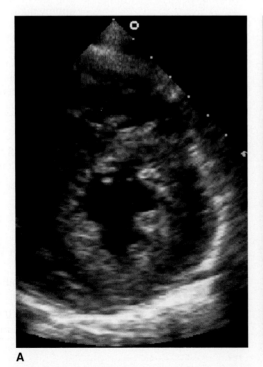 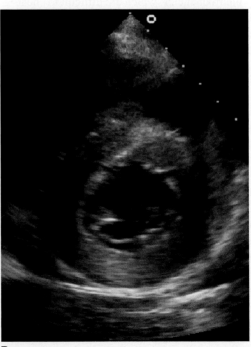

A B

FIGURE 3.1 From Armstrong WF, Ryan T. *Feigenbaum's Echocardiography.* 7th ed. Philadelphia, PA: Lippincott Williams & Wilkins, 2010.

10. Which of the following relationships regarding the creation of a 2D image is least accurate?

A. The PRF (pulse repetition frequency) is dependent on the depth of the image.

B. Increasing the 2D sector angle from 60 to 90 degrees requires more raster lines to maintain image quality.

C. A line density (# lines/degree) of at least 200 lines/degree is necessary for maintaining high-quality 2D images.

D. Increasing the frame rate will lower the line density and worsen the image quality.

E. To include color-flow images on the same display as 2D images, the entire velocity spectrum cannot be measured, and only the mean frequency (and frequency spread—"variance") is calculated.

11. You are asked to assist in the performance of an intraoperative TEE as the surgeon is coming off bypass. When you arrive on the scene, the anesthesiologist is frustrated since the US system just "shut down" after an error message about "heating." Upon further questioning, the same midesophageal image was being viewed by medical students throughout the entire 45-minute operation. Which of the following statements is most accurate?

A. Heating is so rare; this likely represents a malfunction of the ultrasound system or TEE probe. This patient is at potential risk for severe injury, and the probe should not be used again until checked.

B. This likely could have been avoided by maintaining a transgastric view instead of an esophageal view.

C. This likely could have been avoided by using the freeze button or reducing the mechanical index.

D. This is a normal US system process and is likely due to a febrile patient. It requires the operator to "dial up" the "patient temperature" to match the probe temperature.

E. Restarting the US system and continuing to image as before are safe and do not place this patient at an increased risk.

12. Match the common 2D artifact highlighted on each figure with the most likely artifact description:

Figure 3.2	A. Ring-down artifact
Figure 3.3	B. Side-lobe artifact
Figure 3.4	C. Reverberation artifact
Figure 3.5	D. Shadowing artifact
Figure 3.6	E. Enhancement artifact
	F. Mirror-image artifact
	G. Not an artifact—real pathology

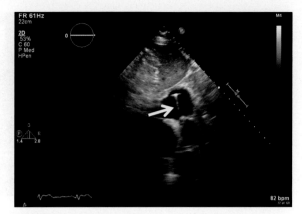

FIGURE 3.2

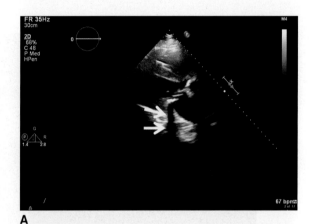

A

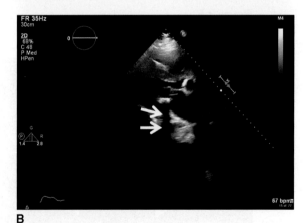

B

FIGURE 3.3

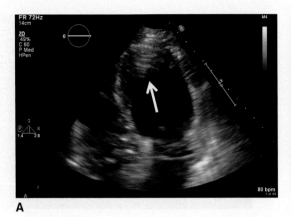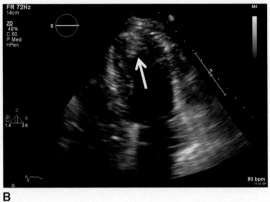

A   **B**

FIGURE 3.4

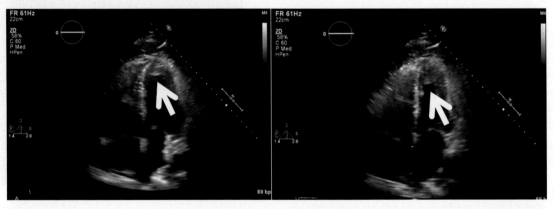

FIGURE 3.5

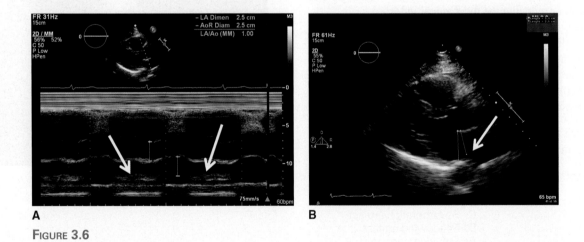

A   **B**

FIGURE 3.6

Answer 1: C. This question assesses the basic understanding of ultrasound waves, specifically those used for medical imaging. Ultrasound frequency is above the human hearing spectrum (hence the nomenclature), which usually ranges from 20 to 20,000 Hz. Ultrasound waves technically may have any frequency of >20,000 Hz, but most echo probes are in the 1- to 12-MHz ranges (1,000,000- to 12,000,000-Hz range). For ease of visualization, ultrasound waves are often depicted as sinusoidal waves where the sounds waves amplify perpendicular to the direction of the wavefront, but sound waves actually amplify parallel to the direction of the wavefront (longitudinal). This leads to vibration of particles in the direction of the ultrasound wavefront. Similar to peaks (or crests) and troughs in sinusoidal waves, longitudinal waves have areas of compression (oscillations are close together/particles are closely related to one another) and areas of rarefaction (oscillations are further apart/particles are loosely related to one another). Within the medium, these minor particle oscillations correspond to subtle changes in pressure, but no genuine particle motion transpires.

The wavelength is measured from the beginning of one compression to the beginning of the next compression. Similar to any other wave, the frequency of emission of an ultrasound wave is inversely related to the wavelength and the product of both equals the speed of sound. The speed of sound in a specific medium is fixed, and does not vary. The speed of sound is different in different mediums though (i.e., muscle different than water, which is different than the speed of sound in air).

Unlike audible frequency sound, ultrasound has several unique characteristics that contribute to its diagnostic use. Ultrasound can be directed as a beam and focused. Ultrasound adheres to the rules of reflection (straight target) and refraction (angled target). Small targets will reflect ultrasound and can be characterized. Unfortunately, when ultrasound hits a gaseous medium, attenuation is severe. This is worse with higher frequencies.

The degree of reflection, refraction, and attenuation depend on the acoustic properties of the media. The lungs reflect most of the ultrasound energy resulting in poor penetration. However, when the material property of the lungs changes (e.g., pulmonary edema), the ultrasound characteristics predictably change and provide an opportunity for diagnostic imaging. Soft tissues (and blood) reflect much less of the ultrasound energy allowing increased penetration and greater diagnostic value.

Option A is incorrect since sounds will travel at a fixed speed through a specific medium and not a variable speed. In the body, speed will vary as it interacts with different media.

Option B is incorrect since human hearing ranges from 20 to 20,000 Hz, so "ultrasound" is higher than 20,000 Hz (infrasound is <20 Hz).

Option D is incorrect since most cardiac imaging probes are between 1 and 12 MHz (or 1,000,000 and 12,000,000 Hz).

Option E is incorrect since ultrasound, unlike audible sounds, is less likely to diffract and more likely to travel in a straight line.

Suggested Reading
Wells PNT. Physics. In: Leech G, Sutton G, eds. *An Introduction to Echocardiography*. London, UK: MediCine Ltd., 1978.

Answer 2: *A.* The degree of reflection, refraction, and attenuation will vary on the acoustic properties of the tissue it is traveling through. If there is much air (or other gaseous material), such as the lung and bone (with its interfaces), then most of the sound is reflected, and attenuation occurs rapidly. Very dense media reflect most of the ultrasound energy, and less dense media (soft tissues and blood) allow much more ultrasound energy to propagate and create a diagnostic image.

All of the answer choices (except for option E) are true statements. This question intends to separate out characteristics of ultrasound that are advantageous and leveraged to generate useful data versus characteristics of ultrasound that result in potential artifacts. These factors often influence the clinical acquisition of images and therefore can be manipulated.

Option B is an advantage of ultrasound. Since particles vibrate parallel to the line of propagation, longitudinal waves are created allowing for the creation of an adequate 2D image.

Option C is also an advantage of ultrasound since this acoustic mismatch within the medium is what is responsible for creating a diagnostic ultrasonic image.

Option D is important and an advantage of ultrasound since this variable property within the media is predictable and consistent. Therefore, the degree of reflection, refraction, and attenuation leads to differences in tissue appearance on ultrasound.

Option E is an incorrect statement. Importantly, the particle oscillation is very tiny, and no actual particle motion occurs. It would be extremely rare for tissue heating to occur with routine medical ultrasound.

Suggested Readings
Kisslo JA, vonRamm OT, Thurstone FL. Cardiac imaging using a phased array ultrasound system. II. Clinical technique and application. *Circulation* 1976;53:262–267.

Roelandt J, van Dorp WG, Bom N, et al. Resolution problems in echocardiology: a source of interpretation errors. *Am J Cardiol* 1976;37:256–262.

Answer 3: *D.* This question assesses the different velocities of sound in different media. The velocity of sound varies depending on the density of tissue as it travels through the medium. TABLE 3.1 represents the velocity of sound and various tissues.

Velocity is fastest in bone (>4,000 m/s) and slowest in air (<350 m/s). Most soft tissue organs and blood are the same, and blood travels at 1,540 m/s (or 1.54 km/s).

Suggested Readings
King DL. Cardiac ultrasonography. Cross-sectional ultrasonic imaging of the heart. *Circulation* 1973;47:843–847.

vonRamm OT, Thurstone FL. Cardiac imaging using a phased array ultrasound system. I. System design. *Circulation* 1976;53:258–262.

Table 3.1 **Velocity of Sound and Various Tissues**

TISSUE TYPE	VELOCITY (M/S)
Air	330
Fat	1,450
Soft tissues	1,540
Blood	1,570
Muscle	1,580
Bone	4,080

Answer 4: Correct pairings:

A—3
B—5
C—4
D—1
E—2

This question assesses the basic understanding of commonly used terms in clinical echocardiography (and frankly all clinical ultrasound modalities). See TABLE 3.2 of basic definitions related to ultrasound. While matching is not a common method for testing these concepts, these concepts are readily tested.

Suggested Readings

Armstrong WF, Ryan T. *Feigenbaum's Echocardiography*. 7th ed. Philadelphia, PA: Lippincott Williams & Wilkins, 2010.

Pye SD, Wild SR, McDicken WN. Adaptive time gain compensation for ultrasonic imaging. *Ultrasound Med Biol* 1992;18:205–212.

Answer 5: D. This question assesses the impact of wavelength and frequency on the axial spatial resolution and attenuation. For a given medium, the speed of sound is constant (for muscle and blood, this is around 1,540 m/s). $V = \lambda \times f$ (where V = speed of sound, λ = wavelength, and f = frequency). Therefore, increasing the frequency of the probe would decrease the wavelength and vice versa. The axial spatial resolution is usually described as the minimum distance between two points to accurately discriminate them (smaller distance means better spatial resolution) and is determined by the equation:

$$\text{Axial spatial resolution} = \text{Spatial pulse length}/2$$

or

$$\text{Axial spatial resolution} = (\text{\# of cycles per pulse} \times \text{wavelength of pulse})/2$$

Therefore, decreasing the wavelength or increasing the frequency would improve the axial spatial resolution. Higher-

---

Table 3.2   **Basic Definitions Related to Ultrasound**

TERM	DEFINITION
Absorption	The transfer of ultrasound energy to the tissue during propagation
Acoustic impedance	The product of the density of the medium and the velocity of sound; differences in acoustic impedance between two media determine the ratio of transmitted vs. reflected sound at the interface
Amplitude	The magnitude of the pressure changes along the wave; also, the strength of the wave (in decibels)
Attenuation	The net loss of ultrasound energy as a wave propagates through a medium
Cycle	The combination or sum of one compression and one rarefaction of a propagating wave
Dead time	The time in between pulses that the ultrasound is not emitting ultrasound
Decibel	A logarithmic measure of the intensity of sound, expressed as a ratio to a reference value (dB)
Duty factor	The fraction of time that the transducer is emitting ultrasound; a unit-less number between 0 and 1
Far field	The diverging conical portion of the beam beyond the near field
Frequency	The number of cycles per second, measured in hertz (Hz)
Gain	The degree, or percentage, of amplification of the returning ultrasound signal
Half-layer value	The distance an ultrasound beam penetrates into a medium before its intensity has attenuated to one-half the original value
Intensity	The concentration or distribution of power within an area, often the cross-sectional area of the ultrasound beam, analogous to loudness
Longitudinal wave	A cyclic disturbance in which the energy propagation is parallel to the direction of particle motion
Near field	The proximal cylindrical-shaped portion of the ultrasound beam before divergence begins to occur
Period	The time required to complete one cycle, usually expressed in microseconds (μs)
Piezoelectricity	The phenomenon of changing shape in response to an applied electric current, resulting in vibration and the production of sound waves; the ability to produce an electric impulse in response to a mechanical deformation; thus, the interconversion of electrical and sound energy
Power	The rate of transfer over time of the acoustic energy from the propagating wave to the medium, measured in watts
Pulse	A burst or packet of emitted ultrasound of finite duration, containing a fixed number of cycles traveling together
Pulse length	The physical length or distance that a pulse occupies in space, usually expressed in millimeters (mm)
Pulse repetition frequency	The rate at which pulses are emitted from the transducer, that is, the number of pulses emitted within a period of time, usually 1 s
Resolution	The smallest distance between two points that allows the points to be distinguished as separate
Sensitivity	The ability of the system to image small targets at a given depth
Ultrasound	A mechanical vibration in a physical medium, characterized by a frequency >20,000 Hz
Velocity	The speed at which sound moves through a given medium
Wavelength	The length of a single cycle of the ultrasound wave; a measure of distance, not time

From Armstrong WF, Ryan T. *Feigenbaum's Echocardiography*. 7th ed. Philadelphia, PA: Lippincott Williams & Wilkins, 2010.

frequency probes improve spatial resolution because the higher the frequency, the shorter the wavelength.

So why not use high-frequency probes for all imaging? Unfortunately, the physics of diagnostic imaging is robust with trade-offs. The improvement of one aspect of diagnostic imaging is often wrought with another aspect that must worsen for this improvement. In this case, the higher the frequency probe, the more attenuation one gets at a given distance. Attenuation represents the net loss of signal from all sources (absorption, scattering, and reflection) and is directly related to depth of imaging and emitted frequency for any given tissue. Attenuation can be estimated by the following formula: 0.5 dB/cm/MHz. Given than relationship, it can be assumed that the attenuation for a 3.5-MHz transducer imaging an object at 20 cm depth will be $0.5 \times 20 \times 3.5 = 35$ dB. A 5-MHz transducer will undergo much greater attenuation: $0.5 \times 20 \times 5 = 50$ dB. This is a prime reason why transthoracic imaging probes have a lower frequency than transesophageal probes do. Transthoracic imaging probes are usually imaging at a greater depth from the ultrasound source, and therefore are prone to more attenuation due to depth alone (as well as other attenuating tissue, such as bone and air). Transesophageal echocardiograms can image closer to the heart and therefore are subject to less attenuation due to depth (and less attenuating tissue interference).

Option A: The shorter the wavelength, the lower the spatial pulse length, and therefore the smaller the distance between two objects that can be resolved (higher spatial resolution).

Option B: Similarly, the higher the frequency, the shorter the wavelength, leading to improved axial spatial resolution.

Option C: Lower emitted frequency results in lower axial spatial resolution, but at the benefit of increased tissue penetration.

Option E: This statement is also true, and is best reflected at the interface between blood and myocardium where the high acoustic mismatch leads to increased reflection of signal back to the transducer and a "bright" myocardial wall.

Suggested Readings

Kisslo JA, vonRamm OT, Thurstone FL. Dynamic cardiac imaging using a focused, phased-array ultrasound system. *Am J Med* 1977;63:61–68.
Vogel J, Bom N, Ridder J, et al. Transducer design considerations in dynamic focusing. *Ultrasound Med Biol* 1979;5:187–193.

Answer 6: B. This question assesses the role of ultrasound gel in image generation. Acoustic mismatch creates ultrasound echoes. These echoes obey the rules of optics (absorption, reflection, and refraction), and depend on the angle of incidence and the magnitude of the acoustic impedance. Given incomplete contact of a flat ultrasound transducer plate and the more irregular skin surface, pockets of air interfere with the signal. The use of an acoustic coupling gel is necessary to reduce the air–tissue interface at the skin surface (otherwise, >99% of the ultrasonic energy would be lost). This is due to the low acoustic impedance of air. Gel increases the percentage of energy transmitted into the body.

Option B is the correct answer. Due to the very low acoustic impedance of air, gel is necessary to minimize this intervening air layer.

Option A: Gel is not used to modify injury. There is a very limited risk of heating, and this is not due to friction between the transducer footprint and the skin.

Option C: The use of gel decreases the reflection and increases the penetration of ultrasound energy.

Option D: Gel is necessary to create an ultrasound image.

Option E is incorrect. Although ultrasound gel results in increased penetration of energy, this effect is not due to an alteration of the ultrasound frequency.

Answer 7: B. This question requires an understanding of the different type of reflectors. As ultrasound passes through the body, it encounters multiple small and large interfaces that alter the transmission of energy. Specular reflectors are created by targets that are large relative to the ultrasound wavelength. These are generally large structures. This type of interaction is seen in endocardial and epicardial surfaces, cardiac valves, and the pericardium.

Scattered reflectors are created by targets that are small relative to the transmitted wavelength. Only a very tiny portion of the ultrasound energy is reflected back to the transducer. This type of interaction results in the "speckle" pattern that creates the texture within the myocardium. Without this type of interaction, also referred to as Rayleigh scatterers, the myocardial wall would instead appear as two solid lines (endocardium and epicardium/pericardium) with an echo-free space in between.

Options A, C, D, and E are large structures compared to the sub-millimeter wavelength typical of cardiac ultrasound imaging.

Suggested Readings

Kisslo JA, vonRamm OT, Thurstone FL. Cardiac imaging using a phased array ultrasound system. II. Clinical technique and application. *Circulation* 1976;53:262–267.
Morgan CL, Trought WS, Clark WM, et al. Principles and applications of a dynamically focused phased array real time ultrasound system. *J Clin Ultrasound* 1978;6:385–391.

Answer 8: D. This question illustrates the impact transducer frequency changes will have on 2D image quality. It requires recognition that the image on the right has better spatial resolution. The parasternal short-axis image on the left was recorded using a 3.0-MHz transducer, while the image on the right, a similar image, was obtained with a 5.0-MHz probe. The higher-frequency image has superior spatial resolution, which is very noticeable within the myocardium where the lower-frequency image appears more "grainy" and the higher-frequency image is more "smooth." This smooth appearance is due to the ability of the higher spatial resolution to separate "two points very close together" into "two points" as opposed to "one point." The "points" or targets on this image reside within the heterogeneity of the normal LV myocardium. This is also noticeable at the LV endocardial border, where the lower-resolution image on the left has a highly irregular appearance with some areas that inexplicably extend into the cavity (at around the 12 o'clock position in the image).

Option A: Changing the gain affects the overall "loudness" of the image. Turning up the gain is analogous to turning the volume up to listen. While it increases the signal of the structure of interest, it also turns up the background noise and has no effect on spatial resolution. It would not explain the difference in resolution.

Option B: The focal point really affects the lateral resolution more than it does axial resolution, and will cause different lateral resolution within an image. Changing the focus (or focal depth) will cause a portion of the image to appear sharper at the expense of the rest of the image. Changing the focal depth would not explain the overall decreased resolution in the image on the left.

Option C: While it is true that harmonic imaging improves signal to noise compared to fundamental frequency, it does not have a direct effect on axial spatial resolution (the distance that two points need to be for the ultrasound to resolve them as two separate points). Typically, the role of switching to harmonic imaging is to reduce artifact from near-field structures. This is often tested by showing an image with a bright reflector in the near field (chest wall or bright pericardium) with artifact followed by an image with the artifact minimized due to the use of harmonic imaging.

Option E: The LV myocardial image on the *right* has a noticeably higher spatial resolution, which correlates with a higher frequency probe.

Suggested Reading
Pye SD, Wild SR, McDicken WN. Adaptive time gain compensation for ultrasonic imaging. *Ultrasound Med Biol* 1992;18:205–212.

Answer 9: B. This question assesses the role of pulse repetition rate or frequency (PRF) on image generation in different modes. To create either a 2D ultrasound image or an M-mode image, the fundamental approach is similar. Excitation (now, usually electrical excitation) of a piezoelectric crystal generates an ultrasound pulse that travels through the body while the transducer waits to receive returning signals that have been reflected. The rate at which the pulses are generated is known as a pulse repetition rate or frequency (PRF). This has nothing to do with the fundamental frequency of an ultrasound probe but instead has to do with the depth of imaging. It has to wait for the pulse to return before sending out another pulse. The deeper the structure of interest, the longer it takes for the signal to return given a fixed velocity of sound through a specific medium. Therefore, PRF decreases with increasing depth.

Another consideration is the amount of "data" needed to be acquired. The pulse repetition rate (frequency) of M-mode echocardiography is typically 1,000 to 2,000 pulses/s and 3,000 to 5,000 pulses/s to create the 90-degree sector scan associated with 2D. Although the pulse repetition rate is lower for M-mode, all of the pulses are devoted to a single raster line providing a temporal resolution (TR) that is much higher for M-mode compared with 2D echocardiography. To improve the TR of 2D, one can narrow the image sector, and this will greatly improve the TR. Also, decreasing the depth will quicken the time of the transmitted energy to return to the receiver and also improve the TR. Transducers must have very sensitive receivers that can detect signals that are markedly attenuated since <1% of the emitted ultrasound energy is typically reflected.

Option A: All ultrasonic imaging requires energy to be transmitted, reflected, and received, and the transducer must act as both a sender and a receiver of bursts or pulses of ultrasound.

Option C: 2D scanning must have a higher pulse repetition rate needed to create an image over a large (90-degree) sector. Since M-mode has all of its pulses dedicated to a single raster line, the temporal resolution is far greater, despite having slower pulse repetition rates.

Option D: Much more than 50% of the emitted energy is attenuated (99%).

Option E: 2D requires higher pulse repetition rates to maintain an adequate temporal resolution despite creating such a large sector of data.

Answer 10: C. This question focuses on image generation of a 2D ultrasound image. A number of variables must be considered when creating a 2D image. The depth of the examination, the pulse repetition frequency (PRF—related to the depth of examination), the line density, the sector width, and the desired frame rate all conspire to result in a high-quality image. After sending in a burst of ultrasound, the returning signal must be received, and this is mostly a function of the depth of transmission. Each ultrasound pulse provides a single raster line of data, and the rate that the pulses are transmitted is the PRF. An M-mode image represents that single raster line of data over time. The PRF for M-mode is ~1,000 to 2,000 pulses/s. To obtain a 2D image (as opposed to a single-dimensional M-mode image), the ultrasound beam needs to sweep through an angle, obtaining multiple raster lines. Remember, a single pulse gives a single line of information, and the more the lines needed, the longer it would take to get that whole image. Therefore, even with a higher PRF of 3,000 to 5,000 pulses/s, 2D images have a lower temporal resolution than M-mode. This temporal resolution in 2D imaging is driven largely by the number of lines that need to be acquired. The two factors that influence the number of lines acquired are the line density and the sector width. The greater the line density (lines per degree of coverage), the higher the spatial resolution and image quality, but the longer it takes to get a full 2D image (lower temporal resolution). More data lines are needed to fill larger sectors. A line density of approximately two lines per degree is usually adequate to construct a high-quality image. Line density can be increased by decreasing the sector width (same # lines per smaller region), reducing the frame rate (more time for building lines/frame), and reducing the depth (shorter lines = shorter time to build).

The total ultrasonic data recorded during one complete sweep of the ultrasound beam are termed a "field." The sum of imaging data recorded is a frame. Two fields are interlaced (to improve line density) to produce one frame, and therefore, the frame rate is half of the sweep rate.

Option A is a true statement since the PRF is greatly dependent on the time to transmit and receive an ultrasound burst. Since the speed of sound is relatively fixed, the most important variable is the depth of the image.

Answer B is a true statement since more lines of data are necessary to create and maintain an adequate image quality as the sector increases.

Answer D is a true statement. To increase the frame rate, the line density is compromised, and therefore, the image quality degrades.

Answer E is a true statement. This concept is increasingly important as one tries to compare tissue Doppler velocities obtained from two distinct techniques. Since color coding measures mean velocities, these measures will be inherently lower than if pulsed-wave Doppler measures were obtained.

Suggested Readings

Griffith JM, Henry WL. A sector scanner for real time two-dimensional echocardiography. *Circulation* 1974;49:1147–1152.

King DL. Cardiac ultrasonography. Cross-sectional ultrasonic imaging of the heart. *Circulation* 1973;47:843–847.

Wells PNT. Physics. In: Leech G, Sutton G, eds. *An Introduction to Echocardiography*. London, UK: MediCine Ltd., 1978.

Answer 11: C. Ultrasound is one of the safest diagnostic tools available. Despite millions of examinations, no single serious adverse event has been reported in routine clinical studies. However, in animal exams and possibly in newer therapeutic ultrasound techniques, this may change. Since the biologic impact of ultrasound will depend on the total energy (joules) applied, the amount of tissue exposed to this energy, and the duration of the exposure, these are the ultrasound parameters most relevant to discuss further.

1 Watt = 1 joule of energy produced in 1 second. A milliwatt = 0.001 W. Intensity = W/m^2. This concept becomes very confusing in the human since ultrasound is sent in pulses ("duty factor" defines time of US emission), tissues in biologic systems are highly variable, and the power varies within both the ultrasound beam (highest in center) and the medium. The single most relevant biologic effect of acoustic energy is tissue heating.

Heating is dependent on tissue properties, duration of exposure (duty factor), US intensity (power), and inversely on blood flow (which acts to dampen heating by "carrying" heat away from the tissue exposed to US).

Intraoperative TEE imaging is a potential concern since the probe has higher energy and the imaging scan may image the same tissue over and over without manipulation, creating greater likelihood for heating and tissue injury. Thus, TEE probes have a "warning" shutdown that may alert the operator of increased TEE probe temperature and should result in steps to reduce injury (e.g., reduction in imaging power, repositioning the probe often, limiting the imaging time [use freeze button when not actually using US image data]).

Beyond heating, there are very little data to suggest that US has a significant biologic effect on patients. Early in echo development, much concern was raised about the potential for "cavitation." Cavitation is the production of gas bubbles when US energy penetrates tissues, but this has not been demonstrated in vivo. Cyclical variation in the size of injected manufactured microbubbles occurs within the US field and with high power will result in microbubble destruction. This interaction has yet to have demonstrated an important biologic effect. In fact, some investigators have taken advantage of this interaction and have demonstrated more rapid clot lysis with thrombolytic therapy if performed simultaneously with microbubble injection and US imaging.

Option A is incorrect since it is not the single best answer. Although a system malfunction may have occurred, in this situation, a malfunction was not necessary since the students kept the high-frequency TEE probe imaging for 45 minutes at a single location. This invokes a potential risk of esophageal burn. Although not reported in the literature, esophageal perforation has been demonstrated, and the role of localized heating cannot be excluded as a contributing factor.

Option B is incorrect since although the gastric mucosa is thicker (and risk of injury likely less), probe heating will still occur if left imaging in a stationary position for this long.

Option C is the single best answer. Steps to reduce localized heating include limiting the overall imaging time (use freeze button when not actually using US image data) and reduction in imaging power (mechanical index). See discussion below.

Option D is incorrect. Although a febrile patient may actually result in a higher temperature being registered on the TEE probe and US system, assuming this is the cause and increasing the "patient temperature" setting risks potential mucosal injury from heating.

Option E is incorrect since it would pose potential risk to continue to "image as before," which already resulted in the system's warning mechanism to operate as designed and shut down once before.

Suggested Readings

Carstensen EL, et al. Bioeffects in echocardiography. *Echocardiography* 1992;9:605–623.

Hitchcock KE, et al. Ultrasound-assisted thrombolysis for stroke therapy: better thrombus break-up with bubbles. *Stroke* 2010;41:S50–S53.

Min JK, et al. Clinical features of complications from transesophageal echocardiography: a single-center case series of 10,000 consecutive examinations. *J Am Soc Echocardiogr* 2005;18(9):925–929.

Skorton DJ, et al. Ultrasound bioeffects and regulatory issues: an introduction for the echocardiographer. *J Am Soc Echocardiogr* 1988;1:240–251.

Answer 12

Figure 3.2—E. Enhancement artifact. Subcostal short-axis 2D echo demonstrating an example of a hyperechoic enhancement (or comet-tail) artifact. See text for details. See Video 3.1.

Figure 3.3—D. Shadowing artifact. Parasternal long-axis 2D echo in diastole (A) and in systole (B) demonstrating an example of a shadowing artifact. See text for details. See Video 3.2.

Figure 3.4—A. Ring-down artifact. Apical four-chamber 2D echo in diastole (A) and in systole (B) demonstrating an example of a ring-down artifact. In B, note the apical wall motion abnormality, which is not uncommon and makes the recognition of this as an artifact more clinically relevant. See text for details. See Video 3.3.

Figure 3.5—G. Not an artifact—real pathology. Apical four-chamber 2D echo in diastole (left panel) and systole (right panel) demonstrating an example of a large apical thrombus in a patient with hypereosinophilic syndrome. Unlike a ring-down artifact, this echo-bright apical mass is well defined and does not "cross tissue borders." Also note the normal apical wall motion, which is associated with this pathology. See text for details. See Video 3.4.

Figure 3.6—B. Side-lobe artifact. Parasternal long-axis 2D and M-mode echo (A) demonstrating an example of a side-lobe artifact. Note the inaccurate LA dimension measure that underestimates the true LA cavity. See text for details. See accompanying movie. Parasternal long-axis 2D echo (B) demonstrating an example of a side-lobe artifact. Note the inaccurate LA dimension measure (blue line) that underestimates the true LA cavity and was measured in the M-mode image. The green line is the true LA cavity dimension. See text for details. See Video 3.5.

One of the more important aspects of diagnostic cardiovascular imaging, and cardiac ultrasound in particular, is the recognition of artifacts—which are common. Understanding their origin helps in identifying these as artifacts and not inadvertently labeling a finding as pathology.

All artifacts are errors (noise) on the image display. They are universally due to interruptions in basic rules made by the ultrasound system. These "rules" include the following:

1. Ultrasound will only travel in a straight line.
2. All reflections result from targets seen within the central portion of the US (main) beam.
3. The US signal will travel directly to and from the target source.
4. Sound within the human medium travels at exactly 1,540 m/s.
5. Each target (reflector) contributes to a single echo.

Unfortunately, ultrasound treats these rules as guidelines, and there are many examples where these assumptions do not apply. Importantly, there are some common aspects of artifacts that help to identify them as such. These include the fact that most artifacts are less bright than their original target, may move independently from the adjacent myocardial structure, and may "pass through" adjacent tissue planes. Remember, the *distance* of a reflector is determined by the *time* it takes the US signal to return and does not always represent the actual *location* within the imaging field. Furthermore, US systems will always ascribe the returning sound in the same direction it is "looking" (sending in the ultrasound).

Some of the more commonly identified artifacts are listed below.

Reverberation artifacts are very common and may cause reduced image quality or impact diagnosis (Figs. 3.7 and 3.8, Video 3.6). They occur due to the returning ultrasound wave hitting the transducer (or another near-field reflector) and "reverberating" back into the ultrasound medium. This "reverberating" signal is not as intense as the original signal sent

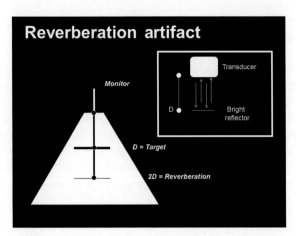

Figure 3.7

from the transducer but is able to be returned to the receiving transducer and create an "additional" image. The "reverberation image" (taking twice as long to be returned) will be displayed twice the distance from the actual target. Also, having reflected off a bright near-field, nonmoving object (e.g., the transducer casing), it will likely not move with the heart. If, however, the near-field object was not fixed (e.g., two strong reflectors within the medium like the aortic walls), then the "reverberating artifact" will be hypermobile, and the signal will move twice as far as its original target. If this signal "reverberation" continues, a series of bright echos that are equidistant from each other will be created, and each "band" will be less intense than the next. It is also important to note that reverberation artifacts may be the result of defective equipment.

Side-lobe artifacts are also very common (Fig. 3.9). Although the majority of the ultrasound beam will be localized in the center, some of the energy is located outside this central beam. A "side lobe" is the noncentral ultrasound beam associated with a single piezoelectric element, as opposed to a "grating lobe" that is associated with an array of piezoelectric elements. This "edge effect" results in noise within the image. Some of the peripheral energy will create an image, but

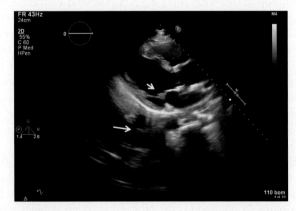

Figure 3.8 Parasternal long-axis 2D echo in systole demonstrating an example of a reverberation artifact (*long arrow*). Note that the native mitral valve (*small arrow*) is reproduced in the extracardiac posterior lung field. See text for details. See Video 3.6.

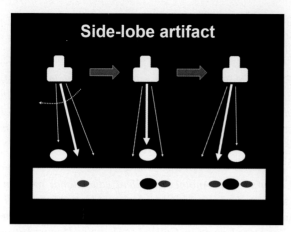

FIGURE 3.9

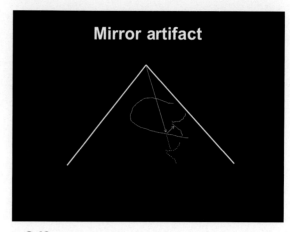

FIGURE 3.10 Cartoon showing the creation of the listed artifact.

this will be significantly less bright than the original signals returning from the central beam. Since all ultrasound will be displayed as if received from the central beam, this may create an artifact within the image display. To create an image from the "side lobe," rather than the central beam, a bright target (strong specular reflector) must generate this, and it needs to be near a much less bright object to be seen as anything other than noise. The posterior wall, left AV groove, and pericardial reflection create such a bright "side-lobe" image, and if the left atrium is dilated, an image will be created within the echo-free LA cavity.

Shadowing artifacts are relatively easy to understand. Essentially, these are severe attenuation (greater than the expected 0.5 dB/cm/MHz) artifacts that are created by very bright (calcific, metallic) targets. These objects mask any ultrasound signal from continuing beyond their reflection, and most of the energy is returned to the transducer. They are helpful in distinguishing the tissue characterization of bright tissues and will always be present from calcium (mitral annulus, coronary artery, etc.).

Ring-down artifacts were extremely common with early transducer technology, but less so with modern imaging employing multiband frequency technology and harmonic imaging. The source of this "near-field" artifact is vibration of the piezoelectric elements that create high-amplitude oscillations near the surface of the transducer. Given the very high frequencies required for certain ultrasound technologies, these linear, "ring-down" artifacts may be more common in intravascular imaging (IVUS) and intracardiac ultrasound (ICE).

Enhancement artifacts, in distinction to attenuation, are hyperechoic artifacts parallel to the US main axis. When these are very thin and long, they are often referred to as "comet tails" for obvious reasons. These are a series of echoes created by multiple reflections within a small but highly reflective object. Like all images, these are due to acoustic mismatch, and the greater the mismatch, the greater the possibility of a "comet-tail" artifact. Common causes include prosthetic clips, staples, sutures, or heart valves.

Mirror-image artifacts are one of the more elegant artifacts seen in cardiac imaging and may provide the reader with many hours of educational material (beating heart within the lung field, two mitral valves, etc.) (Fig. 3.10). These are commonly seen during ultrasound acquisition, but the sonographer is able to alter the image alignment to reduce these, so the interpreting physician sees this much less often than does the sonographer.

As the US signal reflects off a strong, smooth target (e.g., diaphragm), the surface of the target essentially acts as a mirror and reflects the returning signal to another tissue interface. The ultrasound system believes the second interface is beyond the first surface, and this is where it appears on the scan. In Figure 3.11, the *arrow* shows the real object, which appears as if reflected in a mirror.

Lastly, similar to mirror artifacts, *refraction (or lens) artifacts* are also fun for the novice echocardiographer providing numerous examples that seem to defy logic (two aortic valves, six leaflets, two left ventricles, etc.) (Fig. 3.12).

In summary, artifacts may be categorized as appearing more distant than their original target (e.g., reverberation [parallel motion] or mirror [opposite motion]) or at the same location (e.g., side lobe or refraction [lens]).

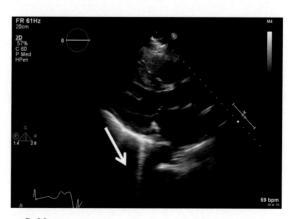

FIGURE 3.11 Parasternal long-axis 2D echo demonstrating a common location for a reverberation artifact.

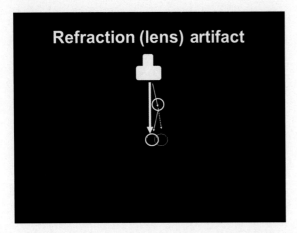

FIGURE 3.12 Cartoon showing the creation of the listed artifact. (VIDEO 3.7 is an excellent example of a lens artifact creating two short axis left ventricles from refraction off the intervening hyperechoic diaphragm.)

Suggested Reading/Watching

Feldman MK, et al. Ultrasound artifacts. *Radiographics* 2009;29:1179–1189.

Editor's Note: This is an outstanding article that addresses most of the potential artifacts created with ultrasound. Although written for radiology with minimal echocardiographic focus, it is well worth reading if this is an area of difficulty.
http://www.youtube.com/watch?v=3k3L4ZNAZqk

Editor's Note: Another excellent educational program exists on YouTube. This is a series of lectures of the Ultrasound Physics Lecture Series brought to you by the Ohio State University College of Medicine Honors Ultrasound Project. There is a four-part topic on ultrasound image artifacts that is outstanding and worth listening to in preparation for the echo boards.

Chapter 4

Basic Principles of Doppler Ultrasound

Vincent L. Sorrell

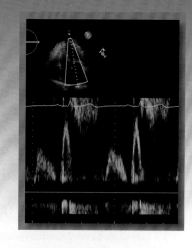

1. Which of the following statements is correct regarding the relationship between the Doppler frequency shift and the velocity of the object?

    A. Velocity is directly proportional to the angle between the Doppler ultrasound interrogating beam and the direction of the blood flow being interrogated.

    B. The change of speed of sound within the medium is an important factor contributing significantly to the measured Doppler velocity.

    C. The small difference in the transmitted and received frequencies is assumed to be twice the actual transducer frequency.

    D. A decrease in the Doppler frequency shift will decrease the recorded velocity.

    E. Velocity is equal to the frequency shift divided by a speed of sound constant times the cosine of the interrogating beam angle.

2. Doppler deviation from a parallel intercept angle to 20 degrees results in which of the following?

    A. Velocity 7% less than actual velocity
    B. Velocity 10% less than actual velocity
    C. Velocity 14% less than actual velocity
    D. Velocity 20% less than actual velocity

3. What modification could be done to improve the interrogation of the site-specific systolic Doppler signal (Fig. 4.1)?

    A. Decrease the size of the sample volume.
    B. Reduce the Nyquist limit.
    C. Increase the depth.
    D. Switch from pulsed-wave to continuous-wave Doppler.
    E. Increase the pulse repetition frequency (PRF).

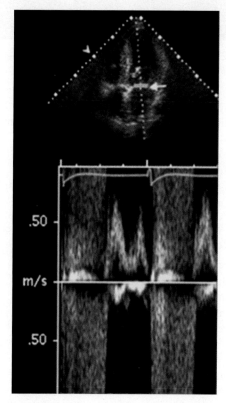

FIGURE 4.1 From Feigenbaum H, Armstrong WF, Ryan T. *Feigenbaum's Echocardiography*. 6th ed. Philadelphia, PA: Lippincott Williams & Wilkins, 2005.

4. Aliasing of the pulsed-wave Doppler spectrum occurs when the frequency is:

    A. Greater than twice the pulse repetition frequency
    B. Greater than one-half the pulse repetition frequency
    C. Greater than one-fourth the pulse repetition frequency
    D. Less than one-half of the pulse repetition frequency

5. What modification should be done to improve this spectral Doppler display (Fig. 4.2)?

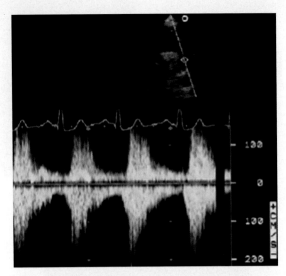

FIGURE 4.2 From Feigenbaum H, Armstrong WF, Ryan T. *Feigenbaum's Echocardiography.* 6th ed. Philadelphia, PA: Lippincott Williams & Wilkins, 2005.

   A. Increase the power output.
   B. Optimize the alignment of the Doppler beam with the flow direction.
   C. Use continuous-wave Doppler.
   D. Increase the frequency.
   E. This image represents aortic stenosis and aortic regurgitation and thus cannot be corrected.

6. Which will occur if you decrease the pulse repetition frequency during color Doppler flow acquisition?

   A. Improves flash artifact
   B. Reduces color Doppler aliasing
   C. Improves sensitivity to slow flow
   D. Increases the frame rate

7. Aliasing artifact is a problem with pulsed-wave Doppler due to which of the following?

   A. High pulse repetition frequency
   B. High Nyquist limit
   C. Sampling signal instead of continuous recording
   D. Higher frequency

8. What should be adjusted to improve the Doppler spectral signal (Fig. 4.3)?

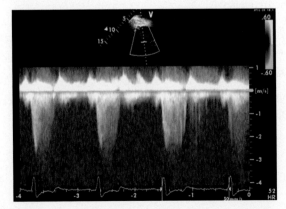

FIGURE 4.3

   A. Wall filter
   B. Gain
   C. Pulse repetition frequency
   D. Sampling rate

9. What should be adjusted to improve the Doppler spectral signal (Fig. 4.4)?

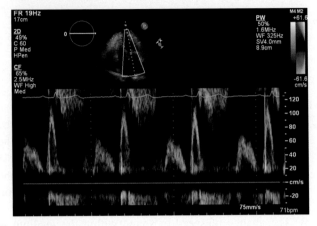

FIGURE 4.4

   A. Increase the wall filter.
   B. Reduce the wall filter.
   C. Increase the gain.
   D. Reduce the gain.
   E. Increase the frequency.

10. With the development of the digital echo examination, the audio signal is heard by the operator but rarely heard by the echo reader. Which of the following concepts related to the audio signal is most accurate?

   A. In clinical practice with a blood flow velocity range of 0.5 to 6.0 m/s, this range represents Doppler frequency shifts between 5% and 60% of the transmitted frequency.
   B. Doppler audio is not possible because the ultrasound frequency is too high to be heard.
   C. The audio signal is no longer utilized in clinical echocardiography since there is no benefit of this practice.
   D. A whistling musical sound would indicate that the frequencies contained in the Doppler signal have similar blood flow velocities and uniform direction of motion characteristic of laminar flow.
   E. Both narrow band– and broadband-shifted frequencies result in harsh audio Doppler sounds.

11. Which of the following steps would not reduce the aliasing artifact when a measured velocity is found to be too high for pulsed-wave Doppler?

   A. Use either continuous-wave Doppler or high PRF techniques.
   B. Set the zero baseline at either the top or the bottom of the spectral display.
   C. Use a higher-frequency transducer.
   D. Increase the intercept angle.
   E. Reduce the depth from the sample volume to the transducer.

Answer 1: D. Velocity of flow as determined by Doppler echocardiography honors the following equation:

$$V = \Delta f \times c/2f_o \times \cos \theta$$

where V = velocity in m/s; Δf = the difference in the transmitted and received frequencies (shifted frequencies expressed in kHz); c = velocity of sound in the medium (which for blood is assumed to be 1,560 m/s); $2f_o$ = twice the frequency transmitted by the transducer (expressed in kHz); $\cos \theta$ is the cosine formed by the angle between the Doppler ultrasound interrogating beam and the actual true direction of the blood flow being interrogated.

Answer A is incorrect. Velocity is *inversely* proportional to the angle between the Doppler ultrasound interrogating beam and the direction of the blood flow being interrogated.

Answer B is incorrect. The speed of sound within the medium is not an important factor contributing significantly to the measured Doppler velocity, and blood flow is assumed to be 1,560 m/s. Since the actual Doppler frequency shift is very small and this is multiplied to such a proportionally large value, it is the change in frequency shift that primarily determines the velocity.

Answer C is incorrect. The small difference in the transmitted and received frequencies, or the *Doppler frequency shift*, is multiplied by the speed of sound and divided by twice the actual transducer frequency.

Answer D is correct. The measured velocity of blood flow is directly proportional to the Doppler shift, and, therefore, a decrease (or increase) in the Doppler frequency shift will decrease (or increase) the recorded velocity.

Answer E is incorrect. Velocity is equal to the frequency shift *multiplied by, not divided by*, a speed of sound constant times the cosine of the interrogating beam angle (and also times $2f_o$).

This formula is important and one of many the readers need to recite. It provides the basic understanding of the relationships between Doppler ultrasound frequency shifts and the subsequently determined blood flow velocity. This velocity is then converted to pressure using the Bernoulli equation, which is essential in nearly every echo examination.

Suggested Readings

Hatle L, Angelsen B. *Doppler Ultrasound in Cardiology: Physical Principles and Clinical Applications.* Philadelphia, PA: Lea & Febiger, 1985:32.
Hoskins PR. A review of the measurement of blood velocity and related quantities using Doppler ultrasound. *Proc Inst Mech Eng H* 1999;213:391–400.

Answer 2: A. The Doppler shift (Δf) depends on the transmitted frequency of the ultrasound, the speed of sound, the intercept angle between the interrogating beam and the flow, and, finally, the velocity of the target (FIG. 4.5).

Red blood cells are moving toward the transducer at a given velocity (v), the reflected frequency (F_r), and emitted frequency (F_0). Cos θ is the cosine of the angle between blood flow and the incidence of the ultrasound beam.

It is evident from this figure, with increasing angle of Doppler transmitted frequency to the direction of blood flow,

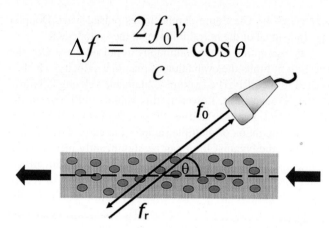

$$\Delta f = \frac{2f_0 v}{c} \cos \theta$$

FIGURE 4.5 From Feigenbaum H, Armstrong WF, Ryan T. *Feigenbaum's Echocardiography.* 6th ed. Philadelphia, PA: Lippincott Williams & Wilkins, 2005.

that there will be reduction in the actual velocity interpreted. Between 0 and 20 degrees, the error is less, but with angle > 20 degrees, there is a significant reduction in the velocity interpreted compared to the actual velocity (TABLE 4.1).

Doppler with angle correction is a common universal technique in vascular ultrasound, which has narrow flow variations within small-caliber vessels. Unfortunately, this same technique cannot be applied to large-caliber chambers assessed with cardiac ultrasound.

With current instrumentation, it is not possible to accurately measure the angle theta (degrees), and therefore it is not possible to use mathematical angle correction algorithms to adjust for flow based upon the accompanying 2D image. The direction of flow in the azimuthal plane (into or out of the monitor screen) is never known and only coincidentally along the line of the 2D flow pattern. For this reason, the operator must compensate for this inability to predict optimal flow alignment by obtaining multiple 2D imaging planes in the hope of coming as close as possible to the true flow (the narrowest angle; cosine = 1.00).

Table 4.1	Values for Cosine for Selected Angles
ANGLE (DEGREE)	**COSINE**
0	+1.00
5	+1.00
10	+0.98
20	+0.94
30	+0.87
40	+0.77
50	+0.64
60	+0.50
90	0.00
180	−1.00

Suggested Reading

Haskins PR. Accuracy of maximum velocity estimates made using Doppler ultrasound systems. *Br J Radiol* 1996;69:172–177.

Answer 3: E. The figure demonstrates pulsed-wave Doppler spectral signal of the mitral inflow and the systolic MR.

Since sampling is not continuous in pulsed-wave Doppler imaging, it limits the evaluation of maximal velocity, which is related to the PRF. The maximal obtainable velocity is known as the Nyquist limit. Lowering this value would worsen the alias artifact demonstrated on the figure (answer B is incorrect). Interrogation of multiple samples increases the PRF, and therefore, the Nyquist limit can be significantly increased. In FIGURE 4.6, multiple samples have been applied with hPRF, which increases the Nyquist limit and allows one to record a much higher velocity. Increasing the depth will lower the Nyquist limit (answer C is incorrect). Changing the sample volume does not significantly alter the Nyquist limit. Although switching to continuous-wave Doppler would certainly eliminate the alias artifact and allow display of the highest velocity, it is not a "site-specific" technique as requested in the prompt. High PRF is also less site specific since it interrogates from multiple gates; it is far more site specific than is CWD.

Suggested Reading

Quinones MA, et al. Recommendations for quantification of Doppler echocardiography: a report from the Doppler Quantification Task Force of the Nomenclature and Standards Committee of the American Society of Echocardiography. *J Am Soc Echocardiogr* 2002;15(2):167–184.

Answer 4: B. An important limitation of pulse Doppler imaging is aliasing. Aliasing occurs if frequency is greater than the Nyquist limit. The number of pulses transmitted from a Doppler transducer each second is called the PRF. Nyquist limit is equal to PRF/2. Sampling rate is an important determinant of how accurately the system resolves frequency. In order

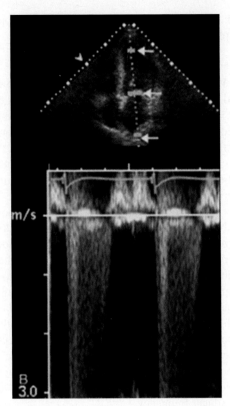

FIGURE 4.6 From Feigenbaum H, Armstrong WF, Ryan T. *Feigenbaum's Echocardiography.* 6th ed. Philadelphia, PA: Lippincott Williams & Wilkins, 2005.

to accurately determine frequency, it must be sampled at least twice PRF = 2 × frequency (1).

Additional definitions that are important when discussing Doppler principles can be seen in TABLE 4.2.

Table 4.2	Doppler Terms and Definitions
TERM	**DEFINITION**
Aliasing	Ambiguous velocities resulting from frequencies exceeding the PRF sampling limit with pulsed-wave (and color-flow) Doppler. The high velocity "wraps around" and is displayed negatively.
Baseline shift	Repositioning of the zero flow velocity line upward or downward to overcome aliasing
Carrier frequency	The frequency emitted by the transducer
Continuous wave	A method of Doppler interrogation to measure the highest Doppler velocity that uses two crystals—one each to constantly transmit and receive frequency shifts. Advantage: no aliasing with high velocities. Disadvantage: no depth localization
Frequency shift	The difference between the transmitted and received frequencies, which is directly proportional to the velocity of blood flow
hPRF	High pulse repetition frequency Doppler is a method to achieve high sampling rates by incorporating multiple sample volumes (and multiple pulses) that allows Doppler shifts to be summed to provide a single output.
Mirror artifact	Also commonly referred to as "cross talk," this spectral Doppler artifact results from the spectrum analyzer to separate positive (forward) and negative (reverse) Doppler signals.
Pulsed wave	A method of Doppler interrogation to measure discrete velocity at a specific region (sample) along the ultrasound beam that uses one crystal to transmit and then pause and wait to receive the localized frequency shift. Advantage: depth localization and site-specific interrogation. Disadvantage: aliasing with high velocities
Spectral broadening	An increase in the number of frequency components in a pulsed-wave Doppler signal indicating disorganized or high-velocity flow
Wall filter	A control that rejects low-velocity ultrasound information such as wall motion. For tissue Doppler interrogation, the filter (and gain) must be set very low.

Reference

1. Feigenbaum H, et al. *Feigenbaum's Echocardiography*. 6th ed. Philadelphia, PA: Lippincott Williams & Wilkins, 2005.

Suggested Reading

Quinones MA, et al. Recommendations for quantification of Doppler echocardiography: a report from the Doppler Quantification Task Force of the Nomenclature and Standards Committee of the American Society of Echocardiography. *J Am Soc Echocardiogr* 2002;15(2):182–184.

Answer 5: *B.* This is the mirror image of a symmetric spectral image on the opposite side of the baseline from the true signal. These artifacts can be reduced by decreasing the power output and optimizing the alignment of the Doppler beam with the flow direction.

Answer 6: *C.* Slow flow produces low-frequency shifts. Setting PRF lower increases sensitivity to low-frequency shifts. Changing PRF has negligible effect on frame rate or flash artifact.

Answer 7: *C.* The number of pulses transmitted from a Doppler transducer each second is called the PRF. Sampling rate is an important determinant of how accurately the system resolves frequency information. The upper limit of frequency that can be detected by a given pulsed system is the Nyquist limit, which is defined as one-half the PRF. To accurately represent a given frequency, it must be sampled at least twice. Aliasing occurs if the signal is not adequately sampled. With continuous-wave Doppler rather than sending out intermittent pulses of information, the ultrasound signal is continuously transmitted and received, and thus prevents aliasing. High Nyquist limit and high PRF prevent aliasing.

Answer 8: *B.* There is noise in the background as well in the spectral display due to high gain. Gain should be reduced to adjust this image.

Answer 9: *B.* Wall filter or high-pass filter eliminates frequency shifts below the set threshold. This definitely helps in eliminating low-frequency tissue movements from the spectral display but may also eliminate low-frequency shifts from slow flow. Increasing the wall filter threshold decreases the sensitivity to detect slow flow (Fig. 4.7).

Suggested Reading

Armstrong WF. *Feigenbaum's Echocardiography*. 7th ed. Philadelphia, PA: Lippincott Williams & Wilkins, 2009.

Answer 10: *D.* Answer A is incorrect. In Doppler echo, the frequency shift (Δf) between the transmitted (solid line) and received frequency (dotted line) is very little (<1%). For typical clinical ranges of velocity between 0.5 and 6.0 m/s, this range represents frequency shifts between 0.03% and 0.76% of the transmitted frequency (Fig. 4.8).

Answer B is incorrect. Although the transmitted frequency is the megahertz range (inaudible), it is transposed to the audible range for humans (<20 kHz).

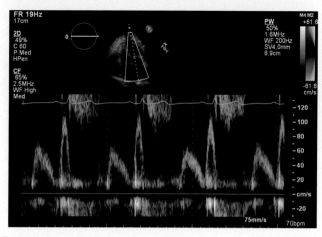

Figure 4.7 Proper wall filter setting.

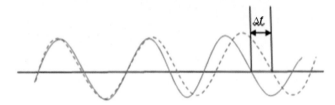

Figure 4.8

Answer C is incorrect. The echo operator and the interpreter used to value this audio signal as it could be used as guidance in the performance of the Doppler examination.

Answer D is correct. A narrow band of shifted frequencies produces a whistling musical audio sound. This is classically noted in laminar, or nondisturbed, blood flow.

Answer E is incorrect. Broadband-shifted frequencies, characteristic of turbulent or disturbed flow, typically produce a harsh audio sound. This is indicative of frequencies within the region of sampling that are heterogeneous with respect to the direction of motion and velocity of the sampled blood.

Suggested Readings

Hatle L. Noninvasive assessment and differentiation of left ventricular outflow obstruction with Doppler ultrasound. *Circulation* 1981;64:381–387.

Spencer MP, Reid JM. Quantitation of carotid stenosis with continuous-wave. *Stroke* 1979;10(3):326–330.

Answer 11: *C.* Prior to the availability of continuous-wave (and high PRF) Doppler techniques, since pulsed-wave Doppler techniques were developed first, the operator had to learn a number of methods to reduce the commonly found aliasing artifact. Currently, the most common technique to reduce this artifact is to switch to CWD or hPRF (answer A is therefore incorrect). Another commonly employed technique is to move the baseline. This will effectively double the velocity range because the entire velocity range is reset relative to the baseline (answer B is therefore incorrect). A lower, not higher, frequency transducer allows a higher velocity range to be obtained. For example, if a 3-MHz transducer permits a measurement of X cm/s, a 1.5-MHz transducer will increase the maximal velocity to 2X (answer C is therefore the correct choice). Increasing the intercept angle will obviously reduce the maximal velocity and will therefore reduce the aliasing artifact (Option D is incorrect). In clinical practice, this should not be done since the angle of flow in the azimuthal (elevational) direction is unknown and the actual velocity remains underestimated. Finally, the operator should always record velocity closest to the transducer as increased depth will reduce the velocity that aliasing occurs (answer E is incorrect).

Suggested Reading

Baker DW, et al. Doppler principles and techniques. In: Fry FJ, ed. *Methods and Phenomena 3: Ultrasound: Its Application in Medicine and Biology. Part I.* Amsterdam, The Netherlands: Elsevier Scientific, 1978: Chapter III.

Chapter 5

Instrumentation and Knobology

Vedant A. Gupta

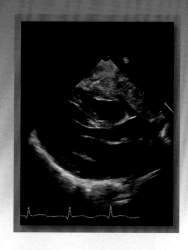

1. An overgained 2D image can be caused by all of the following EXCEPT:

   A. TGCs
   B. Gain
   C. Power Doppler
   D. Monitor

2. The monitor should be adjusted according to:

   A. Ambient light
   B. Transducer frequency
   C. Second harmonics
   D. Patient selection

3. Steps to improve the 2D image quality in an obese adult include all of the following EXCEPT:

   A. Increase frequency
   B. Increase power
   C. Decrease compress and/or dynamic range
   D. Increase gain and adjust TGC

4. One way to reduce the appearance of a grainy 2D image is to:

   A. Turn persistence off
   B. Lower fundamental frequency
   C. Increase compress and/or dynamic range
   D. Foreshorten imaging plane

5. Nonstandard views are useful in all of the following situations EXCEPT:

   A. Prior cardiac surgeries
   B. Congenital anomalies
   C. Stress echo
   D. Difficult body habitus

6. Strategies to optimize the following image to a more conventional parasternal long-axis orientation would include all of the following EXCEPT:

   A. Move the transducer up an intercostal space.
   B. Slide the transducer closer to the sternum.
   C. Lower the head of the bed.
   D. Turn the patient more toward the left side.

7. Suggestions to optimize an off-axis apical four-chamber view (left ventricular apex angled to the right side of monitor) include all of the following EXCEPT:

   A. Move the transducer more laterally.
   B. Lean the patient back slightly.
   C. Utilize bed cutout.
   D. Have the patient sit upright.

8. Spectral Doppler modalities include all of the following EXCEPT:

   A. Pulsed wave
   B. Continuous wave
   C. High-pulse repetition frequency mode
   D. Power Doppler

9. Standard pulsed wave Doppler measures velocities that are:

   A. Sample site specific.
   B. Averaged over multiple heart beats.
   C. Perpendicular to the beam.
   D. Aliased by continuous wave.

10. When acquiring the mitral inflow Doppler pattern for diastolic function, which of the following describes the optimal location and volume sample size?

    A. Place <1-mm pulse wave sample volume at least 1 to 2 cm distal to the mitral valve leaflet tips (Fig. 5.1, Video 5.1).
    B. Place >3-mm pulse wave sample volume at the mitral valve annulus (Fig. 5.2, Video 5.2).
    C. Place 1- to 3-mm pulse wave sample volume at the mitral valve leaflet tips (Fig. 5.3, Video 5.3).
    D. Place 1- to 3-mm pulse wave sample volume at the mitral valve annulus (Fig. 5.4, Video 5.4).

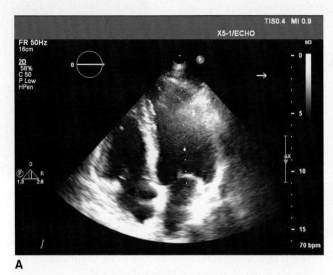
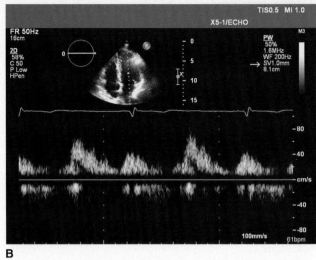

A

B

FIGURE 5.1

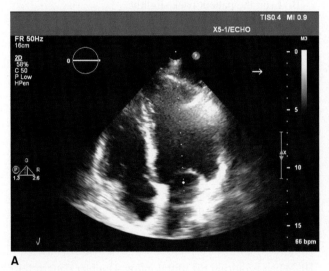
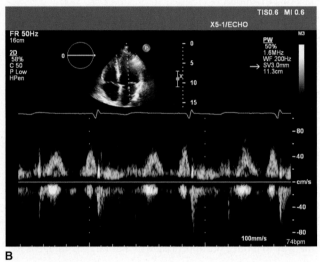

A

B

FIGURE 5.2

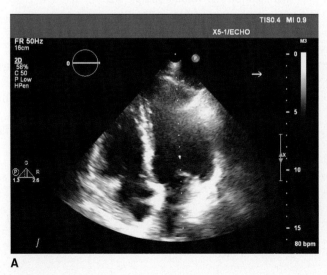
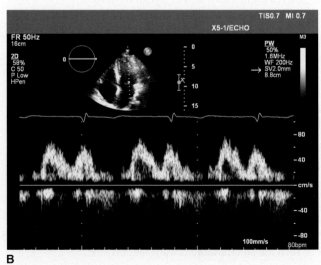

A

B

FIGURE 5.3

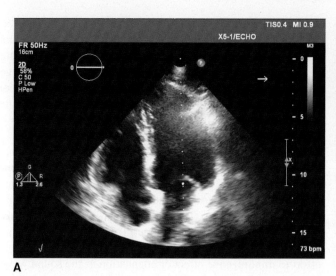

A

FIGURE 5.4

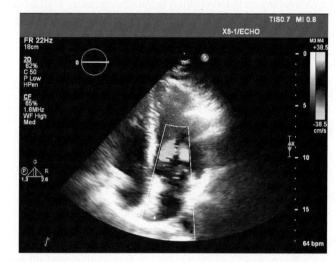

FIGURE 5.6

11. Which of the following describes the optimal technique for obtaining pulmonary vein flow?

A. Utilize color Doppler in apical four-chamber view and angle posterior while placing sample volume at the base of the pulmonary vein with sample volume size of 1 to 2 mm (FIG. 5.5, VIDEO 5.5).

B. Utilize color Doppler in apical four-chamber view and angle anterior while placing sample volume 1 cm into the pulmonary vein with sample volume size of 3 to 4 mm (FIG. 5.6, VIDEO 5.6).

C. Utilize color Doppler in apical four-chamber view and angle anterior while placing sample volume 1 cm into the pulmonary vein with sample volume size of 1 to 2 mm (FIG. 5.7, VIDEO 5.7).

D. Utilize color Doppler in apical four-chamber view and angle anterior while placing sample volume at the base of the pulmonary vein with sample volume size of 3 to 4 mm (FIG. 5.8, VIDEO 5.8).

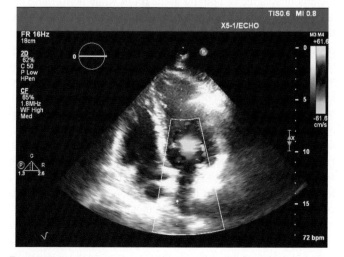

FIGURE 5.5

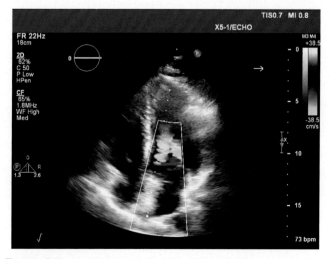

FIGURE 5.7

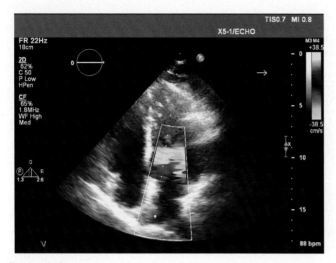

FIGURE 5.8

12. According to the simplified Bernoulli equation, high flow velocities can result in significant underestimation of a gradient when there is/are:

A. Small deviations in beam angulation.
B. Decreased lateral resolution.
C. Increased signal-to-noise correlation.
D. Lack of time gain compensation.

13. The recommended Nyquist limit or aliasing velocity for color flow Doppler is between:

A. 30 and 40 cm/s.
B. 40 and 50 cm/s.
C. 50 and 60 cm/s.
D. 60 and 70 cm/s.

14. You are scanning a patient on the neurology service due to concern about an embolic stroke. You acquire the following apical views (VIDEOS 5.9A AND B). You decide to use an echocardiographic contrast agent. All of the following are appropriate considerations to maintain optimal image quality EXCEPT:

A. Position patient prior to injection and identify optimal imaging window.
B. Lower the frame rate.
C. Bring the focus to the near field.
D. Increase power output.

15. Optimizing a color flow Doppler (CFD) image to resolve aliasing can potentially be achieved by which of the following maneuvers:

A. Decreasing the pulse repetition frequency
B. Imaging at a shallower depth (potentially by switching imaging window)
C. Become better aligned to the direction of flow
D. Not necessary as there is no aliasing in CFD

Answer 1: C. This question requires an understanding of factors that influence gain. Gain is the strength of the receiving signal of the image. A good way to think about gain is the "loudness of the image." The best image is one where the receiving signal from true structures is very strong with other signal (noise) being much weaker. Keeping with the analogy of the image to a recording, increasing the gain is like turning up the volume. The song will get louder, but so will the background noise. Time Gain Compensation (or TGC) is increasing the gain differentially along the axis of the ultrasound beam. Finally, the monitor influences not only settings during image acquisition but also viewing afterward.

Power Doppler (color angio) is a nondirectional color Doppler application for which the strength of the reflected signal is processed without regard to direction or speed as noted in typical Doppler applications. Additionally, Power Doppler is a Doppler setting and not related to the overall gain of a 2D ultrasound image.

Option A: This is a true statement. Time Gain Compensation (TGC) is directly related to amplification of the image in an effort to minimize the effect of attenuation as the sound waves travel deeper into the far field.

Option B: This is a true statement. Gain (receiver gain) alters the strength of the voltages in the ultrasound receiver after reception from the transducer. Gain is different from power since power increases the strength of the ultrasound transmitted, whereas gain simply increases the strength once received.

Option D: This is a true statement. The monitor has a brightness and contrast setting and should always be adjusted according to ambient lighting.

Suggested Readings

Edelman SK. *Understanding Ultrasound Physics*. 3rd ed. Canada: KnowledgeMasters, 2004.
Geiser EA. Echocardiography: physics and instrumentation. In: Skorton DJ, et al., eds. *Marcus Cardiac Imaging: A Companion to Braunwald's Heart Disease*. 2nd ed. Philadelphia, PA: WB Saunders, 1996:273–291.
Kremkau FW. *Sonography Principles and Instruments*. 8th ed. China: Jeanne Olson, 2011.
Pye SD, Wild SR, McDicken WN. Adaptive time gain compensation for ultrasonic imaging. *Ultrasound Med Biol* 1992;18:205–212.

Answer 2: A. This question requires understanding of environmental factors that influence image acquisition. **Ambient light** is the amount/degree of lighting in the room while performing the scan. Prior to imaging, the monitor needs to be adjusted according to the ambient light within the room. Failure to do so can lead to poor-quality real-time images and/or digital recording. Depending on the individual preference, the monitor can be adjusted to provide either a smooth or a crisp image simply by adjusting the contrast level on the monitor. To achieve a smoother appearance, decrease the contrast level on the monitor; for a more crisp appearance, increase the contrast. In addition, the brightness level should be adjusted according to the room brightness. Typically, begin with the brightness level in the middle range and increase or decrease with respect to background preference (black or gray) and according to ambient light. In addition, it is a good idea to periodically check the reading room monitor as well (FIG. 5.9).

Option B: The frequency of the transducer is dependent on the object being imaged and what depth is needed. However, this does not influence the monitor settings during image acquisition.

Option C: Second harmonics or harmonic imaging is a method of imaging in which the sending frequency is half of the receiving

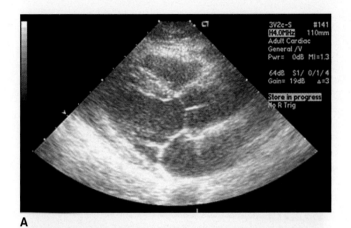

A

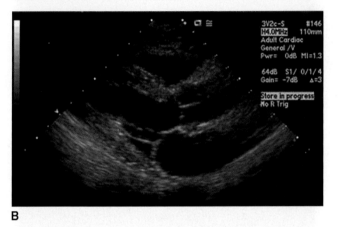

B

FIGURE 5.9 A: Parasternal long-axis view exemplifying too much gain. Note the degradation in image resolution and lack of distinction between echoes. **B:** Parasternal long-axis view with the correct amount of gain setting. Note the differences between echoes.

frequency. Harmonic imaging allows for utilization of nonlinear variation created by ultrasound and, as a result of multiples of the tissue harmonics, can be used to create a cleaner image.

Option D: Patient selection depends on the indication for the diagnostic procedure. However, the patient specific factors do not influence monitor settings.

Suggested Readings

Edelman SK. *Understanding Ultrasound Physics*. 3rd ed. Canada: KnowledgeMasters, 2004.
Kremkau FW. *Sonography Principles and Instruments*. 8th ed. China: Jeanne Olson, 2011.
McCulloch ML, Davis R. Practical scanning tips and considerations: a review of the basics. *Cardiac Ultrasound Today* 2003;9/10(9):171–199.
Thomas JD, Rubin DN. Tissue harmonic imaging: why does it work? *J Am Soc Echocardiogr* 1998;11:803–808.

Answer 3: *A.* This question requires understanding of impact of different settings on 2D image quality in the obese patient. Increasing frequency does lead to better spatial resolution, however, at the expense of decreased depth of imaging (more attenuation). Obese adult patients tend to have more tissue to penetrate through in an effort to image the heart and need lower-frequency transducers with lesser spatial resolution, but the ability to penetrate deeper depth ranges.

Option B: This is a true statement. Power is the rate at which energy is transferred and describes the magnitude of the wave, which in turn affects the brightness of the image. The unit value of power is noted in watts; however, on ultrasound systems, power is noted by the MI or thermal index (TI).

Option C: This is a true statement. Compression/dynamic range adjusts the images of the grayscale map by increasing or decreasing the number of shades of gray. Increasing the compression/dynamic range will enhance small differences in weak signals as different grayscale levels and, with obese or difficult images, there will be a wide range of signal noise that will be tagged as a shade of gray for which reducing the compression/dynamic range is beneficial.

Option D: This is a true statement. Obese adults typically need to be scanned at deeper depths for which it is critical to increase the overall gain and TGC in an effort to enhance the backscatter in far field.

Suggested Readings

Carlsen EN. Ultrasound physics for the physician. A brief review. *J Clin Ultrasound* 1975;3:69–75.
Edelman SK. *Understanding Ultrasound Physics*. 3rd ed. Canada: KnowledgeMasters, 2004.
Kremkau F. Ultrasound physics. *Ultrasound Med Biol* 1991;17:411.
Kremkau FW. *Sonography Principles and Instruments*. 8th ed. China: Jeanne Olson, 2011.
McCulloch ML, Davis R. Practical scanning tips and considerations: a review of the basics. *Cardiac Ultrasound Today* 2003;9/10(9):171–199.

Answer 4: *C.* This question requires understanding the impact of compress on image quality. Increasing compress and/or dynamic range will add shades of gray to the grayscale map and provide a softer or smoother image appearance. Conversely, lowering the compress and/or dynamic range will enhance the raw or grainy appearance of the image in which the image will appear darker without a wide range of shades of gray.

Option A: Persistence refers to temporal averaging and will cause the image to have a smoother or blurry appearance. Turning off the persistence will provide a raw unprocessed image that will appear grainy or nonsmoothed.

Option B: Lowering fundamental frequency decreases the overall image resolution, which would not improve the grainy appearance of an image.

Option D: Foreshortening the image plane will have no effect on the grainy appearance of the image but will impact appropriate visualization of the true apex.

Suggested Readings

Carlsen EN. Ultrasound physics for the physician. A brief review. *J Clin Ultrasound* 1975;3:69–75.
Edelman SK. *Understanding Ultrasound Physics*. 3rd ed. Canada: KnowledgeMasters, 2004.
Kremkau F. Ultrasound physics. *Ultrasound Med Biol* 1991;17:411.
Kremkau FW. *Sonography Principles and Instruments*. 8th ed. China: Jeanne Olson, 2011.
McCulloch ML, Davis R. Practical scanning tips and considerations: a review of the basics. *Cardiac Ultrasound Today* 2003;9/10(9):171–199.

Answer 5: *C.* Stress echo mandates that a select set of standardized views be used consistently throughout the stress exam so that a 17-segment model can be correlated to associated coronary beds. All of the standard views need to be consistent with respect to depth, gain, and image orientation throughout all comparative image acquisitions.

Option A: This is a true statement. Off-axis views are often necessary in patients with prior cardiac surgeries and can be beneficial in patients with valve disease and myocardial disease in order to fully visualize the heart structure and function.

Option B: This is a true statement. Patients with congenital heart disease often rely on nonstandard views. A complete examination may require that custom, or in-between, planes be used to investigate or display an abnormality.

Option D: This is a true statement. Difficult body habitus refers to patients with structural abnormalities that impede the acquisition of traditional standard views and include but are not limited to concave or convex mediastinum, breast implants, and lung resection.

Suggested Readings

Lang RM, Bierig M, Devereux RB, et al. Recommendations for chamber quantification: a report from the American Society of Echocardiography's Guidelines and Standards Committee and the Chamber Quantification Writing Group, developed in conjunction with the European Association of Echocardiography, a branch of the European Society of Cardiology. *J Am Soc Echocardiogr* 2005;18:1440–1463.

Lopez L, Colan SD, Frommelt PC, et al. Recommendations for quantification methods during the performance of a pediatric echocardiogram: a report from the Pediatric Measurements Writing Group of the American Society of Echocardiography Pediatric and Congenital Heart Disease Council. *J Am Soc Echocardiogr* 2010;23:465–495.

Pellikka PA, Nagueh SF, Elhendy AA, et al. American Society of Echocardiography recommendations for performance, interpretation, and application of stress echocardiography. *J Am Soc Echocardiogr* 2007;20:1021–1041.

Picard MH, Adams D, Bierig SM, et al. American Society of Echocardiography recommendations for quality echocardiography laboratory operations. *J Am Soc Echocardiogr* 2011;24:1–10.

Answer 6: *C.* This question requires an understanding of strategies for image acquisition. This is a common issue that arises during image acquisition. This figure represents an off-axis parasternal long-axis view, where the LV apex is pointed up and to the left of the screen. This is usually because the transducer is an interspace too low. This is further evidenced by the sharp angle between the interventricular septum and the aorta. The goal is to move the image plane higher up in relation to the cardiac silhouette. This can be accomplished by moving either the imaging plane "up" or the cardiac silhouette "down." Either of these maneuvers will help to rotate the LV apex lower in the screen and "flatten" the angle between the interventricular septum and aorta. Lowering the head of the bed would move the cardiac silhouette "up," which would make the apex point further up toward the transducer. The resulting image would look more in between a parasternal long-axis and apical long-axis view. The benefit of having an on-axis parasternal long includes improved spatial resolution with respect to the septum and posterior since the tissue is perpendicular to the ultrasound beam (Fig. 5.10).

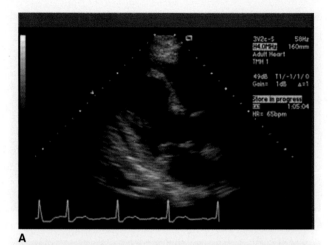

A

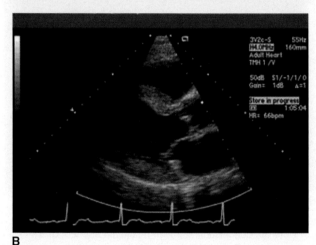

B

FIGURE 5.10 A: Off-axis parasternal long-axis view. Note how the angle of the LV apex is tilted toward the upper left side of the screen, which sometimes occurs when the image is acquired in a low parasternal window. **B:** Same heart but now on-axis. The transducer has been moved up an intercostal space, closer to the sternum, and angled back toward the heart, thereby shifting the heart in the center of the screen. In addition, the patient was moved more on the left side with the head flat down.

Option A: This is a true statement. Moving up an interspace would move the imaging plane higher in relation to the heart, further away from the apex.

Option B: This is a true statement. These images are generally acquired from the left parasternal window, and moving closer to the sternum would move away from the LV apex.

Option D: This is a true statement. Moving into the left lateral decubitus not only shifts the heart closer to the chest wall but also lowers it down and more lateral. This also helps to "pull" the LV apex away from the transducer.

Suggested Readings

Edelman SK. *Understanding Ultrasound Physics*. 3rd ed. Canada: KnowledgeMasters, 2004.

Kremkau FW. *Sonography Principles and Instruments*. 8th ed. China: Jeanne Olson, 2011.

Reynolds T, Abate K, Abate J. "Rib-hooks," "pressure points," and "hugs"—technical hints for improving two-dimensional echocardiographic imaging. *J Am Soc Echocardiogr* 1993;6(3):312–318.

Walsh CA, Wilde P. *Practical Echocardiography*. London, UK: Greenwich Medical Media Limited, 1999.

Answer 7: D. This question requires an understanding of strategies for image acquisition. **Having the patient sit upright** shifts the heart and the apex more medially. The most optimal scenario is to have a cooperative patient that can lie in the left lateral decubitus with their left arm raised toward the head of the bed. This will allow for wider rib spacing and greater imaging access. In addition, due to the effect of gravity, the apex of the heart will shift laterally, thereby allowing for an on-axis view of the apical four chambers.

Option A: This is a true statement. When the apex is pointing toward the right side of the screen, the transducer is not on the apex and needs to be moved laterally in an effort to aim directly at the apex.

Option B: This is a true statement. If there is difficulty in aiming at the apex and there is not a cutout, try leaning the patient back in an effort to point the transducer directly at the apex, which will then align the apical four-chamber view upright and on-axis.

Option C: This is a true statement. Customized beds with sectional dropouts or cutouts are great for allowing the transducer access to the true apex while the patient is in a left lateral position.

Suggested Readings

McCulloch ML, Davis R. Practical scanning tips and considerations: a review of the basics. *Cardiac Ultrasound Today* 2003;9/10(9):171–199.

Reynolds T, Abate K, Abate J. "Rib-hooks," "pressure points," and "hugs"—technical hints for improving two-dimensional echocardiographic imaging. *J Am Soc Echocardiogr* 1993;6(3):312–318.

Walsh CA, Wilde P. *Practical Echocardiography*. London, UK: Greenwich Medical Media Limited, 1999.

Answer 8: D. This question requires an understanding of spectral Doppler. Spectral Doppler typically refers to the output where different velocities are plotted out over time. Therefore, any spectral Doppler display would need to be able to quantify velocities and direction. Range ambiguity (difference between pulsed wave and continuous wave Doppler) is not a deciding factor as to whether a modality is a spectral Doppler modality. **Power Doppler** (color angio) is a nondirectional color Doppler application for which the strength of the reflected signal is processed without regard to direction or speed as noted in typical Doppler applications. Therefore, power Doppler cannot be displayed in a spectral format with velocity over time.

Option A: This is a true statement. PW Doppler is sample site specific and offers a spectral display with velocity over time.

Option B: This is a true statement. CW Doppler samples velocities continuously along the line of the Doppler angle and is not sample site specific. The spectral display is velocity over time.

Option C: This is a true statement. HPRF is a hybrid between PW and CW. In an effort to obtain higher velocities and still have some sample site specificity, the machine will use a higher PRF to get a higher Nyquist limit. However, there is some range ambiguity, as the velocity recorded could be from multiple areas. Fortunately, in most clinical scenarios, the other sample sites are in locations where such high velocities are usually not seen.

Suggested Readings

Edelman SK. *Understanding Ultrasound Physics*. 3rd ed. Canada: KnowledgeMasters, 2004.

Kremkau FW. *Sonography Principles and Instruments*. 8th ed. China: Jeanne Olson, 2011.

McCulloch ML, Davis R. Practical scanning tips and considerations: a review of the basics. *Cardiac Ultrasound Today* 2003;9/10(9):171–199.

Answer 9: A. This question requires an understanding of pulsed wave Doppler modality. Pulsed Doppler fundamentally sends out a pulse and waits a certain amount of time to hear a returning signal. This waiting time is determined by the distance from the transducer at which a sample volume is placed. Using this approach, pulsed Doppler modality results in a sample site-specific reading that is limited by a velocity limit above which directionality cannot be determined (aliasing above the Nyquist limit). **Sample site specific** refers to the area the pulsed Doppler sample is placed in order to identify and measure velocities in a specific area.

Option B: The temporal resolution all Doppler modalities are high enough to resolve data from each heart beat and display them over time.

Option C: Pulsed Doppler is a velocity measurement and is best utilized when parallel to the Doppler beam. Measuring flow perpendicular to the Doppler beam would result in no Doppler velocity signal.

Option D: Pulsed Doppler will alias because it is sample site specific and needs to wait to receive information in an effort to identify distances, whereas CW Doppler measures continuously along the line of the Doppler beam. CW Doppler measures every velocity along the beam and is not sample site specific.

Suggested Readings

Edelman SK. *Understanding Ultrasound Physics*. 3rd ed. Canada: KnowledgeMasters, 2004.

Kremkau FW. *Sonography Principles and Instruments*. 8th ed. China: Jeanne Olson, 2011.

McCulloch ML, Davis R. Practical scanning tips and considerations: a review of the basics. *Cardiac Ultrasound Today* 2003;9/10(9):171–199.

Picard MH, Adams D, Bierig SM, et al. American Society of Echocardiography recommendations for quality echocardiography laboratory operations. *J Am Soc Echocardiogr* 2011;24:1–10.

Answer 10: C. This question requires basic understanding of optimal image acquisition. **Placing 1- to 3-mm pulse wave sample volume at mitral valve leaflet tips** is the ideal location for measuring mitral inflow velocities in an effort to estimate diastolic function.

Option A: Placing the sample volume 1 to 2 cm distal to the mitral valve leaflet tips will cause underestimation of velocities, as the sample volume is too far in the ventricle.

Option B: Greater than 3 mm is too large of a sample size, and placing the sample volume at the annulus is not the appropriate location for estimating diastolic filling pressures. However, using a 1- to 3-mm sample volume at the annulus can be used for estimating cardiac output.

Option D: The sample size is correct; however, the location of the annulus is wrong for mitral inflow patterns in estimating diastolic function.

Suggested Readings

Picard MH, Adams D, Bierig SM, et al. American Society of Echocardiography recommendations for quality echocardiography laboratory operations. *J Am Soc Echocardiogr* 2011;24:1–10.

Quinones MA, Otto CM, Stoddard M, et al. Recommendations for quantification of Doppler echocardiography: a report from the Doppler Quantification Task Force of the Nomenclature and Standards Committee of the American Society of Echocardiography. *J Am Soc Echocardiogr* 2002;15:167–184.

Walsh CA, Wilde P. *Practical Echocardiography*. London, UK: Greenwich Medical Media Limited, 1999.

Answer 11: B. This question requires understanding of pulmonary venous anatomy. Imaging pulmonary veins with transthoracic imaging is challenging, and even with the best technique, one may not be visualize them all. Left-sided pulmonary veins are notoriously difficult to see and, more importantly, difficult to sample due to direction of flow compared to transducer. Remember, the primary reason to sample pulmonary veins is to add in assessment of diastolic function and mitral valve disease, both of which require Doppler assessment. This requires pulmonary vein flow to be parallel to the transducer, and the only one that reliably does so is the right lower (inferior) pulmonary vein. Fortunately, this is the one best seen in a typical four-chamber view. **Angling anterior while placing the sample volume 1 cm into the pulmonary vein with sample volume size of 3 to 4 mm** allows for best placement of the Doppler sample volume, and utilizing a sample volume size of 3 to 5 mm allows for optimal Doppler flow acquisition. The inferior pulmonary veins enter more in the middle third of the atria and therefore usually do not require significant posterior angulation to find (Fig. 5.12).

Option A: Pointing posterior is not the best way to bring in the pulmonary vein, and a sample volume 1 to 2 mm is not optimal (Fig. 5.11).

Option C: Angling the transducer anterior and placing the sample volume 1 cm into the pulmonary vein are correct; however, using a sample volume of 1 to 2 mm is not optimal (Fig. 5.13).

Option D: Placing the sample volume at the base of the pulmonary vein is not optimal; however, using a sample volume size of 3 to 4 mm is correct (Fig. 5.14).

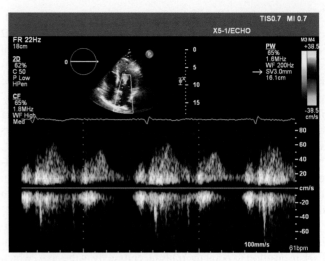

FIGURE 5.12

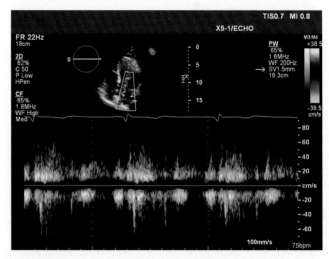

FIGURE 5.13

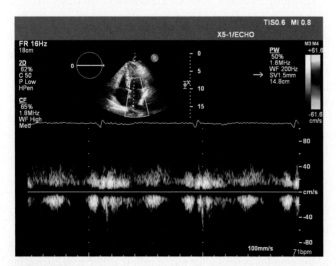

FIGURE 5.11

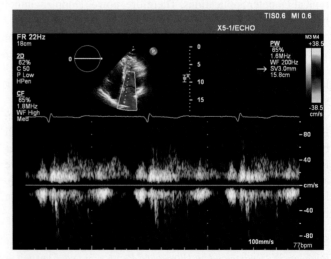

FIGURE 5.14

Suggested Readings

Henry WL, Demaria A, Gramiak R, et al. The ASE committee on Nomenclature and Standards in Two-dimensional Echocardiography. *Circulation* 1980;62:212–227.

Picard MH, Adams D, Bierig SM, et al. American Society of Echocardiography recommendations for quality echocardiography laboratory operations. *J Am Soc Echocardiogr* 2011;24:1–10.

Quinones MA, Otto CM, Stoddard M, et al. Recommendations for quantification of Doppler echocardiography: a report from the Doppler Quantification Task Force of the Nomenclature and Standards Committee of the American Society of Echocardiography. *J Am Soc Echocardiogr* 2002;15:167–184.

Walsh CA, Wilde P. *Practical Echocardiography*. London, UK: Greenwich Medical Media Limited, 1999.

Answer 12: A. This question requires an understanding of the impact of angle of incidence of ultrasound beam to the direction of flow on flow measurement. **Small deviations in beam angulation** can result in significant differences in gradients, and there should be a concerted effort to align the Doppler beam parallel to flow for maximal velocities (FIG. 5.15).

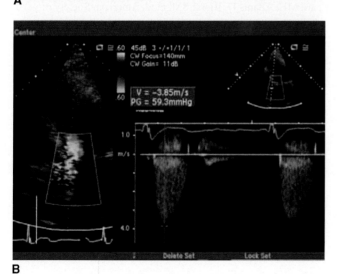

A

B

FIGURE **5.15 A:** Spectral Doppler across the aortic valve in the apical window. Note that the angle of the Doppler beam is not quite parallel to flow and that the peak gradient is measured at 51.3 mm Hg. **B:** Spectral Doppler across the aortic valve in the apical window. The transducer was moved up an intercostal, so the angle of the Doppler beam was more parallel to flow. Note the increase in the peak gradient from 51.3 to 59.3 mm Hg.

This is represented in the Doppler shift equation by cosine θ. This gives a measured velocity (Doppler frequency shift) that is a predictable fraction of the true maximal velocity. Higher velocities will be reduced by the same percentage based on the angle, but a higher absolute velocity.

Option B: Lateral resolution is related to a 2D image and not spectral Doppler velocities.

Option C: Increased signal to noise would correlate with an overestimation as opposed to an underestimation.

Option D: TGC affects a 2D image but not spectral Doppler velocities.

Suggested Readings

Bonow RO, Carabello B, de La ELH. Guidelines for the management of patients with valvular heart disease; executive summary. A report of the American College of Cardiology/American Heart Association Task Force on Practice Guidelines (Committee on Management of Patients with Valvular Heart Disease). *Circulation* 1998;98:1949–1984.

Henry WL, Demaria A, Gramiak R, et al. Report of the ASE committee on Nomenclature and Standards in Two-dimensional Echocardiography. *Circulation* 1980;62:212–227.

Zoghbi WA, Enriquez-Sarano M, Foster E, et al. Recommendations for evaluation of the severity of native valvular regurgitation with two-dimensional and Doppler echocardiography. *J Am Soc Echocardiogr* 2003;16:777–802.

Answer 13: C. The Nyquist limit for cardiac imaging should be between 50 and 60 cm/s and is the recommended setting according to the American Society of Echocardiography (ASE) guidelines. The range between 50 and 60 cm/s is the most optimal for cardiac imaging; however, it may be adjusted higher for faster heart rates or increased hemodynamic flows or lower in an attempt to visualize lower flow velocities.

Option A: A color Nyquist limit between 30 and 40 cm/s is too low for cardiac imaging and will overestimate quantification of regurgitant flows.

Option B: A color Nyquist limit between 40 and 50 cm/s is high enough for cardiac imaging but will overestimate regurgitant flow.

Option D: A color Nyquist limit between 60 and 70 cm/s is too high and may underestimate quantification of regurgitant flow.

Suggested Readings

Bonow RO, Carabello B, de La ELH. Guidelines for the management of patients with valvular heart disease; executive summary. A report of the American College of Cardiology/American Heart Association Task Force on Practice Guidelines (Committee on Management of Patients with Valvular Heart Disease). *Circulation* 1998;98:1949–1984.

Henry WL, Demaria A, Gramiak R, et al. Report of the ASE committee on Nomenclature and Standards in Two-dimensional Echocardiography. *Circulation* 1980;62:212–227.

Klein AL, Burstow DJ, Tajik AJ, et al. Age-related prevalence of valvular regurgitation in normal subjects: a comprehensive color flow examination of 118 volunteers. *J Am Soc Echocardiogr* 1990;3:54–63.

Zoghbi WA, Enriquez-Sarano M, Foster E, et al. Recommendations for evaluation of the severity of native valvular regurgitation with two-dimensional and Doppler echocardiography. *J Am Soc Echocardiogr* 2003;16:777–802.

Answer 14: D. This question requires an understanding of optimal imaging settings when using intravenous echocardiographic contrast agents. In the evaluation of cardiac source of emboli, the LV apex is an important source to interrogate. In this patient, the LV apex is not well visualized, and this would be a reasonable indication for an intravenous contrast agent to opacify the LV cavity. However, it is important to understand that imaging during contrast infusion is fundamentally a little different. It is important to position the patient adequately and identify optimal windows given that timing is not only important, but more time imaging leads to more destruction of the microbubbles. Also, given the field of view is in the near field, it is appropriate to move the focal depth into the near field. Finally, a major source of error during contrast use is a swirling artifact due to destruction of microbubbles. This is due to using a high power output (represented by mechanical index, MI), imaging more than needed (either with a high frame rate or while searching for an optimal window). Therefore, it is important to use a low MI setting (usually MI < 0.3) and identify important landmarks early. Also, lowering the frame rate minimizes ultrasound pulses delivered and limits destruction of microbubbles. All of the proposed strategies are appropriate except for increasing the power output, given that we would want to lower power output to minimize microbubble destruction and swirling. A practical approach if there is a lot of swirling is to "freeze" the image for about 5 to 10 seconds to allow recirculation of contrast agent, "unfreeze" the image, and immediately acquire the image. Destruction of microbubbles will start right away but should be able to get a usable image before significant swirling occurs.

Option A: This is an appropriate intervention, as optimizing patient position and image windows will allow for rapid image acquisition.

Option B: Lowering the frame rate will minimize destruction of microbubbles.

Option C: Bringing the focus to the near field will allow optimal visualization of the LV apex, which is the focus in this image.

Suggested Reading

Porter TR, Abdelmoneim S, Belcik JT, et al. Guidelines for the cardiac sonographer in the performance of contrast echocardiography: a focused update from the American Society of Echocardiography. *J Am Soc Echocardiogr* 2014;27:797–810.

Answer 15: B. This question requires an understanding of principles of color flow Doppler (CFD). CFD is fundamentally a pulse wave modality that uses autocorrelation to identify directionality of flow based on surrounding pixel information. Given that it is a pulse wave modality, it offers site-specific information at the expense of limits on velocities that can be measured (risk of aliasing). Strategies to minimize aliasing are the same as in pulsed wave Doppler, except for that high PRF is not a mode typically used in CFD like it is in pulsed wave Doppler. A corollary to high PRF is power Doppler, where a higher Nyquist limit can be achieved by increasing the pulse repetition frequency (PRF), but this would introduce range ambiguity. In color flow, this is manifested as removal of directional information, just peak velocities displayed on a color scale. As with other pulse wave modalities, the closer the area being sampled is to the transducer, the higher the Nyquist limit that can be sampled. Therefore, of all of the answer choices, this is the best option. Sometimes, this is not possible, or frankly enough, but should initially be tried. While being better aligned with flow should always be a goal, this would increase the maximal velocity sampled and worsen aliasing.

Option A: Decreasing PRF would lower the Nyquist limit, and worsen aliasing.

Option C: Better alignment with the flow in question would increase the maximal velocity sampled, which would also worsen aliasing.

Option D: Given that CFD is essentially a pulsed wave modality, it is at risk of aliasing.

Suggested Readings

Griffith JM, Henry WL. An ultrasound system for combined cardiac imaging and Doppler blood flow measurement in man. *Circulation* 1978;57:925–930.

Henry WL, Demaria A, Gramiak R, et al. Report of the ASE committee on Nomenclature and Standards in Two-dimensional Echocardiography. *Circulation* 1980;62:212–227.

Picard MH, Adams D, Bierig SM, et al. American Society of Echocardiography recommendations for quality echocardiography laboratory operations. *J Am Soc Echocardiogr* 2011;24:1–10.

Zoghbi WA, Enriquez-Sarano M, Foster E, et al. Recommendations for evaluation of the severity of native valvular regurgitation with two-dimensional and Doppler echocardiography. *J Am Soc Echocardiogr* 2003;16:777–802.

Chapter 6

Understanding Spatial and Temporal Resolution

Vedant A. Gupta and Vincent L. Sorrell

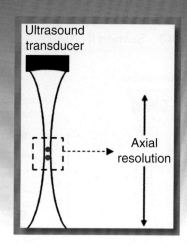

Ultrasound transducer

Axial resolution

1. The axial resolution at the focus of a single-element ultrasound transducer depends the least on which of the following variables?

A. Center frequency of the ultrasound transducer
B. Diameter of the ultrasound transducer
C. Backing material of the ultrasound transducer
D. Speed of sound of the medium

2. The lateral resolution at the focus of a single-element ultrasound transducer depends on all of the following variables except the:

A. Duration of the excitation pulse
B. Center frequency of the ultrasound transducer
C. Diameter of the ultrasound transducer
D. Focal length of the ultrasound transducer

3. Why might a sonographer switch from a 5-MHz to a 1-MHz ultrasound transducer during a scan?

A. To improve axial spatial resolution
B. To improve lateral spatial resolution
C. To increase the range (or imaging depth)
D. To increase the frame rate

4. Which of the following maneuvers might help resolve the following artifact during PW Doppler imaging (FIG. 6.1)?

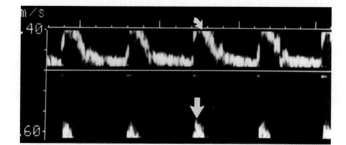

FIGURE 6.1

A. Reduce the pulse repetition frequency.
B. Increase the transmitted ultrasound frequency.
C. Adjust the baseline.
D. Add extra focal zones.

5. You want to measure blood velocity using color Doppler imaging. Which situation in FIGURE 6.2 produces the largest Doppler shift, assuming differences in the size of the vessels are negligible and other physical parameters are similar (e.g., speed of sound, ultrasound frequency).

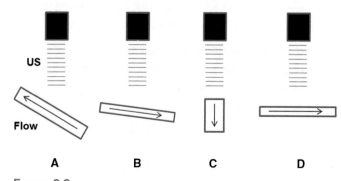

US

Flow

A   B   C   D

FIGURE 6.2

6. Compared to a linear ultrasound array, a planar array for 3D imaging has:

A. Better elevational resolution
B. Smaller *spacing (or pitch)* between the elements
C. Higher frame rates
D. Superior axial spatial resolution

7. Which of the following statements is the least accurate regarding tissue harmonic imaging?

A. Harmonic imaging improves contrast between fat and muscle tissues.
B. Higher-frequency components are attenuated in deeper structures.
C. Harmonic imaging improves axial spatial resolution.
D. The amplitude of the detected harmonic frequency is larger than that of the fundamental frequency.

Answer 1: B. This question requires identification of factors that influence axial resolution. The *axial resolution* (as opposed to lateral resolution) refers to the ability to resolve structures along (or parallel to) the axis of ultrasound propagation (FIG. 6.3).

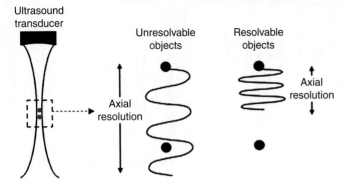

FIGURE 6.3 Axial resolution depends on the duration of the transmitted pulse. In this example, a single-element focused ultrasound transducer has an ultrasound beam that passes over two objects shown inside the *box* (**left**). A low ultrasound frequency produces a relatively long transmitted ultrasound pulse, such that the two objects are unresolvable (**middle**). The shorter pulse with higher ultrasound frequency (and shorter wavelength) is able to resolve the two objects (**right**).

Given depth z, speed of sound c, and propagation time t, the following relations are helpful in understanding spatial resolution along the propagation axis of the ultrasonic wave:

$$z = (c/2)(t) \, [\text{range equation relates } z \text{ to } c \text{ and } t]$$

$$\Delta z = (c/2)(\Delta t) \, [\text{axial resolution } \Delta z \text{ related to the duration}$$
$$\text{of the transmitted pulse } \Delta t]$$

$$\Delta z = (\lambda/2)(f_0/\Delta f) \, [\text{relates } \Delta z \text{ to wavelength,}$$
$$\text{center frequency } f_0, \text{ and bandwidth } \Delta f]$$

The axial resolution is usually represented as the minimum distance between two objects needed to resolve them as separate. Therefore, the smaller the distance, the better the resolution. By convention, if increasing a variable leads to a decrease in the distance needed to resolve two structures, it is said to be inversely proportional to axial resolution (even though the axial resolution actually improves). Axial resolution is inversely related to the center frequency and the bandwidth (higher frequency/larger bandwidth = smaller distance that can be resolved = better axial resolution). Conversely, increasing the speed of sound and keeping frequency the same is directly proportional to axial resolution (increases the wavelength, leading to an increase in the distance needed to resolve two structures). From the last equation, it is clear that the diameter of the ultrasound transducer is not a factor in determining the axial spatial resolution.

Option A: True. The axial resolution is inversely proportional to the ultrasound center frequency.

Option C: True. The backing material affects the bandwidth of the transducer, which is inversely proportional to the axial resolution (i.e., larger bandwidth = better resolution).

Option D: True. The speed of sound is proportional to axial resolution.

Suggested Readings

Hedrick WR, Hykes DL, Starchman DE. *Ultrasound Physics and Instrumentation*. 4th ed. St. Louis, MO: Elsevier/Mosby, 2005.
Szabo TL. *Diagnostic Ultrasound Imaging: Inside Out*. Boston, MA: Boston University Academic Press, 2004:Chapters 6 and 7.

Answer 2: A. This question requires identification of factors that influence lateral resolution. The lateral resolution refers to the ability to resolve two adjacent structures that appear perpendicular to the axis of the ultrasound beam (as opposed to axial resolution, which is the ability to resolve structures that appear parallel to the axis of the ultrasound beam). Similar to axial resolution, lateral resolution is represented as minimum distance needed to resolve two structures (perpendicular to the axis of the ultrasound beam). Therefore, increasing variables that lead to a decrease in the distance needed to resolve two structures are said to be inversely proportional to lateral resolution (even though lateral resolution actually improves). The lateral resolution is related to the bandwidth w of the ultrasound beam, which has the following relationship:

$$w = 1.4 \times Fc/(2af),$$

where F = focal length, c = speed of sound, a = aperture (or radius of the crystal), and f = ultrasound frequency. Therefore, lateral resolution improves (gets smaller) with increasing ultrasound frequency and increasing aperture (e.g., larger diameter). It also improves with a shorter focal length and in a medium with a slower speed of sound.

Option B: True. The lateral resolution is proportional to the acoustic wavelength, which is inversely proportional to the ultrasound center frequency.

Option C: True. The lateral resolution is inversely proportional to the diameter of the ultrasound transducer.

Option D: True. The lateral resolution is proportional to the focal length of the ultrasound transducer (Fig. 6.4).

Suggested Readings

Hedrick WR, Hykes DL, Starchman DE. *Ultrasound Physics and Instrumentation*. 4th ed. St. Louis, MO: Elsevier/Mosby, 2005.
Szabo TL. *Diagnostic Ultrasound Imaging: Inside Out*. Boston, MA: Boston University Academic Press, 2004:Chapters 6 and 7.

Answer 3: C. This question requires understanding of the impact of central frequency on image generation. The loss of intensity of the ultrasonic wave as it travels through tissue is determined by the attenuation coefficient μ expressed in dB/cm/MHz, the ultrasound frequency f, and the distance traveled z.

Intensity loss (dB) = $\mu f z$.

Therefore, an ultrasound transducer that produces 1-MHz ultrasound will penetrate much further than an equivalent transducer producing 5-MHz ultrasound. This is at the expense of axial and lateral resolution, but with minimal impact on temporal resolution (frame rate). The depth of imaging will affect temporal resolution, but the central frequency by itself does not.

Option A: False. The axial resolution is proportional to the acoustic wavelength, which is greater at 1 MHz.

Option B: False. The lateral resolution is also proportional to the acoustic wavelength.

Option C: *True.* The *attenuation coefficient* of tissue is lower at 1 MHz than 5 MHz. This effectively increases the imaging depth.

Option D: False. There is minimal or no effect on frame rate, which is primarily effected by the range.

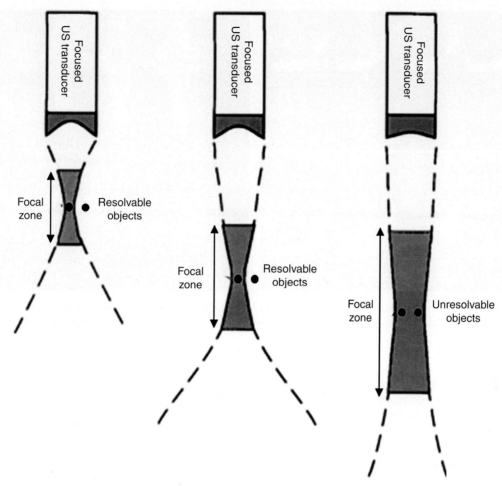

FIGURE 6.4 This figure illustrates a decreasing lateral focus (and smaller focal zone) with a shorter focal length and the transducer's ability to resolve objects perpendicular to the US beam. (Modified from Hedrick WR, Hykes DL, Starchman DE. *Ultrasound Physics and Instrumentation.* 4th ed. St. Louis, MO: Elsevier/Mosby; 2005:75. Reprinted by permission of Dr. Wayne Hedrick.)

Suggested Reading

Hedrick WR, Hykes DL, Starchman DE. *Ultrasound Physics and Instrumentation.* 4th ed. St. Louis, MO: Elsevier/Mosby, 2005:Chapter 9.

Answer 4: C. This question requires an understanding of factors that lead to aliasing in PW Doppler imaging. The artifact seen is an aliasing artifact. If the velocity of the structure in question is higher than two times the Nyquist limit, there is no maneuver (other than increasing the Nyquist limit) that would resolve the artifact. However, in this case, to accurately measure the Doppler signal, the pulse repetition frequency must be at least twice the frequency of the Doppler echo, according to the Nyquist limit for sampling, and this is directly related to the maximum blood flow velocity that can be measured for a particular setting on the ultrasound machine. Aliasing artifacts occur when the sampling rate is not high enough to capture the fastest flow velocities. Adjusting the baseline shifts the Doppler scale to cover the entire range of flow velocities. Increasing the scale also increases the pulse repetition frequency, enabling a wider range of flow velocities to be detected. FIGURE 6.5 portrays typical PW Doppler artifacts and their remedies.

Option A: False. *Increasing* the PRF might help reduce an aliasing artifact, but decreasing the PRF would decrease the Nyquist limit and exacerbate the artifact.

Option B: False. Increasing the transmitted frequency will not remove the aliasing artifact.

Option D: False. Adding extra focal zones will reduce the PRF, but not remove the artifact.

Suggested Readings

Brant WE. *The Core Curriculum: Ultrasound.* 1st ed. Philadelphia, PA: Lippincott Williams & Wilkins, 2001.
Hedrick WR, Hykes DL, Starchman DE. *Ultrasound Physics and Instrumentation.* 4th ed. St. Louis, MO: Elsevier/Mosby, 2005:Chapter 15.
Mitchell DG. Color Doppler imaging: principles, limitations, and artifacts. *Radiology* 1990;177:1–10.

Answer 5: C. This question requires an understanding of the impact of flow direction on the Doppler shift equation. The Doppler shift equation provides the foundation for Doppler echocardiography (FIG. 6.6).

The Doppler shift (f_D) is dependent on the angle (θ) between the incident acoustic wave and the flow direction. According to the equation in FIGURE 6.6, this shift is proportional to the flow

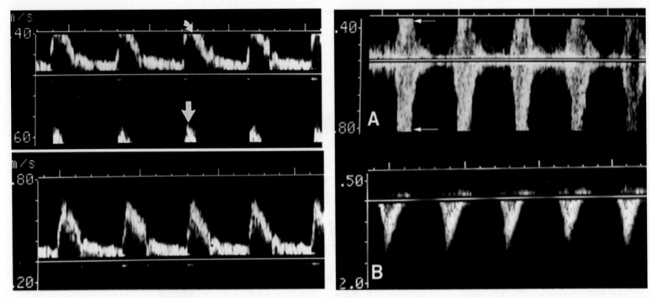

FIGURE 6.5 **Left column:** An aliasing artifact corrected by adjusting the baseline. **Right column:** *A different* aliasing artifact corrected by adjusting the baseline and increasing the scale. (Modified from Brant WE. *The Core Curriculum: Ultrasound.* 1st ed. Philadelphia, PA: Lippincott Williams & Wilkins, 2001.)

velocity (*v*) and frequency (*f*) of the transmitted ultrasound. It is also inversely proportional to the speed of sound (*c*). The cos (*θ*) relation indicates that the maximum Doppler shift occurs when most or all of the flow is in the direction of the propagating acoustic wave. Increasing the angle of incidence between the direction of maximal flow and the ultrasound transducer will predictably decrease the maximal detectable Doppler shift (Table 4.1). This leads to an underestimation of the maximal velocity. The sign of the shift depends on the direction of flow (by convention, toward = positive and away = negative). For this question, Option C will have the maximum Doppler shift given the angle of incidence (*θ*) is 0.

Option A: The angle of incidence to the direction of flow is approximately 45 degrees. The cosine of 45 degrees is approximately 0.7. The maximal Doppler shift detected will only be approximately 70% of the true maximal Doppler shift (and therefore detected velocity).

Option B: This angle of incidence is almost 90 degrees and the cosine of 90 degrees is 0. Therefore, the maximal detected Doppler shift will be a fraction of the true Doppler shift (<30%).

Option D: The direction of flow is perpendicular to the ultrasound beam and will not produce any Doppler shift (*f*$_D$). Cosine of 90 degrees is 0.

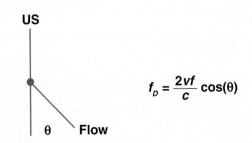

$$f_D = \frac{2vf}{c}\cos(\theta)$$

FIGURE 6.6

Suggested Readings

Foley WD, Erickson SJ. Color Doppler flow imaging. *AJR Am J Roentgenol* 1991;156:3–13.

Hedrick WR, Hykes DL, Starchman DE. *Ultrasound Physics and Instrumentation.* 4th ed. St. Louis, MO: Elsevier/Mosby, 2005:Chapter 14.

Hoskins PR. Accuracy of maximum velocity estimates made using Doppler ultrasound systems. *Br J Radiol* 1996;69:172–177.

Tahmasebpour HR, Buckley AR, Cooperberg PL, et al. Sonographic examination of the carotid arteries. *Radiographics* 2005;25(6):1561–1575.

Answer 6: *A.* This question requires an understanding of different orientations of piezo electrode crystals in ultrasound transducers. A 1D linear array depends on a fixed-focus acoustic lens to determine the elevational focus (or "slice thickness"). The lens typically has a *high f-number* (e.g., 4), indicating that the slice thickness is on the order of several acoustic wavelengths. Three-dimensional ultrasound imaging with a planar array, on the other hand, exploits electronic focusing in both the azimuthal (lateral) and elevational directions. Because the spacing between elements of a planar array is typically less than one wavelength, much better focusing is possible with this arrangement. FIGURE 6.7 compares array types and focusing capability.

Option B: This statement is false. The spacing on a planar probe is similar or worse compared to a linear array due to limitations in the total number of *elements/channels.*

Option C: This statement is false. Three-dimensional imaging, which requires scanning the US beam in an extra dimension, is typically slower than 2D imaging with a linear array.

Option D: This statement is false. The axial resolution is primarily related to the US frequency and should not be affected by switching probes with equivalent center frequency and bandwidth.

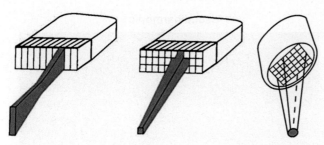

FIGURE 6.7 Displays the beam profile for three different array configurations. **Left:** A standard 1D linear array with the slice thickness determined by an acoustic lens. **Middle:** A 1.5D array that includes a few elements in the elevation direction to improve the focusing in this direction. **Right:** A full 2D planar array for 3D volume imaging provides similar focusing in both the azimuthal and elevational directions using electronic focusing. (Modified from Hedrick WR, Hykes DL, Starchman DE. *Ultrasound Physics and Instrumentation.* 4th ed. St. Louis, MO: Elsevier/Mosby; 2005:125. Reprinted by permission of Dr. Wayne Hedrick.)

Suggested Reading

Hedrick WR, Hykes DL, Starchman DE. *Ultrasound Physics and Instrumentation.* 4th ed. St. Louis, MO: Elsevier/Mosby, 2005:Chapter 8.

Answer 7: D. This question requires an understanding of differences between fundamental and harmonic imaging. In tissue harmonic imaging, the fundamental frequency (f_0) is transmitted and the second harmonic ($2 \times f_0$) is detected. Only nonlinear structures, such as fat or microbubbles, produce harmonic signals.

Tissue harmonic imaging is different than standard B-mode ultrasound imaging in that it detects the harmonic frequencies created by an ultrasound beam as it propagates through tissue. Harmonic frequencies appear due to the nonlinear properties of certain types of structures, such as fat and microbubbles, that serve to distort the sinusoidal waveform of the ultrasound pulse. These harmonic signals are much weaker than the fundamental frequency and can only be detected by proper filtering of the received echoes (FIG. 6.8). Also, because the harmonic signal is at a higher frequency than the fundamental, it is attenuated more quickly as the sound wave propagates through tissue. Consequently, harmonic imaging of deep structures is more difficult.

Tissue harmonic imaging suppresses artifacts associated with the fundamental frequency, enhances nonlinear structures for better contrast, and provides higher spatial resolution due to the higher-frequency harmonic. FIGURE 6.9 provides two examples of tissue harmonic imaging in comparison with the fundamental B-mode image.

Option A: This is a true statement and therefore is an incorrect answer (question asks for least accurate statement). Fat has a larger *nonlinear response* than muscle.

Option B: This is a true statement and therefore is an incorrect answer (question asks for least accurate statement). Acoustic attenuation is stronger at higher frequencies, which affects deeper structures.

Option C: This is a true statement and therefore is an incorrect answer (question asks for least accurate statement). Because the detected frequencies are two times the fundamental, higher spatial resolution is expected, although the signal-to-noise ratio will be lower than standard B-mode imaging.

Suggested Readings

Hedrick WR, Hykes DL, Starchman DE. *Ultrasound Physics and Instrumentation.* 4th ed. St. Louis, MO: Elsevier/Mosby, 2005:Chapter 9.

Tranquart F, Grenier N, Eder V, et al. Clinical use of ultrasound tissue harmonic imaging. *Ultrasound Med Biol* 1999;25(6):889–894.

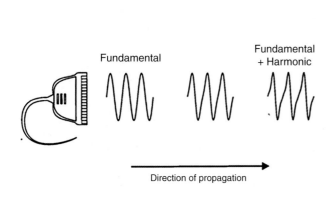

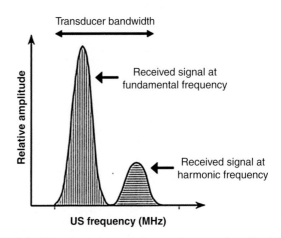

FIGURE 6.8 Left: Harmonic frequencies appear due to absorption and scatter of the US pulse as it travels in a nonlinear medium. The initial frequency exiting the transducer is at the fundamental frequency, but the waveform becomes distorted as harmonic appears in the waveform. The frequency spectrum of the received pulse **(right)** reveals both the fundamental and harmonic frequencies, both within the receiving frequency band of the US transducer. However, in tissue harmonic imaging, only the harmonic frequencies are displayed in the image. (Reprinted from Hedrick WR, Hykes DL, Starchman DE. *Ultrasound Physics and Instrumentation.* 4th ed. St. Louis, MO: Elsevier/Mosby; 2005. Reprinted by permission of Dr. Wayne Hedrick.)

Standard B-mode   **Tissue harmonic**

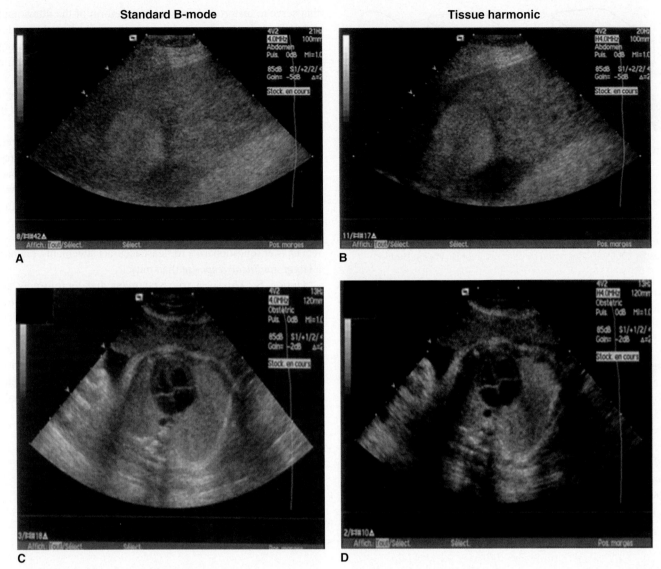

FIGURE 6.9 **A and B:** Standard B-mode and tissue harmonic images of liver metastasis. Tissue harmonic image more clearly reveals posterior ascites and halo around the lesion. **C and D:** Standard B-mode and tissue harmonic images of the heart from a 35-month-old fetus. The tissue harmonic image displays more clarity of the four chambers.

Chapter 7

Microbubbles

Vincent L. Sorrell

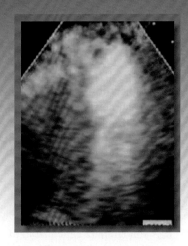

1. Which of the following statements on the differences between manufactured microbubble echo contrast agents and agitated saline contrast is *false*?

   A. Manufactured microbubble echo contrast agents have shells to protect gas from diffusion to blood.
   B. Manufactured microbubble echo contrast agents (2 to 3 μm) are generally smaller than agitated saline microbubbles.
   C. Manufactured microbubble echo contrast agents reliably pass through the pulmonary circulation; agitated saline microbubbles do not.
   D. According to the U.S. FDA, presence of a known or suspected fixed right-to-left shunt is a contraindication for administration of manufactured microbubble echo contrast agents.
   E. The size of agitated saline microbubbles is more uniform than manufactured microbubbles.

2. Which of the following statements regarding the impact of ultrasound on microbubbles are *false*?

   A. Ultrasound increases the rate of destruction of microbubbles.
   B. In response to ultrasound (pressure), microbubbles oscillate and the size of the microbubble may change dynamically in radius in sympathy with the oscillations of the incident ultrasound wave.
   C. Resonant oscillation produces both harmonic and subharmonic frequencies.
   D. Ultrasound mechanical index has no significant impact on microbubble destruction.

3. Which of the following concepts regarding the interaction of microbubbles with ultrasound is *false*?

   A. This interaction results in the reflection of fundamental ultrasound frequency.
   B. This interaction results in the scatter of fundamental ultrasound frequency.
   C. The amplitude of the reflection of ultrasound is related to the diameter of bubble size.
   D. High mechanical index will create harmonic frequency.
   E. Harmonic frequency emitted by microbubbles is lower than the fundamental transmitted frequency.

4. Which of the following is a current indication for commercially manufactured echo contrast agents by the U.S. Food and Drug Administration?

   A. Myocardial perfusion to detect ischemia
   B. Chamber opacification and endocardial border detection
   C. Therapeutic drug delivery
   D. Tumor- or tissue-specific targeted imaging
   E. Shunt detection

5. A sonographer presents the image in Figure 7.1 to you. You found that the left ventricular apex is not well opacified. There is inadequate microbubble filling in the apex with "swirling" seen. The first approach to this condition should be to:

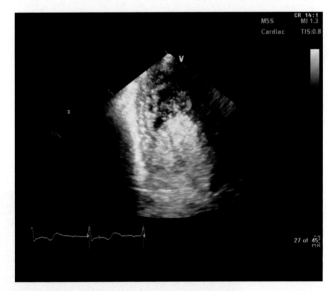

Figure 7.1 Apical four-chamber view with a microbubble contrast agent.

   A. Ask a sonographer to immediately inject more contrast agent.
   B. Look for LV apical systolic dysfunction, since in this setting, contrast "swirling" is unavoidable.
   C. Have the sonographer increase the gain to enhance the brightness of image.
   D. Have the sonographer decrease the mechanical index to reduce microbubble destruction.
   E. Have the sonographer lower the ultrasound frequency to reduce microbubble destruction.

6. Which of the following ultrasound imaging techniques is subject to the effect of myocardial motion generating a Doppler shift to be overlapped with the Doppler shift produced by microbubbles that may artifactually be misinterpreted as myocardial perfusion?

A. Fundamental B-mode imaging
B. Harmonic B-mode imaging
C. Harmonic power Doppler imaging
D. Power pulse inversion imaging

7. A sonographer called from the intensive care unit and asked your permission to give echo contrast to the patient with a poor image quality (Fig. 7.2). The sonographer reported that the patient was an 87-year-old female with history of recent myocardial infarction and two coronary drug-eluting stents. She presented with shortness of breath with oxygen saturation of 92% in room air.

A. Do not give permission because the patient is very elderly and in the ICU, and the risks outweigh the likely benefits.
B. Do not give permission because the image shown, although suboptimal, is adequate for interpretation.
C. Do not give permission because the patient had history of recent myocardial infarction and coronary intervention, especially if the ischemic event was <2 months ago.
D. Do not give permission because the patient had shortness of breath and oxygen saturation of 92%.
E. Give permission with close monitoring in the intensive care unit setting.

8. Which microbubble contrast agent side effect is the *least* common?

A. Headache
B. Nausea and/or vomiting
C. Dizziness
D. Warm sensation/flushing
E. Anaphylaxis

9. Which of the following conditions is *least* likely to benefit from the administration of a manufactured microbubble contrast agent?

A. Unable to identify two or more than two regional myocardial wall segments by regular transthoracic echocardiography due to poor image quality
B. Suspicion of a left ventricular thrombus
C. Suspicion of a cardiac source of emboli in a patient with a large lower extremity deep venous thrombosis
D. Suspicion of LV myocardial noncompaction
E. Improvement in image quality during stress echocardiography

10. A patient who is 32 weeks' pregnant was seen in her physician's office for severe dysphagia. She was subsequently referred to the echocardiography laboratory to assess the left ventricular structure and function, since she also had severe shortness of breath and her obstetrician was suspicious of a cardiomyopathy. The sonographer had difficulty getting optimal images, and the nurse suggested intravenous microbubble contrast use. Which of the following is *true*?

A. You tell the nurse never to give microbubble contrast agents to a woman who is pregnant.
B. You weigh benefits against risks and inform the patient of her options.
C. Call the obstetrician to inform the inability to obtain adequate images.
D. Given the lack of published data in pregnant patients, you should instead perform a routine transesophageal echocardiogram.

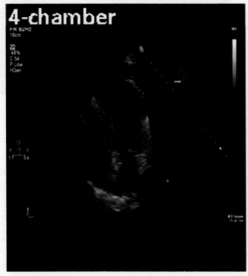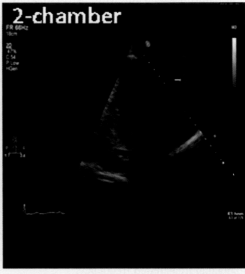

Figure 7.2 Apical four- and two-chamber view without contrast.

11. Which the following statements is true regarding micro-bubbles substantially enhancing backscatter of ultrasound?

    A. Backscatter of ultrasound is substantially enhanced by microbubbles because there is protein in the microbubble shells.

    B. Backscatter of ultrasound is substantially enhanced by microbubbles because there is lipid in the microbubble shells.

    C. Backscatter of ultrasound is enhanced by microbubbles *solely* due to difference in acoustic impendence between the blood and microbubbles.

    D. Backscatter of ultrasound is substantially enhanced by microbubble oscillation when they are exposed to ultrasound beam.

12. For which of the following clinical scenarios is agitated saline microbubble contrast most definitely preferable to manufactured microbubble contrast?

    A. Enhancing the Doppler signal to assess aortic valve gradient

    B. Enhancing the endocardial borders of the left ventricle

    C. Evaluation of left ventricular apical thrombus

    D. Enhancing the Doppler signal to assess mitral regurgitant severity

    E. Detection of right-to-left interatrial shunting

Answer 1: E. **Echo contrast agents:** The structure of the microbubble can be categorized into two types—free gas microbubbles (also called microcavitation) produced most commonly by agitating normal saline and commercially manufactured shelled microbubbles. An advantage of agitated saline microbubbles is that they are low cost and ready to use in clinical setting. However, the size of free gas microbubbles (agitated saline) is not uniform and is usually larger than a red blood cell (7 μm). Therefore, option E is *false* and the correct answer. Agitated saline microbubbles are filtered by lungs and are usually completely cleared by the pulmonary circulation. Therefore, agitated saline microbubbles administered into a systemic vein are not seen in the systemic circulation unless there is a right-to-left shunt between the pulmonary and systemic circulation. The gas in saline microbubbles diffuses rapidly, and therefore, these microbubbles have a short duration in the blood pool. Manufactured echo contrast microbubble agents have special shells. Therefore, option A is true. Shells may be made from a variety of materials. The two agents currently approved by the U.S. FDA have shells comprised of albumin (perflutren type A microspheres or Optison) or lipid (perflutren lipid microsphere or Definity). The shells reduce gas diffusion that enables microbubble contrast agents to persist in the blood pool much longer than free gas microbubbles. The gas (perflutren) used in both of these agents has a low partition coefficient with low diffusion rate that also facilitates persistence in the circulation. Manufactured microbubble echo contrast agents reliably pass through the pulmonary circulation. Therefore, option C is true. The manufacturing process produces a microbubble size that is relatively uniform and small (2 to 3 μm in diameter, which is smaller than a red blood cell). Therefore,

option B is true. Shelled echo microbubble contrast agents are approved and used clinically for chamber opacification and, in investigative settings, are also used as to assess myocardial perfusion. By adding biologic binding receptors, microbubbles can potentially be used for targeted imaging. By adding a drug into the inner layer of shells, microbubbles may potentially be used for drug delivery. Free gas, agitated saline contrast is used to primarily detect right-to-left shunt but can also enhance Doppler signals from tricuspid regurgitation and to opacify the right atrium and right ventricle. According to the U.S. FDA label, the two approved manufactured echo microbubble contrast agents are contraindicated in the presence of a known or suspected right-to-left or bidirectional, even if transient, shunt. Therefore, option D is true. Manufactured echo microbubbles have not been approved for intra-arterial administration.

Suggested Readings

Armstrong WF, Ryan T. *Feigenbaum's Echocardiography*. Philadelphia, PA: Lippincott Williams & Wilkins, 2010.

Becher H, Burns PN. *Handbook of Contrast Echocardiography*. New York: Springer-Verlag Berlin Heidelberg, 2000.

Mulvagh SL, Rakowski H, Vannan MA, et al. American Society of Echocardiography Consensus Statement on the clinical applications of ultrasonic contrast agents in echocardiography. *J Am Soc Echocardiogr* 2008;21:1179–1201.

Answer 2: D. **Impact of ultrasound on microbubbles:** Ultrasound increases the rate of destruction of microbubbles. Therefore, option A is true. With reduction in population of microbubbles, opacification decreases. The effect of micro-bubble disruption by ultrasound largely depends on the pressure produced by ultrasound energy or power of ultrasound. The power of ultrasound in a commercial echocardiography machine is often expressed as the mechanical index (MI), which is defined by peak rarefactional pressure divided by the square root of the ultrasound frequency. Therefore, option D is a false and is the correct answer. In clinical practice, MI usually ranges from 0.1 to 2.0. MI varies throughout the image depending on ultrasound impendence. In the absence of attenuation, the MI is maximal at the focus of the beam. Attenuation shifts the maximum of MI toward the ultrasound transducer. The MI is one of the most important machine settings in a contrast study. It is usually controlled by means of the output power. Its display varies among vendors, and values between different echocardiography machines are not precisely comparable. In response to ultrasound (pressure), microbubbles oscillate and the size of microbubbles may change dynamically in radius in sympathy with the oscillations of the incident ultrasound wave. Therefore, option B is true. A microbubble resonating in the ultrasound field depends on ultrasound frequency, the size of microbubbles, and mechanical properties of the bubble capsule. This resonant oscillation (often nonlinear motion) produces harmonic and subharmonic frequencies, which are two or four times higher than the fundamental ultrasound frequency emitted by a transducer (Fig. 7.3). Therefore, option C is true. By using a selected bandpass filter, echoes returning from solid tissue and red blood cells can be suppressed, and the second harmonic imaging between 3 and 6 MHz (based on

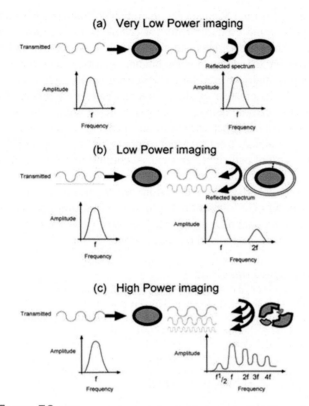

(a) Very Low Power imaging

Transmitted

Reflected spectrum

Amplitude

Frequency

Amplitude

Frequency

(b) Low Power imaging

Transmitted

Reflected spectrum

Amplitude

Frequency

Amplitude

Frequency

(c) High Power imaging

Transmitted

Amplitude

Frequency

Amplitude

Frequency

FIGURE 7.3 With a very low mechanical index, microbubbles reflect fundamental frequency, and tissue generates no harmonics. With low power, microbubbles reflect fundamental frequency and generate harmonic frequency; tissue generates little harmonics. With high power (high mechanical index), microbubbles burst and generate strong harmonics, and tissue also generates harmonics. (Modified from Moir S, Marwick TH. Combination of contrast with stress echocardiography: a practice guide to methods and interpretation. *Cardiovasc Ultrasound* 2004;2:15.)

fundamental frequencies of 1.5 to 3 MHz) can be received and processed. This significantly enhances the image quality.

Suggested Readings

Becher H, Burns PN. *Handbook of Contrast Echocardiography*. New York: Springer-Verlag Berlin Heidelberg, 2000.
Shohet RV, Chen S, Zhou TY, et al. Echocardiographic detection of albumin microtubules directs gene delivery to the myocardium. *Circulation* 2002;101:2554–2556.
Stride E, Saffari N. Microbubble ultrasound contrast agents: a review. *Proc Inst Mech Eng* 2003;217:429–447.

Answer 3: E. **Interaction of microbubbles and ultrasound:** Microbubbles have several interactions with ultrasound. They reflect fundamental ultrasound frequency due to different acoustic impendence between blood and gas in a microbubble. Therefore, option A is the correct statement and true. The greater the difference in impedance between the ultrasound mediums forming the interface, the greater the amount of energy that is reflected back. A more regular and larger object will reflect more ultrasound; particularly, the reflecting surface is perpendicular to the ultrasound beam. Amplitude of reflection of ultrasound depends on the diameter of microbubbles. The larger the diameter of microbubbles, the amplitude of the reflection is more. Sonographers may experience

more sparkles in Optison-enhanced contrast imaging (mean diameters of microbubbles of 3 to 4.5 μm) than Definity-enhanced contrast imaging (mean diameters of microbubbles of 1.1 to 3.3 μm). Therefore, the machine setting for Optison contrast imaging may be slightly different from Definity contrast imaging.

Microbubbles also scatter ultrasound. Since a microbubble is small, it may have more scatter than reflection. Therefore, option B is true. Microbubbles oscillate in the ultrasound field. The oscillation and resonation of microbubbles produce harmonic frequency, especially with high mechanical index (high power). Harmonic frequency is higher than fundamental frequency. For example, if fundamental frequencies of 1.5 to 3 MHz are emitted from a transducer, the second harmonic frequencies are 3 to 6 MHz. Option E is false and is the correct answer.

Suggested Readings

Becher H, Burns PN. *Handbook of Contrast Echocardiography*. New York: Springer-Verlag Berlin Heidelberg, 2000.
Steward VR, Sidhu P. New direction in ultrasound: microbubble contrast. *Br J Radiol* 2006;79:188–194.
Stride E, Saffari N. Microbubble ultrasound contrast agents: a review. *Proc Inst Mech Eng* 2003:217:429–447.

Answer 4: B. **Clinical applications:** In past decades, numerous studies have investigated the potential clinical application of microbubbles contrast echo agents in myocardial perfusion. Some academic centers reported the use of microbubble echo contrast for detection of coronary artery disease with reasonable sensitivity and specificity. Guidelines and consensus from the European Association of Echocardiography discussed potential application of microbubble contrast agents in stress echocardiography tests. Theoretically, coronary stenosis may affect the volume of blood within the perfusion bed as well as blood flow. Measurement of intravascular blood volume can be used for qualification of myocardial perfusion. Shelled microbubbles (commercially manufactured echo contrast agents) will travel to the capillary bed of myocardium following intravenous injection. Microbubble contrast agents may therefore function as an intravascular tracer. However, due to microbubble destruction, gas diffusion, and dilution, only small amounts of venously injected microbubbles reach the capillary bed. Therefore, myocardial contrast signals are weak compared to those in the LV chamber. This nature imposes a significant challenge for myocardial contrast echo imaging. Myocardial contrast imaging often requires specific machine settings and a substantial learning curve. Myocardial perfusion with microbubbles has not been widely applied in the clinical practice due to the length of the learning curve and unresolved issues regarding reproducibility, artifacts, and suboptimal image quality in some patients (severe COPD and obesity). Further investigation is under way. Microbubble drug delivery and targeted imaging are still under investigation. At the present time, chamber opacification and border detection are approved by the FDA for clinical indications based on phase III studies in resting echocardiography primarily using fundamental imaging. Therefore, option B is the correct answer. Options A, C, and D represent potential clinical applications that are still under investigation and are not formally approved by the U.S. Food and Drug Administration. Option E is a contraindication for manufactured microbubble contrast agents, according to the U.S. FDA.

Suggested Readings

Becher H, Burns PN. *Handbook of Contrast Echocardiography*. New York: Springer-Verlag Berlin Heidelberg, 2000.

Kitzman DW, Goldman ME, Gillam LD, et al. Efficacy and safety of the novel ultrasound contrast agent perflutren (Definity) in patients with suboptimal baseline left ventricular echocardiographic images. *Am J Cardiol* 2000;86:669–674.

Porter T, Li S, Kricsfeld D, et al. Detection of myocardial perfusion in multiple echocardiographic windows with one intravenous injection of microbubbles using transient response second harmonic imaging. *J Am Coll Cardiol* 1997;29:791–799.

Tsutsui J, Elhendy A, Anderson JR, et al. Prognostic value of dobutamine stress myocardial contrast perfusion echocardiography. *Circulation* 2005;112:1444–1450.

Answer 5: D. **Ultrasound destroys microbubbles in echo contrast agents:** Administering an additional bolus of a contrast agent may sometimes increase filling of the apex. However, the first step should be to optimize echocardiograph settings. Therefore, option A is *not* the signal best answer. As discussed above, ultrasound destroys bubbles. This phenomenon is more evident at lower ultrasound frequencies and higher acoustic power. The latter is often represented as the mechanical index in commercial echocardiograph. In order to reduce microbubble destruction, minimization of exposure of microbubbles to ultrasound and use of low mechanical index are recommended. Choosing appropriate machine settings is the first step. Therefore, option D is the correct answer. In this case, the mechanical index is 1.3, which is much higher than the current recommendation for routine contrast studies (MI 0.1 to 0.5). Higher mechanical index settings may enhance two-dimensional images. However, it destroys more microbubbles. Increase in gain may increase brightness of contrast image, but will not acutely increase LV cavity filling by microbubbles. Therefore, option C is an incorrect answer. Lowering ultrasound frequency increases ultrasound penetration. However, the apex is in the near field, which is unlikely to benefit from a lower frequency of ultrasound. Furthermore, a lower ultrasound frequency increases destruction of microbubbles (because the power output is inversely proportional to the square root of the frequency). Therefore, option E is an incorrect statement and *not* the best signal answer. For this case, the first step is to decrease mechanical index to <0.8. Reduction in microbubble destruction may be achieved by adjustment of the focal point of ultrasound beam (moving the focus away from swirling area) since the mechanical index is maximal at the focus of the beam. Patients with LV apical aneurysms and severe wall motion abnormalities are more prone to contrast "swirling," but this is not unavoidable and may still be adequately imaged following the above guidelines. Therefore, option B is an incorrect answer.

Suggested Readings

Mulvagh SL, Rakowski H, Vannan MA, et al. American Society of Echocardiography Consensus Statement on the clinical applications of ultrasonic contrast agents in echocardiography. *J Am Soc Echocardiogr* 2008;21:1179–1201.

Skyba DM, Price RJ, Linka AZ, et al. Direct in vivo visualization of intravascular destruction of microbubbles by ultrasound. *Circulation* 1998;98:290–293.

Wei K, Skyba DM, Firschke C, et al. Interaction between microbubbles and ultrasound: in vitro and in vivo observations. *J Am Coll Cardiol* 1997;29:1081–1088.

Answer 6: C. **Image methods:** Contrast-specific imaging technologies include fundamental B-mode imaging, harmonic B-mode imaging, harmonic power Doppler imaging, and power pulse inversion imaging. Rationales of the use of different imaging techniques are to increase signal-to-noise ratio and to attempt to overcome some limitations of microbubble contrast agents. When fundamental B-mode imaging is used, a low mechanical index (0.1 to 0.4) is often used to avoid bubble destruction. Although myocardial texture may not be seen well on gray scale, the LV can be opacified due to the strong scatter from microbubbles (Fig. 7.4).

Harmonic B-mode imaging exploits nonlinear responses of microbubble to ultrasound to generate harmonic imaging. When a low mechanical index is used, tissue (myocardium) generates little harmonics, and the myocardium may not be well visualized (Fig. 7.5A). After injection of microbubbles, the LV can be opacified due to harmonics generated by microbubbles (Fig. 7.5B). This helps to generate LV opacification images without much tissue interference. With appropriate settings, both fundamental B-mode and harmonic B-mode imaging can produce reasonable real-time images for LV opacification. However, propagation of ultrasound through the myocardium results in harmonic signals, which are reflected back

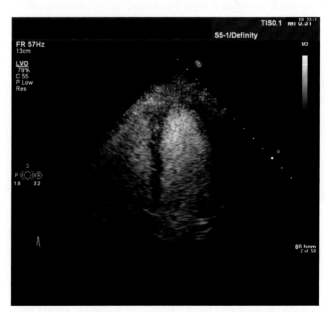

FIGURE 7.4 Fundamental B-mode image of microbubble contrast shows left ventricular opacification. Mechanical index is 0.31 with a transducer frequency of 3.2 MHz.

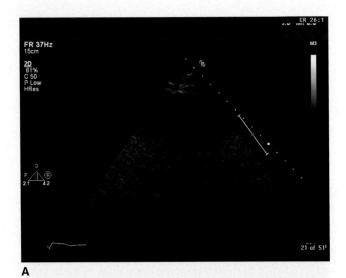

A

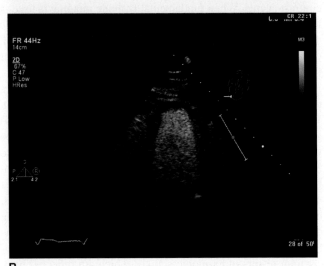

B

FIGURE 7.5 Harmonic B-mode imaging with a low mechanical index of 0.30 and transducer frequency of 4.2 MHz. Myocardium and LV is not well seen with this low mechanical index **(A)**. After injection of microbubbles LV is opacified **(B)**.

from tissue. The signal-to-noise ratio after administration of ultrasound contrast agents with B-mode harmonic imaging is not as high as expected. With an increased mechanical index, myocardial tissue generates harmonics, which may potentially mask myocardial perfusion defects by the microbubble contrast agent. Therefore, use of appropriate echocardiography settings for myocardial perfusion study is important, since this is not related to myocardial motion. Option B is not the correct answer.

Conventional Doppler displays the frequency shift of the received signals (velocity). Harmonic power Doppler imaging displays the amplitude of the received signals, which are associated with the number of scatters (no direction of velocity). Power Doppler imaging offers some advantage over B-mode imaging. It increases the sensitivity of harmonic power imaging. An important limitation of power Doppler imaging is that tissue movement may produce a Doppler shift that may be overlapped with the Doppler shift produced by microbubbles.

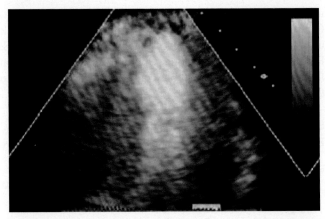

FIGURE 7.6 Harmonic power Doppler imaging shows the microbubble contrast agent. The myocardium is perfused, and the left ventricle is opacified. (Modified from Moir S, Marwick TH. Combination of contrast with stress echocardiography: a practice guide to methods and interpretation. *Cardiovasc Ultrasound* 2004;2:15.)

FIGURE 7.6 illustrates that microbubbles in the LV cavity, myocardium, and surrounding tissue are all displayed by harmonic power Doppler imaging. The overlaps between the Doppler shifts generated by tissue motion and microbubbles may lead to artifactually misinterpreting tissue Doppler signal as microbubble perfusion. Therefore, option C is the correct answer. Power pulse inversion imaging and power pulse inversion flash imaging are other ultrasound imaging techniques. Using a deliberate alternation of transmitted ultrasound pulse forms (inversed ultrasound pulse from transducer), the tissue (myocardial) signal is reduced, and the cavity (microbubble contrast agent) signal is amplified. These techniques are often used in microbubble perfusion studies.

Suggested Readings

Becher H, Burns PN. *Handbook of Contrast Echocardiography*. New York: Springer-Verlag Berlin Heidelberg, 2000.

Heinle SK, Noblin J, Goree-Best P, et al. Assessment of myocardial perfusion by harmonic power Doppler imaging at rest and during adenosine stress. *Circulation* 2000;102:55–60.

Main ML, Magalski A, Chee NK, et al. Full-motion pulse inversion power Doppler contrast echocardiography differentiates stunning from necrosis and predicts recovery of left ventricular function after acute myocardial infarction. *J Am Coll Cardiol* 2001;38(5):1390–1394.

Moir S, Marwick TH. Combination of contrast with stress echocardiography: a practice guide to methods and interpretation. *Cardiovasc Ultrasound* 2004;2:15.

***Answer 7: E.* Safety of microbubble contrast agents:** In 2007, the Food and Drug Administration placed black box warnings for microbubble contrast agents of Definity and Optison after reports of a dozen deaths and nearly 200 cases of cardiopulmonary events. The warning required that the patient's vital signs, cardiac rhythm, and oxygen saturation be monitored during contrast administration and for at least 30 minutes afterward. Most serious reactions occur within 30 minutes of administration. The initial warnings also listed high-risk patients as contraindications such as those who have pulmonary hypertension, unstable cardiopulmonary conditions, acute myocardial infarction, and acute coronary syndromes. Since the FDA warning was placed, several clinical studies were performed. All the studies demonstrated microbubble contrast agents had excellent safety profiles. Review of reported cardiac arrest cases after injection of microbubble contrast could not establish a direct cause–effect relationship between microbubble contrast agents and fatal events. In 2011, based on substantial safety data, the FDA updated the black box warning. Many contraindications were removed, including worsening or clinical unstable congestive heart failure, acute myocardial infarction, acute coronary syndrome, serious ventricular arrhythmias, or high risk of arrhythmia. Therefore, options A, B, C, and D are not correct answers. For Definity, 30 minutes of monitoring of ECG and vital signs and oxygen was removed, and precaution was recommended. For the Optison contrast agent, 30 minutes or longer monitoring is required only in patients with pulmonary hypertension or unstable cardiopulmonary conditions. There is no evidence to support that age or gender would have adverse impact on adverse incidences of microbubble contrast agents. FDA requires resuscitation equipment and trained personnel readily available when microbubble contrast agents are used. In this case, although the patient has a history of MI, stent placement, and advanced age, these are not contraindications for microbubble contrast agents. Shortness of breath could be cardiac or noncardiac. Optimal echocardiographic imaging was helpful for accurately assessing LV function and differentiating a cardiac from noncardiac source of dyspnea. As the patient was in the intensive care unit, ECG and oxygen monitoring was part of routine care. Resuscitation equipment and training personnel were already available. A contrast agent was given and no adverse effects were encountered. High-quality images were obtained (Fig. 7.7). Therefore, option E is the correct answer. It should be remembered that microbubble contrast agents can only be given with the physician's approval (FDA requirement). Pulmonary hypertension is listed as caution for use of microbubble contrast agents. Recent studies have proven

that conventional use of either Definity or Optison is safe in patients with pulmonary hypertension, and the contrast agents did not increase pulmonary artery pressure.

Suggested Readings

Abdelmoneim SS, Bernier M, Scott CG, et al. Safety of contrast agent use during stress echocardiography in patients with elevated right ventricular systolic pressure. *Circ Cardiovasc Imaging* 2010;3:240–248.

Khawaja OA, Shaikh KA, Al-Mallah MH. Meta-analysis of adverse cardiovascular events associated with echocardiographic contrast agents. *Am J Cardiol* 2010;106:742–747.

Shaikh K, Chang SM, Rosendahl-Garcia K, et al. Safety of contrast administration for endocardial enhancement during stress echocardiography: observations from a large cohort and comparison to non-contrast stress. *J Am Soc Echocardiogr* 2008;21:571.

Wever-Pinzon O, Suma V, Ameeta Ahuja A, et al. Safety of echocardiographic contrast in hospitalized patients with pulmonary hypertension: a multi-center study. *Eur Heart J Cardiovasc Imaging* 2012;13:857–862.

Answer 8: E. **Side effects of microbubble contrast agents:** Clinical symptoms associated with microbubble contrast agents were observed in clinical trials and practice. The most common symptoms reported are headache, nausea and/or vomiting, dizziness, and warm sensation/flushing. Severe adverse events such as respiratory distress or potentially hemodynamic instability were rare. Side effects usually occur within 30 minutes after injection of microbubble contrast agents. The black box warning of the FDA recommends monitoring patients with pulmonary hypertension and unstable cardiopulmonary condition after use of Optison. Optison has albumin, which is a blood product. Patients who have adverse reactions to blood products may not receive Optison. Both Definity and Optison have perflutren. They should not be administrated in patients with known or suspected hypersensitivity to the inert gas perflutren. Anaphylaxis is very rare and is the least side effect. Therefore, option E is the correct answer. Anaphylaxis may be a reaction to perflutren, albumin, the lipid shell, or the material in the

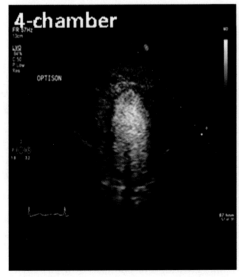 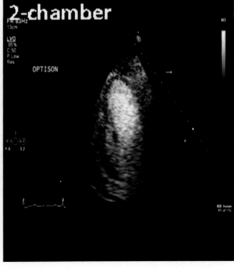

FIGURE 7.7 Apical four- and two-chamber view with contrast.

IV cannula or tubing. Shock, bronchospasm, throat tightness, angioedema, facial swelling, rash, urticaria, and pruritus were reported. Sudden back pain that can be severe but is usually brief and resolves spontaneously has been observed clinically.

Editor's Note: Flank pain occurs in 0.5% to 1.0% of patients receiving a manufactured ultrasound contrast agent (UCA). This is usually self-limited and has not been reported to be associated with subsequent renal damage. A recent study in mice and a small number of humans confirmed that while there is commonly renal cortical microbubble retention, there is no impairment in renal blood flow (Liu YN, Khangura J, Xie A, et al. J Am Soc Echocardiogr 2013;26:1474–1481.) This study also found evidence of complement-mediated interactions between the lipid-based microbubbles tested and the glomerular microvascular endothelium. This interaction generates complement-related intermediates that are known to mediate nociception, suggesting a potential mechanism for UCA-associated flank pain.

Suggested Readings

Dijkmans PA, Juffermans LJ, Musters RJ, et al. Microbubbles and ultrasound: from diagnosis to therapy. *Eur J Echocardiogr* 2004;5:245–256.

Miller DL, Averkiou MA, Brayman AA, et al. Bioeffects considerations for diagnostic ultrasound contrast agents. *J Ultrasound Med* 2008;27:611–632.

Mulvagh SL, Rakowski H, Vannan MA, et al. American Society of Echocardiography Consensus Statement on the clinical applications of ultrasonic contrast agents in echocardiography. *J Am Soc Echocardiogr* 2008;21:1179–1201.

Wei K. Future applications of contrast ultrasound. *J Cardiovasc Ultrasound* 2011;19:107–114.

Answer 9: C. **Indications of contrast agents:** The primary indication for microbubbles is to improve image quality in patients with a suboptimal echocardiogram. Microbubble contrast agents are used to opacify the left ventricle and to improve the delineation of the left ventricular endocardial border. They can be used in regular echocardiography or stress echocardiography, including exercise and dobutamine echocardiography. The American Society of Echocardiography recommends consideration of microbubble contrast if two or more than two LV myocardial segments cannot be adequately visualized. Microbubble contrast agents are used to identify left ventricular thrombus (FIG. 7.8). Several studies reported the usefulness of microbubble contrast agents for the diagnosis of myocardial noncompaction. In a stroke patient with DVT, a paradoxical emboli should be considered if there is suspiciousness of a large atrial septal defect or patent foramen ovale. This is evaluated using agitated saline contrast to exclude an intracardiac shunt. According to the U.S. FDA–approved labels, the presence of known right-to-left shunt, bidirectional shunt, or transient right-to-left shunt is contraindication for microbubble contrast agents. Therefore, option C is an incorrect statement and is the correct answer. Sonographers should be given instructions to routinely ask patients if they have a history of congenital heart disease or cardiac surgery.

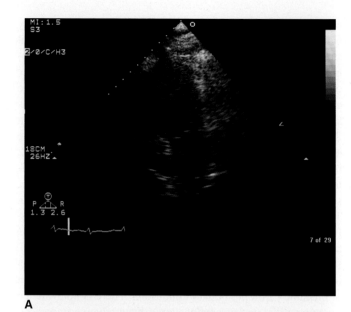

A

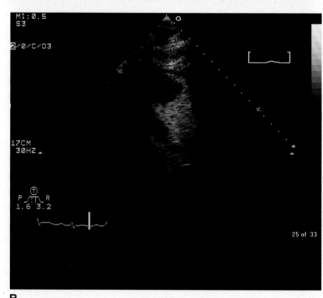

B

FIGURE 7.8 *Left ventricle* of a patient with a history of myocardial infarction. Image quality was suboptimal **(A)**. A large apical thrombus was demonstrated after administration of microbubble contrast **(B)**.

Suggested Readings

Becher H, Burns PN. *Handbook of Contrast Echocardiography*. New York: Springer-Verlag Berlin Heidelberg, 2000.

Mulvagh SL, Rakowski H, Vannan MA, et al. American Society of Echocardiography Consensus Statement on the clinical applications of ultrasonic contrast agents in echocardiography. *J Am Soc Echocardiogr* 2008;21:1179–1201.

Stewart MJ. Contrast echocardiography. *Heart* 2003;89:342–348.

Answer 10: C. **Microbubble contrast agents in special conditions:** Bioeffect of microbubble contrast agents has been studied in vitro. Microbubble disruption by ultrasound may release energy. Cavitation caused by ultrasound (formation, growth, and collapse of a gas cavity in fluid as a result of ultrasound exposure) could raise the temperature. However, there is no evidence of bioeffects from conventional imaging at the current mechanical index level. Blockage of capillary bed was observed in an experimental model. Safety and efficiency of Definity and Optison have not been established in pediatric patients according to the manufacturer's package insert, although clinical use of microbubble contrast agents was reported in children. Currently, Definity and Optison are listed under the pregnancy categories of B and C, respectively. Animal studies have not revealed any evidence of impaired fertility or harm to the fetus caused by Definity. The manufacturer's label suggests Definity should be used during pregnancy only when clearly needed. Therefore, option C is the correct answer. Animal studies showed that Optison has fetotoxicity, which was characterized by a decrease in fetal body weight and an increase in embryo–fetal death in a significantly higher dose than in clinical use. Optison should be used during pregnancy only if the potential benefit justifies the potential risk for the fetus (the manufacturer's label). Performing a TEE in a pregnant woman is not without risks due to conscious sedation. In addition, this patient had a complaint of severe dysphagia. Therefore, option E is incorrect.

Suggested Readings

Denbow ML, Welsh AW, Taylor MJ, et al. Twin fetuses: intravascular microbubble US contrast agent administration-early experience. *Radiology* 2000;214:724–728.
Hua X, Zhu LP, Li R, et al. Effects of diagnostic contrast-enhanced ultrasound on permeability of placental barrier: a primary study. *Placenta* 2009;30:780–784.
McCarville MB. Contrast-enhanced sonography in pediatrics. *Pediatr Radiol* 2011;41(suppl 1):S238–S242.

Answer 11: D. **Microbubble contrast property:** Both agitated saline contrast and microbubble contrast agents produce significant backscatter during echocardiographic examination. Ultrasound backscatters are displayed as bright "sparkles" in two-dimensional echocardiographic images on gray scales and high-density signals in Doppler study. Currently, licensed microbubble contrast agents in the United States include a protein-shelled microbubble contrast agent (Optison) and a lipid-shelled microbubble contrast agent. Neither protein nor lipid shells play a significant role in generation of backscatter of ultrasound. Therefore, options A and B are not correct. The shell functions to reduce gas diffusion, which enables microbubble contrast agents to persist in the blood pool much longer than free gas microbubbles. The shells also protect microbubbles and prevent microbubbles from clearing via the lungs. Significant differences in acoustic impendence between the blood and gas in microbubbles generate strong reflection and scatter of ultrasound. However, it is not a sole mechanism of

backscatters of ultrasound-generated microbubbles. Therefore, option C is not the correct answer. In fact, when microbubbles are exposed to ultrasound, microbubbles will resonate by expanding and contracting. At low ultrasound power, the expansion and contraction are symmetrical, and the bubbles oscillate in a "linear" fashion. The frequency of the scattered signal is similar to fundamental frequency. At higher power, the microbubbles oscillate in "nonlinear" fashion since they resist contraction under positive pressures more than expansion under negative pressures. Oscillation of microbubbles may increase the backscatter by more than 300-fold. Therefore, option D is the correct answer.

Suggested Readings

Becher H, Burns PN. *Handbook of Contrast Echocardiography*. New York: Springer-Verlag Berlin Heidelberg, 2000.
Steward VR, Sidhu P. New direction in ultrasound: microbubble contrast. *Br J Radiol* 2006;79:188–194.

Answer 12: E. Manufactured microbubbles are small and uniform and reliably cross the pulmonary circulation in large numbers. They are thus well suited to evaluation of left-sided pathology, including the left ventricular endocardial borders and intracavitary masses. All microbubbles (agitated saline and an echocardiography contrast agent) can markedly enhance Doppler signals. Prior studies reported that an echocardiography contrast agent was used to enhance the Doppler signal to assess aortic valve gradient and mitral regurgitation. Use of microbubbles for this purpose must deal with the initial "flooding" of the signal and potential overestimation of Doppler velocities. Therefore, this technique has not been routinely applied in clinical setting. Agitated saline is not available in the LV unless there is the presence of a large amount of right-to-left shunting. Therefore, options A, B, C, and D are not correct answers. Detection of interatrial shunting, as in the presence of an atrial septal defect or a patent foramen ovale, depends on detection of microbubbles in the left atrium and the left ventricle. Since manufactured microbubbles are designed to transit into the LV via the pulmonary circulation, they are definitively inferior to agitated saline contrast for detecting atrial shunts. Therefore, option E is correct.

Suggested Readings

Smith LA, Cowell SJ, White AC, et al. Contrast agent increases Doppler velocities and improves reproducibility of aortic valve area measurements in patients with aortic stenosis. *J Am Soc Echocardiogr* 2004;17:247–252.
von Bibra H, Becher H, Firschke C, et al. Enhancement of mitral regurgitation and normal left atrial color Doppler flow signals with peripheral venous injection of a saccharide-based contrast agent. *J Am Coll Cardiol* 1993;22:521–528.

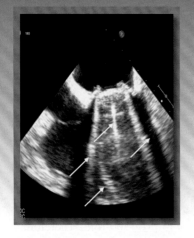

Chapter 8

Common and Uncommon 2D Artifacts

Vedant A. Gupta and Vincent L. Sorrell

1. The image shown in FIGURE 8.1 is taken from a 57-year-old asymptomatic male with a lung nodule referred for preoperative stress testing. Which of the following statements is true? Choose only one correct answer.

A. Discrimination between two point reflectors lying along the longitudinal path of the US beam describes axial resolution.

B. Discrimination between two point reflectors lying perpendicular to the US beam describes axial resolution.

C. Axial resolution is primarily dependent on beam width.

D. Axial resolution is directly proportional to transducer frequency and spatial pulse length.

E. Axial resolution is an echocardiographic technique that allows detection of intracavitary thrombus formation.

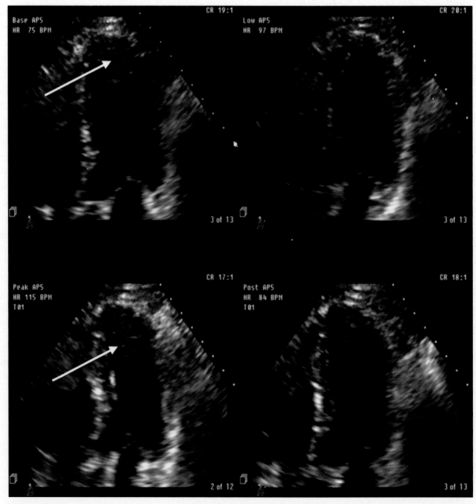

FIGURE 8.1

2. Wave interference in the US beam occurring near the transducer surface causing degradation of image and contrast resolution is known as this type of artifact:

A. Section thickness artifact
B. Speckle artifact
C. Side lobe artifact
D. Misregistration artifact

3. Bright echoes of diminishing intensity created in succession as a result of large differences in impedance between interfaces are known as reverberation. This artifact arises because of which of the following? Select the one best answer.

A. The simultaneous arrival of signals from multiple strong reflectors at varying depths from the transducer
B. The simultaneous arrival of signals from multiple strong reflectors of differing physical properties at varying depths from the transducer
C. The differing arrival times of signals from a strong reflector at a specific depth from the transducer
D. The differing arrival times of signals from multiple weak reflectors at the same depth from the transducer
E. Signals arriving from multiple strong moving reflectors independent of reflector depth

4. The artifact created by the calcified tricuspid valve annulus seen in FIGURE 8.2:

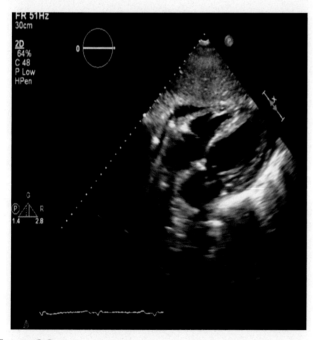

FIGURE 8.2

A. Results from multiple short path reverberations between elements within the reflector
B. Results from the reduction in the amplitude of reflections from an object positioned behind a highly reflective surface
C. Results from an increase in the amplitude of reflections from an object positioned behind a weakly attenuating surface
D. Is specific for calcium-containing structures
E. Can be reduced by adjusting the gain output and increasing the frame rate

5. Which of the following statements is false? Choose the one best answer.

A. Axial resolution improves as the ultrasound frequency increases.
B. Attenuation is directly related to ultrasound frequency.
C. The range of ultrasound frequency useful for diagnostic purposes is typically restricted to 1 to 100 MHz.
D. Ultrasound frequencies <1 MHz increase depth of penetration.

6. Lateral resolution can be improved by which of the following techniques?

A. Reducing the spatial pulse length
B. Increasing the wavelength
C. Increasing the focal zone
D. Aligning more parallel to the direction of flow
E. Increasing the ultrasound frequency

7. Several physical assumptions are made in the creation of ultrasound images by the imaging system. Violation of these assumptions results in imaging artifacts. The image shown in FIGURE 8.3 displays which of the following artifacts?

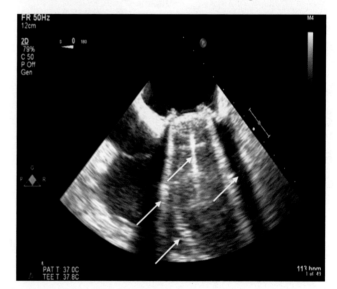

FIGURE 8.3

A. Reverberation artifact only
B. Duplication (multipath) artifact only
C. Reverberation and speckle artifacts
D. Reverberation artifact, side lobe artifact, and duplication artifact
E. Side lobe artifact, reverberation artifact, and attenuation

8. Side lobe artifacts are:

A. More likely to occur as a far-field artifact as a result of beam width enlargement
B. Less likely to occur as a far-field artifact as a result of beam width enlargement
C. More likely to occur as a near-field artifact as a result of greater variability in beam intensity
D. Less likely to occur as a near-field artifact as a result of greater variability in beam intensity

9. Which of the following statements regarding near-field lateral resolution is NOT true? Select the one best answer.

  A. Lateral resolution is related to the beam width.
  B. Lateral resolution is indirectly related to the spatial pulse length.
  C. Lateral resolution denotes the ability to distinguish between two separate reflectors when the incident ultrasound beam is perpendicular to the reflectors.
  D. Lateral resolution is affected by transducer size.
  E. Lateral resolution is improved by increasing the ultrasound beam frequency and sound beam focusing.

10. The image shown in Figure 8.4 and Video 8.1 demonstrates the following (please select the single best answer):

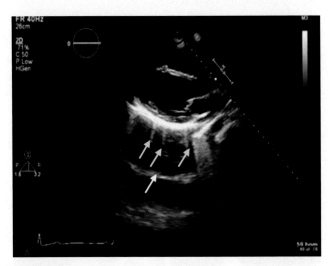

FIGURE 8.4

  A. Mirror artifact
  B. Pericardial effusion
  C. Mirror artifact and pleural effusion
  D. Mirror artifact, reverberation artifact, and a pericardial effusion
  E. Mirror artifact, enhancement, and reverberation artifact

11. Ring-down is a term applied to describe:

  A. The appearance of circular artifacts on an echocardiographic image
  B. The persistence of sound waves after the source of the sound has become silent, resulting from the continuous reverberation or "ringing" of gas bubbles and causing indiscrete echoes associated with reverberation artifacts
  C. Artifacts originating from strong reflectors outside of the body
  D. The propagation of discrete, bright reverberation artifacts throughout the echocardiographic view
  E. The potential artifact created by the damping material used in transducers

12. A 23-year-old woman presented with worsening dyspnea and palpitations over 1 month. Physical exam findings demonstrated a BP of 124/60 mm Hg in the right arm and 127/65 mm Hg in the left arm and an irregular pulse of 130 bpm. She was afebrile, breathing 22 respirations per minute, and maintained normal oxygen saturation on room air. She appeared anxious, but without evidence of JVD. Lung exam was clear. CV exam revealed a normal PMI, dullness to percussion over the left chest, an irregular rate associated with a normal S_1, a split S_2, no gallops, and a 2/6 systolic murmur over the left sternal edge. Carotid, radial, femoral, and pedal pulses were all normal. The abdomen was soft and nontender, without bruits or evidence of organomegaly. CXR demonstrated right atrial enlargement. A 12-lead ECG showed atrial fibrillation, 125 bpm, RBBB, and a mean QRS axis at 120 degrees. A procedure was performed. The images from the TTE performed on initial evaluation are shown in Figure 8.5 and Video 8.2 and demonstrate which of the following?

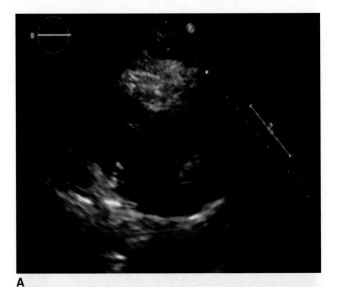

A

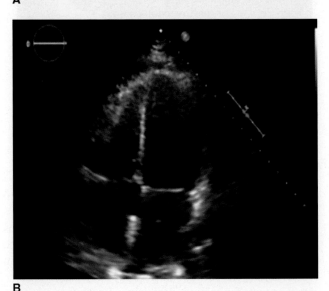

B

FIGURE 8.5

A. RA thrombus
B. LA thrombus
C. Atrial myxoma
D. Interatrial septal closure device
E. MV vegetation

13. A 60-year-old obese male with a remote h/o IVDA presents with symptomatic atrial fibrillation and is referred for elective DC cardioversion. The four-chamber TEE image in FIGURE 8.6 and VIDEO 8.3 shows which of the following?

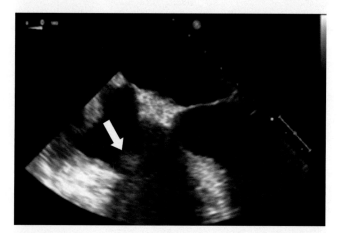

FIGURE 8.6

A. Thickening of the tricuspid valve annulus
B. A tricuspid valve vegetation
C. Lipomatous hypertrophy of the interatrial septum
D. Chiari network
E. All of the above

14. What should be the next appropriate course of action?

A. Begin IV antibiotic therapy.
B. Refer the patient for a CT surgery consultation.
C. Proceed to DC cardioversion if no intracardiac thrombus is seen and continue systemic anticoagulation.
D. A and B.
E. None of the above.

15. The structure shown in FIGURE 8.6 (arrow) and best seen on VIDEO 8.3 is caused by which of the following explanations?

A. Misregistration of the returning ultrasound wave resulting from either deflection by an adjacent interface (multipath) or reflection from a strong reflector (duplication) and incorrect timing assumptions of the imaging system
B. Patient movement during the acquisition of echocardiographic images
C. Near-field side lobes emanating from the ultrasound beam
D. Reverberation and ring-down effects from a highly reflective source object

16. The image in FIGURE 8.7 and VIDEO 8.4 shows which of the following? Choose the one best answer.

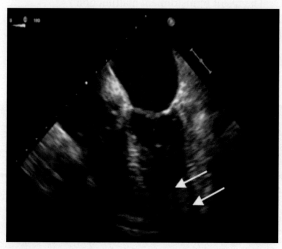

FIGURE 8.7

A. Reverberation artifact originating from the mitral annulus
B. Side lobe artifact from the interatrial septum in the RV free wall
C. Shadowing artifact from the mitral valve chordae
D. Duplication artifact from the interventricular septum

17. The M-mode tracing in FIGURE 8.8 depicts which of the following? Choose one best answer.

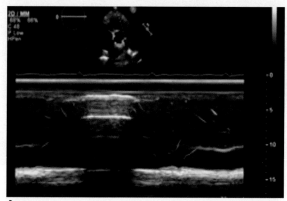

A

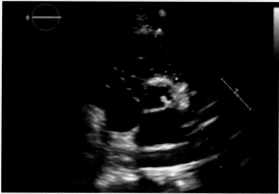

B

FIGURE 8.8

A. A flail PV leaflet
B. Torn MV chordae
C. The result of instrument malfunction
D. The path of infused microbubbles
E. Whip artifact from a Swan-Ganz catheter

18. Match the following imaging artifacts (Figs. 8.9 to 8.13) with the best description.

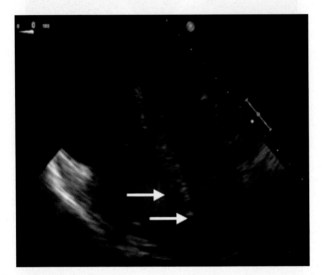

FIGURE **8.9**

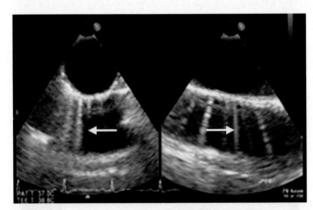

FIGURE **8.10**

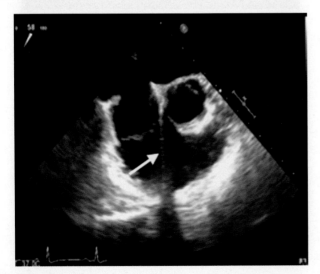

FIGURE **8.11**

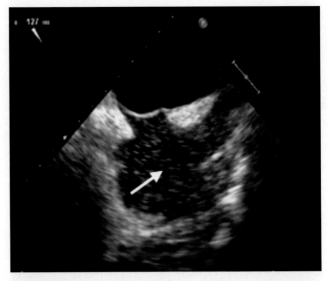

FIGURE **8.12**

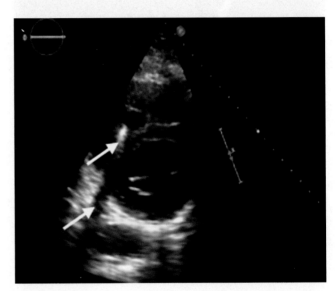

FIGURE **8.13**

A. Comet tail (reverberation)
B. Mirror (duplication) artifact and scatter
C. Reverberation and ring-down
D. Reverberation artifact and attenuation artifact
E. Lateral resolution artifact

19. A 45-year-old male with cardiogenic shock requires extracorporeal membrane oxygenation (ECMO). While adjusting the position of the ECMO catheter using ultrasound guidance, the following image was captured (Fig. 8.14). Which of the following best describes what the image shows?

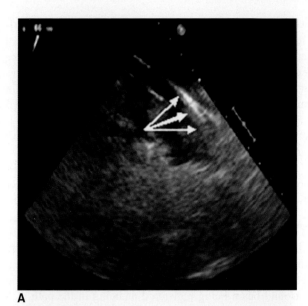

A

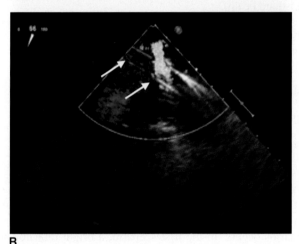

B

FIGURE 8.14

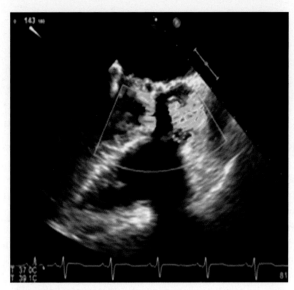

FIGURE 8.15

A. Fill-in correction performed during image processing to handle missing ultrasonographic information.
B. Tissue continuity gaps resulting from inadequate gain adjustment.
C. Patient movement, patient respiration, and arrhythmias can result in this artifact.
D. The presence of a mechanical valvular prosthesis.
E. The US beam encountering attenuators on the body surface such as ECG wires.

Answer 1: *A.* Axial resolution as applied to ultrasonography describes the ability to distinguish between two physical points lying along the longitudinal path of the ultrasound (US) beam. It is strictly defined as the minimum distance required between two objects along the direction of the US beam such that separate reflections are produced. Since the image created is dependent on the ability of the US beam to penetrate the soft tissue, and since the depth of penetration is defined by the US frequency, axial resolution is directly proportional to the transducer frequency. It should be remembered that the higher the frequency, the less the depth of penetration, while the lower the frequency, the greater the depth of penetration (due to increase in attenuation coefficient with frequency). Therefore, a higher transducer frequency will improve resolution but will result in reduced tissue penetration. In addition, axial resolution is indirectly proportional to the spatial pulse length. Spatial pulse length is directly related to the wavelength and number of wavelengths in each pulse. The greater the spatial pulse length, the less the US beam will be able to distinguish two closely apposed objects as separate objects, and vice versa. Axial resolution is also known as longitudinal resolution, range resolution, or depth resolution. Axial resolution has units of distance and is mathematically defined as

A. A kink is present, causing flow turbulence and the appearance of an enhancement artifact on 2D echocardiographic imaging.
B. A break in the ECMO catheter is present, causing scatter artifact.
C. The large difference in impedance between the walls of the ECMO catheter and the surrounding fluid/tissue interface results in the appearance of reverberation artifact.
D. The ECMO catheter is causing significant shadow artifact in the image.

20. The following three-dimensional echocardiographic image (FIG. 8.15) demonstrates a stitch artifact. This artifact arises because of which of the following?

$$\text{Axial resolution (mm)} = \frac{\text{Spatial pulse length (mm)}}{2}$$

For soft tissues, this becomes

$$\text{Axial resolution (mm)} = \frac{1.54 \,(\text{mm}/\mu s) \times \text{Number of cycles}}{2 \times \text{Frequency (MHz)}}$$

$$= (0.77 \times \text{number of cycles})/\text{Frequency}$$

Keep in mind that the larger the numerical value, the less is the actual resolution, while the lesser the numerical value, the greater the resolution.

In contrast, lateral resolution refers to the ability to distinguish between two reflectors lying perpendicular to the US beam path as the beam is scanned across the reflectors. Lateral resolution is equal to beam width. The image in FIGURE 8.1 shows four images of the LV acquired during a typical dobutamine stress protocol. An artifact of axial resolution is noted in the first image at the LV apex, giving the impression of a large apical thrombus or mass. This was not seen in other views. Short-range imaging at a high frame rate often results in the misinterpretation of distant echoes from earlier pulses as occurring in the near field.

Option B: The ability to distinguish between two objects perpendicular to the ultrasound beam is the definition of lateral resolution (not axial resolution).

Option C: Lateral resolution is dependent on beam width, not axial resolution.

Option D: Axial resolution is directly proportional to ultrasound frequency but inversely related to spatial pulse length.

Option E: Generally, injection of echocardiographic contrast agent is the strategy used to identify an intracardiac thrombus. Axial resolution is not a technique, but a property of the ultrasound system and specific settings being used.

Suggested Readings

Baun J. *Physical Principles of General and Vascular Sonography.* San Francisco, CA: California Publishing Company, 2004: Chapter 14. ISBN 940471-35-3.
Kremkau FW. *Diagnostic Ultrasound: Physical Principles and Exercises.* New York, NY: Grune & Stratton, 1980. ISBN 0-8089-1233-X.
Ragland MM, Tak T. The role of echocardiography in diagnosing space-occupying lesions of the heart. *Clin Med Res* 2006;4(1):22–32.

Answer 2: B. Speckle artifact refers to the poorly defined pattern of interference originating from reflectors near the transducer surface. Such interference results in image degradation and suboptimal contrast resolution distal to the proximal "high-resolution" image from the increased speckles near the transducer. These bright reflectors are often small and lead to degradation of the entire far-field image.

The remaining incorrect options are all examples of misregistration artifacts (registering something not truly in the path of the ultrasound beam as being in the path of the ultrasound beam, multipath reflection of the US beam, or artifacts of axial/lateral resolution). Misregistration refers to the malposition of objects in the path of the US beam due to side lobes emanating from the US beam.

Option A: Section thickness artifact is sometimes referred to as elevational width artifact. Similar to side lobes in the lateral direction, elevational width artifact refers to misregistration artifacts in the azimuthal direction. Bright reflectors that are actually "in front" or "behind" the slice of interest are being incorrectly registered as being in the slice itself. True section thickness artifacts are generally hazy artifacts. This has become more common with 3D probes as the 3D probes have an increased thickness to the face plate.

Option C: Side lobe artifacts refer to bright reflectors in the plane perpendicular to the ultrasound beam being incorrectly registered as being in the path of the ultrasound beam. This will be discussed in detail in later questions.

Option D: Misregistration artifacts are a large collection of different artifacts (side lobes and section thickness artifact being two of them) that lead to objects incorrectly being registered in the image (often objects that are not in the path of the ultrasound beam being registered as being in the path of the ultrasound beam).

Suggested Readings

Baun J. *Physical Principles of General and Vascular Sonography.* San Francisco, CA: California Publishing Company, 2004: Chapter 14. ISBN 940471-35-3.
Hedrick WR, Petersen CL. Image artifacts in real time ultrasound. *J Diagn Med Sonogr* 1995;11:300–308.
Kremkau FW, Taylor KJ. Artifacts in ultrasound imaging. *J Ultrasound Med* 1985;5:227–237.
Scanlan KA. Sonographic artifacts and their origins. *Am J Radiol* 1991;156:1267–1272.

Answer 3: C. Reverberation artifacts are commonly seen artifacts in ultrasound imaging and therefore frequently tested. Fundamentally, reverberation artifacts occur when one of two scenarios occurs. In the first scenario, a bright reflector perpendicular to the path of the ultrasound beam sends a signal that is so strong back to the ultrasound transducer that instead of absorbing that entire signal (or dampening the signal), it allows a certain amount of signal to return back into the tissue being imaged. This signal then essentially bounces between the bright reflector and the ultrasound transducer. The second scenario is that there are two bright reflectors perpendicular to the path of the ultrasound beam, and the part of the returning signal from the more distal bright structure hits the more proximal bright structure and bounces back while part of the signal gets through to the ultrasound transducer. The signal that bounces back then hits the distal bright reflector and bounces back again (repeating the cycle). In either of these situations, two things happen: (1) the bright reflector gets reproduced in the imaging field further down from the true structure and (2) given that the reflected signal always loses some intensity, the reverberation artifacts get progressively weaker (and therefore less echogenic). Given that the speed of sound is fixed in soft tissue, the distance between the true structure and the reverberation artifacts would also be fixed and will be a multiple of the distance between the two structures between which the signal is bouncing (either distance from the structure to the transducer or the two bright structures). See FIGURE 8.16.

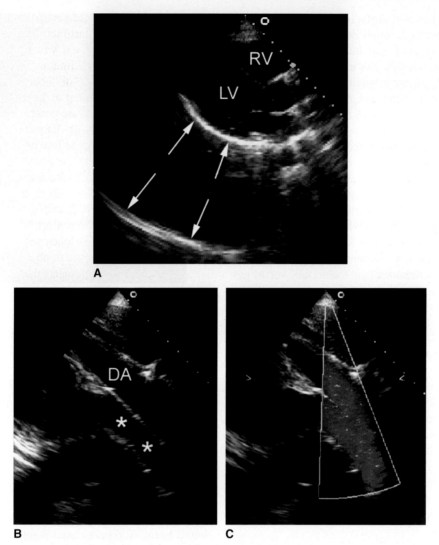

FIGURE 8.16 Reverberation artifacts are demonstrated. **A:** The source of the artifact is the posterior pericardium, which is a very strong reflector. This creates the illusion of a second structure behind the heart. In this case, the second line of echoes (*far arrows*) is twice the distance from the transducer as the actual pericardial echoes. **B:** A second lumen appears just distal to the descending aorta (DA) in this subcostal view. The illusion of a second vessel was apparent with two-dimensional imaging (*, **B**) and color Doppler imaging **(C)**.

Option A: Given that the artifact is being registered at a different depth, the signals received from the artifact have to be coming at different times. Remember, the ultrasound can only figure out time and assumes depth based on the time it takes to receive the returning signal and a fixed speed of sound.

Option B: Again, the image is registering arrival of signals at different times.

Option D: Reverberation artifacts come about due to a strong reflecting signal from a strong reflector. Weak reflectors would not produce a strong enough signal to cause reverberation artifacts.

Option E: Reverberation artifacts are tied to the depth of the original structure (the bright reflector), and near-field structures are more likely to produce reverberation artifacts than are far-field structures. Also, reverberation artifacts are usually seen at a distance related to the distance between the structure and the transducer.

Suggested Readings

Feldman MK, Katyal S, Blackwood MS. US artifacts. *Radiographics* 2009;29:1179–1189.
Hedrick WR, Petersen CL. Image artifacts in real time ultrasound. *J Diagn Med Sonogr* 1995;11:300–308.
Scanlan KA. Sonographic artifacts and their origins. *Am J Radiol* 1991;156:1267–1272.

Answer 4: A. The type of artifact demonstrated in FIGURE 8.2 is commonly known as a "comet tail" artifact and results from multiple short path reverberations between elements within the reflector or between two or more reflectors. Grossly speaking, it is a type of reverberation artifact, but usually, the structure itself (in this case the calcified tricuspid annulus) has multiple small reflectors between which the signal bounces. Similar to reverberation artifacts, part of the signal makes it back to the transducer while some of the signal hits the other highly reflective structure more proximal and sends it back to the original reflector distal. Given the two structures are so close in proximity, the reverberation artifacts are difficult to completely make out, but multiple small lines can be seen if one looks closely. In addition, given that the multiple reflectors are in close proximity to one another, this usually tends to affect a single raster line in a 2D image acquisition (although multiple can be affected) and creates a thin line of duplication or reverberation. This gives the look of a tail, hence the "comet tail" artifact.

Ring-down artifact can be associated with this as well and will often look like a "tail." However, ring-down artifacts are due to issues with gas bubbles within another medium (liquid or solid) creating a "tail" of reverberations. It is thought to be due to constant "ringing" of the piezoelectrode crystals. These artifacts tend to be linear as well but do not always clearly have multiple linear reverberation lines that "comet tail" artifacts do (although they can). The major differentiation comes from the source of the artifact (calcium/metal for "comet tail" versus gas bubbles for ring-down artifacts).

Option B: A reduction in the amplitude of reflections from an object positioned behind a reflective surface is known as attenuation artifact and would appear as a shadowing effect beyond the bright structure.

Option C: An increase in amplitude of reflections from an object located behind a weakly attenuating surface is known as enhancement artifact.

Option D: This artifact is not unique to structures containing calcium but can result any time the ultrasound beam encounters complex and/or multiple strong reflectors.

Option E: The artifact is unlikely to be eliminated simply by adjusting the gain or frame rate. Often, imaging from a different imaging window would allow for visualization of the structures obscured by the comet tail artifact.

Suggested Readings
Feldman MK, Katyal S, Blackwood MS. US artifacts. *Radiographics* 2009;29:1179–1189.
Scanlan KA. Sonographic artifacts and their origins. *Am J Radiol* 1991;156:1267–1272.

Answer 5: *C.* Axial resolution is dependent on transducer frequency and spatial pulse length (which is in turn dependent on wavelength and duration of pulse). Higher-frequency probes have a shorter wavelength and, for the same pulse duration, have a shorter spatial pulse length. This in turn leads to improved axial resolution (Fig. 8.17). The trade-off unfortunately with imaging with higher-frequency probes is an increase in attenuation as attenuation is directly proportional to frequency of probe. This leads to a decrease in depth of imaging possible. At lower frequencies, the depth of penetration is greatest, but the axial resolution suffers. Ultrasound frequencies useful for diagnostic purposes are usually in the range of 1 to 10 MHz.

Option A: This is a true statement. Axial resolution improves as frequency increases. Given that axial resolution is usually described as a minimum distance between two objects for them to be resolved, the smaller the distance, the higher the axial resolution. Axial resolution (as a distance) is, therefore, inversely proportional to transducer frequency.

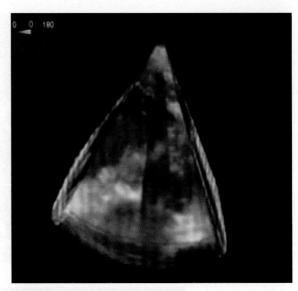

FIGURE 8.17

Option B: This is a true statement. Attenuation is directly proportional to transducer frequency.

Option D: This is a true statement. The lower the transducer frequency, the higher the penetration, but at the expense of axial resolution.

Suggested Reading
Kremkau FW. *Diagnostic Ultrasound: Physical Principles and Exercises.* New York, NY: Grune & Stratton, 1980. ISBN 0-8089-1233-X.

Answer 6: *E.* Lateral resolution refers to the ability to resolve structures that are perpendicular to the direction of the ultrasound beam. Similar to axial resolution, lateral resolution is described as the minimum distance needed to resolve two distinct structures as distinct. Therefore, the smaller the distance reported, the better the lateral resolution. Lateral resolution is slightly more complex in that lateral resolution in the near field is different than lateral resolution in the far field. Similar to a flashlight, the ultrasound beam diverges after a certain distance. This more compact near field is termed Fresnel zone and is where lateral resolution is the best. A longer Fresnel zone will improve lateral resolution in the far field. Lateral resolution is dependent on beam width, transducer frequency, and the speed of sound in a medium. Classically, lateral resolution improves with a higher frequency (inversely related—as frequency increases, the distance needed to resolve two objects decreases). Also, the higher the width or the aperture of the piezoelectrode element, the longer the Fresnel zone and therefore the better the far-field lateral resolution. Larger aperture crystals also have less divergence of the ultrasound beam in the far field. Sometimes the aperture of the piezoelectrode element will be equated to the width of the transducer, and therefore, the wider the transducer, the better the lateral resolution in the far field. This can be a little confusing as intuitively, the narrower the crystal, the narrower the ultrasound beam, and therefore, one would be more likely to separate out two structures close to one another. While this is true in the near field, the ultrasound beam would diverge

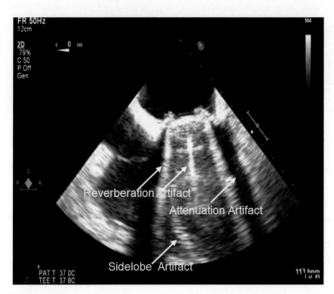

FIGURE 8.18

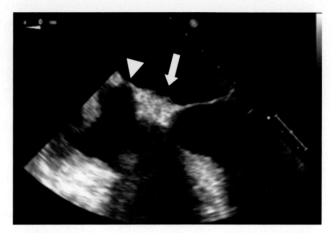

FIGURE 8.19

more quickly, and therefore lateral resolution would degrade rapidly. Similar to ultrasound frequency's impact on axial resolution, narrower transducer width (and therefore beam width) may improve lateral resolution in the near field, but at the cost of depth. Also, shortening the focal zone also improves lateral resolution. Option A: Spatial pulse length is related to axial resolution but has limited impact on lateral resolution.

Option B: Increasing the wavelength would decrease the ultrasound frequency and worsen both axial and lateral resolution.

Option C: Increasing the focal zone degrades the lateral resolution in the focal zone (Fig. 8.18).

Option D: Aligning parallel to flow is important in preventing underestimation of velocity in Doppler echocardiography but has no significant impact on lateral resolution in 2D echocardiography.

Suggested Readings

Baun J. *Physical Principles of General and Vascular Sonography.* San Francisco, CA: California Publishing Company, 2004: Chapter 14. ISBN 940471-35-3.

Kremkau FW. *Diagnostic Ultrasound: Physical Principles and Exercises.* New York, NY: Grune & Stratton, 1980. ISBN 0-8089-1233-X.

Answer 7: E. Ultrasound images are created based on several assumptions. First, US waves emitted from the transducer travel along a straight path to the target object. Second, US waves reflected from an object return to the transducer along a straight path. Third, the US beam is infinitely small in all directions. Fourth, US waves returning to the transducer are derived from the most recent pulse. Fifth, the distance of the object from the transducer is derived from the time it takes for the US wave to leave the transducer, strike the object, and return back to the transducer. The image in FIGURE 8.19 shows a mechanical prosthetic mitral valve. Several artifacts are displayed here and include attenuation (shadowing) by the mechanical prosthesis, reverberation from strong reflector components of the mechanical prosthesis, and side lobe artifacts arising from

incident "stray" ultrasound beams in the near field coming into contact with the components of the mechanical MV prosthesis. Since it is assumed that the image is derived from US waves reflected in line with the US beam, structures "sensed" by side lobes are assumed to be part of the target image.

Suggested Readings

Baun J. *Physical Principles of General and Vascular Sonography.* San Francisco, CA: California Publishing Company, 2004: Chapter 14. ISBN 940471-35-3.

Feldman MK, Katyal S, Blackwood MS. US artifacts. *Radiographics* 2009;29:1179–1189.

Scanlan KA. Sonographic artifacts and their origins. *Am J Radiol* 1991;156:1267–1272.

Answer 8: C. The greatest variability in beam intensity occurs in the near field, and this is the source of side lobes. Side lobes are essentially the result of a "spill-over" effect in the near field in which stray US beams leave the central propagation path. Since it is assumed that all returning US waves are in line with the emitted US beam, these objects are incorrectly assumed to be part of the original target. Side lobe artifacts are generally seen in the raster lines adjacent to a very bright object (i.e., annular calcification or lead).

Suggested Reading

Kremkau FW. *Diagnostic Ultrasound: Physical Principles and Exercises.* New York, NY: Grune & Stratton, 1980. ISBN 0-8089-1233-X.

Answer 9: B. Although lateral resolution can be improved by increasing the US frequency, it is not related to spatial pulse length (this affects axial resolution). One of the main factors that determine the lateral resolution is the length of the near field, where lateral resolution is optimized. The lateral resolution is improved with a longer near-field zone (Fresnel zone). In the Fresnel zone, the lateral resolution can be focused by changing the focal zone. The lateral resolution worsens substantially in the far field (also known as the Fraunhofer zone), because the ultrasound signal diverges dramatically after that. The near-field length can be calculated with the following equation:

$$1 = r^2/\lambda$$

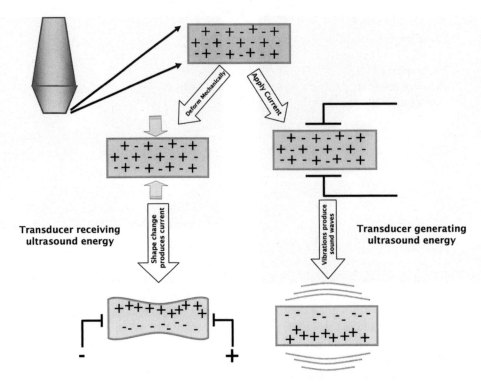

FIGURE 8.20 The length of the near field depends on transducer frequency and transducer size, as illustrated in these four examples. On the left, a transducer with a 10-mm diameter emits ultrasound at 2.0 MHz. This determines both the length of the near field and the rate of divergence in the far field. If the same size transducer emits energy at 4 MHz, the length of the near field increases and the rate of dispersion is less. A transducer half that size (5 mm) transmitting at 4.0 MHz will have a shorter near field. Finally, a 5-mm transducer that transmits at 2 MHz will have the shortest near field and the greatest rate of dispersion in the far field.

Where l = length of the near field, r = radius of the transducer, and λ = wavelength of the ultrasound beam. The impact of changing ultrasound frequency and transducer diameter can be seen in FIGURE 8.20.

Option A: This is a true statement. Lateral resolution is related to beam width (which is in turn related to ultrasound frequency and diameter of the transducer).

Option C: This is a true statement. This is the definition of lateral resolution (the minimum distance needed to distinguish two objects in a plane perpendicular to the direction of the ultrasound beam).

Option D: This is a true statement. Lateral resolution improves as the transducer width increases largely by increasing the length of the near-field zone as well as minimizing divergence of the ultrasound beam in the far field.

Option E: This is a true statement. Lateral resolution improves with increasing ultrasound frequency and focusing of the ultrasound beam.

Suggested Readings

Baun J. *Physical Principles of General and Vascular Sonography.* San Francisco, CA: California Publishing Company, 2004: Chapter 14. ISBN 940471-35-3.

Kremkau FW. *Diagnostic Ultrasound: Physical Principles and Exercises.* New York, NY: Grune & Stratton, 1980. ISBN 0-8089-1233-X.

***Answer 10:** E.* Several artifacts are shown in FIGURE 8.4. The entire image of the left ventricle, mitral valve, and left atrium is duplicated and appears below the actual image. This mirror artifact (*white arrow*) occurs as a result of US waves that are reflected back from the transducer rather than being registered as a returning signal. The distance at which the mirror image appears is proportional to the length of time it takes for the US waves to be detected by the transducer after bouncing back and forth between the transducer and the target. Thus, if the returning signal takes twice as long to be registered as the original pulsed wave, the object is placed at twice the distance from the original object. Mirror image artifacts will mimic the movement of moving structures in the original image. In this example, the "mirrored" mitral valve can be seen moving in the pleural effusion. The inferolateral wall and pericardium are strongly reflective and exhibit an enhancement artifact (*red arrow*) as the US beam leaves an area of relatively lower attenuation within the LV cavity and strikes the soft tissue of the inferolateral wall. The strong reflective surface of the inferolateral wall and pericardium also causes the comet tailing reverberation artifact seen as stripes emanating below the inferolateral wall border (*yellow arrows*). In real time, a reflection of the movement of the mitral valve can clearly be seen within the duplicated LV cavity. The line below the duplicated LV cavity represents a reflection of the anteroseptal wall while the space below this is likely the RV cavity based on mirrored movement of the surrounding soft tissue with the RV free wall. Based on a still frame alone, a pleural effusion would have a similar appearance and could therefore not be excluded as a part of the image.

Option A: A mirror image artifact is seen; however, this answer does not acknowledge the other artifacts seen.

Option B: There is no pericardial effusion. The fluid collection is outside of the pericardial space (in the same plane as the descending aorta).

Option C: Again, while a mirror image artifact and pleural effusion are seen, it does not acknowledge the presence of other artifacts, such as reverberation artifact.

Option D: This is incorrect as there is no evidence of a pericardial effusion.

Suggested Readings

Baun J. *Physical Principles of General and Vascular Sonography.* San Francisco, CA: California Publishing Company, 2004: Chapter 14. ISBN 940471-35-3.

Hedrick WR, Petersen CL. Image artifacts in real time ultrasound. *J Diagn Med Sonogr* 1995;11:300–308.

Scanlan KA. Sonographic artifacts and their origins. *Am J Radiol* 1991;156:1267–1272.

Answer 11: B. Similar to the persistent ringing of a bell after being struck, ring-down describes the excessive ringing of the transducer crystal after the sound wave has been generated. The result is the production of indiscrete echoes appearing at some distance from the reflector. These are usually associated with reverberation artifacts that mimic comet tail artifacts. However, the source is different in comet tail reverberations (usually multiple bright reflectors within a structure), whereas ring-down artifacts typically occur in the presence of air/gas bubbles or particulates. Therefore, the reverberations in comet tail artifacts are more discrete and easier to identify. In ring-down artifacts, the "reverberations" are very fine and often indistinguishable. Transducers are equipped with a damping material to reduce (or eliminate) ring-down effects.

Suggested Readings

Feldman MK, Katyal S, Blackwood MS. US artifacts. *Radiographics* 2009;29:1179–1189.

Kremkau FW. *Diagnostic Ultrasound: Physical Principles and Exercises.* New York, NY: Grune & Stratton, 1980. ISBN 0-8089-1233-X.

Scanlan KA. Sonographic artifacts and their origins. *Am J Radiol* 1991;156:1267–1272.

Answer 12: D. The image in FIGURE 8.5A is an RA/RV view showing the presence of an interatrial septal device. The patient apparently had an atrial septal defect that was repaired in adulthood using a percutaneously placed atrial septal closure device. Unfortunately, this did not prevent the development of atrial fibrillation in this patient. FIGURE 8.5B shows the echogenic interatrial septal closure device well seated. Choice A is incorrect since this would represent an unusual location for an RA thrombus, which is usually seen in areas of blood stasis such as near the entrance of the vena cavae or right atrial appendage and usually in association with an indwelling catheter or pacemaker wire. Additionally, no mass is seen in the apical four-chamber view to suggest the presence of a thrombus. RA thrombus is also not usually associated with atrial fibrillation. Rather, LA thrombus, specifically within the left atrial appendage, is associated with atrial fibrillation. Since the image in FIGURE 8.5A depicts an RA–RV view, choices B and E

cannot be correct. Atrial myxoma is possible but typically can be seen as a pedunculated mass attached to the interatrial septum. Most atrial myxomas (~80%) are located within the LA. If large enough, it may impede flow into and out of the RA or affect the movement of the TV leaflets. The brightness of the interatrial septum suggests that this patient underwent a corrective procedure for her ASD, its morphology in orthogonal views most suggestive of a percutaneous implantation of an ASD closure device. The procedure alluded to was a TEE followed by DC cardioversion.

Suggested Readings

Gatzoulis MA, Freeman MA, Siu SC, et al. Atrial arrhythmia after surgical closure of atrial septal defects in adults. *N Engl J Med* 1995;340:839–846.

Giardini A, Donti A, Sciarra F, et al. Long-term incidence of atrial fibrillation and flutter after transcatheter atrial septal defect closure in adults. *Int J Cardiol* 2009;134:47–51.

Hedrick WR, Petersen CL. Image artifacts in real time ultrasound. *J Diagn Med Sonogr* 1995;11:300–308.

Ragland MM, Tak T. The role of echocardiography in diagnosing space-occupying lesions of the heart. *Clin Med Res* 2006;4(1):22–32.

Answer 13: C. See answer 15.

Answer 14: C. See answer 15.

Answer 15: A. FIGURE 8.21 shows a lipomatous hypertrophy of the interatrial septum (arrow) with the classic pathognomonic sparing at the fossa (arrowhead). Reflective echoes partially reproduce the interatrial septum in the vicinity of the tricuspid annulus, giving the impression of a TV anatomic abnormality, such as a valvular vegetation. Imaging from multiple other angles did not reveal any anatomic abnormalities of the

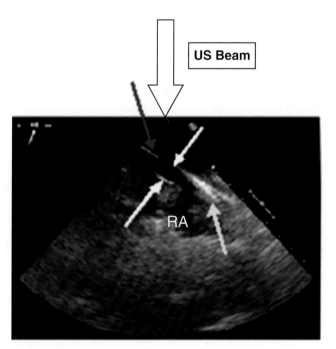

US Beam

RA

FIGURE 8.21

TV or any other heart valve. Since there is no valvular vegetation, treatment with IV antibiotics or referral for surgery is not indicated. Large differences in impedance encountered by the US beam (in this case between the blood pool and the hypertrophied interatrial septum and RA wall) can result in several artifacts including reverberation, duplication, acoustic shadowing, and enhancement.

Suggested Readings

Baun J. *Physical Principles of General and Vascular Sonography*. San Francisco, CA: California Publishing Company, 2004: Chapter 14. ISBN 940471-35-3.

Kremkau FW. *Diagnostic Ultrasound: Physical Principles and Exercises*. New York, NY: Grune & Stratton, 1980. ISBN 0-8089-1233-X.

Answer 16: C. Two-dimensional echocardiography allows optimal visualization of cardiac structures when the US beam is directed perpendicular to those structures. Structures arranged parallel to the US beam are not visible but can result in the production of acoustic attenuation, or shadowing as illustrated by the MV chordae in this image. The shadows created by the MV chordae result in black stripes that can be seen in the background of the LV wall, representing an attenuated US signal.

Option A: Reverberation artifact would be expected to produce increased signal as the US beam bounces between strong reflectors such as a calcified mitral annulus and the transducer, not the absence of signal as shown here.

Option B: Side lobe artifacts involving the interatrial septum are usually seen in the same plane as the original structure (in this case, interatrial septum), oftentimes in the atrial cavity. That is not appreciated here.

Option D: Duplication artifacts from the interventricular septum would cause "extra structures" often in the LV cavity. It would not explain the loss of signal from the distal septum or the apex.

Suggested Readings

Baun J. *Physical Principles of General and Vascular Sonography*. San Francisco, CA: California Publishing Company, 2004: Chapter 14. ISBN 940471-35-3.

Hedrick WR, Petersen CL. Image artifacts in real time ultrasound. *J Diagn Med Sonogr* 1995;11:300–308.

Kremkau FW. *Diagnostic Ultrasound: Physical Principles and Exercises*. New York, NY: Grune & Stratton, 1980. ISBN 0-8089-1233-X.

Answer 17: D. The superior temporal resolution of M-mode echocardiography is sensitive enough to detect and track microbubbles infused through a central venous catheter. This does not represent a machine malfunction. The randomness of the signal is a clue that it does not originate from an anatomic structure. Enhancement artifact is also clearly appreciated from strong proximal and distal reflectors. FIGURE 8.8B demonstrates the microbubbles as seen by 2D imaging. Note the lateral resolution artifact caused by the microbubbles, resulting in the bubbles appearing wider than expected.

Option A: A flail PV might result in similar M-mode artifact but would not show the degree of chaos demonstrated by the infused microbubbles seen here.

Option B: The MV is not seen in this image, given that it is a parasternal SAX at the level of the aortic valve. Torn chordae can have a chaotic path noted on M-mode.

Option C: This is a real finding (microbubbles) and not a result of instrument malfunction.

Option E: An indwelling catheter is not visualized in the 2D view, making choice E incorrect.

Suggested Reading

Hedrick WR, Petersen CL. Image artifacts in real time ultrasound. *J Diagn Med Sonogr* 1995;11:300–308.

Answer 18: FIGURE 8.9 = C, FIGURE 8.10 = B, FIGURE 8.11 = A, FIGURE 8.12 = E, FIGURE 8.13 = D.

The FIGURE 8.9 depicts the ring-down phenomenon that results from the persistent ringing of the crystal within the transducer, causing the appearance of indiscrete echoes along lines of reverberation near the transducer. FIGURE 8.10 shows duplication of the aorta in orthogonal views. Also shown are bright lines of scatter emanating from the echogenic aortic wall. FIGURE 8.11 demonstrates the typical comet tail reverberation artifact. This artifact results in a diminishing trail of reverberations as the distance from the strongly reflective origin increases. FIGURE 8.12 depicts a splaying pattern of injected microbubbles, causing the bubbles to assume an elongated rather than spherical shape. The artifact results from the intrinsic limitations of ultrasound lateral resolution. FIGURE 8.13 shows a catheter located within the right ventricle. The catheter is a strongly reflective object and causes the appearance of reverberation artifact seen as the bright, trailing pattern of echoes. It also causes attenuation of the distal soft tissue, specifically the basal inferoseptal LV wall, pericardium, and lung tissue.

Suggested Readings

Baun J. *Physical Principles of General and Vascular Sonography*. San Francisco, CA: California Publishing Company, 2004: Chapter 14. ISBN 940471-35-3.

Hedrick WR, Petersen CL. Image artifacts in real time ultrasound. *J Diagn Med Sonogr* 1995;11:300–308.

Kremkau FW. *Diagnostic Ultrasound: Physical Principles and Exercises*. New York, NY: Grune & Stratton, 1980. ISBN 0-8089-1233-X.

Scanlan KA. Sonographic artifacts and their origins. *Am J Radiol* 1991;156:1267–1272.

Answer 19: C. The image is of a venovenous ECMO catheter (shown between the *white arrows* in FIG. 8.21) within the right atrium with portions of the catheter lying perpendicular to the direction of the US beam and others lying at more oblique angles. Differences in impedance between the walls of the catheter and fluid interface within the catheter can result in reverberation artifact. The finger-like projections emanating from the catheter (*yellow arrow*) are also reverberations, but these arise from discontinuities in the inner surface of the catheter produced by the presence of inflow and outflow ports. The outflow port (*red arrow*) is correctly positioned within the RA in this case. No physical damage to the catheter is noted. Discontinuities produced by breaks or kinking can also result in similar artifacts but are associated with disturbances in flow at the site of the break or kink, and the defect would also be expected to be seen on the 2D image. In the case of a structural defect, no amount of transducer manipulation is likely to eliminate the aberrant US signal.

Option A: The presence of a kink or break in the catheter would be anticipated to result in significant turbulence of flow or absence of flow depending on the location of the defect.

Option B: In the case of a break in the catheter, more than one jet of flow would also be expected. Additionally, manipulation of the transducer so as to normalize the angle of incidence would demonstrate that the artifact disappears and only reappears when the angle of incidence is once again tangential.

Option D: No significant attenuation or shadowing is imparted by the ECMO catheter.

Suggested Readings

Baun J. *Physical Principles of General and Vascular Sonography*. San Francisco, CA: California Publishing Company, 2004: Chapter 14. ISBN 940471-35-3.

Kremkau FW. *Diagnostic Ultrasound: Physical Principles and Exercises*. New York, NY: Grune & Stratton, 1980. ISBN 0-8089-1233-X.

Platts DG, Sedgwick JF, Burstow DJ, et al. The role of echocardiography in the management of patients supported by extracorporeal membrane oxygenation. *J Am Soc Echocardiogr* 2012;25:131–41.

Answer 20: C. A demarcation line occurring between acquired subvolumes that results in image distortion is called a stitch artifact. Stitch artifact is usually the result of patient motion such as during respiration, movement of the probe during acquisition, arrhythmias, and electrocautery. Breath holding during image acquisition is useful to limit the contribution from patient movement. Gating acquisition can reduce stitch artifacts produced by cardiac arrhythmias. Tissue continuity gaps may be created if the gain is set too low. Finally, there is no fill-in correction associated with 3D image reconstruction.

Option A: This is an issue with malalignment of different subvolumes of data due to some intrinsic difference between the acquisition of each of those subvolumes. There is no mechanism to fill in missing data.

Option B: Gain adjustments may be useful to create a clearer image but would not cause the artifact seen above.

Option D: The presence of mechanical valvular prostheses usually is not associated with significant artifact in 3D echocardiographic imaging provided that proper gain adjustment is used in contrast to 2D imaging.

Option E: When the US beam encounters objects on the body surface such as ECG wires, there is a void in the image resulting from attenuation of the US signal caused by objects in front of the imaging target. This may lead to a distortion of the 3D reconstruction of the image, but not a stitch artifact.

Suggested Readings

Feldman MK, Katyal S, Blackwood MS. US artifacts. *Radiographics* 2009;29:1179–1189.

Hung J, Lang R, Flachskampf F, et al. 3-D echocardiography: a review of the current status and future directions. *J Am Soc Echocardiogr* 2007;20:213–233.

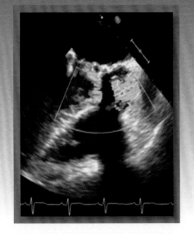

Chapter 9

Artifact with Doppler Echo

Vedant A. Gupta and Vincent L. Sorrell

1. Which of the following statements is NOT true concerning the image shown in FIGURE 9.1?

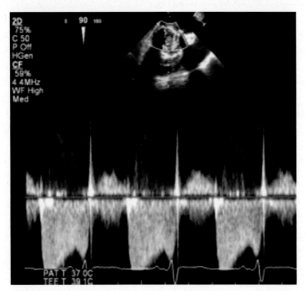

FIGURE 9.1

A. The Doppler process contains information regarding both the absolute frequency difference and direction of the signal.

B. Directionality of a Doppler signal is determined by instrument processing, which includes sideband filtering and demodulation.

C. The Doppler shift occurring between a source and a moving target is proportional to the cosine of the angle between them. This may result in an underestimation of the true velocity of the moving target.

D. The bidirectional flow is an artifact. Reducing the gain on the instrument will likely eliminate this artifact.

2. A 45-year-old male with cardiogenic shock requires extracorporeal membrane oxygenation (ECMO). While adjusting the position of the ECMO catheter using ultrasound guidance, the following image was captured (FIG. 9.2). Which of the following best describes what the image shows?

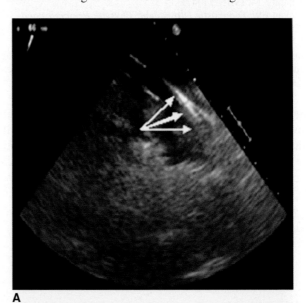

A

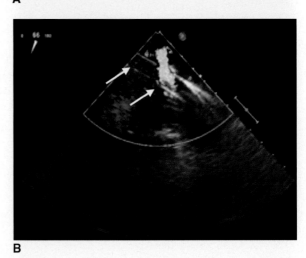

B

FIGURE 9.2

A. A kink is present, causing flow turbulence and the appearance of an enhancement artifact on 2D echocardiographic imaging.

B. A break in the ECMO catheter is present, causing scatter artifact.

C. The large difference in impedance between the walls of the ECMO catheter and the surrounding fluid/tissue interface results in the appearance of reverberation artifact.

D. The ECMO catheter is causing significant shadow artifact in the image.

3. The image shown in FIGURE 9.3 was obtained from a 35-year-old woman with a mechanical prosthetic aortic valve. The image demonstrates which of the following?

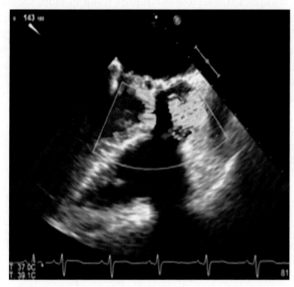

FIGURE 9.3

A. A change in the direction of flow with the angle of incidence occurring perpendicular to the direction of flow

B. Shadowing from the mechanical prosthetic aortic valve preventing the Doppler signal from being registered

C. Interruption of flow due to obstruction through the mechanical prosthetic aortic valve

D. Aberrant image production due to a cracked transducer

E. Shadowing from an object on the surface of the patient's body

4. Which of the following principle as stated is correct regarding the major differences between conventional 2D echocardiography and Doppler echocardiography?

A. The primary target of 2D is the myocardium, whereas the primary target for Doppler is cardiac the valves.

B. Whereas Doppler imaging provides greater information on LV function, 2D is considered complementary.

C. Doppler is considered complimentary to 2D but not essential for comprehensive echo.

D. 2D is best when the US beam is aligned with the target, but Doppler prefers right angles.

E. Both 2D and Doppler are essential tools for myocardial assessment.

5. Which of the following is most accurate when considering the Doppler shift?

A. If the source of the reflected sound wave is stationary, then the returning sound wave has a lower frequency relative to the time necessary to return.

B. If the source of the reflected sound wave is moving away from the origin, then the returning frequency is higher.

C. The frequency and wavelength of the emitted and reflected ultrasound are identical regardless of whether the target is moving or stationary.

D. If the target is approaching the ultrasound source, the reflected frequency is shifted upward.

E. If the RBC is moving away from the probe, the frequency is shifted downward as perceived by the target.

6. Using a 3.0-MHz transducer from the apical window to measure flood flow in the LVOT at 1.0 m/s (assuming a zero angle of incidence), the received frequency is shifted from 3.0 MHz to:

A. 3.4 MHz

B. 3.004 MHz

C. 2.6 MHz

D. 2.996 MHz

E. Not enough information to determine

7. In what manner does the transducer frequency impact the Doppler shift?

A. A high-velocity flow is better recorded using a high-frequency transducer.

B. There is a bimodal relationship—higher-frequency transducers improve the detection of both very high and very low velocities.

C. A 1.0-MHz probe will be superior to a 3.4-MHz probe in the detection of blood flow traveling at 5.0 m/s.

D. 2D and Doppler imaging both prefer higher-frequency transducers for optimal quality imaging.

E. The transducer frequency does not really impact the spectral Doppler display.

Answer 1: A. The Doppler shift that occurs in response to how moving objects reflect US waves registers the absolute difference between the frequency of the transmitted US wave and the returning wave. It is proportional to the cosine of the angle between the source and moving object. The difference in frequency allows the observer to determine whether the object is moving closer or further away from the source of the sound wave but does not contain information regarding the direction of the signal. Directionality is determined by instrument processing that includes demodulation and sideband filtering. Reducing the gain on the acquired image could reduce this artifact.

Suggested Readings

Baun J. *Physical Principles of General and Vascular Sonography.* San Francisco, CA: California Publishing Company, 2004, Chapter 14. ISBN 940471-35-3.

Kremkau FW. *Diagnostic Ultrasound: Physical Principles and Exercises.* New York, NY: Grune & Stratton, 1980. ISBN 0-8089-1233-X.

Answer 2: C. The image is of a venovenous ECMO catheter (shown between the *white arrows* in Fig. 9.4) within the right atrium with portions of the catheter lying perpendicular to the direction of the US beam and others lying at more oblique angles. Differences in impedance between the walls of the catheter and fluid interface within the catheter can result in reverberation artifact. The finger-like projections emanating from the catheter (*yellow arrow*) are also reverberations, but these arise from discontinuities in the inner surface of the catheter produced by the presence of inflow and outflow ports. The outflow port (*red arrow*) is correctly positioned within the RA in this case. No physical damage to the catheter is noted. Discontinuities produced by breaks or kinking can also result in similar artifacts but are associated with disturbances in flow at the site of the break or kink, and the defect would also be expected to be seen on the 2D image. No significant attenuation or shadowing is imparted by the ECMO catheter. The presence of a kink or break in the catheter would be anticipated to result in significant turbulence of flow or absence of flow depending on the location of the defect. In the case of a break in the catheter, more than one jet of flow would also be expected. Additionally, manipulation of the transducer so as to normalize the angle of incidence would demonstrate that the artifact disappears and only reappears when the angle of incidence is once again tangential. In the case of a structural defect, no amount of transducer manipulation is likely to eliminate the aberrant US signal.

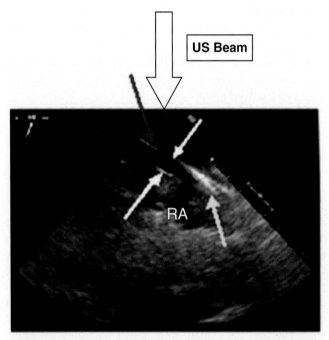

US Beam

RA

FIGURE 9.4

Suggested Readings

Baun J. *Physical Principles of General and Vascular Sonography.* San Francisco, CA: California Publishing Company, 2004, Chapter 14. ISBN 940471-35-3.
Kremkau FW. *Diagnostic Ultrasound: Physical Principles and Exercises.* New York, NY: Grune & Stratton, 1980. ISBN 0-8089-1233-X.
Platts DG, Sedgwick JF, Burstow DJ, et al. The role of echocardiography in the management of patients supported by extracorporeal membrane oxygenation. *J Am Soc Echocardiogr* 2012;25:131–141.

Answer 3: B. In this case, shadowing from the mechanical prosthetic valve creates a wedge-shaped artifact as if flow has been interrupted. Flow into the aorta is visible in this TEE despite the almost perpendicular path of the blood flow in relation to the US beam because of the turbulence created by the mechanical prosthesis. Blood flow through the aortic arch can also appear this way, but in that case, it is due to the oblique course of the aorta relative to the US beam resulting in blood flow that is perpendicular to the path of the US beam. Flow toward the US probe from the LVOT is easily seen to the left of the image as a homogeneous red hue. There is no evidence of flow obstruction through the mechanical aortic valve prosthesis in this view given that incident flow is laminar and, immediately beyond the mechanical prosthesis, occupies the entire lumen of the aortic root. Obstructed flow would typically result in more focal turbulence sometimes associated with an eccentric flow pattern within the aortic root. It is important to see other views before concluding that there is an obstruction of the mechanical prosthetic valve. Interfering objects on the patient's body, such as ECG wires or tape, can attenuate US signals from the heart, but generally, this attenuation is more uniformly distributed.

Suggested Readings

Feldman MK, Katyal S, Blackwood MS. US artifacts. *Radiographics* 2009;29:1179–1189.
Hedrick WR, Petersen CL. Image artifacts in real time ultrasound. *J Diagn Med Sonogr* 1995;11:300–308.
Scanlan KA. Sonographic artifacts and their origins. *Am J Radiol* 1991;156:1267–1272.

Answer 4: E. The primary target of 2D echo is the myocardium and valves. For Doppler imaging, the primary target is the red blood cells. 2D echo provides greater information on structure, and Doppler imaging provides more physiologic information on valve function and cardiovascular hemodynamics. Whereas 2D echo is optimal when the beam and the target are at right angles, the Doppler equation requires a parallel alignment between the beam and blood target. 2D echocardiography and Doppler imaging provide diagnostic data that are complementary and both necessary for a comprehensive study. With the advent of Doppler tissue imaging, the myocardium is only completely studied using both 2D and Doppler.

Suggested Readings

Le HT, Hangiandreou N, Timmerman R, et al. Imaging artifacts in echocardiography. *Anesth Analg* 2016;122(3):633–646.
Rubens DJ, Bhatt S, Nedelka S, et al. Doppler artifacts and pitfalls. *Radiol Clin North Am* 2006;44:805–835.

Answer 5: D. Austrian physicist Christian Doppler (1842) is credited with reporting the phenomenon that the apparent pitch of sound was affected by motion either toward or away from the listener. If the source of sound were stationary, then the pitch or frequency of that sound was constant. If, however, the source of sound moved toward the listener, the frequency increased and the pitch appeared to rise. Conversely, if the sound source was moving away from the listener, the frequency of the sound decreased relative to the listener and the pitch appeared lower.

Ultrasound is emitted from a transducer and reflected from a moving target (red blood cell). If target is stationary, the frequency and wavelength of the emitted and reflected ultrasound are identical. For a target moving toward the transducer source, the reflected frequency is "shifted" upward (higher frequency) proportional to the velocity of the target relative to the transducer. Conversely, movement of the target away from the transducer results in the reflected ultrasound having a lower frequency than the emitted ultrasound, a downward shift in frequency. This increase or decrease in frequency is the *Doppler shift*. From the perspective of the target, the frequency is unchanged and not shifted.

Suggested Readings

Le HT, Hangiandreou N, Timmerman R, et al. Imaging artifacts in echocardiography. *Anesth Analg* 2016;122(3):633–646.

Rubens DJ, Bhatt S, Nedelka S, et al. Doppler artifacts and pitfalls. *Radiol Clin North Am* 2006;44:805–835.

***Answer 6:** B.* It is critical to know this equation: $\Delta F = 2f_0 v/C \times \cos\theta$.

It can be seen that the actual Doppler shift is quite small. For example, using a 3-MHz transducer to sample blood flowing toward the transducer at 1.0 m/s, the received frequency is increased up by only 4 kHz, from 3.0 to 3.004 MHz. Of course, the Doppler shift depends not only on blood velocity but also on the angle of incidence, θ.

Suggested Readings

Le HT, Hangiandreou N, Timmerman R, et al. Imaging artifacts in echocardiography. *Anesth Analg* 2016;122(3):633–646.

Rubens DJ, Bhatt S, Nedelka S, et al. Doppler artifacts and pitfalls. *Radiol Clin North Am* 2006;44:805–835.

***Answer 7:** C.* An important component of the Doppler equation is the transducer frequency—a primary determinant of the maximal blood flow velocity that can be resolved. The relationship between the Doppler shift and blood flow velocity at four different transmitted frequencies is illustrated in FIGURE 9.5.

A high-flow velocity such as 5 m/s is more readily recorded using a low carrier frequency such as 1 MHz compared with a high transducer frequency such as 5 or 10 MHz because of the corresponding Doppler shift. With 2D echo, a higher transducer frequency is desirable because it is associated with a higher spatial resolution. With Doppler imaging, a lower frequency is advantageous because it allows high-flow velocity to be optimally recorded.

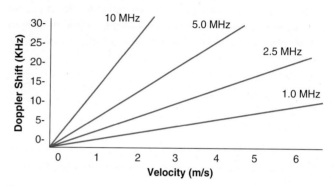

FIGURE 9.5

Chapter 10

Biologic Effects of Ultrasound

Vedant A. Gupta

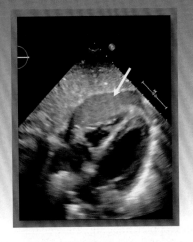

1. The American Institute of Ultrasound Medication (AIUM) states that there are no confirmed biologic effects with ultrasound beam intensity for an unfocused beam below:

    A. 100 mW/cm²
    B. 100 W/cm²
    C. 200 mW/cm²
    D. 200 mW/mm²
    E. 400 mW/cm²

2. Which of the following is true regarding biologic effects of ultrasound?

    A. The two primary mechanisms of biologic effects of ultrasound are sound and thermal effect.
    B. Stable cavitation is potentially more harmful than is transient cavitation.
    C. An unfocused beam carries more potential harm than does a focused beam.
    D. The risk of cavitation is not related to the mechanical index.
    E. The most effective method during scanning to reduce biologic effect is to increase scan time.

3. It is advised that all ultrasound system users are knowledgeable of biologic effects and the ALARA (As Low as Reasonably Achievable) principle. Which of the following is least accurate in regard to ultrasound safety?

    A. Gas-containing organs such as the lung and digestive tract are at a relatively higher risk for harm by mechanical mechanisms than are solid organs.
    B. Addition of ultrasound contrast agents increases the potential for cavitation.
    C. Ultrasound contrast agents have been shown to increase the risk of microvascular damage and capillary rupture in preclinical models.
    D. Avoidance of a high mechanical index can prevent thermal effects with contrast agents.
    E. There is no confirmed harm by biologic effects in human beings with diagnostic ultrasound use.

4. The _____ is an output display standard of the relative potential of ultrasound to induce a nonthermal adverse bioeffect:

    A. TIS
    B. TIC
    C. TIB
    D. MI
    E. None of the options

5. In regard to the likelihood of resulting in thermal bioeffects, which of the following are listed in the correct descending order (*continuous-wave Doppler [CWD], pulsed-wave Doppler [PWD], color-flow Doppler [CFD], 2-dimensional scanning [2D])?

    A. 2D, CWD, PWD, CFD
    B. CFD, PWD, CWD, 2D
    C. CFD, CWD, PWD, 2D
    D. CWD, PWD, CFD, 2D
    E. PWD, CWD, 2D, CFD

6. Which of the following statements is **least accurate** regarding mechanical index?

    A. Mechanical index represents a risk of nonthermal adverse biologic effects in the body and is a part of the ODS (output display standard).
    B. The risk of tissue damage from cavitation is higher in gas-filled organs than in solid organs for any given mechanical index.
    C. There are clinical applications leveraging the cavitation properties of high MI imaging.
    D. Mechanical index is directly related to peak rarefaction pressure (degree of compression/rarefaction).
    E. Contrast agents are more likely to rupture, and therefore lead to potential tissue damage at a MI < 0.4.

Answer 1: A. The AIUM in 1976 made a statement that no biologic effect with ultrasound beam intensity for an unfocused beam below 100 mW/cm² was confirmed. There has been no update to this limit within the last three decades.

Suggested Reading

Shankar H, Pagel PS. Potential adverse ultrasound-related biological effects: a critical review. *Anesthesiology* 2011;11(115):1109–1124.

Answer 2: C. Clinical ultrasound systems are primarily unfocused beams (the ultrasound pulse spreads out like a flashlight). This is generally true, even with focal zones (the width of any typical 2D sector in the near field is smaller than the width in the far field). Unfocused ultrasound beams deliver the ultrasound energy to a larger amount of tissue, and any heat generation is unable to dissipate to surrounding tissue (as the surrounding tissue is also experiencing that ultrasound energy). As a contrast, focused ultrasound beams deliver ultrasound energy to a small area of tissue, and the heat can then dissipate to surrounding tissue, which minimizes the risk of thermal damage to that tissue. Therefore, unfocused ultrasound beams have a higher risk of thermal damage than do focused ultrasound beams.

The two primary biologic effects of ultrasound are the aforementioned thermal effects and mechanical effects (primarily cavitation). Cavitation is directly related to the mechanical index on the output monitor. Cavitation can be either stable or transient. In stable cavitation, gas-filled microbubbles expand and contract consistently (compression and rarefaction) with no subsequent rupture of the bubble. However, in transient cavitation, a stable gas-filled microbubble is expanded or contracted transiently, which increases the risk of rupture with possible injury to the surrounding tissue. Therefore, transient cavitation is potentially more harmful than is stable cavitation. Sound, or noise, which is ultrasound produced during diagnostic scanning, is not known to be harmful to humans. The most effective method during scanning to reduce biologic effect is to decrease scan time.

Option A: The two most common biologic effects of ultrasound are thermal and mechanical (cavitation). Sound does not have a significant biologic effect.

Option B: Transient cavitation (transient compression and rarefaction) is more likely to cause rupture of gas-filled structures and therefore lead to injury.

Option D: Cavitation is directly related to mechanical index. The higher the MI, the higher the risk of mechanical effects from ultrasound.

Option E: Decreasing scan time is the most effective way to reduce all biologic effects of ultrasound.

Answer 3: *D*. This question requires an understanding of the biologic effects of ultrasound. ALARA stands for as low as reasonably achievable, which is a universally accepted acronym for safety in ultrasound and radiation exposure. The two main biologic effects of ultrasound are thermal and mechanical effects (primarily cavitation). In simple terms, thermal effects are related to heating of tissue by ultrasound, and mechanical effects are related to rupture of gas-filled bubbles with damage of surrounding tissue.

Cavitation is the primary mechanical effect of concern, and since rupture of gas-filled microbubbles is the underlying basis, gas-filled organs are at a higher risk of cavitation. Addition of contrast agents causes a fluid-filled chamber such as the ventricle to be filled with gas microbubbles, which then increases the risk of cavitation. The risk of mechanical effects is measured by the mechanical index (MI), while the risk of thermal effects to a tissue is measured by the thermal index (TI). Mechanical

index does not reflect the risk of thermal injury (and therefore is the least accurate statement).

While no biologic harmful effects of ultrasound or contrast agents have been reported in humans, animal studies have reported rupture of capillaries in the lungs of small mammals and induction of premature ventricular contractions (PVCs) with high mechanical indices > 0.4.

Most modern ultrasound machines would reduce the MI to <0.3 when contrast settings are applied. However, contrast agents do not affect thermal effects, and therefore, a reduced MI with contrast use would prevent mechanical effects and not thermal effects.

Currently, there are no biologic harmful effects in human beings with ultrasound use. However, due to animal data, judicial use is recommended with ultrasound, especially in the subspecialty of fetal imaging.

Option A: This is a true statement. Given the primary mechanical effect is cavitation, and the risk is primarily of rupture of gas-filled microbubbles, gas-filled organs are at a higher risk of mechanical effects than are solid organs.

Option B: This is a true statement. Addition of gas-filled microbubbles (ultrasound contrast agents) increases the risk of cavitation.

Option C: This is a true statement. In animal studies, rupture of the gas-filled microbubbles has led to pulmonary capillary rupture especially at higher MI (>0.4). While there have been no adverse events in humans, judicious use of ultrasound contrast agents is recommended.

Option E: This is also a true statement. As previously mentioned, ultrasound is generally safe with no adverse events of ultrasound in general or contrast use in humans.

Suggested Reading
Deng CX, Lizzi FL. A review of physical phenomena associated with ultrasonic contrast agents and illustrative clinical applications. *Ultrasound Med Biol* 2002;28(3):277–286.

Answer 4: *D*. Thermal index (TI) is the ratio of the power used to that required to produce a temperature rise of 1°C. A TI of 1.5 would indicate conditions under which the rise in temperature would be 1.5°C at a specific point along the ultrasound beam. However, due to complexities of tissue and heating, the actual measured change in temperature is variable.

The tissue-specific thermal indices are the following:

Thermal index in soft tissue (TIS)

Thermal index in bone (TIB)

Thermal index in the cranium (TIC)

The mechanical index (MI) is the only listed nonthermal bioeffect.

Mechanical index gives a relative indication of the potential for mechanical effects, such as cavitation.

TI and MI are both included in the output display standard (ODS), which are numbers displayed on the screen during ultrasound scanning (Fig. 10.1).

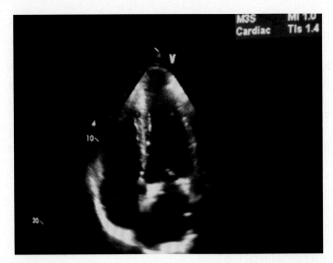

FIGURE **10.1**

Answer 5: *D.* This question requires an understanding of scanning parameters' impact on thermal bioeffects. Modalities that continuously send ultrasound pulses in the same direction are considered "nonscanned" modalities. Modalities that send ultrasound pulses along multiple axis are considered "scanned" modalities. Nonscanned modalities and higher duty factors carry the highest risk for bioeffects. Nonscanned modalities transmit repeatedly in the same direction (i.e., CW, PW), allowing for heat to build up, increasing the risk of thermal bioeffects. CW and PW are nonscanned modalities, while 2D is a scanned modality.

Continuous-wave Doppler transmits and receives 100% of the time with a duty factor of 100%, while pulsed-wave Doppler carries a duty factor of <3% (transmits <3% of the time). Therefore, CWD carries a higher risk of bioeffects than does PWD.

Color-flow Doppler has properties of both scanned and non-scanned modalities.

2D carries the lowest risk, while CWD and PWD have a higher risk with color-flow Doppler being intermediate.

Hence, the correct descending order is CWD, PWD, CFD, and 2D.

Answer 6: *E.* This question assesses nonthermal or mechanical risk potential of ultrasound. The two primary biologic effects of ultrasound can be broken up into thermal and nonthermal risk (via cavitation). Thermal risk has to do with tissue heating with ultrasound (via a focused or an unfocused ultrasound beam), and the potential for thermal injury is displayed on the output display standard (or ODS) via a thermal index (TI). Given that the risk of thermal injury is different for different tissue, this risk is manifest as thermal index in different tissue.

A similar concept is true for nonthermal or mechanical risk potential of ultrasound. This risk is largely conferred from cavitation of gas-filled structures or organs. Mechanical index is calculated with the following equation:

$$\text{MI} = \text{Peak rarefaction (negative) pressure}/\sqrt{\text{frequency}}$$

It is directly related to the degree of compression and rarefaction and inversely related to central frequency. As an ultrasound pulse passes through the body with areas along the ultrasound wave of compression and rarefaction, gas-filled structures will compress and expand as well. This compression and expansion of these gas-filled structures or organs is known as cavitation. The risk of continuously compressing and expanding these structures is rupture of the structure, and that risk is higher with transient cavitation versus stable cavitation. The potential of an ultrasound to induce this rupture is captured via a mechanical index (MI). The higher the mechanical index, the greater the degree of compression and rarefaction and the higher the risk of rupture of gas-filled structures (also known as cavitation nucleation). Naturally, the more gas, the higher the risk of cavitation, and gas-filled organs (lungs, intestine) are at a higher risk of adverse effects from cavitation than are solid organs. In animal models, the risk of pulmonary hemorrhage (a gas-filled structure in the lungs) could be seen with an MI of approximately 0.4, while intestinal injury did not occur until an MI of approximately 1.4. Solid organs did not appear to have any nonthermal adverse events at an MI below 1.9 (the limit of diagnostic ultrasound). It is important to note that this has not been systematically studied in humans.

The most important parameter to manipulate during the routine clinical use of manufactured contrast agents is the mechanical index. Ultrasound contrast media are gas-filled structures surrounded by a protein, fatty acid, or lipid shell. At higher MIs, they are at risk of rupturing, which can lead to theoretical injury to surrounding structures and which limits the effectiveness of contrast agents to opacify the structure of interest. Interestingly, myocardial contrast echocardiographic techniques have tried to leverage this by intermittently imaging to destroy microbubbles and allowing for microbubbles to refill the structure of interest.

Option A: Option A is an accurate statement. MI does reflect the nonthermal effects of ultrasound, and MI is reported as a part of the ODS.

Option B: Option B is an accurate statement. The primary risk of cavitation is in gas-filled structures, and therefore, the risk of nonthermal injury is highest in gas-filled organs, such as lung or intestine. In animal models, these were seen at varying MIs, while injury to solid organs has not been seen up to an MI of 1.9.

Option C: Option C is an accurate statement. Leveraging microbubble rupture (the risk of cavitation) has been used in myocardial contrast echocardiography.

Option D: Option D is an accurate statement. Based on the above equation, mechanical index is directly related to the degree of compression and rarefaction (measured by peak rarefaction pressure).

Suggested Readings

American Institute of Ultrasound in Medicine. AIUM statement on mammalian in vivo ultrasound biologic effects. August 1976. Reapproved in March 25, 2015.

Church CC, Carstensen EL, Nyborg WL, et al. The risk of exposure to diagnostic ultrasound in postnatal subjects: nonthermal mechanisms. *J Ultrasound Med* 2008;27:565–592.

Miller DL, Averkiou MA, Brayman AA, et al. Bioeffects consideration for diagnostic ultrasound contrast agents. *J Ultrasound Med* 2008;27:611–632.

Chapter 11

Understanding the AUC Guidelines

Sasanka Jayasuriya

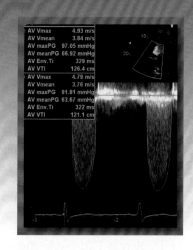

1. According to the 2011 Appropriate Use Criteria (AUC) for Echocardiography, which of the following clinical scenarios would be considered an "appropriate" indication to order a transthoracic echocardiogram (TTE) in an asymptomatic patient?

   A. Routine preoperative evaluation prior to noncardiac surgery

   B. Sinus bradycardia with an otherwise normal ECG

   C. Occasional premature atrial contractions without other signs of heart disease

   D. Initial evaluation of a soft diastolic murmur heard at the left upper sternal border

   E. Initial evaluation of ventricular function (e.g., screening) with a normal ECG

2. According to the 2011 AUC for Echocardiography, which of the following defines an "appropriate" imaging test?

   A. An appropriate imaging test is one that will be reimbursed by both governmental and private payers >80% of the time.

   B. An appropriate imaging test is one that will provide important additional clinical information that is assured to prompt a change in the patient's clinical management, while exposing the patient no real or perceived risks.

   C. An appropriate imaging test is one that provides important clinical information and is a useful first step to guide subsequent history and physical examination.

   D. An appropriate imaging test is one for which there is established evidence that performance of the test improves patient outcomes.

   E. An appropriate imaging study is one in which the expected incremental information, combined with clinical judgment, exceeds the expected negative consequences by a sufficiently wide margin for a specific indication that the procedure is generally considered acceptable care and a reasonable approach for the indication.

3. According to the 2011 AUC for Echocardiography, it is expected that transesophageal echocardiography (TEE) will be performed as an adjunct or subsequent test to TTE only if necessary for most clinical scenarios. However, the 2011 AUC for Echocardiography recognize that there are a few clinical scenarios where a TEE as the initial echocardiographic test would be reasonable. Which of the following clinical scenarios would NOT be an "appropriate" indication for the initial use of TEE?

   A. To evaluate suspected aortic pathology such as aortic dissection

   B. For a patient with a clear indication for TTE, but in whom there is a high likelihood of nondiagnostic TTE due to patient habitus/positioning

   C. To evaluate the etiology of a holosystolic murmur loudest at the apex

   D. To guide decision-making regarding cardioversion in a patient with atrial fibrillation

   E. To evaluate for endocarditis in a patient with a prosthetic heart valve and bacteremia

4. According to the 2011 AUC for Echocardiography, in which of the following patients with established valvular heart disease would a follow-up TTE be considered "rarely appropriate"*?

   A. ≥3 years after initial TTE in a patient with mild aortic stenosis with no change in clinical status or physical examination

   B. 2 years after initial TTE showing mild mitral regurgitation in a patient with no new symptoms and no change in clinical status

   C. 6 months after initial TTE showing moderate aortic regurgitation in a patient with new-onset dyspnea and lower extremity edema

   D. 1 year after initial TTE showing severe aortic stenosis in an asymptomatic patient without any change in clinical status

   E. 9 months after initial TTE showing normal function of a mechanical prosthetic aortic valve in a patient with new-onset shortness of breath

5. Which of the following patients with known or suspected heart failure would NOT have an "appropriate" indication for TTE according to the 2011 AUC for Echocardiography?

A. Repeat TTE in a patient with long-standing systolic left ventricular dysfunction (left ventricular ejection fraction = 40%), last TTE 11 months ago, now New York Heart Association Class 1 on a stable medication regimen.

B. Initial evaluation of a patient with shortness of breath and mild lower extremity edema.

C. Repeat TTE 6 months after prior TTE demonstrating new left ventricular dysfunction (left ventricular ejection fraction = 25%) obtained during acute coronary syndrome for which percutaneous revascularization was performed. The patient is now improved on an optimal medical therapy regimen, and the TTE was ordered to reassess left ventricular ejection fraction to determine candidacy for implantable cardiac defibrillator.

D. Repeat TTE 1 year after initial TTE showing mild left ventricular dysfunction (left ventricular ejection fraction 45%) and mild mitral regurgitation, now on a stable medication regimen and diet with no new symptoms but found to have a louder pansystolic apical murmur and new appreciable third heart sound.

E. Initial evaluation of a patient with long-standing hypertension, ECG with voltage criteria for left ventricular hypertrophy with a strain pattern, and lower extremity edema.

6. Which of the following statements regarding the incorporation of AUC into the echocardiography laboratory accreditation procedures as outlined in the Intersocietal Commission for the Accreditation of Echocardiography Laboratories (ICAEL) Standards and Guidelines for Echocardiography Laboratory Accreditation is FALSE?

A. As part of an ongoing quality improvement program, echo laboratories must incorporate the measurement of AUC.

B. Echo labs must apply AUC for a minimum of 30 consecutive TTE, TEE, and stress echo examinations annually.

C. The average number of appropriate, inappropriate, and uncertain, for each modality (TTE, TEE, and stress echo), must be documented and included in the facility's quality improvement program annual summary.

D. AUC tracking and reporting have been required as part of the ICAEL accreditation since January 2012.

E. Echo laboratories can "opt out" of AUC tracking as part of the laboratory accreditation if they have never received a quality-related citation in prior accreditation cycles.

7. Which of the following risk profiles would have an "appropriate" indication to perform a stress echocardiogram in an asymptomatic patient for the purpose of coronary artery disease detection/cardiovascular risk prediction according to the 2011 AUC for Echocardiography?

A. Low global coronary artery disease risk

B. Intermediate global coronary artery disease risk, with an interpretable ECG (for exercise testing)

C. Intermediate global coronary artery disease risk, with an uninterpretable ECG (for exercise testing)

D. High global coronary artery disease risk

E. None of the above

8. Which of the following less common clinical scenarios would be deemed "rarely appropriate"* for TTE by the 2011 AUC for Echocardiography?

A. Repeat TTE in a stable patient with a history of surgically repaired membranous VSD 18 months after prior study demonstrating no residual structural or hemodynamic abnormality

B. Screening TTE in an asymptomatic 18-year-old with the first-degree relative with confirmed hypertrophic cardiomyopathy

C. Screening TTE for assessment of proximal ascending aorta in a patient with Marfan syndrome

D. Screening TTE in a potential heart transplant donor

E. Repeat TTE, 3 months after a normal initial TTE, in a patient with breast cancer who has since received doxorubicin (Adriamycin) therapy

9. In which of following acute settings would a TTE be "rarely appropriate"* according to the 2011 AUC for Echocardiography?

A. A 56-year-old male with ongoing acute-onset chest pain suspicious for myocardial infarction, but with a nondiagnostic ECG

B. A 49-year-old inpatient with a new drop in blood pressure to 82/50 without clear etiology

C. A 29-year-old with respiratory failure and unexplained hypoxemia

D. A 33-year-old with suspected pulmonary embolism to establish the diagnosis and help guide therapy for PE

E. A 75-year-old with new murmur 3 days after large anterior wall myocardial infarction

10. According to clinical implementation studies of the AUC for Echocardiography, which of the following statements is TRUE regarding the likelihood of a TTE being deemed "rarely appropriate"*?

A. Inpatient TTEs are more likely to be deemed "rarely appropriate"* than are outpatient TTEs.

B. Initial TTEs are more likely to be deemed "rarely appropriate"* than is follow-up or repeat TTEs.

C. Asymptomatic patients are more likely to have a "rarely appropriate"* indication than are patients with new symptoms or a "change in clinical status."

D. A majority of TTEs ordered in clinical practice are deemed "inappropriate."

E. Normal TTEs are always deemed "inappropriate."

*Editor's Note: *In 2013, the previously published AUC documents referenced in these questions were updated, changing the wording of the previous designation "inappropriate" to "rarely appropriate." Details of these changes may be found in "Hendel RC, et al. JACC 2013;61(12):1305–1317." It is likely that this new terminology will be incorporated in* *future published AUC revisions, and therefore, this nomenclature was used in these questions. However, readers must be prepared for the possibility that the term "inappropriate" may be used on the National Echo Board Exam and should consider these terms synonymous. (Hendel RC, Patel MR, Allen JM, et al. 2013 ACCF appropriate use criteria methodology update: a report of the American College of Cardiology Foundation appropriate use criteria task force. J Am Coll Cardiol 2013;61(12):1305–1317.)*

11. A cardiology consult team was asked to see a 72-year-old patient who had a right hip fracture after a mechanical fall. The patient has diabetes mellitus type 2 and has been relatively active and admittedly walks 30 minutes on the treadmill with no complaints of shortness of breath, chest discomfort, or lower extremity edema. On auscultation, there is a normal S1 and S2 and no murmur. An echocardiogram was ordered to evaluate left ventricular function preoperatively. This echo study is:

A. Appropriate, due to the patient's age and the past medical history of diabetes
B. Appropriate, due to the urgency of the patient's surgery
C. Appropriate since the cardiology consult team requested the study
D. Inappropriate, due to the absence of symptoms and request for preoperative evaluation
E. Inappropriate, due to the type of surgery

12. If the following were new patient consultations in your office, which of the following clinical scenarios would be considered an "appropriate" indication for transthoracic echocardiography in a currently asymptomatic patient?

A. Sinus bradycardia with an HR of 46 beats per minute in a patient undergoing hernia surgery
B. A 32-year-old female with palpitations and Holter monitor revealing 2% atrial premature contractions (APCs) with concurrent symptoms
C. A 54-year-old patient with a family history of premature coronary artery disease

D. A 42-year-old patient, active male, presenting because his brother suffered premature sudden cardiac death a few weeks ago
E. A 75-year-old lady with an episode of presyncope 2 days after up-titration of antihypertensive regimen

13. A 45-year-old male with diabetes mellitus, hypertension, and dyslipidemia presents with substernal chest pain of 1 hour duration. His vital signs are recorded as temperature 99.8°F, HR of 120 bpm, and BP 147/92 mm Hg. The invasive cardiac team was called for management of the patient with ST-elevation myocardial infarction. Which of the following is the most appropriate diagnostic test?

A. Transthoracic echocardiography
B. Exercise stress echocardiography
C. Transesophageal echocardiography
D. Pulmonary CTA
E. Emergent coronary angiography

14. According to the 2011 AUC for Echocardiography, which of the following defines an "appropriate" imaging test?

A. An appropriate imaging test is one that will be reimbursed by both governmental and private payers >80% of the time.
B. An appropriate imaging test is one that will provide important additional clinical information that is assured to prompt a change in the patient's clinical management, while exposing the patient to no real or perceived risks.
C. An appropriate imaging test is one that provides important clinical information and is a useful first step to guide subsequent history and physical examination.
D. An appropriate imaging test is one for which there is established evidence that performance of the test improves patient outcomes.
E. An appropriate imaging study is one in which the expected incremental information may or may not change the treatment course.

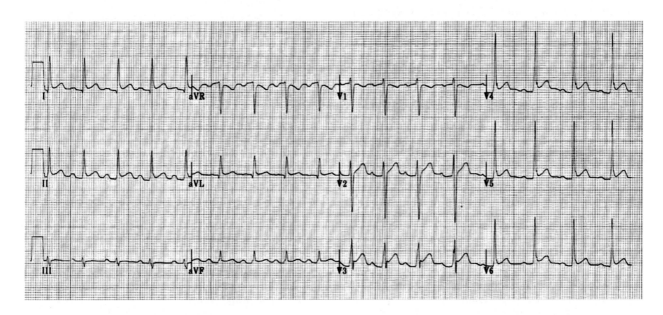

15. Which of the following would be an "appropriate" indication for the initial use of transesophageal echocardiography?

A. A 50-year-old previously healthy female who presents with difficulty of speaking since this morning

B. A 75-year-old male with a history of moderate COPD and obesity, now presenting with chest pain

C. Intraprocedural guidance of a left main percutaneous coronary intervention in a 52-year-old male

D. An 85-year-old male presenting with fever and blood cultures positive for *Candida albicans*

E. A 48-year-old male with paroxysmal atrial fibrillation anticoagulated with Coumadin and a history of congestive heart failure presenting with urinary tract infection with an INR of 1.4.

16. According to the 2011 AUC for Echocardiography, in which of the following patients with established valvular heart disease would a follow-up TTE be considered "rarely appropriate"?

A. An 80-year-old male noted to have aortic stenosis with an aortic valve area of 1.7 cm^2 and a mean gradient of 18 mm of mercury 4 years ago, who is currently asymptomatic

B. A 42-year-old female with mild mitral regurgitation and anterior leaflet prolapse 1 year ago presenting for follow-up

C. A 75-year-old female with moderate aortic regurgitation noted 6 months ago presenting with dyspnea on exertion.

D. An 80-year-old female noted to have aortic stenosis with an aortic valve area of 1.0 cm^2 and a mean gradient of 42 mm of mercury 1 year ago without any change in functional status

E. A 68-year-old male whose postoperative transthoracic echocardiogram 9 months ago revealed normal valve function of the mechanical prosthetic aortic valve now presenting with shortness of breath

17. Which of the following patients with known or suspected heart failure would be an appropriate indication for TTE?

A. A 42-year-old patient with a diagnosis of dilated cardiomyopathy since age 25, on a stable medical regimen currently with NYHA class 1 symptoms with the last echocardiogram revealing an LV ejection fraction of 40%, 11 months ago.

B. A 45-year-old patient who suffered an anterior myocardial infarction and underwent successful primary PCI 1 month ago with LV ejection fraction of 25% noted prior to discharge on a stable medical regimen.

C. A 56-year-old patient with a familial cardiomyopathy who underwent biventricular ICD placement for cardiac resynchronization therapy 12 months ago with a prior ejection fraction of 20% with stable symptoms on an appropriate medical regimen.

D. A 56-year-old female referred by her primary care physician due to a recent diagnosis of hypertension controlled on a 2-drug regimen. Physical examination and electrocardiogram are normal.

E. A 45-year-old female undergoing chemotherapy for treatment of HER2-positive breast cancer within normal echocardiogram 3 months ago.

18. Which of the following risk profiles would have an "appropriate" indication to perform a stress echocardiogram in an asymptomatic patient for the purpose of coronary artery disease detection/cardiovascular risk prediction according to the 2011 AUC for Echocardiography?

A. A 35-year-old male with no cardiac risk factors or family history of coronary artery disease and a normal electrocardiogram

B. A 45-year-old male with diabetes and hypertension and a normal electrocardiogram

C. A 45-year-old African American male with long-standing hypertension and electrocardiogram with left ventricular hypertrophy and strain

D. A 65-year-old Caucasian male with diabetes mellitus, hypertension, dyslipidemia, and current smoking history and a normal electrocardiogram

E. A 58-year-old gentleman who underwent an "executive physical" with an Agatston calcium score of 482

19. The following patients underwent Holter monitoring due to presyncope and palpitations. According to the 2011 appropriate use criteria, which of the following patients would have an appropriate indication for stress echocardiography?

A. A 65-year-old woman with premature ventricular contractions recorded as 3% of the total QRS complexes

B. A 72-year-old female with paroxysmal atrial fibrillation with heart rate ranging from 85 to 130 beats per minute

C. A 68-year-old male with nonsustained ventricular tachycardia

D. A, B, and C

E. A and C

20. The first year Cardiology fellow had performed many "stat echocardiograms" overnight and questioned the appropriateness of these studies. Which of the following was a "rarely appropriate" or "inappropriate" indication to perform echocardiography?

A. A 56-year-old male with ongoing acute-onset chest pain suspicious for myocardial infarction, but with a nondiagnostic ECG

B. A 49-year-old inpatient with a new drop in blood pressure to 82/50 without clear etiology

C. A 29-year-old with respiratory failure and unexplained hypoxemia

D. A 33-year-old with a pulmonary embolism

E. None of the above

21. Which of the following is an "appropriate" indication for stress echocardiography in an asymptomatic patient with coronary arteriosclerosis, in keeping with the 2011 appropriate use criteria?

A. 3 years after coronary artery bypass grafting

B. 1 year after percutaneous coronary intervention

C. 30% stenosis of the distal right coronary artery by coronary angiography

D. Chronic total occlusion of the left anterior descending artery with LV ejection fraction of 25% and anterior scar by myocardial perfusion imaging

E. None of the above

Answer 1: D.

A. This is "rarely appropriate"* according to the 2011 AUC (indication #13).

B. This is "rarely appropriate"* according to the 2011 AUC (indication #6).

C. This is "rarely appropriate"* according to the 2011 AUC (indication #3).

D. This is "appropriate" according to the 2011 AUC (indication #34).

E. This is "rarely appropriate"* according to the 2011 AUC (indication #10).

While the initial TTE examination for evaluation of symptomatic patients or patients with a "change in clinical status" is frequently deemed "appropriate" by the 2011 AUC for Echocardiography, there are very few "appropriate" indications for asymptomatic patients. This is particularly true for asymptomatic patients without other signs that might suggest an underlying cardiovascular disease. TTE is considered "appropriate" to evaluate asymptomatic patients with cardiac murmurs, provided there is a "reasonable suspicion of valvular or structural heart disease." TTE has a Class 1 indication in the updated 2008 ACC/AHA Guidelines for the Management of Patients with Valvular Heart Disease for "asymptomatic patients with diastolic murmurs, continuous murmurs, holosystolic murmurs, late systolic murmurs, murmurs associated with ejection clicks, or murmurs that radiate to the neck or back."

Suggested Readings

Bonow RO, Carabello BA, Chatterjee K, et al.; American College of Cardiology/American Heart Association Task Force on Practice Guidelines. 2008 focused update incorporated into the ACC/AHA 2006 guidelines for the management of patients with valvular heart disease. *J Am Coll Cardiol* 2008;52(13):e1–e142.

Douglas P, Garcia M, Haines D, et al.; ACCF/ASE/ACCP/AHA/ASNC/HFSA/HRS/SCAI/SCCT/SCMR 2011. Appropriate use criteria for echocardiography. *J Am Coll Cardiol* 2011;57(9):1126–1166.

Answer 2: E. Answer E is the definition of an "appropriate imaging test" as listed in all the AUC documents, including the 2011 AUC for Echocardiography. The appropriateness of an imaging test is not defined by likelihood of reimbursement, though increasingly the AUC are being employed by private and governmental payers to help aid in reimbursement protocols and decisions. It is not required that an "appropriate" imaging test has no risks, only that expected benefits of doing the test exceed any "negative consequences" such that the test represents "acceptable care and a reasonable approach for the indication." Standard evaluation of a patient including history and physical examination should always precede any imaging test so that the most useful imaging test is obtained. There are surprisingly few clinical trials that have proven the performance of any imaging test directly leads to improved patient outcomes, and thus, this standard has not been applied to the definition of an appropriate imaging test.

Suggested Reading

Douglas P, Garcia M, Haines D, et al.; ACCF/ASE/ACCP/AHA/ASNC/HFSA/HRS/SCAI/SCCT/SCMR 2011. Appropriate use criteria for echocardiography. *J Am Coll Cardiol* 2011;57(9):1126–1166.

Answer 3: C.

A. This is "appropriate" according to the 2011 AUC (indication #104).

B. This is "appropriate" according to the 2011 AUC (indication #99).

C. This is "rarely appropriate"* according to the 2011 AUC (indication #100).

D. This is "appropriate" according to the 2011 AUC (indication #112).

E. This is "appropriate" according to the 2011 AUC (indication #108).

In a patient with a holosystolic murmur suggestive of mitral regurgitation, a TTE would be "reasonably anticipated to resolve all diagnostic and management concerns," and thus, initial use of TEE would be "rarely appropriate"* according to the 2011 AUC for Echocardiography (indication #100). If severe mitral regurgitation is identified, supplemental TEE may become "appropriate" to assess for suitability of an intervention (AUC indication #106), such as to assess the candidacy/approach for mitral valve surgery. But in this scenario, the findings on the TTE would guide the decision to proceed to TEE and thus should be done first.

Suspected aortic dissection (indication #104), guiding cardioversion in a patient with atrial fibrillation (indication #112), and a moderate to high pretest probability of endocarditis in patient with a prosthetic valve (indication #108) all would have "appropriate" indications for initial use of TEE.

Initial use of TEE in patients with a high likelihood of nondiagnostic TTE is considered "appropriate" according to the 2011 AUC for Echocardiography (indication #99).

Suggested Reading

Douglas P, Garcia M, Haines D, et al.; ACCF/ASE/ACCP/AHA/ASNC/HFSA/HRS/SCAI/SCCT/SCMR 2011. Appropriate use criteria for echocardiography. *J Am Coll Cardiol* 2011;57(9):1126–1166.

Answer 4: B.

A. This is "appropriate" according to the 2011 AUC (indication #39).

B. This is "rarely appropriate"* according to the 2011 AUC (indication #43).

C. This is "appropriate" according to the 2011 AUC (indication #37).

D. This is "appropriate" according to the 2011 AUC (indication #41).

E. This is "appropriate" according to the 2011 AUC (indication #50).

Routine surveillance TTE of mild valvular heart disease <3 years after initial TTE in patients with no new symptoms or change in clinical status is considered to be "rarely appropriate"* according to the 2011 AUC for Echocardiography (indications #38 and #43). In any patient with established valve disease or a prosthetic valve that develops new symptoms or a change in clinical status, a repeat TTE is considered "appropriate" at any time interval (indications #37 and #50).

Routine surveillance of severe valvular stenosis or regurgitation ≥1 year after initial TTE is considered "appropriate" even in the absence of a change in clinical status.

Suggested Readings

Bonow RO, Carabello BA, Chatterjee K, et al.; American College of Cardiology/American Heart Association Task Force on Practice Guidelines. 2008 focused update incorporated into the ACC/AHA 2006 guidelines for the management of patients with valvular heart disease. *J Am Coll Cardiol* 2008;52(13):e1–e142.
Douglas P, Garcia M, Haines D, et al.; ACCF/ASE/ACCP/AHA/ASNC/HFSA/HRS/SCAI/SCCT/SCMR 2011. Appropriate use criteria for echocardiography. *J Am Coll Cardiol* 2011;57(9):1126–1166.

Answer 5: A.

A. This is "rarely appropriate"* according to the 2011 AUC (indication #74).
B. This is "appropriate" according to the 2011 AUC (indication #70).
C. This is "appropriate" according to the 2011 AUC (indication #76).
D. This is "appropriate" according to the 2011 AUC (indication #71).
E. This is "appropriate" according to the 2011 AUC (indication #67).

In stable patients with a history of congestive heart failure (systolic or diastolic) with no change in clinical status or cardiac examination, routine surveillance TTE is "rarely appropriate"* within 1 year after the initial TTE (indication #74) and "uncertain" ≥1 year after initial TTE, according to the 2011 AUC for Echocardiography.

Initial TTE in any patient with new signs or symptoms of heart failure (systolic or diastolic) is considered "appropriate" (indication #70).

Repeat TTE for "reevaluation after revascularization and/or optimal medical therapy to determine candidacy for device therapy" is an "appropriate" indication in the AUC (indication #76).

Repeat TTE in a patient with known heart failure (systolic or diastolic) with new symptoms or signs, including new cardiac exam findings, would be an "appropriate" indication for TTE (indication #71).

In patients with hypertension, initial TTE examination when there is a suspicion of hypertensive heart disease is also deemed "appropriate" in the 2011 AUC for Echocardiography (indication #67).

Suggested Reading

Douglas P, Garcia M, Haines D, et al.; ACCF/ASE/ACCP/AHA/ASNC/HFSA/HRS/SCAI/SCCT/SCMR 2011. Appropriate use criteria for echocardiography. *J Am Coll Cardiol* 2011;57(9):1126–1166.

Answer 6: E. Since January 1, 2012, tracking and reporting of AUC have been a requirement as part of echocardiography laboratory accreditation procedures by the Intersocietal Commission for the Accreditation of Echocardiography Laboratories (ICAEL).

Answers A to C above are all specifically listed as required elements in the IAC/ICAEL Standards and Guidelines for Echocardiography Laboratory Accreditation. All laboratories are subject to these requirements, and there are no "opt out" provisions.

Suggested Reading

IAC/ICAEL Standards and Guidelines for Adult Echocardiography Accreditation. Updated 8/2012. http://intersocietal.org/echo/main/echo_standards.htm. Accessed November 19, 2012.

Answer 7: E. There are no indications for asymptomatic patients listed in the 2011 AUC for Echocardiography that are deemed "appropriate" for stress echocardiography for the purpose of coronary artery disease detection/cardiovascular risk assessment.

Answers A and B are both deemed "rarely appropriate"* (indications #124 and #125), as both would be candidates for routine ECG stress testing if stress testing is required.

Answers C and D are deemed to be of "uncertain" appropriateness (indications #126 and #127). In the AUC, "uncertain" for specific indication suggests that a "test *may be* generally acceptable and *may* be a reasonable approach for the indication" and also "implies that more research and/or patient information is needed to classify the indication definitively."

Suggested Reading

Douglas P, Garcia M, Haines D, et al.; ACCF/ASE/ACCP/AHA/ASNC/HFSA/HRS/SCAI/SCCT/SCMR 2011. Appropriate use criteria for echocardiography. *J Am Coll Cardiol* 2011;57(9):1126–1166.

Answer 8: A.

A. This is "rarely appropriate"* according to the 2011 AUC (indication #95).
B. This is "appropriate" according to the 2011 AUC (indication #90).
C. This is "appropriate" according to the 2011 AUC (indication #63).
D. This is "appropriate" according to the 2011 AUC (indication #85).
E. This is "appropriate" according to the 2011 AUC (indication #91).

In patients with repaired adult congenital heart disease without residual structural or hemodynamic abnormality and no change in clinical status, routine surveillance TTE is considered to be "rarely appropriate"* <2 years after prior TTE (indication #95) and "uncertain" ≥2 years after prior TTE, according the 2011 AUC for Echocardiography. Answers B to E are less common clinical scenarios in clinical practice, but all are "appropriate" indications for TTE.

Suggested Reading

Douglas P, Garcia M, Haines D, et al.; ACCF/ASE/ACCP/AHA/ASNC/HFSA/HRS/SCAI/SCCT/SCMR 2011. Appropriate use criteria for echocardiography. *J Am Coll Cardiol* 2011;57(9):1126–1166.

Answer 9: *D.*

A. This is "appropriate" according to the 2011 AUC (indication #21).
B. This is "appropriate" according to the 2011 AUC (indication #19).
C. This is "appropriate" according to the 2011 AUC (indication #26).
D. This is "rarely appropriate"* according to the 2011 AUC (indication #28).
E. This is "appropriate" according to the 2011 AUC (indication #23).

TTE is deemed "appropriate" in many acute care settings according to the 2011 AUC for Echocardiography. These include any patients with unexplained hypotension or hypoxemia. In addition, TTE is "appropriate" in a variety of clinical scenarios involving acute myocardial infarction/acute coronary syndromes, including ongoing chest pain with a nondiagnostic ECG to exclude a regional wall motion abnormality and for evaluation of suspected acute mechanical complications after myocardial infarction.

While TTE would be considered "appropriate" to help guide therapy after a documented pulmonary embolus (looking for right heart strain to guide thrombolytics or thrombectomy—indication #29), TTE is "rarely appropriate"* when used as the definitive test to "establish the diagnosis" of pulmonary embolus (indication #28).

Suggested Reading

Douglas P, Garcia M, Haines D, et al.; ACCF/ASE/ACCP/AHA/ASNC/HFSA/HRS/SCAI/SCCT/SCMR 2011. Appropriate use criteria for echocardiography. *J Am Coll Cardiol* 2011;57(9):1126–1166.

Answer 10: *C.* Since the publication of the initial AUC for Echocardiography, numerous clinical implementation studies have been performed to assess the appropriateness of current clinical practice of echocardiography. From these studies, themes have emerged. For example, outpatient TTE studies, follow-up or repeat TTEs, and TTEs ordered for asymptomatic patients are more likely to be deemed "rarely appropriate"* than inpatient studies, initial TTEs, or TTEs ordered for patients with new symptoms, respectively. This is largely because the majority of these later groups have a "change in clinical status," a key feature to determine appropriateness in the AUC. Follow-up TTEs in particular are frequently deemed "rarely appropriate"* in the absence of change in clinical status or new symptoms.

While the vast majority of TTEs in current practice are "appropriate," being aware of clinical settings where "rarely appropriate"* studies are more common may help providers improve the appropriateness of their practice.

Abnormal findings on TTE are more likely to be found on TTEs ordered for "appropriate" indications compared to "rarely appropriate"* indications. However, many "appropriate" TTEs are found to be normal, and thus, TTE findings are not a relevant gauge of appropriateness. For example, consider a patient with new-onset dyspnea (an "appropriate" indication for TTE according to the 2011 AUC) who is found to have a normal TTE. This TTE may prompt pulmonary workup, which may identify the cause of dyspnea and thus meets every reasonable definition of clinical appropriateness of a diagnostic test.

Suggested Readings

Douglas P, Garcia M, Haines D, et al.; ACCF/ASE/ACCP/AHA/ASNC/HFSA/HRS/SCAI/SCCT/SCMR 2011. Appropriate use criteria for echocardiography. *J Am Coll Cardiol* 2011;57(9):1126–1166.
Mansour IN, Razi RR, Bhave NM, et al. Comparison of the updated 2011 appropriate use criteria for echocardiography to the original criteria for transthoracic, transesophageal, and stress echocardiography. *J Am Soc Echocardiogr* 2012;25(11):1153–1161.
Ward RP, Mansour I, Lemieux N, et al. Prospective evaluation of the ACCF/ASE appropriateness criteria for echocardiography. *J Am Coll Cardiol Imaging* 2008;1:663–671.

Answer 11: *D.* Option A is incorrect. Though the patient may have risk factors for coronary artery disease, the patient is asymptomatic and does not require an echocardiogram for these risk factors. Option B is incorrect. This patient was able to walk 30 minutes on the treadmill without any cardiac symptoms; hence, an evaluation of a baseline echocardiogram does not adequately evaluate this person's risk for surgery, and a hip fracture is not a high-risk surgery.

Option C is incorrect. Regardless of who orders the test, this is not an appropriate reason to order an echocardiogram.

Option D is correct. This is an inappropriate test since the patient was asymptomatic and did not have any cardiac findings on examination. Requesting an echocardiogram prior to surgery as a "preoperative evaluation" is deemed inappropriate.

Option E is incorrect. Regardless of the surgery, an echocardiogram prior to surgery is not indicated.

Echocardiography is a noninvasive, safe, ubiquitous imaging modality, which gives very useful information in addition to our clinical assessment. However, with limited resources, appropriate use of technology is paramount. This patient has two cardiac risk factors, no murmurs on auscultation, and no signs of heart failure and is without symptoms, which do not warrant an echocardiographic study. In addition, routine perioperative evaluation of ventricular function without cardiac symptoms is an inappropriate indication for an echocardiographic study.

Suggested Reading

Douglas PS, Khandheria B, Stainback RF, et al. ACCF/ASE/ACEP/ASNC/SCAI/SCCT/SCMR 2007 appropriateness criteria for transthoracic and transesophageal echocardiography: a report of the American College of Cardiology Foundation Quality Strategic Directions Committee Appropriateness Criteria Working Group, American Society of Echocardiography, American College of Emergency Physicians, American Society of Nuclear Cardiology, Society for Cardiovascular Angiography and Interventions, Society of Cardiovascular Computed Tomography, and the Society for Cardiovascular Magnetic Resonance endorsed by the American College of Chest Physicians and the Society of Critical Care Medicine. *J Am Coll Cardiol* 2007;50:187–204.

Answer 12: *D.* While the initial TTE examination for evaluation of symptomatic patients or patients with a "change in clinical status" is frequently deemed "appropriate" by the 2011

AUC for Echocardiography, there are very few "appropriate" indications for asymptomatic patients.

In 2013 appropriateness criteria methodology update, the term "rarely appropriate" was used replacing "inappropriate." Test takers should take note that these two terms may be used in an interchanging fashion to describe the same appropriateness criterion.

The correct answer to this question is D. While further details surrounding the cause of death of his brother including history and autopsy details would be of value, in the absence of this, a familial cardiomyopathy should be excluded. The 2011 guidelines on diagnosis and treatment of hypertrophic cardiomyopathy recommend echocardiographic evaluation as a class 1 indication in the initial evaluation of all patients with suspected HCM. Further, up to one-third or one-half of cases of dilated cardiomyopathy are familial. Echocardiography would be of benefit in diagnosing familial syndromes of aortopathy and ARVC. Hence, screening this patient for a familial cardiomyopathy would be appropriate.

Asymptomatic isolated sinus bradycardia and infrequent APCs or infrequent VPCs without other evidence of heart disease were inappropriate indications for screening echocardiograms according to the 2011 appropriate use criteria for echocardiography. Hence, answers A and B are incorrect.

Resting echocardiography is not a diagnostic study for premature coronary artery disease. This patient would ideally undergo aggressive risk factor management with evidence in favor of coronary calcium score testing. Hence, answer C is incorrect.

The history provided in answer E gives a clear reason for presyncope, which is likely hypotension related to up-titration of therapy. Hence, an echocardiogram is rarely indicated. However, it should be noted that when there are clinical symptoms or signs consistent with a cardiac diagnosis known to cause lightheadedness, presyncope, or syncope, echocardiographic evaluation is considered appropriate.

Suggested Readings

Burkett EL, Hershberger RE. Clinical and genetic issues in familial dilated cardiomyopathy. *J Am Coll Cardiol* 2005;45:7969–7981.

Gersh BJ, Maron BJ, Bonow RO, et al.; American College of Cardiology Foundation/American Heart Association Task Force on Practice Guidelines. 2011 ACCF/AHA Guideline for the Diagnosis and Treatment of Hypertrophic Cardiomyopathy: a report of the American College of Cardiology Foundation/ American Heart Association Task Force on Practice Guidelines. Developed in collaboration with the American Association for Thoracic Surgery, American Society of Echocardiography, American Society of Nuclear Cardiology, Heart Failure Society of America, Heart Rhythm Society, Society for Cardiovascular Angiography and Interventions, and Society of Thoracic Surgeons. *J Am Coll Cardiol* 2011;58(25):e212–e260.

Douglas PS, Garcia MJ, Haines DE, et al.; ACCF/ASE/AHA/ASNC/ HFSA/HRS/SCAI/SCCM/SCCT/SCMR. ACCF/ASE/AHA/ ASNC/HFSA/HRS/SCAI/SCCM/SCCT/SCMR 2011 appropriate use criteria for echocardiography. *J Am Soc Echocardiogr* 2011;24(3):229–267.

Hendel RC, et al. Appropriate use of cardiovascular technology: 2013 ACCF appropriate use criteria methodology update: a report of the American College of Cardiology Foundation appropriate use criteria task force. *J Am Coll Cardiol* 2013;61(12):1305–1317.

Answer 13: *A.* The patient discussed in this vignette has definite risk factors for coronary artery disease. However, low-grade fever, stable blood pressure, and an electrocardiogram with global ST elevation and subtle PR depression in leads II and V6 as well as ST-elevation aVR is diagnostic of pericarditis. With the current guidelines for management of patients with STEMI recommending a door-to-device time of <90 minutes, very often patients are rolled away for coronary angiography without much time for a complete history and physical examination. At the same time, in the rare instance a "wrap around LAD" was acutely occluded causing anterior and inferior ST elevation, emergent revascularization is key. Hence, to differentiate between these two diagnoses, a "stat echocardiogram" would be of value. In the absence of regional wall motion abnormalities, acute coronary syndrome could be excluded. The current AUC recommend echocardiography in presentations with acute chest pain with suspected MI and nondiagnostic ECG when a resting echocardiogram can be performed during pain. Hence, Answer A is correct.

There are no indications for exercise stress echocardiography or transesophageal echocardiography with this clinical presentation. A pulmonary embolus is less likely with the presenting electrocardiogram. While an emergent coronary angiogram was requested by the emergency department treatment team, when the diagnosis is questionable echocardiogram could often be used for definitive diagnosis. Hence, answers B, C, D, and E are incorrect.

Suggested Readings

Douglas PS, Garcia MJ, Haines DE, et al.; ACCF/ASE/ACCP/ AHA/ASNC/HFSA/HRS/SCAI/SCCT/SCMR. ACCF/ASE/ ACCP/AHA/ASNC/HFSA/HRS/SCAI/SCCT/SCMR 2011 appropriate use criteria for echocardiography. *J Am Coll Cardiol* 2011;57(9):1126–1166.

O'Gara PT, Kushner FG, Ascheim DD, et al. 2013 ACCF/AHA guideline for the management of ST-elevation myocardial infarction: a report of the American College of Cardiology Foundation/ American Heart Association Task Force on Practice Guidelines. *J Am Coll Cardiol* 2013;61(4):e78–e140.

Answer 14: *E.* E is a simplified definition of an "appropriate imaging test" as listed in all the AUC documents, including the 2011 AUC for Echocardiography. The appropriateness of an imaging test is not defined by likelihood of reimbursement. It is not required that an "appropriate" imaging test has no risks, only that expected benefits of doing the test exceed any "negative consequences" such that the test represents "acceptable care and a reasonable approach for the indication." Standard evaluation of a patient including history and physical examination should always precede any imaging test so that the most useful imaging test is obtained. There are surprisingly few clinical trials that have proven that the performance of any imaging test directly leads to improved patient outcomes, and thus this standard has not been applied to the definition of an appropriate imaging test.

Suggested Reading

Douglas PS, Garcia MJ, Haines DE, et al.; ACCF/ASE/ACCP/ AHA/ASNC/HFSA/HRS/SCAI/SCCT/SCMR. ACCF/ASE/ ACCP/AHA/ASNC/HFSA/HRS/SCAI/SCCT/SCMR 2011 appropriate use criteria for echocardiography. *J Am Coll Cardiol* 2011;57(9):1126–1166.

Answer 15: D. According to the 2011 AUC guidelines, transesophageal echocardiography is rarely the first imaging test recommended. However diagnosis of infective endocarditis with a moderate to high pretest probability with Staph bacteremia, fungemia prosthetic heart valve areintracardiac device is deemed an appropriate indication.

Hence the patient with *Candida albicans* bacteremia could directly proceed for transesophageal echocardiography.

Answer A is incorrect as the patient should have a transthoracic echocardiography as the initial diagnostic study. If this were to be negative, a transesophageal echocardiogram would be a reasonable second option for evaluation of cardiac source of emboli.

Answer B describes a patient whose imaging could be technically difficult due to body habitus and comorbidities. While an appropriate indication for initial transesophageal echocardiography includes a high likelihood of a nondiagnostic TTE due to patient characteristics, the vignette does not provide sufficient information to determine that transthoracic echocardiography was not possible.

Intraprocedural guidance with transesophageal echocardiography is commonplace today. Transesophageal echocardiography is used for imaging guidance during transcatheter valve repair and replacement, closure device placement, and ablation for arrhythmias. However, TEE is not utilized during percutaneous coronary intervention. Hence answer C is incorrect.

The patient described in answer E presents with a subtherapeutic INR and an unrelated clinical presentation. There are no data suggesting that cardioversion should be undertaken. Therefore, a transesophageal echocardiography is not indicated. While it is quite possible that the patient does have thrombi in the left atrial appendage, the treatment would include appropriate anticoagulation.

Suggested Reading

Douglas PS, Garcia MJ, Haines DE, et al.; ACCF/ASE/ACCP/ AHA/ASNC/HFSA/HRS/SCAI/SCCT/SCMR. ACCF/ASE/ ACCP/AHA/ASNC/HFSA/HRS/SCAI/SCCT/SCMR 2011 appropriate use criteria for echocardiography. *J Am Coll Cardiol* 2011;57(9):1126–1166.

Answer 16: B. Answer B describes a patient with mild valvular regurgitation and no mention of change in clinical status who presents 1 year later for follow-up. The current appropriate use criteria consider routine surveillance transthoracic echocardiography of mild valvular heart disease <3 years after initial TTE in patients with no new symptoms or change in clinical status "rarely appropriate."

Answer A describes a patient with mild aortic stenosis who underwent echocardiography more than 3 years ago. Hence, a follow-up TTE would be appropriate.

Answer C describes a patient who developed new symptoms. According to the 2011 AUC for echocardiography, it is appropriate to repeat echocardiography in any patient with established valve disease and a change in clinical status.

Answer D describes an asymptomatic patient with severe aortic stenosis. Routine surveillance of severe valvular stenosis or regurgitation 1 year after initial TTE is considered appropriate even in the absence of change in clinical status.

Answer E describes a patient with a mechanical valve with a change in clinical status. In any patient with a prosthetic valve that develops new symptoms, a repeat transthoracic echocardiogram is considered appropriate at any time interval.

Suggested Readings

Nishimura RA, et al. 2014 AHA/ACC guideline for the management of patients with valvular heart disease: executive summary: a report of the American College of Cardiology/American Heart Association Task Force on Practice Guidelines. *J Am Coll Cardiol* 2014;63(22):2438–2488.

Douglas PS, Garcia MJ, Haines DE, et al.; ACCF/ASE/ACCP/ AHA/ASNC/HFSA/HRS/SCAI/SCCT/SCMR. ACCF/ASE/ ACCP/AHA/ASNC/HFSA/HRS/SCAI/SCCT/SCMR 2011 appropriate use criteria for echocardiography. *J Am Coll Cardiol* 2011;57(9):1126–1166.

Answer 17: E. In stable patients with a history of congestive heart failure, systolic or diastolic, with no change in clinical status or cardiac examination, routine surveillance with transthoracic echocardiography is rarely appropriate within 1 year after the initial evaluation and uncertain >1 year after initial TTE according to the 2011 AUC for echocardiography. Hence, answer A is incorrect.

Repeat transthoracic echocardiography for reevaluation after revascularization and optimal medical therapy to determine candidacy for device therapy in patients with the ejection fraction <35% is an appropriate indication after 3 months of treatment. Therefore performing an echocardiogram within 1 month is rarely appropriate, and answer B is incorrect.

Routine surveillance of an implanted device without any change in clinical status or examination is rarely appropriate according to the appropriate use criteria, and therefore answer C is incorrect. However, initial evaluation for CRT device optimization after implantation is an appropriate indication for echocardiography.

Answer D describes the patient with a recent diagnosis of hypertension without symptoms or signs of hypertensive heart disease. Routine evaluation of systemic hypertension without symptoms or signs of hypertensive heart disease is a rarely appropriate indication. Therefore, answer D is incorrect.

Answer E is the correct answer, as this is a patient who is undergoing cardiotoxic chemotherapy. Baseline and serial reevaluations in a patient undergoing therapy with cardiotoxic agents are an appropriate indication. The U.S. FDA and the National Comprehensive Cancer Network recommendations include echocardiography every 3 months for patients treated with cardiotoxic chemotherapy such as trastuzumab for treatment of HER2-positive breast cancer.

Suggested Readings

Douglas PS, Garcia MJ, Haines DE, et al.; ACCF/ASE/ACCP/ AHA/ASNC/HFSA/HRS/SCAI/SCCT/SCMR. ACCF/ASE/ ACCP/AHA/ASNC/HFSA/HRS/SCAI/SCCT/SCMR 2011 appropriate use criteria for echocardiography. *J Am Coll Cardiol* 2011;57(9):1126–1166.

National Comprehensive Cancer Network. NCCN clinical practice guidelines in oncology: breast cancer, version 3; 2015. http://www.nccn.org

Wang TJ, Evans JC, Benjamin EJ, et al. Natural history of asymptomatic left ventricular systolic dysfunction in the community. *Circulation* 2003;108:977–982.

Answer 18: *E.* There are no indications for asymptomatic patients listed in the 2011 AUC for Echocardiography that are deemed "appropriate" for stress echocardiography for the purpose of coronary artery disease detection/cardiovascular risk assessment except an Agatston calcium score of >400.

Answer A with a low global coronary artery disease risk and answer B with an intermediate global coronary artery disease risk with an interpretable ECG are both deemed "rarely appropriate" as both would be candidates for routine ECG stress testing if stress testing is required.

Answers C and D are deemed to be of "uncertain" appropriateness. In the AUC, "uncertain" for specific indication suggests that a "test *may* be generally acceptable and *may* be a reasonable approach for the indication" and also "implies that more research and/or patient information is needed to classify the indication definitively."

An Agatston score of >400 is considered an "appropriate" indication for stress echocardiography. A score of <100 is considered inappropriate or rarely appropriate. A score between 100 and 400 is of uncertain appropriateness. Hence, answer E is the correct answer.

Suggested Reading

Douglas PS, Garcia MJ, Haines DE, et al.; ACCF/ASE/ACCP/AHA/ASNC/HFSA/HRS/SCAI/SCCT/SCMR. ACCF/ASE/ACCP/AHA/ASNC/HFSA/HRS/SCAI/SCCT/SCMR 2011 appropriate use criteria for echocardiography. *J Am Coll Cardiol* 2011;57(9):1126–1166.

Answer 19: *C.* According to the 2011 appropriate use criteria, frequent PVCs, exercise-induced ventricular tachycardia, nonsustained ventricular tachycardia, and sustained ventricular tachycardia are considered appropriate indications for stress echocardiography.

Infrequent PVCs are a rarely appropriate or inappropriate indication. New-onset atrial fibrillation is of uncertain significance.

Therefore, the only appropriate indication is C. Answer A has a low burden of premature ventricular contractions and would not be an indication.

Suggested Reading

Douglas PS, Garcia MJ, Haines DE, et al.; ACCF/ASE/ACCP/AHA/ASNC/HFSA/HRS/SCAI/SCCT/SCMR. ACCF/ASE/ACCP/AHA/ASNC/HFSA/HRS/SCAI/SCCT/SCMR 2011 appropriate use criteria for echocardiography. *J Am Coll Cardiol* 2011;57(9):1126–1166.

Answer 20: *E.* TTE is deemed "appropriate" in many acute-care settings according to the 2011 AUC for Echocardiography. These include any patients with unexplained hypotension or hypoxemia. In addition, TTE is "appropriate" in a variety of clinical scenarios involving acute myocardial infarction/acute coronary syndromes, including ongoing chest pain with a nondiagnostic ECG to exclude a regional wall motion abnormality and for evaluation of suspected acute mechanical complications after myocardial infarction.

TTE would be considered "appropriate" to help guide therapy after a documented pulmonary embolus for consideration of thrombectomy or catheter-directed thrombolysis. However, it would be rarely appropriate for diagnosis of pulmonary embolism.

Therefore, answers A through D were appropriate indications for echocardiography and the correct answer is E.

Suggested Reading

Douglas PS, Garcia MJ, Haines DE, et al.; ACCF/ASE/ACCP/AHA/ASNC/HFSA/HRS/SCAI/SCCT/SCMR. ACCF/ASE/ACCP/AHA/ASNC/HFSA/HRS/SCAI/SCCT/SCMR 2011 appropriate use criteria for echocardiography. *J Am Coll Cardiol* 2011;57(9):1126–1166.

Answer 21: *E.* According to the current appropriate use criteria, stress testing <5 years after coronary artery bypass grafting and <2 years after percutaneous coronary intervention, in the absence of symptoms, is determined to be inappropriate or rarely appropriate. After this stated time line, stress testing in the absence of symptoms is noted as an "uncertain" indication. Therefore, answers A and B are incorrect.

While stress testing to evaluate for ischemia in an intermediate stenosis is acceptable, a 30% stenosis in the distal right coronary artery in an asymptomatic patient is not an indication for stress testing. Hence, answer C is incorrect.

Dobutamine stress testing may be carried out to evaluate for viability in the setting of a low ejection fraction. However, in this clinical scenario, myocardial perfusion has confirmed an anterior scar and therefore, there is no utility in presenting with dobutamine stress. Answer D is incorrect.

Therefore the correct answer is E, in which none of the above are appropriate indications.

Suggested Readings

Douglas PS, Garcia MJ, Haines DE, et al.; ACCF/ASE/ACCP/AHA/ASNC/HFSA/HRS/SCAI/SCCT/SCMR. ACCF/ASE/ACCP/AHA/ASNC/HFSA/HRS/SCAI/SCCT/SCMR 2011 appropriate use criteria for echocardiography. *J Am Coll Cardiol* 2011;57(9):1126–1166.

Mansour IN, Razi RR, Bhave NM, et al. Comparison of the updated 2011 appropriate use criteria for echocardiography to the original criteria for transthoracic, transesophageal, and stress echocardiography. *J Am Soc Echocardiogr* 2012;25(11):1153–1161.

Ward RP, Mansour I, Lemieux N, et al. Prospective evaluation of the ACCF/ASE appropriateness criteria for echocardiography. *J Am Coll Cardiol Imaging* 2008;1:663–671.

Chapter 12

Common TTE Anatomy

Sasanka Jayasuriya

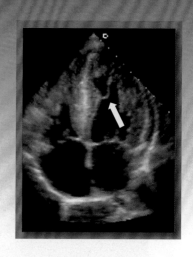

1. A 47-year-old female is referred for a TTE to evaluate dyspnea. The sonographer informs you of a mass near the left atrium (FIG. 12.1, VIDEO 12.1). Which of the following is the least likely explanation?

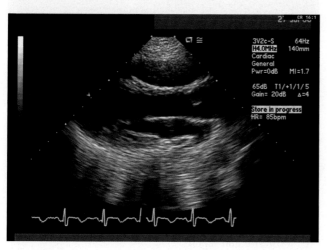

FIGURE 12.1

A. CHF
B. Ebstein anomaly
C. Persistent left superior vena cava
D. Anomalous left coronary artery from the pulmonary artery
E. Pulmonary hypertension

2. What echo maneuver or additional procedure would best aide in the diagnosis of the patient in Question 1?

A. Inject the manufactured ultrasound contrast agent in the right arm.
B. Inject agitated saline microbubbles in the left arm.
C. Inject agitated saline microbubbles in the right arm.
D. Inject agitated saline microbubbles in the right leg.
E. Inject agitated saline microbubbles in the left leg.

3. Which structure is highlighted in this view (FIG. 12.2, VIDEO 12.2)?

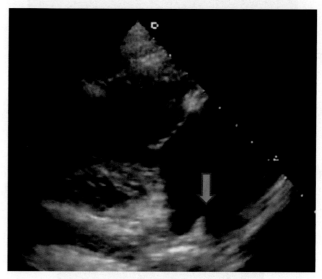

FIGURE 12.2

A. Superior vena cava
B. Inferior vena cava
C. Eustachian valve
D. Coronary sinus
E. Transverse sinus

4. What are the leaflets of the pulmonic valve?

A. Right, left, posterior
B. Right, left, anterior
C. Anterior, posterior, right
D. Anterior, posterior, left

5. Which aortic valve coronary cusp is starred in FIGURE 12.3?

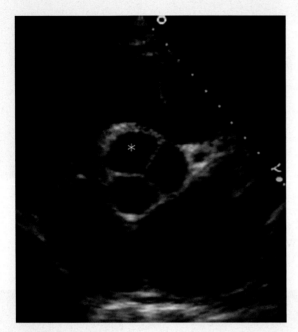

Figure 12.3

A. Septal
B. Right
C. Left
D. Noncoronary
E. Anterior

6. A 75-year-old admitted with a TIA is referred for a bubble study. What structure is seen in the right atrium (Fig. 12.4, Video 12.3)?

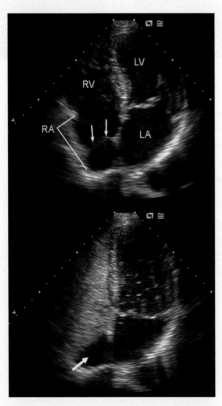

Figure 12.4 From Armstrong WF, Ryan T. *Feigenbaum's Echocardiography.* 7th ed. Philadelphia, PA: Lippincott Williams & Wilkins, 2010.

A. Cor triatriatum
B. Eustachian valve
C. Crista terminalis
D. Myxoma
E. Side lobe artifact

7. Which leaflets are seen in this view (Fig. 12.5)?

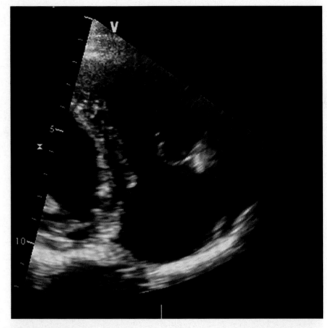

Figure 12.5

A. Anterior and posterior
B. Anterior and septal
C. Posterior and septal
D. Anterior and right
E. Posterior and right

8. A 56-year-old female with dyspnea was referred for an echocardiogram. What is the most likely explanation for the echogenic mass (Video 12.4)?

A. Thrombus
B. Flail leaflet
C. Vegetation
D. Chiari network
E. Crista terminalis

9. Which vessel is marked in this suprasternal view (Fig. 12.6)?

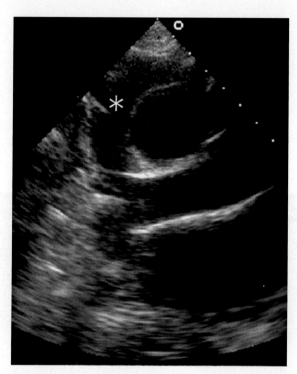

Figure 12.6

A. Superior vena cava
B. Left atrium
C. Aorta
D. Right pulmonary artery
E. Left pulmonary artery

10. Which vessel is starred in this view (Fig. 12.7)?

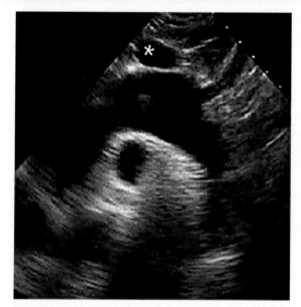

Figure 12.7

A. Left atrium
B. Right brachiocephalic vein
C. Right pulmonary artery
D. Left pulmonary artery
E. Left brachiocephalic vein

11. Which structure is the arrow pointing to in Figure 12.8, Video 12.5?

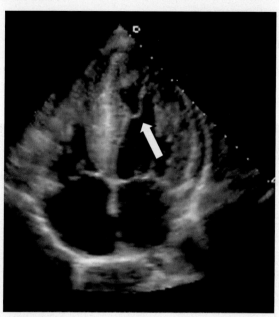

Figure 12.8

A. The structure associated with housing the right bundle branch
B. A congenital abnormality rarely seen in adults
C. A component of the mitral valve apparatus
D. Is more commonly seen in patients with idiopathic VT
E. Is very common and present in 50% or more of autopsies

12. A 75-year-old male with congestive heart failure was admitted with pulmonary edema. An echocardiogram was ordered to evaluate his ventricular function. What structure is highlighted (Fig. 12.9)?

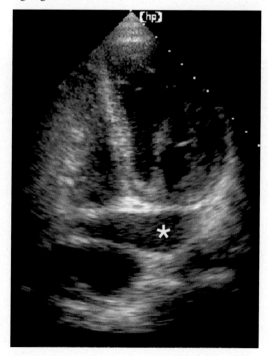

Figure 12.9 From Armstrong WF, Ryan T. *Feigenbaum's Echocardiography.* 7th ed. Philadelphia, PA: Lippincott Williams & Wilkins, 2010.

A. Anomalous pulmonary vein
B. Primum atrial septal defect
C. Coronary sinus
D. Circumflex artery
E. Transverse sinus

13. A 52-year-old female who is visiting her family became acutely short of breath. An echocardiogram demonstrates an abnormality in which structure (Fig. 12.10)?

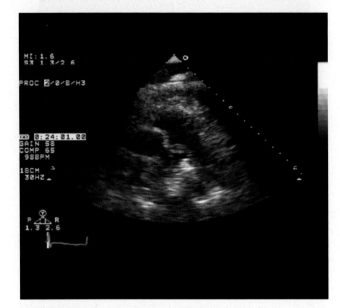

FIGURE 12.10

A. Aorta
B. Right pulmonary artery
C. Left pulmonary artery
D. Both right and left pulmonary arteries
E. Superior vena cava

14. Which papillary muscle is identified in Figure 12.11?

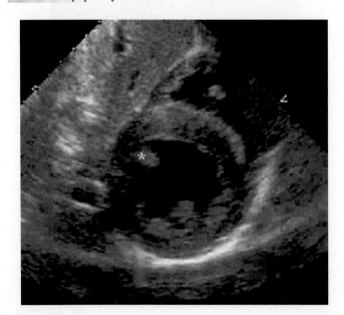

FIGURE 12.11

A. Anterolateral
B. Posterolateral
C. Anteromedial
D. Posteromedial
E. Accessory papillary muscle

15. A 62-year-old female with a long history of tobacco use and hypertension was referred for an echocardiogram following the detection of atrial fibrillation. What structure is the arrow pointing to in Figure 12.12?

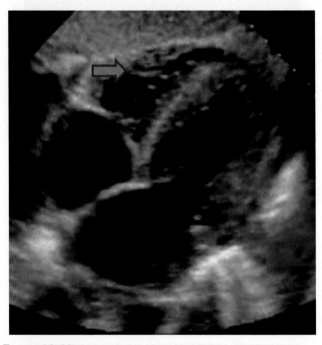

FIGURE 12.12

A. Accessory band
B. Papillary muscle
C. Moderator band
D. Chordae tendineae

Answer 1: D. Dilation of the coronary sinus (CS) can result from congenital abnormalities that lead to increase venous drainage to the CS or from conditions leading to increased right atrial pressure. Examples of anomalous communication with either the venous system or the right atrium include PLSVC with drainage into the CS, total anomalous pulmonary venous return with CS drainage, coronary AV fistula with drainage into the CS, and an unroofed CS leading to a CS ASD. Dilation of the CS as a result of increased RA pressure/volume includes right ventricular dysfunction, right atrial hypertension, Ebstein anomaly, ASD with large shunt leading to RV volume overload, and severe pulmonary hypertension. Anomalous origin of the left coronary artery arising from the pulmonary artery (ALCAPA) requires surgical repair upon diagnosis. The adult form leads to coronary steal into the PA from right coronary artery collateralization, but does not specifically affect venous return. Adults may have chronic ischemia and develop LV dysfunction and heart failure, which might indirectly cause a dilated CS, but this would be the least likely option of the choices provided.

Suggested Readings

Andrade J, Somerville J, Carvalho A, et al. Echocardiographic routine analysis of the coronary sinus by an apical view. *Tex Heart Inst J* 1982;13(2):197–202.

Feigenbaum H, Armstrong WF, Ryan T. Contrast echocardiography. In: Feigenbaum H, Armstrong WF, Ryan T, eds. *Feigenbaum's Echocardiography*. 6th ed. Philadelphia, PA: Lippincott Williams & Wilkins, 2005.

Kowalski M, Maynard R, Ananthasubramaniam K. Imaging of persistent left sided superior vena cava with echocardiography with multi-slice computed tomography: implications for daily practice. *Cardiol J* 2011;18:1–5.

Pena E, Nguyen E, Merchant N, et al. ALCAPA syndrome, not just a pediatric disease. *Radiographics* 2009;29:553–565.

Answer 2: B. A PLSVC can be identified by injection of agitated saline or echo contrast from the left peripheral arm veins. Agitated saline injected from either peripheral arm vein will normally enter the right atrium from a single SVC and opacify the right heart. Agitated saline microbubbles are large and mostly destroyed during transpulmonary passage and are therefore not normally seen in the CS and certainly not before appearing in the right atrium. In the setting of PLSVC, agitated saline injected into the left arm drains through the abnormal connection between the left-sided venous return and the CS. The agitated saline microbubbles can clearly be seen first in the CS, followed by right heart opacification. Injection of a contrast agent into either of the femoral veins will normally return to the right atrium via the IVC.

Suggested Readings

Andrade J, Somerville J, Carvalho A, et al. Echocardiographic routine analysis of the coronary sinus by an apical view. *Tex Heart Inst J* 1982;13(2):197–202.

Feigenbaum H, Armstrong WF, Ryan T. Contrast echocardiography. In: Feigenbaum H, Armstrong WF, Ryan T, eds. *Feigenbaum's Echocardiography*. 6th ed. Philadelphia, PA: Lippincott Williams & Wilkins, 2005.

Kowalski M, Maynard R, Ananthasubramaniam K. Imaging of persistent left sided superior vena cava with echocardiography with multi-slice computed tomography: implications for daily practice. *Cardiol J* 2011;18:1–5.

Answer 3: C. On the right ventricular inflow view, the posterior structures of the right atrium are seen. The coronary sinus (CS) enters the right atrium adjacent to the tricuspid annulus, more inferior is the inferior vena cava is seen. At the inferior cavoatrial junction, a prominent eustachian valve is seen. The SVC is best seen on transthoracic echo in the suprasternal view. The transverse sinus is a pericardial space between the aorta and pulmonary artery that would not be seen in this view (FIG. 12.13).

Suggested Readings

Netter FH. *Atlas of Human Anatomy*. 2nd ed. Teterboro, NJ: Icon Learning Systems, 2001:200–217.

Otto C. Normal anatomy and flow patterns on transthoracic echocardiography. In: *Textbook of Clinical Echocardiography*. 5th ed. Elsevier Saunders, 2013:31–59.

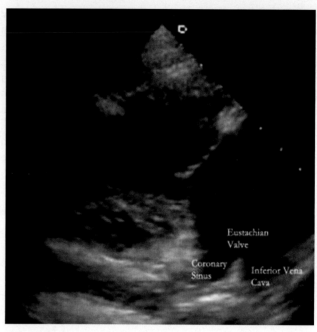

FIGURE 12.13

Answer 4: B. The pulmonic valve is a tricuspid semilunar valve comprised of the right, left, and anterior leaflets. The pulmonic valve is out of plane relative to the aortic valve and rarely seen en face with TTE. With TEE, however, all three leaflets may be seen in short axis similar to the common AV en face view. This requires much anteflexion of the TEE probe to see the more superiorly located pulmonic valve. Both AV and PV have an RC (right cusp) and LC (left cusp), but can be differentiated by the NCC (noncoronary posterior cusp) of the AV and the AC (anterior cusp) of the PV.

Suggested Readings

Gilliam L, Otto C. *Advanced Approaches in Echocardiography*. 1st ed. Philadelphia, PA: Elsevier, 2011:158–170.

Netter FH. *Atlas of Human Anatomy*. 2nd ed. Teterboro, NJ: Icon Learning Systems, 2001:200–217.

Answer 5: B. The basal short-axis view allows for visualization of the aortic annulus. The aortic valve is trileaflet, comprised of the left, right, and noncoronary cusps. The noncoronary cup is easily recognized since it is intersected by the interatrial septum. ED comment: It is important to remember that the interatrial septal cusp is the NCC since this helps to identify anatomic leaflets regardless of view or type of echo (TTE or TEE). The right coronary cusp is the most anterior and adjacent to the right ventricular outflow tract. The left coronary cusp is the only one remaining. Superior angulation occasionally will allow visualization of the left main and right coronary arteries.

Suggested Readings

Netter FH. *Atlas of Human Anatomy*. 2nd ed. Teterboro, NJ: Icon Learning Systems, 2001:200–217.

Otto C. Transthoracic views, normal anatomy and flow patterns. In: *Textbook of Clinical Echocardiography*. 3rd ed. Philadelphia, PA: Elsevier Saunders, 2004:70–95.

Answer 6: B. The linear echo traversing the right atrium is the eustachian valve (EV). The EV is an embryologic structure in the right atrium that redirects blood away from the underdeveloped pulmonary system across the foramen ovale. In this example, injected saline contrast fills the inferior atrium; an echo-free space is seen in the area adjacent to the IVC. Bubbles are seen entering the left atrium via a right-to-left shunt. The cor triatriatum membrane is usually seen in the left atrium. Atrial myxoma is most frequently seen attached to the fossa ovalis in the left atrium. A prominent crista terminalis ridge would not redirect blood flow. Thrombi also have a characteristic echogenic appearance and are usually mobile.

Suggested Readings

Carson W, Chiu SS. Image in cardiovascular medicine. Eustachian valve mimicking intracardiac mass. *Circulation* 1998;97:2188.
Limacher MC, Gutgesell HP, Vick GW, et al. Echocardiographic anatomy of the Eustachian valve. *Am J Cardiol* 1986;57:363–365.
Schuchlenz HW, Saurer G, Weihs W, et al. Persisting Eustachian valve in adults: relation to patent foramen ovale and cerebrovascular events. *J Am Soc Echocardiogr* 2004;17:231–233.

Answer 7: B. The right ventricular inflow is obtained by starting in the parasternal long-axis view; medial angulation of the probe allows for visualization of the right side of the heart. The scan plane courses through (as in this example) the posterior segment of the interventricular septum. The septal and anterior tricuspid valve leaflets are seen. Further clockwise rotation is necessary to remove the left ventricle (RV inflow is not parallel to LV), leaving only the right atrium and right ventricle. Now the anterior and posterior TV leaflets will be seen as well as the posterior structures of the right atrium (eustachian valve and IVC) (Fig. 12.14).

Suggested Readings

Anwar A, Geleijnse M, Soliman O, et al. Assessment of normal tricuspid valve anatomy in adults by real-time three-dimensional echocardiography. *Int J Cardiovasc Imaging* 2007;23(6):717–724.
Badano L, Agricola E, Perez L, et al. Evaluation of the tricuspid valve morphology and function by transthoracic real-time three-dimensional echocardiography. *Eur J Echocardiogr* 2009;10:477–484.
Feigenbaum H, Armstrong WF, Ryan T. The echocardiographic examination. In: Feigenbaum H, Armstrong WF, Ryan T, eds. *Feigenbaum's Echocardiography*. 7th ed. Philadelphia, PA: Lippincott Williams & Wilkins, 2010:91–122.

Answer 8: D. The Chiari network is an embryologic remnant seen in 2% to 3% of the population. They are best seen in the right parasternal long axis, RVOT sax, and four-chamber views—described as a bright, rotary, and highly mobile linear structures that can be seen in several locations in the right atrium. They do not move in the RV in diastole (typical of TV vegetation). Identification of three normal tricuspid valve leaflets is necessary to differentiate from a flail leaflet. The crista terminalis is located at the junction of the trabeculated right atrial appendage with the smooth left atrium and runs from the SVC to IVC. It appears as an echo-dense linear ridge in the posterior right atrial wall extending laterally from the atrial septum. Right atrial thrombi are highly mobile and usually

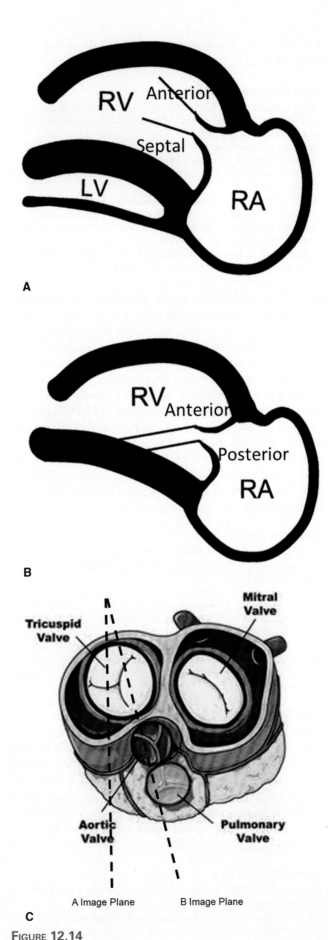

FIGURE 12.14

have a cylindrical shape from being casted in the veins prior to embolization.

Suggested Readings

Cloez JL, Neimann JL, Chivoret G, et al. Echographic rediscovery of an anatomical structure: the Chiari network. Apropos of 16 cases. *Arch Mal Coeur Vaiss* 1983;76:1284–1292.
McKay T, Thomas L. Prominent crista terminalis and Eustachian ridge in the right atrium. *Eur J Echocardiogr* 2007;8(4):288–291.
Oh J, Seward J, Tajik A. Pulmonary hypertension and pulmonary vein stenosis. In: Oh J, Seward J, Tajik A, eds. *The Echo Manual*. 3rd ed. Philadelphia, PA: Lippincott Williams & Wilkins, 2007:143–154.
Werner JA, Cheitlin MD, Gross BS, et al. Echocardiographic appearance of the Chiari network: differentiation from right-heart pathology. *Circulation* 1981;63:1104–1109.

Answer 9: A. This view is obtained at the suprasternal notch by rotating the probe perpendicular to the aortic arch. The superior vena cava (SVC), ascending aorta (AA), right pulmonary artery (RPA), and left atrium (LA) are all seen in this imaging plane (Fig. 12.15). The left pulmonary artery is not seen.

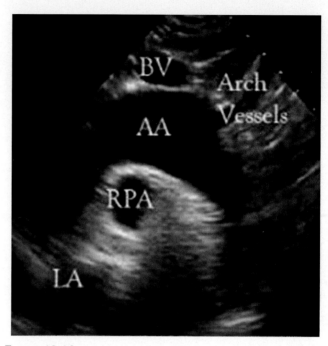

FIGURE 12.16

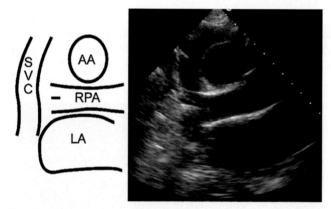

FIGURE 12.15

Suggested Readings

Feigenbaum H, Armstrong WF, Ryan T. The echocardiographic examination. In: Feigenbaum H, Armstrong WF, Ryan T, eds. *Feigenbaum's Echocardiography*. 7th ed. Philadelphia, PA: Lippincott Williams & Wilkins, 2010:91–122.
Otto C. Transthoracic views, normal anatomy and flow patterns. In: *Textbook of Clinical Echocardiography*. 3rd ed. Philadelphia, PA: Elsevier Saunders, 2004:70–95.

Answer 10: E. The suprasternal notch view is obtained with the probe pointed at the left shoulder and tilted down to parallel the aortic arch (Fig. 12.16, AA). Structures that can be visualized in this view include the left brachiocephalic vein (BV) emptying into the SVC, right pulmonary artery (RPA) coursing under the arch, left atrium, and arch vessels. The arch vessels are difficult to identify unless all three are seen. The left pulmonary artery and right common carotid artery (branch of innominate artery) are not seen in this view.

In Figure 12.17, the right (RBV) and left (LBV) brachiocephalic veins are seen joining the SVC.

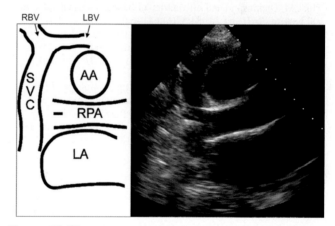

FIGURE 12.17

Suggested Readings

Feigenbaum H, Armstrong WF, Ryan T. The echocardiographic examination. In: Feigenbaum H, Armstrong WF, Ryan T, eds. *Feigenbaum's Echocardiography*. 7th ed. Philadelphia, PA: Lippincott Williams & Wilkins, 2010:91–122.
Otto C. Transthoracic views, normal anatomy and flow patterns. In: *Textbook of Clinical Echocardiography*. 3rd ed. Philadelphia, PA: Elsevier Saunders, 2004:70–95.

Answer 11: E. This is an apical four-chamber view (Fig. 12.18). The left ventricle is identified by recognizing the papillary muscles, increased wall thickness, and more basal mitral valve. A left ventricular band, known by several names including false tendon, are fibromuscular structures in the left ventricle that cross the cavity joining nearby trabeculations or papillary muscles. Chordae tendineae connect the papillary muscles to the mitral valve. The moderator band is located in the right ventricle.

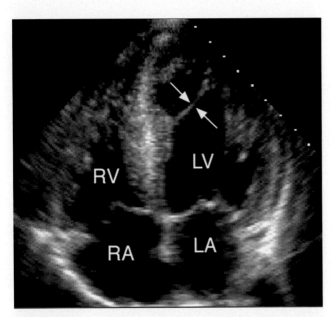

FIGURE 12.18

Suggested Readings

Gerlis LM, Dickinson DF. Left ventricular bands: a normal anatomical feature. *Br Heart J* 1984;52(6):641–647.

Gualano SK, Bolling SF, Gordon D, et al. High prevalence of false chordae tendinae in patients without left ventricular tachycardia. *Pacing Clin Electrophysiol* 2007;30(suppl 1):S156–S159.

Kenchaiah S, Benjamin EJ, Evans JC, et al. Epidemiology of left ventricular false tendons: clinical correlates in the Framingham heart study. *J Am Soc Echocardiogr* 2009;22(6):739–745.

Sugiyama M. Echocardiographic features of false tendons in the left ventricle. *Am J Cardiol* 1981;48(1):177–183.

Answer 12: *C.*

A. Anomalous pulmonary vein is incorrect. Anomalous pulmonary veins are not well seen on TTE. The most common abnormality is a right superior venous attachment to the SVC (sinus venosus defect). TEE is more helpful to visualize posterior structures.

B. Primum atrial septal defect is incorrect because the septum primum is intact. Also, this abnormality is frequently part of a spectrum of endocardial cushion defects that are not present on this example.

C. Coronary sinus: See discussion.

D. Circumflex artery is incorrect; the vessel courses in lateral AV grove and is not well seen on a four-chamber view.

E. Transverse sinus is incorrect. It is a pericardiac space between the aorta and pulmonary artery seen best on a basal short-axis view or by TEE.

The coronary sinus (CS) runs in the posterior AV groove and enters the right atrium adjacent to the tricuspid annulus. The coronary sinus is best seen on transthoracic imaging in the long-axis view of the right ventricle and a posterior angulated four-chamber view.

Suggested Readings

Andrade J, Somerville J, Carvalho A, et al. Echocardiographic routine analysis of the coronary sinus by an apical view. *Tex Heart Inst J* 1986;13(2):197–202.

Gilliam L, Otto C. *Advanced Approaches in Echocardiography*. 1st ed. Philadelphia, PA: Elsevier, 2011:158–170.

Netter FH. *Atlas of Human Anatomy*. 2nd ed. Teterboro, NJ: Icon Learning Systems, 2001:200–217.

Answer 13: *D.* A high parasternal short-axis view with superior angulation will show the pulmonary artery and sometimes past the bifurcation. In this case example, the patient has a saddle embolism that extends into both the right and left pulmonary artery. The right pulmonary is identified adjacent to the aortic annulus and courses under the aortic arch.

Suggested Readings

Feigenbaum H, Armstrong WF, Ryan T. The echocardiographic examination. In: Feigenbaum H, Armstrong WF, Ryan T, eds. *Feigenbaum's Echocardiography*. 7th ed. Philadelphia, PA: Lippincott Williams & Wilkins, 2010:91–122.

Otto C. Transthoracic views, normal anatomy and flow patterns. In: *Textbook of Clinical Echocardiography*. 3rd ed. Philadelphia, PA: Elsevier Saunders, 2004:70–95.

Answer 14: *D.* The two papillary muscles in the left ventricle are the anterolateral and posteromedial. In the short-axis subcostal view, the right ventricle can be used as an anatomic reference for orientation (FIG. 12.19). The inferior wall is adjacent to the liver.

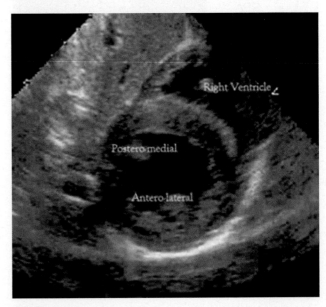

FIGURE 12.19

Suggested Readings

Feigenbaum H, Armstrong WF, Ryan T. The echocardiographic examination. In: Feigenbaum H, Armstrong WF, Ryan T, eds. *Feigenbaum's Echocardiography*. 7th ed. Philadelphia, PA: Lippincott Williams & Wilkins, 2010:91–122.

Otto C. Transthoracic views, normal anatomy and flow patterns. In: *Textbook of Clinical Echocardiography*. 3rd ed. Philadelphia, PA: Elsevier Saunders, 2004:70–95.

Answer 15: C. In the subcostal four-chamber view, the right ventricle is identified adjacent to the liver and by the presence of a trabeculated myocardium, moderator band, and tricuspid valve (apically displaced relative to mitral annulus). The moderator band is located in the right ventricular apex and connects the interventricular septum to the anterior papillary muscle. Accessory bands are seen in the left ventricle. Chordae tendineae are identified by attachments to the papillary muscles and valve leaflets. It is thought that the moderator band is responsible for carrying the major portion of the right bundle branch and, being muscular, contributes to RV contraction. This structure also helps to prevent sudden distension of the RV.

Suggested Readings

Feigenbaum H, Armstrong WF, Ryan T. The echocardiographic examination. In: Feigenbaum H, Armstrong WF, Ryan T, eds. *Feigenbaum's Echocardiography*. 7th ed. Philadelphia, PA: Lippincott Williams & Wilkins, 2010:91–122.

Ho S. Anatomy, echocardiography, and normal right ventricular dimensions. *Heart* 2006;92:i2–i13.

Otto C. Transthoracic views, normal anatomy and flow patterns. In: *Textbook of Clinical Echocardiography*. 3rd ed. Philadelphia, PA: Elsevier Saunders, 2004:70–95.

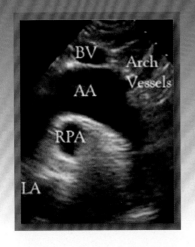

Chapter 13

Normal TEE Anatomy

Vincent L. Sorrell

1. During multiplanar examination, the full extent of the aortic arch is best examined by a plane that is oriented at:

  A. 0 degree

  B. 45 degrees

  C. 120 degrees

  D. 90 degrees

2. Examination of the left carotid bulb may be feasible in some individuals using:

  A. A standard midesophageal level approach.

  B. An upper esophageal approach with the probe positioned very high in the esophagus.

  C. Probe withdrawal into the pharynx.

  D. The carotid bulb cannot be visualized during the transesophageal echocardiographic examination.

3. A high-resistance spectral Doppler flow pattern is identified in the:

  A. Left common carotid artery

  B. Right internal carotid artery

  C. Left subclavian artery

  D. Left vertebral artery

4. The venous structure imaged beneath the aortic arch during upper transesophageal echo examination commonly represents the:

  A. Left innominate vein

  B. Hemiazygos vein

  C. Left subclavian vein

  D. Left pulmonary artery

5. A large venous structure imaged beneath the descending thoracic aorta points to the diagnosis of:

  A. Dilated venous collaterals resulting from coarctation of the aorta

  B. Lymphatic obstruction, most commonly seen in patients with breast cancer metastases

  C. Dilated intercostal veins of any etiology

  D. An interrupted inferior vena cava with azygos continuation

6. The "Coumadin" ridge ("Q" tip) is:

  A. Formed by infolding of the left inferior pulmonary vein

  B. Formed by infolding of the left atrial appendage

  C. Formed by infolding of the left superior pulmonary vein

  D. A vestigial structure of no clinical significance

7. A 2D TEE may be supplemented by 3D TTE in excluding a clot in the LAA in patients with atrial fibrillation undergoing ablation. A 3D TTE:

  A. Always demonstrates all lobes of LAA

  B. May differentiate pectinate muscles from thrombi

  C. Provides a higher-quality study because of its three-dimensional nature

  D. All of the options

8. A normal systolic velocity in a nonstenotic intercostal artery will not exceed the following maximal Doppler flow value:

  A. <0.5 m/s.

  B. <1.0 m/s.

  C. <2 m/s.

  D. <3 m/s.

  E. The intercostal artery is too small to be seen with routine TEE imaging of the aorta.

9. During transesophageal echo examination, the true left ventricular apex is best visualized in the:

  A. Four-chamber view

  B. Two-chamber view

  C. Transgastric short-axis view

  D. Deep transgastric (reverse four-chamber view)

10. 2D TEE is generally inferior to a good quality 2D TTE in assessing the:

  A. Mitral and aortic valves

  B. Tricuspid and pulmonary valves

  C. Left atrium

  D. Descending aorta

11. A 35-year-old male is admitted with fever. A transesophageal echocardiogram is performed with the findings in Video 13.1 and Figure 13.1. Which of the following is correct regarding the view and chamber visualized?

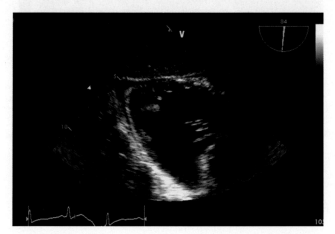

FIGURE 13.1

A. Midesophageal, left ventricle
B. Transgastric, left ventricle
C. Midesophageal, right ventricle
D. Transgastric, right ventricle
E. Midesophageal, left atrium

12. Which of the following is true regarding the findings (Video 13.1, Fig. 13.2) in the same patient from question 1?

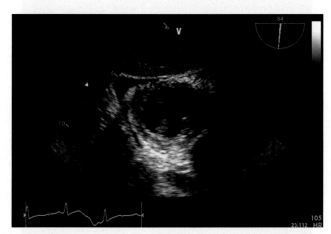

FIGURE 13.2

A. There is evidence of a pathologic mass.
B. A large pericardial effusion is present.
C. The degree of tricuspid regurgitation is probably severe.
D. The chambers are dilated.
E. A foreign body is present and needs further evaluation.

13. Figure 13.3 (Video 13.2) is a bicaval view obtained by transesophageal echocardiography. Which of the following is the most likely reason for the thrombus visualized in the right atrium?

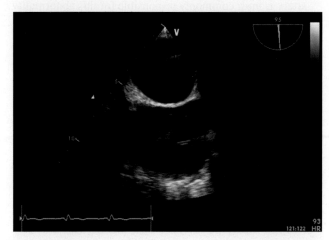

FIGURE 13.3

A. Thrombus in transit
B. Malignancy
C. Central line
D. Patent foramen ovale (PFO)
E. Atrial fibrillation

14. Which of the following are completely or partially visualized in Figure 13.4 (Video 13.3)?

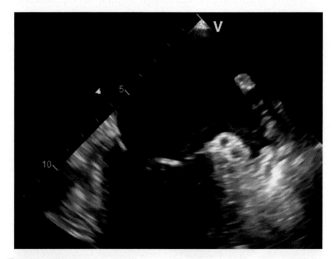

FIGURE 13.4

A. Right upper pulmonary vein
B. Ligament of Marshall
C. Thrombus in the left atrial appendage (LAA)
D. Left circumflex artery
E. Cardiac vein

15. A 76-year-old patient who has a history of coronary artery disease presents for a transesophageal echocardiogram. A regional wall motion abnormality is noted in the segments marked in red (Fig. 13.5). Disease in which coronary artery is *most* commonly responsible for this abnormality?

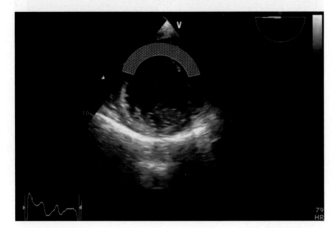

FIGURE **13.5**

A. Left anterior descending artery
B. Left circumflex artery
C. Right coronary artery
D. Left main artery
E. Ramus intermedius

16. A 65-year-old patient underwent hip surgery. The day following discharge, he developed sudden severe shortness of breath and presented to the emergency department. On examination, he is afebrile with significant tachypnea and tachycardia (Figs. 13.6 and 13.7, Videos 13.4 and 13.5). The most likely etiology of this presentation is:

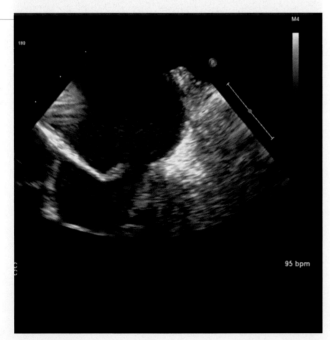

FIGURE **13.6**

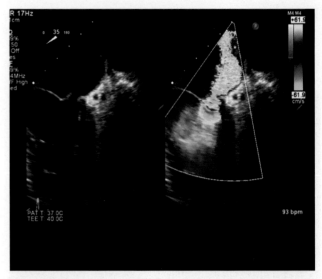

FIGURE **13.7**

A. Pulmonary embolism
B. Chronic severe mitral regurgitation
C. Severe LV systolic dysfunction
D. Endocarditis
E. Flail A2 segment of mitral valve

17. A 30-year-old patient is referred for evaluation of cryptogenic stroke. Which of the following is correct regarding the images (Fig. 13.8, Video 13.6)?

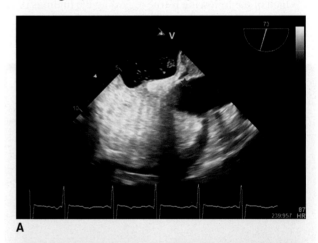

A

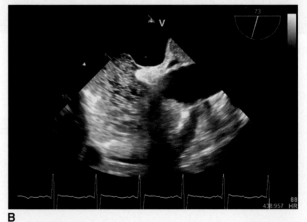

B

FIGURE **13.8**

A. This is a false-negative study as the patient is sedated.

B. The atrial septum is aneurysmal.

C. The opacified area marked by a red star is the right atrial appendage.

D. Commercially produced microbubble contrast was used for this study.

E. Percutaneous closure is the first line of therapy.

Questions 18 and 19

A patient undergoes transesophageal echocardiography prior to cardiothoracic surgery. A midesophageal view is recorded (Fig. 13.9, Video 13.7; main pulmonary artery [MPA], right pulmonary artery [RPA], left pulmonary artery [LPA]).

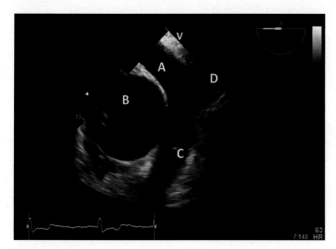

Figure 13.9

18. Which statement identifies structures labeled from A through D in correct sequence?

A. Aortic arch, MPA, aortic valve, subclavian artery

B. LPA, ascending aorta, MPA, RPA

C. Aortic arch, RV outflow tract, aortic valve, subclavian artery

D. RPA, ascending aorta, pulmonary valve, LPA

19. The most likely indication for CT surgery in this patient is:

A. Williams syndrome

B. Ascending aortic aneurysm

C. Coarctation of aorta

D. Pulmonary atresia

20. Choose the best statement that applies to the image (Fig. 13.10, Video 13.8):

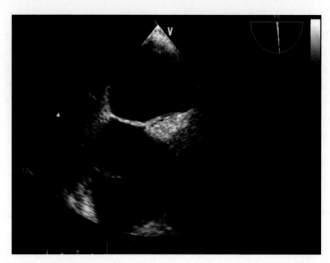

Figure 13.10

A. To obtain this view from the short-axis view of the aortic valve, the probe should be rotated in a counterclockwise direction.

B. Advancing the probe would better visualize the superior vena cava.

C. Advancing the probe will better visualize the origin of the structure marked with an asterisk.

D. Clockwise rotation of the probe from this position will better evaluate the left atrium.

E. The probe should be withdrawn to visualize the coronary sinus.

Answer 1: *D.* The aortic arch is best examined by a vertical or a 90-degree planar angle and rotating the probe clockwise to examine the right side of the arch and in a counterclockwise direction to assess the left side of the arch. In this manner, the whole of the arch can be examined in most individuals.

Suggested Readings

Agrawal G, LaMotte LC, Nanda NC, et al. Identification of the aortic arch branches using transesophageal echocardiography. *Echocardiography* 1997;14:461–466.

Nanda NC, Domanski M. *Atlas of Transesophageal Echocardiography*. 2nd ed. Baltimore, MD: Lippincott Williams & Wilkins, 2007:560.

Answer 2: *C.* In a patient in whom the pharynx is well anesthetized, the left common carotid artery is identified using the upper transesophageal approach by first examining the left side of the aortic arch with 90-degree plane angulation and then rotating and withdrawing the probe slowly. Subsequently, the probe is further withdrawn very slowly into the pharynx, keeping the left common carotid artery continuously in view. The carotid bulb is recognized as a localized dilation of the left common carotid artery. At this point, bifurcation of the left common carotid artery into external and internal branches may also be visualized. Including color-flow Doppler may assist in optimal visualization. It is important to ask the patient not to move his/her tongue during this maneuver; otherwise, the probe will lose contact with the pharyngeal wall.

Suggested Reading

Nanda NC, Biederman RW, Thakur AC, et al. Examination of left external and internal carotid arteries during transesophageal echocardiography. *Echocardiography* 1998;15:755–758.

Answer 3: C. The left subclavian artery, which supplies the face and left upper limb, demonstrates high-resistance flow signals with conventional spectral Doppler. This means flow signals are oriented in one direction in systole and in the opposite direction in diastole. The other vessels named supply the brain and characteristically show low-resistance flow; that is, flow signals are oriented in the same direction in both systole and diastole. Both internal and external carotid arteries show low-resistance flow signals. However, the external carotid artery generally shows sharper systolic velocity waveforms and lower velocity diastolic velocities as compared to the internal carotid vessel. Also, the internal carotid artery frequently has a more vertically oriented course compared to the external branch. This facilitates parallel placement of the Doppler beam resulting in accurate recording of velocities and is a potential advantage over the surface approach where it is impossible to align the Doppler beam parallel to flow direction. The external carotid is also differentiated from the internal carotid by the presence of branches. On the other hand, no branches originate from the initial carotid in its extracranial course.

Suggested Readings

Nanda NC, Biederman RW, Thakur AC, et al. Examination of left external and internal carotid arteries during transesophageal echocardiography. *Echocardiography* 1998;15:755–758.
Nanda NC, Thakur AC, Thakur D, et al. Transesophageal echocardiographic examination of left subclavian artery branches. *Echocardiography* 1999;16:217–277.

Answer 4: A. The left innominate vein is typically visualized beneath the aortic arch. Hemiazygos and left subclavian veins are not usually anatomically present in this region. The left pulmonary artery is not a venous structure.

Suggested Reading

LaMotte LC, Nanda NC, Thakur ACC, et al. Transesophageal echocardiographic identification of neck veins: value of contrast echocardiography. *Echocardiography* 1998;15:259–267.

Answer 5: D. Congenital or acquired interruption of the inferior vena cava often results in a dilated hemiazygos vein, which appears as a large structure behind the descending thoracic aorta. Normally, these veins are small and not very conspicuous. Collaterals from coarctation of the aorta are arterial in nature. Dilated lymphatics do not produce Doppler signals because of the paucity of scatterers. Dilated intercostal veins beneath the descending thoracic aorta have never been reported.

Suggested Reading

Blanchard DG, Sobel JL, Hope J, et al. Infrahepatic interruption of the inferior vena cava with azygos continuation: a potential mimicker of aortic pathology. *J Am Soc Echocardiogr* 1998;11:1078–1083.

Answer 6: C. Insertion of the left superior pulmonary vein into the left atrium results in its invagination in that chamber, producing a ridge commonly called the "Coumadin" ridge. The left inferior pulmonary vein does not insert into the left atrium in the region of the left atrial appendage. It is formed by infolding of the left superior pulmonary vein.

Suggested Readings

Nanda NC, Domanski M. *Atlas of Transesophageal Echocardiography.* 2nd ed. Baltimore, MD: Lippincott Williams & Wilkins, 2007:36–40.
Pinheiro L, Nanda NC, Jain H, et al. Transesophageal echocardiographic imaging of the pulmonary veins. *Echocardiography* 1991;8:741–748.

Answer 7: B. Since any 2D TEE image represents only a thin slice through the appendage, a prominent pectinate muscle viewed in short axis can easily mimic a clot. This can be clarified by 3D TTE cropping, which provides both long- and short-axis views of pectinate muscles and hence can ascertain whether the structure in question is related to pectinate musculature. In certain patients, but not in all, 3D TTE may delineate all the lobes of the appendage. The 3D TTE image quality is inferior to 2D TEE and also 2D TTE, and hence, it is useful as a supplement to 2D TEE only in patients with good acoustic windows.

Suggested Reading

Karakus G, Kodali V, Inamdar V, et al. Comparative assessment of left atrial appendage by transesophageal and combined two and three-dimensional transthoracic echocardiography. *Echocardiography* 2008;25(8):918–927.

Answer 8: C. The intercostal artery on 2D/3D imaging and its flow pattern with color-flow and conventional Doppler are commonly seen during TEE, and these should be recognized as a normal arterial branches arising from the descending thoracic aorta. Therefore, Option E is incorrect. Maximal Doppler flow velocities >2.0 m/s indicate stenosis, which usually occurs at their origin from the aorta and is commonly due to involvement with the atherosclerotic process.

Suggested Reading

Ravi BS, Nanda NC, Htay T, et al. Transesophageal echocardiographic identification of normal and stenosed posterior intercostal arteries. *Echocardiography* 2003;20:609–615.

Answer 9: B. This view generally provides the maximum length between the mitral annulus and the apex and is the view with the least foreshortening. In general, TEE is inferior to TTE for comprehensive examination of the left ventricular apex. The other views often provide a foreshortened image of the left ventricle, resulting in nonvisualization or partial visualization of the apex.

Suggested Reading

Nanda NC, Domanski M. *Atlas of Transesophageal Echocardiography*. 2nd ed. Baltimore, MD: Lippincott Williams & Wilkins, 2007:304–325.

Answer 10: B. The tricuspid and pulmonary valves represent structures in the far field of the transducer as compared to other structures mentioned above and hence may not be fully evaluated by 2D TEE. The transducer used for 2D TEE is a higher-frequency transducer that has a limited capability for resolving structures located in the far field, that is, at a greater distance from the probe.

Suggested Reading

Nanda NC, Domanski M. *Atlas of Transesophageal Echocardiography*. 2nd ed. Baltimore, MD: Lippincott Williams & Wilkins, 2007:191–204.

Answer 11: D. The image is a transgastric, RV inflow view as the liver is visualized between the probe and the pericardium, and the closest chamber to the probe is a ventricle. In the midesophageal views, the chamber closest to the probe is the left atrium. Hence, answers A, C, and E are incorrect as it is not a midesophageal view.

Answer 12: A. See FIGURE 13.11. The arrow points to a mass with mixed echogenicity attached to the anterior wall of the right ventricle, which is better visualized on the video than in the still image. Given the clinical scenario, this is very likely endocarditis. Therefore, answer A is correct. The pericardial effusion visualized is small. Hence, answer B is incorrect. There is no evidence of severe tricuspid regurgitation as the structure of the tricuspid valves is preserved. Since there is no evidence of malcoaptation noted on the 2D images, there are no findings supportive of severe tricuspid regurgitation. Hence, answer C is incorrect. There are no standardized measurements for chamber size in transesophageal echocardiography. However, visually, there is no chamber enlargement in this patient. Hence, answer D is incorrect. There is no evidence of a foreign body in this image. Answer E is therefore incorrect.

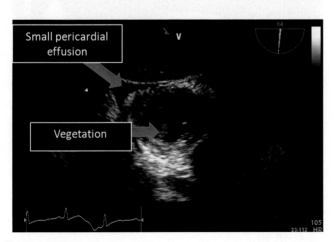

FIGURE 13.11

Suggested Reading

Reeves ST, et al. Basic perioperative transesophageal echocardiography examination: a consensus statement of the American Society of Echocardiography and the Society of Cardiovascular Anesthesiologists. *J Am Soc Echocardiogr* 2013;26:443–456.

Answer 13: C. The image shows a central line protruding to the right atrium through the superior vena cava (FIG. 13.12). The central line is identified by the echodense "tram track"–like parallel lines. On careful review, the video shows a round thrombus attached to this central catheter. Thrombus attachment is a known complication of central venous catheters protruding to the right atrium. Hence, answer C is correct, and if a catheter is seen in the right atrium during cardiac imaging, the ordering provider should be notified as there is a risk of thrombus formation and atrial arrhythmias.

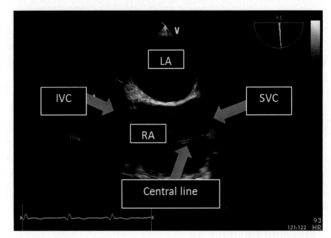

FIGURE 13.12

The thrombus is fixed to the central line and is therefore unlikely to be thrombus in transit. Hence, answer A is incorrect. There is no evidence of malignancy in this patient. In patients with ovarian cancer and renal cancer, metastasis may be visualized through the IVC, which is not seen in this image. Hence, answer B is incorrect. There is no evidence of a PFO on this image, which does not have color Doppler or saline bubble contrast. The rhythm seems to be sinus rhythm in the three beats recorded on the rhythm strip. Further, since there is a central line evident, answer C would be the most likely reason for thrombus formation.

Suggested Reading

Gilon D, Schechter D, Rein AJJT, et al. Right atrial thrombi are related to indwelling central venous catheter position: insights into time course and possible mechanism of formation. *Am Heart J* 1998;135(3):457–462.

Answer 14: A. The image is a midesophageal view around 60 degrees. The left atrial appendage is in view, and dense spontaneous echo contrast (smoke) with a mobile thrombus in the LAA is present (FIG. 13.13). This is more obvious on the video image where the thrombus has a "jello-like" appearance. Therefore, answer C is not the correct answer.

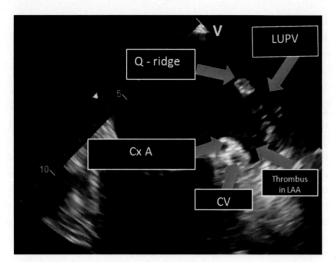

FIGURE 13.13

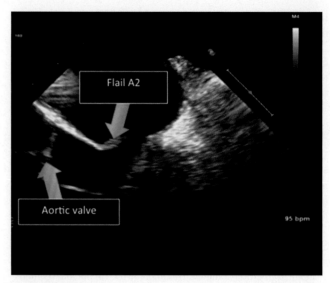

FIGURE 13.14

Immediately superior to the left atrial appendage is the Coumadin ridge or Q-ridge (also known as the Ligament of Marshall), which demarcates the left atrial appendage from the left upper pulmonary vein (LUPV). The right upper pulmonary vein is not seen in this view and enters the left atrium adjacent to the interatrial septum (IAS). Therefore, answer A is the correct answer to this question.

Two vessels are seen in cross-section in the atrioventricular groove. The smaller vessel is the circumflex artery (Cx A), and the larger, irregular, more superficial vessel is a coronary vein (CV) as it drains into the coronary sinus. Hence, answers D and E are not the correct answer.

Suggested Reading

Reeves ST, et al. Basic perioperative transesophageal echocardiography examination: a consensus statement of the American Society of Echocardiography and the Society of Cardiovascular Anesthesiologists. *J Am Soc Echocardiogr* 2013;26:443–456.

http://pie.med.utoronto.ca/TEE/TEE_content/TEE_spectral_leftAtrialAppendage.html

Answer 15: C. The image is a transgastric view. The marked segments are the midinferior and inferior septal segments, which are commonly supplied by the right coronary artery. Rarely, a dominant circumflex artery may also supply these segments. It is important to be cognizant of the fact that the segments will be reversed in the transgastric short-axis view in TEE when compared to transthoracic short-axis views (VIDEO 13.9).

Suggested Reading

Lang RM, et al. Recommendations for chamber quantification: a report from the American Society of Echocardiography's Guidelines and Standards Committee and the Chamber Quantification Writing Group, developed in conjunction with the European Association of Echocardiography, a branch of the European Society of Cardiology. *J Am Soc Echocardiogr* 2005;18(12):1440–1463.

Answer 16: E. The still image and the video images show that the edge of the anterior mitral leaflet moves beyond the coaptation point (flail) during systole, giving rise to severe mitral regurgitation. Therefore, the most likely reason for sudden severe shortness of breath is chordal rupture giving rise to a flail anterior mitral leaflet.

It is important for the echocardiographer to be familiar with the Carpentier classification for mitral scallops, as this would be the terminology commonly used when describing diseased mitral valves.

In the given image, the aortic valve is visible in a "reverse long-axis" image. When the aortic valve is seen in long axis, the mitral scallops visualized are usually the A2 and P2 segments. Therefore, the flail segment is the A2 segment, and answer E is the correct answer (FIGS. 13.14 AND 13.15, VIDEOS 13.4 AND 13.10).

Although PE should always be suspected in the postoperative orthopedic patient who has sudden severe shortness of breath, there is no indirect evidence of a pulmonary embolism (RV dilation or abnormal septal motion) on this echocardiogram. Hence, answer A is incorrect and not the best option.

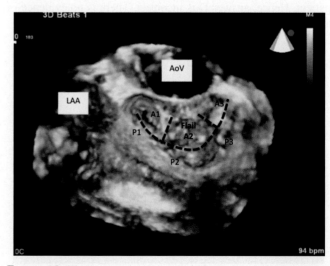

FIGURE 13.15

The presentation is unlikely to be due to chronic severe mitral regurgitation as the flail leaflets usually cause acute severe mitral regurgitation. Therefore, answer B is not the most correct option.

The images show the LV is small in size. The video image clearly excludes severe LV dysfunction as the LV systolic function is hyperdynamic. Hence, answer C is incorrect.

This patient was afebrile on presentation. Considering there is no clinical picture suggestive of endocarditis, answer D is a less correct option. Endocarditis is a clinical diagnosis with confirmatory echocardiographic findings.

Suggested Readings

Himelman RB. The flail mitral valve: echocardiographic findings by precordial and transesophageal imaging and Doppler color flow mapping. *J Am Coll Cardiol* 1991;17(1):272–279.

Pearson AC, St Vrain J, Mrosek D, et al. Color Doppler echocardiographic evaluation of patients with a flail mitral leaflet. *J Am Coll Cardiol* 1990;16(1):232–239.

Answer 17: B. The video shows a midesophageal view that optimizes the septum secundum of the interatrial septum during a saline bubble study. The images show that the interatrial septum is aneurysmal with a bidirectional movement of more than 20 mm (evident in the still images as well as the video). Therefore, the correct answer is B.

A small amount of bubbles is seen crossing the interatrial septum immediately after the leftward shift and following the peak opacification. Hence, this study is abnormal and commonly referred to as "positive" for the presence of a patent foramen ovale. Therefore, answer A is incorrect. While it could be challenging to get a patient to perform a Valsalva maneuver during a TEE study, minimal sedation enabling better patient cooperation and applying abdominal pressure are ways of improving the sensitivity of the test. To confirm that an adequate maneuver is performed, one should monitor the atrial septal motion for a transient leftward shift. In patients with aneurysmal motion, additional shifting may not be necessary to "open" the PFO, and bubbles often pass through despite poor patient cooperation or prior to Valsalva.

The area opacified marked by a red star is the pulmonary artery. This could be identified as it is parallel to the ascending aorta and is densely opacified confirming it is a right-sided structure. Answer C is therefore wrong. The transverse sinus is the small echo-free pericardial space between the aorta and the pulmonary artery.

The contrast used for this study is saline microbubbles. Commercially available microbubbles are commonly used for opacification of left-sided chambers. Hence, answer D is incorrect.

According to the current recommendations, first-line therapy for a PFO in the setting of a cryptogenic stroke is antiplatelet therapy followed by anticoagulation. Percutaneous closure at present is recommended in the setting of failure of the above treatment options.

Hence, answer E is incorrect. Patients with a cryptogenic stroke and PFO are encouraged to enroll in ongoing trials that further examine optimum treatment options.

Suggested Readings

Attaran R, Ata I, Kudithipudi V, et al. Protocol for optimal detection and exclusion of a patent foramen ovale using transthoracic echocardiography with agitated saline microbubbles. *Echocardiography* 2006;23(7):616–622.

Cabanes L, Coste J, Derumeaux G, et al. Interobserver and intraobserver variability in detection of patent foramen ovale and atrial septal aneurysm with transesophageal echocardiography. *J Am Soc Echocardiogr* 2002;15:441–446.

Lansberg MG, O'Donnell MJ, Khatri P, et al. Antithrombotic and thrombolytic therapy for ischemic stroke: antithrombotic therapy and prevention of thrombosis, 9th ed: American College of Chest Physicians Evidence-Based Clinical Practice Guidelines. *Chest* 2012;141:e601S–e636S.

Answer 18: D. The image is the midesophageal ascending aortic short-axis view of the aorta in cross-section. The pulmonary trunk is present to the left of the ascending aorta (B). Following the pulmonary valve (C), the MPA bifurcates to the left (D) and right (A) pulmonary arteries.

In a normal heart, the pulmonary valve is anterior and to the left of the aorta. The RPA "hugs" the ascending aorta and aortic valve.

Therefore, A to D is as follows: A, right pulmonary artery; B, ascending aorta; C, pulmonary valve; and D, left pulmonary artery.

Answer 19: B. The scale to the left of the image shows that the ascending aorta is dilated to almost 7 cm. Surgical intervention is recommended when an ascending aortic aneurysm is dilated >5.0 to 5.5 cm. Hence, this patient was referred for aortic aneurysm repair.

Williams syndrome is a genetic disorder in which supravalvular aortic stenosis is present. Answer A is incorrect as the ascending aorta is aneurysmal in this case.

There is no evidence of coarctation since the aortic arch is not visualized. Hence, answer C is incorrect. The visualized segments of the pulmonary trunk are of normal caliber, and there is no pulmonary atresia. Therefore, answer D is incorrect.

Suggested Readings

http://www.echobasics.de/tee-en.html

Collins RT II. Cardiovascular disease in Williams syndrome. *Circulation* 2013;127(21):2125–2134.

Svensson LG. Aortic valve and ascending aorta guidelines for management and quality measures: executive summary. *Ann Thorac Surg* 2013;95(4):1491–1505.

Answer 20: C. The image is close to a midesophageal bicaval view.

As noted in the image (Fig. 13.16), the left atrium (LA), right atrium (RA), and the interatrial septum (IAS) are visualized in this view. The SVC is to the right of the screen, while the IVC is to the left. In this patient, the structure marked with an asterisk is the eustachian valve, which is an embryologic remnant, attached to the IVC to RA junction. To better visualize this structure, the probe should be advanced toward the IVC. Therefore, answer C is correct.

To obtain this view, from a view of the short-axis aortic valve, the probe should be rotated, so the ultrasound beam is

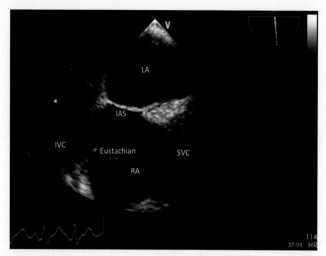

FIGURE 13.16

directed more to the right of the patient. Clockwise rotation enables structures on the right side to be better visualized. Hence, answer A is incorrect in stating that counterclockwise rotation would obtain this view.

To visualize the SVC, the probe should be withdrawn from this position as the SVC is a superior structure. Further advancing the probe would help to better study the IVC and not the SVC. Hence, answer B is incorrect. In the video accompanying this question, a central catheter is seen in the SVC.

Clockwise rotation of the probe would not help to better evaluate the LA since the ultrasound beam needs to be focused to the left of the patient for this purpose. Hence, counterclockwise rotation would help to better evaluate the LA. Answer D is therefore incorrect.

The coronary sinus is best seen when the probe is advanced to the gastroesophageal junction. When advancing the probe to a transgastric position, the coronary sinus could be well seen. Hence, answer E is incorrect in stating that withdrawing the probe would help to visualize the coronary sinus.

Suggested Readings

http://pie.med.utoronto.ca/TEE/TEE_content/TEE_probeManipulation_intro.html

Peters PJ, Reinhardt S. The echocardiographic evaluation of intracardiac masses: a review. *J Am Soc Echocardiogr* 2006;19(2):230–240.

Chapter 14

Abnormal TEE Anatomy

Sasanka Jayasuriya

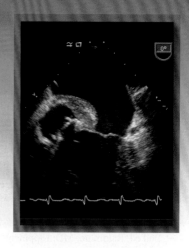

1. Which of the following 2D echo findings is most typical of an aortic dissection?

    A. A linear echo with irregular motion (mimicking a worm wiggling) in the aorta

    B. A linear echo roughly parallel to the walls of the aorta

    C. A linear echo perpendicular to the aortic walls

    D. None of the above

2. During the immediate postbypass period after mitral valve surgery, which of the following findings on transesophageal color-flow Doppler is **LEAST** likely to represent severe residual mitral regurgitation?

    A. Systolic MR flow noted in the left atrial appendage.

    B. MR flow seen in the left inferior but not left superior pulmonary vein.

    C. MR flow area within the LA cavity measures >8 cm².

    D. The MR jet has multiple origins.

    E. Each of these is consistent with severe MR.

3. Aortic transection is characterized by:

    A. A linear echo in the aortic lumen parallel to the aortic walls

    B. A linear echo not parallel but perpendicular to the aortic walls

    C. Multiple linear echoes in the aorta

    D. Absence of any linear echo in the aorta since the patient has transection, not dissection

4. A 72-year-old female develops pulmonary edema 5 days following a nonrevascularized inferior wall myocardial infarction and also has a 5/6 grade harsh pansystolic murmur heard throughout the precordium and a new palpable thrill. The TTE echo was extremely limited due to COPD. Which 2D TEE window will most likely visualize the suspected pathologic finding?

    A. Four-chamber view

    B. Short-axis view at the level of the papillary muscles

    C. Two-chamber view

    D. Transgastric views

5. A 45-year-old African American male presented with dysarthria and weakness of the left side of the body with complete recovery in 15 minutes. Past history was significant for mild systemic hypertension, well controlled with a thiazide diuretic and an ACE inhibitor. Physical examination was essentially unremarkable with a BP of 128/82 mm Hg. Routine 2D TTE was normal except for borderline left ventricular hypertrophy. A TEE with a bubble study was next performed. During intravenous saline injection, no shunt was initially detected, but a repeat study with manual abdominal pressure showed bubbles crossing the atrial septum into the left atrium (VIDEO 14.1). Since the patient was well sedated during the TEE study, it was not possible for him to do a Valsalva maneuver, and hence, abdominal pressure was applied. This case illustrates the importance of raising the right atrial pressure above the left atrial pressure using abdominal pressure during saline injection without which the patent foramen ovale (PFO) would not have been diagnosed. Normally, the PFO is closed because the left atrial pressure is higher than the right atrial pressure, which keeps both the septum primum and septum secundum in close apposition with each other. When the right atrial pressure is increased, the septum primum separates from the septum secundum opening up the PFO. The effectiveness of abdominal compression is judged by noting the movement or bulge of the atrial septum toward the left atrium. A PFO cannot be excluded with certainty if no bulge is noted during a bubble study because this would mean that the right atrial pressure was not elevated above the left atrial pressure. In this patient, it was decided not to close the PFO since this was the first occurrence and a DVT screen was negative. The patient was sent home on aspirin.

In which of the following conditions would the TEE bubble study with abdominal pressure be negative even if a PFO was present?

    A. Severe tricuspid stenosis and regurgitation

    B. Mild aortic regurgitation

    C. Severe mitral regurgitation

    D. Chronic obstructive pulmonary disease

6. During a transthoracic bubble study, contrast bubbles were seen in the left heart chambers. This patient was diagnosed to have an intrapulmonary shunt because:

    A. Bubbles appeared in the left heart after seven cardiac beats.

    B. Bubbles were noted in the left ventricle but not in the left atrium.

    C. Bubbles were noted only with the Valsalva maneuver.

    D. Bubbles appeared to be smaller in size than with a PFO.

Answer 1: A. A linear echo with irregular motion like a wiggling worm is most diagnostic of aortic dissection. An echo parallel to the walls of the aorta may, in many instances, be due to an artifact. An echo perpendicular to the walls of the aorta is not typical of aortic dissection.

Suggested Readings

Ballal RS, Nanda NC, Gatewood R, et al. Usefulness of transesophageal echocardiography in the assessment of aortic dissection. *Circulation* 1991;84:1903–1914.

Nanda NC, Domanski M. *Atlas of Transesophageal Echocardiography.* 2nd ed. Baltimore, MD: Lippincott Williams & Wilkins, 2007: 145–160.

Answer 2: D. Mitral regurgitation is considered severe if it extends into *any pulmonary vein* in systole or *left atrial appendage* in the immediate postbypass period. Therefore, answers A and B are incorrect options. It is also severe if the MR color-flow area by planimetry measures more than 8 cm². A large PISA or vena contracta of the regurgitant jet may also provide a clue to severe mitral regurgitation especially when the jet is eccentric and abutting the mitral leaflets or adjacent left atrial wall. This will reduce its area considerably because the impact of the eccentric jet against another structure will diminish its velocity, resulting in decreased turbulence. The presence of multiple jets on color-flow Doppler is not a marker of MR severity and would be expected to be seen on the vertical, 90-degree (intercommissural) TEE view. Therefore, Option D is the correct answer.

Suggested Reading

Nanda NC, Domanski M. *Atlas of Transesophageal Echocardiography.* 2nd ed. Baltimore, MD: Lippincott Williams & Wilkins, 2007: 71–78.

Answer 3: B. The transected internal or intimal–medial layer protrudes into the aortic lumen, and hence, the linear echo mimicking a dissection flap is roughly perpendicular to the walls of the aorta. On the other hand, with aortic dissection, the flap often has a very irregular motion (like a "worm wiggling" in the aorta) but still tends to be generally parallel to the aortic walls. Also, in transection, the perpendicular linear echo is often localized to the aortic isthmus (junction of the aortic arch with the descending thoracic aorta). The isthmus is relatively fixed compared to other aortic segments and hence has a greater tendency to transect during traumatic injury.

The reference discusses this aspect well.

Suggested Reading

Galvin IF, Black IW, Lee CL, et al. Transesophageal echocardiography in acute aortic transection. *Ann Thorac Surg* 1991;51:310–311.

Answer 4: D. This patient most likely has a postinfarct acute ventricular septal defect (VSD). Because these defects occur in the posterior ventricular septum, they are often not detected during examination performed with the probe positioned in the esophagus. Therefore, Options A and C are incorrect. They are best visualized with the transgastric approach that images the LV inferior wall and the posterior and inferior portions of the ventricular septum. Examination should be performed with the color Doppler turned on to visualize flow signals moving from the left ventricle to the right ventricle through the rupture site. The four-chamber view generally visualizes the anterior, not posterior, portion of the ventricular septum. The two-chamber view images the inferior and anterior walls of the left ventricle, not the septum. It is difficult to obtain a short-axis view at the level of the papillary muscles with the transducer positioned in the esophagus, but it is much easier to do this with the probe positioned in the stomach. Although a mid–short-axis image (at the level of the papillary muscles) may identify the VSD, it would be more likely from a basal short-axis view since most VSDs occur at this location. Therefore, Option B is incorrect.

Suggested Readings

Balal RS, Sanyal RS, Nanda NC, et al. Usefulness of transesophageal echocardiography in the diagnosis of ventricular septal rupture secondary to acute myocardial infarction. *Am J Cardiol* 1993;71:367–370.

Kishon Y, Iqbal A, Oh JK, et al. Evolution of echocardiographic modalities in detection of post myocardial infarction ventricular septal defect and papillary muscle rupture: study of 62 patients. *Am Heart J* 1993;126:667–675.

Nanda NC, Domanski M. *Atlas of Transesophageal Echocardiography.* 2nd ed. Baltimore, MD: Lippincott Williams & Wilkins, 2007: 290–293.

Answer 5: C. In patients with severe mitral regurgitation, the left atrial pressure would be expected to be elevated, making it unlikely to elevate the right atrial pressure above the high left atrial pressure with abdominal compression. Left atrial pressure would not be elevated in patients with mild aortic regurgitation, and hence, the bubble study with abdominal compression would still be positive. Severe tricuspid stenosis and regurgitation and COPD may result in raised right atrial pressure, which would facilitate bubbles crossing over into the left atrium.

> *Editor's Note: A common testing practice is to provide clinical scenarios that cause common hemodynamic alterations rather than listing the actual hemodynamics. In this situation, the reader must recognize the "focus" of the question (the teaching point) in order to select the most likely clinical scenario.*

Suggested Reading

Attaran RA, et al. Protocol for optimal detection and exclusion of a patent foramen ovale using transthoracic echocardiography with agitated saline microbubbles. *Echocardiography* 2006; 23(7):616–622.

Answer 6: A. Bubbles with a PFO usually appear within three beats following arrival in the right atrium or appear with the Valsalva maneuver, which would be expected to raise the right atrial pressure above that in the left atrium. On the other hand, bubbles from an intrapulmonary shunt appear typically much later because of the longer circulation time taken by the bubbles to travel to the lungs from the right atrium. The "size" of the bubbles has no relation to the presence of a PFO or intrapulmonary shunt. Bubbles may not be noted in the left atrium with either a PFO or intrapulmonary shunt because of the slice-like nature of a 2D section that could transect a portion of the left atrium that has no bubbles. Moving and angling the transducer would bring into view different sections of the left atrium and increase the chances of observing the bubbles in that chamber as well.

Suggested Readings

Attaran RR, Ata I, Kudithipudi V, et al. Protocol for optimal detection and exclusion of a patent foramen ovale using transthoracic echocardiography with agitated saline microbubbles. *Echocardiography* 2006;23:616–622.

Gupta V, Yesilbursa D, Huang WY, et al. Patient foramen ovale in a large population of ischemic stroke patients: diagnosis, age distribution, gender and race. *Echocardiography* 2008;25:217–227.

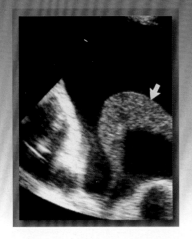

Chapter 15

Noncardiac Findings on Echocardiograms

Vincent L. Sorrell

1. What is the estimated incidence of management-altering non-cardiac findings on routine transthoracic echocardiograms?

A. Very rare and reported at 0.5% to 1.0%

B. More common in outpatient requests compared to inpatient requests

C. Very common, occurring at an incidence of >20.0% in most outpatient clinics

D. Relatively common, occurring at a reported incidence of 9% in the hospital setting

E. Very common, occurring at a reported incidence of 15.5% and requiring a critical evaluation of noncardiac structures in all patients

2. A 65-year-old male with cirrhosis is seen in clinic for evaluation of liver transplant. An echo is done as a preoperative screening exam. On the subcostal view, a mobile structure is seen in FIGURE 15.1. The echo noted by the arrow is due to:

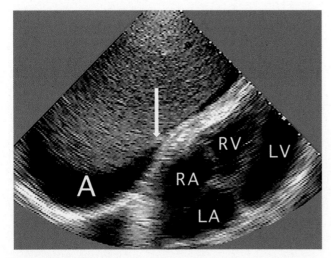

FIGURE 15.1

A. Falciform ligament

B. Pericardial fibrinous material

C. Ascites fibrinous material

D. Pericardial cyst

3. A 68-year-old male with diabetes, hypertension, and prior myocardial infarction presents with a chief complaint of difficulty in breathing. Physical exam showed decreased breath sounds at bilateral lung bases, cardiomegaly, and lower extremity edema. Electrocardiogram showed old anterior myocardial infarction. Chest x-ray showed moderate bilateral pleural effusions and mild prominence of pulmonary vasculature. Echocardiogram showed mild dilation of the left ventricle and moderate reduction in left ventricular function with regional wall motion abnormalities, and the image is shown in FIGURE 15.2.

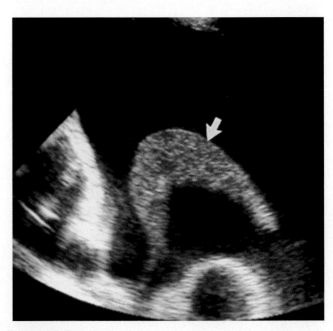

FIGURE 15.2

What is the large echo-dense mass shown?

A. Pericardial tumor

B. Left ventricular pseudoaneurysm

C. Atelectatic lung segment

D. Extramural cardiac tumor

4. Which of the following would be the most serious noncardiac finding on transthoracic echo?

   A. Well-demarcated echo-lucent circular area within the liver parenchyma on the subcostal view

   B. Echo-free space posterior to the heart in a patient in supine or left lateral position

   C. Highly reflective echo areas within the gallbladder, with mobility upon repositioning the patient, and marked posterior acoustic shadowing

   D. Mobile lobulated echo-dense structure seen in the inferior vena cava extending into the right atrium

   E. Echo-free space located between the liver and diaphragm, outside the pericardial sac

5. Which of the following would be a typical associated finding on transthoracic subcostal echocardiography in a patient with a large mass invading and filling the lumen of the inferior vena cava and extending into the right atrium?

   A. Turbulent color Doppler flow entering the right atrium

   B. Bowing of the intra-atrial septum toward the left atrium

   C. Hepatic vein flow reversal in inspiration

   D. Echo-lucent mass seen in the inferior vena cava entering the right atrium

   E. Elevated tricuspid regurgitation jet velocity

6. A 64-year-old female with hypertension and obesity presents with substernal chest pain and rapid onset of dyspnea. Stat echocardiogram showed the following (Fig. 15.3 and Video 15.1):

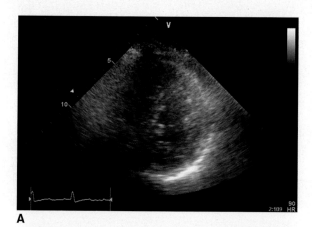

A

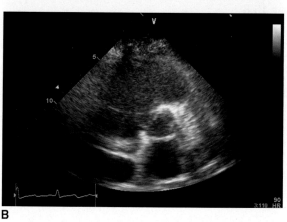

B

Figure 15.3

What is the most likely etiology of the patient's chest pain and dyspnea and most optimal immediate course of management?

   A. Acute right ventricular infarction; urgent coronary angiography

   B. Left ventricular failure; IV furosemide

   C. Saddle pulmonary embolus; consider urgent thrombolysis

   D. Chronic pulmonary hypertension; urgent left and right heart catheter

7. What is the structure denoted by the arrow in Figure 15.4?

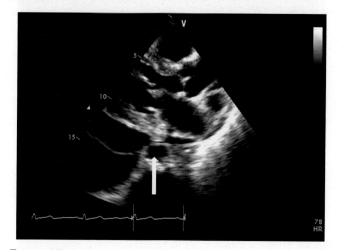

Figure 15.4

   A. Dilated coronary sinus

   B. Thoracic descending aorta

   C. Thoracic ascending aorta

   D. Hepatic cyst

   E. Pericardial cyst

8. A patient with weight loss and dyspnea is sent to the echo lab for evaluation. A mass is noted in the inferior vena cava on subcostal view. Which is *most* likely to be the source (Fig. 15.5, Videos 15.2 and 15.3)?

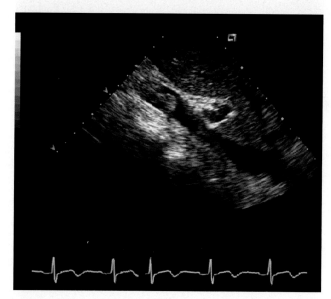

Figure 15.5

A. Renal cell carcinoma
B. Melanoma
C. Colon carcinoma
D. Leiomyosarcoma

9. A 75-year-old female presents for a transesophageal echo-cardiogram prior to a procedure for inserting an atrial occluder device. The images obtained immediately after insertion of the occluder are shown. What is the structure seen in FIGURES 15.6 AND 15.7?

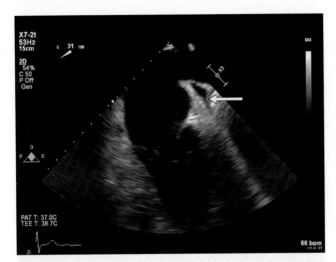

FIGURE 15.6

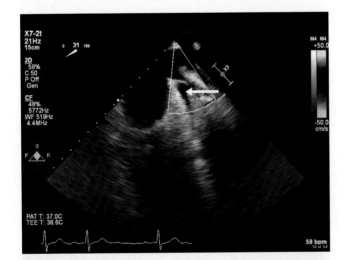

FIGURE 15.7

A. Right superior pulmonary vein
B. Transverse sinus
C. Oblique sinus
D. Coumadin ridge

10. A 72-year-old female with hypertension and hyperlip-idemia was referred for a transthoracic echocardiogram for atypical chest pain. What structure is identified by the arrow in FIGURE 15.8A?

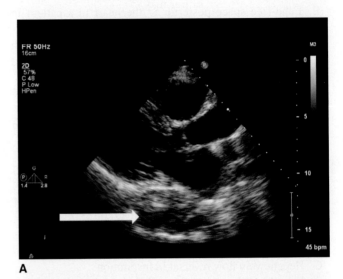

A

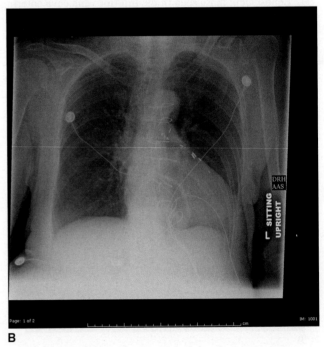

B

FIGURE 15.8

A. Descending aortic aneurysm
B. Dilated coronary sinus
C. Aortic dissection
D. Hiatal hernia
E. Pericardial tumor

11. A 55-year-old male with a recent diagnosis of esophageal cancer is referred from the oncology service for evaluation of LV function prior to therapy. A TTE suggests a mass posterolateral to the LA as shown by the arrow (Fɪɢ. 15.9). The most likely cause of this mass is:

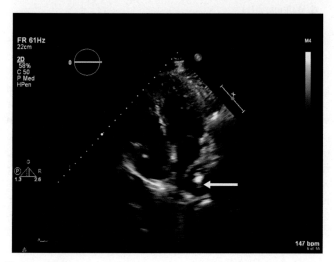

Fɪɢᴜʀᴇ 15.9

A. Thoracic vertebra
B. Coronary calcification
C. Dilated coronary sinus
D. Esophageal mass
E. Artifact from reverberation

Answer 1: D. The prevalence of noncardiac findings on routine TTE has largely been based on case reports and small series. The largest study, a retrospective study of >1,000 consecutive clinical comprehensive transthoracic echocardiograms (TTE) performed during a month at a tertiary academic medical center, showed 7.5% of patients had noncardiac findings (NCF). There was increased prevalence of NCF among inpatient TTE studies as compared to outpatient studies (10.6% versus 5.3%, $P = 0.003$) and an increased prevalence of potentially management-altering NCF on inpatient studies as compared to outpatient studies (9.0% versus 3.0%, $P = 0.002$). Management-altering findings were defined as pleural effusions, ascites, cholelithiasis, metastasis, or venous thromboses.

Suggested Reading

Manning WJ, et al. Prevalence of noncardiac pathology on clinical transthoracic echocardiography. *J Am Soc Echocardiogr* 2012;25(5):553–560.

Answer 2: A. The falciform ligament is an important finding on TTE to determine the presence of ascites. The falciform ligament is a thin peritoneal fold that runs anterior–posterior. It connects the liver to the posterior aspect of the anterior abdominal wall just to the right of the midline and represents a remnant of the umbilical vein and the in vitro vitelline circulation. The falciform ligament is usually not seen on TTE unless ascites is present. It is best seen on the subdiaphragmatic view. Pericardial fibrinous material is incorrect as it would be seen

in the pericardial space and contained within the pericardium. Ascites fibrinous material is seen in the intra-abdominal space and would be thinner and more filamentous on echo. A pericardial cyst would be a round cystic-like structure located adjacent to the pericardium. It would not appear linear on echo.

Suggested Readings

Cardello FP, et al. The falciform ligament in the echocardiographic diagnosis of ascites. *J Am Soc Echocardiogr* 2006;19:1074. e3–1074.e4.
Kerut EK, et al. Utility of identification of the falciform ligament in the echocardiography laboratory. *Echocardiography* 2007;24(8):887–888.

Answer 3: C. Atelectatic lung segments are seen frequently in cross-sectional imaging of the heart but not well described in the literature. They are usually seen as free-floating echo-bright well-delineated objects lateral to the heart, and they are almost always seen in the presence of moderate to large pleural effusions. Atelectatic lung segments may be differentiated from extracardiac pericardial tumors or cysts as they are not attached to the pericardium, and they often have a ground-glass appearance. They will be sharply delineated from the sonolucent area of the pleural effusion. The mass would likely resolve after thoracentesis. CT is the ideal ancillary imaging modality to verify the diagnosis. A pericardial cyst would be a round cystic-like structure located adjacent to the pericardium, and it (as well as an extramural cardiac tumor) would not be seen within the abdominal cavity. A left ventricular pseudoaneurysm would be seen best in apical views. It represents a contained rupture of the left ventricular free wall. The wall of a pseudoaneurysm is composed of organized thrombus and varying portions of the epicardium. It is best differentiated from a true aneurysm by a "narrow neck."

Suggested Reading

Mann DL, et al. Cross-sectional echocardiographic characterization of atelectatic lung segments: differentiation from extracardiac tumors. *Chest* 1990;92(2):404–406.

Answer 4: D. Option A represents a simple liver cyst; option B represents left pleural effusion; option C represents cholelithiasis; option D represents venous thrombosis; and option E represents ascites. Noncardiac findings (NCF) are generally classified as benign, indeterminate, or worrisome on transthoracic echo (TTE). Benign NCF include simple hepatic cysts, hemangiomas, or cholelithiasis; these are findings that would not generally alter management or require follow-up assessment. Indeterminate NCF might require some follow-up assessment such as pleural effusions or ascites. Worrisome NCF include metastases or venous thrombosis; findings that would prompt urgent follow-up imaging and greatly impact patient management.

Suggested Readings

Khosa F, et al. Prevalence of non-cardiac findings on clinical cardiovascular MRI. *AJR Am J Roentgenol* 2011;1996:380–386.
Manning WJ, et al. Prevalence of non-cardiac pathology on clinical transthoracic echocardiography. *J Am Soc Echocardiogr* 2012;25(5):553–560.

Answer 5: *A.* A large mass seen at the inferior vena cava (IVC, right atrial junction) would potentially cause flow obstruction into the right atrium. Thus, there would be turbulent color Doppler flow seen into the right atrium similar to a stenosis. With obstruction to right atrial inflow, there is the possibility for lower right atrial pressures, and thus, the intra-atrial septum would not bow to the left. A renal cell mass would be echo-dense and not echo-lucent such as a cystic structure. There should be no elevation in the velocity of the tricuspid regurgitant jet and thus no elevation in peak systolic pulmonary pressures (unless there is evidence of large pulmonary emboli present). This is a common presentation of renal cell carcinomas. Hepatic vein flow reversal in inspiration is seen with restrictive cardiomyopathies and not with masses in the IVC.

Suggested Reading

Ananthasubramaniam K, et al. Metastatic renal cell cancer detected by transoesophageal echocardiography. *Heart* 2000;83:708–710.

Answer 6: *C.* The images demonstrate hyperdynamic left ventricular function and a freely mobile echo-dense structure seen in the right pulmonary artery just near the bifurcation of the main pulmonary artery. This is an acute pulmonary embolism. In addition, there is right ventricular dilation, right ventricular dysfunction, and right ventricular pressure overload as noted by the "D-shaped" intraventricular septum. The clinical scenario is consistent with right ventricular strain due to a massive pulmonary embolus.

> ***Editor's Note:*** *The final decision to use thrombolytic therapy (in addition to immediate IV anticoagulation) is individually determined after weighing the benefits versus risks. In the absence of any overt contraindications, the greatest benefit of lytic therapy will be in patients with evidence of shock, respiratory failure, or moderate to severe RV strain (defined by marked RV hypokinesis [as seen in this patient], RV systolic pressure >40 mm Hg, and/or elevated cardiac biomarkers). Therefore, Option C is correct and thrombolysis should be considered.*

Suggested Readings

Feigenbaum H, Armstrong WF, Ryan T, eds. *Feigenbaum's Echocardiography*. 7th ed. Philadelphia, PA: Lippincott Williams & Wilkins, 2011.

Jaff MR, et al. Management of massive and submassive pulmonary embolism, iliofemoral deep vein thrombosis, and chronic thromboembolic pulmonary hypertension. A scientific statement from the American Heart Association. *Circulation* 2011;123:1788–1830.

Otto C. *Textbook of Clinical Echocardiography*. 3rd ed. Philadelphia, PA: Elsevier, 2004:39–70.

Answer 7: *B.* The structure denoted by the arrow is the thoracic descending aorta. The thoracic descending aorta is not contained within the pericardial sac, as seen in this image. The pericardium is anterior to the thoracic descending aorta. In this image, there are both a pericardial effusion as well as a pleural effusion. A dilated coronary sinus would be contained within the pericardium and seen adjacent to the atrioventricular grove. Similarly, a pericardial cyst would be seen within the pericardial space. The liver is not seen in this view, and thus, a hepatic cyst would not be visualized in this view.

Suggested Reading

Feigenbaum H, Armstrong WF, Ryan T, eds. *Feigenbaum's Echocardiography*. 7th ed. Philadelphia, PA: Lippincott Williams & Wilkins, 2011.

Answer 8: *A.* Tumor metastases from renal cell carcinomas and hypernephromas are several times more common to involve the heart than primary tumors. However, renal cancers, hepatomas, and leiomyosarcomas can all present on echocardiography as echo-dense structures in the inferior vena cava. Leiomyosarcomas are a rare type of sarcoma that results from smooth tissue. Leiomyosarcomas can spread via transvenous route with extension of tumor thrombus into the right atrium via the superior or inferior vena cava. It is quite rare that adenocarcinoma of the colon presents with transvenous metastatic tumor advancement in the inferior vena cava. Colon cancer is more likely to metastasize via direct mediastinal/thoracic invasion of the pericardium and epicardium.

Suggested Readings

Abraham KP, Reddy V, Gattuso P. Neoplasms to the heart: review of 3314 consecutive autopsies. *Am J Pathol* 1990;3:195–198.

Chiles C, Woodard PK, Gutierrez FR, et al. Metastatic involvement of the heart and pericardium: CT and MR imaging. *Radiographics* 2001;21:439–449.

Makhija Z, Deshpande R, Desai J. Unusual tumours of the heart: diagnostic and prognostic implications. *J Cardiothorac Surg* 2009;4:4.

Moreno-Vega AL, Fuentes-Pradera J, Gordón-Santiago Mdel M, et al. Intraventricular metastases from rectal-sigmoid adenocarcinoma. *Clin Transl Oncol* 2006;8(4):296–297.

Martin JL, Boak JG. Cardiac metastasis from uterine leiomyosarcoma. *J Am Coll Cardiol* 1983;2(2):383–386.

Answer 9: *C.* The arrow points to the oblique sinus, which represents the pericardial space between the left atrium and posterior pericardial sac and is easily seen when there is pericardial fluid present. The atrial appendage is not seen in these images since the occluder has been deployed. The color still frame identifies the right superior pulmonary vein and the adjacent "Coumadin ridge."

Answer A is incorrect since the small echo-free space is adjacent to the border of the LA appendage, too small for a pulmonary vein, and close to the *left*, but not *right*, superior pulmonary vein course.

The transverse sinus is the space posterior to the great arteries. The *"Coumadin ridge"* (*so-called because it was historically misinterpreted as an atrial thrombus*) separates the left superior pulmonary vein from the left atrial appendage. The oblique sinus is often seen in transesophageal studies of the left atrial appendage.

Suggested Readings

Maltagliati A, Pepi M, Tamborin G, et al. Usefulness of multiplane transesophageal echocardiography in the recognition of artifacts and normal anatomical variants that may mimic left atrial thrombi in patients with atrial fibrillation. *Ital Heart J* 2003;4(11):797–802.

Otto C. *Textbook of Clinical Echocardiography*. 3rd ed. Philadelphia, PA: Elsevier, 2004:39–70.

Veinot JP, Harrity PJ, Gentile F, et al. Anatomy of the normal left atrial appendage: a quantitative study of age-related changes in 500 autopsy hearts: implications for echocardiographic examination. *Circulation* 1997;96(9):3112–3115.

Answer 10: D. The arrow is pointing to an echo-free space behind the left side of the heart that is partially compressing the left atrium and is consistent with the common location and echo appearance of a hiatal hernia. The chest radiograph (Fig. 15.8B) also demonstrates a large hiatal hernia. Hiatal hernias can compress the left atrium and are often mistaken for left atrial masses on TTE. Ingestion of a carbonated beverage will produce a contrast effect in the stomach and aid to better diagnose a hiatal hernia. Short-axis and subcostal imagings are additional views to visualize a hernia. Hiatal hernias typically displace the descending aorta posteriorly, and thus, the aorta is not seen in the parasternal long-axis view. A dilated coronary sinus is best seen in the atrioventricular groove. Although a saccular aortic aneurysm may be seen in this location and should be considered in the differential diagnosis, this echo and CXR is not typical for an aortic dissection. Pericardial tumors are usually associated with pericardial effusions and rarely this large.

Suggested Readings

D'Cruz IA, Hancock HL. Echocardiographic characteristics of diaphragmatic hiatus hernia. *Am J Cardiol* 1995;75:308–310.

Hunley SO, et al. Thoracic aortic aneurysm presenting as pulmonary vein stenosis: a case presentation and review of the literature. *Echocardiography* 1998;15(5):493–498.

Koskinas K, Oikonomou K, Karapatsoudi E, et al. Echocardiographic manifestation of hiatus hernia simulating a left atrial mass. *Cardiovasc Ultrasound* 2008;6:46.

Answer 11: D. The patient has a history of cancer in the esophagus and the mass is located in the region of the left midposterior thorax, between the LA and descending aorta. This is most likely an image from the tumor itself. The spine may be imaged in thin patients as a bright surface but posteriorly produces shadowing. Although it is possible to see coronary artery calcification during routine echocardiography, this would not be a location where the coronary might be seen. The mass seen here is irregular but generally round but not in a typical location of the descending aorta. The coronary sinus is seen as horizontal and posterior to the mitral valve in this imaging plane. An artifact is not likely since there is not nearby echo-reflective structure in the lateral or near fields.

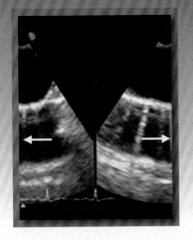

Chapter 16

Image Acquisition (from Here to There)

Vincent L. Sorrell

For each of the pairs of images described in the questions, select the maneuver (or maneuvers) from the following list that is (are) necessary to be performed by the operator to move from image A to image B (may select up to two answers).

Options

A. Insert TEE probe
B. Withdrawal TEE probe
C. Rotate clockwise
D. Rotate counterclockwise
E. Superior tilt TTE probe
F. Inferior tilt TTE probe
G. Anteflex TEE probe
H. Retroflex TEE probe
I. Rotate TEE imaging sector to larger angle
J. Rotate TEE imaging sector to smaller angle
K. Move probe to a new window

1.
  A. Apical four-chamber view
  B. Apical two-chamber view

2.
  A. Apical three-chamber view
  B. Apical two-chamber view

3.
  A. Parasternal long-axis view
  B. Parasternal short-axis view

4.
  A. Parasternal long-axis view
  B. Right ventricular inflow view

5.
  A. Apical four-chamber view
  B. Apical five-chamber view

6.
  A. Subcostal short-axis image
  B. Subcostal long-axis image

7.
  A. TEE four-chamber view
  B. TEE three-chamber view

8.
  A. TEE RUPV
  B. TEE LUPV

9.
  A. TEE aortic valve leaflet tips short-axis orientation
  B. TEE LVOT view short-axis orientation

10.
  A. TEE bicaval view
  B. TEE hepatic vein

11.
  A. TEE apical four-chamber foreshortened view
  B. TEE apical four-chamber optimized view

12.
  A. TEE RVOT view
  B. TEE pulmonary artery bifurcation view

13.
  A. TEE main pulmonary artery long-axis view
  B. TEE right pulmonary artery long-axis view

14.
  A. Transgastric apical four-chamber view
  B. Coronary sinus long-axis view

15.
  A. Right pulmonary artery long-axis view
  B. Left atrium optimized view

16.
  A. Low descending thoracic aorta short-axis centered image
  B. High descending thoracic aorta short-axis centered image

112

17.

A. TEE apical four-chamber view
B. TEE apical five-chamber view

18.

A. TEE apical four-chamber view; LV centered
B. TEE apical four-chamber view; RV centered

19.

A. TEE bicaval view
B. TEE two-chamber view

20.

A. TEE LV short-axis papillary muscle level
B. TEE LV short-axis apical level

21.

A. Descending thoracic aorta TEE short-axis orientation
B. Descending thoracic aorta TEE long-axis orientation

22.

A. TEE apical long-axis view focused on ascending aorta
B. TEE distal ascending aorta maximal visualization

23.

A. TEE long-axis ostial left subclavian artery view
B. TEE short-axis optimized innominate artery view

Answers

Answer 1: D.

Answer 2: C.

Answer 3: C.

Answer 4: F and C.

Answer 5: E.

Answer 6: C.

Answer 7: I.

Answer 8: D.

Answer 9: A.

Answer 10: A.

Answer 11: H and B.

Answer 12: B and G.

Answer 13: B and C.

Answer 14: B.

Answer 15: A and J.

Answer 16: B and D.

Answer 17: B and J.

Answer 18: C.

Answer 19: D.

Answer 20: H and or A.

Answer 21: I.

Answer 22: B and J.

Answer 23: J and C.

It is critically important that you understand how to optimally image (and center in your image display) the anatomic or pathologic structure of interest. It is now a common approach on Echo Boards to assess this skill in a similar manner to the questions in this chapter. It is equally likely that instead of text, you may have a clinical scenario with images to recognize and then demonstrate your understanding of their interrelationship.

At most times, there is never a "single" manipulation required as suggested by these "simple" single answers. However, there is usually a single major maneuver required to get near to your selected image display and then a series of more subtle, minor maneuvers to "fine-tune" the image and optimize the display. There is no way short of practice to become truly competent, and only through continued experience, to become expert.

A couple of minor points regarding TEE manipulation: since the image sector originates from a specific point on the TEE transducer, any significant amount of ante-flexion will by default, slightly withdrawal the image origin. Without simultaneous, albeit slight, probe insertion, the image will have changed its superior to inferior orientation. Similarly, retroflexion will demand a tiny bit of withdrawal to keep the image origin from moving inferiorly.

No option for lateral (small knob) manipulation of the TEE probe was offered as an answer. That is not because this option is not available, but simply because it is less often required. This is still valuable for "lateral" and "medial" structures (or anterior/posterior structures at 90-degree angles) and may be extremely valuable to optimize the LA appendage or pulmonary veins.

Suggested Reading

Lang RM, Goldstein SA, Kronzon I, et al. *ASE Comprehensive Echocardiography*. 2nd ed.; Chapters 6 and 12, 2015.

Chapter 17

Aortic Stenosis

John R. Kotter

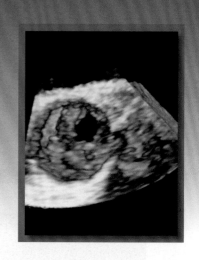

1. Which of these M-mode images is suggestive of valvular aortic stenosis?

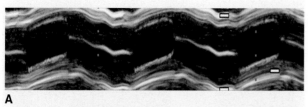

A

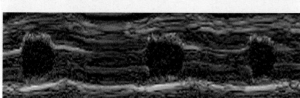

B

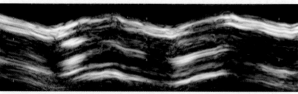

C

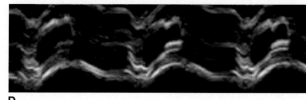

D

FIGURE 17.1

A. FIGURE 17.1A
B. FIGURE 17.1B
C. FIGURE 17.1C
D. FIGURE 17.1D

2. Which of these continuous-wave spectral Doppler tracings is most suggestive of aortic stenosis?

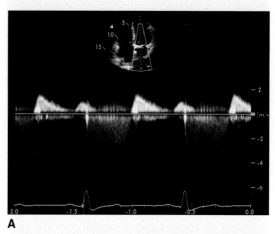

A

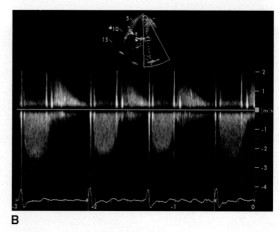

B

FIGURE 17.2

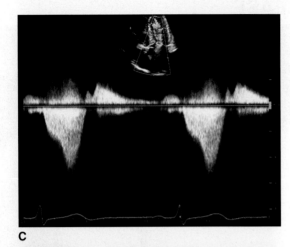

C

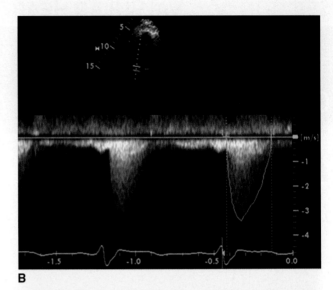

B

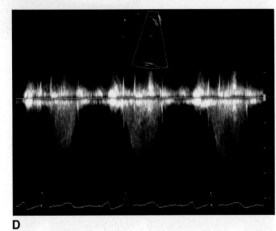

D

FIGURE 17.2 (*Continued*)

   A. FIGURE 17.2A
   B. FIGURE 17.2B
   C. FIGURE 17.2C
   D. FIGURE 17.2D

3. Assessment of aortic stenosis severity by the continuity equation (using TVI) here suggests (FIG. 17.3):

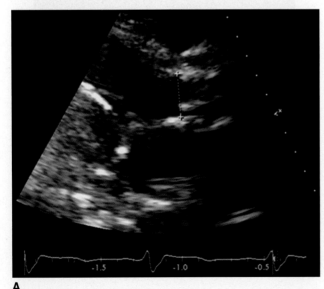

A

FIGURE 17.3

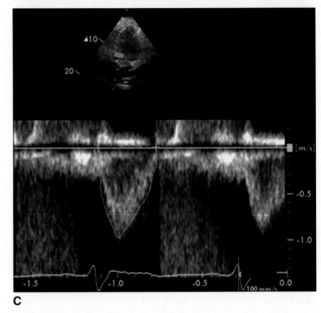

C

FIGURE 17.3 (*Continued*)

   A. Normal aortic flow
   B. Mild aortic stenosis
   C. Moderate aortic stenosis
   D. Severe aortic stenosis

4. Which of the following comorbid conditions will most impact the accuracy of the simplified Bernoulli equation ($p = 4v^2$) to measure transaortic valve gradients?

   A. Severe aortic regurgitation
   B. Mitral regurgitation
   C. Hypothyroidism
   D. Severe mitral stenosis

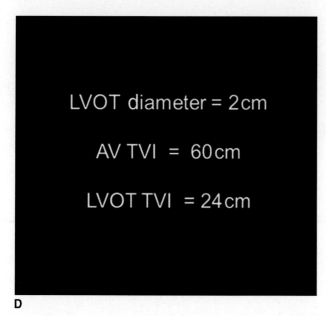

LVOT diameter = 2 cm

AV TVI = 60 cm

LVOT TVI = 24 cm

D

FIGURE 17.3 (Continued)

5. The largest source of error in calculation of aortic valve area by the continuity equation is:

   A. Peak velocity across the aortic valve
   B. LVOT diameter
   C. Peak velocity across the LVOT
   D. Time–velocity integral of aortic valve CW spectral Doppler display
   E. Time–velocity integral of LVOT PW spectral Doppler display

6. Which of the following statements regarding calculation of the dimensionless index is most appropriate?

   A. A dimensionless index of 0.30 or less is consistent with severe aortic stenosis.
   B. Dimensionless index can be calculated by V_{max} LVOT/V_{max} AV or VTI LVOT/VTI AV.
   C. Dimensionless index is not useful if LVOT velocities are elevated.
   D. Dimensionless index is affected by the error in measurement of LVOT diameter.

7. A patient has severe mitral stenosis (MVA 0.9 cm², mean gradient 11 mm Hg), severe aortic stenosis (AVA 0.9 cm², mean gradient 44 mm Hg), and no significant valvular regurgitation. The difference between transaortic and transmitral gradients is explained by:

   A. Relative differences in flow rates across each valve
   B. Relative differences in blood velocities across the aortic and mitral valves
   C. Relative difference in pressures between the left atrium/ left ventricle in diastole and that of the left ventricle/ aorta in systole
   D. Mild to moderate aortic regurgitation

8. Which of the following statements is most correct regarding aortic valve gradients?

   A. Aortic valve peak gradients by echo are instantaneous and overestimate the true gradient.
   B. Catheter-based aortic valve peak-to-peak gradients are generally lower than echo-based peak gradients.
   C. Increased cardiac output is more likely to affect measurement of catheter-based gradients rather than echo-based gradients.
   D. Catheter-based aortic valve mean gradients are generally higher than echo-based mean gradients.

9. With regard to pseudosevere aortic stenosis:

   A. This phenomenon relates to calculation of a falsely reduced aortic valve area due to reduced excursion of the aortic valve leaflets in the setting of low cardiac output.
   B. It can be distinguished from severe aortic stenosis using high-dose dobutamine infusion.
   C. It is suggested by a mean gradient of <40 mm Hg and change in valve area of ≤0.3 cm² with dobutamine echocardiography.
   D. It is suggested by a mean gradient of >40 mm Hg and change in valve area of ≥0.3 cm² with dobutamine echocardiography.

10. With regard to low-output low-gradient severe aortic stenosis:

    A. This diagnosis relates to the presence of low gradients despite the presence of severe aortic stenosis directly as a result of reduced stroke volume.
    B. It is suggested by a mean gradient of >40 mm Hg and change in valve area of ≥0.3 cm² with dobutamine echocardiography.
    C. The presence of contractile reserve is a marker of good prognosis following surgical repair and refers to an increase in stroke volume by 10% or more.
    D. The presence of contractile reserve is a marker of increased patient survival and improved functional class following surgical repair.

11. A patient has a calculated AVA of 0.6 cm², a mean trans- aortic valve gradient of 20 mm Hg, a stroke volume index of 30 mL/m², and a systolic blood pressure of 190 mm Hg. Which of the following statements is least correct?

    A. Global hemodynamic load in aortic stenosis is limited to the degree of valvular obstruction.
    B. Quantification of the global hemodynamic load (Z) can be performed by dividing LV systolic pressure plus mean transaortic valve gradient by the stroke volume index.
    C. A global hemodynamic load Z value > 4.5 mm Hg/mL/ m² reflects low impedance.
    D. Pseudonormalization of blood pressure refers to the fact that blood pressure may be normal despite low impedance, particularly if stroke volume is increased.

12. A patient has a calculated AVA of 0.6 cm² and a mean transaortic valve gradient of 20 mm Hg. Such discrepant findings could be accounted for by which of the following?

A. Measurement error involving overestimation of LVOT diameter

B. Severe aortic stenosis and incorrect measurement of the CW Doppler signal

C. Severe aortic stenosis and high cardiac output

D. Severe aortic stenosis and increased LVOT velocity

13. A patient has a calculated AVA of 0.6 cm², a mean transaortic valve gradient of 20 mm Hg, a stroke volume index of 30 mL/m², and an ejection fraction of 55%. Which of the following statements is true?

A. Low flow (stroke volume) cannot be present with a preserved ejection fraction.

B. A stroke volume index of <35 mL/m² reflects low flow.

C. Gradients are flow independent.

D. Surgery is not indicated here as outcomes are likely to be better with medical treatment.

14. With regard to pressure recovery:

A. This is defined as the variable decrease in pressure downstream from the vena contracta.

B. This is due to the conversion of a certain amount of potential energy (static pressure) to kinetic energy (dynamic pressure).

C. This can account for falsely elevated prosthetic valve gradients, particularly bileaflet mechanical valves.

D. This can account for falsely elevated native valve gradients particularly in the presence of a low-output state and a large aortic size.

15. Which of the following is a predictor of outcome (death or need for valve replacement due to symptoms) in patients with severe, asymptomatic aortic stenosis?

A. Patient sex

B. Diabetes mellitus

C. Bicuspid aortic valve morphology

D. The presence of moderate to severe calcification

16. Which of the following statements regarding etiology of aortic stenosis is most appropriate?

A. Calcific degenerative stenosis of a trileaflet valve is a more common indication for aortic valve replacement than bicuspid aortic valve disease with supraimposed calcification.

B. Radiation damage typically involves severe aortic valve thickening without calcification.

C. Commissural fusion is suggestive of an autoimmune etiology.

D. A preserved second heart sound and a normal pulse typically do not exclude hemodynamically significant calcific degenerative aortic stenosis.

17. Which of the following regarding fixed subvalvular aortic stenosis is most appropriate?

A. It is rarely associated with other cardiac malformations.

B. It is less common than supravalvular aortic stenosis.

C. It more commonly manifests as a tunneled stenosis rather than a discrete membrane.

D. It can be an unrecognized cause of persistently high gradients after aortic valve surgery.

18. Which of the following statements regarding aortic flow in the presence of fixed subvalvular aortic stenosis is most appropriate?

A. Increased flow and gradients are seen following a Valsalva maneuver.

B. Decreased flow and gradients are seen following an ectopic beat.

C. Valsalva effects on flow and gradients are different than with valvular aortic stenosis.

D. Valsalva effects on flow and gradients are different than with hypertrophic cardiomyopathy.

19. Which of the following is a typical finding associated with the image in FIGURE 17.4 and VIDEO 17.1?

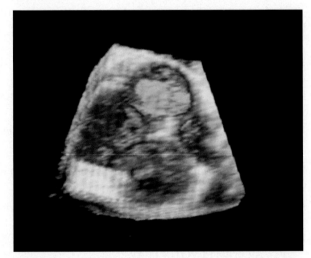

FIGURE 17.4

A. Absence of associated hemodynamic abnormalities in over half of the cases

B. Aortic stenosis more commonly than aortic regurgitation

C. Concomitant congenital cardiac defects

D. Four equal cusps

20. Which of the following is a typical finding associated with the demonstrated image in FIGURE 17.5?

A. Fusion of all three cusps.

B. Associated aortic regurgitation more commonly than aortic stenosis.

C. Most common presentation is an incidental finding in adulthood.

D. The eccentric opening variety shown here is less common than a single, central opening.

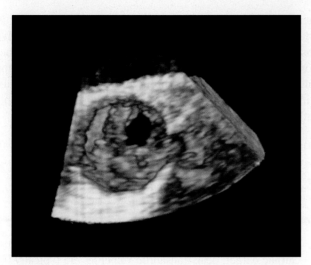

FIGURE 17.5

21. An asymptomatic 45-year-old female is noted on clinical examination to have a loud crescendo–decrescendo murmur at the base of the heart radiating to both carotids. Palpation of the carotids is notable for a slow-rising plateau pulse, while auscultation reveals a soft second heart sound. ECG shows a pattern consistent with pressure overload left ventricular hypertrophy with strain. Echocardiography reveals calcific aortic stenosis, an aortic valve area by continuity of 0.8 cm^2, a peak transaortic velocity of 4.5 m/s, peak/mean gradients of 75/45 mm Hg, and a preserved left ventricular ejection fraction. Aortic valve morphology is shown in VIDEO 17.2.

Which of the following statements regarding this valve morphology is true?

A. Is found in 0.1% to 0.2% of the population.
B. Is more commonly found in women than in men.
C. Is associated with aortic root dilation and aortic coarctation.
D. Yearly echo is recommended if the aorta is >5 cm.

22. A 72-year-old male undergoes a low-dose dobutamine infusion protocol with echocardiography to evaluate aortic stenosis. The LVOT is measured at 2.0 cm. The following results were obtained:

DOBUTAMINE DOSE (μg/kg/min)	LVOT VTI (cm)	AORTIC VALVE VTI (cm)	AORTIC VALVE MEAN GRADIENT (mm Hg)	LVEF (%)
0 (Baseline)	18	60	24	30
10	26	68	37	45

Which of the following is the most correct interpretation of the procedure?

A. Pseudosevere (moderate) aortic stenosis
B. Low-flow, low-gradient severe aortic stenosis
C. Severe aortic stenosis with low contractile reserve
D. Mild aortic stenosis

Answer 1: C.

A. False. This M-mode appearance is consistent with a normal aortic valve.
B. False. This M-mode appearance is consistent with a normal aortic valve in the setting of reduced cardiac output.
C. True. See discussion below.
D. False. This M-mode appearance is consistent with a normal aortic valve in the setting of hypertrophic cardiomyopathy.

M-mode in aortic stenosis reveals multiple dense echoes consistent with thickened cusps and reduced valve opening (FIG. 17.6C). Normal aortic cusps are thin, have a maximal separation of around 2 cm, and taper a little in midsystole (FIG. 17.6A). In the presence of reduced cardiac output, aortic valve opening may be limited in duration with blunted cusp separation (FIG. 17.6B). Partial closure of the aortic valve in midsystole is a classic feature of subvalvular obstruction with the exaggerated taper caused by either the dynamic gradient of hypertrophic cardiomyopathy (FIG. 17.6D) or fixed obstruction in the presence of a subaortic membrane.

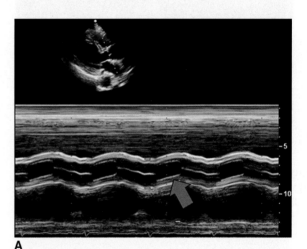

A

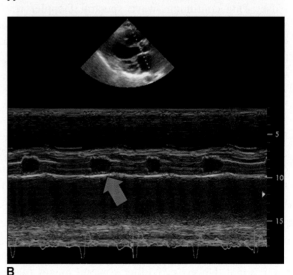

B

FIGURE 17.6

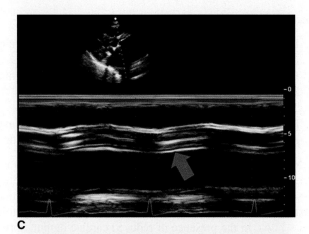

C

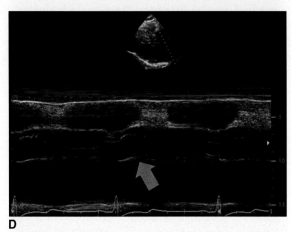

D

Figure 17.6 (*Continued*)

Suggested Reading

Oh JK, Seward JB, Tajik AJ. *The Echo Manual*. Philadelphia, PA: Lippincott Williams & Wilkins, 2006.

Answer 2: *B.*

A. False. This continuous-wave spectral Doppler tracing demonstrates velocities (flow) that start before aortic valve opening and end after aortic valve closure and thus cannot represent aortic stenosis. Given the Doppler alignment, this is mitral regurgitation.

B. True. See discussion below.

C. False. This gradient appears dynamic consistent with hypertrophic cardiomyopathy.

D. False. Again, this continuous-wave spectral Doppler tracing demonstrates velocities (flow) that start before aortic valve opening and end after aortic valve closure and thus cannot represent aortic stenosis. Given the Doppler alignment, this is tricuspid regurgitation.

The timing of aortic stenosis is obviously limited by valve opening and closure, which can sometimes be seen as abrupt bright spikes in the continuous-wave spectral Doppler signal thereby providing a useful means (particularly if using a nonimaging probe) to distinguish aortic stenosis flow (see Fig. 17.6B) from either mitral or tricuspid regurgitation. Option C is incorrect because it demonstrates

increased velocities (flow) in a dynamic pattern worse in late systole, which would not be typical for fixed valve obstruction. Rather, this pattern is seen with LVOT obstruction due to systolic anterior motion of the mitral valve in the setting of hypertrophic cardiomyopathy, which correlates clinically to the classic mid- to late systolic peaking of this pathology.

Suggested Reading

Baumgartner H, Hung J, Bermejo J, et al. Echocardiographic assessment of valve stenosis: EAE/ASE recommendations for clinical practice. *Eur J Echocardiogr* 2009;10(1):1–25.

Answer 3: *C.*

A. False. In the setting of normal LV function and normal cardiac output, peak transaortic velocities are typically 0.5 to 1.5 m/s, and normal aortic valve area is 3 to 4 cm². Peak transaortic velocities of up to 2.5 m/s may be related to aortic sclerosis.

B. False. Mild aortic stenosis is typically suggested by peak transaortic velocities of 2.6 to 2.9 m/s and an aortic valve area of 1.5 to 3.0 cm².

C. True. See discussion below.

D. False. Severe aortic stenosis is typically suggested by peak transaortic velocities of >4 m/s and an aortic valve area <1.0 cm².

A peak transaortic velocity of 3.5 m/s and an aortic valve area of 1.3 cm² typically suggest that the severity of aortic stenosis is in the moderate range. When using continuous-wave Doppler to assess valve disease severity as part of the continuity equation (Fig. 17.7), it is important to image in multiple windows (apical/right sternal border/subcostal/right parasternal/suprasternal) to find the maximum velocity. Using the simplified Bernoulli equation, the gradient across the aortic valve can be estimated by $4v^2$ where v = maximal velocity as measured by continuous-wave Doppler.

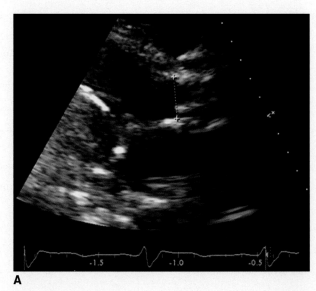

A

Figure 17.7

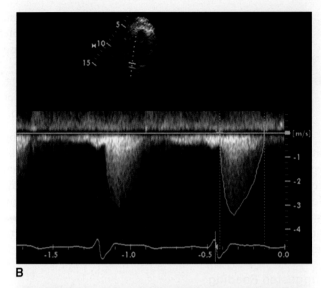

B

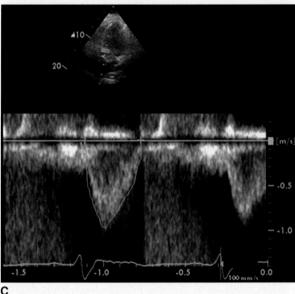

C

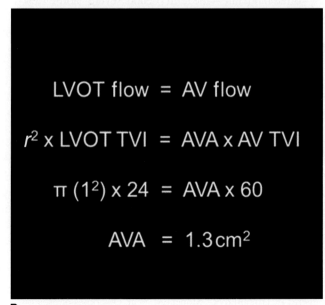

LVOT flow = AV flow

r^2 x LVOT TVI = AVA x AV TVI

π (1^2) x 24 = AVA x 60

AVA = 1.3 cm^2

D

FIGURE 17.7 *(Continued)*

Suggested Reading

Dennig K, Kraus F, Rudolph W. Doppler echocardiography determination of the orifice area in aortic valve stenosis using a continuity equation. *Herz* 1986;11:309–317.

Answer 4: A.

A. True. See discussion below.
B. False. The stroke volume across the aortic valve is not increased and the simplified Bernoulli equation can be applied.
C. False. As in B.
D. False. As in B.

This simplified version of the Bernoulli equation makes several assumptions that need to be considered in certain clinical scenarios. The most clinically relevant assumption is that LVOT velocity is negligible compared to transaortic valve velocity. Thus, in conditions where LVOT velocity is increased (>1 m/s) such as in options A, a longer version of the formula ($\Delta p = 4(VAV^2 - VLVOT^2)$) should be used. Other assumptions include lack of a significant friction factor (viscosity) and the absence of a significant inertial or convective component to flow across a restrictive orifice.

Suggested Reading

Rijsterborgh H, Roelandt J. Doppler assessment of aortic stenosis: Bernoulli revisited. *Ultrasound Med Biol* 1987;13:241–248.

Answer 5: B.

A. False. Error in measuring peak velocity across the aortic valve can be limited by imaging in multiple windows to ensure that true maximum velocities are obtained.
B. True. See discussion below.
C. False. Errors in measuring peak velocity across the LVOT can be limited by imaging in multiple windows were imaged and that true maximum velocities were obtained.
D. False. Once a true transaortic valve Doppler signal is obtained, measurement error in the aortic valve VTI is generally not significant.
E. False. Once the PW sample volume is carefully located, measurement error in LVOT VTI is generally not significant.

The largest source of error in the continuity equation is measurement of LVOT diameter. There are two main reasons for this: firstly, there is an inherent difficulty involved in obtaining this measurement; secondly, this value is squared in the equation. Such errors can be avoided by calculation of the dimensionless index, a useful marker of aortic valve stenosis severity, which does not necessitate measurement of LVOT diameter. The dimensionless index is simply a ratio of either the LVOT velocity (be it peak or mean) or the LVOT VTI over the equivalent measure recorded across the aortic valve with values below 0.25 representing severe stenosis.

Suggested Reading

Baumgartner H, Hung J, Bermejo J, et al. Echocardiographic assessment of valve stenosis: EAE/ASE recommendations for clinical practice. *Eur J Echocardiogr* 2009;10(1):1–25.

Answer 6: *B.*

A. False. A dimensionless index of 0.25 or less is consistent with severe aortic stenosis.
B. True. See discussion below.
C. False. The dimensionless index remains valid in the setting of elevated LVOT velocities, unlike the simplified version of the Bernoulli equation, which assumes LVOT velocities are negligible.
D. False.

Dimensionless index can be calculated by V_{max} LVOT/V_{max} AV or VTI LVOT/VTI AV or indeed V_{mean} LVOT/V_{mean} AV. The dimensionless index inversely reflects how much faster (or further) blood travels as it crosses the narrowed aortic valve. A dimensionless index of 0.25 or less is consistent with severe aortic stenosis and means that blood velocity speeds up (or would travel further) by a factor of four or more as it crosses the stenosis. One of the advantages of this index is that it avoids the error associated with LVOT diameter measurement.

Suggested Reading
Finegold JA, Manisty CH, Cecaro F, et al. Choosing between velocity-time-integral ratio and peak velocity ratio for calculation of the dimensionless index (or aortic valve area) in serial follow-up of aortic stenosis. *Int J Cardiol* 2013;167:1524–1531.

Answer 7: *C.*

A. False. In the absence of significant valvular regurgitation, flow rates across the mitral and aortic valves should be roughly equivalent.
B. False. Blood velocities are a consequence of and not a cause of pressure gradients per se.
C. True. See discussion below.
D. False. For a given aortic valve area, the presence of concomitant aortic regurgitation will result in an increase in aortic valve gradient, but this is not the primary underlying explanation here.

Gradients in aortic stenosis are generated in systole and by the left ventricle, which is capable of generating high pressures even relative to aortic pressures to drive blood across the stenosed aorta valve. In contrast, gradients in mitral stenosis are generated in diastole and by the left atrium in which case the pressure differential is relatively lower compared to aortic stenosis as described.

Suggested Reading
Thomas JD, Popovic ZB. Intraventricular pressure differences: a new window into cardiac function. *Circulation* 2005;112:1684–1686.

Answer 8: *B.*

A. False. Echocardiography by its nature can detect the actual maximal peak gradient at the vena contracta (location of the narrowest orifice, highest velocity, and lowest pressure) "in an instantaneous fashion" with negligible time lag and theoretically characterizes the true degree of stenosis.
B. True. See discussion below.
C. False. Without consideration of the increase in LVOT velocity, echo-based pressure gradients will typically be overestimated in the setting of increased cardiac output. Here, LVOT velocity would likely not be negligible compared to transaortic valve velocity and prohibit the use of the simplified version of the Bernoulli equation.
D. False. Unlike peak gradients, which are measured at one time point only, mean pressure gradients are averaged over systole and tend to be similar by catheterization and echo.

During measurement of peak aortic valve gradients by catheterization, the time lag involved in catheter "pullback" typically results in submaximal values being recorded that are typically lower than those measured by echocardiography. However, it has also been argued that the net pressure drop as obtained by distal pressure measurements including pressure recovery may serve as a better physiologic indicator of the hemodynamic significance of the stenosis.

Suggested Reading
Baumgartner H, Stefenelli T, Niederberger J, et al. "Overestimation" of catheter gradients by Doppler ultrasound in patients with aortic stenosis: a predictable manifestation of pressure recovery. *J Am Coll Cardiol* 1999;33:1655–1661.

Answer 9: *A.*

A. True. See discussion below.
B. False. Low-dose dobutamine echocardiography is useful in this regard with typical protocols involving 5 µg/kg increments up to 20 µg/kg.
C. False. It is suggested by an increase in mean gradient to <40 mm Hg and change in valve area of ≥0.3 cm^2 (peak valve area of ≥1.0 cm^2) with dobutamine echocardiography.
D. False. As in (C).

Pseudosevere aortic stenosis is a condition in which calculated aortic valve area falsely overestimates the severity of aortic stenosis when the aortic valve area is calculated at a low-flow state. Since most of these patients have some degree of AS—often moderate—the term pseudo"severe" aortic stenosis is preferred.

For patients with contractile reserve (inducible increase in stroke volume ≥20%) and pseudosevere aortic stenosis, low-dose dobutamine infusion results in an increase in the ratio of VTI LVOT/VTI AV and a normalization of the estimated aortic valve area as measured using the continuity equation. Here, VTI LVOT increases due to increased cardiac output, while VTI AV does not change (or may even reduce) as a result of less impedance (increased excursion of the aortic valve leaflets) despite the increase in flow. Aortic valve gradients do not increase to the same extent in pseudosevere aortic stenosis following dobutamine infusion as they do in patients with low-output low-gradient "true" severe aortic stenosis and contractile reserve because reduced transaortic valve impedance offsets an increase in gradients due to the increase in flow.

Suggested Reading
Fougeres E, Tribouilloy C, Monchi M, et al. Outcomes of pseudo-severe aortic stenosis under conservative treatment. *Eur Heart J* 2012;33:2426–2433.

Answer 10: A.

A. True. See discussion below.
B. False. It is suggested by an increase in mean gradient to >40 mm Hg and change in valve area of ≤0.3 cm^2 (peak valve area of ≤1.0 cm^2) with dobutamine echocardiography.
C. False. Contractile reserve means significant augmentation of stroke volume following dobutamine administration and is a marker of good prognosis. However, contractile reserve refers to an increase in stroke volume of 20% or more (and not 10%).
D. False. While the presence of contractile reserve is a marker of increased postoperative patient survival, the effect of aortic valve replacement on functional class in this setting is unaffected by contractile reserve.

Low-dose dobutamine infusion in the setting of low-output low-gradient severe aortic stenosis with contractile reserve (where stroke volume increases by >20%) results in the estimated aortic valve area (using the continuity equation) remaining low. Here, the ratio of VTI LVOT/VTI AV does not change—VTI LVOT increases due to an increase in stroke volume as does VTI AV reflecting increased flow across a fixed stenosis. Furthermore, aortic valve gradients increase in true low-output low-gradient aortic stenosis with contractile reserve as impedance also increases in response to augmented flow across the true stenosis. Although absence of contractile reserve is a predictor of a high surgical mortality and poor long-term outcome, valve replacement may still result in improved LV function and outcome in such patients.

Suggested Reading

Fougeres E, Tribouilloy C, Monchi M, et al. Outcomes of pseudo-severe aortic stenosis under conservative treatment. *Eur Heart J* 2012;33:2426–2433.

Answer 11: B.

A. False. Systemic vascular resistance and arterial compliance should also be considered.
B. True. See discussion below.
C. False. By definition, high impedance is defined as "Z values" > 4.5 mm Hg/mL/m^2.
D. False. Pseudonormalization of blood pressure refers to the fact that blood pressure may be normal despite high impedance particularly if stroke volume is decreased.

In this case, global hemodynamic load equals the sum of LV systolic pressure (190 mm Hg) plus mean transaortic valve gradient (20 mm Hg) divided by the stroke volume index (30 mL/m^2), which translates to a Z value of 7 mm Hg/mL/ m^2. In patients with aortic stenosis and a high global hemodynamic load (Z value > 4.5 mm Hg/mL/m^2), the left ventricle has to deal with increased afterload from an additional source, namely, decreased systemic arterial compliance. Recent studies have suggested that such patients with a high global hemodynamic load even in the setting of moderate to severe aortic stenosis may benefit from valve surgery.

Of note, this patient has a low output (stroke volume index < 35 mL/m^2), and if the above measurements are true, a low-dose dobutamine infusion may help further distinguish between pseudosevere aortic stenosis, low-gradient "true" severe aortic stenosis, or absent contractile reserve.

Suggested Reading

Dumesnil JG, Pibarot P, Carabello B. Paradoxical low-flow and/or low-gradient severe aortic stenosis despite preserved left ventricular ejection fraction: implications for diagnosis and treatment. *Eur Heart J* 2010;31(3):281–289.

Answer 12: B.

A. False. Overestimation of LVOT diameter would result in overestimation of aortic valve area.
B. True. See discussion below.
C. False. These findings would be typical of low-output low-gradient severe aortic stenosis.
D. False. Use of the simplified Bernoulli equation without consideration of increased LVOT velocity would result in overestimation of the transaortic valve gradient.

In the continuity equation, estimated aortic valve area increases in direct proportion to (the square of half) the LVOT diameter. Thus, underestimation of LVOT diameter would result in underestimation of aortic valve area in comparison to the true measured gradient. Correct angulation and the use of multiple windows for imaging are important in order to avoid missing the presence of severe aortic stenosis.

Suggested Reading

Baumgartner H, Hung J, Bermejo J, et al. Echocardiographic assessment of valve stenosis: EAE/ASE recommendations for clinical practice. *Eur J Echocardiogr* 2009;10(1):1–25.

Answer 13: B.

A. False. Left ventricular hypertrophy related to aortic stenosis not uncommonly results in small left ventricular cavity size and thus a low flow (stroke volume) despite the presence of a preserved ejection fraction.
B. True. See discussion below.
C. False. Gradients are highly flow dependent. An analogous relationship is seen in electromechanics where voltage gradients equal resistance times current (flow).
D. False. Surgical outcomes in this scenario may be preferable to medical therapy.

Multiple reasons exist as to why echocardiographic measurements of aortic valve area and gradients may be discrepant. Firstly, measurement error may play a role—aortic valve area calculations are derived from multiple measurements and are prone to error (especially LVOT measurements), while gradient calculations require an optimal window to obtain peak values. A second reason that relates to a potential inconsistency within the guidelines for aortic stenosis severity is that an aortic valve area of 0.8 cm^2 or less (not 1.0 cm^2) is necessary as per the Gorlin formula to yield a gradient of >40 mm Hg (assuming a normal cardiac output). A third reason relates to the fact that gradients are flow dependent and up to 35% of patients with severe aortic stenosis may have low flow (stroke volume < 35 mL/m²) even despite a normal EF. A fourth reason relates to pressure recovery, defined as the variable increase in pressure downstream from the vena contracta (site of lowest pressure/highest velocity) due to the conversion of a certain amount of kinetic energy (dynamic pressure) to potential energy (static pressure).

Suggested Reading

Baumgartner H, Stefenelli T, Niederberger J, et al. "Overestimation" of catheter gradients by Doppler ultrasound in patients with aortic stenosis: a predictable manifestation of pressure recovery. *J Am Coll Cardiol* 1999;33:1655–1661.

Answer 14: C.

A. False. The vena contracta is the site of lowest pressure/ highest velocity slightly downstream of the stenotic orifice.
B. False. The opposite is true—it relates to conversion of kinetic energy (dynamic pressure) to potential energy (static pressure) downstream from the vena contracta.
C. True. See discussion below.
D. False. In native aortic valve disease, pressure recovery typically is only clinically relevant in the presence of either a high-output state and/or small aortic size.

Pressure recovery can be defined as the variable increase in pressure downstream from the vena contracta (site of lowest pressure/highest velocity) due to the conversion of a certain amount of kinetic energy (dynamic pressure) to potential energy (static pressure). Aortic valve area by continuity can be adjusted for the effects of pressure recovery as follows: $(EOA \times A)/(A - EOA)$ where EOA = continuity orifice area, and A = aortic cross-sectional area measured at the sinotubular junction. The concept of pressure recovery is also incorporated into a recently described parameter called the energy loss index, a measure of the left ventricular workload as a result of the aortic stenosis. Calculation of the energy loss index is given by $[4V^2(1 - EOA/A)^2]/BSA$ with values <0.5 cm²/m² suggesting a high left ventricular workload where V = peak trans-aortic velocity and BSA = body surface area.

Suggested Reading

Garcia D, Pibarot P, Dumesnil JG, et al. Assessment of aortic valve stenosis severity: a new index based on the energy loss concept. *Circulation* 2000;101:765–771.

Answer 15: D.

A. False. Patient gender has not been demonstrated to predict clinical outcomes in this setting.
B. False. Equally, diabetes mellitus has not been demonstrated to predict clinical outcomes in this setting.
C. False. The underlying aortic valve morphology in severe aortic stenosis typically does not provide useful additional prognostic information and may even be ambiguous in the presence of moderate to severe calcification.
D. True. See discussion below.

The question of when to refer a patient with asymptomatic severe aortic stenosis for aortic valve replacement can be difficult. Requiring an individualized approach, the risk of watchful waiting needs to be considered in light of the surgical risk. Current guidelines suggest that patients with asymptomatic severe aortic stenosis undergoing heart surgery for another indication should undergo concomitant aortic valve replacement. Other factors that should be considered include the presence of impaired systolic left ventricular function, exercise-induced hypotension, ventricular tachycardia, marked left ventricular hypertrophy, or rapidly increasing velocities across the aortic valve (>0.3 m/s/y) and increased gradients (a peak transvalvular velocity of ≥5 m/s, and/or a mean gradient of ≥60 mm Hg). Importantly, the extent of aortic valve calcification has been demonstrated as a strong predictor of subsequent events (namely, death or need for valve replacement due to symptoms). In the absence of aortic valve calcification, the likelihood of occurrence of adverse events is very low. In contrast, once the aortic valve becomes at least moderately calcified, event rates increase significantly where about half of patients likely experience events in 2 years, regardless of patient age.

Aortic valve calcification is identified by echocardiography by the presence of dense echogenicities and/or the presence of acoustic shadowing. The severity of aortic valve calcification is generally graded semiquantitatively, as illustrated in Figure 17.8. A noncalcified aortic valve has normal echogenicity and no acoustic shadowing (A). A mildly calcified aortic valve has few areas of dense echogenicity with little acoustic shadowing (B). A moderately calcified aortic valve has more pronounced focal areas of dense echogenicity and acoustic shadowing (C). A severely calcified aortic valve has globally increased echogenicity with prominent acoustic shadowing and is also usually extensively thickened (D).

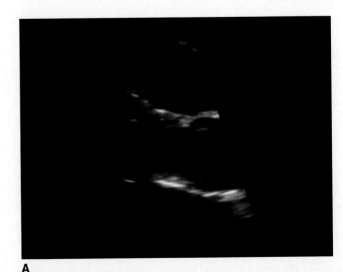

A

Figure 17.8

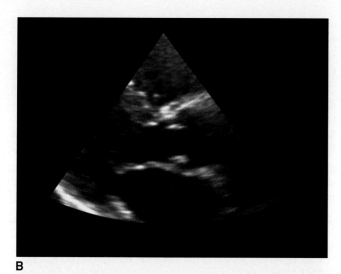

B

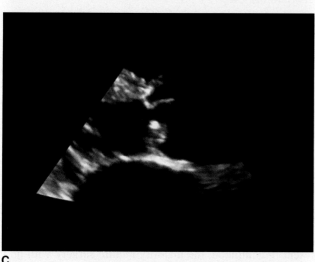

C

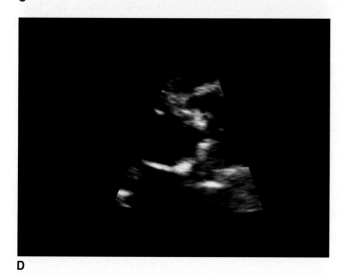

D

FIGURE 17.8 (Continued)

Suggested Readings

Nishimura RA, Otto CM, Bonow RO. 2014 AHA/ACC guideline for the management of patients with valvular heart disease: a report of the American College of Cardiology/American Heart Association Task Force on Practice Guidelines. *J Am Coll Cardiol* 2014;63(22):2438–2488.

Rosenhek R, Binder T, Porenta G, et al. Predictors of outcome in severe, asymptomatic aortic stenosis. *N Engl J Med* 2000;343(9):611–661.

Zamorano JL, Badano LP, Bruce C, et al. EAE/ASE recommendations for the use of echocardiography in new transcatheter interventions for valvular heart disease. *Eur Heart J* 2011;32:2189–2214.

Answer 16: C.

A. False. More than 50% of all valve replacements in Europe and the United States relate to bicuspid aortic valve disease although calcification of a trileaflet valve accounts for most of the remainder.

B. False. Radiation is typically associated with severe aortic valve leaflet calcification and also calcification of other structures such as the aorta and the mitral–aortic valve curtain.

C. True. See discussion below.

D. False. The clinical examination remains an important part of the assessment of a patient with suspected aortic stenosis. Signs that may help distinguish aortic sclerosis from hemodynamically significant aortic stenosis include preservation of the second heart sound, a normal pulse, and the absence of a mid to late peak intensity of the murmur.

Rheumatic disease, suggested by commissural fusion and systolic doming, rarely affects the aortic valve in isolation and typically also involves the mitral valve. Radiation-induced aortic stenosis occurs as part of a spectrum of extracardiac and cardiac lesions ("pancarditis") that include radiation-induced atherosclerosis; pericardial, myocardial, and valvular disease; as well as conduction abnormalities. However, concomitant manifestations of atherosclerosis and some degree of mitral regurgitation are commonly seen in patients with degenerative aortic stenosis.

Suggested Reading

Baumgartner H, Hung J, Bermejo J, et al. Echocardiographic assessment of valve stenosis: EAE/ASE recommendations for clinical practice. *Eur J Echocardiogr* 2009;10(1):1–25.

Answer 17: D.

A. False. Fixed subvalvular aortic stenosis is associated with other cardiac malformations in over half of cases. This most commonly includes a patent ductus arteriosus, aortic coarctation, or ventricular septal defect.

B. False. The incidence of subvalvular aortic stenosis is estimated to be 6 in 10,000 live births (versus 1 in 25,000 live births of supravalvular aortic stenosis).

C. False. The most common manifestation subvalvular aortic stenosis is as a discrete subvalvular membrane either that is attached to the interventricular septum or that completely encircles the LVOT. Far less commonly, there may be a diffuse, "tunnel-like" narrowing of the LVOT that may be associated with aortic annular hypoplasia.

D. True. See discussion below.

Fixed subvalvular aortic stenosis is associated with a harsh murmur, progressive aortic valve scarring and regurgitation, a high risk of endocarditis, and recurrence postsurgical correction.

If unrecognized, it can be a cause of persistently high gradients after aortic valve replacement. Supravalvular aortic stenosis is the least common form of left ventricular outflow tract obstruction and is associated with Williams syndrome (part deletion of chromosome 7 resulting in elastin gene abnormalities). Here, the level of obstruction is typically just above the sinuses of Valsalva but can also manifest as aortic coarctation or renal artery stenosis.

Suggested Readings

Ewart AK, Jin W, Atkinson D, et al. Supravalvular aortic stenosis associated with a deletion disrupting the elastin gene. *J Clin Invest* 1994;93:1071–1077.

Kitchiner D, Jackson M, Malaiya N, et al. Incidence and prognosis of obstruction of the left ventricular outflow tract in Liverpool (1960–91): a study of 313 patients. *BMJ* 1994;71:588–595.

Answer 18: D.

A. False. Following a Valsalva maneuver, flow across a fixed aortic obstruction is reduced, and thus, there is a corresponding decrease in flow-dependent gradients.
B. False. Following an ectopic beat, flow across a fixed aortic obstruction is increased, and there is a corresponding increase in flow-dependent gradients.
C. False. Similar effects are seen post-Valsalva maneuver in the setting of any fixed aortic obstruction.
D. True. See discussion below.

In the presence of fixed aortic obstruction, hemodynamic effects typically contrast with those seen in the setting of a dynamic obstruction. For example, following the Valsalva maneuver, flow across a fixed aortic obstruction is reduced, and thus, there is a corresponding decrease in flow-dependent gradients. In contrast, the Valsalva maneuver results in increased gradients in hypertrophic cardiomyopathy as the degree of obstruction is generally greater when left ventricular volumes are reduced. A second example of contrasting findings between fixed and dynamic obstruction is seen following an ectopic beat. With fixed obstruction, after a premature ventricular contraction, the following ventricular contraction will be more forceful, and the pressure generated in the left ventricle and ascending aortic pressure will be higher. In contrast, a higher gradient and a drop in aortic pressure are seen postectopic in dynamic obstruction (the Brockenbrough–Braunwald–Morrow sign) due mainly to increased inotropy and rest potentiation.

Suggested Reading

Faber L, Heemann A, Surig M, et al. Outflow acceleration assessed by continuous-wave Doppler echocardiography in left ventricular hypertrophy: an analysis of 103 consecutive cases. *Cardiology* 1998;90:220–226.

Answer 19: A.

A. True. See discussion below.
B. False.
C. False.
D. False.

The congenital aortic valve demonstrated in the video is a quadricuspid AV. Quadricuspid aortic valve morphology is associated with hemodynamic abnormalities in fewer than half of cases, but when present, aortic regurgitation (44%) is a more common finding than aortic stenosis (VIDEO 17.1). Quadricuspid aortic valve is not generally associated with other congenital cardiac defects, although concomitant patent ductus arteriosus, subvalvular aortic stenosis, ventricular septal defect, and mitral valve abnormalities have been described. The most common morphology is three equal large cusps and one smaller cusp. It has been suggested that the greater the degree of cusp asymmetry, the higher the risk of complications such as aortic regurgitation or endocarditis due to increased flow disturbance (VIDEO 17.3).

Suggested Reading

James KB, Centorbi LK, Novoa R. Quadricuspid aortic valve. Case report and review of the literature. *Tex Heart Inst J* 1991;18:141–143.

Answer 20: A.

A. True. See discussion below.
B. False. Associated aortic stenosis is more common than aortic regurgitation.
C. False. The typical presentation is in infancy or early childhood.
D. False. The single opening is typically eccentric or unicommissural (as shown).

Unicuspid aortic valve morphology results from congenital fusion of all three cusps and is more commonly associated with aortic stenosis than with aortic regurgitation (VIDEO 17.4A). These valves are typically stenotic at birth, and patients typically present in infancy or early childhood. Of those cases that present in adulthood, the majority require surgery with up to half of patients having associated aortic dilation. The single opening is typically eccentric or unicommissural (VIDEO 17.4B) but may be central without a true commissure.

Suggested Reading

Krishnamoorthy KM. Images in cardiology: unicuspid aortic valve. *Heart* 2001;85:217.

Answer 21: C.

A. False. This woman has bicuspid aortic valve disease, found in 1% to 2% of the population.
B. False. There is a male to female predominance of 3:1 with bicuspid aortic valve disease.
C. True. See discussion below.
D. False. Yearly echo is advised once the aortic root size is >4 cm with bicuspid aortic valve disease.

Bicuspid aortic valve is a common inheritable abnormality occurring in 1% to 2% of the population with familial clustering noted in over a third of cases (VIDEO 17.2). Peak incidence of symptomatic disease is 40 to 60 years of age. Importantly, this pathology is not isolated to the aortic valve alone but rather is associated with aortic pathology in addition as described (VIDEO 17.5). The presence of associated aortic coarctation should always be considered particularly in the setting of concomitant hypertension. Aortic dilation is also an important consideration with yearly echo advised once the aortic root size is >4 cm. Surgery is usually advised under different scenarios. One, if aortic size is >5.5 cm. Two, if aortic size is >5.0 cm and additional risk factor for dissection is present and/or the patient is low surgical risk and being treated at a center of expertise. Or, three, the aortic size is >4.5 cm and aortic valve surgery is needed.

Suggested Readings

Nishimura RA, Bonow RO, Guyton RA. Surgery for aortic dilation in patients with bicuspid aortic valves: a statement of clarification from the American College of Cardiology/American Heart Association Task Force on Clinical Practice Guidelines. *Circulation*. 2016;133(7):680–686.

Siu SC, Silversides CK. Bicuspid aortic valve disease. *J Am Coll Cardiol* 2010;55:2789–2800.

Answer 22: A.

A. True. See discussion below
B. False. See discussion below
C. False. See discussion below
D. False. See discussion below

Low-dose dobutamine stress echocardiography can be utilized to differentiate pseudosevere aortic stenosis for low-flow, low-gradient aortic stenosis. With pseudosevere stenosis, the valve area appears reduced (as calculated using the continuity equation) as the low stroke volume does not fully open the aortic valve. However, following administration of dobutamine, the stroke volume increases and the peak and mean gradients will likewise increase. The calculated valve area will also increase. With low-gradient, low-flow severe aortic stenosis, the gradients will increase in response to dobutamine but the calculated valve area will not increase.

Suggested Readings

deFilippi C, Willett D, Brickner M, et al. Usefulness of dobutamine echocardiography in distinguishing severe from nonsevere valvular aortic stenosis in patients with depressed left ventricular function and low transvalvular gradients. *Am J Cardiol* 1995;75:191–194.

Nishimura R, Grantham J, Connolly H, et al. Low-output, low-gradient aortic stenosis in patients with depressed left ventricular systolic function: the clinical utility of the dobutamine challenge in the catheterization laboratory. *Circulation* 2002;106:809–813.

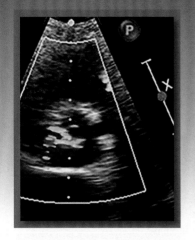

Chapter 18

Aortic Regurgitation

John R. Kotter

1. Which of the following aortic valve findings is most consistent with the M-mode displayed in FIGURE 18.1?

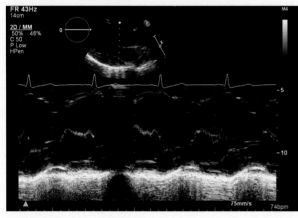

FIGURE 18.1

A. Aortic stenosis
B. Mild or moderate aortic regurgitation
C. Aortic valve vegetation
D. Aortic fibroelastoma
E. Early closure from severe AR

Questions 2 and 3

2. What is the most likely diagnosis of the patient with the M-mode displayed in FIGURE 18.2?

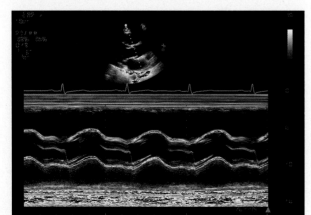

FIGURE 18.2

A. Severe aortic stenosis
B. Large aortic valve vegetation
C. Bicuspid aortic valve
D. Severe LV systolic dysfunction
E. Severe mitral stenosis

3. Which of the following is the most common congenital anomaly associated with this M-mode finding?

A. Mitral valve cleft
B. Ventricular septal defect
C. Subaortic membrane
D. Atrial septal defect
E. Coarctation

4. What is the severity of the aortic regurgitation in FIGURE 18.3?

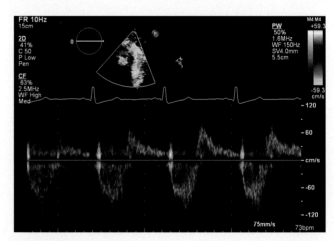

FIGURE 18.3

A. None
B. None or mild
C. Mild to moderate
D. Moderate to severe
E. Unable to quantify

5. Parameters that meet criteria for severe aortic regurgitation include:

A. Jet width/LVOT diameter ratio = 70%.
B. Vena contracta width = 0.5 cm.
C. Aortic regurgitation PHT = 260 ms.
D. Regurgitant fraction = 40%.
E. Effective regurgitant orifice area = 0.27 cm².

6. Which of the following indications for the echocardiographic evaluation of aortic regurgitation is considered as rarely appropriate/inappropriate or uncertain or may be appropriate indication according to 2017 AUC for multimodality imaging in valvular heart disease?

A. Diagnosis and assessment of severity
B. Evaluation of left ventricular size and function in severe aortic regurgitation
C. Reevaluation of a patient with mild or moderate aortic regurgitation when new symptoms occur
D. Reevaluation (<1 year) of moderate aortic insufficiency without change in clinical status or physical exam

7. An echocardiographic study should be performed to evaluate aortic regurgitation for which of the following clinical scenarios?

A. Routine evaluation of a patient who used anorectic drugs and who has mild aortic regurgitation
B. Follow-up evaluation of a patient with severe aortic regurgitation with an LV systolic diameter of 5.5 cm
C. Routine evaluation of a patient with asymptomatic severe aortic regurgitation
D. Routine surveillance (>3 years) of mild valvular insufficiency without a change in symptoms or physical exam

8. A patient with asymptomatic severe aortic regurgitation has an echocardiogram to reassess left ventricular size and function. On the 2D echo evaluation, the left ventricular ejection fraction is 45% using a biplane Simpson method. What do you recommend?

A. Continuation of medical therapy
B. Surgical replacement
C. Cardiac rehabilitation
D. Transcutaneous aortic valve replacement (TAVR)

9. What is the most likely etiology of the acute aortic regurgitation based upon the 2D and color-flow Doppler images shown in FIGURE 18.4?

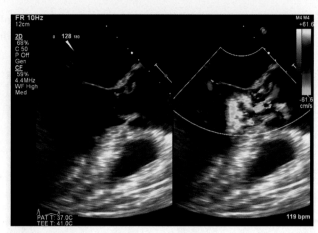

FIGURE 18.4

A. Degenerative aortic valve disease
B. Aortic valve endocarditis
C. Aortic aneurysm
D. Aortic dissection

10. What is the most likely etiology of the chronic aortic regurgitation based upon the 2D and color-flow Doppler images shown in FIGURE 18.5?

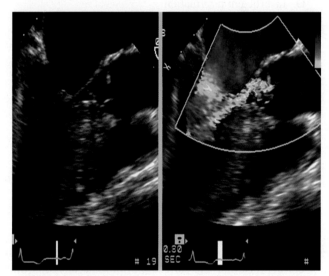

FIGURE 18.5

A. Subaortic membrane
B. Aortic valve endocarditis
C. Aortic aneurysm
D. Aortic dissection

11. What is typically the most appropriate view utilized in order to measure a vena contracta to estimate aortic valve insufficiency?

A. Parasternal long axis
B. Parasternal short axis
C. Apical 5 chamber
D. Apical 3 chamber
E. Suprasternal

12. In this M-mode echo (Fig. 18.6), what is the severity of aortic regurgitation (LVOT width is 3.8 cm and the width of the aortic regurgitation is 0.7 cm)?

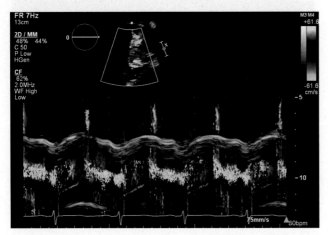

FIGURE **18.6**

   A. Mild
   B. Moderate
   C. Severe
   D. Insufficient information

13. To quickly determine the severity of aortic regurgitation, color-flow Doppler is an established, but imperfect, technique. Which of the following is most accurate regarding the use of qualitative characteristics of the color-flow display?

   A. The overall gain will not significantly alter the appearance of the AR color display unless the jet severity is severe.
   B. The temporal resolution has no impact on the color-flow jet appearance.
   C. Jet eccentricity is important and often results in overestimation of the AR severity.
   D. Color gain is best optimized by studying the color-flow pattern outside of the cardiac chamber.

14. Which of the following hemodynamic scenarios is most correct regarding the correlation of the deceleration time (DT) of the continuous-wave Doppler spectral display of aortic regurgitation (AR) and severity of AR?

   A. The DT indirectly correlates with the difference in pressure between the left atrium and left ventricle during diastole.
   B. The DT indirectly correlates with the difference in pressure between the aorta and left ventricle during diastole.
   C. The DT is not influenced by the difference in pressure between the left ventricle and right ventricle during diastole.
   D. The DT is not influenced by the summation of pressure between the aorta and left ventricle during diastole.
   E. The pressure half-time is an important variable that correlates with the severity of AR, but the DT is less correlative and therefore not used.

15. Based on the 2D image in Figure 18.7 (Video 18.1), the most likely mechanism of aortic regurgitation in this immunosuppressed patient with fungal endocarditis is:

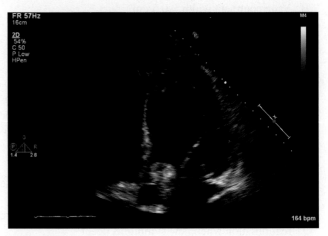

FIGURE **18.7**

   A. Perforation.
   B. Aortic rupture.
   C. Aortic dissection.
   D. Dilation of the sinus of Valsalva.

16. A 43-year-old female with mitral stenosis also has severe aortic regurgitation. Which of the following is most accurate regarding the use of the pressure half-time method to calculate her mitral valve area?

   A. The PHT method remains accurate and is not affected by the severity of aortic regurgitation.
   B. This will result in the overestimation of the mitral valve area.
   C. This will result in the underestimation of the mitral valve area.
   D. For best accuracy, you will need to adjust your measure by using an angle factor correction.
   E. In the setting of severe AR, the PHT of the AR jet can be subtracted from the mitral inflow PHT to obtain the correct value.

17. A 55-year-old female recently had a "general" physical examination by a new primary care physician who noted a systolic ejection murmur graded 2/6 and radiating to her neck and also a diastolic murmur graded 2/6 best heard at the cardiac apex. She was sent for an echocardiogram. Based upon the 3D echo image in Figure 18.8, which of the following is the most correct diagnosis?

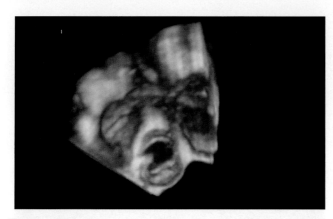

FIGURE **18.8**

A. Aortic valve endocarditis
B. Unicuspid aortic valve
C. Bicuspid aortic valve
D. Calcific degenerative senile aortic valve

Questions 18 to 20

18. A 70-year-old female patient is referred for echocardiography for evaluation of a diastolic murmur. Based upon the color-flow Doppler images in FIGURE 18.9 and the calculated effective regurgitant orifice of 38 mm², what will you report as the severity of aortic regurgitation?

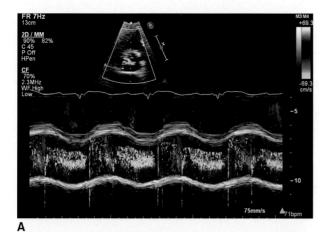

A

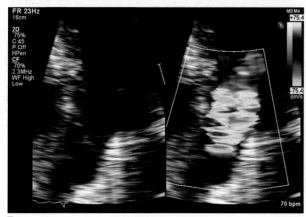

B

FIGURE **18.9**

A. Mild aortic regurgitation due to the color M-mode display
B. Moderate aortic regurgitation based on quantitative ERO
C. Moderate to severe aortic regurgitation based upon discrepant color-flow Doppler (severe) and quantitative (moderate) findings
D. Severe aortic regurgitation

19. FIGURE 18.10 demonstrates a continuous-wave Doppler through the aortic valve of this patient. Given a blood pressure recorded at the time of the study of 148/50 mm Hg, what is her estimated LVEDP?

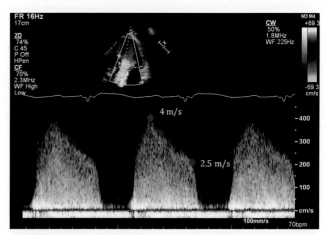

FIGURE **18.10**

A. 44 mm Hg
B. 25 mm Hg
C. 14 mm Hg
D. 40 mm Hg

20. Because of her reported abnormal echocardiogram, she is now referred to your clinic for subsequent evaluation and treatment recommendations. She informs you that she has experienced increased shortness of breath with climbing stairs and occasionally has lower extremity swelling on hot summer days. Her LVEDD is 5.5 cm, and her calculated LVEF = 65%. There are no wall motion abnormalities. She denies regular exercise and admits to smoking one pack of cigarettes/day, and her blood pressure in the office is recorded as 180/92 mm Hg. Your advice to her:

A. Admit for urgent aortic valve replacement.
B. Initiate a trial medical therapy with vasodilators to improve symptoms due to reduced LV systolic function.
C. Smoking cessation; optimize antihypertensive therapy; recommend a structured exercise regimen; return for clinical evaluation in 3 to 6 months and planned repeat echocardiography in 1 year, assuming symptoms do not worsen.
D. Smoking cessation; optimize antihypertensive therapy; recommend structured exercise regimen; return for repeat echocardiography in 3 months, assuming symptoms do not worsen.

Answer 1: B. The figure is an M-mode of the mitral valve leaflets, which demonstrates "fluttering" (high-frequency chaotic motion) of the anterior mitral leaflet during diastole (white arrow). This is indicative of aortic regurgitation, but is not a representation of the actual severity of regurgitation. Features of severe AR, such as LV cavity dilation or early valve closure, are not seen, and therefore, the single best option is answer B.

A papillary fibroelastoma or vegetation of the aortic valve is often associated with aortic regurgitation, but without visualizing the actual pathologic mass, which would not likely be seen on the mitral valve M-mode, this diagnosis cannot be made. Therefore, answers C and D are incorrect.

Aortic stenosis does not cause specific M-mode changes of the mitral valve. Therefore, answer A is incorrect.

Early closure of the mitral valve is a finding in acute severe aortic regurgitation when the mitral valve is noted to close prior to the end of the diastolic period marked by the rhythm strip ECG tracing. This occurs as the LVEDP rises to equalize LA pressure in a very short time due to the severe AR, forcing the mitral leaflets to close prior to the end of diastole. Note that in this image, the MV closure occurs after the onset of the QRS complex (beat 3, Fig. 18.11). Since early MV closure is not seen in this M-mode image, answer E is incorrect.

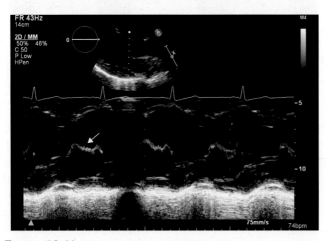

FIGURE 18.11 *Arrow* pointing to diastolic fluttering of the anterior mitral leaflet. Vertical line represents QRS onset (immediately prior to MV closure).

Suggested Readings

Eusebio J, Louie EK, Edwards LC III, et al. Alterations in transmitral flow dynamics in patients with early mitral valve closure and aortic regurgitation. *Am Heart J* 1994;128:941–947.

Louie EK, et al. Determinants of anterior mitral leaflet fluttering in pure aortic regurgitation from pulsed Doppler study of the early diastolic interaction between the regurgitant jet and mitral inflow. *Am J Cardiol* 1988;61(13):1085–1091.

Answer 2: C. This is an M-mode across the aortic valve and aorta. In this image, the coaptation line of the aortic valve in diastole demonstrates significant eccentricity and is closer to the anterior border of the aorta (straight arrow, Fig. 18.12). This is a common characteristic finding in a bicuspid aortic valve. Therefore, answer C is the most correct answer.

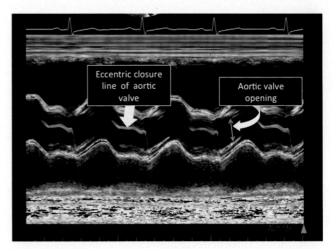

FIGURE 18.12

A stenotic aortic valve would have reduced valve opening, which is not the case in this patient (blue arrow). Although M-mode is not able to directly correlate with the severity of AS, an opening >1.0 cm is not possible in a patient with an area <1.0 cm^2. Therefore, answer A is incorrect.

Although a small vegetative mass may be missed on M-mode echo, a large mass should be evident. There is no evidence of a high-frequency (independently mobile) echo-dense mass (vegetation) on this M-mode image. Answer B is therefore incorrect.

The motion of the aorta demonstrates a normal anterior–posterior motion, and the aortic valve opening is persistent through the entire systolic ejection. Both findings suggest a normal LV stroke volume. Therefore, answer D is incorrect.

Likewise, a normal-sized LA cavity (slightly >4.0 cm on this M-mode) rules out severe mitral stenosis. Answer E is incorrect.

Suggested Readings

Corya BC, Rasmussen S, Phillips JF, et al. Forward stroke calculated from aortic valve echocardiograms in normal subjects and patients with mitral regurgitation secondary to left ventricular dysfunction. *Am J Cardiol* 1981;47:1215.

Nanda MC, Gramiak R, Manning J, et al. Echocardiographic recognition of the congenital bicuspid aortic valve. *Circulation* 1974;49:870–875.

Answer 3: E. Bicuspid aortic valve (BAV) is the most common congenital valve anomaly affecting approximately 1% of the population. Coarctation of the aorta is the most common associated anomaly affecting up to 10% of patients with bicuspid aortic valve. BAV is also associated with other left-sided anomalies, including aortic aneurysms, supra-aortic and sub-aortic membranes, hypoplastic left heart syndrome, and ventricular and atrial septal defects.

Cleft mitral valve is usually associated with AV canal defects. Therefore, the most correct answer to this question is answer E, and answers A to D are incorrect.

Suggested Readings

Cripe L, Andelfinger G, Martin LJ, et al. Bicuspid aortic valve is heritable. *J Am Coll Cardiol* 2004;44:138.

Lewin MB, Otto CM. The bicuspid aortic valve: adverse outcomes from infancy to old age. *Circulation* 2005;111:832–834.

Answer 4: *D.* The pulsed-wave spectral Doppler pattern obtained from the descending thoracic aorta shows holodiastolic reversal of flow (blue arrow, FIG. 18.13), which is specific for moderate to severe aortic regurgitation. No single Doppler feature is without limitation, and therefore, multiple parameters must be combined for final clinical interpretation.

In addition to being holodiastolic, the early (>60 cm/s) and late (>20 cm/s) maximal velocity flow profiles are further evidence that the AR is likely severe, where a diastolic flow reversal >18 cm/s is indicative of a cath-derived regurgitant volume ≥40% with a sensitivity of 89% and a specificity of 96%.

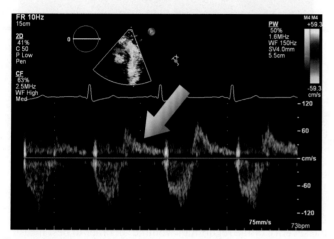

FIGURE **18.13**

Suggested Readings

Messika-Zeitoun D, Detaint D, Leye M, et al. Comparison of semiquantitative and quantitative assessment of severity of aortic regurgitation: clinical implications. *J Am Soc Echocardiogr* 2011;24(11):1246–1252.
Tribouilloy C, Avinee P, Shen WF, et al. End diastolic flow velocity just beneath the aortic isthmus assessed by pulsed Doppler echocardiography: a new predictor of the aortic regurgitant fraction. *Br Heart J* 1991;65:37–40.
Zoghbi WA, Enriquez-Sarano M, Foster E, et al. Recommendations for evaluation of the severity of native valvular regurgitation with two-dimensional and Doppler echocardiography. *J Am Soc Echocardiogr* 2003;16:777–802.

Answer 5: *A.* The assessment of aortic regurgitation consists of multiple echocardiographic parameters, which are qualitative and quantitative.

Qualitative Parameters

- Dilated left ventricle (chronic aortic regurgitation) >7.5 cm
- Flail aortic leaflet
- Dense continuous-wave Doppler spectrum of the AR signal
- Pressure half-time <200 ms
- Prominent holodiastolic reversal in the descending aorta

Quantitative Parameters

- Vena contract width > 0.6 cm
- Jet width/LVOT width ≥ 65%
- Jet CSA/LVOT CSA ≥ 60%
- Regurgitant volume ≥ 60%
- Regurgitant fraction ≥ 50%
- EROA ≥ 0.3 cm²

Suggested Reading

Zoghbi WA, Enriquez-Sarano M, Foster E, et al. Recommendations for evaluation of the severity of native valvular regurgitation with two-dimensional and Doppler echocardiography. *J Am Soc Echocardiogr* 2003;16:777–802.

Answer 6: *D.* It is rarely appropriate to repeat echocardiography in the absence of symptoms or change in cardiac exam if echocardiography has been performed in the prior year. Therefore, option D is correct as this is a rarely appropriate indication if less than severe AR. If AR is severe and the patient is VHD Stage C1, the repeat echo in 6 to 12 months is considered "may be appropriate" (score = 6). Appropriate use of echo in the evaluation of aortic insufficiency include:

A. Confirmation of the diagnosis of aortic regurgitation with equivocal signs based on physical examination
B. Confirmation of the presence, severity, and cause of acute or chronic aortic regurgitation
C. Assessment of left ventricular size and function in asymptomatic patients with severe aortic regurgitation or re-evaluation of mild, moderate, or severe aortic regurgitation in patients with new or changing symptoms
D. Assessment of the aortic root size

Suggested Reading

Doherty JU, et al. ACC/AATS/AHA/ASE/ASNC/HRS/SCAI/SCCT/SCMR/STS 2017 Appropriate Use Criteria for Multimodality Imaging in Valvular Heart Disease. *JACC* 2017. https://doi.org/10.1016/j.jacc.2017.07.732.

Answer 7: *C.* Routine assessment of mild aortic regurgitation is inappropriate particularly if there has not been a change in symptoms or new symptoms. Therefore, a follow-up echocardiogram should not be performed in the scenario described in answer A and D.

A patient with an LV systolic diameter of 5.5 cm and chronic severe aortic regurgitation should be referred for aortic valve surgery. Hence, performing a follow-up echocardiogram would not be appropriate.

It is appropriate for patient with asymptomatic severe aortic regurgitation to undergo echocardiographic assessment every 6 to 12 months to evaluate for LV size and function.

Suggested Reading

Nishimura RA, Otto CM, Bonow RO, et al. 2017 AHA/ACC Focused Update of the 2014 AHA/ACC Guideline for the Management of Patients With Valvular Heart Disease: A Report of the American College of Cardiology/American Heart Association Task Force on Clinical Practice Guidelines. *J Thorac Cardiovasc Surg* 2014;64(16):1763.

Answer 8: *B.* Medical therapy with vasodilators has limited indications. It is indicated in patients with symptomatic severe aortic regurgitation or left ventricular dysfunction when valve replacement is not recommended (class I). Aortic valve replacement is indicated for symptomatic severe aortic regurgitation, asymptomatic severe aortic regurgitation, and LV systolic dysfunction (EF < 50%) and in those with severe aortic regurgitation while undergoing CABG or aortic surgery. Therefore, the single best choice to the above question is answer B.

Suggested Reading

Nishimura RA, Otto CM, Bonow RO, et al. 2017 AHA/ACC Focused Update of the 2014 AHA/ACC Guideline for the Management of Patients With Valvular Heart Disease: A Report of the American College of Cardiology/American Heart Association Task Force on Clinical Practice Guidelines. *J Thorac Cardiovasc Surg* 2014;64(16):1763.

Answer 9: *D.* This image shows a case of aortic dissection with a prolapsing intimal flap (blue arrow, FIG. 18.14). There are several mechanisms for aortic regurgitation in the setting of dissection of the ascending aorta, which include dilation of the aortic root, pressure from a dissection causing flail, or prolapsed aortic leaflets and torn annular causing reduced leaflet support. As there is a dissection flap in this image, the correct answer is D. Of the choices, aortic dissection is the most acute etiology.

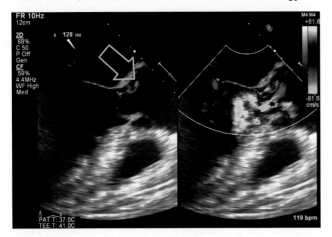

FIGURE 18.14

Suggested Reading

Stout KK, Verrier ED. Acute valvular regurgitation. *Circulation* 2009;119:3232.

Answer 10: *A.* The images show an echo-dense linear structure (arrow, FIG. 18.15) in the left ventricular outflow tract and eccentric aortic regurgitation. Of the choices offered, the most likely diagnosis is a subaortic membrane causing aortic regurgitation—*answer A.* 2D and 3D transthoracic and transesophageal echocardiography is utilized to diagnose this condition. Careful attention should be applied, and a subaortic membrane should be suspected when aortic regurgitation is seen and the valve appears structurally normal and the etiology remains obscure. Three-dimensional echo is valuable as this "membrane" is often more of a "muscular ridge-like" structure rather than a true "membrane" and can be more completely visualized using this tool.

A subaortic membrane is an acquired condition with a genetic predisposition in which a membranous or muscular growth occurs in the left ventricular outflow tract. This membrane causes turbulent blood flow in the LVOT and over time leads to aortic regurgitation due to an unclear mechanism.

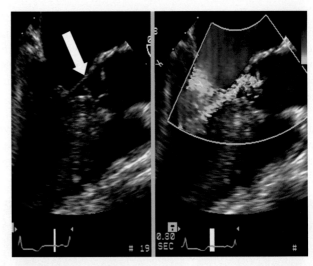

FIGURE 18.15

Suggested Readings

Carr JA, Sugeng L, Weinert L, et al. Images in cardiovascular medicine. Subaortic membrane in the adult. *Circulation* 2005;112:e347.

Leichter DA, et al. "Acquired" discrete subvalvular aortic stenosis: natural history and hemodynamics. *JACC* 1989;14:1539–1544.

Answer 11: *A.* The width of the vena contracta corresponds to the severity of the regurgitant volume. In order to best measure the width, one should image perpendicular to flow. The parasternal long axis usually provides this orientation. The other imaging windows usually do not provide this advantage.

Suggested Reading

Tribouilloy CM, Enriquez-Sarano M, Bailey KR, et al. Assessment of severity of aortic regurgitation using the width of the vena contracta. *Circulation* 2000;102:558–564.

Answer 12: *A.* The image given is a color M-mode display near the level of the LVOT. In FIGURE 18.16, the diameter of the LVOT (large white arrow) and the maximal height/width of the color jet of aortic regurgitation (small black arrow) are shown.

In this demonstration of the jet width/LVOT width ratio, the resulting ratio is clearly <25%, and the degree of aortic regurgitation is most consistent with answer A, mild.

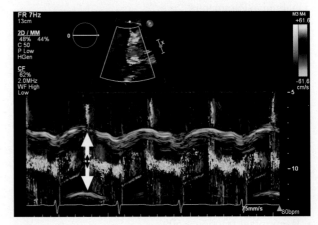

FIGURE 18.16

Suggested Reading

Zoghbi WA, Enriquez-Sarano M, Foster E, et al. Recommendations for evaluation of the severity of native valvular regurgitation with two-dimensional and Doppler echocardiography. *J Am Soc Echocardiogr* 2003;16:777–802.

Answer 13: D. Color-flow Doppler is a qualitative (eyeball) as well as a semiquantitative method to assess the severity of aortic regurgitation. Due to the influence from nonphysiologic (technical) factors, it is recommended as a modality to compliment other more quantitative parameters of assessing severity of valvular regurgitation such as regurgitant volume and fraction.

Answer A is incorrect since overall gain may markedly alter the appearance of the color-flow display and may result in either an overestimation of mild AR or an underestimation of severe AR. Therefore, color-flow Doppler must be consistently optimized. This is best done by increasing the color gain until the color is noted outside of the cardiac chambers and carefully decreased until this is eliminated. Therefore, answer D is correct. Temporal resolution (TR) is an important factor that will impact the appearance of the color display, and therefore, a narrow color sector should always be used to maximize TR. Answer B is incorrect. Answer C is incorrect since jet eccentricity frequently results in a visually narrow display from the rapid deceleration along the ventricular septum or mitral leaflet (the Coanda effect), and this leads to underestimation of AR severity.

Suggested Reading

Messika-Zeitoun D, Detaint D, Leye M, et al. Comparison of semiquantitative and quantitative assessment of severity of aortic regurgitation: clinical implications. *J Am Soc Echocardiogr* 2011;24:1246.

Answer 14: A. In a compliant left ventricle, the aortic deceleration time reflects the transaortic gradient in diastole. However, conditions that affect left ventricular loading and compliance negatively affect the correlation between deceleration time and degree of aortic regurgitation. Pressure half-time (PHT) is the product of $0.29 \times DT$ and indirectly correlates with the severity of AR (shorter the PHT, more severe the AR). Answer E is therefore incorrect since these values have equal correlation. Answer B is incorrect since the DT (and PHT) directly correlates with the difference in pressure between the aorta and left ventricle during diastole. Since the DT (and PHT) is also influenced by the difference in pressure between the left ventricle and right ventricle during diastole and also by the summation of pressure between the aorta and left ventricle during diastole, answers C and D are incorrect.

Suggested Reading

Griffin BP, Flachskampf FA, Siu S, et al. The effects of regurgitant orifice size, chamber compliance, and systemic vascular resistance on aortic regurgitant velocity slope and pressure half-time. *Am Heart J* 1991;122(4 Pt 1):1049–1056.

Answer 15: A. Of the choices provided, only answer A is a specific leaflet pathology. There is a large aortic valve echodensity protruding into the ventricular surface and a linear echo-free space within this density. This is fungal endocarditis, which caused leaflet perforation and severe aortic regurgitation. The lack of demonstrated findings to support an aortic pathology lowers the likelihood for an aortic etiology for the AR; therefore, answers B, C, and D are incorrect.

Suggested Reading

Sarma R, Prakash R, Kaushik VS, et al. Reliability of two-dimensional echocardiography in diagnosing fungal endocarditis. *Clin Cardiol* 1983;6(1):37–40.

Answer 16: B. Pressure half-time (PHT) is the duration of time taken for the peak diastolic mitral gradient to fall to half its value. Mitral valve area (MVA) can then be estimated by the formula that is measured by taking an initial point at peak velocity by continuous-wave Doppler. A line is drawn from this peak diastolic pressure gradient along the slope of descent. A second point is determined at the velocity at which the pressure gradient falls to 50% of the peak value and the time to reach this velocity is measured:

$$MVA\ (cm^2) = 220/PHT$$

In the setting of moderate to severe aortic regurgitation, increase in left ventricular end-diastolic pressure (LVEDP) results in a decreased transmitral gradient and therefore a shorter pressure half-time. This results in an overestimation of mitral valve area. Answer B is therefore most correct, and answers A and C are incorrect.

Answers D and E are completely fictitious.

Suggested Reading

Moro E, et al. Influence of aortic regurgitation on the assessment of the pressure half time and derived mitral valve area in patients with mitral stenosis. *Eur Heart J* 1988;9(9):1010–1017.

Answer 17: C. This is a three-dimensional echo of a bicuspid aortic valve viewed from the perspective of the aorta (Fig. 18.17). AoV, aortic valve; RVOT, right ventricular outflow tract; and LA, left atrium. Note the well-visualized, nearly equal-sized, AV leaflets in systole and the complete extension across the aortic annulus (only seen in congenital BAV).

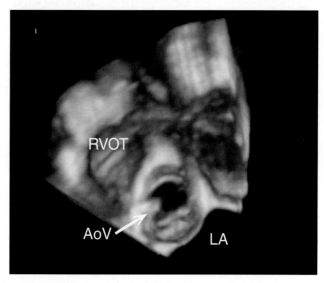

Figure 18.17

Suggested Reading

Muraru D, Badano LP, Vannan M, et al. Assessment of aortic valve complex by three-dimensional echocardiography: a framework for its effective application in clinical practice. *Eur Heart J Cardiovasc Imaging* 2012;13(7):541–555. doi:10.1093/ehjci/jes075.

Answer 18: *D.* The color M-mode shows a jet width/LVOT width >65% (answer A is incorrect). The A5C view demonstrates a wide vena contracta >8 mm as well as a readily visualized proximal flow convergence. The calculated ERO is provided and significantly >30 mm^2 (answer B is incorrect). It is important to note that a smaller ERO than typically required for MR (where >0.4 cm^2 is necessary) will result in a severe regurgitant volume >60 mL (likely due to the longer duration of diastolic aortic regurgitation).

Therefore, this patient has multiple concordant color-flow Doppler and quantitative features to report severe aortic regurgitation (answer C is incorrect). Answer D is the single most correct option (TABLE 18.1).

Suggested Reading

Zoghbi WA, Enriquez-Sarano M, Foster E, et al. Recommendations for evaluation of the severity of native valvular regurgitation with two-dimensional and Doppler echocardiography. *J Am Soc Echocardiogr* 2003;16:777–802.

Answer 19: *B.* The left ventricular end-diastolic pressure (LVEDP) can be calculated from the end-diastolic velocity from a well-aligned continuous-wave Doppler spectrum of the aortic regurgitant jet. Using the Bernoulli equation to estimate the AO to an LV end-diastolic gradient at a velocity of 2.5 m/s, then $4 \times (2.5)2$ results in an end-diastolic gradient of 25 mm Hg. The LVEDP is the difference between the diastolic BP and this estimated gradient: LVEDP = 50 − 25 = 25 mm Hg.

Table 18.1 ERO and Jet/Height Ratios to Evaluate the Degree of Aortic Regurgitation

	ERO	JET/HEIGHT RATIO
Mild	<0.1	<25%
Moderate	0.1–0.3	25%–65%
Severe	>0.3	>65%

Suggested Reading

Nagueh SF, et al. Recommendations for the evaluation of left ventricular diastolic function by echocardiography. *Eur J Echocardiogr* 2009;10(2):165–193.

Answer 20: *C.* Her shortness of breath could be due to many factors including diastolic dysfunction, persistent smoking, and lack of exercise. Therefore, the best clinical recommendation would be smoking cessation; optimize antihypertensive therapy (vasodilator Rx may be preferred); initiate a structured, preferably supervised, exercise regimen; and return for clinical evaluation in 3 to 6 months to confirm symptomatic improvement and importantly confirm no clinical worsening. A repeat echocardiogram in 1 year assuming symptoms do not worsen is also considered appropriate: routine surveillance (>1 year) of moderate or severe valvular regurgitation without a change in clinical status or cardiac exam (appropriate use score A [8]). Therefore, answer C is the single best option, and answers D and E are incorrect.

Aortic valve replacement is indicated for symptomatic patients with severe AR regardless of LV function and size (class I, level of evidence B). So in this patient with multiple causes of her symptoms, it is critical to follow closely and demonstrate that her symptoms will improve. If they do not, then AVR should be considered. However, there are no reasons for urgent hospitalization and emergent AVR given the normal LV size and function. Therefore, answer A is incorrect.

Answer B is incorrect since initiation of vasodilator therapy, which may be indicated for chronic therapy in patients with severe AR and symptoms (class I, level of evidence B), would not be expected to improve the LV systolic function in this patient with normal heart size and LVEF. Should her symptoms improve with other listed clinical recommendations, vasodilator therapy would be a class IIb recommendation for an asymptomatic patient with severe AR despite LV dilation but normal systolic function (level of evidence B).

Suggested Reading

Nishimura RA, Otto CM, Bonow RO, et al. 2014 AHA/ACC Guideline for the Management of Patients With Valvular Heart Disease: Executive Summary: A Report of the American College of Cardiology/American Heart Association Task Force on Practice Guidelines. *Circulation* 2014;129(23):2440–2492.

Chapter 19

Mitral Stenosis

John R. Kotter

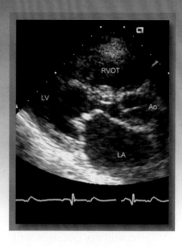

1. The most common etiology of mitral stenosis in industrialized countries is:

   A. Rheumatic
   B. Degenerative
   C. Connective tissue disease
   D. Congenital

2. In which of the following circumstances is pressure half-time the MOST appropriate method to use for calculating the mitral valve area?

   A. Acute severe aortic regurgitation
   B. Severe left ventricular diastolic dysfunction
   C. Severe tricuspid regurgitation
   D. Within the first 48 hours after balloon mitral commissurotomy

3. A patient with mitral stenosis undergoes a TEE for evaluation of possible mitral balloon valvuloplasty. Pathology in which of the following structures will not affect the calculated Wilkins score?

   A. Leaflet mobility
   B. Subvalvular calcification
   C. Subvalvular thickening
   D. Leaflet calcification
   E. Leaflet thickening

4. Which of the following changes will increase the radius of the proximal isovelocity surface area (PISA) when this method is used in estimating the mitral valve area in the apical four-chamber view on a transthoracic echocardiogram?

   A. Shifting the baseline of the velocity scale away from direction of diastolic MV inflow.
   B. Shifting the baseline of the velocity scale in the direction of mitral regurgitant flow.
   C. Increasing the Nyquist limit.
   D. Radius of PISA is determined by the transvalvular gradients and cannot be changed.

5. You are asked to calculate the mitral valve area by the pressure half-time method. The V_{max} of mitral inflow is 1.41 m/s. Without knowing the slope of deceleration of the mitral inflow velocity, it is possible to calculate P t½ by measuring the time interval from 1.41 m/s to:

   A. 1.0 m/s
   B. 0.7 m/s
   C. 0.35 m/s
   D. Pressure half-time cannot be assessed with velocity data alone

6. Which of the following methods for the estimation of mitral valve area is least accurate and most likely to have the poorest reproducibility?

   A. Direct planimetry of the mitral valve opening
   B. 220/pressure half-time
   C. Maximal MV gradient/mitral valve resistance
   D. Proximal isovelocity surface area determined by flow rate/maximal MV inflow velocity
   E. LVOT VTI × LVOT area/MV VTI

7. Which of the following is the least accurate variation of the Hatle equation (pressure half-time method) for calculating mitral valve area?

   A. 220/pressure half-time
   B. 190/mitral valve inflow VTI
   C. 759/deceleration time
   D. 220/0.29 deceleration time

8. You are performing a transesophageal echocardiogram for the evaluation of mitral valve pathology. From a probe position high in the esophagus, you insert the probe deeper while keeping the imaging plane at 0 degrees (horizontal). The most common MV leaflet segments (scallops) seen initially are:

   A. A1P1
   B. A2P2
   C. A3P3
   D. A3P1

9. Which of the following statements in the transthoracic echocardiographic evaluation of mitral stenosis is correct?

   A. Commissural fusion is best assessed in the parasternal long-axis view.
   B. Leaflet thickening and mobility are identified best in the apical two-chamber view.
   C. Chordal shortening and thickening are best measured in the parasternal long-axis and apical four-chamber views.
   D. In the presence of significant mitral regurgitation, the continuity equation will be accurate.

10. Which of the following is the most appropriate indication for percutaneous valvuloplasty repair of mitral stenosis?

    A. A symptomatic patient with mitral valve area of <1.5 cm^2 and baseline resting pulmonary artery systolic pressure of 60 mm Hg and Wilkins score = 12
    B. An asymptomatic patient with mitral valve area of >1.5 cm^2, but the pulmonary capillary wedge pressure increases during exercise testing to >25 mm Hg
    C. A symptomatic patient with mitral valve area of >1.5 cm^2 and exercise-induced mean gradient of <15 mm Hg
    D. An asymptomatic patient with mitral valve area of <1.0 cm^2 and Wilkins score of 6

11. Which of the following statements is most accurate in the clinical setting of combined mitral stenosis and atrial fibrillation?

    A. There is no need for anticoagulation to decrease the risk of embolic events.
    B. When measuring the mean pressure gradient, the shortest three R–R intervals should be averaged.
    C. As the heart rate increases, the mean gradient across the mitral valve will increase.
    D. Mean ΔP and end-diastolic ΔP are directly proportional to the duration of the cardiac cycle.

12. You are evaluating two patients with mitral stenosis. Patient A has peak early diastolic transmitral gradient of 9 mm Hg and mean gradient of 6 mm Hg. Patient B has peak early diastolic gradient of 27 mm Hg and mean gradient of 7 mm Hg. Which of the following clinical scenarios least likely explains the echo Doppler findings of patient B compared to A?

    A. Associated mitral regurgitation
    B. Pregnancy
    C. Thyrotoxicosis
    D. Nonrestrictive ventricular septal defect
    E. Delayed left ventricular relaxation

13. Which of the following is most likely found on M-mode echocardiography in patients with mitral stenosis?

    A. Diastolic anterior motion of the posterior mitral leaflet
    B. "Hockey stick" deformity of the anterior mitral leaflet
    C. Increased EF slope
    D. Diastolic fluttering of the anterior mitral valve leaflet

14. The mitral valve area is most likely to be measured correctly when using the pressure half-time method in which of the following conditions?

    A. Acute severe aortic regurgitation
    B. Restrictive LV function
    C. Left-to-right shunt at atrial level
    D. Severe mitral regurgitation

15. When measuring the mitral valve area by the PISA method, determining the flow rate at the PISA hemisphere without angle correction for the diminished opening of the mitral leaflets would result in:

    A. Overestimation of the flow rate.
    B. Underestimation of the mitral valve area.
    C. Underestimation of the flow volume.
    D. Angle correction is NOT dependent on the Nyquist limit.

16. Mitral inflow velocities demonstrate grade I diastolic dysfunction. If you calculate the mitral valve area using the P t½ method in this patient:

    A. The mitral valve area will be underestimated.
    B. The mitral valve stenosis will be severely underestimated.
    C. The pressure half-time will be short relative to other grades of diastolic dysfunction.
    D. The mitral valve area calculation will not change.

Answer 1: *A.* Mitral stenosis is the most frequent valvular complication of rheumatic fever. Although the incidence of rheumatic heart disease is decreasing, it still remains the most frequent cause of mitral stenosis worldwide. Other causes are much less common.

Degenerative diseases result from physiologic and/or pathologic wear and tear of tissues. The structure and function of the affected tissue/organ deteriorate over time. Degenerative valve disease is a consequence of fibrosis and calcification on the valve leaflets and the annulus. Degenerative mitral valve disease is seen in elderly patients with hypertension, elderly patients with atherosclerotic disease, or elderly patients with aortic stenosis. Mitral annular calcification can uncommonly cause mitral stenosis but more often causes mitral regurgitation.

Connective tissue disorders can affect the heart valves. For example, Marfan syndrome and Ehlers-Danlos syndrome can cause mitral valve prolapse. However, these disorders do not cause mitral stenosis. Congenital mitral stenosis is rare and involves abnormalities within the subvalvular apparatus.

Suggested Readings

Iung B, Baron G, Butchart EG, et al. A prospective survey of patients with valvular heart disease in Europe: the Euro Heart Survey on Valvular Heart Disease. *Eur Heart J* 2003;24:1231–1243.

Soler-Soler J, Galve E. Worldwide perspective of heart disease. *Heart* 2000;83:721–725.

Answer 2: C. Pressure half-time (P t½) is defined as the time interval, in milliseconds, between the maximal mitral pressure gradient in early diastole and the time when the pressure gradient is half the maximum value.

The rate of decline in velocity of transmitral flow, after the peak velocity of early diastolic filling, is directly proportional to mitral valve area. Mitral stenosis slows the rate of fall of mitral inflow velocity. The left ventricular diastolic filling rate, which is reflected in the deceleration slope of the E wave, depends not only on mitral valve area but also on mitral pressure gradient in early diastole, left atrial compliance, and left ventricular diastolic compliance.

Aortic regurgitation increases the rate of left ventricular diastolic filling because blood enters the LV from both the mitral valve and the aortic valve. This shortens the P t½. In acute severe aortic regurgitation, the diastolic LV volume and hence the pressure rise rapidly, which in turn rapidly reduces the transmitral gradient. This shortens the P t½, which would then underestimate the severity of the mitral stenosis. Therefore, P t½ cannot be used when there is an associated acute severe aortic regurgitation.

Impairment of left ventricular diastolic compliance shortens the P t½ (measured as the mitral deceleration time) so that this value is not an accurate measure of mitral valve area.

Tricuspid regurgitation does not affect mitral P t½.

There are abrupt changes in mitral gradient and left atrial compliance within the first 48 hours after balloon mitral commissurotomy. In addition, the atrial septostomy that is performed as a part of the balloon valvuloplasty procedure leads to a decrease in the transmitral gradient. These combined effects make the P t½ method an inaccurate measure of mitral valve area immediately after mitral commissurotomy.

Suggested Readings

Karp K, Teien D, Bjerle P, et al. Reassessment of valve area determinations in mitral stenosis by the pressure half-time method: impact of left ventricular stiffness and peak diastolic pressure difference. *J Am Coll Cardiol* 1989;13:594–599.

Messika-Zeitoun D, Meizels A, Cachier A, et al. Echocardiographic evaluation of the mitral valve area before and after percutaneous mitral commissurotomy: the pressure half-time method revisited. *J Am Soc Echocardiogr* 2005;18:1409–1414.

Thomas JD, Wilkins GT, Choong CY, et al. Inaccuracy of mitral pressure half-time immediately after percutaneous mitral valvotomy. Dependence on transmitral gradient and left atrial and ventricular compliance. *Circulation* 1988;78:980–993.

Answer 3: B. The Wilkins score is used in determining the suitability of candidates for mitral balloon valvuloplasty. Patients considered suitable for valvuloplasty are those with a Wilkins score (also known as splitability index or Abascal score) of 8 or less, with less than moderate mitral regurgitation, and with no left atrial thrombus. Balloon valvuloplasty is considered successful when mitral valve area increases by >50%, or increases to >1.5 cm², and with less than moderate mitral regurgitation after the procedure (TABLE 19.1).

Answer 4: B. As the blood from the left atrium converges toward the stenotic mitral valve during diastole, blood velocity gradually increases forming a series of hemispheres. The velocity is equal along the surface of any one hemisphere, hence the name isovelocity.

Color-flow imaging can be used to identify the isovelocity hemisphere. The red–blue aliasing interface (blue–red on TEE orientation) identifies one hemisphere. The velocity along this hemisphere is equal to the aliasing velocity. For all hemispheres, the surface velocity multiplied by the surface area is constant, for any valve. When the aliasing velocity is lower, the hemisphere is larger and farther away from the stenotic valve. The aliasing velocity can be altered by shifting the baseline. Generally, the baseline should be shifted in the direction of jet flow. Since diastolic flow is toward the left ventricular cavity or toward the transducer in TTE, the baseline should be shifted in

Table 19.1	Assessment of Mitral Valve Anatomy According to the Wilkins Score			
GRADE	MOBILITY	THICKENING	CALCIFICATION	SUBVALVULAR THICKENING
1	Highly mobile valve with only leaflet tips restricted	Leaflets near normal in thickness (4–5 mm)	A single area of increased echo brightness	Minimal thickening just below the mitral leaflets
2	Leaflet mid- and base portions have normal mobility	Midleaflets normal, considerable thickening of margins (5–8 mm)	Scattered areas of brightness confined to leaflet margins	Thickening of chordal structures extending to one-third of the chordal length
3	Valve continues to move forward in diastole, mainly from the base	Thickening extending through the entire leaflet (5–8 mm)	Brightness extending into the midportions of the leaflets	Thickening extended to distal third of the chords
4	No or minimal forward movement of the leaflets in diastole	Considerable thickening of all leaflet tissue (>8–10 mm)	Extensive brightness throughout much of the leaflet tissue	Extensive thickening and shortening of all chordal structures extending down to the papillary muscles

The total score is the sum of the four items and ranges between 4 and 16.

Reproduced from Wilkins GT, Weyman AE, Abascal VM, et al. Percutaneous balloon dilatation of the mitral valve: an analysis of echocardiographic variables related to outcome and the mechanism of dilatation. *Br Heart J* 1988;60(4):299–308, with permission from BMJ Publishing Group Ltd.

this direction to obtain an optimally visualized and contoured hemispheric PISA. If TEE is used, then the baseline will have to be shifted downward ("away" from the transducer, in the direction of blood flow). Note that the reverse is true in mitral regurgitation. Answer B is therefore correct.

Aliasing velocity should be decreased in order to increase the radius of PISA. Answer C is therefore not true. Answer D is incorrect since it is possible to change the PISA radius as explained above.

Suggested Reading

Messika-Zeitoun D, Fung Yiu S, Cormier B, et al. Sequential assessment of mitral valve area during diastole using color M-mode flow convergence analysis: new insights into mitral stenosis physiology. *Eur Heart J* 2003;24:1244–1253.

Answer 5: *A.* Pressure half-time can be conveniently measured from the deceleration slope of the diastolic mitral inflow. The height of the E wave is the maximum inflow velocity (V_{max}), and the corresponding pressure gradient is the peak instantaneous pressure gradient.

Using the simplified Bernoulli equation, $P = 4V^2$, we can calculate $V^2 = P/4$, and therefore, $V = \sqrt{P}/2$ (square root of P, divided by 2). Pressure half-time is the time required for the maximal pressure (P_{max}) to decrease by half. The maximal pressure gradient can be calculated from the given maximal velocity of 1.41 m/s:

$$P_{max} = 4V^2$$
$$= 4(1.41)^2$$
$$= 4(2) = 8\,\text{mm Hg}$$

Therefore, the P t½ is the time between the maximum gradient of 8 and 4 mm Hg. When the pressure gradient is 4 mm Hg, the velocity is.

$$P = 4V^2$$
$$4 = 4V^2$$
$$1 = V^2$$
$$V = 1\,\text{m/s}$$

Hence, the correct answer is (A).

Suggested Readings

Hatle L, Bruback A, Tromsdal A, et al. Noninvasive assessment of pressure drop in mitral stenosis by Doppler ultrasound. *Br Heart J* 1978;40:131.

Thomas JD, Weyman AE. Doppler mitral pressure half-time: a clinical tool in search of theoretical justification. *J Am Coll Cardiol* 1987;10:923–929.

Answer 6: *C.* While no one technique to measure mitral valve area is always accurate and reproducible, mitral valve resistance is the least accurate of the given techniques. Mitral valve resistance is the ratio of mean mitral diastolic gradient to mitral diastolic flow rate. The value obtained is dependent on flow conditions. This method is not recommended for clinical use by the ASE.

Planimetry is recommended as a method to assess the severity of mitral stenosis. Planimetry has the advantage of directly measuring the orifice area, so that the value is independent of heart rate, cardiac output, chamber compliance, and associated valve lesions. When the mitral valve leaflets open in diastole, a cone-shaped passage is created from the base to the tip of the leaflets. The narrowest part of the orifice is the tip of the cone, which is usually at the level of the tip of mitral leaflets. It is imperative to ensure that the cross-sectional cut obtained by the sonographer is precisely at the tip, or else, the valve area would be overestimated (Fig. 19.1). Appropriate gain adjustment and image magnification may be needed for best results. The accuracy of planimetry is diminished when there is severe mitral valve calcification. The reproducibility may be enhanced by 3D echo and 3D-guided biplane imaging.

Pressure half-time is defined above (see the answer to question 2). The mitral valve area can be calculated as 220/P t½, where P t½ is measured in milliseconds. This method is not accurate when other factors alter the rate of decline of mitral inflow velocity. These factors include severe aortic regurgitation, severely reduced LV diastolic compliance, decreased left atrial compliance, and within 48 hours following mitral balloon commissurotomy. When these conditions are not present, the P t½ method is recommended (Fig. 19.2).

Proximal isovelocity surface area (PISA) method measures transmitral diastolic volumetric flow rate (in cm³/s). This value divided by the maximum velocity of mitral diastolic flow equals mitral valve area. However, this area should be multiplied by angle α/180 degrees. Angle α is the angle subtended by the opening of leaflets at end diastole. The value is in the range of 118 ± 15 degrees. This is to account for the leaflet opening, which is generally smaller than 180 degrees, so the PISA flow is not a complete hemisphere. This method is technically demanding and is inaccurate if the mitral orifice is grossly irregular. This method is considered appropriate only in selected cases.

The continuity equation is the law of conservation of mass applied to valve area. Specifically, the antegrade flow across all four heart valves must be the same in each cardiac cycle, in the absence of more than trivial valve insufficiency or an intracardiac shunt lesion. For any cardiac valve, the velocity–time integral of antegrade flow during one cardiac cycle, multiplied by the valve area, is the antegrade volumetric flow across that valve during one cardiac cycle. This must be the same for all four valves, in the absence of regurgitation or intracardiac shunt. Thus, mitral valve area can be calculated as left ventricular outflow tract (LVOT) area (calculated from the diameter of the LVOT) multiplied by left ventricular outflow tract systolic velocity–time integral (VTI), divided by mitral valve diastolic VTI:

Mitral valve VTI × mitral valve area = aortic valve VTI × aortic valve area = LVOT VTI × LVOT area.

Therefore, MVA = LVOT VTI × LVOT area/MV VTI. This method involves multiple measurements, so it is appropriate only for selected cases.

Suggested Reading

Baumgartner H, Hung J, Bermejo J, et al. Echocardiographic assessment of valve stenosis: EAE/ASE recommendations for clinical practice. *J Am Soc Echocardiogr* 2009;22:1–25.

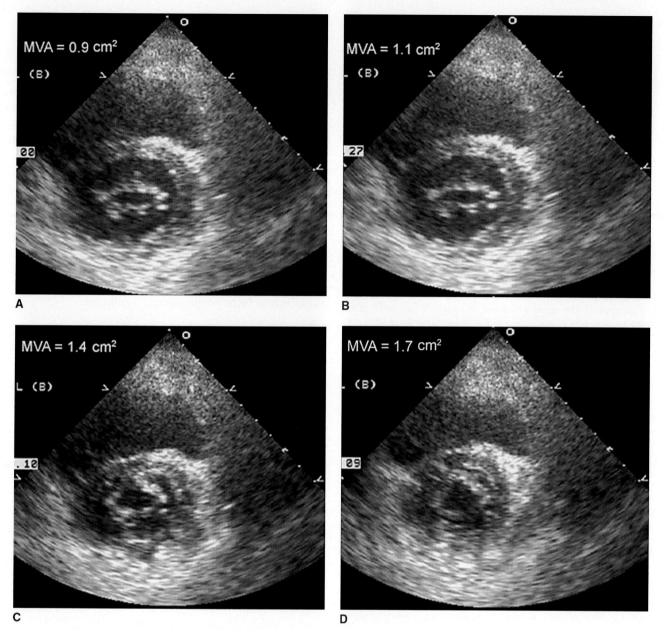

FIGURE 19.1 Series of parasternal short-axis views in a patient with rheumatic MS. The smallest and therefore most accurate orifice is in **(A)**. Images **(B)** to **(D)** were obtained from the same patient; each image was progressively closer to the annulus, and therefore, the orifice appears to be progressively larger. (From Armstrong WF, Ryan T. *Feigenbaum's Echocardiography.* 7th ed. Philadelphia, PA: Lippincott Williams & Wilkins, 2010.)

Answer 7: B. Answers A, C, and D are all modifications of Hatle equation. Although the relationship between mitral valve area and pressure half-time was originally described by Libanoff and Rodbard (*Circulation* 1966;33:218 and *Circulation* 1968;38:144), it was popularized by Hatle et al. The relationship has been simplified using the formula, MVA = 220/P t½. One can derive the same results using the deceleration slope of the mitral inflow: P t½ = 0.29 × MDT (mitral deceleration time). Substituting the above relationship into the equation, MVA = 220/P t½ = 220/0.29 × mitral deceleration time = 759/mitral deceleration time.

Suggested Reading

Hatle L, Angelsen L, Tromsdal A. Noninvasive assessment of atrioventricular pressure half-time by Doppler ultrasound. *Circulation* 1979;60(5):1096–1104.

Answer 8: A. Mitral annulovalvular apparatus has saddle-shaped geometry. This results in leaflet cusp attachment height discrepancy. This unique orientation leads to lateral aspect being at a higher position than the medial aspect. The nomenclature of mitral leaflet segments is based on their proximity to the left atrial appendage, with A1/P1 being the most

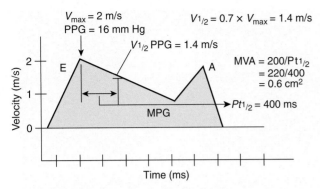

$V_{max} = 2$ m/s
PPG = 16 mm Hg

$V_{1/2} = 0.7 \times V_{max} = 1.4$ m/s

$V_{1/2}$ PPG = 1.4 m/s

MVA = $200/Pt_{1/2}$
    = 220/400
    = 0.6 cm^2

$Pt_{1/2} = 400$ ms

Figure 19.2 Schematic representation of mitral valve inflow depicting different parameters that can be extracted for determination of the severity of mitral stenosis. In the schematic, note the relatively flat decay of pressure from the E point. Parameters that can be measured include integration of the overall pressure gradient beneath the spectral display to calculate the pressure half-time method. For the pressure half-time method, the time required for the pressure to decay from its peak value (16 mm Hg in this example) to one-half of that value (8 mm Hg) is determined. The velocity at which the gradient has declined to one-half its peak can be calculated as $0.7 \times V_{max}$. This value (400 ms in this example) is then entered into the equation MVA = 220/P t½. In the schematic, the MVA calculates to 0.6 cm^2. PPG, peak pressure gradient. (From Armstrong WF, Ryan T. *Feigenbaum's Echocardiography.* 7th ed. Philadelphia, PA: Lippincott Williams & Wilkins, 2010.)

superior and A3/P3 being the most inferior. Therefore, as the transesophageal probe is inserted, the first MV segments seen in the apical four-chamber orientation (0 degrees) are most commonly A1/P1.

Suggested Reading

Salcedo EE, Quaife RA, Seres T, Carroll JD. A framework for systematic characterization of the mitral valve by real time three-dimensional transesophageal echocardiography. *J Am Soc Echocardiogr* 2009;22(10):1087–1099.

Answer 9: *C.* Mitral commissures are located at medial and lateral edges where A3/P3 and A1/P1 cusps meet. The best TTE view to visualize all the cusps and commissures is the parasternal short-axis view at the level of mitral leaflets. Commissural fusion can thus be demonstrated best in this view. The typical appearance in this view is described as the "fish-mouth" appearance.

To assess the mobility and thickness of the MV leaflets, the parasternal long-axis view is the best. The reason for this is that the ultrasound beam is perpendicular to the leaflets in the parasternal long-axis view.

Chordal structures are best assessed in either the parasternal long-axis view or the apical four-chamber view.

The continuity equation relies on the law of conservation of mass. It is valid when the flow is the same across the mitral and aortic valves. In the presence of mitral regurgitation, a fraction of forward diastolic mitral flow regurgitates back during systole. This results in higher forward flow across the mitral valve than across the aortic valve. The continuity equation cannot be used in such situations.

Suggested Reading

Baumgartner H, Hung J, Bermejo J, et al. Echocardiographic assessment of valve stenosis: EAE/ASE recommendations for clinical practice. *J Am Soc Echocardiogr* 2009;22:1–25.

Answer 10: *D.* According to current ACC/AHA, indications for mitral balloon valvuloplasty is indicated in symptomatic patients with severe mitral stenosis and favorable valve morphology in the absence of contraindications. It is also indicated in asymptomatic patients with very severe mitral stenosis (mitral valve area < 1 cm^2) in the absence of contraindications. Option A is incorrect as favorable valve morphology is consistent with a Wilkins score ≤ 8. Option B is incorrect as the valve area should be ≤1.5 cm prior to balloon valvuloplasty. Option C is incorrect as PMBC may be considered for symptomatic patients with MVA > 1.5 cm^2 if there is evidence of hemodynamically significant MS during exercise. A pulmonary capillary wedge pressure < 15 mm Hg following exercise is unlikely to be hemodynamically significant.

Suggested Reading

Nishimura RA, Otto CM, Bonow RO. 2014 AHA/ACC guideline for the management of patients with valvular heart disease: a report of the American College of Cardiology/American Heart Association Task Force on Practice Guidelines. *J Am Coll Cardiol* 2014;63(22):2438–2488.

Answer 11: *C.* Atrial fibrillation is usually characterized by variable R–R intervals. This produces beat-to-beat variation in the diastolic flow duration. One of the important determinants of mean pressure gradient across the mitral valve is the duration of diastolic flow.

Mean and end-diastolic pressure gradients are inversely proportional to the duration of diastolic flow. Shorter cycles therefore result in higher gradients. During shorter cardiac cycles, there is less time available for ventricular filling and, consequently, less time to allow for the equilibration of transmitral pressure gradients. In such situations, mean pressure gradient should be reported as the average of several cardiac cycles. Avoid measuring short cycles (Fig. 19.3).

Faster heart rates result in decreased diastolic filling period, thereby causing an increase in transmitral gradient. In patients with moderate to severe mitral stenosis, rapid atrial fibrillation can precipitate acute pulmonary edema by suddenly increasing the transmitral gradient.

Suggested Reading

Kim HK, Kim YJ, Chang SA, et al. Impact of cardiac rhythm on mitral valve area calculated by the pressure half time method in patients with moderate or severe mitral stenosis. *J Am Soc Echocardiogr* 2009;22(1):42–47.

Answer 12: *E.* Peak transmitral gradient at the onset of diastole represents the early diastolic pressure difference between the left atrium and the left ventricle. Increased left atrial volume is associated with increased left atrial pressure and, therefore, increased velocity of flow across the mitral valve in early

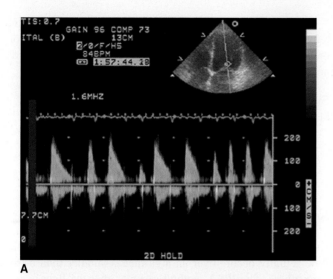

A

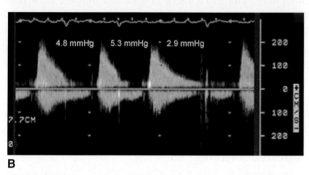

B

FIGURE 19.3 Transmitral continuous-wave Doppler image recorded in a patient with mitral stenosis in atrial fibrillation with an irregular ventricular response. **A:** Note the marked variation in diastolic filling time and the obvious variation in the spectral profile. **B:** Recorded in the same patient, revealing three different diastolic filling profiles. Note the marked variation in the mean pressure gradient, dependent on diastolic filling time. MVA, mitral valve area. (From Armstrong WF, Ryan T. *Feigenbaum's Echocardiography.* 7th ed. Philadelphia, PA: Lippincott Williams & Wilkins, 2010.)

diastole. Other important causes of increased left atrial pressure are mitral stenosis and severe diastolic dysfunction.

In the presence of a hyperdynamic circulation, an increase in the left atrial volume leads to increased early transmitral pressure gradient. The severity of mitral stenosis correlates with the mean gradient and not the peak gradient (FIG. 19.4).

Pregnancy, thyrotoxicosis, and nonrestrictive VSD are all causes of a hyperdynamic circulation. In mitral regurgitation, regurgitated blood leads to volume overload of the left atrium, thereby increasing the LA pressure.

In the presence of delayed relaxation of the LV (grade I diastolic dysfunction), the left atrial pressure is usually not elevated. Therefore, the velocity of the E wave is generally not increased. On occasion, grade I diastolic dysfunction may be associated with an increased LAP and, in this situation, is sometimes referred to as grade Ib. The more classical form of mild LV diastolic dysfunction (LV relaxation abnormality with normal LAP) is then referred to as grade Ia.

Suggested Reading

Thomas JD, Newell JB, Choong CY, et al. Physical and physiological determinants of transmitral velocity: numerical analysis. *Am J Physiol* 1991;260(5 Pt 2):H1718–H1731.

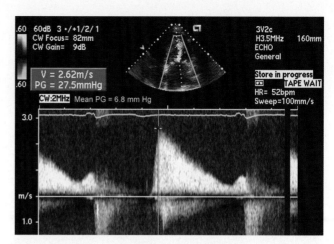

FIGURE 19.4 Transmitral Doppler image recorded in a patient with concurrent mitral stenosis and mitral regurgitation. Note the high peak early gradient (27.5 mm Hg) but the rapid decay and a negligible pressure gradient at end diastole. Compare the peak early gradient of 27.5 mm Hg with the mean gradient of only 6.8 mm Hg. This discrepancy between peak and mean pressure gradient is often seen in patients with concurrent mitral regurgitation. (From Armstrong WF, Ryan T. *Feigenbaum's Echocardiography.* 7th ed. Philadelphia, PA: Lippincott Williams & Wilkins, 2010.)

Answer 13: A. The anterior mitral leaflet is larger and more mobile and has a greater diastolic excursion than the posterior leaflet. The commissural fusion causes the smaller posterior leaflet to move anteriorly, with the anterior leaflet, during diastole. This is well demonstrated on M-mode echo. It is paradoxical, as one would expect posterior motion of the posterior leaflet during diastole.

Classic rheumatic mitral stenosis affects the mitral valve from tip to base in a centripetal fashion. Commissural fusion is one of the earliest manifestations of the rheumatic affliction of the mitral valve (FIG. 19.5).

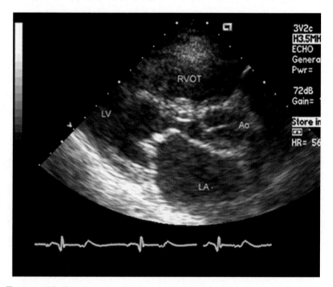

FIGURE 19.5 Transthoracic parasternal long-axis view in a patient with rheumatic MS. There is restricted motion of the leaflet tips creating a "hockey stick" appearance of the anterior mitral leaflet in diastole. (From Armstrong WF, Ryan T. *Feigenbaum's Echocardiography.* 7th ed. Philadelphia, PA: Lippincott Williams & Wilkins, 2010.)

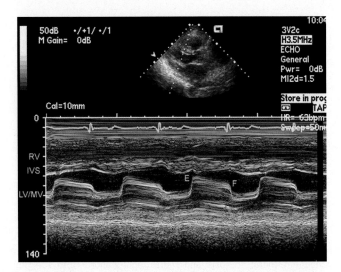

FIGURE 19.6 M-mode echocardiographic findings in a patient with rheumatic MS. Note the thickened mitral leaflets, reduced EF slope, and diastolic anterior motion of posterior mitral leaflet. (From Armstrong WF, Ryan T. *Feigenbaum's Echocardiography*. 7th ed. Philadelphia, PA: Lippincott Williams & Wilkins, 2010.)

In early stages of rheumatic mitral stenosis, the body and base of the valve leaflets may remain pliable, while there is fusion of the commissures. This leads to a "hockey stick"–shaped deformity of the anterior leaflet during diastole. This is a classic and very specific 2D echo finding for rheumatic mitral stenosis. This is not directly seen on the M-mode echo.

Reduced (not increased) EF slope is classically seen in mitral stenosis and could be seen on M-mode echo. Leaflet thickening is a recognizable M-mode finding as well (Fig. 19.6).

Diastolic fluttering of the anterior mitral valve is most commonly seen in aortic regurgitation, not mitral stenosis.

Suggested Reading

Nichol PM, Gilbert BW, Kisslo JA. Two-dimensional echocardiographic assessment of mitral stenosis. *Circulation* 1977;55:120.

Answer 14: D. Valve area estimation by P t½ is based on the rate of decline of pressure across the mitral valve during diastole. Factors affecting LA and LV pressure changes during diastolic flow can change this value. A rapid rise in LV diastolic pressure, rapid fall in left atrial pressure, or decreased left atrial compliance can lead to short P t½. A short P t½ results in an overestimation of the calculated mitral valve area.

Severe aortic regurgitation increases the LV volume precipitously. This in turn leads to early equalization of LA–LV pressures. Similarly, a stiff ventricle due to severe diastolic dysfunction leads to rapid increase in the LV diastolic pressure. In cases of left-to-right atrial shunts, the left atrium empties more rapidly than normal due to the shunt flow. This leads to a decrease in driving pressure from LA to LV and early pressure equalization.

Severe mitral regurgitation leads to volume overload of the left atrium. This will lead to increased early diastolic peak gradient (elevated E), but mean gradient and deceleration slope do not change. Therefore, P t½ should be unaltered.

Suggested Readings

Flachskampf FA, Weyman AE, Guerrero JL, et al. Calculation of atrioventricular compliance from the mitral flow profile: analytic and in vitro study. *J Am Coll Cardiol* 1992;19:998–1004.

Thomas JD, Weyman AE. Doppler mitral pressure half-time: a clinical tool in search of theoretical justification. *J Am Coll Cardiol* 1987;10:923–929.

Answer 15: A. PISA method presumes that the flow occurs through a perfect hemisphere. Normally, the mitral valve leaflets open at an angle that is <180 degrees. This means that the flow actually occurs over an area that is smaller than a true hemisphere. The PISA method assumes that the flow occurs along a hemisphere. Angle correction helps correct this discrepancy. If the flow rates are calculated without making this correction, then the measured value would *overestimate* the flow and thus result in erroneous calculation of mitral valve area.

When the aliasing velocity (Nyquist limit) is high (>40 cm/s), the PISA becomes very small and angle correction is less mandatory.

Suggested Reading

Messika-Zeitoun D, Fung Yiu S, Cormier B, et al. Sequential assessment of mitral valve area during diastole using colour M-mode flow convergence analysis: new insights into mitral stenosis physiology. *Eur Heart J* 2003;24:1244–1253.

Answer 16: A. Grade I diastolic dysfunction results in mitral inflow E/A ratio reversal and denotes the presence of mildly impaired left ventricular relaxation. Consequently, more time is required for pressure equalization to take place between the LA and the LV. Both mitral stenosis and mildly impaired LV relaxation prolong the deceleration time and the pressure half-time. This results in an overestimation of the severity of mitral stenosis and an underestimation of mitral valve area.

The pressure half-time will be prolonged due to combination of delayed relaxation and mitral stenosis.

Suggested Readings

Karp K, Teien D, Bjerle P, et al. Reassessment of valve area determinations in mitral stenosis by the pressure half-time method: impact of left ventricular stiffness and peak diastolic pressure difference. *J Am Coll Cardiol* 1989;13:594–599.

Thomas JD, Wilkins GT, Choong CY, et al. Inaccuracy of mitral pressure half-time immediately after percutaneous mitral valvotomy. Dependence on transmitral gradient and left atrial and ventricular compliance. *Circulation* 1988;78:980–993.

Chapter 20

Mitral Regurgitation

John R. Kotter

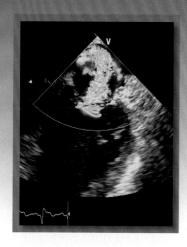

1. What is the most common cause of pathologic mitral regurgitation?

   A. Acute ischemic papillary muscle
   B. Annular dilation
   C. Degenerative mitral valve disease
   D. Rheumatic mitral regurgitation

2. A 76-year-old male undergoes single-vessel coronary artery bypass grafting with left internal mammary artery (LIMA) to the left anterior descending coronary artery. During weaning from bypass, the surgeon called the echocardiographer to the operating room to review the TEE before closing the chest. The images in FIGURE 20.1 and VIDEO 20.1 were acquired. The patient's preoperative echo had mild to moderate (2+) MR with preserved left ventricular ejection fraction. The surgeon reported all his vessels have good flow including the new LIMA graft by Doppler.

What is the etiology of mitral regurgitation in this patient?

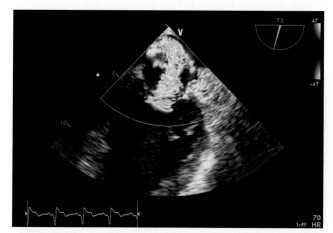

FIGURE 20.1

   A. Occlusion of the LIMA graft.
   B. Stunned myocardium.
   C. The preoperative echo was likely misread.
   D. Ischemic papillary muscle.

3. What is the etiology of MR in this patient (FIG. 20.2)?

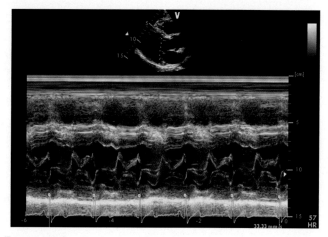

FIGURE 20.2

   A. Restricted anterior leaflet
   B. Restricted posterior leaflet
   C. Prolapse of the anterior leaflet
   D. Prolapse of the posterior leaflet
   E. Systolic anterior motion (SAM) of the anterior MV leaflet

4. Based on the M-mode image in FIGURE 20.2, which of the following descriptions would best describe the regurgitant jet?

   A. Early systolic posteriorly directed
   B. Midsystolic posteriorly directed
   C. Late systolic central jet
   D. Late systolic anteriorly directed
   E. Early systolic anteriorly directed

5. What is the Carpentier classification for the image in FIGURE 20.2?

   A. Type I
   B. Type II
   C. Type IIIa
   D. Type IIIb
   E. Type IV

6. A 72-year-old female is referred for evaluation of shortness of breath. Echocardiography reveals mitral regurgitation. The following measurements were obtained with transthoracic echocardiography:

MR continuous-wave Doppler velocity = 5 m/s.

Nyquist limit scale = 35 cm/s.

Blue to red color-flow Doppler transition = 1 cm.

What is the severity of mitral regurgitation based on the following parameters?

A. Mild (ERO < 0.2 cm^2)
B. Mild to moderate (ERO 0.2 to 0.3 cm^2)
C. Moderate to severe (ERO 0.3 to 0.4 cm^2)
D. Severe (ERO > 0.4 cm^2)
E. Cannot be determined with the information provided

7. Which of these patients with severe MR from a type II, P2 etiology would benefit most with mitral valve surgery?

A. A 60-year-old asymptomatic male with a left ventricular ejection fraction (EF) of 65% to 70% and end-systolic diameter of 3.8 cm.
B. A 68-year-old asymptomatic female with an EF of 65% and end-diastolic diameter of 5.1 cm.
C. A 55-year-old asymptomatic female who runs 3 miles every day and an EF of 55% and end-systolic diameter of 3.4 cm.
D. A 70-year-old asymptomatic male and an EF of 70% and end-systolic diameter of 2.9 cm.
E. None of these asymptomatic patients have an indication for MV repair.

8. A 42-year-old male is referred for transesophageal echocardiography to further evaluate mitral regurgitation. What is the etiology of MR in this patient, and what is the anticipated direction of the regurgitant jet (VIDEO 20.2)?

A. Systolic anterior motion (SAM) of the MV leaflet with posteriorly directed MR
B. Flail anterior MV leaflet with posteriorly directed MR
C. Anterior mitral valve leaflet prolapse with posteriorly directed MR
D. SAM with anteriorly directed MR
E. Posterior mitral valve leaflet prolapse with anteriorly directed MR

9. The previous patient continues to be symptomatic despite maximal medical therapy and surgical myectomy is recommended. Based on the information provided, which of the following statements is most accurate concerning this operation?

A. Some surgeons consider intraoperative TEE to be helpful, but this is not required.
B. The mitral valve will most likely require replacement.
C. Residual SAM and mild MR after surgery will likely require mitral valve replacement.
D. In most circumstances, the MV apparatus is intact, and myectomy will resolve MR.
E. An annuloplasty ring is usually all that is required should the MR persist post myectomy.

10. A 65-year-old female is admitted to the coronary care unit following an acute myocardial infarction. She has a known history of obstructive multivessel coronary artery disease based upon coronary angiography performed 2 months prior. Following her acute myocardial infarction, an invasive strategy was offered, but this was declined by the patient. She was continued on optimal medical therapy including dual antiplatelet therapy. Two days later, the patient became acutely dyspneic and hypotensive. A transesophageal echocardiogram was ordered (see VIDEO 20.3A AND B). What is the next most appropriate course of action assuming the patient is agreeable with the recommendation?

A. Percutaneous coronary intervention
B. Emergent cardiac surgery
C. Obtain blood cultures and start antibiotic therapy
D. Wait 5 to 7 days until platelet function has recovered and proceed with coronary artery bypass grafting

11. Which papillary muscle is most commonly associated with acute ischemic MR?

A. Anterolateral papillary muscle
B. Anteromedial papillary muscle
C. Posteromedial papillary muscle
D. Posterolateral papillary muscle
E. Inferior papillary muscle

12. A 58-year-old African American male with a history of hypertension is admitted to the hospital due to dyspnea on exertion and lower extremity edema. An echocardiogram is performed on the day of admission and 2 days later. Spectral Doppler signals of the mitral regurgitant jet from the two studies are given in FIGURE 20.3A. Assuming that the CW Doppler cursor alignment and all other echo variables are consistent between exams, FIGURE 20.3B was most likely acquired after which of the following noninvasive interventions?

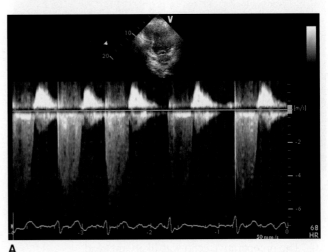

A

FIGURE 20.3

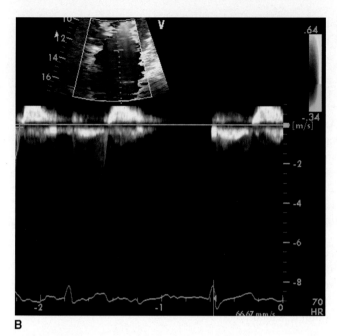

B

FIGURE 20.3 (*Continued*)

A. Lisinopril was added to improve BP control.

B. Diltiazem was discontinued due to borderline low BP.

C. The Valsalva release was performed prior to FIGURE 20.3B.

D. Dobutamine therapy was initiated prior to FIGURE 20.3B.

E. None of the options would have any influence on the MR spectral Doppler display.

13. A patient with known severe aortic stenosis (AS) presents for a follow-up echocardiogram. The sonographer uses a nonimaging CW Doppler probe at both the apical and suprasternal positions to optimize the spectral Doppler signal. While reading the study, you suspect the Doppler signal obtained from the apical region is an MR signal because:

A. The peak velocity of the signal was 3.9 m/s.

B. The spectral signal includes isovolumic contraction and relaxation phases in addition to the ejection phase.

C. A faint shadow of LVOT signal overlaying the spectral Doppler signal could be seen.

D. The peak velocity of the signal was 5.4 m/s.

14. A 48-year-old male with a history of IV drug abuse presents with fever and chills for 1 week and sudden-onset severe shortness of breath. Examination reveals a heart rate of 102 bpm. His echocardiogram reveals the continuous wave spectral Doppler recording in FIGURE 20.4 with the cursor aligned through the MV annulus and the LV apex. The peak velocity is 5 m/s.

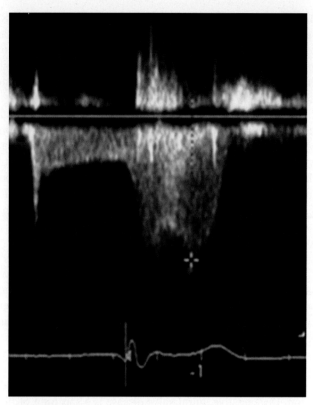

FIGURE 20.4

What is the most likely etiology of his symptoms?

A. Complete heart block

B. Acute severe aortic regurgitation

C. Severe systolic heart failure

D. Acute severe mitral regurgitation

E. Acute severe tricuspid regurgitation

15. A 72-year-old male presents for a second opinion prior to double-valve surgery of the aortic and mitral valves, which is being recommended for new-onset shortness of breath. The echo images are not available. The report states the following:

LVEF = 60%–65%.

Relative wall thickness = 0.45; LV mass index = 132 g/m².

Aortic valve area = 0.8 cm²; mean gradient = 38 mm Hg.

Moderate mitral regurgitation.

Mild mitral annular calcification.

Which of the following is the best recommendation as the next step in management?

A. Proceed with aortic and mitral valve replacement surgery.

B. Refer for aortic valve balloon valvuloplasty.

C. Recommend aggressive medical management.

D. Replace the mitral valve and intraoperatively reassess aortic valve gradients.

E. Perform preoperative transesophageal echocardiogram.

Answer 1: C. Option A is incorrect. Mitral regurgitation (MR) due to acute ischemia of the papillary muscle, also known as acute ischemic MR, occurs due to tethering of the leaflet during ischemia or due to rupture of the papillary muscle. Both these conditions are rare as they occur only during the acute ischemic phase.

Option B is incorrect as annular dilation is associated with left ventricular chamber enlargement and mitral regurgitation, which is also an infrequent cause when considering all patients with MR. Although the architectures of the mitral leaflets, chordae, and papillary muscles are preserved in this condition, apical dislocation of papillary muscles leads to tenting of the leaflets and malcoaptation leading to regurgitation. Therefore, some authors believe that annular dilation has only an adjunct role and is not the causative mechanism.

Option C is correct. See discussion below.

Option D is incorrect as rheumatic MR is not a common cause of primary mitral regurgitation. Rheumatic MR is not an uncommon manifestation of rheumatic heart disease. However, given the decreasing incidence of rheumatic heart disease, this is not a leading cause of primary mitral insufficiency.

The most frequent cause of primary MR is degenerative mitral valve disease and is seen in 20% to 40% of all patients with mitral regurgitation and in 2% to 3% of the general population. Degenerative mitral valve disease is a spectrum of diseases ranging from fibroelastic deficiency seen in older patients to Barlow disease, which is redundant tissue causing bileaflet prolapse and MR seen mostly in younger patients.

Suggested Readings

Chikwe J, et al. Degenerative mitral valve disease. *Heart Lung Circ* 2009;18:319–329.
Edmunds LH Jr, ed. *Cardiac Surgery in the Adult.* New York, NY: McGraw-Hill, 1997.
Foster E. Clinical practice. Mitral regurgitation due to degenerative mitral-valve disease. *N Engl J Med* 2010;363(2):156–165.
Osman O, Al-Radi, et al. Understanding the pathophysiology of mitral regurgitation: the first step in management. *Geriatr Aging* 2003;6(10):42–45.

Answer 2: B. The images show severe global hypokinesis and severe mitral regurgitation. There is global hypokinesis likely due to myocardial stunning, leading to papillary muscle dysfunction and worsening of the degree mitral regurgitation. Myocardial stunning could be seen in varying degrees in patients coming off bypass. Hence, this is the most likely etiology of severe mitral regurgitation in this patient. Occlusion of the LIMA graft would cause segmental wall motion abnormalities. Therefore, Option A is incorrect. Considering the preoperative echo had normal LV systolic function, which has now deteriorated, it is more likely that the degree of MR has also significantly worsened. Hence, Option C is less likely to be correct. While an ischemic papillary muscle could certainly cause severe MR in the postoperative CABG patient, this would also be associated with segmental wall motion abnormalities and an eccentric MR jet (toward the ischemic region). Hence, Option D is less likely to be the etiology.

Suggested Readings

Kloner RA, Przyklenk K, Kay GL. Clinical evidence for stunned myocardium after coronary artery bypass surgery. *J Card Surg* 1994;9(suppl 3):397–402.
Leung JM. Clinical evidence of myocardial stunning in patients undergoing CABG surgery. *Card Surg* 1993;8(suppl 2):220–223.

Answer 3: D. The M-mode image shown is across the mitral valve. The abnormal finding of this image is systolic bowing of the posterior mitral valve leaflet where the posterior leaflet clearly moves posterior to the line of coaptation in systole (Fig. 20.5, *blue arrow*). Hence, the etiology of the mitral leaflet here is posterior mitral valve prolapse. Restricted leaflet function would not be well visualized by M-mode. Hence, Options A and B are not correct. The anterior leaflet is clearly visualized and is not seen prolapsing. Hence, Option C is incorrect. In SAM of the anterior MV leaflet, the anterior MV leaflet would be seen in contact with the interventricular septum during systole, which is not the case in the above image. Hence, Option E is incorrect.

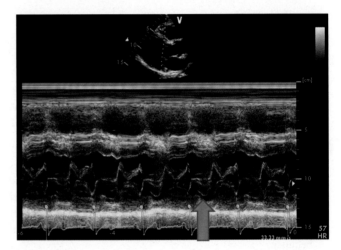

Figure 20.5

Suggested Readings

Bonow RO, et al. 2008 focused update incorporated into the ACC/AHA 2006 guidelines for the management of patients with valvular heart disease. *J Am Coll Cardiol* 2008;52(13):e1–e142.
Feigenbaum H. Role of M-mode technique in today's echocardiography. *J Am Soc Echocardiogr* 2010;23(3):240–257, 335–337.

Answer 4: D. A prolapsed mitral leaflet causes regurgitation in the opposite direction of the leaflet affected. Hence, isolated posterior leaflet prolapse would cause anteriorly directed mitral regurgitation. Therefore, Options A, B, and C are incorrect.

MR of the prolapsed mitral valve initially occurs in the mid-to-late systolic phase and progresses to holosystolic regurgitation as the condition worsens. Therefore, Option E is incorrect. It is important to understand for clinical management that consideration of timing of the regurgitation jet is important as calculation of regurgitant volume and effective regurgitant orifice presuming holosystolic flow may overestimate the severity of MR, when regurgitation is present only in mid- to late systole in mitral valve prolapse.

Suggested Readings

Armstrong WF, Ryan T. *Feigenbaum's Echocardiography.* 7th ed. Philadelphia, PA: Lippincott Williams & Wilkins, 2010.

Carpentier A, et al. Reconstructive surgery of the mitral valve incompetence: ten year appraisal. *J Thorac Cardiovasc Surg* 1980;79:338–348.

Topilsky Y, Michelena H, Bichara V, et al. Mitral valve prolapse with mid-late systolic mitral regurgitation: pitfalls of evaluation and clinical outcome compared with holosystolic regurgitation. *Circulation* 2012;125(13):1643–1651.

Answer 5: B. Dr. Alain Frédéric Carpentier was one of the first persons to describe and categorize MR based on anatomic lesions and the resultant pathophysiology of MV leaflets. This categorization helped standardize MV nomenclature for the surgeon and cardiologist.

The original classification included three types:

Type I: Normal leaflet motion
Type II: Excessive leaflet motion
Type III: Restricted motion

Later, Type III was modified and subdivided into two further types:

Type IIIa: Restricted motion in diastole and systole
Type IIIb: Restricted motion of leaflets in systole
Type IV has been added to describe systolic anterior motion of the mitral valve.

See TABLE 20.1 and FIGURE 20.6.

The M-mode image in FIGURE 20.2 is suggestive of mitral valve prolapse in which regurgitation is caused by increased leaflet motion. Hence, this is categorized under Carpentier type II. There is no evidence of type I or type III dysfunction. Therefore, Options A, C, D are E are incorrect.

Suggested Readings

Carpentier A, et al. Reconstructive surgery of the mitral valve incompetence: ten year appraisal. *J Thorac Cardiovasc Surg* 1980;79:338–348.

Chikwe J, et al. State of the art: degenerative mitral valve disease. *Heart Lung Circ* 2009;18:319–329.

Zoghbi WA, Adams D, Bonow RO, et al. Recommendations for Noninvasive Evaluation of Native Valvular Regurgitation: A Report from the American Society of Echocardiography Developed in Collaboration with the Society for Cardiovascular Magnetic Resonance. *J Am Soc Echocardiogr* 2017;30:303–371.

Table 20.1 **Anatomical Lesions and Resultant Leaflet Dysfunction Causing Mitral Regurgitation**

LEAFLET DYSFUNCTION	ANATOMICAL LESION	REPAIR TECHNIQUES
Type I Normal leaflet motion	Annular dilation	Annuloplasty
	Leaflet perforation	Pericardial patch repair
Type II Leaflet prolapse	Chordal rupture	Gore-Tex neochordae
	Chordal elongation	Chordal transfer
	Papillary muscle rupture	Triangular resection
		Quadrangular resection
		Resection and sliding plasty
		Commissural suture
Type III A: Restricted leaflet opening	Commissural fusion	Commissurotomy
	Leaflet thickening	
	Leaflet calcification	
	Chordal fusion	Chordal fenestration
B: Restricted leaflet closure	Chordal thickening	Chordal division
	Chordal shortening	Annuloplasty
	Ventricular dilation	

Reprinted from Carpentier A, Chauvaud S, Fabiani JN, et al. Reconstructive surgery of mitral valve incompetence: ten-year appraisal. *J Thorac Cardiovasc Surg* 1980;79(3):338–348. Copyright © 1980 Elsevier. With permission.

Answer 6: D. Severe based on the ERO = 0.44 cm². This question tests the proximal isovelocity surface area (PISA) method to calculate the effective regurgitant orifice and the severity of mitral regurgitation. In addition to being helpful in clinical practice to evaluate the severity of MR, it is an easily tested method on the ASC Exam boards.

During systole, the mitral regurgitant flow accelerates from the left ventricle toward the regurgitant orifice. This

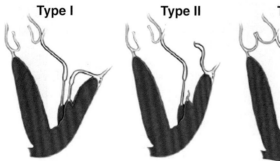
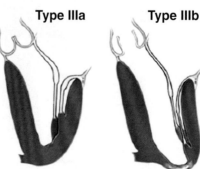

Type I   **Type II**   **Type IIIa**   **Type IIIb**

FIGURE 20.6 Reprinted from Carpentier A, Chauvaud S, Fabiani JN, et al. Reconstructive surgery of mitral valve incompetence: ten-year appraisal. *J Thorac Cardiovasc Surg* 1980;79(3):338–348. Copyright © 1980 Elsevier. With permission.

acceleration occurs in concentric isovelocity hemispheres of decreasing surface area and increasing velocity to reach a maximum velocity at the orifice.

According to the concept of law of conservation of mass, using the area of a hemisphere (PISA) and velocity of flow at this hemisphere (aliasing velocity) and the peak mitral regurgitant velocity ($Vmax_{MR}$), the effective regurgitant orifice (ERO) could be calculated:

PISA surface area × aliasing velocity (Va) = ERO × peak MR velocity ($Vmax_{MR}$)

$$ERO = \frac{\text{PISA surface area} \times Va}{Vmax_{MR}}$$

Therefore, three measurements should be obtained to calculate the ERO by this method:

1. PISA surface area
2. Aliasing velocity (Va)
3. Peak MR velocity

PISA surface area: If r is the radius of the hemisphere, the surface area of a hemisphere is calculated as $2\pi r^2$.

However, to increase the accuracy of this measurement, the baseline of the Nyquist scale is moved in the direction of the regurgitant jet as shown in the schematic below. This increases the radius of the hemispheres. The radius is measured from the red to blue aliasing boundary to the ERO (Fig. 20.7).

The aliasing velocity is obtained from the Nyquist limit seen on the display screen, and the peak MR velocity is measured as the peak velocity on a continuous-wave Doppler recording across the regurgitant jet. All measurements should be converted to centimeter values.

In the above patient,

MR continuous-wave Doppler velocity = $Vmax_{MR}$ = 5 m/s = 500 cm/s

Nyquist limit scale = alias velocity (Va) = 35 cm/s

Blue to red color-flow Doppler transition = PISA radius (r) = 1.0 cm

ERO = (PISA surface area × Va)/$Vmax_{MR}$
ERO = ($2\pi r^2$ × Va)/$Vmax_{MR}$
ERO = (6.28 × 35 cm/s)/500 cm/s
ERO = 0.44 cm^2

An effective regurgitant orifice >0.4 cm^2 is indicative of severe regurgitation, and <0.2 cm^2 is indicative of mild regurgitation. As this patient's ERO was 0.44 cm^2, she suffers from severe mitral regurgitation, which is likely the cause of shortness of breath.

Suggested Readings

Bargiggia GS, Tronconi L, Sahn DJ, et al. A new method for quantification of mitral regurgitation based on color flow Doppler imaging of flow convergence proximal to regurgitant orifice. *Circulation* 1991;84:1481–1489.

Zoghbi WA, Adams D, Bonow RO, et al. Recommendations for Noninvasive Evaluation of Native Valvular Regurgitation: A Report from the American Society of Echocardiography Developed in Collaboration with the Society for Cardiovascular Magnetic Resonance. *J Am Soc Echocardiogr* 2017;30:303–371.

Answer 7: C. Current data suggest that patients with chronic severe mitral regurgitation and an EF of 30% to 60% and/or and LVESD > 40 mm be recommended for mitral valve surgery even in the absence of symptoms. This patient likely is a good candidate for mitral valve repair. Reparability of the mitral valve depends on the surgeon's experience as well as the underlying pathology. Mitral valve prolapse (type II) of the posterior leaflet, middle scallop (P2) is considered a repairable lesion. Therefore, Option C is correct as the patient's EF is <60%, and in spite of an excellent exercise capacity, she would have a better outcome with surgery at this time (Fig. 20.8).

Option A is incorrect as the EF is >60% and the LVESD is <4.0 cm and the patient is asymptomatic.

Guidelines for chronic mitral regurgitation recommend using LVESD not LVEDD. Furthermore, the LVEDD is not enlarged, the EF is >60%, and the patient is asymptomatic, so Option B is not the best answer.

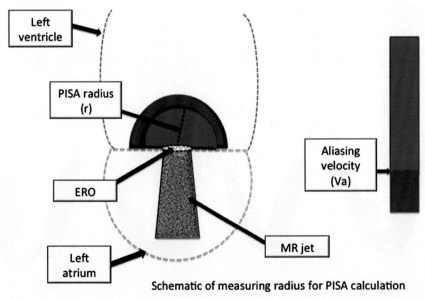

Schematic of measuring radius for PISA calculation

Figure 20.7

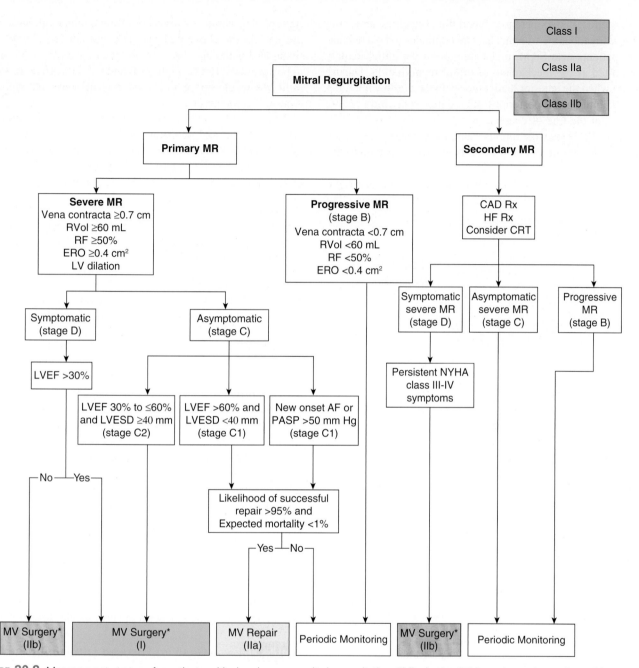

FIGURE 20.8 Management strategy for patients with chronic severe mitral regurgitation. *Mitral valve (MV) repair may be performed in asymptomatic patients with normal left ventricular (LV) function if performed by an experienced surgical team and if the likelihood of successful MV repair is >90%. AF, atrial fibrillation; Echo, echocardiography; EF, ejection fraction; ESD, end-systolic dimension; eval, evaluation; HT, hypertension; MVR, mitral valve replacement. (Reproduced from Bonow RO, et al. 2008 focused update incorporated into the ACC/AHA 2006 guidelines for the management of patients with valvular heart disease. *J Am Coll Cardiol* 2008;52(3):e1–e142.)

Option D is incorrect as the EF is >60% and the LVESD is <4.0 cm and the patient is asymptomatic.

Suggested Readings

Kang DH, Kim JH, Rim JH, et al. Comparison of early surgery versus conventional treatment in asymptomatic severe mitral regurgitation. *Circulation* 2009;119(6):797–804.

Nishimura RA, Otto CM, Bonow RO, et al. 2017 AHA/ACC focused update of the 2014 AHA/ACC guideline for the management of patients with valvular heart disease: a report of the American College of Cardiology/American Heart Association Task Force on Clinical Practice Guidelines. *J Thorac Cardiovasc Surg* 2014;64(16):1763.

***Answer 8:* A.** The video shows systolic anterior motion (SAM) of the mitral valve. Systolic anterior motion of the MV leaflet leads to posteriorly directed MR (VIDEO 20.4). Therefore, Option A is correct. Anteriorly directed mitral regurgitation is not associated with systolic anterior motion unless there is an additional pathology causing MR.

SAM is most commonly associated with hypertrophic cardiomyopathy (HCM) as was the case in this patient. However, it is also seen in post-MV surgery, following myocardial infarctions and hypertensive cardiomyopathy. Many theories have been proposed as to the mechanism of SAM including a

Venturi effect due to increased blood flow velocities across the outflow tract, but the true mechanism continues to be a debate.

In patients with SAM, malcoaptation of the mitral leaflets is reported as the mechanism of mitral regurgitation. During systole when the anterior leaflet moves to the outflow tract, the limited ability of the posterior leaflet to move anteriorly results in a gap at the line of coaptation, which leads to posteriorly directed MR. Hence, the mobility and leaflet length of the posterior leaflet are predictors of degree of MR in patients with SAM (Fig. 20.9).

The video has no evidence of prolapse in which case the line of coaptation would be displaced more than 2 mm or a flail leaflet in which the leaflet tip is displaced beyond the line of coaptation. Hence, Options B, C, and E are incorrect.

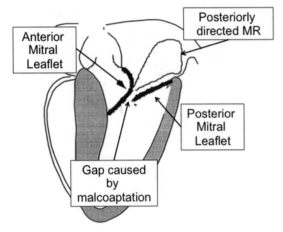

FIGURE 20.9 Schematic on mechanism of MR with SAM. (Modified from Schwammenthal E, Nakatani S, He S, et al. Mechanism of mitral regurgitation in hypertrophic cardiomyopathy: mismatch of posterior to anterior leaflet length and mobility. *Circulation* 1998;98(9):856–865, with permission.)

Suggested Readings

Freed LA, et al. Prevalence and clinical outcome of mitral-valve prolapse. *N Engl J Med* 1999;341(1):1–7.
Himelman RB, et al. The flail mitral valve: echocardiographic findings by precordial and transesophageal imaging and Doppler color flow mapping. *J Am Coll Cardiol* 1991;17(1):272–279.
Luckie M, et al. Systolic anterior motion of mitral valve—beyond hypertrophic cardiomyopathy. *Heart* 2008;94:1383–1385.
Schwammenthal E, et al. Mechanism of mitral regurgitation in hypertrophic cardiomyopathy. Mismatch of posterior to anterior leaflet length and mobility. *Circulation* 1998;98:856–865.

Answer 9: D. In most patients with HCM, the intrinsic architecture of the mitral valve is preserved. Hence, myectomy and relief of the dynamic gradient alone would eliminate MR. In a study by Yu et al. (1), in a series of 93 patients who underwent myectomy for HCM, in the absence of independent mitral valve disease, none of the patients required mitral valve surgery. In this study population, approximately 50% of patients had moderate or severe MR on preoperative assessment. Early postoperative MR was mild or less in degree in 99% of the patients and moderate in 1%. Therefore, Option D is correct in stating that myectomy would resolve MR.

In most cases when further mitral valve surgery is required, additional pathology such as mitral valve prolapse, chordal rupture, degenerative disease, or mitral annular calcification is present. As the above patient's TEE did not reveal any additional MV pathology, valve replacement or repair is not likely to be necessary. Hence, Options B and E are incorrect. Residual mild MR would not require valve replacement, and therefore, Option C is incorrect.

Intraoperative TEE is essential during surgical myectomy for assessment and decision-making of residual LVOT gradients and severity of MR. There is no alternative method of obtaining this information during cardiac surgery; hence, Option A is incorrect in stating that TEE is not required.

Reference

1. Yu EH. Mitral regurgitation in hypertrophic obstructive cardiomyopathy: relationship to obstruction and relief with myectomy. *J Am Coll Cardiol* 2000;36(7):2219–2225.

Suggested Reading

McIntosh CL, et al. Current operative treatment of obstructive hypertrophic cardiomyopathy. *Circulation* 1988;78:487–495.

Answer 10: B. The transesophageal images demonstrate a torn papillary muscle with severe mitral regurgitation. In this rare complication of a myocardial infarction, prompt diagnosis, supportive treatment, and emergency cardiac surgery are all required for a successful outcome. Considering papillary muscle rupture is a rare complication of myocardial infarction, the available data are limited by observational case series and nonrandomized clinical and surgical reports. In a case series of 22 patients (1), the operative mortality was 25% and long-term survival was approximately 50%. Simultaneous coronary revascularization improved outcomes.

Option A is incorrect as percutaneous coronary intervention will not improve the mitral regurgitation.

Option C is incorrect as the clinical history and echocardiographic images are not consistent with endocarditis and definitive treatment should not be delayed.

Option D is incorrect as ruptured papillary muscle is a surgical emergency and treatment should not be delayed (Table 20.2).

Table 20.2	**Goals of Focused Ultrasound (FOCUS)**

Assessment for the presence of pericardial effusion
Assessment of global cardiac systolic function
Identification of marked right ventricular and left ventricular enlargement
Intravascular volume assessment
Guidance of pericardiocentesis
Confirmation of transvenous pacing wire placement

Reprinted from Labovitz AJ, Noble VE, Bierig M, et al. Focused cardiac ultrasound in the emergent setting: a consensus statement of the American Society of Echocardiography and American College of Emergency Physicians. *J Am Soc Echocardiogr* 2010;23(12):1225–1230. Copyright © 2010 Elsevier. With permission.

Reference

1. Kishon Y, Oh JK, Schaff HV, et al. Mitral valve operation in postinfarction rupture of a papillary muscle: immediate results and long-term follow-up of 22 patients. *Mayo Clin Proc* 1992;67:1023.

Answer 11: C. The two papillary muscles are anterolateral and posteromedial. Therefore, Options B, D, and E are incorrect. The posteromedial papillary muscle has a single coronary artery supply (posterior descending artery), while the anterolateral has dual coronary artery supply. Therefore, the posteromedial papillary muscle is more vulnerable to be ischemic in patients who suffer an inferior MI in comparison to the anterolateral papillary muscle. This should be suspected in patients with acute decompensation despite the absence of a murmur on exam due to the acuity of the large regurgitant volume, small, noncompliant LA, and minimal LV to LA gradient.

Suggested Reading
Czarnecki A, et al. Acute severe mitral regurgitation: consideration of papillary muscle architecture. *Cardiovasc Ultrasound* 2008;6:5.

Answer 12: A. Comparing the continuous-wave Doppler images from the initial and follow-up echocardiograms, there is a significant decrease in the density of the spectral envelopes and the recorded maximal velocity. Considering all other variables were unchanged between the two studies, density of the spectral display is a qualitative index of severity, and the maximal velocity represents the LV to LA gradient. Therefore, it can be assumed that the degree of mitral regurgitation and the LV to LA gradient has decreased. Considering the given options, the only intervention that might decrease the severity of MR is the addition of lisinopril. Reduction of systolic blood pressure would decrease the LV pressure in systole and hence the LV to LA gradient and likely also reduce the MR regurgitant volume. Hence, Option A is the single best answer. Options B, C, and D would increase blood pressure, which would result in an increased MR spectral Doppler V_{max}. Option E is incorrect given the above discussion.

This demonstrates the importance of interpreting MR in the clinical setting as it can fluctuate with changes in hemodynamics. It is recommended to record the patient's blood pressure and medications at the time of echocardiography and to take that into account when comparing serial echocardiograms over a period of time. The impact of BP on MR severity is highly relevant in the operating room where the BP is dramatically variable and the MR severity is frequently underestimated when the BP is lowered.

Suggested Reading
Zoghbi WA, et al. Recommendations for evaluation of the severity of native valvular regurgitation with two-dimensional and Doppler echocardiography. *J Am Soc Echocardiogr* 2003;16:777–802.

Answer 13: B. The MR spectral Doppler signal usually has a higher peak velocity as the systolic gradient between the left ventricle and left atrium is higher than that between the left ventricle and the aortic pressure. However, critical AS can also reach a peak velocity of 5.4 m/s. Hence, Options A and D do not help differentiate MR from AS and are incorrect. One of

the key findings of an MR signal is the longer duration encompassing isovolumic contraction and relaxation phases, which is not seen with the aortic stenosis signal. Therefore, Option B is the correct answer (Fig. 20.10). On occasion, one might see a faint outline of an LVOT signal overlying the aortic stenosis spectral Doppler signal and not the MR Doppler envelope, making Option C incorrect.

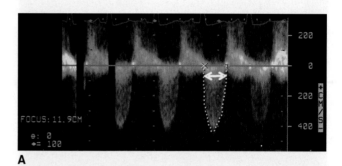

A

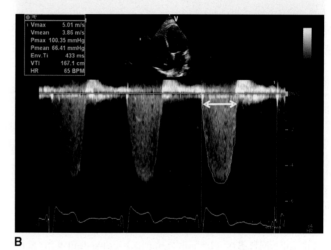

B

Figure 20.10 AS spectral. **A:** AS spectral Doppler (spectral duration, *double arrow*, is shorter in AS than in MR). **B:** MR spectral Doppler (spectral duration, *double arrow*, is longer in MR than in AS).

Suggested Readings
Baumgartner H, et al. EAE/ASE recommendations. Echocardiography assessment of valve stenosis: EAE/ASE recommendations for clinical practice. *Eur J Echocardiogr* 2009;10:1–15.

Oh JK, et al. Differentiation of the aortic stenosis jet from mitral regurgitation by analysis of continuous-wave Doppler spectrum: illustrative cases. *Echocardiography* 1986;3(1):55–60.

Answer 14: B. The spectral Doppler flow pattern is likely across the mitral valve considering it is pansystolic flow with a peak velocity of 5 m/s. In addition to the systolic flow, there also is regurgitant flow during diastole, which is indicative of diastolic mitral regurgitation (Fig. 20.11, *blue arrow*).

Diastolic MR occurs when LV diastolic pressure exceeds LA pressure in mid-to-late diastole leading to premature closure of the mitral valve. Usually, diastolic MR has a low velocity of <2 m/s.

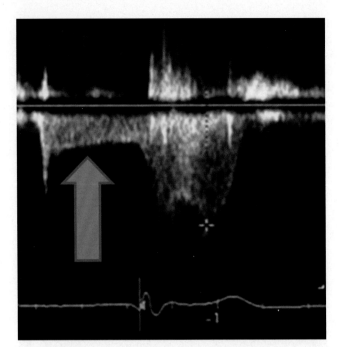

FIGURE 20.11

Causes for diastolic mitral regurgitation include:

1. Acute severe aortic regurgitation
2. Severe left ventricular (LV) dysfunction leading to elevated LV end-diastolic pressure (LVEDP)
3. Severe diastolic dysfunction leading to elevated LVEDP
4. AV dissociation
5. Ectopic ventricular beats
6. Significant first-degree AV block

Of the given answers, Options A, B, and C could give rise to diastolic MR. The clinical scenario is consistent with acute severe aortic regurgitation leading to diastolic MR in the setting of infective endocarditis. Therefore, Option B is the most likely etiology for the given image. It is unlikely to be complete heart block with a heart rate of 102 bpm. Hence, Option A is an incorrect answer. While sudden-onset shortness of breath could be reported in acute systolic heart failure, the history of fever and chills leads to Option B being more likely than C.

In severe MR, the jet is dense with a triangular, early peaking of the maximal velocity. The given Doppler recording is more parabolic in shape, incomplete, and not as dense as the inflow. Also, acute severe MR does not cause diastolic MR. Therefore, Option D is wrong.

The clinical scenario of an IV drug user with fever and chills is suggestive of tricuspid valve endocarditis, which could lead to acute severe tricuspid regurgitation (TR). This Doppler recording is not consistent with severe TR. Similar to that seen with severe MR, in severe TR, the jet is dense with a triangular, early peaking of the maximal velocity. Also, the peak velocity of TR is normally much less than the demonstrated 5.0 m/s. With a maximum velocity of 5 m/s, the estimated pulmonary artery systolic pressure would be approximately 100-mm Hg + RA pressure, which would indicate severe pulmonary hypertension. Acute severe TR or pulmonary hypertension does not

cause diastolic regurgitation of the tricuspid or mitral valves. Hence, Option E is incorrect.

Suggested Readings

Downes TR, et al. Diastolic mitral regurgitation in acute but not chronic aortic regurgitation: implications regarding the mechanism of mitral closure. *Am Heart J* 1989;117(5):1106–1112.

Schnittger I, et al. Diastolic mitral and tricuspid regurgitation by Doppler echocardiography in patients with atrioventricular block: new insight into the mechanism of atrioventricular valve closure. *J Am Coll Cardiol* 1988;11(1):83–88.

Answer 15: E. Mitral regurgitation is a frequent finding in patients with severe aortic stenosis. The etiology of MR in these patients could be due to valvular pathology such as mitral valve prolapse and rheumatic disease or functional due to LV remodeling and increased LVEDP, where the mitral valve apparatus is intact.

It is of vital importance to understand the mechanism of mitral regurgitation prior to valve surgery for which a transesophageal echocardiogram should be performed. Depending on the etiology of MR and severity of residual MR following aortic valve replacement, the surgeon may opt to replace, repair, or not intervene on the mitral valve. Each of these approaches poses very different surgical risks and long-term outcomes. The surgeon and patient should have a candid discussion of these options prior to surgery. Option E is therefore correct as a preoperative TEE is imperative to obtain information on valvular pathology.

Option A is incorrect in stating both valves should be replaced, as mitral valve repair is preferable to replacement with an amenable valve.

Option B is incorrect as aortic valve balloon valvuloplasty has only a short-term benefit and carries a procedural mortality of >10%.

There is no role in medical management for symptomatic severe aortic stenosis. Hence, Option C is incorrect.

The main valvular lesion in this patient is severe AS; therefore, the aortic valve should be replaced first. Hence, Option D is incorrect. MR may "falsely" lower the gradients across the aortic valve, but does not interfere with valve area calculation by continuity equation. Mitral regurgitation may also mask LV dysfunction. The reverse of Option D is correct where the aortic valve should be replaced and mitral regurgitation reassessed intraoperatively. In more than 50% of patients, the severity of MR improved after aortic valve replacement.

Suggested Readings

Baumgartner H, et al. EAE/ASE recommendations. Echocardiography assessment of valve stenosis: EAE/ASE recommendations for clinical practice. *Eur J Echocardiogr* 2009;10:1–15.

Bonow RO, et al. 2008 focused update incorporated into the ACC/AHA 2006 guidelines for the management of patients with valvular heart disease. *J Am Coll Cardiol* 2008;52(13):e1–e142.

Caballero-Borrego J, Gómez-Doblas JJ, Cabrera-Bueno F, et al. Incidence, associated factors and evolution of non-severe functional mitral regurgitation in patients with severe aortic stenosis undergoing aortic valve replacement. *Eur J Cardiothorac Surg* 2008;34(1):62–66.

Chapter 21

Tricuspid and Pulmonic Pathology

John R. Kotter

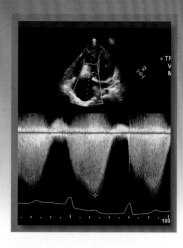

1. Which of the following is true regarding tricuspid valve involvement in carcinoid syndrome?

- A. It occurs primarily in the presence of isolated pulmonary carcinoid.
- B. Valvular involvement in carcinoid disease predominantly affects the tricuspid and aortic valves.
- C. Carcinoid involvement of the tricuspid valve may manifest as isolated tricuspid stenosis.
- D. The typical appearance of a tricuspid valve in carcinoid disease is a thickened, retracted valve with limited mobility and incomplete coaptation.

2. Which of the following is true regarding the condition present in FIGURE 21.1 and VIDEO 21.1?

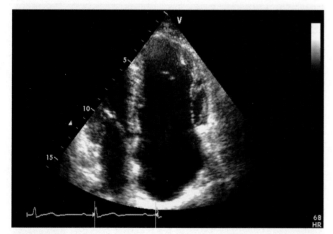

FIGURE 21.1

- A. Is an abnormality, which affects the tricuspid valve only.
- B. More than 50% of patients have a shunt at the atrial level with either a patent foramen ovale or secundum ASD, which results in varying degrees of cyanosis.
- C. The posterior leaflet of the tricuspid valve is usually sail-like and larger than normal.
- D. The most reliable echocardiographic indicator is reduced apical displacement of the septal insertion of the tricuspid valve.
- E. A displacement index of 8 mm is invariably associated with this abnormality.

3. Which of the following is inconsistent with the diagnosis of chronic, severe tricuspid regurgitation?

- A. Normal tricuspid regurgitation CW velocity jet of 2.0 m/s
- B. Normal right atrial size
- C. Systolic reversal of hepatic vein flow on subcostal imaging
- D. A regurgitation vena contracta width of 0.8 cm
- E. Triangular, early peaking of tricuspid regurgitation

4. Which of the following represents the best method to grade the severity of pulmonary stenosis?

- A. Planimetry of the pulmonic valve area
- B. Calculation of the pulmonary valve area via the continuity equation
- C. Proximal isovelocity surface area method
- D. Measurement of systolic pressure gradient via pulsed-wave spectral Doppler measurement from the parasternal short-axis view
- E. Measurement of the maximal systolic pressure gradient via continuous-wave spectral Doppler measurement from the subcostal view

5. A patient with Noonan syndrome presents for transthoracic echocardiographic evaluation. She has excellent quality echo images and is noted to have right ventricular hypertrophy with a dilated right ventricle. She has moderate tricuspid regurgitation, with a TR systolic velocity of 4.2 m/s. The IVC is enlarged. The pulmonary valve appears dysplastic with flow acceleration through the valve, poststenotic dilation, and moderate pulmonary regurgitation. The maximal measured systolic transvalvular velocity is 2.7 m/s from several views. What is the most likely explanation for the difference in pulmonic and tricuspid valve velocities?

- A. Increased right ventricular filling pressure from pulmonary regurgitation.
- B. A left-to-right shunt from an undetected atrial septal defect.
- C. A serial, distal pulmonary branch artery stenosis is present in addition to the PV stenosis.
- D. The pulmonary transvalvular velocities are severely underestimated.

6. Which of the following is true regarding pulmonary and tricuspid regurgitation flow signal evaluation?

  A. Mean pulmonary artery pressure can be estimated from the pulmonary RVOT systolic continuous-wave signal.

  B. Pulmonary diastolic pressure can be estimated from the peak diastolic regurgitation velocity.

  C. Pulmonary vascular resistance can be evaluated by dividing the peak tricuspid regurgitation velocity by the RVOT time–velocity integral.

  D. When augmenting the tricuspid regurgitation flow signal with agitated saline, the addition of blood or plasma to the air–saline concentration degrades the signal.

7. A 57-year-old patient presents to clinic with a history of isolated severe tricuspid regurgitation and normal pulmonary pressures, associated with moderate RV dilation and normal function. Except for mild peripheral edema controlled with diuretics, she has had no interval change in her symptoms. Her last echocardiogram was 14 months ago. You decide to order a repeat surveillance transthoracic echo. Which is the most correct answer considering the current Appropriate Use Criteria for Transthoracic Echocardiography guidelines?

  A. Appropriate (score 7 to 9).

  B. Inappropriate (score 4 to 6).

  C. Uncertain (score 1 to 3).

  D. This topic is unclassified (score 0).

8. Which of the following is **not** ideal with regard to the measurement of tricuspid stenosis gradients?

  A. Measurements should be made at sweep speed of 25 mm/s.

  B. Measurement of tricuspid inflow velocities should be performed at end-inspiration.

  C. Care should be taken to trace the modal velocity of the PW Doppler right ventricular inflow spectral display.

  D. Averaging measurements in patients with atrial fibrillation over a maximum of three cardiac cycles.

  E. Assess the severity of tricuspid stenosis at heart rates between 70 and 80 bpm.

9. Which of the following causes of tricuspid stenosis is demonstrated in Video 21.2 and Figure 21.2?

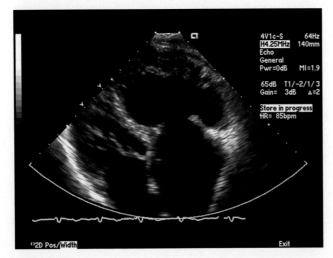

Figure 21.2

  A. Rheumatic heart disease

  B. Carcinoid syndrome

  C. Ebstein abnormality

  D. Lupus valvulitis

  E. Pacemaker-induced adhesions

10. Which of the following is the **most** correct statement regarding the Doppler features of tricuspid regurgitation in patients with a history of tricuspid valve resection for bacterial endocarditis, as demonstrated in Figure 21.3?

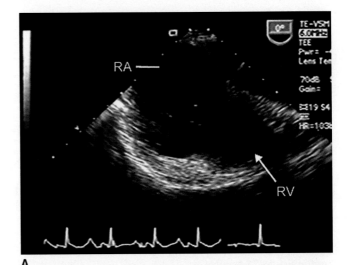

A

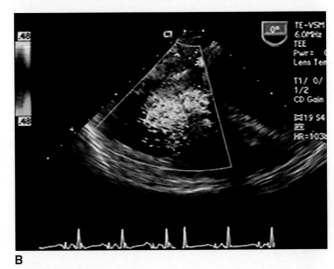

B

Figure 21.3 From Feigenbaum H, Armstrong WF, Ryan T. *Feigenbaum's Echocardiography.* 6th ed. Philadelphia, PA: Lippincott Williams & Wilkins, 2004.

  A. There is organized flow from the right ventricle to the right atrium.

  B. The regurgitant jet flow velocity is high.

  C. It can be mistaken for the absence of significant tricuspid regurgitation.

  D. There is usually an easily visualized convergent zone.

11. What is the likely etiology of tricuspid regurgitation in FIGURE 21.4 and VIDEO 21.3?

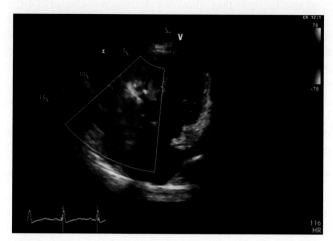

FIGURE 21.4

A. Carcinoid heart disease
B. Ebstein anomaly
C. Biopsy-induced, postcardiac transplant
D. Pacemaker associated
E. Endocarditis

12. Which of the following findings would you expect to be associated with this finding in FIGURE 21.5?

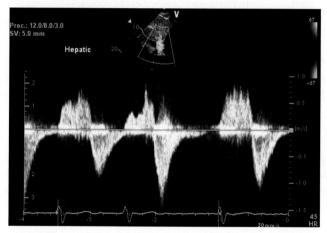

FIGURE 21.5

A. A normal-appearing tricuspid valve morphology with 2D or 3D echo
B. A PISA radius of 0.7 cm at a Nyquist limit setting of 28 cm/s
C. A vena contracta width of 0.8 cm at a Nyquist limit of 60 cm/s
D. A dense, parabolic CW Doppler spectrum
E. A central color-flow Doppler jet area of ≥ 8.0 cm^2

13. Which of the following is the most correct option with regard to the evaluation of pulmonary regurgitation as demonstrated in FIGURE 21.6?

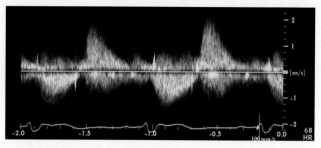

FIGURE 21.6

A. There are few validation studies in the evaluation of pulmonary regurgitation severity.
B. Pulsed-wave Doppler evaluation of RVOT pulmonic flow allows for consistent, accurate evaluation of right-sided stroke volume.
C. Transesophageal echocardiography is better at evaluating pulmonary regurgitation compared to transthoracic echocardiography.
D. Termination of pulmonary regurgitation flow in middiastole is specific for severe pulmonary regurgitation.
E. Color-flow Doppler pulmonary regurgitation jet length is a reliable indicator of pulmonary regurgitation severity.

14. VIDEO 21.4 and FIGURE 21.7 were obtained in an adult patient post tetralogy of Fallot repair. Which of the following is most correct in regard the patient's management?

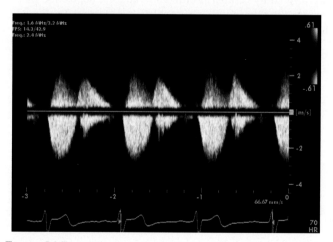

FIGURE 21.7

A. Assessment for anomalous coronary course is indicated, to rule out coronary origin from the pulmonary artery, the most common coronary anomaly in the tetralogy of Fallot patients, in anticipation of pulmonary valve replacement.
B. Continue observation in the presence of recent onset, symptomatic persistent atrial fibrillation with a rapid ventricular response.
C. Continue observation in the presence of serially documented, progressive moderate RV dilation and dysfunction in an asymptomatic patient.
D. Consider pulmonary valve replacement in the presence of progressive dyspnea on exertion with normal RV size and function.

15. What is the most common cause of acquired pulmonary stenosis?

    A. Rheumatic heart disease
    B. Fenfluramine use
    C. Carcinoid syndrome
    D. Intracardiac tumors compressing the RV outflow tract
    E. Chest radiation

Answer 1: D. The typical appearance of a tricuspid valve in carcinoid disease is a thickened, retracted valve with limited mobility and incomplete coaptation.

The cardiac effects of carcinoid tumors are mediated by substances released by the tumor such as serotonin and bradykinin, which are predominantly inactivated by the lung. Therefore, right-sided carcinoid valve pathology is almost exclusively seen in hepatic involvement, with left-sided pathology seen uncommonly, in the presence of pulmonary metastases or right-to-left shunting via a patent foramen ovale. Therefore, Options A and B are incorrect. Carcinoid effects on the tricuspid valve most commonly manifest as pure tricuspid regurgitation. When tricuspid stenosis is present, it is always associated with tricuspid regurgitation, which commonly predominates, increasing the flow through the valve, increasing the transvalvular gradient, and resulting in a greater elevation of right atrial pressure. The morphologic changes of the tricuspid valve are due to the presence of carcinoid plaques, which are formed by cellular proliferation and the deposition of the extracellular matrix, causing a thickened, retracted valve with limited mobility and incomplete coaptation.

Suggested Readings

Pellikka PA, Tajik AJ, Khandheria BK, et al. Carcinoid heart disease: clinical and echocardiographic spectrum in 74 patients. *Circulation* 1993;87:1188–1196.

Simula DV, Edwards WD, Tazelaar HD, et al. Surgical pathology of carcinoid heart disease: a study of 139 valves from 75 patients spanning 20 years. *Mayo Clin Proc* 2002;77:139–147.

Thatipelli MR, Uber PA, Mehra MR. Isolated tricuspid stenosis and heart failure: a focus on carcinoid heart disease. *Congest Heart Fail* 2003;9:294–296.

Answer 2: B. More than 50% of patients have a shunt at the atrial level with either a patent foramen ovale or secundum ASD, which results in varying degrees of cyanosis.

The image shows a patient with the typical characteristics of Ebstein anomaly. Although the orientation is not aligned as a standard ASE alignment (and has the RV on the right side of the display), the reader must be able to distinguish echo features to recognize this common variation. Of these features, apical displacement of the tricuspid valve is the most reliable indicator of an anatomic RV. Ebstein anomaly is a malformation of the tricuspid valve and right ventricle characterized by (a) adherence of the septal and posterior tricuspid leaflets to the underlying myocardium (failure of delamination); (b) apical displacement of the functional annulus; (c) dilation of the "atrialized" portion of the right ventricle with various degrees of hypertrophy and thinning of the wall; (d) redundancy, fenestrations, and tethering of the anterior leaflet with sail-like enlargement; and (e) dilation of the right atrioventricular junction. Note that clear diagnostic criteria are commonly tested in exams because they allow for decreased ambiguity of the answers. Answer A is incorrect as the findings are not limited to the tricuspid valve. Answer C is incorrect as the anterior leaflet is usually sail-like and larger. Echocardiography is the diagnostic test of choice for Ebstein anomaly and allows accurate evaluation of the tricuspid valve leaflets and size and function of the cardiac chambers. The principal echocardiographic feature is apical displacement of the septal leaflet of the tricuspid valve from the insertion of the anterior leaflet of the mitral valve by at least 8 mm/m^2 body surface area. Answer D is incorrect, as increased, and not decreased, apical displacement is characteristic, and answer E is incorrect as the tester needs to show awareness of the need to adjust the septal displacement for body surface area. Associated anatomic lesions include a shunt at the atrial level (>50%), ventricular septal defect, varying degrees of anatomic and physiologic RVOT obstruction, mitral valve prolapse, and left ventricular morphologic abnormalities.

Suggested Readings

Attenhofer Jost CH, Connolly HM, Dearani JA, et al. Ebstein's anomaly. *Circulation* 2007;115(2):277–285.

Shiina A, Seward JB, Edwards WD, et al. Two-dimensional echocardiographic spectrum of Ebstein's anomaly. Detailed anatomic assessment. *J Am Coll Cardiol* 1984;3:356–370.

Warnes CA, Williams RG, Bashore TM, et al. ACC/AHA 2008 guidelines for the management of adults with congenital heart disease: executive summary: a report of the American College of Cardiology/American Heart Association Task Force on Practice Guidelines. *Circulation* 2008;118(23):2395–2451.

Answer 3: B. Evaluation of tricuspid regurgitation severity is limited by the lack of quantitative standards and is mainly derived of a combination of semiquantitative parameters (TABLE 21.1). The presence of normal right atrial and ventricular size suggests milder degrees of tricuspid regurgitation in chronic tricuspid regurgitation, but similar to mitral regurgitation, atrial and ventricular enlargement may not be manifested in acute regurgitation. Therefore, Option B is the correct answer as it is inconsistent with chronic severe TR. The presence of a vena contracta width > 0.7 cm identifies severe TR with a sensitivity of 89% and a specificity of 93%, although the method is not as accurate in eccentric TR jets compared to central jets. Therefore, Option D is incorrect. Although the tricuspid regurgitation CW velocity allows for quantitative assessment of pulmonary pressures, the presence, degree, and severity of pulmonary hypertension do not necessarily correlate with the severity of tricuspid regurgitation. Hence, Option A is incorrect. Massive tricuspid regurgitation is often associated with a low jet velocity secondary to equalization of RV and right atrial pressures. Features of a TR jet visualized by CW Doppler that suggest severe regurgitation include a dense, triangular, early peaking of the velocity due to rapid right atrial pressure equalization. Hence, Option E is incorrect. Systolic hepatic vein flow reversal is also a well-described feature of severe tricuspid regurgitation and explains why Option C is incorrect.

Table 21.1 Echocardiographic and Doppler Parameters Used in the Evaluation of Tricuspid Regurgitation Severity: Utility, Advantages, and Limitations

PARAMETER	UTILITY/ADVANTAGES	LIMITATIONS
RV/RA/IVC size	Enlargement sensitive for chronic significant TR. Normal size virtually excludes significant chronic TR.	Enlargement seen in other conditions May be normal in acute significant TR
TV leaflet alterations	Flail valve specific for significant TR	Other abnormalities do not imply significant TR.
Paradoxical septal motion (volume overload pattern)	Simple sign of severe TR	Not specific for TR
Jet area, color flow	Simple, quick screen for TR	Subject to technical and hemodynamic factors Underestimates severity in eccentric jets
Vena contracta width	Simple, quantitative, separates mild from severe TR	Intermediate values require further confirmation.
PISA method	Quantitative	Validated in only a few studies
Flow quantitation, PW	Quantitative	Not validated for determining TR regurgitant fraction
Jet profile, CW	Simple, readily available	Qualitative, complementary data
Peak tricuspid E velocity	Simple, usually increased in severe TR	Depends on RA pressure and RV relaxation, TV area, and atrial fibrillation; complementary data only
Hepatic vein flow	Simple; systolic flow reversal is sensitive for severe TR.	Influenced by RA pressure, atrial fibrillation

CW, Continuous-wave Doppler; EROA, effective orifice regurgitant area; IVC, inferior vena cava; PISA, proximal isovelocity surface area; PW, pulsed-wave Doppler; RA, right atrium; RV, right ventricle; TV, tricuspid valve; TR, tricuspid regurgitation.
Zoghbi WA, Enriquez-Sarano M, Foster E, et al. Recommendations for evaluation of the severity of native valvular regurgitation with two-dimensional and Doppler echocardiography. *J Am Soc Echocardiogr* 2003;16:777–802.

Suggested Reading

Zoghbi WA, Enriquez-Sarano M, Foster E, et al. Recommendations for evaluation of the severity of native valvular regurgitation with two-dimensional and Doppler echocardiography. *J Am Soc Echocardiogr* 2003;16:777–802.

Answer 4: *E.* Measurement of the maximal systolic pressure gradient via continuous-wave spectral Doppler measurement from the subcostal view.

Calculation of pulmonary stenosis severity is based mainly on the transpulmonary pressure gradient, with moderate severity defined as a peak gradient through the valve of 36 to 64 mm Hg and severe stenosis as >64 mm Hg. Therefore, Option E is the best answer. Continuous-wave Doppler is used to assess the gradient from the best view yielding the highest velocity, which in adults is usually the parasternal short-axis view and occasionally the subcostal or modified apical five-chamber view. Pulsed-wave Doppler can be used to detect sites of varying levels of stenosis in cases of multiple levels of obstruction. Option A is incorrect as the pulmonic valve is very difficult to image in a short-axis plane, making Option A technically unviable. Unlike the aortic stenosis continuity equation valve area calculation, measurement of the RVOT is subject to significant inter- and intraobserver variability and yields inconsistent results. Therefore, Option B is incorrect. The PISA method is used for regurgitant valves and is less validated for assessment of stenotic valves, making Option C incorrect. Option D is incorrect as the gradient is measured via continuous-wave and not pulsed-wave Doppler.

Suggested Readings

Baumgartner H, Hung J, Bermejo J, et al. Echocardiographic assessment of valve stenosis: EAE/ASE recommendations for clinical practice. *J Am Soc Echocardiogr* 2009;22(1):1–23.
Lima CO, Sahn D, Valdes-Cruz LM, et al. Noninvasive prediction of transvalvular pressure gradient in patients with pulmonary stenosis by quantitative two-dimensional echocardiographic Doppler studies. *Circulation* 1983;67:866–871.

Answer 5: *C.* Pulmonic stenosis is a relatively common congenital defect, occurring in 10% of children with congenital heart disease. It occurs at the valvular, subvalvular, and supravalvular levels. In Noonan syndrome, the valve tends to be markedly dysplastic with prominent leaflet thickening and little commissural fusion. Peripheral pulmonary artery stenosis may coexist with pulmonary stenosis such as in Noonan syndrome and Williams syndrome and can occur in the main pulmonary artery or its branches. The possibility of serial stenosis should be considered when the RV systolic pressure estimation (estimated from tricuspid regurgitant velocity and right atrial pressure estimate) is not accounted for by the measured pulmonary valve gradient. Options B, C, and D are possibly correct, but C is the single best answer. The total pressure estimated from the tricuspid systolic velocity + CVP should be equal to the pulmonary transvalvular pressure gradient + the downstream pulmonary artery pressure. The right ventricular end-diastolic pressure should not affect the systolic pressure measurements; hence, Option A is incorrect. In this scenario, the unaccounted pulmonary pressure is equal to $(4 \times [4.2 \text{ m/s}]^2)$ + estimated CVP of 15 mm Hg (dilated IVC) − $(4 \times [2.7 \text{ m/s}]^2)$ = 57 mm Hg. If a left-to-right shunt of significant magnitude via an atrial septal defect were present, sufficient to cause pulmonary hypertension, it would be unlikely to have been missed on "excellent quality" imaging; hence, B is unlikely. Option D is unlikely secondary to the low likelihood of underestimating the transpulmonary gradient to this degree; hence, Option C is the single best answer.

Suggested Reading

Baumgartner H, Hung J, Bermejo J, et al. Echocardiographic assessment of valve stenosis: EAE/ASE recommendations for clinical practice. *J Am Soc Echocardiogr* 2009;22(1):1–23.

Answer 6: *C.* Mean PA pressure can be calculated from the Doppler determination of both PA systolic pressure and diastolic pressure, but this technique is dependent on the accuracy of two independent Doppler variables. Peak diastolic pressure gradient between the PA and the RV approximates mean PA pressure and can be used to estimate mean PA pressure. Therefore, answer A is incorrect. Diastolic PA pressure can be estimated by measuring the end-diastolic pulmonary regurgitant spectral Doppler signal, not the peak diastolic pulmonary regurgitant velocity; hence, Option B is incorrect. Quantitative estimation of pulmonary vascular resistance can be obtained by the simplified equation of PVR Wood units = 10 × tricuspid regurgitant velocity (ms^{-1})/RVOT TVI (cm). This relationship is less reliable in patients with very high PVR (>6 Woods units). Therefore, Option C is correct. The addition of blood or plasma to the air–saline concentration improves the signal; hence, Option D is incorrect.

Suggested Readings

Lee KS, Abbas AE, Khandheria BK, et al. Echocardiographic assessment of right heart hemodynamic parameters. *J Am Soc Echocardiogr* 2007;20:773–782.

Rudski LG, Lai WW, Afilalo J, et al. Guidelines for the echocardiographic assessment of the right heart in adults: a report from the American Society of Echocardiography. *J Am Soc Echocardiogr* 2010;23:685–713.

Answer 7: *A.* The current AUC guidelines for transthoracic echocardiography define routine surveillance (≥1 year) of moderate or severe valvular regurgitation without a change in clinical status or cardiac exam as an appropriate indication with an appropriate use score of 8 (1 to 9). It is, however, arguable, as routine surveillance echocardiography in such a patient is unlikely to result in a change in management unlike in patients with severe mitral regurgitation who initially do not meet surgical intervention criteria. A similar request <1 year from the last study would be considered inappropriate with an appropriate use score of 3 (1 to 9).

> ***Editor's Note:*** *The topic of Appropriateness Use Criteria for Echocardiography is extensively covered elsewhere in this textbook. This is an important area given the current health care reform, and the echo AUC has already undergone a formal revision. This topic will remain an important, and potentially difficult, subject for individuals sitting for the echocardiographic ASE board examination.*

Even the terminology is changing and future AUC revisions will now use *appropriate, maybe appropriate, and rarely appropriate* instead of these older terms.

Suggested Reading

Douglas PS, Garcia MJ, Haines DE, et al. ACCF/ASE/AHA/ASNC/HFSA/HRS/SCAI/SCCM/SCCT/SCMR 2011 appropriate use criteria for echocardiography. *J Am Soc Echocardiogr* 2011;24:229–267.

Answer 8: *E.* Tricuspid inflow velocity is best recorded with CW Doppler either from a low parasternal right ventricular inflow view or from the apical four-chamber view. All measurements should be made at a sweep speed of 100 mm/s thus making Option A incorrect. Secondary to the effects of respiration on right heart hemodynamics, measurements should be averaged throughout the respiratory cycle or recorded at end-expiratory (not end-inspiration, making Option B incorrect) apnea. CW not PW should be utilized as PW Doppler may miss the maximal velocity through the valve, thus making Option C incorrect. In patients with irregular rhythms or atrial fibrillation, a minimum of five-cardiac cycle measurements should be averaged making Option D incorrect. Measurements should not be made at high heart rates (>100 bpm) if possible secondary to the effect of tachycardia on transvalvular gradient and should preferably be at heart rates between 70 and 80 bpm. As with mitral regurgitation, faster heart rates make it impossible to appreciate the deceleration time (or pressure half-time). If faster heart rates persist, the patient should still undergo a CW Doppler evaluation, although the interpretation should be modified to reflect the lower gradients that will likely be derived during normal heart rate evaluation.

Suggested Reading

Zoghbi WA, Adams D, Bonow RO, et al. Recommendations for Noninvasive Evaluation of Native Valvular Regurgitation: A Report from the American Society of Echocardiography Developed in Collaboration with the Society for Cardiovascular Magnetic Resonance. *J Am Soc Echocardiogr* 2017;30(4):303–371.

Answer 9: *B.* Tricuspid stenosis is the least common of the valvular stenosis lesions in the developed world given the low incidence of rheumatic heart disease. In carcinoid syndrome, the classic appearance of carcinoid involvement of the tricuspid valve involves severe immobility of the leaflets with a thickened, retracted valve and incomplete coaptation, as demonstrated in this clip (Option B). Rheumatic tricuspid valve disease echocardiographic features include similar features to mitral valve changes with leaflet thickening, commissural fusion, and variable degrees of calcification. Ebstein anomaly (Option C) is associated with tricuspid regurgitation and not stenosis in addition to the following morphologic features: (a) adherence of the septal and posterior tricuspid leaflets to the underlying myocardium (failure of delamination); (b) apical displacement of the functional annulus; (c) dilation of the "atrialized" portion of the right ventricle with various degrees of hypertrophy and thinning of the wall; (d) redundancy, fenestrations, and tethering of the anterior leaflet with sail-like enlargement; and (e) dilation of the right atrioventricular junction. Lupus valvulitis causes endocarditis-like vegetations on the valve and is an exceedingly rare and, hence, an unlikely cause of tricuspid stenosis (Option D). No pacemaker lead is present; hence, Option E is incorrect.

Suggested Readings

Baumgartner H, Hung J, Bermejo J, et al. Echocardiographic assessment of valve stenosis: EAE/ASE recommendations for clinical practice. *J Am Soc Echocardiogr* 2009;22(1):1–23.

Zoghbi WA, Adams D, Bonow RO, et al. Recommendations for Noninvasive Evaluation of Native Valvular Regurgitation: A Report from the American Society of Echocardiography Developed in Collaboration with the Society for Cardiovascular Magnetic Resonance. *J Am Soc Echocardiogr* 2017;30(4):303–371.

Answer 10: *C.* Tricuspid valve resection used to be performed as treatment of tricuspid valve bacterial endocarditis. This results in free, wide-open tricuspid regurgitation. No organized flow is seen across the atrioventricular annulus in this setting due to the lack of the tricuspid valve, resulting in the absence of a convergence zone. (Hence, Options A and D are incorrect.) The CW Doppler signal will be dense, triangular, early peaking with a low velocity due to rapid right atrial pressure equalization. (Making Option B incorrect.) This may lead to difficulty in recognition of the presence of severe tricuspid regurgitation. (Hence, Option C is incorrect.)

Suggested Reading

Friedman G, Kronzon I, Nobile J, et al. Echocardiographic findings after tricuspid valvectomy. *Chest* 1985;87(5):668–670.

Answer 11: *C.* The image demonstrates findings consistent with a postcardiac transplant state with presence of an atrial suture line in this apical four-chamber view. Moderate to severe tricuspid regurgitation can be noted after heart transplantation secondary to frequent endomyocardial biopsies performed for rejection surveillance that may injure the tricuspid valve leaflets and more commonly its support apparatus. Features of tricuspid leaflet thickening and retraction are absent (Option A). No tricuspid annular apical displacement is seen; hence, Ebstein anomaly is not present (Option B). No pacemaker lead is seen (Option D). No endocarditis vegetations are visible (Option E). Although this does not rule out endocarditis as a possible etiology, given the presence of an atrial suture line, which is a feature of the postcardiac transplant state, Option C is the single best answer.

Suggested Reading

Chan MC, Giannetti N, Kato T, et al. Severe tricuspid regurgitation after heart transplantation. *J Heart Lung Transplant* 2001;20(7):709–717.

Answer 12: *C.* The pulsed-wave spectral Doppler display demonstrates systolic reversal of hepatic vein flow associated with severe tricuspid regurgitation. Other associated findings corresponding to severe tricuspid regurgitation (measured at a Nyquist limit of 50 to 60 cm/s) include a central jet area of >10 cm²; a vena contracta width > 0.7 cm; a dense, triangular, early-peaking CW Doppler spectrum; and flail valve leaflet morphology. Additionally, at a Nyquist limit of 28 cm/s, a PISA radius of >0.9 cm corresponds to severe tricuspid regurgitation (TABLE 21.1).

Suggested Readings

Tribouilloy CM, Enriquez-Sarano M, Bailey KR, et al. Quantification of tricuspid regurgitation by measuring the width of the vena contracta with Doppler color flow imaging: a clinical study. *J Am Coll Cardiol* 2000;36:472–478.

Zoghbi WA, Enriquez-Sarano M, Foster E, et al. Recommendations for evaluation of the severity of native valvular regurgitation with two-dimensional and Doppler echocardiography. *J Am Soc Echocardiogr* 2003;16:777–802.

Answer 13: *A.* Due to the low prevalence of severe, life-threatening pulmonary regurgitation, the difficulties in imaging the pulmonary valve, and infrequent use of other measurement techniques, limited data are available for validation of echocardiographic evaluation of pulmonary regurgitation. Color jet length, rapid deceleration, and termination of flow in middiastole are all dependent on the driving pressure gradient between the pulmonary artery and the RV and are not a reliable index of severity. (Hence, Options D and E are not definitive.) Pulsed-wave Doppler estimation of RV stroke volume is limited by difficulties in accurate estimation of the pulmonic annulus. (Hence, Option B is not true.) The pulmonary artery is an anterior structure and is easily imaged from the transthoracic approach; therefore, the role of TEE in PR severity assessment is limited. (Hence, Option C is not ideal.)

Suggested Reading

Zoghbi WA, Enriquez-Sarano M, Foster E, et al. Recommendations for evaluation of the severity of native valvular regurgitation with two-dimensional and Doppler echocardiography. *J Am Soc Echocardiogr* 2003;16:777–802.

Answer 14: *D.* The images demonstrate the presence of mixed pulmonary stenosis and severe pulmonary regurgitation in a prosthetic valve post tetralogy of Fallot repair with a large, wide color Doppler jet size, dense CW Doppler tracing, steep deceleration, early termination of diastolic flow, and increased systolic flow. Assessment of coronary artery anatomy, specifically the possibility of an anomalous LAD across the RVOT, should be ascertained before operative intervention to avoid damaging this artery. (Option A is incorrect as it incorrectly describes coronary origin from the pulmonary artery as the most common coronary anomaly in the tetralogy of Fallot patients.) Options B and C are both indications to consider surgical revision. Surgical correction of severe pulmonary regurgitation should be considered in **symptomatic** patients with exercise limitation, significant RV dysfunction, significant RV enlargement, or the development of symptomatic or sustained atrial and/or ventricular arrhythmias and significant tricuspid regurgitation. Thus, Option D is the most correct answer.

Suggested Reading

Warnes CA, Williams RG, Bashore TM, et al. ACC/AHA 2008 guidelines for the management of adults with congenital heart disease. *J Am Coll Cardiol* 2008;52(23):e143–e263.

Answer 15: *C.* Acquired pulmonary stenosis is very uncommon. Rheumatic pulmonary stenosis is rare even when the pulmonary valve is affected by the rheumatic process. Carcinoid disease is the most common cause of acquired pulmonary valve disease with combined stenosis and regurgitation with usually predominant regurgitation (Option C).

Suggested Reading

Waller BF, Howard J, Fess S. Pathology of pulmonic valve stenosis and pure regurgitation. *Clin Cardiol* 1995;18:45–50.

Chapter 22

Normal and Abnormal Prosthetic Valve Features

Vincent L. Sorrell

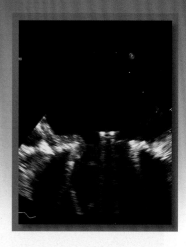

1. Which of the following statements is true about the size of a prosthetic valve?

   A. The valve number (e.g., 23 mm) refers to the internal diameter of the valve ring and can be used as the outflow tract diameter in the continuity equation for calculating effective valve area.

   B. The valve number refers to the outer diameter of the valve sewing ring and is equivalent to the patient's "tissue annulus," indicating the size of the valve that can be implanted.

   C. The valve number is not consistently measured and reported by various manufacturers and thus does not consistently indicate a particular dimension of the valve.

   D. As the valve number increases, the size of the valve increases, and the chance of a false gradient from the pressure recovery phenomenon increases.

2. A 32-year-old female has a 3-year-old bioprosthetic valve and now is 5 months pregnant. Prior to conception, an echocardiogram of her prosthetic aortic valve appeared normal, with normal leaflet motion and a peak continuous-wave Doppler gradient across the valve of 26 mm Hg. Velocity in the left ventricular outflow tract was 1.0 m/s. The repeat study, now that the patient is 5 months pregnant, shows a continuous-wave Doppler gradient of 49 mm Hg (3.5 m/s). The left ventricular outflow tract peak velocity is now 2.0 m/s. Which of the following statements are true?

   A. The increased cardiac output of pregnancy has caused an increase in turbulent flow across the valve, and pressure recovery is now occurring, causing a false increase in the gradient.

   B. The actual peak gradient across the valve is only increased modestly to 33 mm Hg.

   C. The rate of leaflet deterioration on bioprosthetic valves is accelerated by pregnancy. The valve is becoming fibrotic and stenotic.

   D. The patient should be brought back for repeat imaging. This higher flow velocity probably represents contamination from a mitral valve regurgitation signal.

3. A 76-year-old female presents to the emergency department after having a syncopal episode while carrying a box weighing 25 pounds up a flight of stairs. She recently had aortic valve replacement with a #23 bioprosthetic valve about 6 months before this episode. She feels she is fully recovered, and recent evaluation showed normal labs and no evidence of anemia. An echocardiogram is performed. Left ventricular size is normal with mild concentric left ventricular hypertrophy. The ejection fraction is 65%. The following measurements are made: height 175 cm, weight 119 kg, body surface area 2.46 m², and body mass index 38.9 kg/m².

   Left ventricular outflow tract diameter = 22 mm (area = 3.8 cm²)

   Left ventricular outflow tract peak velocity = 104 cm/s

   Left ventricular outflow tract VTI = 29 cm

   Prosthetic valve peak velocity = 406 cm/s

   Prosthetic valve mean velocity = 270 cm/s

   Peak prosthetic valve gradient = 66 mm Hg

   Mean prosthetic valve gradient = 34 mm Hg

   Acceleration time for aortic valve flow = 80 ms

   The bioprosthetic leaflets are difficult to see, but no evidence of aortic valve regurgitation or perivalvular regurgitation is noted. Which of the following statements is most correct about this patient's valve?

   A. The effective orifice area of this valve is 1.0 cm², normal for a bioprosthetic valve of this diameter.

   B. The patient has mild patient–prosthesis mismatch; therefore, the valve is not the cause of her syncope.

   C. Patient–prosthesis mismatch is severe. In order for her to have an appropriate-sized valve, the effective valve area should be at least 2.0 cm².

   D. The valve gradient is increased due to early pannus formation, and the cause of her syncope is prosthetic valve aortic stenosis.

4. FIGURE 22.1 and VIDEO 22.1 show a bileaflet mechanical valve examined by transesophageal echocardiography. Regarding valvular regurgitation, which of the following statements is true?

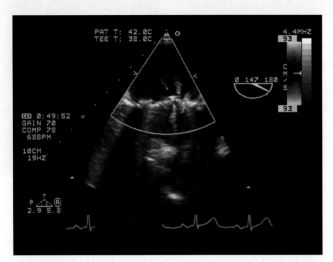

FIGURE 22.1

A. Multiple small regurgitant jets may be detected at the hinge points of mechanical valves.

B. Regurgitant jets are associated with leaflet closure and backwash only in mechanical valves and are not detectable on bioprosthetic valves.

C. Multiple jets are unique to bileaflet valves due to positioning of the hinge points of the two leaflets.

D. Regurgitant jets associated with normal leaflet closure are typically detected originating from outside of the sewing ring.

5. Which of the following statements represents the *least* appropriate use of echocardiography for evaluation of prosthetic valves?

A. Routine follow-up echocardiogram in a stable patient with a bileaflet valve and a normal exam 4 years postoperatively

B. Routine follow-up with a full echocardiogram at the first outpatient clinic visit, 4 weeks following placement of a new bioprosthetic valve

C. An echocardiogram ordered following an annual exam during which an aortic regurgitation murmur was heard for the first time

D. A routine follow-up echocardiogram 6 years postoperatively following placement of a bioprosthetic valve, the last echo having been a normal study performed 6 weeks after placement of the valve

6. A 44-year-old male has had a #19 St. Jude valve for 23 years. He currently is asymptomatic and runs 2 miles, four times per week. On exam, he has a 2/6 systolic ejection murmur with no audible aortic regurgitation, and valve leaflet sounds appear crisp at opening and closure. When the valve was replaced, the patient was a college student weighing 150 pounds. He now weighs 230 pounds. He is in chronic atrial fibrillation, and the maximum gradient from the exam is demonstrated in FIGURE 22.2. Additional findings from the echocardiogram revealed mild aortic valve regurgitation, a normal-sized aorta with a diameter of 3.5 cm above the sinotubular junction, and normal left ventricular function with mild concentric left ventricular hypertrophy. Valve leaflet motion was poorly visualized. Data from the exam

are the following: systolic ejection time 250 ms, aortic valve acceleration time 92 ms, peak aortic valve gradient 108 mm Hg, and mean aortic valve gradient 60 mm Hg.

Regarding the data on this patient's exam, which of the following statements is most accurate?

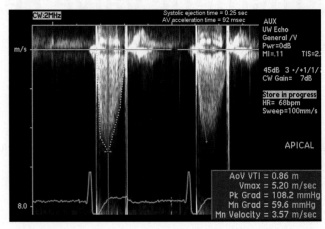

FIGURE 22.2

A. The high gradient across the valve is likely due to thrombosis of one of the two leaflets, allowing the valve to still sound normal.

B. The high gradient is due to gradually worsening patient–prosthesis mismatch, causing increased cardiac output demand combined with pressure recovery downstream from the valve at the level of the central aorta.

C. The aortic ejection time and aortic acceleration times are significantly prolonged, consistent with valvular level stenosis.

D. If a fluoroscopic exam reveals normal leaflet motion, a high gradient is most likely due to a combination of patient–prosthetic mismatch and pressure recovery from flow acceleration through the central orifice of the valve.

7. A 46-year-old male had a #29 bioprosthetic valve replacement 11 years prior to this examination. He remains largely asymptomatic except for shortness of breath with heavy exertion or prolonged walking up stairs. Data from his continuous-wave Doppler exam across the valve are (FIG. 22.3):

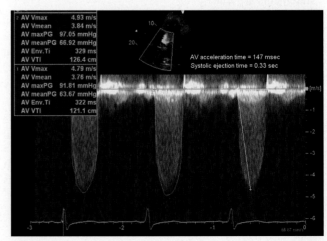

FIGURE 22.3

Peak gradient 94 mm Hg

Mean gradient 65 mm Hg

Valvular velocity time integral 124 cm

Acceleration time 147 ms

Systolic ejection time 330 ms

Of the following choices, which additional findings would be most likely to be expected on the patient's echocardiographic exam?

A. Significant deterioration of the bioprosthetic leaflets with associated severe aortic valve regurgitation, a high flow state across the valve, and thus a high gradient across the valve

B. Heavy calcific and fibrotic changes on the leaflets, severely limiting leaflet motion, causing severe primary bioprosthetic valve stenosis

C. A significantly abnormal Doppler velocity index > 0.35

D. Normal leaflets but evidence of severe patient–prosthetic valve mismatch with an indexed effective valve orifice area > 0.85 cm²/m²

8. The patient is a 34-year-old white female who is 6 months pregnant. She has had known perivalvular aortic valve regurgitation. This study is done to evaluate her valve and ventricular function during pregnancy. Examine the information from FIGURE 22.4 and VIDEO 22.2. Taking into account all the information available, the severity of the patient's perivalvular aortic regurgitation is:

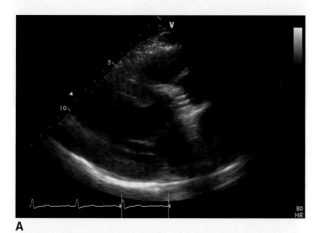

A

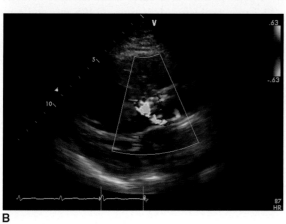

B

FIGURE 22.4

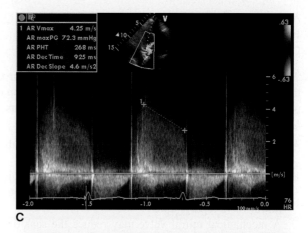

C

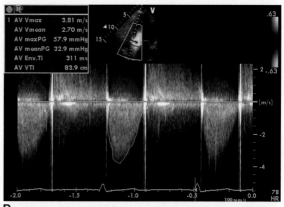

D

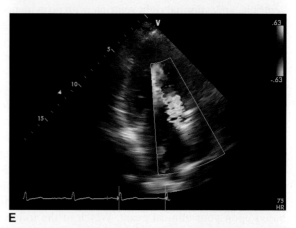

E

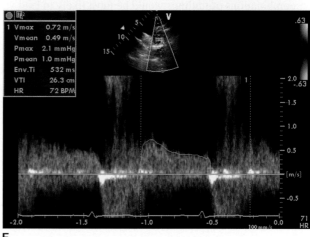

F

FIGURE 22.4 (*Continued*)

A. Mild

B. Moderate

C. Severe

9. Acoustic shadowing from dense structures such as prosthetic valves can reduce the effectiveness of interrogation of portions of the heart. Which of the following statements is *least* correct?

A. Stented bioprosthetic valves cause less shadowing than similar-sized mechanical valves.

B. On a transthoracic exam, the presence of a mechanical aortic valve may reduce the sensitivity for detection of mitral valve regurgitation.

C. A mechanical mitral valve may reduce the sensitivity for detecting mitral regurgitation in both the parasternal long-axis view of a transthoracic study and the apical long-axis view of a transthoracic study.

D. Both a bioprosthetic valve in the mitral position and a mechanical valve in the same location can cause unwanted shadowing of the left ventricle and left atrial appendage on a midesophageal transesophageal long-axis view of the heart.

10. A 67-year-old female returns for an annual visit. She has a 10-year-old bileaflet mitral valve, which was last imaged 5 years ago by two-dimensional echocardiography. At that time, she had normal left ventricular function with an ejection fraction of 60%, a normal-sized left ventricle, and a normal right ventricle with no evidence of pulmonary hypertension. Her mitral prosthetic valve had normal flow characteristics, and there was no evidence of mitral regurgitation by transthoracic exam or by physical exam. Today, she reports some modest increase in shortness of breath over the last 3 months compared to a year ago. On physical exam, there is a new high-pitched blowing systolic murmur at the apex, which extends laterally toward the axilla. There is a questionable soft diastolic rumble also noted. You suspect new mitral regurgitation so you order a transthoracic echocardiogram (FIG. 22.5). The study is performed, and no mitral regurgitation is detectable in any view. However, you remain suspicious based upon your clinical exam. Which of the following combinations of findings would be most likely to lead you to suspect the presence of mitral regurgitation?

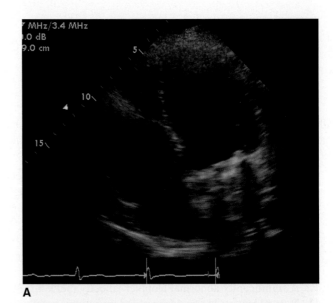

A

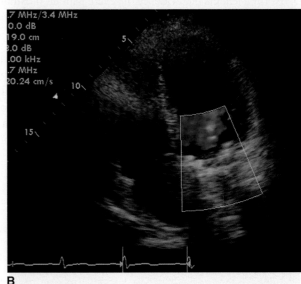

B

FIGURE 22.5

A. Evidence of flow convergence on the left atrial side of the valve using off-axis views, an ejection fraction of 55% in the left ventricle, and a peak forward flow velocity across the prosthetic mitral valve of 1.3 m/s

B. A peak mitral valve early diastolic flow velocity of 2.3 m/s, a pressure half-time of 175 ms, and a mean gradient across the valve of 9 mm Hg

C. A peak mitral valve velocity of 2.3 m/s, a pressure half-time of 90 ms, a mean gradient across the valve of 7 mm Hg, and a left ventricular ejection fraction of 75%

D. A Doppler velocity index of 2.6, a peak mitral valve early diastolic velocity of 1.8 m/s, a left ventricular ejection fraction of 60%, and a mean gradient across the mitral valve of 4 mm Hg

11. A 40-year-old male has a prior history of severe mitral valve myxomatous disease and prolapse. He developed endocarditis with significant valve destruction and underwent prolonged antibiotic therapy and valve replacement with a #29 St. Jude prosthesis approximately 1 year before presentation. He presents to the emergency department with 2 days of fever and malaise. His white blood cell count is found to be 18,900 with a left shift in his erythrocyte sedimentation rate at 88. This is the first fever the patient has had since discharge after valve surgery. The patient is admitted to the hospital. Prosthetic valve sounds appear normal, and no significant regurgitant murmur is appreciated. Images from the transesophageal echocardiogram are shown in FIGURE 22.6 and VIDEO 22.3. Which of the following statements regarding endocarditis is *least correct*?

A. The sensitivity of a transesophageal echocardiogram is markedly better than the sensitivity of a transthoracic echocardiogram for detection of vegetation. This, combined with a strong index of suspicion based on clinical grounds, justifies directly ordering a transesophageal study.

B. This study shows an unusual location of the mass associated with the prosthetic valve. Usually, vegetations are associated with direct attachment to the leaflets of the prosthesis.

C. Distinguishing a vegetation from valve thrombosis is nearly impossible based upon echocardiographic criteria alone.

D. Determining the size of the vegetation or thrombus is important for direction of initial and future therapy.

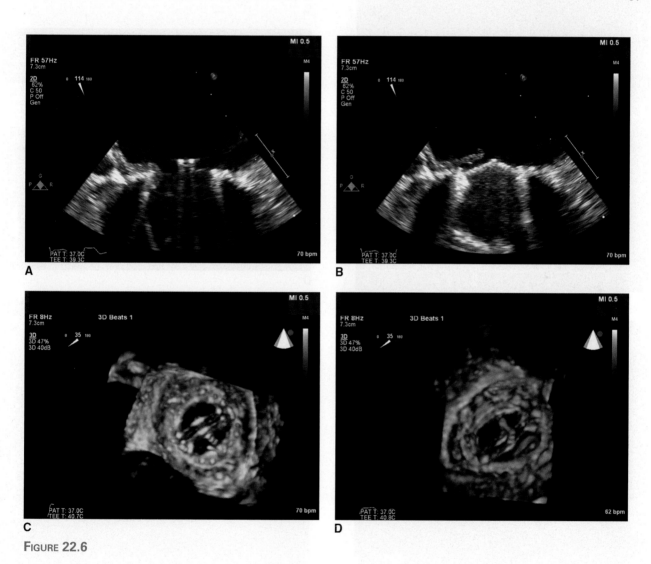

FIGURE 22.6

12. A 70-year-old male with a history of a bioprosthetic mitral valve replacement following a failed valve repair 8 years prior to admission develops a febrile illness. Despite oral antibiotics, the illness progresses with fever and night sweats. Six days prior to transfer, he awakes with a right-sided facial droop and is admitted to an outside hospital, where he has positive blood cultures for *Streptococcus mitis*. Intravenous antibiotics are begun, and he is transferred for further therapy. Images from his admitting echocardiogram are shown in FIGURE 22.7 and VIDEO 22.4. The figures show images from his echo exam. The following averaged Doppler data from his echocardiographic exam were obtained:

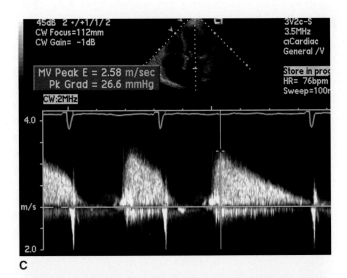

C

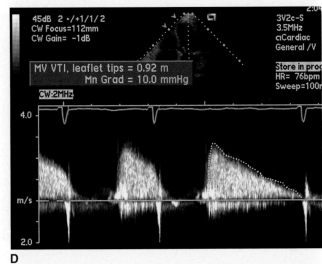

D

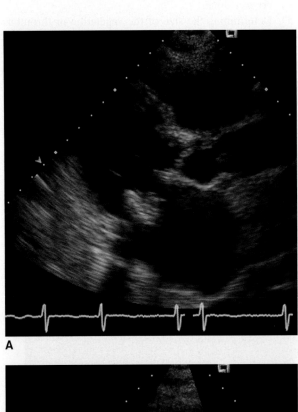

A

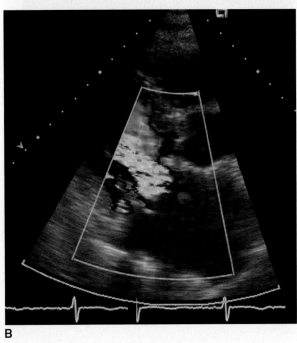

B

FIGURE 22.7

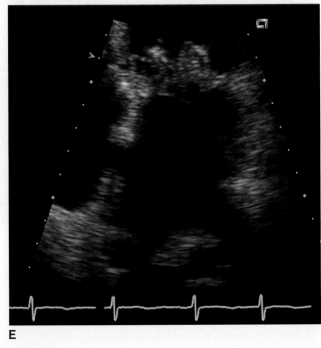

E

FIGURE 22.7 (*Continued*)

Left ventricular outflow tract VTI = 23 cm

Transmitral VTI = 73 cm

Stroke volume = 92 mL

Mitral valve peak early diastolic gradient = 29 mm Hg

Mitral valve mean gradient = 15 mm Hg

Mitral valve pressure half-time = 168 ms

The color-flow Doppler exam detects moderate mitral valve regurgitation.

Considering the information given about this mitral valve, which of the following statements is the most correct option?

A. The data are consistent with significant mitral valve stenosis.

B. The data are consistent with possible mitral valve stenosis.

C. The valve is not stenotic. The data above are consistent with a high volumetric flow rate across the valve because of the fever and mitral valve regurgitation.

D. Pressure half-time is not accurate when mitral valve regurgitation is also present.

13. A 66-year-old male presents to the clinic with new-onset dyspnea over the last 3 weeks. He had a #29 St. Jude mitral valve replacement 10 years ago. He has never had any difficulty with emboli, thrombosis, or bleeding since the valve was placed. Recently, he has had two dental procedures and a screening colonoscopy, with his warfarin being started and stopped on three different occasions. He still has an audible opening click and closure sound from his valve and no definite new murmurs appreciated. A transthoracic echocardiogram is ordered but shows continued normal left and right ventricular function and no evidence of mitral regurgitation. It was difficult to see motion of the leaflets, but forward flow velocities across the valve had changed compared to the prior study 3 years ago. Therefore, a transesophageal study was ordered, and images from that study are demonstrated in FIGURE 22.8 and VIDEO 22.5, with one image being during systole, one image being during diastole, and a Doppler flow signal presented. Which of the following statements are true?

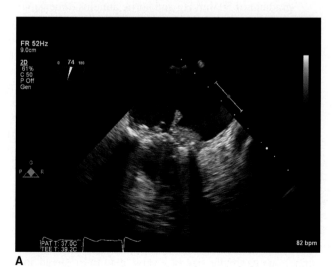

A

FIGURE 22.8

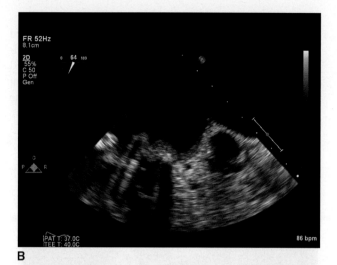

B

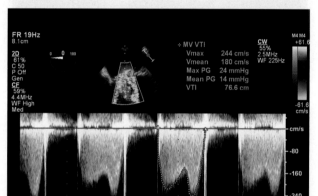

C

FIGURE 22.8 *(Continued)*

A. The lesion visualized is due to chronic pannus formation because pannus is more likely in the mitral position.

B. If a significant thrombus is present on a prosthetic valve, an area of the thrombus at its largest extent of >0.9 cm² confers a low embolic risk for thrombolytic therapy.

C. The data do not indicate significant obstruction to forward flow across the valve.

D. The two most common clinical findings indicating a high risk of embolism during thrombolytic therapy are a history of a previous cerebrovascular event and a thrombus size by TEE of >0.8 cm².

Questions 14 and 15

14. A 56-year-old male is 2 years status post placement of a #25 Medtronic-Hall valve for aortic stenosis caused by a bicuspid valve. His aorta was left intact. Since the surgery, he has had no history of complications of either emboli or bleeding. He recently moved and now presents to the emergency department with complaints of occasional fever and night sweats but otherwise normal functional capacity. Laboratory exam is positive for an erythrocyte sedimentation rate of 44, a white blood count of 12,500, and an INR of 2.6. Blood cultures are pending. A transthoracic echocardiogram is ordered and shows normal left ventricular function with normal flow characteristics across the Medtronic-Hall valve, with the expected central jet of aortic regurgitation. No evidence of a perivalvular regurgitation jet is identified. The patient is scheduled for a transesophageal echocardiogram, and images from that study are shown in FIGURE 22.9 and VIDEO 22.6. Regarding the images shown, what is the most likely diagnosis?

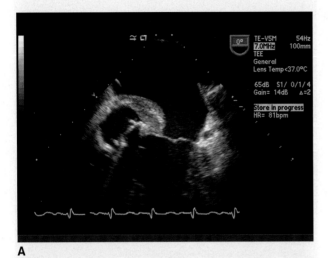

A

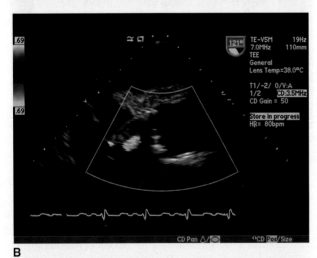

B

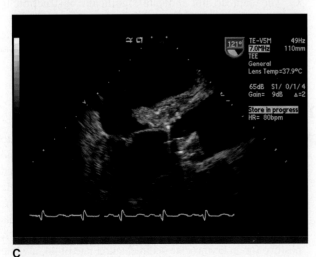

C

FIGURE 22.9

A. The Medtronic-Hall valve is normally positioned and normally functioning, with only a small, expected central jet of aortic regurgitation.

B. The valve appears normally positioned, and there is persistent postoperative thickening in the aortic annulus, an expected finding after this type of surgery.

C. The patient has developed an abscess of the native mitral valve, starting at the base of the anterior leaflet.

D. The patient has developed a periprosthetic aortic valve abscess even though there is no evidence of a perivalvular leak or vegetations.

15. Regarding prosthetic valve infections, which of the following statements is *least correct*?

A. Transesophageal echocardiography is most sensitive for detecting an abscess around a prosthetic valve early in the course of the disease process and early in the postoperative period.

B. The efficacy of transesophageal echocardiography for the diagnosis of an abscess is reduced by the presence of posterior lateral mitral valve annular calcification.

C. An abscess complicating infective endocarditis of the aortic valve starts in the aortic root wall. It may take serial studies to determine if that region is actually thickened.

D. In prosthetic valve infections, vegetative lesions are not necessarily present because the infection typically starts not on the leaflets but at the junction of the sewing ring and the aortic annulus.

16. Currently, the Edwards SAPIEN percutaneously delivered aortic valve is available using FDA-approved #23 and #26 sizes. Which of the following preprocedure echocardiographic findings is *not* a contraindication for the placement of this valve?

A. A calcified bicuspid aortic valve with severe stenosis, mean gradient 45 mm Hg, and calculated aortic valve area 0.7 cm^2.

B. Documented severe calcific aortic stenosis with a mean gradient of 50 mm Hg and aortic annulus dimension of 28 mm measured by transesophageal echocardiography.

C. Moderate left ventricular enlargement with associated mild left ventricular dysfunction, estimated ejection fraction 45%; moderate aortic valve regurgitation and mild ascending aortic enlargement, diameter 36 mm above the sinotubular junction; senile calcific stenosis is present with a mean gradient of 42 mm Hg.

D. Systolic anterior motion of the mitral valve with a left ventricular outflow tract gradient of 60 mm Hg and associated severe mitral valve regurgitation.

Answer 1: *C.* The reported size of a prosthetic valve usually refers to the outer diameter of the valve ring, in millimeters. However, manufacturers do not consistently report this measurement in the same way from valve to valve. Thus, as with clothing, one particular size of a valve may fit inside an annulus, whereas another size of a different manufacturer's valve may be required to fit the same annulus. It has been reported in one study that differences in diameter ranged from 3.5 mm smaller to 3.0 mm larger than the actual labeled size. Thus, the number on a valve should be considered a rough guide to the diameter of the valve, and current guidelines do not recommend using the valve number as a substitute for annulus measurement. Also, some valves, particularly the new percutaneous valves, are capable of being placed into annuli of varying sizes. Thus, the number on the valve indicates the maximum diameter the valve can be expanded to but does not represent the actual diameter that the valve was opened to in a given individual.

Answer A is incorrect because the valve number typically refers to the outer diameter of the valve ring and not the inner diameter. Answer B is incorrect because of the inconsistency in measurement of the outer diameter as noted above. Answer D is also incorrect. The pressure recovery phenomenon refers to increased flow velocities across certain types of mechanical valves. In general, as valve size increases, the chance of pressure recovery goes down, not up. Pressure recovery typically occurs when there are multiple orifices of the valve and is thought to originate, for instance, in a bileaflet valve from the small, middle-third orifice of the valve that may have local increases in velocities because the orifice is small and local jets can be detected by Doppler.

Suggested Readings

Chambers JB, Oo L, Narracott A, et al. Nominal size in six bileaflet mechanical aortic valves: a comparison of orifice size and biologic equivalence. *J Thorac Cardiovasc Surg* 2003;125:1388–1393.
Christakis GT, Buth KJ, Goldman BS, et al. Inaccurate and misleading valve sizing: a proposed standard for valve size nomenclature. *Ann Thorac Surg* 1998;66:1198–1203.

***Answer 2:** B.* Cardiac output has gone up in this woman who is now pregnant. A key factor in this case is that the simplified Bernoulli equation $4V^2$, while valid at baseline when the outflow tract velocity was only 1.0 m/s, is no longer valid because of the higher velocity in the outflow tract of 2.0 m/s. It is recommended that outflow tract velocity be taken into account when calculating the peak gradient if the velocity is >1.5 m/s. Thus, in the current case, using the more complete form of the Bernoulli equation, $p = 4\left(V_2^2 - V_1^2\right)$, gives the value of 33 mm Hg gradient across the valve (where V_2 = velocity across the aortic valve and V_1 = velocity in the LV outflow tract).

Option A is incorrect. Pressure recovery generally does not occur in bioprosthetic valves, so this would be a very unlikely answer.

Option C is incorrect. While valves deteriorate more rapidly in young individuals, it would be highly unlikely that a valve would rapidly deteriorate over a 5-month period, particularly if the leaflets were still normal before pregnancy.

Option D is incorrect. A mitral regurgitation signal of only 3.5 m/s would be unlikely in a healthy, young individual.

Suggested Reading

Zoghbi WA, Chambers JB, Dumesnil JG, et al. Recommendations for evaluation of prosthetic valves with echocardiography and Doppler ultrasound: a report From the American Society of Echocardiography's Guidelines and Standards Committee and the Task Force on Prosthetic Valves, developed in conjunction with the American College of Cardiology Cardiovascular Imaging Committee, Cardiac Imaging Committee of the American Heart Association, the European Association of Echocardiography, a registered branch of the European Society of Cardiology, the Japanese Society of Echocardiography and the Canadian Society of Echocardiography, endorsed by the American College of Cardiology Foundation, American Heart Association, European Association of Echocardiography, a registered branch of the European Society of Cardiology, the Japanese Society of Echocardiography, and Canadian Society of Echocardiography. *J Am Soc Echocardiogr* 2009;22:975–1014.

***Answer 3:** C.* The patient has severe patient–prosthetic mismatch (PPM). Her body habitus is that of significant obesity, and her body surface area is quite increased. A #23 valve was placed and, unfortunately, the surgeon was unable to place a larger valve. In determining patient–prosthesis mismatch, one first needs to calculate effective orifice area. In this case, the effective orifice area is 1.0 cm². The equation for effective orifice area is EOA = stroke volume/prosthetic valve VTI. To determine whether or not there is patient–prosthetic mismatch, the effective orifice area is divided by body surface area to determine an indexed value. In this case, 1.0/2.46 = 0.41 cm²/m². General guidelines from the literature suggest that the effective orifice area should be >0.85 cm/m². Determination of severity of patient–prosthetic mismatch is shown in Table 22.1.

In this case, the patient has severe patient–prosthetic mismatch; thus, the correct answer is C. In circumstances where patients are large, with large body surface areas, preoperatively one can back calculate to a desirable valve area. In this particular case, one would need to place a valve with an effective orifice area of at least 2.1 cm² to achieve an effective orifice area index to body surface area >0.85. Option B is incorrect because mismatch is not mild.

Option A is not correct because an area of 1.0 cm² is not normal for a #23 valve. It could be argued that the effective orifice area calculated in this example is less than expected for a #23 valve. Indeed, reported effective valve areas for #23 prosthetic valves tend to be in the range of 1.3 to 1.7 cm². If this was the case for this patient, it might be less likely she became symptomatic; however, even optimal valve area for a #23 valve would still result in patient–prosthetic mismatch. With regard to choice D, it is unlikely that the patient has rapid formation of pannus. The fact that the patient has an acceleration time of 80 ms across the prosthetic valve suggests that this is a high flow state and not a stenotic valve. A recent study published by Ben Zekry et al. suggests that an acceleration time of 100 ms or greater had a sensitivity and specificity of 86% for identifying stenosis across a prosthetic valve.

Table 22.1	Determination of Severity of Patient–Prosthetic Mismatch
PPM	**EOA/BSA (CM²/M²)**
Desirable	>0.85
Moderate	0.85–0.65
Severe	<0.65

Suggested Readings

Ben Zekry S, Saad RM, Ozkan M, et al. Flow acceleration time and ratio of acceleration time to ejection time for prosthetic aortic valve function. *JACC Cardiovasc Imaging* 2011;4:1161–1170.

Dumesnil JG, Honos GN, Lemieux M, et al. Validation and applications of indexed aortic prosthetic valve areas calculated by Doppler echocardiography. *J Am Coll Cardiol* 1990;16:637–643.

Pibarot P, Dumesnil JG. Hemodynamic and clinical impact of prosthesis-patient mismatch in the aortic valve position and its prevention. *J Am Coll Cardiol* 2000;36:1131–1141.

Answer 4: *A.* This question focuses on physiologic regurgitation of prosthetic valves. Small amounts of regurgitation, typically called physiologic, are present on virtually all valves, including bioprosthetic valves. Therefore, B is incorrect. Indeed, stentless bioprosthetic valves appear to have somewhat more regurgitation than stented bioprosthetic valves.

Regurgitation is caused by the closing motion of the prosthetic valve, which displaces backward toward the ring during the closing sequence. This is true of all mechanical valves regardless of the design. Bileaflet valves typically also have a second series of regurgitant jets that are associated with the hinges of the two leaflets. Other mechanical valves may have multiple jets. The best example is the single leaflet Medtronic-Hall valve that may have small closure jet and a central jet at the central orifice. Therefore, Option C is not correct. These jets occur inside the sewing ring and not outside the sewing ring. Therefore, Option D is incorrect. Most of the time, physiologic regurgitation is of relatively low velocity and nonturbulent, as shown in the example because the velocity is generated by the closing velocity of the leaflet and not the pressure gradient across the valve. Jets that are significantly turbulent should raise a concern about pathologic regurgitation. Different types of mechanical valves tend to have a "signature" that helps define the expected spectrum of physiologic regurgitation. Bioprosthetic valves on the other hand usually display a small central jet.

Suggested Readings

Flachskampf FA, O'Shea JP, Griffin BP, et al. Patterns of normal transvalvular regurgitation in mechanical valve prostheses. *J Am Coll Cardiol* 1991;18:1493–1498.

Temesvari A, Mohl W, Kupilik N. Characterization of normal leakage flow of monostrut tilting disk prosthetic mitral valves by multiplane transesophageal echocardiography. *J Am Soc Echocardiogr* 1997;10:155–158.

Zoghbi WA, Chambers JB, Dumesnil JG, et al. Recommendations for evaluation of prosthetic valves with echocardiography and Doppler ultrasound: a report From the American Society of Echocardiography's Guidelines and Standards Committee and the Task Force on Prosthetic Valves, developed in conjunction with the American College of Cardiology Cardiovascular Imaging Committee, Cardiac Imaging Committee of the American Heart Association, the European Association of Echocardiography, a registered branch of the European Society of Cardiology, the Japanese Society of Echocardiography and the Canadian Society of Echocardiography, endorsed by the American College of Cardiology Foundation, American Heart Association, European Association of Echocardiography, a registered branch of the European Society of Cardiology, the Japanese Society of Echocardiography, and Canadian Society of Echocardiography. *J Am Soc Echocardiogr* 2009;22:975–1014.

Answer 5: *A.* Appropriate use criteria have been established and recently revised in 2011 to define the most appropriate use of echocardiography in valvular heart disease. Currently, there is strong support for a baseline echocardiographic study following valve surgery. This is typically recommended for performance 2 to 6 weeks after hospital discharge if an echocardiogram was not performed during the hospitalization. Therefore, Option B is an incorrect choice since this is an appropriate indication. An echo at this time is actually more desirable as the patient has had a chance to recover and stabilize. The hyperadrenergic state immediately post-op and the anemia typically present at discharge should be less prominent and thus less likely to cause an artificial high output state. Routine follow-up of prosthetic valves generally involves a clinic visit annually and a physical examination. One indication for a repeat echocardiogram is a change in the exam, particularly if a new murmur is detected. Therefore, Option C is incorrect because this type of a follow-up echo also is strongly supported by the appropriateness guidelines. Bioprosthetic valves have a shorter expected life cycle. Generally, bioprosthetic valves do not show substantial deterioration in the first several years after placement. Therefore, routine follow-up of bioprosthetic valves is not recommended during the first 3 years or longer (as long as the physical exam is normal). Routine surveillance of older valves is reasonable to begin to evaluate for evidence of deterioration. Therefore, Option D is incorrect (this is an appropriate indication). Annual routine echocardiograms in otherwise stable patients with no evidence of a change in clinical status are not recommended. Therefore, Option A is the correct choice and is the *least* appropriate indication.

Suggested Reading

Douglas PS, Garcia MJ, Haines DE, et al. ACCF/ASE/AHA/ASNC/HFSA/HR/SCAI/SCCM/SCCT/SCMR 2011 appropriate use criteria for echocardiography. A report of the American College of Cardiology Foundation Appropriate Use Criteria Task Force, American Society of Echocardiography, American Heart Association, American Society of Nuclear Cardiology, Heart Failure Society of America, Heart Rhythm Society, Society for Cardiovascular Angiography and Interventions, Society of Critical Care Medicine, Society of Cardiovascular Computed Tomography, and Society for Cardiovascular Magnetic Resonance endorsed by the American College of Chest Physicians. *J Am Coll Cardiol* 2011;57:1126–1166.

Answer 6: *D.* The phenomenon known as pressure recovery most frequently manifests itself in flow signals across a prosthetic aortic valve. Occasionally, downstream effects may cause mild pressure recovery phenomena when pressure drop in the central aorta is compared to measurements close to the valve. This is most prevalent when the aorta is small, but in this case, the aorta is normal sized. Thus, answer B would be unlikely. The most common form of pressure recovery is that of localized phenomena of increased flow velocity through the small central orifice of a bileaflet valve. This is a localized increase in pressure drop. It is difficult to steer the CW Doppler beam through only a larger orifice, particularly when a transthoracic study is done and particularly when the valve is small, as in this case. This, indeed, may explain part of the high gradient in this particular patient's case. When this valve was replaced, the patient was a relatively thin, normal-sized college student who has gained considerable weight over the years. This would tend to exacerbate patient–prosthetic mismatch. Reported effective orifice areas for a valve of this type are in the range of 1.0 ± 0.2 cm^2, which would certainly lead to the expectation of a significant gradient across the valve. Given the measurements reported for ejection time and acceleration time, it is unlikely that this patient has valve leaflet stenosis. The ejection time is reasonably short, and the acceleration time also falls into a range less consistent with stenosis of the prosthetic valve. Therefore, Option C is incorrect. A recent study published by Ben Zekry et al. (see Suggested Reading) suggests that a cutoff time for acceleration time of 100 ms has a sensitivity and specificity of 86% for identifying prosthetic aortic valve stenosis. This patient's value of 92 ms is somewhat below this level. In addition, the same study evaluated the ratio of acceleration time to ejection time. The cutoff from this study was 0.37. This patient falls right at that level. Patients with values above this level are more likely to have stenosis. In this case, the most sensible thing to do would be also to check leaflet motion fluoroscopically since it was not seen well by echocardiography. This makes D the most correct answer. Option A, while possible, is less likely. One would expect prolongation of the valve acceleration time. Theoretically, valve area would be 0.5 cm^2. It is unlikely he could run 2 miles with no symptoms and that valve area.

Suggested Readings

Baumgartner H, Khan S, DeRobertis M, et al. Discrepancies between Doppler and catheter gradients in aortic prosthetic valves in vitro. A manifestation of localized gradients and pressure recovery. *Circulation* 1990;82:1467–1475.

Baumgartner H, Khan S, DeRobertis M, et al. Effect of prosthetic aortic valve design on the Doppler-catheter gradient correlation: an in vitro study of normal St. Jude, Medtronic-Hall, Starr-Edwards and Hancock valves. *J Am Coll Cardiol* 1992;19:324–332.

Ben Zekry S, Saad RM, Ozkan M, et al. Flow acceleration time and ratio of acceleration time to ejection time for prosthetic aortic valve function. *JACC Cardiovasc Imaging* 2011;4:1161–1170.

Chafizadeh ER, Zoghbi WA. Doppler echocardiographic assessment of the St. Jude Medical prosthetic valve in the aortic position using the continuity equation. *Circulation* 1991;83:213–223.

Answer 7: *B.* This patient has severe bioprosthetic valve aortic stenosis. He has gradually developed significant calcific aortic valve disease over the last several years. The flow velocity signal in the figure is consistent with a very high gradient across the valve. In addition, the flow acceleration time is markedly prolonged at 147 ms, highly consistent with aortic stenosis. The shape of the forward flow signal is rounded, peaking in the middle of systole and not early. Systolic ejection time, combined with the acceleration time, gives a markedly abnormal ratio of 0.44. These values would be highly unlikely given just a high flow state across the valve caused by something such as severe anemia or severe aortic regurgitation. Thus, answer A is not correct. One would expect a markedly abnormal Doppler velocity index; however, the index should be markedly reduced

and substantially <0.35. Recall that the Doppler velocity index is the ratio of the velocity time integral of the left ventricular outflow tract divided by the velocity time integral of the prosthetic valve. Assuming a relatively typical outflow tract velocity time integral of perhaps 28, the Doppler velocity index would be 0.22. Therefore, Option C is incorrect.

Option D is only partially correct. The patient does have severe patient–prosthetic valve mismatch, but the listed value associated with this statement is incorrect. One would expect the value to be substantially <0.85, which is the cutoff for a normal effective orifice area index.

The 2009 American Society of Echocardiography guidelines (see Suggested Reading) suggest the following values for significant prosthetic valve stenosis: peak velocity >4 m/s, mean gradient >35 mm Hg, Doppler velocity index <0.25, effective orifice area <0.8, or an effective orifice area two standard deviations below the reference value for the valve. The guidelines also suggest that the contour of a stenotic valve, as in this case, should be rounded and symmetric and the acceleration time should be >100 ms.

Suggested Reading

Zoghbi WA, Chambers JB, Dumesnil JG, et al. Recommendations for evaluation of prosthetic valves with echocardiography and Doppler ultrasound: a report From the American Society of Echocardiography's Guidelines and Standards Committee and the Task Force on Prosthetic Valves, developed in conjunction with the American College of Cardiology Cardiovascular Imaging Committee, Cardiac Imaging Committee of the American Heart Association, the European Association of Echocardiography, a registered branch of the European Society of Cardiology, the Japanese Society of Echocardiography and the Canadian Society of Echocardiography, endorsed by the American College of Cardiology Foundation, American Heart Association, European Association of Echocardiography, a registered branch of the European Society of Cardiology, the Japanese Society of Echocardiography, and Canadian Society of Echocardiography. *J Am Soc Echocardiogr* 2009;22:975–1014.

Answer 8: *B.* The patient has a perivalvular leak around her St. Jude aortic valve. The first figure shows that the valve continues to be well seated and positioned in the aortic annulus. There is no evidence of dehiscence or rocking motion identifying abnormal movement of the entire valve apparatus. Color Doppler from the parasternal long-axis view was difficult for showing the vena contracta of the jet clearly. This is due to the significant eccentricity of the perivalvular leak, which makes the typical quantification of relative jet width or vena contracta diameter difficult. Thus, the apical long-axis view is also shown. In this view, the jet does not appear to be large enough to occupy >65% of the outflow tract area but certainly is significant; thus, it most likely falls in the moderate range. The continuous-wave Doppler signal is shown twice, once in relationship to the aortic forward flow signal, which is increased as one would expect, and also as an individual signal. The signal is not more dense in relationship to forward flow across the valve (as would be expected in severe AR), again suggesting it is probably moderate. The deceleration slope is indicated. It falls at a fairly steep angle but still falls into the moderate range. The last image is that of a pulsed-wave Doppler signal in the proximal descending aorta. This signal is fairly prominent and actually would fall into the severe range given the velocity and holodiastolic nature of the signal.

These findings show examples of many of the guideline-recommended measurements to be performed for evaluation of severity of prosthetic aortic regurgitation. The guidelines for evaluation of severity are largely applied to prosthetic valves in a fashion similar to that identified over the last several years for evaluating native aortic valve regurgitation. In this case, most of the measurements come out into the moderate range, as noted above. Other parameters not shown, but also commonly utilized, would be a direct measurement of the vena contracta width. In this case, the regurgitation signal simply cannot be isolated in a fashion to allow a direct measurement. A typical moderate jet, however, would be 3 to 6 mm in width. Other parameters that can be calculated include regurgitant volume and regurgitant fraction. In this particular case, data from the right ventricular outflow tract were inadequate to obtain accurate stroke volumes at an alternate site. An indirect sign of the severity of regurgitation would be the degree of enlargement of the left ventricle. In this individual's case, the left ventricle is mildly dilated.

The full criteria for evaluation of aortic regurgitation, as recommended by the American Society of Echocardiography, are published in the guidelines for prosthetic valve evaluation (see Suggested Reading).

Editor's Note: This case demonstrates the importance of utilizing multiple echo and Doppler features to determine the severity of valve regurgitation. Furthermore, the classification of "severe" regurgitation should be reserved for quantitative features that fulfill more than one estimate of severity since the potential ramifications of this incorrect classification are significant.

Suggested Reading

Zoghbi WA, Chambers JB, Dumesnil JG, et al. Recommendations for evaluation of prosthetic valves with echocardiography and Doppler ultrasound: a report From the American Society of Echocardiography's Guidelines and Standards Committee and the Task Force on Prosthetic Valves, developed in conjunction with the American College of Cardiology Cardiovascular Imaging Committee, Cardiac Imaging Committee of the American Heart Association, the European Association of Echocardiography, a registered branch of the European Society of Cardiology, the Japanese Society of Echocardiography and the Canadian Society of Echocardiography, endorsed by the American College of Cardiology Foundation, American Heart Association, European Association of Echocardiography, a registered branch of the European Society of Cardiology, the Japanese Society of Echocardiography, and Canadian Society of Echocardiography. *J Am Soc Echocardiogr* 2009;22:975–1014.

Answer 9: *D.* A major problem with the evaluation of prosthetic mitral valve disease, or even native mitral valve disease, is shadowing from prosthetic devices. The problem is more severe with metal mechanical valves since there is a greater surface area of the ring and the leaflets that are highly reflective. Bioprosthetic valves, however, are not immune to this problem, particularly stented bioprosthetic valves, which

generally have a dense ring and a wire frame that also can cause significant shadowing. Therefore, Option A is incorrect. On a transthoracic echocardiogram, a prosthetic valve in the aortic position may in certain views cause shadowing of the area just below the mitral annulus on the parasternal long-axis view or near the roof of the left atrium in the apical long-axis view. Therefore, Option B is incorrect. These considerations are sometimes important if there is an eccentric mitral valve jet that is difficult to characterize. Similar phenomenon can occur on transesophageal studies, as shown in FIGURE 22.10 of an individual who has a St. Jude aortic valve in place. Shadowing in the mitral position is generally more problematic. The most significant problem occurs when a mitral prosthesis is evaluated in the apical views. In this situation, a considerable portion of the left atrium may be shadowed in all the apical views. Also, areas proximal to the valve, particularly posteriorly, may be shadowed in the parasternal views. Therefore, Option C is incorrect. Thus, a combination of transthoracic and transesophageal images may be necessary in some circumstances to completely interrogate a prosthetic mitral valve. Note that answer D is partially correct and that the mitral valve does shadow the left ventricle from a TEE exam but DOES NOT SHADOW the left atrial appendage. In both types of exams, imaging in multiple off-axis views and incorporating three-dimensional en face imaging combined with color-flow Doppler imaging may help identify difficult-to-find perivalvular leaks.

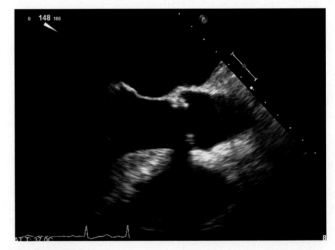

FIGURE 22.10

Suggested Readings

Sprecher DL, Adamick R, Adams D, et al. In vitro color flow, pulsed and continuous wave Doppler ultrasound masking of flow by prosthetic valves. *J Am Coll Cardiol* 1987;9:1306–1310.

Zoghbi WA, Chambers JB, Dumesnil JG, et al. Recommendations for evaluation of prosthetic valves with echocardiography and Doppler ultrasound: a report From the American Society of Echocardiography's Guidelines and Standards Committee and the Task Force on Prosthetic Valves, developed in conjunction with the American College of Cardiology Cardiovascular Imaging Committee, Cardiac Imaging Committee of the American Heart Association, the European Association of Echocardiography, a registered branch of the European Society of Cardiology, the Japanese Society of Echocardiography and the Canadian Society of Echocardiography, endorsed by the American College of Cardiology Foundation, American Heart Association, European

Association of Echocardiography, a registered branch of the European Society of Cardiology, the Japanese Society of Echocardiography, and Canadian Society of Echocardiography. *J Am Soc Echocardiogr* 2009;22:975–1014.

Answer 10: C. In many circumstances, shadowing may cause a total inability to detect a mitral regurgitation flow signal. If one has a high index of suspicion, several other clues on the routine echo exam may help determine if mitral regurgitation is indeed present. Particularly valuable would be evidence of hyperdynamic left ventricular function. In this case, you know that the patient had a normal ejection fraction in the past, so an increase in the ejection fraction might indicate increased processing of volume. This, combined with the left ventricular outflow tract stroke volume calculation or cardiac output calculation that was either normal or low, would indicate that there is a substantial amount of mitral valve regurgitation present. Also using information from the velocity time integral and the left ventricular outflow tract, the Doppler velocity index can be calculated. This is the ratio of the velocity time integral across the prosthetic valve to the velocity time integral in the left ventricular outflow tract. If this ratio is >2.2, one may suspect moderate, or more, mitral regurgitation.

A third consideration is to evaluate peak velocity across the valve. The combination of a high peak early diastolic velocity >2 m/s should raise significant suspicion. One study showed that a peak early diastolic velocity of 1.9 m/s or greater had a 90% sensitivity and 89% specificity for detecting moderate or greater mitral regurgitation. Specificity, however, might be reduced if there are other reasons for the patient to be in a high cardiac output state. Similarly, a mean gradient across the mitral valve of >6 mm Hg also has a reported sensitivity of 90% and a specificity of 70% for detecting mitral regurgitation. Thus, the typical forward flow signal across a nonstenotic prosthetic valve that has a significant regurgitant leak, usually perivalvular, would be a high peak early velocity with an increased gradient but a normal deceleration slope and pressure half-time.

Some studies have also shown that the presence of flow convergence on color Doppler, particularly at the site of a perivalvular leak, may also localize the presence of a significant valve leakage. In answer A, the flow convergence was on the wrong side of the valve, and the other indicators suggested normal flows. Answer B is a combination of findings typical of mitral stenosis across a prosthetic valve. Answer C is the most logical combination of findings, with a high peak early diastolic velocity, a normal pressure half-time for a prosthetic valve, a modest increase in the gradient across the valve, and hyperdynamic left ventricular function. Answer D has conflicting information. While the Doppler velocity index is high, raising suspicion, the rest of the findings don't meet typical criteria for a regurgitant valve.

Suggested Readings

Fernandes V, Olmos L, Nagueh SF, et al. Peak early diastolic velocity rather than pressure half-time is the best index of mechanical prosthetic mitral valve function. *Am J Cardiol* 2002;89:704–710.

Olmos L, Salazar G, Barbetseas J, et al. Usefulness of transthoracic echocardiography in detecting significant prosthetic mitral valve regurgitation. *Am J Cardiol* 1999;83:199–205.

Rahko PS. Assessing prosthetic mitral valve regurgitation by transoesophageal echo/Doppler. *Heart* 2004;90:476–478.

Answer 11: B. A large number of studies performed after transesophageal echocardiography became commonly available demonstrated conclusively a markedly higher sensitivity for detection of vegetations, particularly for the mitral valve. Reported sensitivities for detection of vegetations range from 86% to 94% with equally excellent specificities ranging from 88% to 100%. Thus, TEE is the test of choice, particularly when there is a high clinical index of suspicion for infection. In the case of the current patient, the index of suspicion would be very high given the fact that he already had one episode of endocarditis followed by valve replacement and now has recurrent evidence of infection. Thus, Option A is incorrect.

The imaging characteristics of a mass do not allow distinct differentiation between an active vegetation and a fresh thrombus. Therefore, Option C is incorrect. Vegetations are most frequently attached to the sewing ring of the valve and also may be associated with perivalvular leaks and perivalvular abscesses. Therefore, Option D is incorrect. Thrombi can also be associated with the sewing ring but do not necessarily have to be associated with perivalvular leaks. In many cases, a thrombus may be somewhat more layered and less mobile and also be attached in an obstructing fashion to valve leaflets. Small thrombi or vegetations may be the most difficult to differentiate based on echocardiographic grounds.

Measuring the size of the lesion is important to help determine therapy and embolic risk. It is recommended that the maximal dimensions and area of a suspected vegetative mass attached to the prosthesis be measured and reported.

Suggested Readings

Birmingham GD, Rahko PS, Ballantyne F III. Improved detection of infective endocarditis with transesophageal echocardiography. *Am Heart J* 1992;123:774–781.

Daniel WG, Mugge A, Grote J, et al. Comparison of transthoracic and transesophageal echocardiography for detection of abnormalities of prosthetic and bioprosthetic valves in the mitral and aortic positions. *Am J Cardiol* 1993;71:210–215.

Shively BK, Gurule FT, Roldan CA, et al. Diagnostic value of transesophageal compared with transthoracic echocardiography in infective endocarditis. *J Am Coll Cardiol* 1991;18:391–397.

Zoghbi WA, Chambers JB, Dumesnil JG, et al. Recommendations for evaluation of prosthetic valves with echocardiography and Doppler ultrasound: a report From the American Society of Echocardiography's Guidelines and Standards Committee and the Task Force on Prosthetic Valves, developed in conjunction with the American College of Cardiology Cardiovascular Imaging Committee, Cardiac Imaging Committee of the American Heart Association, the European Association of Echocardiography, a registered branch of the European Society of Cardiology, the Japanese Society of Echocardiography and the Canadian Society of Echocardiography, endorsed by the American College of Cardiology Foundation, American Heart Association, European Association of Echocardiography, a registered branch of the European Society of Cardiology, the Japanese Society of Echocardiography, and Canadian Society of Echocardiography. *J Am Soc Echocardiogr* 2009;22:975–1014.

Answer 12: B. This patient has both mitral stenosis from a deteriorating prosthetic valve and endocarditis. Parameters for evaluating prosthetic valve mitral stenosis have an unusual classification in the American Society of Echocardiography guidelines. Doppler parameters are categorized as normal, consistent with possible stenosis, or consistent with significant stenosis. An examination of the parameters on this patient does represent a mixed picture. Several parameters should be examined when determining severity of mitral stenosis. One parameter is the peak velocity across the valve. For most valves, a peak velocity of 1.9 m/s or less would be considered to fall into the normal range. Possible stenosis ranges from 1.9 to 2.5 m/s, and significant stenosis is considered present when the flow velocity is >2.5 m/s. Similarly, gradients are judged in a very similar fashion to those seen for native mitral stenosis. Normal values are considered to be less than a mean of 5 mm Hg, possible stenosis 6 to 10 mm Hg, and significant stenosis >10 mm Hg. When one examines the data in this case, both parameters actually fall into the significant stenosis range. Therefore, Option C is incorrect. However, a caveat in this case is the fact that the patient has developed moderate mitral valve regurgitation. It is actually perivalvular. This should caution one into automatically jumping to the conclusion that there is severe stenosis because there is also an increased flow state and the patient is febrile. Therefore, Option A is incorrect.

Another parameter to consider is the Doppler velocity index for the mitral valve. This is defined as:

$$DVI = VTI_{\text{prosthetic mitral valve}}/VTI_{\text{LVOT}}$$

Note that the ratio is just the opposite of what one would use for aortic stenosis. Thus, for the mitral valve, the higher the ratio, the more severe is the possible stenosis. In our case, the ratio is quite high at 3.2, but again the patient has a higher flow state.

This should lead one to consider other measures of valve area. The pressure half-time is affected by multiple parameters. Most studies suggest that a pressure half-time >130 suggests some degree of abnormal functioning of a valve prosthesis. A marked increase of pressure half-time >200 ms would suggest significant obstruction. In our patient, the value falls in the intermediate range. One can also calculate effective orifice area. It is not recommended that pressure half-time be used to do this with prosthetic valves. It is recommended that the continuity equation be used. The formula for effective orifice area is:

$$EOA_{\text{prosthetic MV}} = \text{stroke volume}/VTI_{\text{prosthetic MV}}$$

In this case, the continuity equation–calculated effective orifice area also falls in the moderate range.

The pressure half-time is affected by multiple parameters. Atrial chamber and ventricular chamber compliance both can affect pressure half-time, particularly if there are other abnormalities of the left ventricle that might affect the rate of relaxation such as left ventricular hypertrophy or underlying cardiomyopathic or systolic dysfunction. Loading conditions may affect the pressure half-time, and aortic regurgitation has been shown to alter pressure half-time. Mitral regurgitation, however, does not have a significant effect on pressure half-time. Thus, Option D is incorrect.

None of these measurements are definitive in their own right. In evaluating cases such as this patient, all of the parameters

should be calculated as noted and a conclusion reached based upon the preponderance of data, hopefully falling in one of these major categories. In the present case, the patient ended up having obstruction from a combination of a deteriorating bioprosthetic valve and a rather large vegetation burden on the valve apparatus. Ultimately, the patient recovered from his stroke, which was caused by septic emboli, and underwent successful mitral valve replacement.

Suggested Readings

Bitar JN, Lechin ME, Salazar G, et al. Doppler echocardiographic assessment with the continuity equation of St. Jude Medical mechanical prostheses in the mitral valve position. *Am J Cardiol* 1995;76:287–293.

Dumesnil JG, Honos GN, Lemieux M, et al. Validation and applications of mitral prosthetic valvular areas calculated by Doppler echocardiography. *Am J Cardiol* 1990;65:1443–1448.

Fernandes V, Olmos L, Nagueh SF, et al. Peak early diastolic velocity rather than pressure half-time is the best index of mechanical prosthetic mitral valve function. *Am J Cardiol* 2002;89:704–710.

Zoghbi WA, Chambers JB, Dumesnil JG, et al. Recommendations for evaluation of prosthetic valves with echocardiography and Doppler ultrasound: a report From the American Society of Echocardiography's Guidelines and Standards Committee and the Task Force on Prosthetic Valves, developed in conjunction with the American College of Cardiology Cardiovascular Imaging Committee, Cardiac Imaging Committee of the American Heart Association, the European Association of Echocardiography, a registered branch of the European Society of Cardiology, the Japanese Society of Echocardiography and the Canadian Society of Echocardiography, endorsed by the American College of Cardiology Foundation, American Heart Association, European Association of Echocardiography, a registered branch of the European Society of Cardiology, the Japanese Society of Echocardiography, and Canadian Society of Echocardiography. *J Am Soc Echocardiogr* 2009;22:975–1014.

Answer 13: D. The clinical presentation of a thrombus on a prosthetic valve can be highly variable. Smaller thrombi may be asymptomatic and discovered incidentally. Larger, obstructive thrombi tend to cause relatively rapid onset of symptoms, with dyspnea being the most frequent symptom, followed by systemic embolism. Abnormal findings by physical exam such as new regurgitant murmurs or obstructive murmurs or a change in prosthetic valve sounds should prompt immediate imaging evaluation. Initial transthoracic echocardiography, particularly when the valve is in the mitral position, may not visualize an actual thrombus but may show signs of abnormal hemodynamics. Cine fluoroscopy can be of considerable value to analyze motion of metal prosthetic leaflets. Transesophageal echocardiography should be performed to further characterize the nature of the thrombus and the size of the clot burden. The TEE exam should be directed to carefully interrogate the valve by 2D and 3D imaging to determine the degree of immobility or reduction in leaflet motion. The size and location of the thrombus should be carefully evaluated. Note that thrombi can sometimes be in unusual positions on either side of the valve, although as in this case, thrombus on the atrial side of the valve is probably most frequent. When the thrombus is smaller, it may be difficult to differentiate from pannus formation, and in many cases, pannus formation is difficult to visualize. Thrombi tend to have less echogenicity, whereas a pannus has quite dense fibrotic-looking echogenicity. Option A is incorrect because the visualized lesion is large, "soft," and mobile, characteristics more typical of a thrombus. Pannus formation is more common on the aortic rather than mitral valve. TEE is important for guiding therapeutic strategies. For left-sided obstructive thrombi, current guidelines recommend surgery as the first choice, with fibrinolysis as an alternate choice in patients not candidates for repeat surgery. Furthermore, patients who have had a prior cerebrovascular event or have a relatively large thrombus, defined in one study as >0.8 cm², present major risks for embolic complication. Therefore, Option B is incorrect. Patients with a small thrombotic burden may initially be treated with heparinization and followed serially by transesophageal echocardiography, with thrombolysis being considered if the small thrombus does not resolve with more conservative means. Small thrombi should also be differentiated from filamentous strands, which are usually very narrow (<1 mm wide) but can be quite long. The presence of stranding probably carries a much smaller embolic potential. TEE can be limited in its ability to make a diagnosis of thrombosis, particularly if the thrombus is on the ventricular side of the mitral prosthesis. A combination of transthoracic and transesophageal echocardiography may yield the greatest sensitivity. Furthermore, aortic prostheses sometimes are difficult to visualize and determine if there is compromise or an abnormal structure involved.

Option C is incorrect. Review the figure showing forward flow velocity across the valve. The data available from this figure show a mean gradient suggesting significant stenosis and a peak velocity suggesting at least a possible stenosis. While it is recognized that significant valvular regurgitation is also present, the data certainly also suggest an element of stenosis. Option C states that there is no evidence of obstruction, which is not correct.

Suggested Readings

Barbetseas J, Nagueh SF, Pitsavos C, et al. Differentiating thrombus from pannus formation in obstructed mechanical prosthetic valves: an evaluation of clinical, transthoracic and transesophageal echocardiographic parameters. *J Am Coll Cardiol* 1998;32:1410–1417.

Bonow RO, Carabello BA, Chatterjee K, et al. 2008 Focused update incorporated into the ACC/AHA 2006 guidelines for the management of patients with valvular heart disease: a report of the American College of Cardiology/American Heart Association Task Force on Practice Guidelines (Writing Committee to Revise the 1998 Guidelines for the Management of Patients with Valvular Heart Disease). Endorsed by the Society of Cardiovascular Anesthesiologists, Society for Cardiovascular Angiography and Interventions, and Society of Thoracic Surgeons. *J Am Coll Cardiol* 2008;52:e1–e142.

Deviri E, Sareli P, Wisenbaugh T, et al. Obstruction of mechanical heart valve prostheses: clinical aspects and surgical management. *J Am Coll Cardiol* 1991;17:646–650.

Roudaut R, Serri K, Lafitte S. Thrombosis of prosthetic heart valves: diagnosis and therapeutic considerations. *Heart* 2007;93: 137–142.

Zoghbi WA, Chambers JB, Dumesnil JG, et al. Recommendations for evaluation of prosthetic valves with echocardiography and Doppler ultrasound: a report From the American Society of Echocardiography's Guidelines and Standards Committee and the Task Force on Prosthetic Valves, developed in conjunction

with the American College of Cardiology Cardiovascular Imaging Committee, Cardiac Imaging Committee of the American Heart Association, the European Association of Echocardiography, a registered branch of the European Society of Cardiology, the Japanese Society of Echocardiography and the Canadian Society of Echocardiography, endorsed by the American College of Cardiology Foundation, American Heart Association, European Association of Echocardiography, a registered branch of the European Society of Cardiology, the Japanese Society of Echocardiography, and Canadian Society of Echocardiography. *J Am Soc Echocardiogr* 2009;22:975–1014.

Answer 14: D.

Editors' Note: This question is entirely based upon the ability of the test taker to interpret echocardiographic images and provide the most correct option.

Options A and B are incorrect options given the grossly abnormal appearance of the intervalvular fibrosa between the aorta and mitral valves.

Option C is not the best option since it would be exceedingly rare for a native mitral valve to develop an abscess.

Option D is most correct and importantly emphasizes the need for the echo board taker to know that this disease process can occur in the absence of a clearly visualized perivalvular regurgitant AR jet or a prosthetic vegetative lesion.

Suggested Readings

Habib G, Badano L, Tribouilloy C, et al. Recommendations for the practice of echocardiography in infective endocarditis. *Eur J Echocardiogr* 2010;11:202–219.

Habib G, Thuny F, Avierinos JF. Prosthetic valve endocarditis: current approach and therapeutic options. *Prog Cardiovasc Dis* 2008;50:274–281.

Piper C, Korfer R, Horstkotte D. Prosthetic valve endocarditis. *Heart* 2001;85:590–593.

Answer 15: A. This case is an example of the development of postoperative aortic root abscess in a patient with a mechanical prosthetic aortic valve. Abscess formation frequently starts in association with a perivalvular leak, but this is not necessary in all cases. As shown in this particular example, an abscess can start without evidence of vegetation and without evidence of increasing valvular or perivalvular regurgitation. Therefore, Option D is incorrect. The reason for this is that the mechanism of infection usually involves seating of the sewing ring of the valve or the junction between the annulus and the sewing ring. This is particularly true for a mechanical valve but less common for a bioprosthetic valve, where it is also possible for the bioprosthetic leaflet structure to become involved in the infection and develop significant sized vegetative lesions or perforations or tearing of the valve apparatus. Because of this difference in mechanisms, a single negative echocardiogram is not uncommon when prosthetic valve endocarditis is suspected. Thus, a single study does not necessarily exclude the diagnosis of infective endocarditis or abscess. If the first study is negative, a repeat exam should be strongly considered, particularly if the clinical suspicion for infection remains high. Therefore, Option C is incorrect. A second examination 7 to 10 days later may now detect progressive changes, particularly

in the case of an abscess, that were not evident on the first examination. A third echocardiogram has not been shown to be of additional benefit.

The rate of prosthetic endocarditis is about 1% to 6% in various series reported and comprises about 10% to 30% of all cases of infective endocarditis. The actual incidence of endocarditis is similar between mechanical valves and bioprosthetic valves.

Another limitation of both transthoracic and transesophageal echocardiography is reduced sensitivity for detecting an abscess early in the course of disease. Small abscesses forming early on in the disease process are difficult to detect and differentiate from normal tissue. Furthermore, there can be material in and around the aortic annulus, particularly early after placement of the valve that gradually absorbs over the first several months, making differentiation from infection versus normal healing process problematic. Therefore, Option A is the best choice for being "least correct." If mitral calcification was significant on the posterior annulus and leaflet, then the TEE image of the intervalvular fibrosa may be shadowed; hence, Option B is incorrect.

Suggested Readings

Habib G, Badano L, Tribouilloy C, et al. Recommendations for the practice of echocardiography in infective endocarditis. *Eur J Echocardiogr* 2010;11:202–219.

Habib G, Thuny F, Avierinos JF. Prosthetic valve endocarditis: current approach and therapeutic options. *Prog Cardiovasc Dis* 2008;50:274–281.

Piper C, Korfer R, Horstkotte D. Prosthetic valve endocarditis. *Heart* 2001;85:590–593.

Answer 16: C. Echocardiographic assessment of aortic stenosis is critical for screening patients that are potential candidates for percutaneous placement of a bioprosthetic aortic valve. Comprehensive echocardiographic assessment is essential. Particular attention must be paid to qualify the patient first by documenting severe aortic stenosis. The valve area should be <0.8 cm², the mean gradient across the valve should be at least 40 mm Hg, or the peak gradient across the valve should be at least 64 mm Hg. Only trileaflet valves are currently allowed. Bicuspid valves, due to potential asymmetry in placement of the device due to the elliptical valvular orifice and possible increased risk of incomplete or abnormal deployment of the valve, are not recommended. Therefore, Option A is incorrect.

The range of acceptable aortic annular dimensions must meet the range of the two valves currently available. This is expected to increase in the future as more valve sizes become available. Currently, the range for the #23 valve is approximately 18 to 22 mm in diameter, and the range for the #26 valve is approximately 22 to 25 mm. Aortic annulus sizes greater than this are not acceptable for TAVI procedures. Correct selection of size is important. Therefore, Option B is incorrect. Undersizing may result in device migration or significant paravalvular aortic regurgitation following placement of the valve. Oversizing may increase the risk of vascular access complications during the procedure or run the risk of underexpansion of the valve that might cause central aortic leaflet regurgitation following deployment. Currently, ventricular function should be an ejection fraction of 40% or greater; severe ventricular dysfunction is a contraindication, but moderate ventricular enlargement and some reduction in function, along with mild or moderate aortic valve regurgitation or moderate mitral regurgitation, are not contraindications to placement of the valve. The presence of outflow tract obstruction or flow acceleration below the valve could make implantation very difficult and cause prosthesis dislodgement. Therefore, Option D is incorrect. The presence of a thrombus in the left ventricle is also considered a significant contraindication.

Suggested Readings

Holmes DR Jr, Mack MJ, Kaul S, et al. 2012 ACCF/AATS/SCAI/STS expert consensus document on transcatheter aortic valve replacement. *J Am Coll Cardiol* 2012;59:1200–1254.

Zamorano JL, Badano LP, Bruce C, et al. EAE/ASE recommendations for the use of echocardiography in new transcatheter interventions for valvular heart disease. *J Am Soc Echocardiogr* 2011;24:937–965.

Chapter 23

2D Measures

Sasanka Jayasuriya

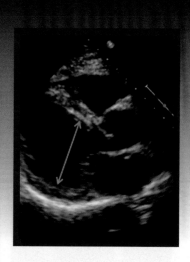

1. Which of the following statements comparing a linear estimate of LV global systolic function (fractional shortening %) and 2D midventricular ratio of diastolic area to systolic area (fractional area change %) is *least* accurate?

A. Both techniques are limited by regional LV function.

B. Both methods have inherent limitations of cursor and image alignment.

C. The correct LV short-axis view for measuring LV mass is located more basally than the view used to calculate the FAC%.

D. The lower limit of normal for fractional shortening is lower in men than women.

E. The papillary muscle should be *excluded* from the endocardial contour tracing.

2. The ASE recommends the use of the Simpson rule (method of disks; MOD) to estimate LV diastolic and systolic volumes and then calculate stroke volume and LV ejection fraction. This technique is recommended over other previous geometric assumption methods. Which of the following statements regarding this technique is *least* accurate?

A. Each disk used to estimate LV volumes is assumed to have the same diameter at its basal and apical margins.

B. The height of each disk is fixed and inherent upon the individual ultrasound system.

C. Individual disk volume is calculated as the product of the individual disk height × the individual disk area.

D. This method often underestimates the true LV volume due to foreshortening of the LV length.

E. Abnormal LV geometry and regional wall motion abnormalities remain a limitation to this technique, and the true LV volume is improved by additional views (biplane or triplane Simpson).

3. Which of the following statements regarding the LV ejection fraction is *false*?

A. Despite the recent knowledge that normal men typically have a higher LVEF than do normal women, these values are assumed to be equal by convention.

B. The single-plane Simpson rule is able to provide an accurate LVEF if there are no wall motion abnormalities and should be used if an orthogonal long-axis view is inadequate.

C. An LVEF of 44% is considered moderately abnormal.

D. An LVEF of 30% is considered moderately abnormal.

E. The LVEF is calculated as the stroke volume/LV diastolic volume.

4. Which of the following statements are most accurate regarding global and regional LV function?

A. Because wall thickening and endocardial motion are intrinsically related, nearly all regional wall motion abnormalities are associated with abnormal thickening as well as abnormal motion.

B. The use of the 17–regional wall segment model is preferred over the 16-segment model since the inclusion of the LV apical cap motion may add 5% to the overall LV ejection fraction.

C. Regional wall motion abnormalities are nearly always due to coronary artery disease even when located beyond conventional coronary artery regional territories.

D. The only difference between the 16– and 17–wall segment models is the expansion of the distal LV wall segments from 4 to 5 radial segments in the 17-segment model.

E. Adding manufactured LV contrast improves the assessment of regional endocardial motion, but has not demonstrated improved calculation of LVEF.

5. In FIGURE 23.1A–E, which is the correct pair of measures used to calculate an accurate LVEF using the single-plane Simpson method of disks? Consider image quality, image acquisition, and quantitative technique.

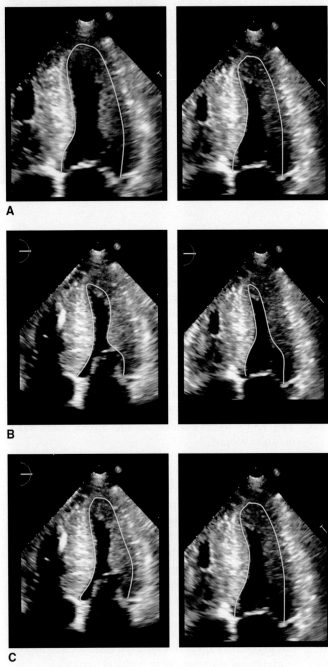

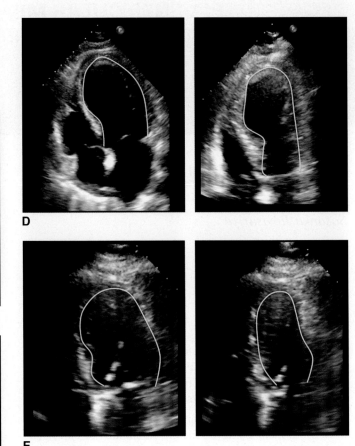

E

FIGURE 23.1 (*Continued*)

A. FIGURE 23.1A
B. FIGURE 23.1B
C. FIGURE 23.1C
D. FIGURE 23.1D
E. FIGURE 23.1E

FIGURE 23.1

6. A 65-year-old male with bicuspid aortic valve has severe aortic regurgitation. He currently is able to exercise regularly on a treadmill for 40 minutes and denies feeling short of breath or fatigue. How would you best follow this patient?

A. LV dimensions using M-mode taken from a short axis at the base of the LV
B. LV dimensions using 2D echo parasternal long-axis view distal to the mitral valve
C. LV dimensions using 2D echo from an apical long-axis view
D. All of the options
E. None of the options

7. A noncontrast echo study was performed on a patient post myocardial infarction. The assessment of wall motion should be based on:

A. A 17-segment model
B. A 16-segment model
C. A 20-segment model
D. None of the options
E. All of the options

8. In a 55-year-old female with breast cancer, left ventricular ejection fraction is being evaluated prior to chemotherapy. Which method of left ventricular assessment of ejection fraction has the most accuracy?

A. Visual assessment
B. Fractional shortening
C. 2D echocardiography using biplane Simpson
D. 3D echocardiography
E. All of the above

9. With regard to linear measurement of left ventricular measurements, which one of the following statements is most accurate?

A. M-mode measurements made in the parasternal long axis are highly reproducible, with high spatial resolution, but beam orientation is often off axis.
B. 2D-guided measurements in the parasternal long-axis view can be made perpendicular to the long axis but have lower frame rate than M-mode.
C. Measurements should be made at the level of the mitral annulus, perpendicular to the LV long axis.
D. The septum measurement should include RV trabeculation.
E. The end-diastolic and end-systolic frames can be from separate cardiac cycles.

10. Regarding different methods of LV volumetric measurements, which one of the following statements is most accurate?

A. The Teicholz and the Quinones methods of deriving LV volumes are derived from linear measurements and can be used in a wide variety of cardiac pathologies.
B. Endocardial border enhancement is limited by acoustic shadowing in the LV apex with excess contrast.
C. Use of 3D images for volumetric analysis has the advantage of better temporal resolution.
D. The biplane summation of disks method corrects for shape distortions better than the area length method for volume calculation.
E. There is inadequate data to report LV volumes indexed to BSA separately in men and women.

11. Which method would accurately measure LV mass in this patient? (See Fig. 23.2.)

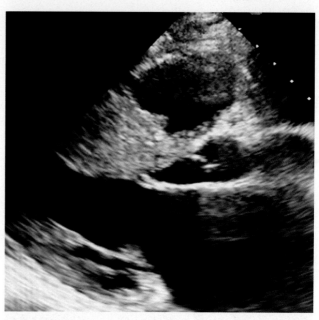

FIGURE 23.2

A. Cube formula using linear M-mode
B. Cube formula using linear 2D measurements
C. Truncated ellipsoid method
D. Area length method
E. 3D-based formula

12a. The measurements of a transthoracic echo study are given in Table 23.1. What is the relative wall thickness in this patient?

A. 0.30
B. 0.55
C. 0.8
D. 1.14
E. 1.6

Table 23.1	Transthoracic Echocardiography Study Measurements
Age	50
Sex	Male
Heart rate	82 bpm
Blood pressure	184/102 mm Hg
BSA	1.9 m²
Interventricular septum in diastole	1.6 cm
LV internal diameter in systole	2.8 cm
LV internal diameter in diastole	4.0 cm
Posterior wall in diastole	1.6 cm
LV mass	258 g

12b. Which of the following is the correct classification regarding the LV mass in Q 12a?

A. Normal
B. Eccentric remodeling
C. Eccentric hypertrophy
D. Concentric hypertrophy
E. Cannot be calculated in the absence of the LV ejection fraction

13. A 75-year-old male is referred for echocardiography (Fig. 23.3, Video 23.1). Severe increase in left atrial volume index (LAVI) is reported. The referring provider is concerned as an increased LAVI is associated with a worse outcome in this patient. Which of the following conditions is the likely etiology of left atrial enlargement?

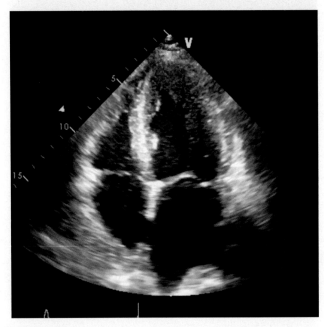

Figure 23.3

A. Apical hypertrophic cardiomyopathy
B. Dilated cardiomyopathy
C. Hypereosinophilic syndrome
D. Mild mitral regurgitation
E. Pulmonary embolus

14. Which of the following is correct in evaluating left atrial volume?

A. LA size is measured at the end of ventricular systole.
B. Pulmonary veins are excluded, but the left atrial appendage is included in the Simpson method.
C. The anterior posterior diameter measured in parasternal long-axis view is a reliable surrogate to LA volume.
D. The cuboid formula is the most accurate method of assessment.
E. The left atrial volume is commonly indexed to body mass index, as body size is known to influence LA volume.

15. A 45-year-old patient with ischemic cardiomyopathy is referred for echocardiography for repeat estimation of systolic function prior to internal defibrillator placement. The left ventricular ejection fraction (LVEF) was estimated as 40% by the biplane modified Simpson method. Figure 23.4 is the frame of the apical four-chamber view used to calculate end-diastolic volume. Which of the following statements is correct?

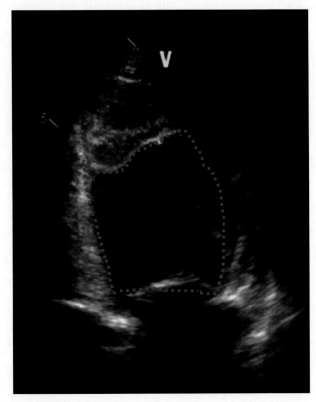

Figure 23.4

A. The LVEF is inaccurate as the apical endocardium is excluded.
B. The LVEF is inaccurate as the papillary muscles are excluded.
C. The biplane method cannot be applied in the setting of a large apical thrombus.
D. End of the T wave on ECG identifies end systole.
E. In the setting of an apical thrombus, transesophageal echocardiography is more accurate for LV function measurement.

Answer 1: *C.* Option C is the single best answer.

Option A is incorrect since this is a correct statement. It is easy to imagine how a large LV apical wall motion abnormality will be missed with these midventricular measures and the resulting estimates will overestimate LV function in both techniques.

Option B is incorrect since this is a correct statement. Single-site measures of LV global function are limited by both regional nonsymmetric contraction patterns and correct alignment of midventricular measures. Using M-mode, the cursor alignment should be confirmed by 2D, and the use of anatomic M-mode is recommended when transducer alignment from patient positioning remains suboptimal. Similarly, a misaligned short-axis 2D view will provide incorrect estimates of both diastolic and systolic areas used to determine the FAC%.

Option C is the single best answer since this statement is incorrect. The same LV mid–short-axis view is used for measuring the FAC% and the LV myocardial mass.

Option D is incorrect since the statement is a correct statement. The normal values for the endocardial fractional shortening are 27% to 45% for women (severely reduced <16%) and 25% to 43% for men (severely reduced <14%).

Option E is incorrect since this is a correct statement. For optimal interstudy reproducibility, the papillary muscles are excluded from measuring areas (and volumes) but may be included when measuring LV mass (especially if large and hypertrophied).

Linear measurements of left ventricular dimension and area measurement change provide an estimate of left ventricular function. However, both methods do not reflect accurate global ventricular function particularly in asymmetric ventricles or in the presence of regional wall motion. A two-dimensional methodology is preferred compared to linear dimensions; nonetheless, fractional area change is dependent on where the image is obtained.

Suggested Reading

Domanski MJ, et al. Analysis of fractional area change at various levels in the normal left ventricle. *Am J Cardiol* 1992;70(15): 1367–1368.

Answer 2: B. The single best answer is B.

Option A is incorrect since this is a correct statement. Multiple disks (typically 20) are included in this technique since each disk is assumed to have the same diameter at its basal and apical margins. Using fewer disks, with this "erroneous" assumption, would be more likely to result in incorrect values since it is unlikely clinically that this "edge assumption" holds true.

Option B is the single best answer since this is an incorrect statement. The height of each disk is *not* fixed and is defined as the LV length from the mitral annulus to LV apex/total number of disks. Therefore, measuring the accurate LV length is critical in estimating LV volumes.

Option C is incorrect since this is a correct statement. Thus, measuring an accurate length is critical in determining the disk height and estimating the correct disk volume.

Option D is incorrect since this is a correct statement. Underestimation of LV volume is common (indeed expected) and is due to incorrect endocardial contours (effort should be made to exclude trabeculation and papillary muscles), cardiac translation (impacts LV systole more than diastole), as well as LV foreshortening.

Option E is incorrect since this is a correct statement. In symmetric LV contraction (no wall motion abnormality, WMA) and normal LV geometry, the single-dimensional apical four-chamber MOD is a reliable measure of LV global systolic function.

However, this single-plane measure would overestimate (isolated regional inferior or anterior WMA) or underestimate (isolated septal or lateral WMA) the global LV function. It has been demonstrated that biplane (A4C and A2C) is a superior global estimate than single plane (A4C view alone), and triplane (A4C, A2C, and A3C views) is slightly more accurate than biplane. To further this logic, 3D measures are superior to 2D (multiplane) measures.

There are several methods used to determine left ventricular volumes and subsequently stroke volume, cardiac output, or ejection fraction. Most of these methodologies use the assumption that the left ventricle is symmetrical. The most common methodology is the Simpson rule or "method of disks." An apical four-chamber and two-chamber view is obtained. The endocardial border is traced in end diastole and end systole. The length of the ventricle is divided into equally spaced disks along the long axis of the ventricle. There are limitations to this methodology due to assumptions of geometrical shape of the ventricle and that the two orthogonal planes are along a common long axis. When foreshortening occurs, common in the four-chamber view, it contributes to overestimation of the left ventricular ejection fraction.

Suggested Reading

Feigenbaum H, Armstrong WF, Ryan T, et al. *Feigenbaum's Echocardiography.* Philadelphia, PA: Lippincott Williams & Wilkins, 2005.

Answer 3: A. Option A is the single best answer.

Option A is a partially correct statement, but not entirely true. Indeed, normal ranges for LVEF in men and women are assumed to be equal, but recent data from both echo and MRI have confirmed that *women*, not *men*, normally have a higher LVEF.

Option B is a correct statement. The single-plane Simpson rule is able to provide a relatively accurate LVEF when the LV shape is normal and there are no wall motion abnormalities. Ideally, an orthogonal long-axis view should be included to improve the estimated LV volumes. However, if the orthogonal image is of poor quality, and the LV geometry and contraction are normal, then including this value may lower the overall accuracy of the determined LVEF.

Option C is a correct statement. An LVEF of 30% to 44% is considered moderately abnormal.

Option D is a correct statement. An LVEF of 30% to 44% is considered moderately abnormal.

Option E is a correct statement. The LVEF is calculated as the LV diastolic volume – LV systolic volume (which equals the LV stroke volume)/LV diastolic volume.

See TABLE 23.2.

Suggested Reading

Lang RM, Bierig M, Devereux RB, et al. Recommendations for chamber quantification: a report from the American Society of Echocardiography's Guidelines and Standards Committee and the Chamber Quantification Writing Group, developed in conjunction with the European Association of Echocardiography, a branch of the European Society of Cardiology. *J Am Soc Echocardiogr* 2005;18:1440–1463.

Table 23.2 Reference Values of LVEF (Men and Women)

NORMAL	MILDLY ABNORMAL	MODERATELY ABNORMAL	SEVERELY ABNORMAL
>55%	45%–54%	30%–44%	<30%

Adapted from Lang RM, Bierig M, Devereux RB, et al. Recommendations for chamber quantification: a report from the American Society of Echocardiography's Guidelines and Standards Committee and the Chamber Quantification Writing Group, developed in conjunction with the European Association of Echocardiography, a branch of the European Society of Cardiology. *J Am Soc Echocardiogr* 2005;18:1440–1463.

Answer 4: *A.* Option A is the single best answer.

Option A is a correct statement. Both wall thickening and endocardial motion are intrinsically interrelated. Nearly all regional wall motion abnormalities are associated with abnormal thickening as well as abnormal motion, and this provides an important avenue for confirmation of regional contraction. When cardiac translation results in abnormal regional motion but myocardial wall thickening is normal, this is likely normal contraction and should not be reported as abnormal.

Option B is incorrect. It is true that the use of the AHA (and multisocietal) 17–regional wall segment model is now preferred over the original ASE 16-segment model. The 17-segment model incorporates the apical cap, which is thin and does not contribute to contraction. Therefore, inclusion of the LV apical cap will neither add nor subtract significantly to the overall calculated LV ejection fraction.

Option C is incorrect. Regional wall motion abnormalities are commonly due to coronary artery disease (CAD), but there are many other causes of regional LV dysfunction. Many dilated cardiomyopathies, in the absence of CAD, have regional contraction patterns.

Option D is incorrect. In the original ASE 16-segment model, the base and midregions included 6 radial segments each, and the distal region included only 4. In the contemporary multisocietal 17-segment model, the base, mid-, and distal regions remain unchanged, and the apical cap (beyond the LV cavity) is added to make 17 total segments. Since this region does not contract, this model is more valuable for perfusion than is wall motion assessment.

Option E is an incorrect statement. It has been demonstrated that adding manufactured LV contrast improves the assessment of regional endocardial motion, as well as the calculation of LV volumes and LVEF compared with cardiovascular MRI.

With multiple imaging modalities (CT, MRI, echo, and nuclear imaging), there have been efforts to standardize left ventricular segmentation and agree on nomenclature of these segments. In echocardiography, a 16-segment model is used for wall motion; however, with myocardial perfusion imaging using contrast echo, a 17-segment model may be appropriate for both wall motion and perfusion, which recognizes the apical cap. To assess regional wall motion, the ventricle is displayed in thirds: basal, midcavity, and apical slices, which are perpendicular to the long axis of the ventricle. Other imaging modalities divide the ventricle in several short-axis slices that are <1 cm thickness (but not <3 to 6 mm) with myocardium present in all 360 degrees.

Suggested Reading
Cerqueira MD, Weissman NJ, Dilsizian V, et al. Standardized myocardial segmentation and nomenclature for tomographic imaging of the heart. A statement for healthcare professionals from the Cardiac Imaging Committee of the Council on Clinical Cardiology of the American Heart Association. *Circulation* 2002;105:539–542.

Answer 5: *A.* Option A is correct. Both end diastole and end systole are appropriate.

Option B is incorrect. Endocardial tracing should include the papillary muscle within the left ventricular volume. The diastolic endocardial tracing (on the left) excludes the papillary muscles.

Option C is incorrect. Choosing the correct diastolic frame is important. The image on the left is not the appropriate diastolic frame since the left ventricular is not the largest and the mitral valve is open.

Option D is incorrect. Both are images of a four-chamber view; however, one is at a higher depth (on the left) and one at a lower depth (on the right). Endocardial tracing of the left ventricle should be done at a lower depth to ensure higher spatial resolution.

Option E is incorrect. The image quality is poor. The endocardial border is not well visualized in at least two contiguous segments; hence, contrast echo should have been used in this case.

The preferred method for the quantitation of left ventricular volumes and ejection fraction is the modified Simpson rule (biplane method of disks). An end-diastolic frame should be chosen at the beginning of the QRS, when the left ventricular chamber is largest or the frame after mitral valve closure. The end-systolic frame is chosen when the left ventricular cavity is smallest just before the mitral valve opens. Visualization of endocardial borders should be optimized; however, when greater than two contiguous segments are poorly seen, then contrast echo should be performed. Tracing of the endocardial border should include trabeculae and papillary muscles in the ventricular cavity.

Suggested Reading
Lang RM, Bierig M, Devereux RB, et al. Recommendations for chamber quantification: a report from the American Society of Echocardiography's Guidelines and Standards Committee and the Chamber Quantification Writing Group, developed in conjunction with the European Association of Echocardiography, a branch of the European Society of Cardiology. *J Am Soc Echocardiogr* 2005;18:1447.

Answer 6: *B.* Option B is the single best answer.

Option A is incorrect. Left ventricular dimensions are usually measured from a parasternal short axis using M-mode from a parasternal long-axis view at the level of the papillary muscle.

Option B is correct. Left ventricular dimensions are measured from a parasternal long axis just distal to the mitral valve tips in diastole and systole. An increase in LV dimensions >75 mm in diastole and >55 mm in systole is an indication to refer this patient to surgery.

Option C is incorrect. Measurements should not be performed from an apical window.

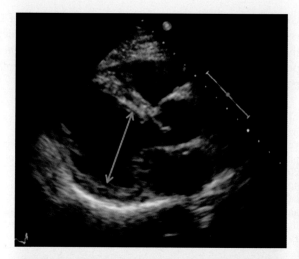

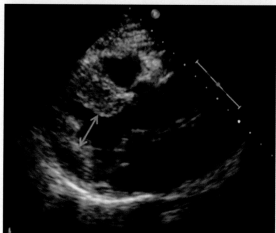

FIGURE 23.5

Though M-mode provides excellent temporal resolution, it should be used in addition to 2D images (FIG. 23.5). Left ventricular internal diameter, interventricular septal wall thickness, and posterior wall thickness are measured at end diastole and end systole on 2D or M-mode images from a parasternal long-axis window at the level of the left ventricular minor axis just distal to the mitral valve leaflet. It should be noted that M-mode tracings should be perpendicular to the long axis of the ventricle; hence, when this is not possible, measurements should not be made on an M-mode tracing.

Suggested Reading

Lang RM, Bierig M, Devereux RB, et al. Recommendations for chamber quantification: a report from the American Society of Echocardiography's Guidelines and Standards Committee and the Chamber Quantification Writing Group, developed in conjunction with the European Association of Echocardiography, a branch of the European Society of Cardiology. *J Am Soc Echocardiogr* 2005;18:1440–1463.

Answer 7: B. Option B is the correct choice.

Option A is incorrect. A 17-segment model is more appropriate for echo contrast perfusion imaging.

Option B is correct. In assessment of wall motion abnormalities, it is appropriate to use a 16-segment model.

Option C is incorrect. SPECT imaging divides the left ventricle into a 20-segment model, which includes the base, midcavity, and apical segment along the long axis of the left ventricle and includes two segments for the apical cap. With this segmentation, there is overrepresentation of the apex.

Options D and E are incorrect.

Wall motion scoring is based on either a 16- or 17-segment model. The left ventricle is divided into thirds along the long axis named the basal, midcavity, and apical. Basal and midcavity are divided into six segments of 60 degrees each named anterior, anteroseptal, inferoseptal, inferior, inferolateral, and anterolateral, whereas the apical segment is divided into four: apical anterior, apical septal, apical inferior, and apical lateral, which make the 16-segment model. Segment 17 represents the tip of the ventricle devoid of cavity, appropriately called the apical cap or apex. However, when assessing wall motion abnormalities, a 16-segment model is appropriate. If a contrast perfusion study was performed, then a 17-segment model could be used and can be compared to other imaging modalities.

Suggested Reading

Cerqueira MD, Weissman NJ, Dilsizian V, et al. Standardized myocardial segmentation and nomenclature for tomographic imaging of the heart. A statement for healthcare professionals from the Cardiac Imaging Committee of the Council on Clinical Cardiology of the American Heart Association. *Circulation* 2002;105:539–542.

Answer 8: D. Option A is incorrect. Visual assessment for the evaluation of ventricular size and function has significant interobserver variability and is dependent on observer experience. When using visual assessment, it should be compared to a quantitative method.

Option B is incorrect. Fractional shortening using M-mode echocardiography when compared to other quantitative methods is particularly inaccurate when there is marked left ventricular dilation or an abnormally shaped ventricle.

Option C is incorrect. Biplane Simpson method is more accurate than M-mode; however, there is a tendency to underestimate volumes compared to 3DE or MRI.

Option D is correct. 3D echocardiography is most accurate and reliable compared with other 2D techniques and is even more accurate in estimation of ventricular volumes when using contrast echo.

Option E is incorrect.

For long-term follow-up in patients undergoing chemotherapy or valvular regurgitation, accurate and reliable estimation of left ventricular volumes and ejection fraction is crucial. 3D echocardiography is the most accurate and reliable method compared to other 2D methods and has good correlation with MRI values.

Suggested Reading

Jenkins C, Bricknell K, Hanekom L, et al. Reproducibility and accuracy of echocardiographic measurements of left ventricular parameters using real-time three-dimensional echocardiography. *J Am Coll Cardiol* 2004;44:878–886.

Answer 9: B. Updated guidelines for measurement of LV dimensions in 2015 from the ASE have emphasized 2D measurements over M-mode measurements. It is important to carefully make measurements that are perpendicular to the long axis of the LV and use electronic caliper points that are placed at the mitral valve leaflet tips accurately at the endocardial boundary of the LV cavity.

Suggested Reading

Lang RM, Badano LP, Mor-Avi V, et al. Recommendations for cardiac chamber quantification by echocardiography in adults: an update from the American Society of Echocardiography and the European Association of Cardiovascular Imaging. *J Am Soc Echocardiogr* 2015;28(1):1–39.e14.

Answer 10: D. The disadvantage of using linear measurements to measure LV volume is the assumptions made of a fixed geometric shape. A wide variety of cardiac pathologies change the LV shape and render these calculations inaccurate.

Current guidelines recommend routine use of 2D to calculate LV volumes by the biplane summation of disks method and 3D in laboratories with expertise. Also, it is recommended to index both linear measurements and volumes to BSA.

Suggested Reading

Lang RM, Badano LP, Mor-Avi V, et al. Recommendations for cardiac chamber quantification by echocardiography in adults: an update from the American Society of Echocardiography and the European Association of Cardiovascular Imaging. *J Am Soc Echocardiogr* 2015;28(1):1–39.e14.

Answer 11: E. 3D-based formula allows measurement of LV mass based on direct visualization of endocardial borders, without making assumptions about LV shape or location of hypertrophy. This is most relevant in patients with eccentric hypertrophy and with regional wall thinning.

Suggested Readings

Mor-Avi V, Sugeng L, Weinert L, et al. Fast measurement of left ventricular mass with real-time three-dimensional echocardiography: comparison with magnetic resonance imaging. *Circulation* 2004;110(13):1814–1818.

Lang RM, Badano LP, Mor-Avi V, et al. Recommendations for cardiac chamber quantification by echocardiography in adults: an update from the American Society of Echocardiography and the European Association of Cardiovascular Imaging. *J Am Soc Echocardiogr* 2015;28(1):1–39.e14

Answer 12a: C. Relative wall thickness (RWT) is a measure that defines increased LV mass index as eccentric or concentric hypertrophy:

$$\text{Relative wall thickness (RWT)} = \frac{2 \times \text{posterior wall in diastole}}{\text{LV internal diameter in diastole}}$$
$$\text{RWT} = \frac{2 \times 1.6}{4}$$
$$= 0.8$$

Answer 12b: D. This patient's LV mass index is 258 g.

Therefore, the LV mass index is LV mass/BSA = 258/1.9 = 136 g/m^2.

The relative wall thickness is 0.8 as calculated in the previous answer.

Suggested Reading

Lang RM, Badano LP, Mor-Avi V, et al. Recommendations for cardiac chamber quantification by echocardiography in adults: an update from the American Society of Echocardiography and the European Association of Cardiovascular Imaging. *J Am Soc Echocardiogr* 2015;28(1):1–39.e14.

Answer 13: A. Option A is correct as the image shows progressive thickening of the left ventricle from base to apex with significant apical hypertrophy, giving the left ventricle a "spade shape" in diastole, which is consistent with apical hypertrophic cardiomyopathy. Thus, this condition is also called spade cardiomyopathy and Yamaguchi cardiomyopathy. Increased LAVI is reported to be a predictor of poor outcomes in patients with apical hypertrophic cardiomyopathy.

Option B is incorrect as the size of the left ventricle is normal.

Video 23.1 demonstrates preserved systolic function, which rules out dilated cardiomyopathy. However, increased LAVI is a marker for poor outcomes in patients with dilated cardiomyopathy as well.

Option C is incorrect as the characteristic finding of hypereosinophilic syndrome (HES) on echocardiography is obliteration of the LV apex with fibrotic and thrombotic material with preserved wall motion. Progressive increase in LV wall thickness and LV hypertrophy are not the characteristics in this condition.

Left atrial enlargement is not concomitant with cardiac involvement in HES; however, thickening of the posterior basal wall could cause tethering of the posterior mitral leaflet and give rise to mitral regurgitation and atrial enlargement in this condition.

Option D is incorrect as there is no definite evidence of mitral regurgitation in the 2D image. Further, it is unlikely that mild mitral regurgitation would cause atrial enlargement.

Severe left atrial enlargement is a supportive finding in chronic severe mitral regurgitation and not mild regurgitation.

Option E is incorrect as an acute pulmonary embolus does not cause left atrial enlargement, but right atrial and right ventricular enlargements are common findings.

Suggested Reading

Moon J. Clinical and echocardiographic predictors of outcomes in patients with apical hypertrophic cardiomyopathy. *Am J Cardiol* 2011;108(11):1614–1619.

Answer 14: A. Option A is correct as the LA size is measured at the end of ventricular systole. This is the timing of the cardiac cycle, immediately prior to mitral valve opening at which time the left atrium has the largest volume. In evaluating options such as option A, attention should be paid to the stated timing of the specific chamber in the cardiac cycle, that is, atrial systole versus ventricular systole.

Option B is incorrect. During planimetry of the LA, the pulmonary veins and the left atrial appendage are excluded.

Option C is incorrect. Measurement of the anterior posterior (AP) diameter of the left atrium was used for many years as LA size. However, current studies evaluating LA volume demonstrate that the AP diameter is a poor reflection of the overall LA volume. During pressure overload of the left atrium, the dimension of the left atrium with the least enlargement is the AP diameter as it is constrained between the spine and thoracic cavity with predominant enlargement seen in the superior–inferior and medial and lateral dimensions. Hence, the AP diameter is a poor surrogate for LA volume.

Option D is incorrect. There are three common methods used to evaluate the LA volume. The cube (or cuboid) formula assumes the LA is a sphere. In this method, the AP diameter is cubed to obtain the LA volume. As explained in option C, as the AP diameter is not a reasonable representation of overall LA volume, a formula using the AP diameter as the index measurement does not accurately calculate LA volume.

The ellipsoid model uses three diameters of the left atrium, obtained from the parasternal long-axis, parasternal short-axis, and apical four-chamber view in calculating LA volume. Hence, it is more accurate than the cube formula.

Finally, the Simpson rule could also be applied to the left atrium, in which the left atrial border is traced in two orthogonal planes to calculate the LA volume. This is an accurate evaluation and stands as the current recommendation. Therefore, option D is incorrect as the cube formula is not the most accurate method.

Option E is incorrect as the common practice is to index LA volume to body surface area and not body mass index.

Reference values currently in use for the left atrial volume index (LAVI) are indexed to body surface area and are similar in males and females.

Suggested Readings

Lester SJ, Ryan EW, Schiller NB, et al. Best method in clinical practice and in research studies to determine left atrial size. *Am J Cardiol* 1999;84:829–832.

Moller JE, Hillis GS, Oh JK, et al. Left atrial volume: a powerful predictor of survival after acute myocardial infarction. *Circulation* 2003;107:2207–2212.

Pritchett AM, Jacobsen SJ, Mahoney DW, et al. Left atrial volume as an index of left atrial size: a population-based study. *J Am Coll Cardiol* 2003;41:1036–1043.

Answer 15: A. The image shows the left ventricle in the apical four-chamber view with a large laminated apical thrombus.

When LVEF is measured using the modified Simpson method, the end-systolic and end-diastolic volumes in the four- and two-chamber views are obtained by tracing the endocardium. The endocardial border is traced contiguously excluding papillary muscles, trabeculations, and ventricular thrombi (Fig. 23.6). In the given image, the endocardium has been inaccurately traced excluding the border with overlying thrombus. As LV thrombi form over myocardial segments with wall motion abnormalities (usually aneurysmal, dyskinetic, or akinetic), excluding such segments in LVEF measurement would lead to an inaccurate assessment of LVEF. Hence, option A is correct.

Suggested Reading

Lang RM, Badano LP, Mor-Avi V, et al. Recommendations for cardiac chamber quantification by echocardiography in adults: an update from the American Society of Echocardiography and the European Association of Cardiovascular Imaging. *J Am Soc Echocardiogr* 2015;28(1):1–39.e14.

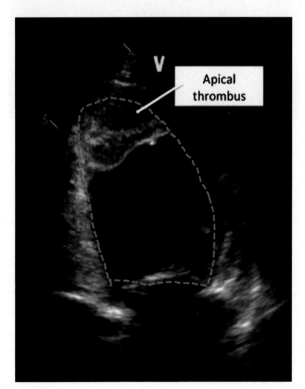

FIGURE 23.6

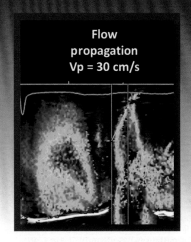

Flow
propagation
Vp = 30 cm/s

Chapter 24

Doppler Measurements

Vidya Nadig

1. A 45-year-old female is being evaluated for progressive shortness of breath over the past 6 weeks. Transthoracic echocardiography (TTE) was performed, and the following continuous-wave spectral Doppler tracing of the mitral regurgitant (MR) jet was obtained from the apical four-chamber view (Fig. 24.1). Letters A through D represent Doppler velocities; corresponding time points are labeled Ta through Td.

Which is the correct formula for calculating left ventricular dP/dT, a measure of systolic function?

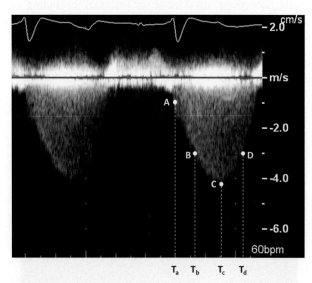

Figure 24.1

A. $(4C^2 - 4A^2)/(Tc - Ta)$
B. $(4B^2 - 4A^2)/(Tb - Ta)$
C. $(4D^2 - 4C^2)/(Td - Tc)$
D. $(4D^2 - 4B^2)/(Td - Tb)$
E. $(4D^2 - 4A^2)/(Td - Ta)$

2. The pulsed-wave Doppler tracing of the left ventricular outflow tract (LVOT) in Figure 24.2 was obtained on TTE. The LVOT velocity time integral (VTI) was measured at 20 cm.

Which of the following patients (labeled A through E) with the above LVOT VTI would have the highest effective systemic cardiac output (CO)?

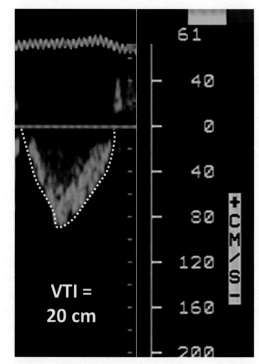

VTI =
20 cm

Figure 24.2

	A	B	C	D	E
Blood pressure (mm Hg)	90/50	120/80	150/60	100/60	110/70
Heart rate (beats/min)	60	60	80	70	85
LVOT diameter (cm)	2.0	2.1	2.1	1.8	1.7
Other findings	Mitral stenosis; mitral valve area of 1.2 cm²	Mitral regurgitation; regurgitant volume of 30 mL	Aortic regurgitation; regurgitant volume of 20 mL	Atrial septal defect with left-to-right shunt; shunt volume of 25 mL	Aortic stenosis; aortic valve area of 1.8 cm²

3. A 67-year-old male undergoes TTE for evaluation of a murmur. The flow across the mitral valve is evaluated using pulsed-wave spectral Doppler (left panel in Fɪɢ. 24.3) as well as by measuring the mitral annular diameter in the apical four-chamber (A4C) view (middle panel) and the apical two-chamber (A2C) view (right panel). At the time of TTE, blood pressure equals 120/70 mm Hg and heart rate 80 beats/min.

Which is the correct statement regarding the assessment of antegrade flow across the mitral valve?

A. To calculate the stroke volume (SV), pulsed-wave spectral Doppler sample volume is placed at mitral leaflet tips.
B. Mitral annular diameters are measured at peak systole as a distance between inner edges of the annulus.
C. In normal individuals, the SV across the mitral valve is always greater than the SV across the LVOT.
D. Patients with severe mitral regurgitation have a lower diastolic SV at the mitral orifice compared to patients with no regurgitation.
E. In patients with patent ductus arteriosus, the mitral SV multiplied by the heart rate represents the pulmonic flow (Qp).

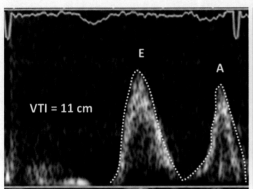 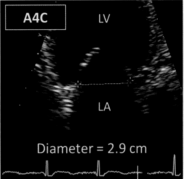 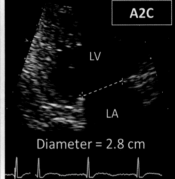

Fɪɢᴜʀᴇ 24.3

4. An 82-year-old female undergoes TTE for follow-up of aortic stenosis. Her aortic valve area is calculated at 1.2 cm², and the mean aortic valve gradient is 32 mm Hg. The pulsed-wave spectral Doppler tracings of the mitral inflow and the right upper pulmonary vein are shown in Fɪɢᴜʀᴇ 24.4.

Which is the correct statement regarding the Doppler assessment of her left ventricular function?

A. The ratio of peak systolic (S) to peak diastolic (D) velocity of pulmonary vein inflow in this patient is indicative of elevated left atrial pressure (LAP).
B. In normal individuals, the atrial reversal (AR) wave lasts at least 30 ms longer than the mitral A wave.
C. In atrial fibrillation, the pulmonary vein diastolic (D) wave disappears.
D. The patient has elevated left ventricular end-diastolic pressure.
E. The peak velocity of the pulmonary vein AR wave is abnormally low.

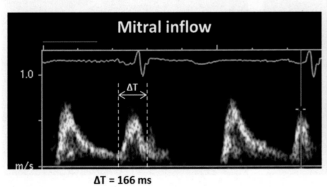 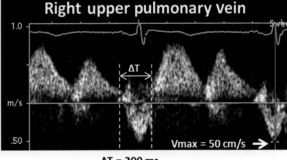

Fɪɢᴜʀᴇ 24.4

5. A 68-year-old male presents with new-onset dyspnea on exertion. TTE revealed moderate aortic stenosis and mild to moderate mitral regurgitation. Spectral Doppler tracings of the mitral and aortic valve are shown in Figure 24.5.

Which of the following is the correct formula for calculating the myocardial performance index (MPI), also known as the Tei index?

A. (A − B)/A
B. A/(A + B)
C. (A − B)/B
D. (A + B)/A
E. B/(A + B)

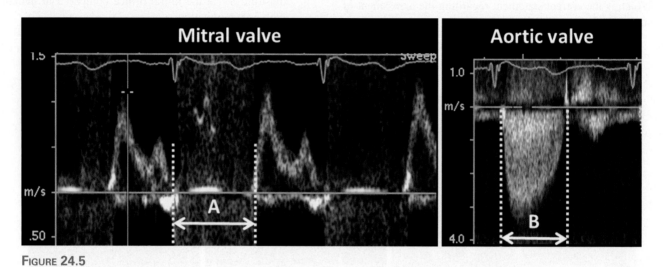

FIGURE 24.5

6. A 45-year-old female presented with chronic lower extremity edema. TTE revealed a left ventricular ejection fraction of 35% and no significant valvular disease. The left ventricular tracings in Figure 24.6 were obtained on this patient.

Which of the following is a correct statement?

A. Pulmonary artery wedge pressure (PAWP) is elevated.
B. Flow propagation tracing was obtained by color B-mode technique.
C. Flow propagation velocity (Vp) is normal.
D. There is a pseudonormal mitral inflow pattern.
E. The patient is in atrial fibrillation.

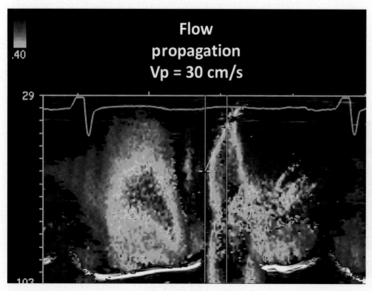

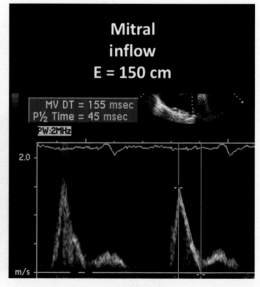

FIGURE 24.6

7. A 67-year-old male underwent intraoperative transesophageal echocardiography (TEE) prior to ventricular septal defect (VSD) repair. There was no significant valvular disease. A month earlier, he presented with an acute myocardial infarction. At the time of this TEE, his blood pressure was 110/50 mm Hg, and the right atrial pressure was invasively measured at 10 mm Hg (Fɪɢ. 24.7).

The panel on the left demonstrates the VSD on color Doppler in a transgastric view. The panel on the right shows the spectral Doppler tracing across the VSD in the same transgastric view.

Which of the following is a correct statement?

A. Findings are consistent with a supracristal VSD.
B. The patient has a very loud diastolic murmur.
C. Pulmonary artery systolic pressure (PASP) is 68 mm Hg.
D. There is a predominant right-to-left shunt.
E. Peak left ventricular systolic pressure (LVSP) is normal.

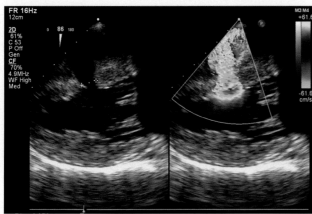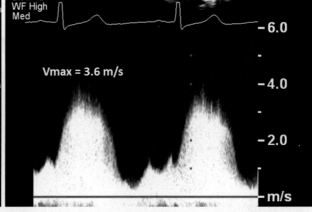

FɪɢURE 24.7

---

8. A 73-year-old female was referred for evaluation of progressive dyspnea on exertion and lower extremity edema over the preceding 3 months. Her exercise tolerance is significantly reduced, and she gets tired after walking only a short distance.

FɪɢURE 24.8 represents the Doppler-based strain curve of the left ventricle (LV) obtained from the apical four-chamber view.

Which of the following is a correct statement?

A. The curve represents the radial strain of the LV.
B. The peak strain value in this patient is normal.
C. All LV segments can be analyzed by Doppler-based strain imaging.
D. Subendocardial fibers are primarily responsible for longitudinal strain.
E. LV ejection fraction in this patient is definitely abnormal.

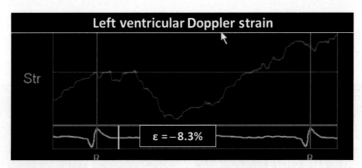

FɪɢURE 24.8

9. A 55-year-old obese female presents with shortness of breath after undergoing right knee replacement. Transthoracic echocardiogram revealed normal left ventricular systolic function and no significant valvular disease, and the right heart findings are depicted in FIGURE 24.9.

The left panel represents tissue Doppler recordings of the tricuspid annulus. The right panel shows M-mode recording of the tricuspid annulus. In addition, spectral Doppler of the tricuspid inflow was obtained (not shown); it revealed a peak E-wave velocity of 45 cm/s, a peak A-wave velocity of 28 cm/sec, and a deceleration time (DT) of the tricuspid E wave of 145 ms.

Which of the following is a correct statement?

A. The findings confirm the diagnosis of massive pulmonary embolism.

B. Tricuspid filling pattern demonstrates abnormal relaxation.

C. There is normal longitudinal RV systolic function.

D. Tricuspid annular tissue peak velocity of S wave is diminished.

E. Tricuspid E-wave DT is abnormally short.

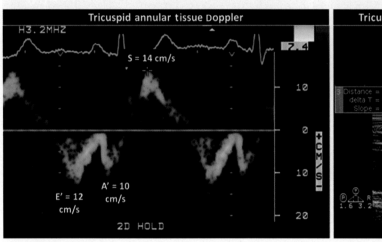
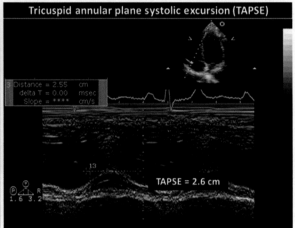

FIGURE 24.9

10. A 62-year-old male with no known past medical history was admitted because of exertional shortness of breath over the preceding 6 weeks. Recently, he also noted he could no longer put on his shoes because of ankle and foot swelling. Transthoracic echocardiogram was performed on admission. VIDEOS 24.1 and 24.2 and FIGURE 24.10 are from that study.

The left panel represents spectral Doppler recordings of the mitral inflow, and the right panel shows spectral Doppler tracings from the right upper pulmonary vein obtained on the apical four-chamber view.

Which of the following is a correct statement?

A. DT of the mitral E wave is prolonged.

B. Mitral tissue Doppler recordings are not required to estimate LA pressure in this patient.

C. After completion of diuresis, the mitral E/A ratio is expected to increase.

D. A decrease of <50% in the E/A after the Valsalva maneuver would confirm that LA pressure is elevated.

E. Recordings are diagnostic of a pseudonormal filling pattern.

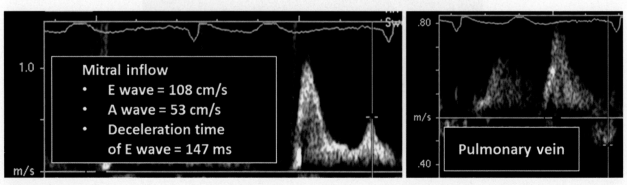

FIGURE 24.10

11. A 75-year-old female with recent-onset syncope is referred to the echo lab for evaluation of an ejection systolic murmur suggestive of aortic stenosis (AS). Precise left ventricular outflow tract (LVOT) diameter measurement is vital for accurate calculation of the aortic valve area (AVA). Which of the following is most correct regarding this measurement?

A. LVOT is measured in midsystole in the parasternal long-axis view.

B. The pulsed wave (PW) should be placed 3 to 4 mm apical to the point of LVOT measurement.

C. Apical displacement of the LVOT PW Doppler measurement overestimates AVA.

D. Measurement should be made 0.5 to 1 mm apical to the aortic valve parallel to the valve plane.

E. An error in the LVOT measurement is doubled when AVA is calculated.

12. The images in FIGURE 24.11 were obtained from the same patient. What are the peak and mean gradients across the aortic valve?

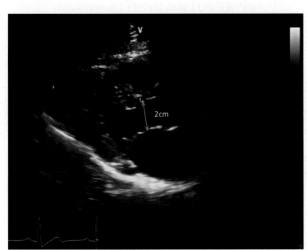

A

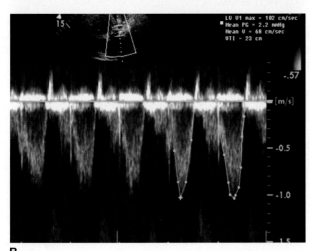

B

FIGURE 24.11

C

FIGURE **24.11** (Continued)

A. 123 and 83.

B. 123 and 43.

C. 135 and 83.

D. 218 and 83.

E. Gradients cannot be calculated from the above images.

13. Which of the following is the least useful maneuver/technique in optimizing the peak Doppler gradient across the aortic valve in the above patient?

A. Nonimaging probe

B. Suprasternal notch imaging

C. Contrast administration

D. Doppler angle correction

E. Optimizing patient position

14. Which of the following Doppler tracings is least likely to mimic the Doppler tracing of aortic stenosis?

A. Supravalvular aortic stenosis

B. Ventricular septal defect

C. Pulmonary stenosis

D. Subclavian artery stenosis

E. Tricuspid stenosis

15. What is the aortic valve area in the patient described in Question 12?

A. 0.4 cm^2.

B. 0.6 cm^2.

C. 0.8 cm^2.

D. 1.2 cm^2.

E. The valve area cannot be calculated, as the LV ejection fraction is not stated.

Questions 16 to 19

Doppler tracings in echocardiography are used to estimate pressure in different cardiac chambers and vascular systems. Which of the following Doppler tracings could be utilized to estimate the pressures listed in each question?

Doppler signals:

Tricuspid regurgitation (TR)
Aortic regurgitation (AR)
Pulmonic regurgitation (PR)
Ventricular septal defect (VSD)

16. Pulmonary artery systolic pressure?

   A. TR only
   B. TR and PR only
   C. TR and VSD only
   D. TR, PR, and VSD only
   E. TR, AR, PR, and VSD

17. PA diastolic pressure?

   A. TR only
   B. PR only
   C. TR and VSD only
   D. TR, PR, and VSD only
   E. TR, AR, PR, and VSD

18. Mean PA pressure?

   A. TR only
   B. TR and PR only
   C. TR and VSD only
   D. TR, PR, and VSD only
   E. TR, AR, PR, and VSD

19. LVEDP?

   A. TR only.
   B. AR only.
   C. AR and VSD only.
   D. AR, PR, and VSD only.
   E. LVEDP cannot be estimated.

20. A patient presents with shortness of breath. The following data are obtained during echocardiography.

   Heart rate = 102 bpm, blood pressure = 92/54 mm Hg, body surface area = 2.0 m^2, LVOT diameter = 2.0 cm, LVOT VTI = 12 cm, aortic valve VTI = 15 cm, and peak TR velocity = 4.2 m/s.

   What is the cardiac output?

   A. 1.8 L/min
   B. 2.8 L/min
   C. 3.8 L/min
   D. 4.8 L/min
   E. 5.8 L/min

Answer 1: B. The rate of left ventricular pressure rise during early systole (dP/dT) is a measure of left ventricular systolic function. dP/dT can be calculated using the continuous-wave Doppler tracing of the MR jet.

dP/dT represents the slope of an MR jet Doppler tracing between two time points in early systole. By convention, the first time point is when the MR jet velocity reaches 1 m/s (point A in Fig. 24.1). The second one is when the MR jet velocity reaches 3 m/s (point B in Fig. 24.1).

One can increase accuracy of these measurements by increasing the sweep speed to make the mitral regurgitant jet Doppler envelope as wide as possible and by decreasing the velocity scale to just above 3 m/s.

Using the simplified Bernoulli equation (dP = 4V^2), the pressure difference between points A and B can be calculated as follows:

$$dP = 4A^2 - 4B^2$$

$$dP = 4 \times (3 \text{ m/s})^2 - 4 \times (1 \text{ m/s})^2$$

$$dP = 36 - 4 = 32 \text{ mm Hg}$$

Thus, to calculate the left ventricular dP/dT, one only needs to measure the time interval (in seconds) between points A and B.

$$dP/dT = 32 \text{ mm Hg}/dT \text{ (in seconds)}$$

In the patient above, dT = Tb − Ta = 0.12 s.

$$dP/dT = 32 \text{ mm Hg}/0.12 \text{ s}$$

$$dP/dT = 267 \text{ mm Hg/s}$$

This patient has markedly diminished left ventricular systolic function (flat slope). Normal dP/dT is typically >1,000 mm Hg/s (steep slope).

Suggested Readings

Bargiggia GS, Bertucci C, Recusani F, et al. A new method for estimating left ventricular dP/dt by continuous wave Doppler-echocardiography. Validation studies at cardiac catheterization. *Circulation* 1989;80(5):1287–1292.

Mason DT, Braunwald E, Covell JW, et al. Assessment of cardiac contractility. The relation between the rate of pressure rise and ventricular pressure during isovolumic systole. *Circulation* 1971;44(1):47–58.

Answer 2: B. The stroke volume (SV) leaving the left ventricle through the left ventricular outflow tract (LVOT) can be calculated as follows:

SV (in mL) = LVOT cross-sectional area (in cm^2) × LVOT VTI (in cm)

Assuming a circular shape of the LVOT, the formula becomes

SV = π × (½ × LVOT diameter)^2 × LVOT VTI

Cardiac output (CO) is then calculated as

CO (in mL/min) = SV (in mL) × heart rate (in beats/min).

The effective CO is defined as the CO seen by the peripheral systemic circulation and may be the same or lower than the left ventricular CO.

Regarding individual answers:

A. Incorrect answer. Effective CO in this patient is 3,800 mL/min; LVOT stroke volume is 63 mL. Mitral stenosis does not impact calculation of CO at the level of the LVOT.

B. Correct answer. Effective CO in this patient is 4,200 mL/min; LVOT stroke volume is 69 mL. Mitral regurgitation does not impact calculation of stroke volume at the level of the LVOT. One has to bear in mind that in mitral regurgitation, the total left ventricular stroke volume is larger than the effective stroke volume across the LVOT and is equal to the sum of the mitral regurgitant volume and the effective stroke volume across the LVOT.

C. Incorrect answer. Effective CO in this patient is 3,900 mL/min; effective LVOT stroke volume is 49 mL. In aortic regurgitation, the stroke volume calculated at the level of the LVOT is the sum of the effective stroke volume and the aortic regurgitant volume:

SV at LVOT = Effective SV + Aortic regurgitant volume
By rearranging the above equation,
Effective SV = SV at LVOT−Aortic regurgitant volume
In this patient,

$$\text{Effective SV} = 69 - 20 = 49 \text{ mL}$$
$$\text{Effective CO} = 49 \text{ mL} \times 80 \text{ bpm} = 3900 \text{ mL/min}$$

D. Incorrect answer. Effective CO in this patient is 3,600 mL/min; LVOT stroke volume is 51 mL. Atrial septal defect does not impact calculation of CO at the level of the LVOT.

E. Incorrect answer. Effective CO in this patient is 3,900 mL/min; LVOT stroke volume is 45 mL. Aortic stenosis does not impact calculation of CO at the level of the LVOT.

Suggested Readings

Lewis, JF, Kuo, LC, Nelson, JG, et al. Pulsed Doppler echocardiographic determination of stroke volume and cardiac output: clinical validation of two new methods using the apical window. *Circulation* 1984;70:425–431.

Zoghbi WA, Quinones MA. Determination of cardiac output by Doppler echocardiography: a critical appraisal. *Herz* 1986;11: 258–268.

Answer 3: E. Diastolic stroke volume (SV) can be calculated at the level of the mitral valve using the following formula:

SV (in mL) = mitral orifice cross-sectional area (in cm²)
× mitral velocity time interval (VTI)

Mitral orifice cross-sectional area can be estimated by one of the following two methods depending on the assumption of the geometric shape of the mitral orifice:

1. Circular mitral orifice—diastolic mitral annular diameter (D) is measured typically in the apical four-chamber view, and the mitral cross-sectional orifice area (MOCSA) is calculated as

$$\text{MOCSA} = \pi \times (\tfrac{1}{2} D)^2$$

In this patient,

$$\text{MOCSA} = 3.14 \times (\tfrac{1}{2} \times 2.9 \text{ cm})^2 = 6.6 \text{ cm}^2$$

2. Ellipsoid mitral orifice—diastolic mitral annular diameters are measured in the apical four-chamber view (D1) and apical two-chamber view (D2). Using the formula for surface area of an ellipse, MOCSA can be calculated as follows:

$$\text{MOCSA} = 3.14 \times (\tfrac{1}{2} \times \text{D1}) \times (\tfrac{1}{2} \times \text{D2})$$

3. In this patient,

$$\text{MOCSA} = 3.14 \times (\tfrac{1}{2} \times 2.9 \text{ cm}) \times (\tfrac{1}{2} \times 2.8 \text{ cm})$$
$$\text{MOCSA} = 6.4 \text{ cm}^2$$

Once MOCSA is known, we can then calculate the stroke volume and the cardiac output across the mitral valve:

SV (in mL) = MOCSA (in cm²) × Mitral VTI (in cm)
CO (in mL/min) = SV (in mL) × Heart rate (in beats/min)

In this patient using the ellipsoid approach,

$$\text{SV} = 6.4 \text{ cm}^2 \times 11 \text{ cm} = 70 \text{ mL}$$
$$\text{CO} = 70 \text{ mL} \times 80 \text{ bpm} = 5600 \text{ mL/min}$$

Regarding individual answers:

A. Incorrect answer. When calculating the stroke volume at the mitral level, the pulsed-wave Doppler sample volume is placed at the level of the mitral annulus (the same level at which the mitral annular diameter is measured). This is in contrast to measurements of mitral inflow for the assessment of left ventricular diastolic function when the sample volume is placed at mitral leaflet tips.

B. Incorrect answer. The diameter of the mitral annulus was measured (inner edge to inner edge) at the base of the leaflets at the time of maximal valvular opening during diastole.

C. Incorrect answer. In the absence of significant mitral or aortic regurgitation, the diastolic stroke volume across the mitral valve is the same as the systolic stroke volume at the level of the left ventricular outflow tract.

D. Incorrect answer. The more severe the mitral regurgitation, the larger is the diastolic stroke volume across the mitral valve. In mitral regurgitation, the diastolic flow across the mitral valve is the sum of the effective stroke volume (as measured at the level of the left ventricular outflow tract) and the mitral regurgitant volume.

E. Correct answer. In patients with patent ductus arteriosus, the cardiac output measured at the mitral valve level represents the pulmonic flow (Qp), while the flow across the right ventricular outflow tract represents the systemic flow (Qs).

Suggested Readings

Enriquez-Sarano M, Bailey KR, Seward JB, et al. Quantitative Doppler assessment of valvular regurgitation. *Circulation* 1993;87(3):841–848.

Lewis JF, Kuo LC, Nelson JG, et al. Pulsed Doppler echocardiographic determination of stroke volume and cardiac output: clinical validation of two new methods using the apical window. *Circulation* 1984;70:425–431.

Answer 4: D.
Regarding individual answers:

A. Incorrect answer. In this patient, the ratio of systolic (S) to diastolic (D) pulmonary vein peak velocity is >1. This is indicative of normal mean left atrial pressure.

B. Incorrect answer. An atrial reversal (AR) wave that lasts 30 ms longer than the mitral A wave is indicative of elevated left ventricular end-diastolic pressure.

C. Incorrect answer. It is the atrial reversal (AR) wave and not the diastolic (D) wave that disappears in atrial fibrillation. In addition, the peak velocity of the systolic (S) wave decreases, and the S/D ratio becomes <1.

D. Correct answer. An atrial reversal (AR) wave that lasts 30 ms longer than the mitral A wave is indicative of elevated left ventricular end-diastolic pressure. In this patient, AR duration – A duration = 200 – 166 = 34 ms.

E. Incorrect answer. Pulmonary vein atrial reversal (AR) velocities may increase with age but usually do not exceed 35 cm/s. Higher AR peak velocities are indicative of increased left ventricular end-diastolic pressure as is the case in this patient (AR = 50 cm/s).

Suggested Readings

Nagueh SF, Appleton CP, Gillebert TC, et al. Recommendations for the evaluation of left ventricular diastolic function by echocardiography. *J Am Soc Echocardiogr* 2009;22(2):107–133.

Rossvoll O, Hatle LK. Pulmonary venous flow velocities recorded by transthoracic Doppler ultrasound: relation to left ventricular diastolic pressures. *J Am Coll Cardiol* 1993;21(7):1687–1696.

Answer 5: C. Myocardial performance index (MPI), proposed in 1995 and also known as the Tei index, is a measure of both systolic and diastolic left ventricular function. Conceptually, MPI is the following ratio:

$$MPI = (IVCT + IVRT)/EP$$

Where IVCT is isovolumic contraction time, IVRT is isovolumic relaxation time, and EP is ejection period. In normal hearts, the sum of the two isovolumic ratios is roughly 1/3 of the ejection period. Normal values of left ventricular MPI are reported as 0.39 +/– 0.05. With systolic and/or diastolic dysfunction, this ratio increases.

Because calculating IVCT and IVRT is technically challenging using mitral and aortic blood flow velocity tracings, one can calculate MPI as follows:

$$MPI = (A - B)/B$$

where A is the time duration between the end of mitral flow in one cardiac cycle to the beginning of mitral flow in the next cardiac cycle and B is the ejection period as measured by the duration of aortic flow.

It is important to emphasize that MPI is preload and afterload dependent. Left ventricular afterload increase and preload reduction are associated with significant increases in the MPI values. In contrast, changes in left ventricular contractility do not seem to alter MPI values significantly.

Regarding individual answers:

A. Incorrect answer. See General Discussion above.
B. Incorrect answer. See General Discussion above.
C. Correct answer. Indeed, the MPI (Tei index) is calculated as (A – B)/B. In this patient, MPI = (410 – 300)/300 = 0.37, which is a normal value.
D. Incorrect answer. See General Discussion above.
E. Incorrect answer. See General Discussion above.

Suggested Readings

Cheung MM, Smallhorn JF, Redington AN, et al. The effects of changes in loading conditions and modulation of inotropic state on the MPI: comparison with conductance catheter measurements. *Eur Heart J* 2004;25(24):2238–2242.

Harada K, Tamura M, Toyono M, et al. Comparison of the right ventricular Tei index by tissue Doppler imaging to that obtained by pulsed Doppler in children without heart disease. *Am J Cardiol* 2002;90(5):566–569.

Pellett AA, Tolar WG, Merwin DG, et al. The Tei index: methodology and disease state values. *Echocardiography* 2004;21(7):669–672.

Tei C, Ling LH, Hodge DO, et al. New index of combined systolic and diastolic myocardial performance: a simple and reproducible measure of cardiac function—a study in normals and dilated cardiomyopathy. *J Cardiol* 1995;26(6):357–366.

Answer 6: A.
Regarding individual answers:

A. Correct answer. In this patient with reduced left ventricular systolic function, the pulmonary artery wedge pressure (PAWP) is elevated as judged by the markedly increased E/Vp ratio (the ratio of the peak velocity of the mitral E wave to the flow propagation velocity, Vp). The full regression equation for calculating PAWP is as follows:

$$PAWP = 4.6 + 5.27 \times E/Vp$$

In this patient,

$$E/Vp = 150/30 = 5$$
$$PAWP = 4.6 + 5.27 \times 5 = 31 \text{ mm Hg}$$

It has been shown that in patients with depressed left ventricular systolic function, an E/Vp >2.5 predicts a PAWP > 15 mm Hg with reasonable accuracy. Patients with normal LV volumes and ejection fraction but elevated left ventricular filling pressures may have a misleadingly normal Vp. Thus, the E/Vp method should be used with caution in individuals without left ventricular systolic dysfunction.

B. Incorrect answer. To obtain Vp, one uses the color M-mode technique. In the apical four-chamber view, a color box is placed over the left ventricle, and the color scale (Nyquist limit) is typically set at 40 cm/s. Then, the M-mode interrogation line is placed in the left ventricle and aligned with the mitral inflow. Flow propagation velocity (Vp) is measured as the slope of the first aliasing velocity during early diastole. Vp slope is measured from the mitral valve plane to 4 cm apically into the left ventricular cavity.

C. Incorrect answer. This patient has diminished Vp; normal values are >50 cm/s. The lower the Vp, the slower the left ventricular relaxation rate and the lower the suction force of the left ventricle.

D. Incorrect answer. The patient's mitral inflow is restrictive as judged by an E/A ratio >2 and a very rapid deceleration time of the E wave (<160 ms). In the presence of left ventricular systolic dysfunction, this is also indicative of elevated pulmonary artery wedge pressure.

E. Incorrect answer. The patient is not in atrial fibrillation as the mitral inflow tracing demonstrates the presence of a mitral atrial (A) wave. This correlates with an organized atrial contraction and argues against atrial fibrillation.

Suggested Readings

Garcia MJ, Ares MA, Asher C, et al. An index of early left ventricular filling that combined with pulsed Doppler peak E velocity may estimate capillary wedge pressure. *J Am Coll Cardiol* 1997;29(2):448–454.

Nagueh SF, Appleton CP, Gillebert TC, et al. Recommendations for the evaluation of left ventricular diastolic function by echocardiography. *J Am Soc Echocardiogr* 2009;22(2):107–133.

Answer 7: *E.*

Regarding individual answers:

A. Incorrect answer. The recent history of myocardial infarction and the location of the ventricular septal defect are typical of an acquired postinfarction muscular VSD. Supracristal VSD is a type of congenital VSD and is close to the aortic root and the pulmonic valve:

$$PASP = RVSP$$

RVSP can be calculated if systolic blood pressure (SBP) and peak systolic gradient across the VSD (ΔP) are known. In the absence of LV outflow obstruction, SBP is equal to the peak left ventricular systolic pressure (LVSP).

AU Response: Agreed.

$$SBP = LVSP$$

Therefore,

$$RVSP = LVSP - \Delta P$$
$$RVSP = SBP - \Delta P$$

In this patient,

$$RVSP = 110 - 4 \times (3.6 \text{ m/s})^2$$
$$RVSP = 58 \text{ mm Hg}$$

It is important to emphasize that this is a direct estimate of RVSP, and there is no need to add right atrial pressure to the pressure gradient. This is in contrast to the RVSP estimate using the tricuspid regurgitant jet.

B. Incorrect answer. Although there is diastolic flow across the VSD on spectral Doppler, this is silent on auscultation. Patients with VSD typically have a holosystolic murmur.

C. Incorrect answer. In the absence of pulmonic stenosis, peak pulmonary artery systolic pressure (PASP) is equal to the peak right ventricular systolic pressure (RVSP).

D. Incorrect answer. Both the color and spectral Doppler are indicative of a predominant left-to-right shunt.

E. Correct answer. Since the patient does not have LVOT or AV obstruction, systolic blood pressure (SBP) is equal to the peak left ventricular systolic pressure (LVSP). Thus, LVSP in this patient is 110 mm Hg, which is a normal value.

Suggested Readings

Hatle L, Rokseth R. Noninvasive diagnosis and assessment of ventricular septal defect by Doppler ultrasound. *Acta Med Scand* 1981;645:47–56.

Murphy DJ, Ludomirsky A, Huhta JC. Continuous wave Doppler in children with ventricular septal defect: noninvasive estimation of interventricular pressure gradient. *Am J Cardiol* 1986;57:428–432.

Answer 8: *D.*

Regarding individual answers:

A. Incorrect answer. There are three major types of myocardial strain: longitudinal, circumferential, and radial. Strain represents a change in myocardial segment length relative to end-diastolic length. Since the myocardium shortens in the longitudinal and circumferential axes, longitudinal and circumferential strain values are negative. In contrast, the myocardium thickens in the radial axis; thus, the radial strain has positive values. In this patient, the peak strain value is −8.3% and thus cannot represent radial strain.

B. Incorrect answer. The Doppler-based strain curve in this patient was obtained from the apical view and represents longitudinal strain. It was obtained from the basal lateral wall but could have been obtained from any nonapical LV segment. Absolute longitudinal strain values of ≤12% are definitely abnormal.

C. Incorrect answer. Doppler-based strain imaging has the same limitation as any other Doppler techniques, namely, the inability to image velocities of structures that are perpendicular to the insonation beam. Thus, the LV apex cannot be well visualized using Doppler-based strain imaging.

D. Correct answer. Longitudinal LV mechanics are predominantly governed by the subendocardial fibers, which are the first to be affected in a wide variety of myocardial disorders.

E. Incorrect answer. All forms of myocardial mechanics (such as strain and twist) contribute to global LV function and ejection fraction (LVEF). A loss of longitudinal strain is often compensated by an increase in other forms of strain or twist, which can result in a normal LVEF despite abnormalities in individual strains.

Suggested Readings

Geyer H, Caracciolo G, Abe H, et al. Assessment of myocardial mechanics using speckle tracking echocardiography: fundamentals and clinical applications. *J Am Soc Echocardiogr* 2010;23(4):351–369.

Mor-Avi V, Lang RM, Badano LP, et al. Current and evolving echocardiographic techniques for the quantitative evaluation of cardiac mechanics: ASE/EAE consensus statement on methodology and indications endorsed by the Japanese Society of Echocardiography. *J Am Soc Echocardiogr* 2011;24(3):277–313.

Answer 9: C.

Regarding individual answers:

A. Incorrect answer. Although the clinical scenario may suggest the diagnosis of pulmonary embolism, the echocardiographic findings are not confirmatory. Massive pulmonary embolism is typically associated with reduced right ventricular systolic function. This patient has normal TAPSE (≥1.6 cm) and peak S-wave velocity (≥10 cm/s) values, which argue against right ventricular systolic dysfunction.

B. Incorrect answer. An abnormal relaxation pattern is characterized by a tricuspid E/A ratio of <0.8. In this patient, E/A = 1.6 (normal 0.8 to 2.1). Furthermore, this patient has a normal tricuspid E/E' ratio of 3.8 (normal ≤ 6); this argues against RV diastolic dysfunction.

C. Correct answer. Tricuspid annular plane systolic excursion (TAPSE) is an M-mode technique that measures systolic displacement of the tricuspid annulus. Normal TAPSE values are ≥1.6 cm and correspond to normal longitudinal right ventricular systolic function.

D. Incorrect answer. The patient has normal S-wave velocity of 12 cm/s (normal ≥10 cm/s). Normal S-wave velocity is indicative of normal RV longitudinal contractility.

E. Incorrect answer. The patient has normal deceleration time (DT) of the tricuspid E wave (145 ms; normal ≥120 ms). Values <120 ms indicate restrictive filling pattern when tricuspid E/A is >2.1. Note the different cutoff values for mitral versus tricuspid restrictive filling pattern (mitral restrictive pattern has DT <150 ms; tricuspid restrictive pattern has DT <120 ms).

Suggested Reading

Rudski LG, Lai WW, Afilalo J, et al. Guidelines for the echocardiographic assessment of the right heart in adults: a report from the American Society of Echocardiography endorsed by the European Association of Echocardiography, a registered branch of the European Society of Cardiology, and the Canadian Society of Echocardiography. *J Am Soc Echocardiogr* 2010;23(7):685–713.

Answer 10: B.

Regarding individual answers:

A. Incorrect answer. The patient's deceleration time (DT) of the mitral E wave is abnormally short (<150 ms) and consistent with a restrictive filling pattern since the E/A ratio is >2.

B. Correct answer. This patient presents with acutely decompensated heart failure due to LV systolic dysfunction. When LV ejection fraction is diminished, left atrial pressure (LAP) can often be estimated from the mitral inflow alone. If mitral E/A is <1 and E is ≤50 cm/s, LAP is normal. In contrast, an E/A >2 and the deceleration time of E wave <150 ms (restrictive filling pattern) as is the case with this patient imply that LAP is elevated. Pulmonary venous flow demonstrating systolic (S) wave less than diastolic (D)-wave peak velocity further indicates that LAP is elevated in this patient. When patients present with heart failure and normal LV ejection fraction, LAP cannot be estimated from the mitral inflow alone, and additional parameters (such as the E/E' ratio) are required.

C. Incorrect answer. Diuretic therapy decreases LV preload and typically leads to lower E-wave velocities compared to prediuretic recordings in patients with acutely decompensated heart failure. A lack of significant decrease in E-wave velocity following adequate diuretic therapy in patients who initially present with a restrictive filling pattern may portend worse survival.

D. Incorrect answer. In cardiac patients, a decrease of ≥50% in the mitral E/A ratio is highly specific for elevated LV filling pressures. However, a change in the E/A ratio of <50% does not always indicate that the LV filling pressures are normal.

E. Incorrect answer. A pseudonormal filling pattern is characterized by a mitral E/A ratio between 1 and 2, a deceleration of the mitral E wave of >150 ms, and a pulmonary venous flow pattern demonstrating systolic (S) wave is less than the diastolic (D)-wave peak velocity. Although the patient has an S/D ratio of <1, his filling pattern is restrictive since the mitral E/A ratio is >2, and the DT of the mitral E wave is <150 ms.

Suggested Reading

Nagueh SF, Appleton CP, Gillebert TC, et al. Recommendations for the evaluation of left ventricular diastolic function by echocardiography. *J Am Soc Echocardiogr* 2009;22(2):107–133.

Answer 11: A.

Answer A is correct as the LVOT is measured in the parasternal long-axis window in midsystole. This is the timing of the cardiac cycle that the velocity is expected to be greatest across the LVOT. However, in critical aortic stenosis, the peak velocity may occur later in systole. In reality, the single-dimensional LVOT measurement varies little throughout the cardiac cycle, and since image quality is the greatest variable for an accurate value, other periods in the cardiac cycle may be used if image quality is vastly superior.

Answer B is incorrect. The LVOT should be measured at the exact point the PW is placed as the flow through that plane is calculated when the continuity equation is applied.

Answer C is incorrect as apical displacement of the LVOT measurement underestimates the AVA. The LVOT has a more elliptical shape toward the apical area and is circular closer to the aortic valve. Assuming an elliptical area is circular would underestimate the cross-sectional area of the LVOT, thereby underestimating the AVA.

Answer D is incorrect as the measurement should be made 5 mm to 10 mm apical to the aortic valve to avoid sampling the elliptical segment of the LVOT. However, attention should be paid to avoid the area of flow acceleration when this measurement is made.

Answer E is incorrect as an error in LVOT measurement is squared (not doubled) when the AVA is calculated.

Answer 12: C. *Peak gradient:* Following interrogation from all available windows, the Doppler envelope with the highest peak velocity and the cleanest envelope, with no previous ectopic beats, are selected. The peak velocity is measured at the outer edge of the dark signal. The higher-velocity fine linear artifacts referred to as "hair" are not included.

The EAE/ASE guidelines recommend three values be averaged for a regular rhythm and more than five values be averaged for an irregular rhythm.

Once the peak velocity is obtained, the Bernoulli equation is applied to calculate the peak pressure gradient between the LV and aorta.

However, if the proximal gradient, which is the LVOT gradient, is >1.5 m/s or the peak velocity is <3.0 m/s, the proximal velocity should be included:

$$\text{Peak gradient} = 4V_{max}^2 - 4V_{proximal}^2$$

Since the LVOT gradient in most cases is <1.0 m/s, the modified Bernoulli equation could be applied:

$$\text{Peak gradient} = 4V_{max}^2$$

In FIGURE 24.11, the peak velocity is 5.8 m/s.

Therefore, the peak gradient = 4 × 5.8² = 134.56 mm Hg = >135 mm Hg.

The mean gradient: The mean gradient is obtained by multiple instantaneous values from the entire envelope. Therefore, the mean gradient is more representative of the severity of AS than the maximum velocity. When the outer margin of the velocity curve is traced, current echocardiography systems are capable of computing the mean gradient.

As seen in FIGURE 19.9, the tissue velocity integral is 123 cm and the mean gradient is 83 mm Hg. Therefore, *answer C* is correct.

Suggested Reading
Lang RM, Bierig M, Devereux RB, et al. Recommendations for chamber quantification. *Eur J Echocardiogr* 2006;7:79–108.

Answer 13: D. Careful attention should be paid to obtaining the highest Doppler velocity across the aortic valve in an echocardiographic evaluation of suspected aortic stenosis. The experienced echocardiographer would utilize many imaging techniques to obtain this value. Obtaining the continuous-wave signal most parallel to the flow and recording a clear Doppler envelope are key in achieving this.

Option A: A nonimaging or Pedoff probe is a continuous-wave probe and has a smaller footprint compared to an imaging probe. Therefore, in comparison with an imaging probe, manipulation and obtaining an acoustic window in between ribs would prove easier to obtain the signal most parallel with the stenotic flow. As 2-D imaging is not available for guidance, one should pay attention to ensure the obtained Doppler signals are due to aortic stenosis and not other pathologies.

Option B: Imaging from all possible windows is important in AS evaluation. In most patients, these include apical, right parasternal, and suprasternal windows. However, right supra-clavicular and subcostal windows also yield the highest velocity in a minority of patients.

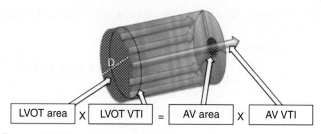

FIGURE 24.12

Option C: In a patient with poor acoustic windows, manufactured contrast administration enhances the Doppler signal significantly (white arrows, FIG. 24.12). Therefore, it is a very useful technique to optimize Doppler recordings. However, it should be noted that use of contrast might slightly increase Doppler velocities.

Option D: Doppler angle correction is not recommended in echocardiography and, in fact, may increase the error and usually underestimates gradients. This is the reason multiple imaging windows are utilized to obtain the beam that is most parallel to the flow. The aim when interrogating the aortic valve by Doppler is that the angle of interrogation would be <15 degrees. Therefore, Doppler angle correction is the least useful in optimizing the Doppler signal.

Option E: Patient positioning should always be optimized during echocardiographic evaluation. Due to considerable anatomic variations, the experienced sonographer would reposition the patient and consider off-axis imaging to obtain the best images.

Suggested Reading
Smith LA. Contrast agent increases Doppler velocities and improves reproducibility of aortic valve area measurements in patients with aortic stenosis. *J Am Soc Echocardiogr* 2004;17(3):247–252.

Answer 14: E. Transthoracic echocardiographic evaluation is the only diagnostic study to evaluate the severity of AS that most patients with symptomatic severe aortic stenosis undergo prior to aortic valve replacement. Therefore, it is imperative that an accurate diagnosis is made and precise gradients are reported. *Answers A, B, C, and D* could each give rise to ejection systolic Doppler signals. The velocities of these conditions could be similar to that seen in aortic stenosis ranging approximately between 2 and 5 m/s. Hence, these signals could mimic that of aortic stenosis. Therefore, answers A to D may be misrepresented as an aortic stenosis gradient.

The Doppler signal of tricuspid stenosis on the other hand is a biphasic diastolic flow, toward the apex. Hence, it is unlikely to mimic the Doppler signal of aortic stenosis. Therefore, *answer E* is the correct answer to the above question.

Answer 15: B. The information could be used to calculate the aortic valve area with the continuity equation.

According to the law of conservation of mass, the stroke volume at the LVOT has to be equal to the stroke volume at the aortic valve. As the stroke volume is the product of area and velocity time integral, this could be applied to calculate the aortic valve area. When the LVOT area, LVOT VTI, and aortic

VTI are known, the aortic valve area is determined as shown in FIGURE 24.12.

In the patient,

$$AV\ area = \frac{LVOT\ area \times LVOT\ VTI}{AV\ VTI}$$

$$LVOT\ area = 2\pi r^2 = 0.785 \times D^2$$

$$AV\ area = \frac{0.785 \times 2^2 \times 23}{123}$$

$$\textbf{Aortic valve area} = 0.59\ cm^2 => 0.6\ cm^2$$

The continuity equation does not require the LV ejection fraction. It also can be applied when concomitant aortic regurgitation is present to calculate the aortic valve area accurately as regurgitant flow is included in LVOT stroke volume and stroke volume through the AV.

Suggested Readings

Baumgartner H, Hung J, Bermejo J. Echocardiographic assessment of valve stenosis. *Eur J Echocardiogr* 2009;10:1–25.

Feigenbaum H, Armstrong AF, Ryan T. *Feigenbaum's Echocardiography*. 6th ed. Philadelphia, PA: Lippincott Williams & Wilkins, 2005.

Answer 16: *C.* PA systolic pressure could be estimated using the peak TR velocity and peak VSD velocity. The Bernoulli equation is applied for this assumption:

$$\textbf{PA systolic pressure} = 4V^2 + RA\ pressure$$

RA pressure is estimated by IVC size and collapsibility.

If the peak TR velocity is 3.5 m/s, then the estimated PA systolic pressure would be

PA systolic pressure = $4V^2$ + RA pressure = 50 mm Hg + RA pressure.

If a VSD is present and an adequate Doppler envelope could be obtained with less than a 15-degree angulation between the angle of interrogation and direction of flow, the peak velocity of the VSD jet could be used to estimate PA systolic pressure.

When the shunt is left to right,

PA systolic pressure = aortic pressure in systole (systolic blood pressure) − $4V^2_{VSD}$.

If the PA pressure has exceeded systemic pressure in the setting of Eisenmenger syndrome and the shunt is right to left, the estimated PA systolic pressure is

PA systolic pressure = aortic pressure in systole (systolic blood pressure) + $4V^2_{VSD}$.

Aortic regurgitation, mitral regurgitation, and pulmonary regurgitant jets cannot be used to estimate PA systolic pressure.

Answer 17: *B.* Diastolic PA pressure could be estimated by using the end PR velocity:

$$\textbf{Diastolic PA pressure (PADP)} = 4 \times end\ PR\ velocity^2 + estimated\ RA\ pressure$$

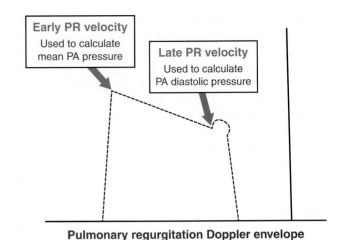

Pulmonary regurgitation Doppler envelope

FIGURE **24.13**

TR, VSD, MR, or AR velocities cannot estimate PA diastolic pressure.

Answer 18: *B.* The mean PA pressure could be estimated by using the early PR velocity from the PR Doppler envelope.

Mahan equation (FIG. 24.13):

$$\textbf{Mean PA pressure} = 4 \times early\ PR\ velocity^2 + estimated\ RA\ pressure$$

Abbas et al. described a method to estimate PA mean pressure by obtaining the mean pressure gradient between the RV and RA by tracing the tricuspid regurgitation (TR) continuous-wave jet and adding RA pressure:

Mean pressure = mean TR pressure + RA pressure

Another method of obtaining PA mean pressure is to estimate the PA systolic and PA diastolic pressures and to calculate the mean arterial pressure by the standard formula for mean pressure:

$$\textbf{Mean PA pressure} = 1/3(PASP) + 2/3(PADP)$$

Mean PA pressure may also be estimated by using pulmonary acceleration time (AT) measured by utilizing the Doppler of the pulmonary artery in systole using the following equation when the heart rate is between 60 and 100 bpm:

$$\textbf{Mean PA pressure} = 79 - (0.45 \times AT)$$

Answer 19: *B.* End-diastolic aortic regurgitant pressure is the pressure gradient between diastolic aortic pressure (DBP) and LVEDP. As the diastolic aortic pressure could be obtained by the blood pressure reading, the following formula would estimate LVEDP:

$$\textbf{LVEDP} = DBP - 4 \times late\ AR\ velocity^2$$

For example, if the patient's blood pressure is 120/80 mm Hg and the end AR velocity is 3.5 m/s, the LVEDP is 80 − 50 = 30 mm Hg.

TR, PR, or VSD has no role in estimating LVEDP.

Answer 20: C. The left ventricular stroke volume is initially calculated to obtain the cardiac output:

Stroke volume = LVOT cross−sectional area × LVOT VTI

Stroke volume = LVOT πr^2 × LVOT VTI

Stroke volume = 3.14 × 12 = 37.6 mL

Cardiac output = heart rate × stroke volume

Cardiac output = 3,835 mL/min = 3.8 L/min

While this is a simple calculation and an easy question, board exams are notorious for providing unnecessary data. There also could be answers to match mistakes that are made. For example, the above question tests calculation of the cardiac output and not the cardiac index. However, answer A is the correct cardiac index (CO/BSA). Therefore, it is up to the exam taker to tease out only the relevant data. An efficient strategy is to read the question stem initially and then the body of the question so as to minimize wasting time comprehending irrelevant information.

Suggested Readings

Abbas AE, Fortuin FD, Schiller NB, et al. Echocardiographic determination of mean pulmonary artery pressure. *Am J Cardiol* 2003;92:1373–1376.

Milan A. Echocardiographic indexes for the non-invasive evaluation of pulmonary hemodynamics. *J Am Soc Echocardiogr* 2010;23(3):225–239.

Sorrell VL, Reeves WC. Noninvasive right and left heart catheterization: taking the echo lab beyond an image-only laboratory. *Echocardiography* 2001;18(1):31–41.

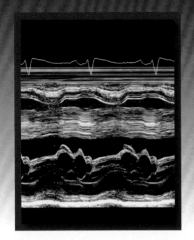

Chapter 25

M-Mode Findings

Sasanka Jayasuriya

1. Which of the following statements regarding M-mode estimates of global LV function is most accurate?

A. In the presence of normal ventricular shape and symmetric systolic function, single linear measurements are an adequate measure of ventricular function.

B. If a true LV minor axis dimension can be obtained, then the estimated fractional shortening is as accurate as are other 2D measures.

C. These measures are valuable for normal or severely reduced LV systolic function, but not adequate for intermediate grades of LV dysfunction.

D. M-mode measures should always use the 2D image for optimal alignment, and accordingly, the Teichholz EF is an adequate estimate of LV global systolic function.

E. 2D measures of LV function are always recommended and more accurate than M-mode estimates regardless of LV geometry, image quality, or technique.

2. See Figure 25.1. What is the fractional shortening?

End-diastolic diameter 50 mm

End-systolic diameter 25 mm

Interventricular septum in systole 1.1 cm

Posterior wall in diastole 1.0 cm

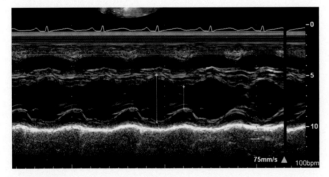

Figure 25.1

A. 35%
B. 24%
C. 50%
D. 30%
E. 23%

3. Which of the following concepts regarding LV systolic function is the most correct?

A. There is an excellent linear correlation between the degree of systolic annular excursion of the base of the LV at the mitral annulus and regional LV systolic function.

B. The magnitude of mitral valve opening (E-wave height) has a strong linear correlation with LV stroke volume, even in patients with mitral regurgitation.

C. The ratio of E-wave height to LV size (E point to septal separation) directly correlates with LV systolic function and is normally within 6 mm.

D. The aortic valve opening on M-mode becomes rounded in early systole in patients with reduced LV systolic function and is another marker of LV systolic dysfunction.

E. Tissue Doppler mitral annular E′ velocities directly reflect the systolic excursion, providing another estimate of LV global systolic function.

4. A 65-year-old male with multivessel CAD, s/p bypass surgery 13 years earlier, now presents with worsening dyspnea on exertion and orthopnea. On exam, BP is 106/62 mm Hg, HR is 80 to 90 bpm, and bilateral crackles are heard half way up the posterior lung fields, with a loud S3 gallop, soft holosystolic murmur of MR, and 2+ bilateral pitting edema. Which of the following figures is most consistent with the above clinical description (Fig. 25.2)?

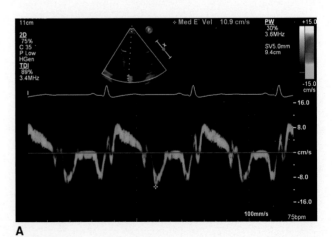

A

Figure 25.2

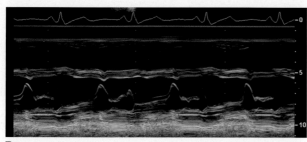

B

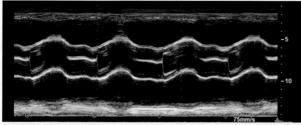

C

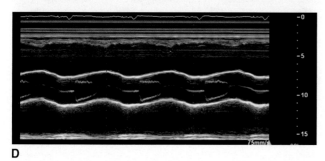

D

FIGURE 25.2 (*Continued*)

A. FIGURE 25.2A
B. FIGURE 25.2B
C. FIGURE 25.2C
D. FIGURE 25.2D
E. None of the options

5. A 53-year-old female presents with dyspnea on exertion and has a loud murmur on exam. Echocardiogram performed shows the following image. Based on this, what is the next best step in the management of this patient (FIG. 25.3)?

A. Schedule for aortic valve replacement.
B. Schedule for mitral valve replacement.
C. Refer her for pericardial stripping.
D. Perform an urgent pericardiocentesis.

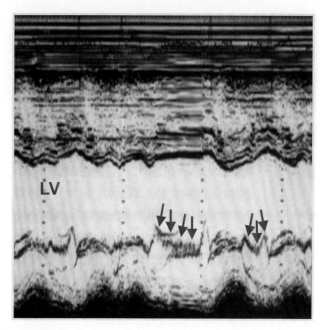

FIGURE 25.3

6. A 62-year-old female with multiple cardiac surgeries, who is a poor historian, presents to establish cardiac care. Presently she is asymptomatic. Echocardiogram is consistent with which of the following pathologies (FIG. 25.4)?

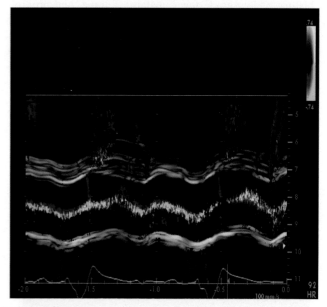

FIGURE 25.4

A. Mechanical aortic valve prosthesis
B. Left ventricular assist device
C. Subaortic membrane
D. Hypertrophic cardiomyopathy
E. Dilated cardiomyopathy

7. A 45-year-old male with hypertension and diabetes presents with pedal edema and dyspnea on exertion. On exam, BP is 145/75 mm Hg, with heart rate of 65 bpm. He has never had an echocardiogram and undergoes the study (FIG. 25.5). What is the most likely cause for his symptoms?

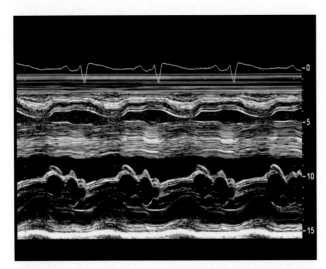

FIGURE 25.5

A. Mitral stenosis
B. Elevated left ventricular filling pressures
C. Systolic anterior motion of the mitral valve leaflet
D. Atrial flutter
E. Pulmonary hypertension

8. A 52-year-old male with diabetes type 2, with coronary artery bypass grafting 8 years ago, presents with a 1-week history of low-grade fever, malaise, fatigue, and progressive dyspnea. He had mild chest pain 10 days ago, which has now resolved. He denies any orthopnea or paroxysmal nocturnal dyspnea. On exam, he is afebrile. BP is 112/75 mm Hg, with HR of 90 bpm. An M-mode image from the patient's echocardiogram is included (FIG. 25.6). What findings are expected on the patient's clinical exam?

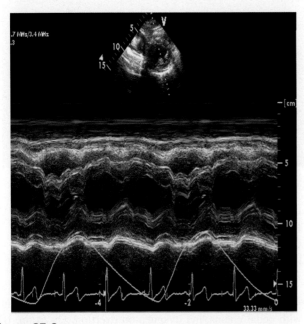

FIGURE 25.6

A. The manual BP demonstrates a higher systolic BP with expiration than inspiration.
B. The manual BP demonstrates a higher systolic BP with inspiration than expiration.
C. The jugular venous pressure rises with inspiration.
D. The jugular venous pressure does not change with respiration.
E. Prominent V wave is present on his jugular venous exam.

9. FIGURE 25.7 is most consistent with which of the following scenarios?

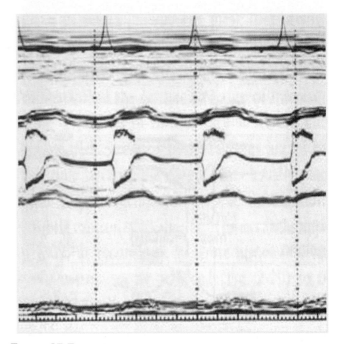

FIGURE 25.7

A. A 59-year-old male with cardiac sarcoidosis and a left ventricular ejection fraction of 10%
B. A 52-year-old male with hypertrophic cardiomyopathy
C. A 81-year-old female with heart failure with preserved ejection fraction
D. A 41-year-old female with breast cancer and a large pericardial effusion
E. A 25-year-old male with bicuspid aortic valve and aortic regurgitation

Answer 1: A. Option A is the single best answer.

Option B is incorrect. Although it is indeed a correct statement that the LV minor axis needs to be obtained, this method remains single dimensional and less accurate than 2D in most patients with acquired heart disease.

Option C is incorrect. All methods of estimating ventricular function are more accurate in normal or severely reduced LV systolic function and have a higher confidence interval for intermediate grades of function. Linear M-mode estimates are more subject to error from abnormal geometry and regional function than grade of LV dysfunction.

Option D is incorrect. Both the Teichholz and Quinones methods of calculating LVEF from LV linear dimensions may result in inaccuracies as a result of the geometric assumptions required to convert a linear measurement to a 3D volume. Accordingly, the use of linear measurements to calculate LV global systolic function is not recommended by the ASE.

Option E is incorrect. In circumstances of poor 2D image quality and normal LV geometry and symmetric function, such as in patients with uncomplicated hypertension, obesity, or valvular diseases, such regional differences are rare, and high-quality linear estimates may provide more useful information than does the 2D estimate.

M-mode echocardiography was the initial technique for estimating LV global systolic function, but since the development of 2D techniques, this is mostly historical. Linear measurements are simple and rapid but subject to significant error since these only evaluate ventricular function along a single line. However, if ventricular shape is normal and the LV contraction pattern is symmetrical, then these linear measures reflect the true global systolic function. For this reason, the fractional shortening estimates remain popular in pediatric (noncongenital) examinations where these parameters often apply. In adult patients with heart disease, abnormal LV shape is common, and regional variation in systolic function exists.

M-mode measurements are inherently limited by the inability to measure the true LV minor axis. Fortunately, 2D echo allows optimal alignment for M-mode measures and can confirm the off-axis alignment when this occurs. Furthermore, 2D provides an area- or volume-based estimate of LV function that, despite the lower temporal resolution to M-mode, is a superior technique, and the biplane Simpson method is now the recommended technique by the ASE guidelines.

Another measure with potential clinical relevance is the midwall fractional shortening (MWFS) instead of the endocardial FS%. LV midwall contraction may reflect intrinsic contractility better than does endocardial fiber contraction, especially in certain circumstances such as concentric LVH. This can be obtained using the following formula:

Inner shell = [(LVIDd + SWTd/2 + PWTd/2)^3 – LVIDd^3 + LVIDs^3]$^{1/3}$ – LVIDs

MWFS = ([LVIDd + SWTd / 2 + PWTd / 2] – [LVIDs + inner shell])/(LVIDd + SWTd / 2 + PWTd / 2) × 100

Suggested Readings

de Simone G, et al. Assessment of left ventricular function by the midwall fractional shortening/end-systolic stress relation in human hypertension. *J Am Coll Cardiol* 1994;23:1444–1451.

Lang RM, Bierig M, Devereux RB, et al. Recommendations for chamber quantification: a report from the American Society of Echocardiography's Guidelines and Standards Committee and the Chamber Quantification Writing Group, developed in conjunction with the European Association of Echocardiography, a branch of the European Society of Cardiology. *J Am Soc Echocardiogr* 2005;18:1440–1463.

Quinones MA, et al. A new, simplified and accurate method for determining ejection fraction with two-dimensional echocardiography. *Circulation* 1981;64:744–753.

Teichholz LE, et al. Problems in echocardiographic volume determinations: echocardiographic angiographic correlations in the presence of absence of asynergy. *Am J Cardiol* 1976;37:7–11.

Answer 2: *C.* Fractional shortening is a method to evaluate LV systolic function with M-mode echocardiography. This is the percentage change in the LV internal dimension during systole in relation to the

$$\textbf{Fractional shortening (FS)} = \frac{\textbf{LVEDD} - \textbf{LVESD}}{\textbf{LVEDD}} \times \textbf{100}$$

Therefore, in the patient

$$\textbf{FS} = \frac{\textbf{LVEDD} - \textbf{LVESD}}{\textbf{LVEDD}} \times \textbf{100}$$
$$\textbf{FS} = \frac{\textbf{50} - \textbf{25}}{\textbf{50}} \times \textbf{100}$$
$$= \textbf{50\%}$$

The parasternal long-axis or short-axis view could be used to obtain the LV end-diastolic and end-systolic diameters. These measurements are obtained at the level of the mitral chordae and should intersect the long axis of the left ventricle. While previously measurements were made from the leading edge to the next leading edge, with improved image quality, it is current practice to measure the distances between true tissue blood interphases. Distances could be obtained from 2D-targeted M-mode images or M-mode images. However, the normal limit for fractional shortening obtained from 2D imaging is 18%, while the value from M-mode is 25% as M-mode overestimates distances.

FS evaluates basal contractility and therefore is not a reliable method for evaluation of global LV function in the setting of regional wall motion abnormalities. FS is also dependent on preload and afterload.

Suggested Readings

Lewis RP, et al. Relationship between changes in the left ventricular dimension and ejection fraction in man. *Circulation* 1971;44:548.

Triulzi MO, Gillam LD, Gentile F, et al. Normal adult cross-sectional echocardiographic values: linear dimensions and chamber areas. *Echocardiography* 1984;1:403–426.

Answer 3: *C.* Option C is the single best answer.

Option A is incorrect since systolic annular excursion of the base of the LV at the mitral annulus reflects *global* and not *regional* LV systolic function.

Option B is incorrect since patients with mitral regurgitation will have a falsely increased forward stroke volume as estimated by the MV stroke volume. In this setting, the magnitude of mitral valve opening may be falsely increased and less correlated with global LV systolic function.

Option C is correct. The E point to septal separation directly correlates with LV systolic function and is normally within 6 mm. With worsening LV function, this value becomes greater.

Option D is incorrect since the aortic valve opening on M-mode becomes rounded in *late*, not *early*, systole in patients with reduced LV systolic function. See Figure 20.8.

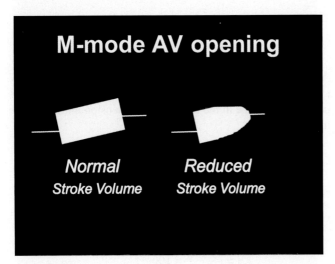

FIGURE 25.8

Option E is incorrect since tissue Doppler mitral annular *systolic* S-wave velocity (and not the *diastolic* E′ velocity) correlates directly with the *systolic* excursion of the LV annulus.

Several M-mode findings provide clues to the presence of systolic dysfunction. The E point to septal separation (EPSS) is a very simple and easily obtained parameter used to gauge left ventricular function, correlating well with LVEF. The left ventricular diameter is proportional to diastolic volume; the mitral excursion during mitral valve opening in diastole correlates with mitral stroke volume. The smaller the mitral opening during diastole, the worse is the left ventricular function. Similarly, in those with decreased cardiac output, the aortic valve closure does not have a sharp opening and closure but becomes rounded at the end of systole (FIG. 25.8). In terms of tissue Doppler imaging, the systolic velocity reflects the degree of systolic function. The systolic velocity of the interventricular septum (Sm) > 7.6 cm/s correlates with LVEF > 50% with a sensitivity of 90%.

Suggested Readings

Feigenbaum H, Armstrong WF, Ryan T, et al. *Feigenbaum's Echocardiography*. Philadelphia, PA: Lippincott Williams & Wilkins, 2005.

Fukuda K, Oki T, Tabata T, et al. Regional left ventricular wall motion abnormalities in myocardial infarction and mitral annular descent velocities studied with pulsed tissue Doppler imaging. *J Am Soc Echocardiogr* 1998;11:841–848.

Answer 4: D. Option A is incorrect. This is a normal tissue Doppler velocity for systole and diastole.

Option B is incorrect. This patient has a normal peak E point to septal separation (EPSS), which is approximately 6 mm for a normal ventricle.

Option C is incorrect. This is a normal systolic anterior motion of the aortic root.

Option D is correct. There is a decrease in systolic anterior motion of the aortic root, which is consistent with this patient's decrease in left ventricular function.

From the clinical presentation, this patient has left ventricular dysfunction. Hence, this patient would have decreased tissue Doppler systolic velocity, increased EPSS (>6 mm), and

decreased systolic anterior motion of the aortic root. The systolic anterior motion of the aortic root is proportional to cardiac output. Also, the diastolic backward motion of the aortic root is determined by the emptying dynamics of the left atrium during left ventricular filling and thus also reflects the left ventricular diastolic filling pattern. In a carefully performed catheterization lab study to determine if aortic root systolic anterior–posterior excursion measured by echo is related to stroke volume, it was determined that the normal aortic motion is 9 ± 1.5 mm (range 7 to 12 mm). In patients with coronary artery disease and congestive heart failure, the authors found significantly smaller values of 4 ± 1.2 ($P < 0.001$). Aortic root motion correlated positively with stroke volume ($r = 0.59$), but not with ejection fraction. By increasing the HR from 75 to 174 bpm (atrial pacing), stroke volume fell from 81 to 34 mL, and the aortic excursion also fell from 10 to 5 mm ($P < 0.001$).

Suggested Readings

Aizawa Y, et al. Stroke volume estimated at aortic root in M-mode echocardiography. *Jpn Heart J* 1981;22(2):185–190.

Burggraf GW, et al. Aortic root motion determined by ultrasound: relation to cardiac performance in man. *Cathet Cardiovasc Diagn* 1978;4(1):29–46.

Answer 5: A. The image represents an M-mode through the mitral valve demonstrating fluttering of the valve leaflets in diastole, secondary to a posteriorly directed jet of aortic regurgitation. The ventricle also appears dilated with an increased E point septal separation, consistent with severe aortic regurgitation resulting in left ventricular dilation. The patient is also symptomatic with dyspnea. Based on this, she should be referred for aortic valve replacement. There is no evidence for primary mitral valve disease, pericardial disease, or pericardial effusion, making the other choices incorrect.

Suggested Reading

Zoghbi W, et al. Recommendations for noninvasive evaluation of native valvular regurgitation: a report from the American Society of Echocardiography Developed in Collaboration with the Society for Cardiovascular Magnetic Resonance. *J Am Soc Echocardiogr* 2017;30(4):303–371.

Answer 6: B. This image represents an M-mode through the aortic valve. The leaflets barely open, and there is constant amount of trace aortic regurgitation. Such findings are present in the setting of an LVAD where the aortic valve is sewn shut, and trivial aortic regurgitation may be present. In the absence of an LVAD, no forward flow through the aortic valve is not compatible with life, making all other choices incorrect. There is no evidence of a mechanical aortic valve (which would also open normally). Furthermore, the left ventricular wall thickness is normal making choice D incorrect. The left ventricle does not appear particularly dilated at present, making choice E incorrect.

Suggested Reading

Stainback RF, et al. Echocardiography in the management of patients with left ventricular assist devices: recommendations from the American Society of Echocardiography. *J Am Soc Echocardiogr* 2015;28:853–909.

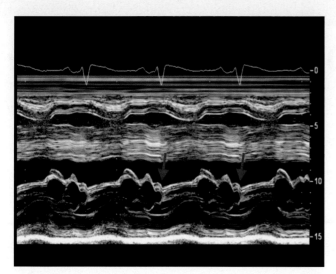

FIGURE 25.9

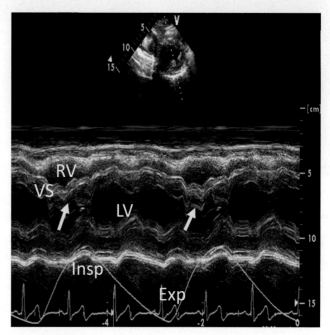

FIGURE 25.10

Answer 7: B. The M-mode image through the mitral valve shows a patient with hypertrophic cardiomyopathy. There is evidence of asymmetric hypertrophy of the septum. However, this is no evidence of systolic anterior motion of the mitral valve leaflet making choice C incorrect. There an extra bump (b bump—see *arrows* on FIG. 25.9) after the mitral valve opening, consistent with high left ventricular filling pressures. The correct answer is B. There is no evidence of mitral valve pathology, and based on the ECG, the patient is having a normal sinus rhythm (choice D is incorrect). There is no evidence of elevated pressures on the right side to suggest pulmonary hypertension, making choice E incorrect as well.

Suggested Reading

Nagueh SF, et al. Recommendations for the evaluation of left ventricular diastolic function by echocardiography: an update from the American Society of Echocardiography and the European Association of Cardiovascular Imaging. *J Am Soc Echocardiogr* 2016;29:277–314.

Answer 8: C. The image represents and M-mode through the short axis of the left ventricle with constrictive physiology (see FIG. 25.10). The respirometer shown at the bottom of the image delineates inspiration and expiration. With inspiration, the right ventricle fills more at the cost of the left ventricle, due to a thickened pericardium surrounding the ventricle. This results in shifting of the interventricular septum toward the left ventricle (arrow) during inspiration. The reverse happens with expiration. There is increased intrathoracic pressure, resulting in decreased filling of the right ventricle. As a result, the left ventricle has a chance to expand as the septum shifts back toward the right ventricle. This interventricular dependence is classic for constrictive physiology. Also note the thickened pericardium both anteriorly and posteriorly. During constriction, JVP rises with inspiration and decreases with expiration

(Kussmaul sign), making choice C correct. Higher arm cuff BP with expiration than inspiration (pulsus paradoxus) as listed in choice A would be consistent with tamponade. There is no pericardial effusion and no evidence of tamponade physiology in the provided images, making choice A incorrect. Choice E of prominent V waves would be seen with tricuspid regurgitation. The remainder of the choices is not consistent with constrictive physiology.

Suggested Reading

Klein AL, et al. American Society of Echocardiography clinical recommendations for multimodality cardiovascular imaging of patients with pericardial disease. *J Am Soc Echocardiogr* 2013;26:965–1012.

Answer 9: A. The image represents M-mode through the aortic valve in a patient with very low cardiac output (choice A). The aortic valve opens normally but closes prematurely (arrows) due to severe left ventricular dysfunction and low cardiac output. This fits best with choice A. Also note the dilated left atrium. There is no evidence of left ventricular wall thickening (choice B), pericardial effusion (choice D), or primary aortic valve pathology (choice E), making these choices incorrect. Choice C is not correct since this option states normal ejection fraction, but the image has a reduced ejection fraction.

Suggested Reading

Porter TR, et al. Guidelines for the use of echocardiography as a monitor for therapeutic intervention in adults: a report from the American Society of Echocardiography. *J Am Soc Echocardiogr* 2015;28:40–56.

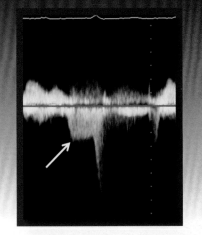

Chapter 26

Diastolic Physiology

Vidya Nadig

1. An ECG with a prolonged PR interval is most likely to be associated with which of the following mitral valve inflow spectral Doppler findings?

    A. Increased E/A ratio

    B. Decreased E/A ratio

    C. Decreased mitral A-wave duration

    D. Prolonged diastasis

    E. Exaggerated mitral L wave

2. What is the most likely LVEDP based upon FIGURE 26.1?

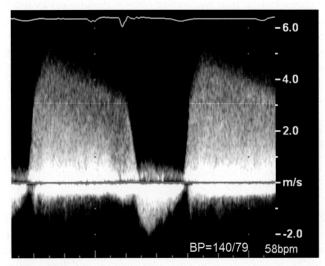

FIGURE 26.1

    A. 10 mm Hg

    B. 20 mm Hg

    C. 30 mm Hg

    D. 5 mm Hg

    E. Cannot be calculated

3. The images in FIGURE 26.2 are consistent with what diagnosis?

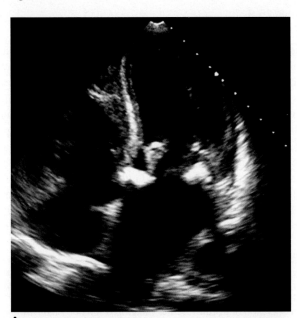

A

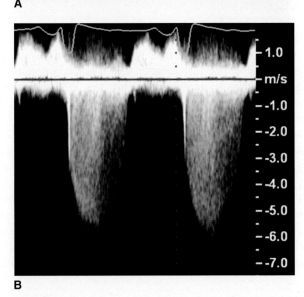

B

FIGURE 26.2

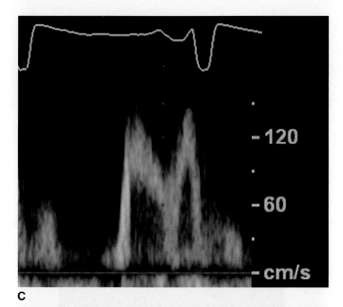

C

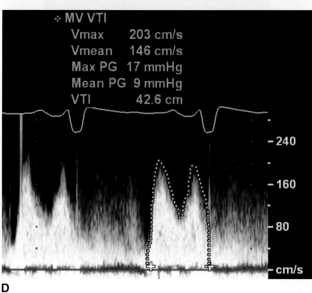

✧ MV VTI
Vmax   203 cm/s
Vmean   146 cm/s
Max PG 17 mmHg
Mean PG 9 mmHg
VTI   42.6 cm

D

FIGURE 26.2 (*Continued*)

A. Severe mitral regurgitation
B. Severe mitral stenosis
C. Grade 1 diastolic dysfunction
D. Severe MR and moderate MS

4. In a patient with a dilated cardiomyopathy, which of the following mitral inflow pulsed-wave Doppler spectral patterns, obtained after a Valsalva maneuver, is associated with a 2-year survival rate of <50%?

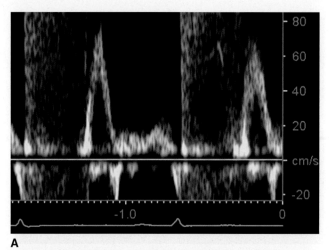

A

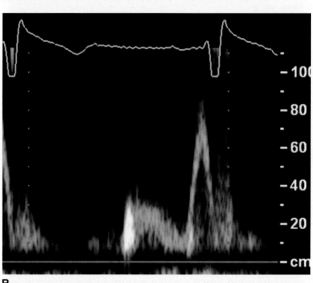

B

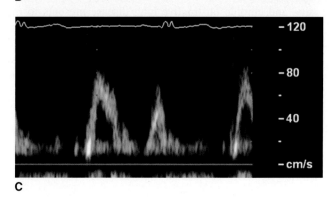

C

FIGURE 26.3

A. FIGURE 26.3A
B. FIGURE 26.3B
C. FIGURE 26.3C
D. Cannot tell

5. The following continuous-wave Doppler tracing across the left heart (Fig. 26.4) is obtained from the apex. The abnormal Doppler finding is least likely to be seen in which of the following conditions?

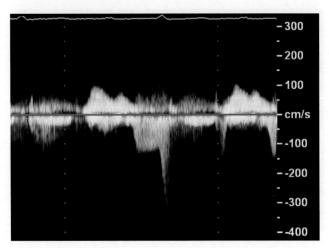

FIGURE 26.4

A. Hyperdynamic LV systolic function and hypovolemia
B. Dilated cardiomyopathy with stage D heart failure and left bundle-branch block
C. Normal LVEF and complete heart block
D. Endocarditis with hypotension and acute severe aortic regurgitation

6. Which of the following is the primary determinant of mitral inflow E-wave and A-wave velocities?

A. LA compliance
B. LV compliance
C. Transmitral pressure gradient
D. Mitral valve area
E. LV relaxation

7. A 62-year-old female with a history of hypertension, obesity, and chronic obstructive lung disease presents to the emergency department with shortness of breath. Vital signs are obtained as follows: HR 75 bpm, BP 114/70 mm Hg, and O_2 saturation 93% on room air. Examination demonstrates distant heart sounds and no audible murmurs. An echocardiogram is obtained, with the Doppler recordings across the left heart (Fig. 26.5). Which of the following is most likely the cause of her symptoms?

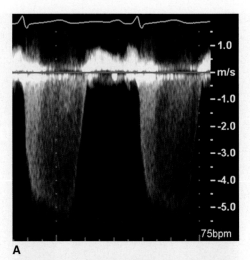

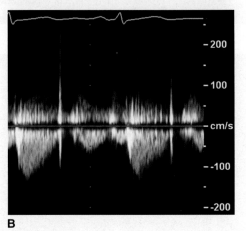

FIGURE 26.5

A. Elevated left atrial pressure
B. Aortic stenosis
C. Severe mitral regurgitation
D. None of the above

8. A 70-year-old male presents with dyspnea, lower extremity edema, and increased abdominal girth. He had undergone CABG and aortic valve replacement 2 months prior. Echocardiogram shows no pericardial effusion. The IVC is dilated, and mitral E/A is 2.5. There is no mitral E-wave respiratory flow variation noted at rest. Which of the following maneuvers during the echocardiogram may be helpful for eliciting respiratory flow variation in the evaluation of suspected constrictive pericarditis?

A. Have the patient sit up
B. Leg raise
C. Handgrip
D. None of the above

9. Which of the following findings suggests markedly elevated left atrial pressure in a 50-year-old female?

A. Deceleration time = 190 ms
B. IVRT = 120 ms
C. Deceleration time = 280 ms
D. IVRT = 50 ms
E. E wave > A wave

10. The mitral valve inflow pulsed-wave spectral Doppler tracing in FIGURE 26.6 is most likely to be seen in which of the following scenarios?

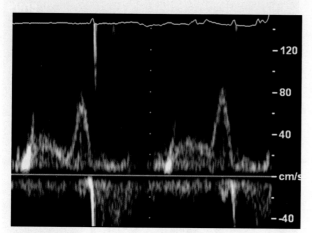

FIGURE 26.6

A. A 45-year-old male with an LVEF = 45%, history of myocardial infarction, and NYHA class I functional status
B. A 20-year-old female with a benign flow murmur and no cardiac symptoms
C. A 70-year-old male with restrictive cardiomyopathy and NYHA class IV functional status
D. A 52-year-old male with idiopathic dilated cardiomyopathy and elevated BNP

11. In a 55-year-old female, which of the following echo/Doppler findings would least indicate that the mitral inflow pattern in FIGURE 26.7 is pseudonormal?

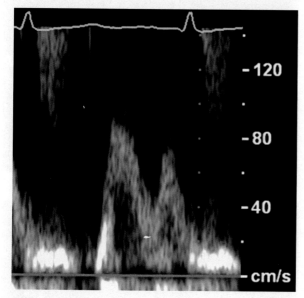

FIGURE 26.7

A. Pulmonary venous flow systolic filling fraction = 0.3
B. E/e′ = 18
C. Left atrial volume index = 42 mL/m²
D. Pulmonary venous atrial reversal duration − mitral A-wave duration = 0 ms
E. Color M-mode propagation rate = 35 cm/s

12. Respiratory flow variation of the mitral valve E wave is least likely to be seen in which of the following clinical scenarios?

A. Cardiac tamponade
B. Pericardial constriction
C. Chronic obstructive lung disease
D. Right ventricular myocardial infarction
E. Restrictive cardiomyopathy

13. A 65-year-old male with a history of hypertension and smoking presents for evaluation of shortness of breath. Vital signs are normal. There is no jugular venous distension. Lungs are clear to auscultation. Cardiac examination demonstrates a regular rate and rhythm, an S4, and no murmurs. He undergoes an echocardiogram with a Doppler tracing shown in FIGURE 26.8. What is the estimated pulmonary artery diastolic pressure?

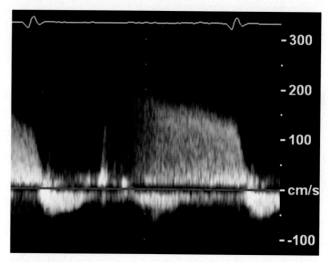

FIGURE 26.8

A. 14 mm Hg
B. 21 mm Hg
C. 9 mm Hg
D. 32 mm Hg
E. 40 mm Hg

14. Which of the following clinical scenarios in a 58-year-old female with hypertension and worsening dyspnea on exertion supports starting with the mitral inflow velocities to assess diastolic function (select all that apply)?

A. Recent onset of atrial fibrillation (AF).
B. Mild mitral stenosis.
C. Moderate mitral annular calcification.
D. Moderate mitral regurgitation.
E. Mitral valve repair.
F. Mitral valve replacement.
G. LV assist devices.
H. Left bundle-branch block.
I. Atrial paced rhythm.
J. None of these clinical scenarios should start with the mitral inflow.

15. Which of the following echo/Doppler findings would be least expected in a patient with typical features of constrictive pericarditis?

A. Preserved e′ velocity in *both* septal and lateral annulus
B. Increased hepatic vein diastolic flow reversal during expiration
C. Exaggerated respiratory flow variation with decreased mitral E-wave velocity during expiration
D. Septal bounce—even during a breath-held image
E. Tissue Doppler "annulus reversus"

16. Which of the following statements is the least correct regarding pulmonary venous flow?

A. Pulmonary venous S1 flow is affected by left atrial relaxation.
B. Decreased pulmonary venous systolic flow velocity and shortened pulmonary venous diastolic flow duration are seen in mitral stenosis.
C. Pulmonary venous systolic flow may be reversed in severe mitral regurgitation.
D. Pulmonary venous D-wave velocity decreases with increasing age.

17. Which of the following statements is the least correct regarding LA size and function?

A. Enlarged left atrial volume may reflect the cumulative effect of elevated filling pressures over time.
B. Left ventricular diastolic compliance influences left atrial contractile function.
C. Left atrial enlargement may be seen in the athlete's heart.
D. In stage 1 diastolic dysfunction, dependence on left atrial conduit function is increased.
E. Left atrial reservoir function is influenced by left atrial compliance.

18. The tracing in Figure 26.9 is a septal annular recording in a 53-year-old male. The mitral E-wave velocity is 100 cm/s, the E-wave deceleration time is 170 ms, A-wave velocity is 80 cm/s, and IVRT is 80 ms.

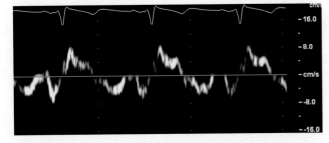

Figure 26.9

A. The findings are consistent with normal diastolic function.
B. The findings are consistent with constrictive pericarditis.
C. The findings are consistent with a cardiomyopathy.
D. The findings are indeterminate.

19. Choose the correct measurements for the Doppler tracings in Figure 26.10:

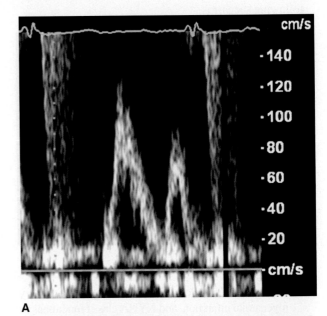

A

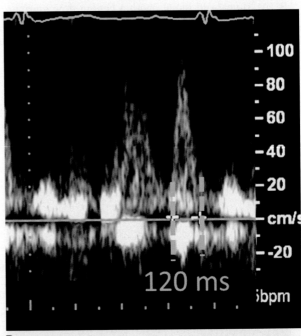

B

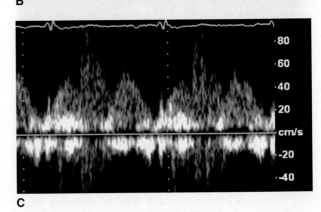

C

Figure 26.10

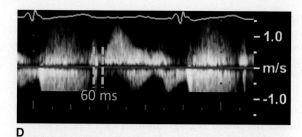

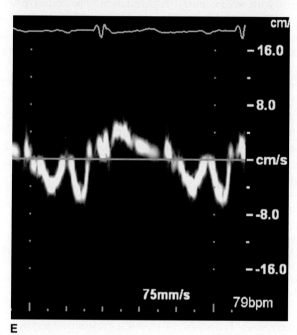

FIGURE 26.10 (Continued)

A. S/D ratio = 0.9; E wave = 120 cm/s; A wave = 85 cm/s; IVRT = 60 ms; e′ = 5 cm/s
B. S/D ratio = 1.4; E wave = 120 cm/s; A wave = 85 cm/s; IVRT = 60 ms; e′ = 5 cm/s
C. S/D ratio = 0.9; E wave = 120 cm/s; A wave = 85 cm/s; IVRT = 120 ms; e′ = 6 cm/s
D. S/D ratio = 1.4; E wave = 80 cm/s; A wave = 50 cm/s; IVRT = 60 ms; e′ = 5 cm/s
E. S/D ratio = 0.9; E wave = 80 cm/s; A wave = 50 cm/s; IVRT = 60 cm; e′ = 6 cm/s

20. Which of the following statements is most accurate?

A. Lateral E/e′ can be used to identify elevated filling pressures in a patient with a mitral valve prosthesis.
B. Lateral e′ velocity is usually lower than septal e′ velocity.
C. E/e′ is unreliable for estimation of LV filling pressures in patients with preserved LVEF and moderate to severe mitral regurgitation.
D. e′ velocities increase with normal aging.
E. E/e′ is independent of preload in normal hearts.

21. An E/A ratio >2.0 would be of greatest concern as a marker of LA pressure elevation in which of the following clinical scenarios:

A. A 60-year-old male patient recently underwent TEE-guided DCCV for atrial fibrillation
B. A 32-year-old female training for her first triathlon
C. An overweight 55-year-old male with dyspnea, normal LV, and an averaged E/e′ ratio <10
D. A 72-year-old female with LVEF 0.30, normal LAVI, and normal TR velocity

Answer 1: *B.*

Option A: False. See discussion for choice "B."

Option B: True. Fusion of the mitral E wave and A waves may occur in the setting of first-degree AV block. In addition, the mitral A-wave velocity may be increased, thereby resulting in reduced E/A.

Option C: False. Since the PR interval is prolonged, the mitral A-wave duration lengthens.

Option D: False. First-degree AV block can cause partial or total fusion of E and A waves and would not prolong diastasis.

Option E: False. The mitral L wave is a middiastolic wave that may be seen in the mitral inflow Doppler interrogation. It has been reported in young, healthy individuals with bradycardia and may also be seen in patients with heart failure and elevated filling pressures. When the velocity is ≥20 cm/s, the L wave often reflects abnormal diastolic function and elevated filling pressures (Fig. 26.11).

Brief Discussion related to the echo Doppler findings of variations in PR interval (editor's note):

If the PR interval is too short, atrial filling is terminated early by ventricular contraction thus reducing mitral A duration, LV end-diastolic volume, and cardiac output. A first-degree AV

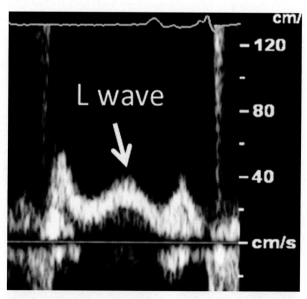

FIGURE 26.11

block of 200 to 280 ms is usually well tolerated if the LVEF and heart rate are normal. However, in patients with shortened diastolic filling periods due to markedly impaired LV relaxation, faster heart rates, bundle-branch block, or ventricular pacing, a first-degree AV block of >280 ms usually results in "fusion" of E and A velocities. If atrial contraction occurs before early diastolic mitral flow velocity has decreased to ≤20 cm/s, the E/A velocity ratio is reduced because of a higher A-wave velocity. This "fusion" of early and late diastolic filling with an E/A velocity ratio of <1 can be misinterpreted as impaired relaxation filling pattern.

In addition, with mitral E and A fusion, the larger atrial stroke volume increases the mitral A-wave duration and pulmonary venous peak systolic velocity and time-velocity integral. Diastolic fusion of filling waves can also limit exercise capacity because LV end-diastolic volume is reduced, lowering maximal cardiac output. At PR values >320 ms, AV synchrony becomes "unphysiologic" because of marked E-wave and A-wave fusion, or filling only with atrial contraction (uniphasic A wave), and diastolic MR is seen. In these patients, exercise tolerance is limited.

Suggested Readings

Ha JW, Oh JK, Redfield MM, et al. Triphasic mitral inflow velocity with middiastolic filling: clinical implications and associated echocardiographic findings. *J Am Soc Echocardiogr* 2004;17:428–431.

Nagueh SF, et al. Recommendations for the evaluation of left ventricular diastolic function by echocardiography: an update from the American Society of Echocardiography and the European Association of Cardiovascular Imaging. *J Am Soc Echocardiogr* 2016;29:277–314.

Answer 2: *C.* The LVEDP can be calculated from the end-diastolic velocity of the aortic regurgitant (AR) jet, because the end-diastolic AR jet velocity is determined by the difference between the aortic diastolic pressure and the LVEDP. Using the simplified Bernoulli equation, the end-diastolic pressure gradient between the aorta and LV is calculated as $4 \times Var2$.

In this case, the end-diastolic velocity of the AR jet is 3.5 m/s, so LVEDP = $79 - 4 \times (3.5)2 = 30$ mm Hg (Fig. 26.12).

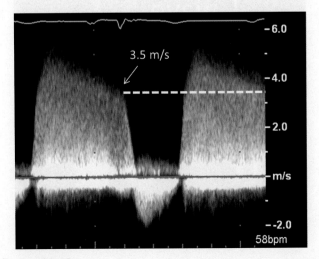

Figure 26.12

Suggested Reading

Grayburn PA, Handshoe R, Smith MD, et al. Quantitative assessment of the hemodynamic consequences of aortic regurgitation by means of continuous wave Doppler recordings. *J Am Coll Cardiol* 1987;10:135–141.

Answer 3: *A.* The intensity of the continuous-wave Doppler signal of the mitral regurgitation jet (see Fig. 26.2B) is consistent with severe mitral regurgitation. The mitral E-wave velocity is increased, and the transmitral gradient is increased (see Fig. 26.2C and D). The increased volume load associated with severe mitral regurgitation results in an increased E-wave velocity (>1.2 m/s) and increased transmitral gradient. The pressure half-time is not significantly increased and, in combination with the 2D image, does not suggest significant (moderate or severe) mitral stenosis. In grade 1 diastolic dysfunction, the mitral E-wave velocity is reduced, not increased; in this case, the E-wave deceleration time is not prolonged, and E/A is not <0.8 and therefore not consistent with grade 1 diastolic dysfunction.

Suggested Readings

Thomas L, Foster E, Schiller NB. Peak mitral inflow velocity predicts mitral regurgitation. *J Am Coll Cardiol* 1998;31:174–179.

Zoghbi WA, Enriquez-Sarano M, Foster E, et al. Recommendations for evaluation of the severity of native valvular regurgitation with two-dimensional and Doppler echocardiography. *J Am Soc Echocardiogr* 2003;16:777–802.

Answer 4: *A.* Figure 26.3A shows a "restrictive physiology" mitral inflow pattern, which is associated with advanced (grade 3) diastolic dysfunction. This pattern is characterized by a high E/A ratio (≥2) and short E-wave deceleration time (<160 ms). This type of pattern can occur when the left atrial and left ventricular diastolic pressures are markedly elevated. In these cases, most of ventricular filling occurs during early diastole, when volume from the high-pressure left atrium flows into the LV; however, the flow decelerates quickly because the LV diastolic pressure rises rapidly in the setting of abnormal LV compliance. In late diastole, the LV pressure is already high, and the amount of additional filling during atrial contraction is small. These factors lead to a high E/A ratio and shortened deceleration time. When this pattern is reversible with hemodynamic maneuvers (such as diuresis), it is referred to as "grade 3A diastolic dysfunction"; when the pattern remains fixed despite preload-reducing maneuvers, it is termed "grade 3B (or grade IV) diastolic dysfunction." Grade 3 diastolic dysfunction has been shown to predict a poor prognosis in both restrictive and dilated cardiomyopathies, with grade 3B having the worst prognosis.

Figure 26.3B shows an "abnormal relaxation" mitral inflow pattern or grade 1 diastolic dysfunction. This pattern may be seen in early stages of diastolic dysfunction, when there is abnormal LV relaxation, but normal LV filling pressures. The E/A ratio is reduced (<0.8), reflecting the decrease in E-wave velocity with impaired early diastolic filling and the increased A-wave velocity with greater contribution of atrial contraction to LV diastolic filling. The E-wave deceleration time is prolonged (>200 ms), because the rate of LV early diastolic pressure change is slowed in the setting of abnormal left ventricular relaxation.

FIGURE 26.3C shows a mitral inflow pattern that can be seen either in normal individuals or in those with grade 2 diastolic dysfunction ("pseudonormal" pattern). The pseudonormal pattern is an intermediate phase of diastolic dysfunction, in which the pattern is a transition between the early dysfunction and advanced dysfunction stages. Other diastolic parameters, such as mitral E/e′, pulmonary venous flow, and left atrial size, may be helpful in distinguishing pseudonormal from normal mitral inflow.

Suggested Readings

Klein A, Hatle L, Taliercio C, et al. Prognostic significance of Doppler measures of diastolic function in cardiac amyloidosis. A Doppler echocardiography study. *Circulation* 1991;83:808–816.

Pinamonti B, Di Lenarda A, Sinagra G, et al. Restrictive left ventricular filling pattern in dilated cardiomyopathy assessed by Doppler echocardiography: clinical, echocardiographic and hemodynamic correlations and prognostic implications. *J Am Coll Cardiol* 1993;22:808–815.

Pozzoli M, Traversi E, Cioffi G, et al. Loading manipulations improve the prognostic value of Doppler evaluation of mitral flow in patients with chronic heart failure. *Circulation* 1997;95:1222–1230.

Xie GY, Berk MR, Smith MD, et al. Prognostic value of Doppler transmitral flow patterns in patients with congestive heart failure. *J Am Coll Cardiol* 1994;24:132–139.

Answer 5: A. The Doppler tracing shows diastolic mitral regurgitation (FIG. 26.13, *arrow*) in a patient with complete heart block. In patients with first-degree AV block, diastolic mitral regurgitation can also occur. In the setting of atrioventricular block, diastolic mitral regurgitation can occur owing to the lack of synchronized ventricular contraction following atrial contraction and consequent incomplete closure of the mitral valve during atrial relaxation. Diastolic mitral regurgitation can also be seen in the setting of markedly elevated LVEDP or severe aortic insufficiency (especially acute severe aortic insufficiency), if left ventricular pressure exceeds left atrial pressure at end diastole. Answer "A" is false.

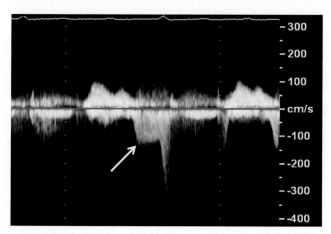

FIGURE 26.13

Suggested Readings

Agmon Y, Freeman W, Oh JK, et al. Diastolic mitral regurgitation. *Circulation* 1999;99:e13.

Panidis IP, Ross J, Munley B, et al. Diastolic mitral regurgitation in patients with atrioventricular conduction abnormalities: a common finding by Doppler echocardiography. *J Am Coll Cardiol* 1986;7:768–774.

Answer 6: C. While a number of variables affect mitral E-wave and A-wave velocities (e.g., preload, LV compliance, LV relaxation properties, LA contractile function, mitral inflow obstruction), the primary single determinant of the mitral inflow velocities is the pressure gradient between the left atrium and the left ventricle during diastolic filling.

Suggested Reading

Appleton CP, Hatle LK, Popp RL. Relation of transmitral flow velocity patterns to left ventricular diastolic function: new insights from a combined hemodynamic and Doppler echocardiographic study. *J Am Coll Cardiol* 1988;12:426–440.

Answer 7: D. None of the above (this patient likely has moderate MR)

Option A: False. FIGURE 26.14 shows mitral regurgitation, with a jet velocity of 5.2 m/s. Using the simplified Bernoulli equation, the systolic pressure gradient between LV and LA is $4 \times V_{max}MR2 = 108$ mm Hg. In the absence of LV or aortic outflow obstruction (no obstruction is seen on the accompanying continuous-wave Doppler tracing in FIG. 26.5B), LV systolic pressure ≈ aortic systolic blood pressure ≈ 114 mm Hg. The LA pressure can be calculated as $LAP = LVSP - 4V_{max}MR2 = 114 - 108 = 6$ mm Hg. Thus, the LA pressure is not elevated.

Option B: False. The continuous-wave Doppler signal across the aortic valve (FIG. 26.5B) is early peaking and has a normal velocity; it is not consistent with aortic stenosis.

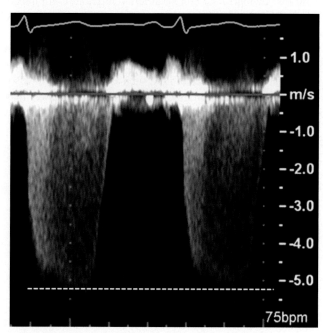

FIGURE 26.14

Option C: False. The intensity of the Doppler signal of the mitral regurgitant jet is not consistent with severe mitral regurgitation. Neither is the E velocity (<1.0 m/s).

Suggested Reading

Gorcsan J III, Snow FR, Paulsen W, et al. Noninvasive estimation of left atrial pressure in patients with congestive heart failure and mitral regurgitation by Doppler echocardiography. *Am Heart J* 1991;121(3 Pt 1):858–863.

Answer 8: A. In some patients with constrictive pericarditis, respiratory flow variation may not be present. In patients who are volume overloaded, maneuvers to decrease loading conditions, such as sitting the patient up, head tilt, or diuresis, may help to elicit latent respiratory flow variation.

Leg raise maneuver would increase preload, rather than decrease it, so it would not be helpful in this scenario. Handgrip would increase afterload and would not decrease preload.

Suggested Reading

Oh J, Tajik A, Appleton C, et al. Preload reduction to unmask the characteristic Doppler features of constrictive pericarditis. *J Am Coll Cardiol* 1997;95:796–799.

Answer 9: D. In early diastolic dysfunction (i.e., grade 1 diastolic dysfunction), IVRT is prolonged (≥100 ms) due to impaired early diastolic ventricular relaxation. In more advanced stages of diastolic dysfunction, with elevated filling pressures, the IVRT is shortened (≤60 ms).

Normal mitral E-wave deceleration time is 160 to approximately 200 ms (some reports have used an upper limit of 240 ms, while others use 200 ms). In early diastolic dysfunction, deceleration time is prolonged due to abnormal LV relaxation in the early phase of diastolic filling. In advanced stages of diastolic dysfunction, the deceleration time shortens (<160 ms) owing to the abnormal left ventricular compliance, high LVEDP, and rapid decline of the LA–LV early diastolic pressure gradient.

Option E is incorrect since an E > A ratio may be a normal finding in patients aged 50 years. If additional detail was provided regarding the degree of E/A, such as a ratio >2.0 or associated with a deceleration time <110 ms, then this answer may be correct. However, as stated, this is not the single best answer.

Suggested Readings

Garcia MJ, Thomas JD, Klein AL. New Doppler echocardiographic applications for the study of diastolic function. *J Am Coll Cardiol* 1998;32:865–875.

Lester SJ, Tajik AJ, Nishimura RA, et al. Unlocking the mysteries of diastolic function: deciphering the Rosetta stone 10 years later. *J Am Coll Cardiol* 2000;51:679–689.

Nagueh SF, et al. Recommendations for the evaluation of left ventricular diastolic function by echocardiography: an update from the American Society of Echocardiography and the European Association of Cardiovascular Imaging. *J Am Soc Echocardiogr* 2016;29:277–314.

Answer 10: A. The Doppler tracing shows an abnormal relaxation mitral inflow pattern. The E/A ratio is <0.8, and

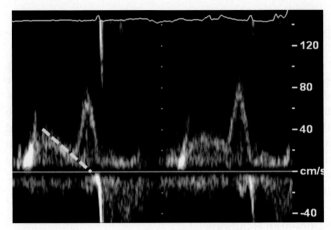

Figure 26.15

deceleration time (Fig. 26.15, *yellow dashed line*) is prolonged. This pattern is typically seen in patients with decreased LV relaxation (e.g., ischemic heart disease or hypertensive heart disease), in the absence of elevated LVEDP. The E-wave deceleration time is prolonged because the abnormal LV relaxation causes prolongation of early diastolic passive filling. E/A is reduced because of decreased contribution of early diastolic passive filling and increased contribution of atrial active contraction toward LV filling.

A young person without cardiac pathology would be expected to have a normal mitral inflow pattern (E/A = 1 to 1.5, deceleration time = 160 to 200 ms).

Patients with either restrictive cardiomyopathy or dilated cardiomyopathy and elevated filling pressures would be expected to have either a pseudonormal (grade 2 diastolic dysfunction) or a restrictive (grade 3 diastolic function) mitral inflow pattern.

It should be noted that in patients with diastolic dysfunction and preserved ejection fraction, mitral inflow parameters do not correlate reliably with LVEDP.

Suggested Readings

Nagueh SF, et al. Recommendations for the evaluation of left ventricular diastolic function by echocardiography: an update from the American Society of Echocardiography and the European Association of Cardiovascular Imaging. *J Am Soc Echocardiogr* 2016;29:277–314.

Yamamoto K, Nishimura RA, Chaliki HP, et al. Determination of left ventricular filling pressure by Doppler echocardiography in patients with coronary artery disease: critical role of left ventricular systolic function. *J Am Coll Cardiol* 1997;30:1819–1826.

Answer 11: D. Pulmonary venous flow is composed of a systolic component *S*, a diastolic component *D* (corresponding to the mitral E wave), and an atrial reversal component *Ar* (occurring during atrial contraction). In young persons, the diastolic component is often prominent, corresponding to the predominance of early diastolic LV filling. The velocity ratio of S/D increases with increasing age, reflecting the decrease in LV filling during early diastole. However, in patients with elevated left atrial pressure (LAP), the S/D ratio decreases, and Ar velocity and duration increase. Thus, S/D < 1 and Ar duration − mitral A duration ≥30 ms both are indicative of elevated LAP. Mitral A-wave durations can be affected by arrhythmias; in patients with sinus tachycardia or first-degree AV block, the mitral A-wave duration may be increased, while in patients with a short PR, the mitral A-wave duration may be truncated. Systolic filling fraction can also be calculated as $S_{VTI}/(S_{VTI} + D_{VTI})$; a value of <40% is suggestive of increased LAP. However, systolic filling fraction and S/D velocity ratio are more reliable as indicators of elevated LAP in patients with reduced LVEF than in those with preserved or hyperdynamic LVEF.

In patients with elevated LVEDP, the ratio of mitral E-wave velocity to mitral annular early diastolic velocity (e′) may be elevated. $E/e'_{septal} ≥ 15$ suggests an elevated LVEDP, while $E/e' ≤ 8$ suggests normal LVEDP.

Left atrial volume index ≥34 mL/m² is a marker of chronically increased left atrial load and may be helpful in identifying abnormal diastolic function, taken together with other parameters.

Reduced color M-mode flow propagation rate (Vp < 50 cm/s) is associated with abnormal diastolic function. In addition, a ratio of E/Vp ≥ 2.5 has been reported to be associated with elevated LA pressure. However, color M-mode flow propagation rate is felt to be less reliable in patients with preserved ejection fraction than in those with reduced LVEF. In patients with heart failure and preserved ejection fraction, normal flow propagation rate may be seen despite an elevation in filling pressures.

Suggested Readings

Garcia MJ, Smedira NG, Greenberg NL, et al. Color M-mode Doppler flow propagation velocity is a preload insensitive index of left ventricular relaxation: animal and human validation. *J Am Coll Cardiol* 2000;35:201–208.

Kelin AL, Tajik AJ. Doppler assessment of pulmonary venous flow in healthy subjects and in patients with disease. *J Am Soc Echocardiogr* 1991;4:379–392.

Kuecherer HF, Muhiudeen IA, Kusumoto FM. Estimation of mean left atrial pressure from transesophageal pulsed Doppler echocardiography of pulmonary venous flow. *Circulation* 1990;82:1127–1139.

Nagueh SF, et al. Recommendations for the evaluation of left ventricular diastolic function by echocardiography: an update from the American Society of Echocardiography and the European Association of Cardiovascular Imaging. *J Am Soc Echocardiogr* 2016;29:277–314.

Nagueh SF, Middleton KJ, Kopelen HA, et al. Doppler tissue imaging: a noninvasive technique for evaluation of left ventricular relaxation and estimation of filling pressures. *J Am Coll Cardiol* 1997;30:1527–1533.

Ommen SR, Nishimura RA, Appleton CP, et al. Clinical utility of Doppler echocardiography and tissue Doppler imaging in the estimation of left ventricular filling pressures: a comparative simultaneous Doppler-catheterization study. *Circulation* 2000;102:1788–1794.

Takatsuji H, Mikami T, Urasawa K, et al. A new approach for evaluation of left ventricular diastolic function: spatial and temporal analysis of left ventricular filling flow propagation by color M-mode Doppler echocardiography. *J Am Coll Cardiol* 1996;27:365–371.

Answer 12: E. Respiratory flow variation is not seen in restrictive cardiomyopathy, but can be seen in constrictive pericarditis (in which there is dissociation between the changes in intrathoracic and intracardiac pressures). Respiratory flow variation can also be seen in pericardial tamponade, right ventricular myocardial infarction, and right ventricular failure associated with acute pulmonary embolus. In patients with chronic obstructive lung disease (COPD), respiratory flow variation may be seen due to the exaggerated change in intrathoracic pressure with the respiratory cycle; however, there is also increased inspiratory forward flow in the superior vena cava, which is not seen in constrictive pericarditis. In addition, patients with COPD are less likely to display a "restrictive" (i.e., grade 3) mitral inflow pattern.

Suggested Readings

Boonyaratavej S, Oh JK, Tajik J, et al. Comparison of mitral inflow and superior vena cava Doppler velocities in chronic obstructive pulmonary disease and constrictive pericarditis. *J Am Coll Cardiol* 1998;32:2043–2048.

Hatle L, Appleton C, Popp R. Differentiation of constrictive pericarditis and restrictive cardiomyopathy by Doppler echocardiography. *Circulation* 1989;79:357–370.

Answer 13: A. The pulmonary artery diastolic pressure can be estimated from the pulmonic regurgitant (PR) jet end-diastolic velocity. The end-diastolic PR jet velocity in this case is 1.5 m/s. Using the simplified Bernoulli equation, $4V_{PR}^2$ yields the diastolic pressure gradient between the PA and RV. The diastolic RV pressure can be estimated to be approximately the same as the RA pressure. In this case, the RA pressure is estimated to be normal (~5 mm Hg), based on the normal jugular venous pulse. The RA pressure can also be estimated echocardiographically, by integrating information regarding IVC size, presence or absence of IVC respiratory collapse, hepatic venous flow signals, and right atrial enlargement. In this case, $PAD = 4V_{PR}^2 + RAP = 9 + 5 = 14$ mm Hg (Fig. 26.16).

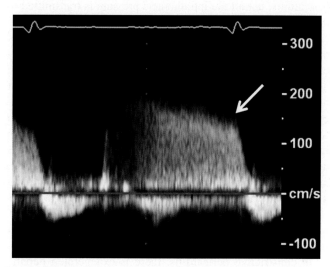

Figure 26.16

Suggested Reading

Rudski LG, Lai WW, Afilalo J, et al. Guidelines for the echocardiographic assessment of the right heart in adults: a report from the American Society of Echocardiography Endorsed by the European Association of Echocardiography, a registered branch of the European Society of Cardiology, and the Canadian Society of Echocardiography. *J Am Soc Echocardiogr* 2010;23:685–713.

Answer 14: I. Given the presence of situations in which LAP and LVEDP are different and because LAP is the pressure that relates better with mean PCWP and thus pulmonary congestion symptoms at the time of the echocardiographic examination, the algorithm is presented with the premise of estimating mean LAP. The *approach starts with mitral inflow velocities* and is applied in the absence of atrial fibrillation (AF), significant mitral valve disease (at least moderate mitral annular calcification [MAC], any mitral stenosis or mitral regurgitation [MR] of more than moderate severity, mitral valve repair or prosthetic mitral valve), LV assist devices, left bundle-branch block, and *ventricular* paced rhythm. Although not specifically studied, atrial pacing should not significantly impact the interpretation of the mitral inflow pattern.

Suggested Reading

Nagueh SF, et al. Recommendations for the evaluation of left ventricular diastolic function by echocardiography: an update from the American Society of Echocardiography and the European Association of Cardiovascular Imaging. *J Am Soc Echocardiogr* 2016;29:277–314.

Answer 15: C. In patients with constrictive pericarditis, annular velocities are preserved, since the myocardium itself is not diseased. In some cases of constrictive pericarditis, the septal annular early diastolic velocity may actually be increased and paradoxically higher than the lateral wall e′ (annulus reversus). In contrast, annular early diastolic velocities are typically decreased in patients with cardiomyopathies.

Patients with constrictive pericarditis may have prominent respiratory flow variation, with a decrease in mitral flows of ≥25% during inspiration. This occurs because, in constrictive pericarditis, not all the intrathoracic pressure is transmitted to the heart. The left atrium (which is not fully encased in pericardium) has an inspiratory decrease in pressure that is not transmitted to LV (which is fully encased in the shell-like pericardium). Left ventricular end-diastolic pressure is therefore not altered by the change in intrathoracic pressure, and left heart filling decreases (because of decreased pressure gradient between the left atrium and left ventricle). Venous return to the right heart normally augments during inspiration, but in constrictive pericarditis, the intrathoracic pressure changes are not fully transmitted to the right atrium or right ventricle, and right ventricular filling is impaired due to the constraining pericardium. However, the decreased filling of the LV allows for increased flow into the RV during inspiration (via displacement of the interventricular septum toward the left heart), manifesting as increased inspiratory right-sided flow velocities.

In constrictive pericarditis, there is exaggerated hepatic flow reversal during expiration because of the dissociation between cardiac and intrathoracic pressures and the worsened impairment to right ventricular filling during expiration. Conversely, in restrictive cardiomyopathy, there is augmented hepatic flow reversal during inspiration, owing to the increased venous return to the right atrium, leading to increased right atrial pressure in the setting of impaired RV compliance and elevated RV filling pressures.

Septal bounce is a classic finding of constrictive pericarditis and is an early diastolic bouncing motion of the interventricular septum that occurs as a result of the tightened ventricular interdependence within the constraining pericardium. Abnormal septal motion is accentuated during inspiration, when augmented filling of the right heart is enabled by the posterior displacement of the interventricular septum; this inspiratory movement of the interventricular septum is seen as an abrupt septal shift on 2D or M-mode imaging. During a breath hold, septal bounce is reduced but is not eliminated.

Suggested Readings

Ha JW, Ommen SR, Tajik AJ. Differentiation of constrictive pericarditis from restrictive cardiomyopathy using mitral annular velocity by tissue Doppler echocardiography. *Am J Cardiol* 2004;94:316–319.

Oh J, Hatle L, Seward J, et al. Diagnostic role of Doppler echocardiography in constrictive pericarditis. *J Am Coll Cardiol* 1994;23:154–162.

Voelkel A, Pietro D, Folland E. Echocardiographic features of constrictive pericarditis. *Circulation* 1978;58:781–775

Answer 16: B. In some patients, two components of pulmonary venous systolic flow may be visible: early systolic flow (S1) and midsystolic to late systolic flow (S2). S1 occurs during atrial relaxation, when the decrease in LA pressure allows forward pulmonary venous flow into the LA. Thus, answer choice "A" is correct. S2 coincides with a rise in pulmonary venous pressure. Following S2, a diastolic forward flow occurs, which coincides with the mitral E wave and left ventricular early diastolic filling. During atrial contraction, a retrograde flow (Ar) is seen. For patients in whom both S1 and S2 are visible, S2 should be used in the calculation of S/D velocity ratio.

In patients with mitral stenosis, the systolic flow velocity is often reduced. Diastolic pulmonary venous flow mirrors changes in mitral E-wave flow; the diastolic flow duration will be prolonged, just as the mitral E-wave pressure half-time is prolonged.

Reversal of pulmonary venous systolic flow is a finding that is seen in severe mitral regurgitation.

Similar to mitral E-wave velocity, diastolic pulmonary venous flow velocity decreases with increasing age, in the setting of decreased early diastolic passive LV filling.

Suggested Readings

Klein AL, Bailey AS, Cohen GI, et al. Effects of mitral stenosis on pulmonary venous flow as measured by Doppler transesophageal echocardiography. *Am J Cardiol* 1993;72:66–72.

Tabata T, Thomas JD, Klein AL. Pulmonary venous flow by Doppler echocardiography: revisited 12 years later. *J Am Coll Cardiol* 2003;41(8):1243–1250.

Thomas L, Levett K, Boyd A, et al. Compensatory changes in atrial volumes with normal aging: is atrial enlargement inevitable? *J Am Coll Cardiol* 2002;40:1630–1635.

Zoghbi WA, Enriquez-Sarano M, Foster E, et al. Recommendations for evaluation of the severity of native valvular regurgitation with two-dimensional and Doppler echocardiography. *J Am Soc Echocardiogr* 2003;16:777–802.

Answer 17: *D.* Increased LA size may be seen in patients who have chronically elevated LA pressures. However, increased LA size may also be seen in elite athletes. LA function can be categorized into three phases: reservoir phase (accommodation of blood from the venous circulation during ventricular systole and isovolumic relaxation), conduit phase (transfer of blood from LA to LV during passive early diastolic LV filling), and contractile phase (atrial contraction).

Atrial contractile function is influenced by left ventricular diastolic compliance and left atrial contractility. LA reservoir function is influenced by LA relaxation and compliance, as well as LV systolic function, mitral annular displacement, and RV function. LA conduit function is affected by LA compliance, LV relaxation, and the presence of mitral inflow obstruction.

In patients with early diastolic dysfunction and impaired LV relaxation, there is increased dependence on reservoir and atrial contraction phases for LV filling and decreased contribution of the conduit phase. However, as left atrial pressures increase and atrial contractile function declines, the contribution of the conduit phase becomes more dominant.

Suggested Readings

Abhayaratna WP, Seward JB, Appleton CP, et al. Left atrial size: physiologic determinants. *J Am Coll Cardiol* 2006; 47:2357–2363.

Pelliccia A, Maron BJ, Di Paolo FM, et al. Prevalence and clinical significance of left atrial remodeling in competitive athletes. *J Am Coll Cardiol* 2005;46:690–696.

To AC, Flamm SD, Marwick TH, et al. Clinical utility of multi-modality left atrial imaging: assessment of size, function, and structure. *J Am Coll Cardiol Imaging* 2011;4:788–798.

Answer 18: *C.* The tracing (FIG. 26.17) shows a mitral annular septal early diastolic (e′) velocity of 6 cm/s, which is reduced (normal mitral septal e′ ≥ 8 cm/s in adults). Reduced e′ velocity is indicative of abnormal myocardial relaxation. In addition, the ratio of E/e′ = 100/6 ≈ 17, which is indicative of elevated left atrial pressure. In this case, the mitral E/A ratio, deceleration time, and IVRT are consistent with a pseudonormal pattern (grade 2 diastolic dysfunction).

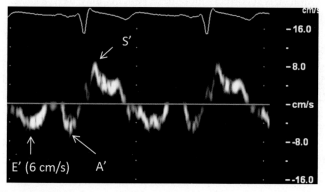

FIGURE 26.17

In patients with constrictive pericarditis, the septal e′ velocity is normal or increased. Typically, the mitral inflow pattern is "restrictive" (high E/A, short deceleration time).

Suggested Readings

Ha JW, Oh JK, Ling LH, et al. Annulus paradoxus: transmitral flow velocity to mitral annular velocity ratio is inversely proportional to pulmonary capillary wedge pressure in patients with constrictive pericarditis. *Circulation* 2001;104:976–978.

Sohn DW, Chai IH, Lee DJ, et al. Assessment of mitral annulus velocity by Doppler tissue imaging in the evaluation of left ventricular diastolic function. *J Am Coll Cardiol* 1997;30:474–480.

Answer 19: *B.* FIGURE 26.18.

FIGURE 26.18A shows mitral inflow early diastolic (E) wave and late diastolic (A) wave obtained at the mitral valve leaflet tips.

FIGURE 26.18B shows measurement of mitral A-wave duration, which is correctly performed at the mitral annulus level.

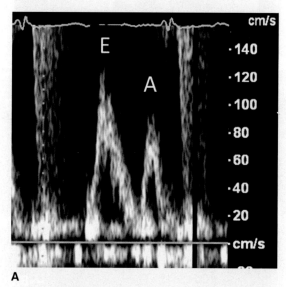

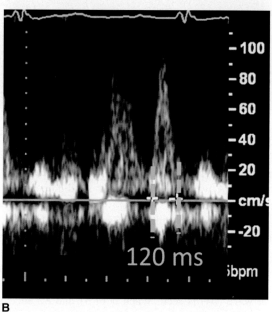

FIGURE 26.18 A: Mitral inflow (PW MV leaflet tips). **B:** Mitral annulus PW: A-wave duration shown in *green dashed lines*. **C:** Pulmonary venous flow. **D:** IVRT (between *green dashed lines*). **E:** TDI medial annulus.

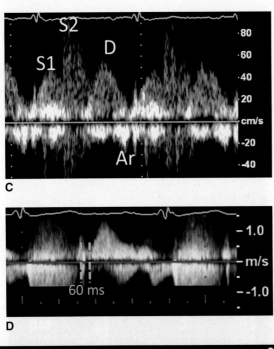

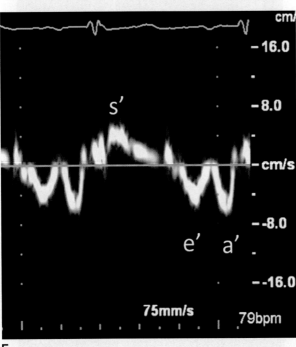

FIGURE 26.18 (Continued)

However, this is not the correct position to measure mitral inflow E- and A-wave velocities, which should be measured at the leaflet tips.

FIGURE 26.18C shows pulmonary venous flow. In some individuals, two systolic waves may be seen: S1 (early systolic, occurring during atrial relaxation) and S2 (late systolic, occurring during a rise in pulmonary venous pressure). In addition, a diastolic wave (D) is seen, and in patients in sinus rhythm, an atrial reversal wave (Ar) is seen. When both S1 and S2 are visible, measurement of S/D ratio should be calculated using the ratio of peak S2 and peak D waves. Thus, in this case, S/D ratio = 1.4.

FIGURE 26.18D shows measurement of IVRT (60 ms), obtained using continuous-wave Doppler positioned in the LVOT so that the end of aortic ejection and beginning of mitral inflow are both visible.

FIGURE 26.18E shows a tissue Doppler recording at the medial mitral annulus. Early diastolic velocity (e′), late diastolic velocity (a′), and systolic velocity (s′) are shown labeled. In this case, e′ is reduced (5 cm/s), consistent with abnormal diastolic function.

Suggested Reading

Nagueh SF, et al. Recommendations for the evaluation of left ventricular diastolic function by echocardiography: an update from the American Society of Echocardiography and the European Association of Cardiovascular Imaging. *J Am Soc Echocardiogr* 2016;29:277–314.

Answer 20: *C.* Mitral annular velocities may be reduced in patients with mitral valve prosthesis, mitral stenosis, or substantial mitral annular calcification; thus, E/e′ is not reliable for estimation of LVEDP in these patients. In patients with moderate to severe mitral regurgitation and preserved LV systolic function, e′ is increased, and E/e′ is therefore unreliable for estimation of filling pressures in this setting. e′ velocities decrease with increasing age. The lateral e′ velocity is usually higher than septal e′ velocity, with the exception of patients who have a lateral wall motion abnormality or constrictive pericarditis, in whom the converse may occur. E/e′ is dependent on preload in structurally normal hearts without heart failure and therefore may not be a reliable tool for evaluation of diastolic function in normal individuals.

Suggested Readings

Little WC, Oh JK. Echocardiographic evaluation of diastolic function can be used to guide clinical care. *Circulation* 2009;120:802–809.

Nagueh SF, et al. Recommendations for the evaluation of left ventricular diastolic function by echocardiography: an update from the American Society of Echocardiography and the European Association of Cardiovascular Imaging. *J Am Soc Echocardiogr* 2016;29:277–314.

Tschöpe C, Paulus WJ. Doppler echocardiography yields dubious estimates of left ventricular diastolic pressures. *Circulation* 2009;120:810–820.

Answer 21: *D.*

Option A is incorrect since these patients may have a falsely increased E/A ratio.

Option B is incorrect since young patients may normally have an E/A ratio >2.0.

Option C is not the best option. Although an overweight 55-year-old male with dyspnea, normal LV, and an averaged E/e′ ratio <10 may also have an elevated TR max velocity and enlarged LAVI, concluding in an elevated LAP, this information is not provided.

Option D is the best option since anyone with a reduced LVEF and E/A > 2.0 should be considered to have an elevated LAP, regardless of a normal LAVI and normal TR velocity.

Brief Discussion

The mitral DT should be used for assessment of LV diastolic function in patients with recent cardioversion to sinus rhythm who can have a markedly reduced mitral A velocity because of LA stunning at the time of the echocardiographic examination, thus leading to an E/A ratio >2 despite the absence of elevated LV filling pressures. In young individuals (<40 years of age), E/A ratios >2 may be a normal finding; therefore, in this age group, other signs of diastolic dysfunction should be sought. Importantly, normal subjects have normal annular e′ velocities.

Suggested Reading

Nagueh SF, et al. Recommendations for the evaluation of left ventricular diastolic function by echocardiography: an update from the American Society of Echocardiography and the European Association of Cardiovascular Imaging. *J Am Soc Echocardiogr* 2016;29:277–314.

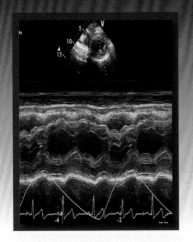

Chapter 27

Right Ventricular Physiology

Vidya Nadig

1. What is the estimated right atrial pressure in the patient in FIGURE 27.1?

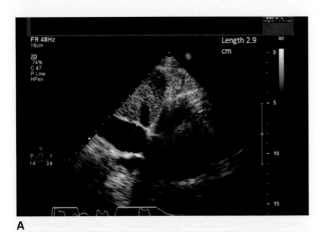

A

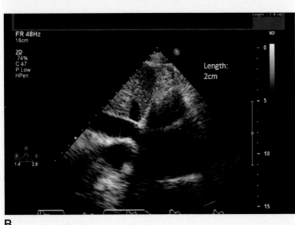

B

FIGURE 27.1 **A:** Normal respiration. **B:** Imaged when the patient was asked to "sniff."

A. 3 mm Hg
B. 5 mm Hg
C. 8 mm Hg
D. 15 mm Hg

2. Which of the following is the correct measurement of the IVC diameter in estimating RA pressure (FIG. 27.2)?

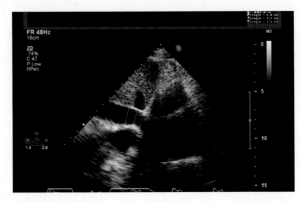

FIGURE 27.2

A. A
B. B
C. C
D. None of the above

3. A ventilated patient undergoes echocardiographic evaluation. The IVC diameter is 10 mm. This suggests an RA pressure of:

A. <10 mm Hg
B. 10 to 15 mm Hg
C. >15 mm Hg
D. Cannot determine the RA pressure as the patient is ventilated

4. Based on the hepatic vein flow pattern in FIGURE 27.3, what is the estimate of the RA pressure?

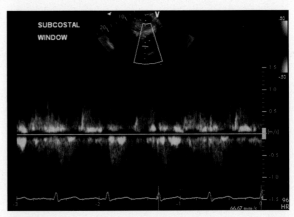

FIGURE 27.3

A. High RA pressure
B. Low RA pressure
C. Normal/low RA pressure
D. Cannot estimate

5. In the RV inflow image displayed in Figure 27.4, which leaflets of the tricuspid valve are referred to by A and B?

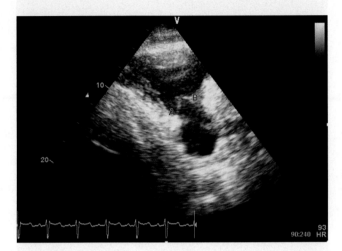

Figure 27.4

A. A, anterior; B, septal
B. A, posterior; B, sepal
C. A, posterior; B, anterior
D. A, anterior; B, posterior
E. Unable to comment

6. Which one of the following is the accurate value of TAPSE (Fig. 27.5)?

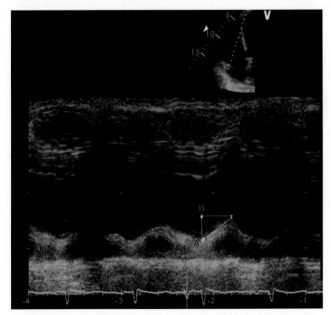

Figure 27.5

A. Distance between A and B.
B. Distance between B and C.
C. Distance between A and C.
D. Any of the above would be correct.
E. None of the above are correct.

7. The findings in a 37-year-old patient (Fig. 27.6) are suggestive of what grade of RV diastolic function?

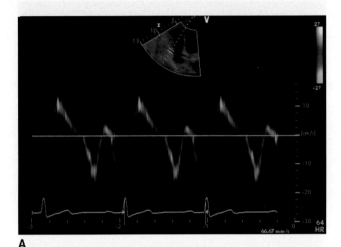

A

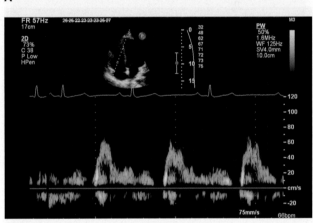

B

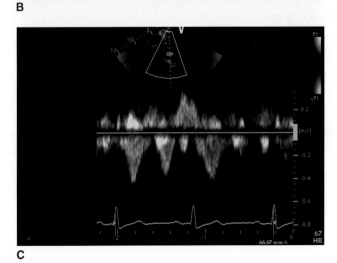

C

Figure 27.6

A. Impaired relaxation
B. Pseudonormal filling
C. Restrictive pattern
D. Normal

8. What is the pulmonary artery systolic pressure in the patient (FIG. 27.7) based on an RA pressure of 10 mm Hg?

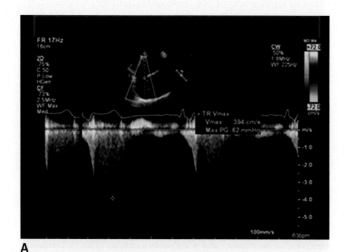

A

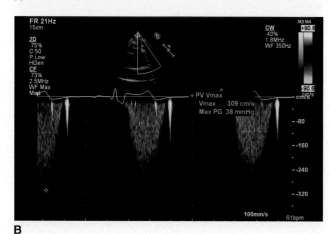

B

FIGURE 27.7

A. 34 mm Hg
B. 24 mm Hg
C. 14 mm Hg
D. 52 mm Hg

9. The end-systolic and end-diastolic parasternal short-axis views of a 75-year-old patient are shown in FIGURE 27.8. Which of the following statements is more likely to be true?

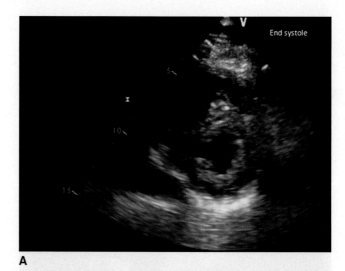

A

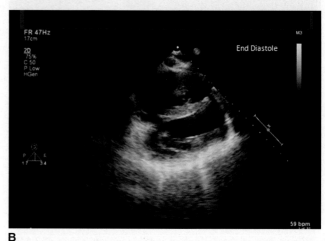

B

FIGURE 27.8

A. This patient likely has carcinoid heart disease.
B. This patient likely has Eisenmenger physiology.
C. There is evidence of a large VSD.
D. Pulmonic stenosis is suspected.
E. These images are classic for Ebstein anomaly.

10. Which of the following statements comparing echo to magnetic resonance imaging (MRI) is correct?

A. The area–length method overestimates the RV volume.
B. The disk summation method overestimates the RV volume.
C. RV volumes and EF may be precisely measured by 3D echocardiography without any risk of underestimation.
D. Manufactured ultrasound contrast agents improve the 2D and 3D echo correlation of RV volumes with MRI.
E. None of the above are accurate statements.

11. Which of the following echo views is recommended to obtain RV measurements, including linear measurements, TAPSE, and tissue Doppler S′ wave?

 A. Traditional apical four-chamber view
 B. Apical four-chamber, RV-focused view
 C. RV-modified apical four-chamber view
 D. Parasternal long-axis view
 E. Subcostal view

12. A 52-year-old male with diabetes type 2 and coronary artery bypass graft surgery 8 years ago, presents with a 1-week history of low-grade fever, malaise, fatigue, and progressive dyspnea. He had mild chest pain 10 days ago that has now resolved. He denies any orthopnea or paroxysmal nocturnal dyspnea. On exam, he is afebrile. BP is 112/75; HR is 90 bpm. An M-mode image from the patient's echocardiogram is included (Fig. 27.9). What findings are expected on the patient's clinical exam?

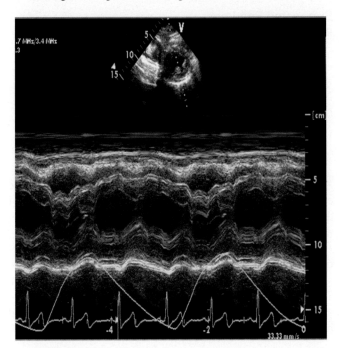

FIGURE 27.9

 A. The manual BP demonstrates a higher systolic BP with expiration than inspiration.
 B. The manual BP demonstrates a higher systolic BP with inspiration than expiration.
 C. The jugular venous pressure rises with inspiration.
 D. The jugular venous pressure does not change with respiration.
 E. The jugular venous exam demonstrates a prominent V-wave.

13. A 52-year-old male underwent atrial flutter ablation and returns 2 weeks later feeling short of breath. On exam, BP is 90/62; heart rate is 92 bpm. The cardiac auscultation is unremarkable. Prompt echocardiogram is performed and an M-mode image is included (Fig. 27.10). Which of the following statements is correct?

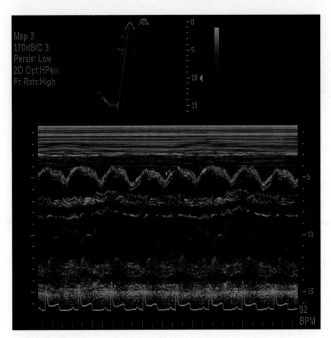

FIGURE 27.10

 A. The patient has a small-sized pericardial effusion with evidence of tamponade.
 B. The patient has a small-sized pericardial effusion with evidence of constriction.
 C. The patient has a small-sized pericardial effusion but there is no evidence of tamponade.
 D. The patient has recurrent atrial flutter, and the ablation was unsuccessful.
 E. The patient now has slow ventricular tachycardia, is unstable, and needs to be cardioverted urgently.

Answer 1: D. According to the most recent guidelines, answer D is correct. This patient had an IVC diameter of 2.9 cm, which collapses <50% with sniff suggestive of an RA pressure of 15 mm Hg (range 10 to 20 mm Hg). IVC diameter <2.1 cm with more than 50% collapse with sniff indicates a normal RA pressure of 3 mm Hg (range 0 to 5 mm Hg). In indeterminate cases, an intermediate value of 8 mm Hg (range, 5 to 10 mm Hg) can be applied.

≤2.1 cm	>50%	3 mm Hg (0–5 mm Hg)
Indeterminate cases		8 mm Hg
>2.1 cm	<50%	15 mm Hg (10–20 mm Hg)

In indeterminate cases, if any of the below mentioned secondary indices for elevated RA pressure are present, the estimated RA pressure is 15 mm Hg. If none of these are present, the RA pressure is estimated at 3 mm Hg.

1. Restrictive right-sided diastolic function
2. Tricuspid E/E′ >6
3. Diastolic flow predominance in hepatic veins

Suggested Readings

Lang RM, et al. Recommendations for cardiac chamber quantification by echocardiography in adults: an update from the American Society of Echocardiography and the European Association of Cardiovascular Imaging. *J Am Soc Echocardiogr* 2015;28:1–39.

Rudski LG, et al. Guidelines for the echocardiographic assessment of the right heart in adults: a report from the American Society of Echocardiography Endorsed by the European Association of Echocardiography, a registered branch of the European Society of Cardiology, and the Canadian Society of Echocardiography. *J Am Soc Echocardiogr* 2010;23:685–713.

Answer 2: A. The measurement should be perpendicular to the long axis of the IVC, just proximal to the hepatic vein junction, which is approximately 0.5 to 3.0 cm proximal to the ostium of the right atrium (RA).

Suggested Readings

Ommen SR, Nishimura RA, Hurrell DG, et al. Assessment of right atrial pressure with 2-dimensional and Doppler echocardiography: a simultaneous catheterization and echocardiographic study. *Mayo Clin Proc* 2000;75:24–29.

Weyman A. *Cross-Sectional Echocardiography.* Philadelphia, PA: Lea & Febiger, 1981.

Answer 3: A. In a patient ventilated with positive pressure, the degree of IVC collapse cannot be used to determine the RA pressure. However, if the IVC diameter is <12 mm Hg, this can be indicative of an RA pressure of <10 mm Hg. In these patients, a collapsed IVC is indicative of hypovolemia.

Suggested Reading

Jue J, Chung W, Schiller NB. Does inferior vena cava size predict right atrial pressures in patients receiving mechanical ventilation? *J Am Soc Echocardiogr* 1992;5:613–619.

Answer 4: C. In this case, the hepatic vein flow pattern is systolic dominant (*red arrow,* Fig. 27.11), which indicates a low/ normal RA pressure. In case of an elevated RA pressure, the systolic predominance is lost. The hepatic vein systolic filling fraction is the ratio Vs/(Vs + Vd), and a value <55% was found to be the most sensitive and specific sign of elevated RA pressure.

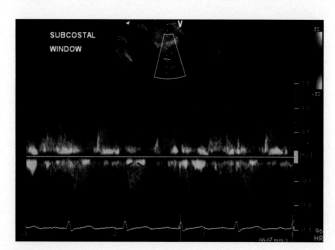

Figure 27.11

Suggested Reading

Nagueh SF, Kopelen HA, Zoghbi WA. Relation of mean right atrial pressure to echocardiographic and Doppler parameters of right atrial and right ventricular function. *Circulation* 1996;93:1160–1169.

Answer 5: C. The RV inflow is the only view that the posterior leaflet of the tricuspid valve can be visualized. Most other views such as the apical four-chamber view, parasternal short-axis view, and subcostal views visualize the anterior and septal leaflets.

> *Editor's Note: Although the RV inflow view is the most commonly used view to visualize the posterior TV leaflet since the image sector passes through the middle of this leaflet, portions of the PTVL may be seen in other views, especially when the leaflet is diseased (endocarditis, redundancy, flail, etc.). Be aware of this possibility when reading echo studies or taking echo examinations.*

Suggested Readings

Rudski LG, et al. Guidelines for the echocardiographic assessment of the right heart in adults: a report from the American Society of Echocardiography Endorsed by the European Association of Echocardiography, a registered branch of the European Society of Cardiology, and the Canadian Society of Echocardiography. *J Am Soc Echocardiogr* 2010;23:685–713.

Lang RM, et al. Recommendations for cardiac chamber quantification by echocardiography in adults: an update from the American Society of Echocardiography and the European Association of Cardiovascular Imaging. *J Am Soc Echocardiogr* 2015;28:1–39.

Answer 6: A. TAPSE stands for tricuspid annular plain systolic excursion, which is a measurement of longitudinal function of the lateral tricuspid annulus. Option A is the correct measurement that demonstrates the longitudinal movement.

Options B and C are measurements dependent on RV function and heart rate and are not accurate measurements of RV systolic function (although option C will also provide the TAPSE value as well since M-mode "distance" will report the "height" between options A and B and not "length" displayed between options A and C).

Suggested Readings

Kaul S, Tei C, Hopkins JM, et al. Assessment of right ventricular function using two-dimensional echocardiography. *Am Heart J* 1984;107:526–531.

Rudski LG, et al. Guidelines for the echocardiographic assessment of the right heart in adults: a report from the American Society of Echocardiography Endorsed by the European Association of Echocardiography, a registered branch of the European Society of Cardiology, and the Canadian Society of Echocardiography. *J Am Soc Echocardiogr* 2010;23:685–713.

Lang RM, et al. Recommendations for cardiac chamber quantification by echocardiography in adults: an update from the American Society of Echocardiography and the European Association of Cardiovascular Imaging. *J Am Soc Echocardiogr* 2015;28:1–39.

Answer 7: D. In this case, the tricuspid E/E′ of < 6 and systolic dominant hepatic vein flow indicate a normal right ventricular diastolic function in this 37-year-old patient. A tricuspid E/A ratio <0.8 suggests impaired relaxation, a tricuspid E/A ratio of

0.8 to 2.1 with an E/e′ ratio >6 or diastolic flow predominance in the hepatic veins suggests pseudonormal filling, and a tricuspid E/A ratio >2.1 with deceleration time <120 ms suggests restrictive filling.

Suggested Readings

Lang RM, et al. Recommendations for cardiac chamber quantification by echocardiography in adults: an update from the American Society of Echocardiography and the European Association of Cardiovascular Imaging. *J Am Soc Echocardiogr* 2015;28:1–39.

Rudski LG, et al. Guidelines for the echocardiographic assessment of the right heart in adults: a report from the American Society of Echocardiography Endorsed by the European Association of Echocardiography, a registered branch of the European Society of Cardiology, and the Canadian Society of Echocardiography. *J Am Soc Echocardiogr* 2010;23:685–713.

Answer 8: A. The pulmonary artery systolic pressure is almost equal to RV systolic pressure if there is no gradient across the RVOT. RV systolic pressure can be determined from TR jet velocity using the Bernoulli equation: RVSP = 4(V)2 + RA pressure, where V is the peak velocity (in meters per second) of the tricuspid valve regurgitant jet and RA pressure is estimated from IVC diameter and respiratory changes. In the case of RVOT obstruction, the gradient between the PA and RV should be subtracted from RVSP to calculate the PA systolic pressure. In the above patient, the RVSP is 72 mm Hg (62 + 10), and as there is a 38 mm Hg gradient across the pulmonic valve, this should be subtracted from 72 mm Hg to estimate the PA systolic pressure: 72 − 38 = 34 mm Hg.

Suggested Readings

Lang RM, et al. Recommendations for cardiac chamber quantification by echocardiography in adults: an update from the American Society of Echocardiography and the European Association of Cardiovascular Imaging. *J Am Soc Echocardiogr* 2015;28:1–39.

Rudski LG, et al. Guidelines for the echocardiographic assessment of the right heart in adults: a report from the American Society of Echocardiography Endorsed by the European Association of Echocardiography, a registered branch of the European Society of Cardiology, and the Canadian Society of Echocardiography. *J Am Soc Echocardiogr* 2010;23:685–713.

Answer 9: A. These views show flattening of the interventricular septum mainly seen in end diastole, which is indicative of RV volume overload (RVVO), which can be seen in significant tricuspid regurgitation (as would be expected in carcinoid heart disease) or an ASD. Flattening of the septum in end systole is more indicative of RV pressure overload situations as seen in pulmonary hypertension (Eisenmenger) or pulmonic stenosis. In VSD, the left-to-right shunting happens in systole, and the RV does not encounter a volume overload situation.

Suggested Readings

Galie N, Hinderliter AL, Torbicki A, et al. Effects of the oral endothelin-receptor antagonist bosentan on echocardiographic and Doppler measures in patients with pulmonary arterial hypertension. *J Am Coll Cardiol* 2003;41:1380–1386.

Louie EK, Rich S, Levitsky S, et al. Doppler echocardiographic demonstration of the differential effects of right ventricular pressure and volume overload on left ventricular geometry and filling. *J Am Coll Cardiol* 1992;19:84–90.

Mori S, Nakatani S, Kanzaki H, et al. Patterns of the interventricular septal motion can predict conditions of patients with pulmonary hypertension. *J Am Soc Echocardiogr* 2008;21:386–393.

Raymond RJ, Hinderliter AL, Willis PW, et al. Echocardiographic predictors of adverse outcomes in primary pulmonary hypertension. *J Am Coll Cardiol* 2002;39:1214–1219.

Ryan T, Petrovic O, Dillon JC, et al. An echocardiographic index for separation of right ventricular volume and pressure overload. *J Am Coll Cardiol* 1985;5:918–927.

Answer 10: E. The area–length method, most commonly based on modified pyramidal or ellipsoidal models of RV, underestimates the RV volume compared to MRI. The disk summation method also underestimates the RV volume due to RVOT exclusion and other limitations of echocardiography. With 3D echocardiography, there is less underestimation, and the RV volumes and EF may be accurately measured. Contrast agents improve the correlation of LV volumes but are not FDA approved nor have they been well studied for RV assessment.

Suggested Readings

Gopal AS, Chukwu EO, Iwuchukwu CJ, et al. Normal values of right ventricular size and function by real-time 3-dimensional echocardiography: comparison with cardiac magnetic resonance imaging. *J Am Soc Echocardiogr* 2007;20:445–455.

Watanabe T, Katsume H, Matsukubo H, et al. Estimation of right ventricular volume with two dimensional echocardiography. *Am J Cardiol* 1982;49:1946–1953.

Answer 11: B. Current guidelines recommend use of the RV-focused view to make linear measurements of the RV and measures of systolic function, including TAPSE, TDI S′, and fractional area shortening based on an RV-focused view. This view is obtained by angling the probe anteriorly from an apical four-chamber position, to maximize the RV minor dimension in the basal segment.

Suggested Reading

Lang RM, et al. Recommendations for cardiac chamber quantification by echocardiography in adults: an update from the American Society of Echocardiography and the European Association of Cardiovascular Imaging. *J Am Soc Echocardiogr* 2015;28:1–39.

Answer 12: C. The image represents and M-mode through the short axis of the left ventricle with constrictive physiology (Fig. 27.12). The respirometer shown at the bottom of the image delineates inspiration and expiration. With inspiration, the right ventricle fills more at the cost of the left ventricle, due to a thickened pericardium surrounding the ventricle. This results in shifting of the interventricular septum toward the left ventricle (arrow) in inspiration. The reverse happens with expiration. There is increased intrathoracic pressure, resulting in decreased filling of the right ventricle. As a result, the left ventricle has a chance to expand the septum shifts back toward the right ventricle. This interventricular dependence is classic for constrictive physiology. Also note the thickened pericardium both anteriorly and posteriorly. During constriction, JVP rises with inspiration and decreases with expiration (Kussmaul sign), making choice C correct. Higher arm cuff BP with expiration than inspiration (pulsus paradoxus) as listed in choice A would be consistent with tamponade. There is no

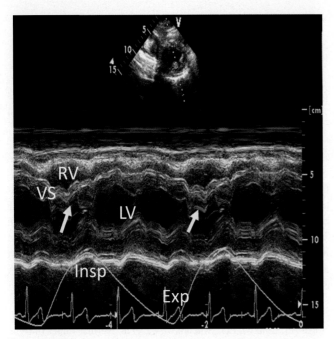

FIGURE 27.12

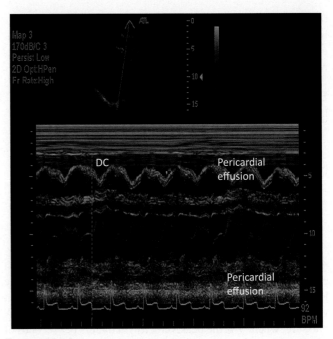

FIGURE 27.13

pericardial effusion and no evidence of tamponade physiology in the provided images, making choice A incorrect. Choice E of prominent V waves would be seen with tricuspid regurgitation. The remainder of the choices are not consistent with constrictive physiology.

Answer 13: *A.* The M-mode image through the parasternal long-axis view demonstrates diastolic collapse of the free wall of the right ventricle consistent with tamponade physiology (choice A) (FIG. 27.13). Note the opening of the mitral valve that suggests the start of diastole (marked by dashed line). At the end of RV systole, the RV relaxes resulting in lower

intracavitary RV pressure compared to the pericardium, and this results in RV collapse in diastole. As the RV fills up, the RV chamber pressure rises, and the myocardial wall moves back toward the parietal pericardium. There is a small amount of pericardial effusion, and the size of the effusion does not predict tamponade. The pericardium can accumulate a large amount of fluid over time, without developing tamponade, and even small effusions that develop rapidly can result in tamponade. There is no evidence of recurrent atrial flutter or ventricular tachycardia, by both the image and ECG, making choices D and E incorrect. There is no evidence of constriction making choice B incorrect.

Chapter 28

Acute Coronary Syndromes and Infarct Complications

Vincent L. Sorrell

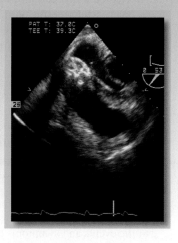

1. The earliest manifestation of myocardial ischemia is:

A. Release of troponin

B. Chest pain

C. Impairment of regional myocardial systolic thickening

D. ST-segment–T-wave abnormalities on ECG

E. Drop in blood pressure

2. Hypokinesis of a myocardial segment is defined as an increase in systolic wall thickness of:

A. More than 70%

B. More than 50%

C. <50%

D. <40%

E. <10%

3. Blood supply to the anterolateral papillary muscle is usually provided by the:

A. Right coronary artery

B. Left anterior descending coronary artery

C. Ramus (intermediate) coronary artery

D. Right coronary and left anterior descending coronary arteries

E. Right coronary and left circumflex coronary arteries

4. Which of the following conditions commonly mimics the echocardiographic findings of acute inferolateral wall myocardial infarction from plaque rupture?

A. Stress-induced cardiomyopathy

B. Type B aortic dissection

C. Acute myocarditis

D. Primary or metastatic cardiac tumors

E. Hypertrophic cardiomyopathy, apical variant

5. Non–ST elevation myocardial infarction (NSTEMI) is usually associated with which of the following echocardiographic findings?

A. Mild and/or limited segmental wall motion abnormalities

B. Pericardial effusion

C. Mitral regurgitation

D. Right ventricular dysfunction

6. Which of the following is the **least correct** option regarding myocardial infarct–related ventricular septal defect?

A. Occurs in the early phase (within the first week) of acute infarct healing.

B. It is more common in elderly women without previous myocardial infarction.

C. Nearly half of the patients have single-vessel coronary artery disease.

D. The defect is always located in the region of the thinned infarcted myocardium.

E. It requires transesophageal echocardiography (TEE) study for diagnosis in the majority of cases.

7. Which of the following statements regarding right ventricular infarction is the **least correct**?

A. It is usually associated with inferior wall myocardial infarction.

B. Hemodynamically significant right ventricular infarct is rare.

C. Patients with right ventricular infarct may develop hypotension after nitroglycerin administration.

D. Peak tricuspid regurgitation velocity is usually over 3 m/s (estimated right ventricular systolic pressure of 41 to 46 mm Hg, assuming right atrial pressure of 5 to 10 mm Hg).

E. Right-to-left shunt may occur through a patent foramen ovale.

8. Which of the following statements regarding myocardial viability is the *least correct*?

A. Regional myocardial function will likely improve after successful reperfusion if the infarcted segment involves <25% of transmural wall thickness.

B. Resting two-dimensional echocardiography can sometimes differentiate between a viable and fibrotic (scarred) segment.

C. Recovery of a stunned myocardium may take days to weeks.

D. Low-dose dobutamine echo can distinguish stunned from hibernating myocardium.

E. Viability of myocardial segments and the presence of collateral blood flow may be detected by contrast echocardiography.

9. Which of the following represents the temporal relationship of the events and symptoms that occur during an acute coronary syndrome?

A. ECG changes, angina, diastolic LV dysfunction, systolic LV dysfunction

B. Diastolic LV dysfunction, systolic LV dysfunction, ECG changes, angina

C. Angina, ECG changes, diastolic LV dysfunction, systolic LV dysfunction

D. Systolic LV dysfunction, ECG changes, diastolic LV dysfunction, angina

10. A 38-year-old female with atypical chest pain and an abnormal ECG at rest presented for an exercise echocardiogram. On her baseline and stress 2D images, she was found to have normal regional LV systolic function. Her exercise wall motion score index (WMSI) is:

A. 0

B. 17

C. 1

D. 16

11. A transthoracic echocardiogram with perflutren protein type A microspheres for left ventricular opacification was performed following a non–Q-wave myocardial infarction to improve left ventricular (LV) cavity opacification and to rule out mural thrombus. Which of the following would not improve the image (VIDEO 28.1)?

A. Lower the mechanical index.

B. Push a larger dose of contrast.

C. Change from harmonic to fundamental imaging.

D. Deliver a faster saline flush.

12. Which of the following is a mechanism for the development of mitral regurgitation during and after an acute coronary syndrome?

A. Papillary muscle dysfunction

B. Segmental wall motion abnormalities

C. Progressive left ventricular dilation

D. All of the options

13. The following statements are true regarding the mass shown on the 2D echocardiogram in VIDEO 28.2 **except:**

A. The incidence of apical left ventricular clots has decreased in the era of thrombolytic therapy.

B. It is associated with severe segmental wall motion abnormality at the distal septal wall and apex.

C. Its appearance suggests a high probability of systemic embolization.

D. Urgent surgical removal is indicated.

E. Anticoagulation with warfarin should be instituted for at least 3 to 6 months.

Questions 14 to 16

An 88-year-old female with a remote history of MI 30 years ago presents as an outpatient with progressive symptoms of congestive heart failure over the past 2 weeks. She was found to have a chronically occluded right coronary artery (RCA) and moderate to severe disease in her left anterior artery (LAD) and circumflex arteries upon catheterization.

14. Transthoracic echocardiography (FIG. 28.1 and VIDEO 28.3) demonstrated a/an:

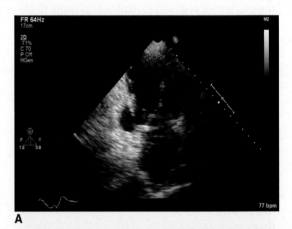

A

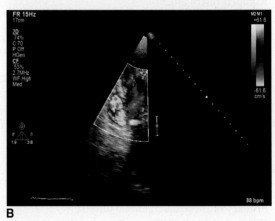

B

FIGURE 28.1

A. Basal anterior ventricular aneurysm
B. Basal inferior ventricular aneurysm
C. Basal inferior pseudoaneurysm
D. Basal anterior pseudoaneurysm
E. Basal inferior ventricular septal defect

15. Right heart catheterization was performed; the patient was noted to have a Qp:Qs of 2.8. Transesophageal echocardiography images (Fig. 28.2 and Video 28.4) also demonstrate a/an:

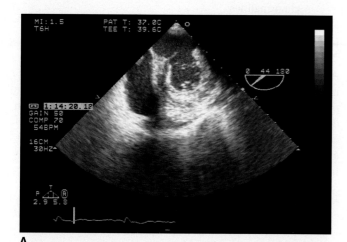

A

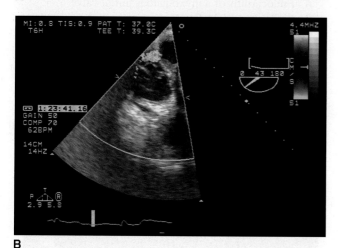

B

Figure 28.2

A. Atrial septal defect
B. Patent ductus arteriosus
C. Supracristal VSD
D. Muscular VSD
E. Membranous VSD

16. Given the significant cardiac shunt and clinical heart failure symptoms, repair of her shunt was attempted. Which of the following procedures did the patient undergo? (See Fig. 28.3 and Video 28.5.)

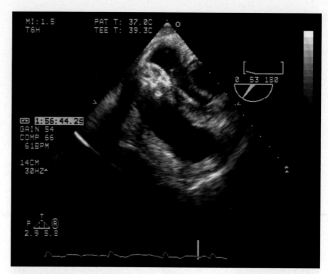

Figure 28.3

A. Sirolimus-coated stent
B. Covered endovascular stent
C. Amplatzer septal occluder
D. Open surgical repair of the ventricular septum

Questions 17 to 19

A 65-year-old female with a history of hypertension and tobacco use had a witnessed collapse at home after developing severe chest pain. The patient was resuscitated, and 12-lead ECG revealed anterior ST-segment elevations, and she was taken emergently to the cardiac catheterization laboratory.

Coronary catheterization was performed (Video 28.6), and subsequently, an emergent transthoracic echocardiogram was performed (Video 28.7).

17. Which of the following is the most appropriate next step in the management of the patient?

A. Percutaneous intervention of the left main artery
B. Spiral CT scan
C. Intra-aortic balloon pump placement (IABP)
D. Immediate cardiovascular surgery consultation
E. Thrombolytic therapy

18. All of the following are true statements regarding the entity above **except:**

A. Involvement of the left main coronary artery is more common than the right coronary artery.
B. Coronary artery occlusion may be secondary to extravasation of blood into the pericardial and perivascular tissues.
C. Coronary artery involvement can be assessed with transesophageal echocardiography.
D. Acute myocardial infarction related to involvement of a dissection flap into the ostium of a coronary artery occurs in <5% of patients with type A aortic dissection.

19. The TEE image in Figure 28.4 illustrates which of the following?

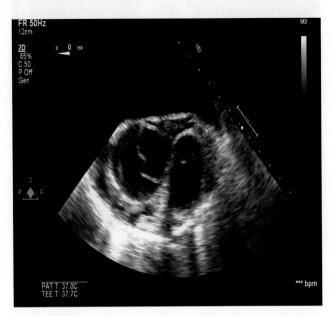

Figure 28.4

A. Fistulous communication between the aorta and pulmonary artery

B. The probable bicuspid aortic valve with visualization of left atrial appendage thrombus

C. Stanford type A aortic dissection with extension into the right coronary artery

D. Stanford type B aortic dissection with aortic arch involvement

E. Stanford type A aortic dissection with extension into the left main artery

Questions 20 and 21

A 66-year-old male presented to the ER with severe chest pain and hypotension. Electrocardiogram revealed acute posterior wall infarction. Echocardiogram revealed no evidence of mitral regurgitation, and inferolateral wall hypokinesis was seen. Transthoracic echocardiogram images from subcostal view are shown in Video 28.8.

20. The clinical scenario and echocardiogram images are most consistent with which of the following?

A. Pericardial mass secondary to metastatic disease

B. Ventricular septal defect

C. Pericardial hematoma

D. Dressler syndrome

E. Right ventricular infarction

21. Regarding echocardiographic findings with myocardial rupture complicating myocardial infarction, all of the following are true **except**?

A. Myocardial constraint can be used to help confirm the diagnosis.

B. A site of rupture is universally seen with Doppler color flow into the pericardial space.

C. Pericardial effusion > 5 mm in size is commonly seen.

D. Associated inferior wall motion abnormalities are less frequently seen than anterior or lateral wall motion abnormalities.

Questions 22 to 24

A 52-year-old patient presents with a history of recently diagnosed pulmonary fibrosis at an outside institution with acute profound shortness of breath. His 12-lead electrocardiogram demonstrates a recent inferoposterior STEMI with possible lateral extension. He has a grade III/VI holosystolic murmur radiating to the axilla on physical examination. Video 28.9 shows his echocardiogram.

22. Upon reviewing the available images, the etiology of the mitral regurgitation appears to be most likely the result of which of the following conditions?

A. Endocarditis of a myxomatous mitral valve

B. Flail posterior leaflet of a myxomatous mitral valve

C. Inferior wall myocardial infarction

D. Flail posterior leaflet

E. Inferior wall myocardial infarction and flail posterior leaflet

23. Using the PISA method, which of the following represents the calculated effective regurgitant office and associated severity of mitral regurgitation? (See Fig. 28.5.)

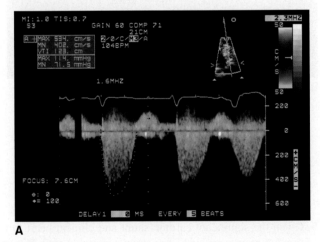

A

Figure 28.5

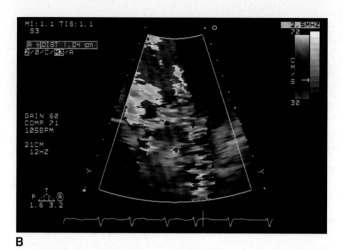

B

FIGURE 28.5 (*Continued*)

A. ERO = 2 cm², moderate mitral regurgitation
B. ERO = 32 cm², moderate mitral regurgitation
C. ERO = 34 cm², severe mitral regurgitation
D. Not enough information provided
E. Unable to accurately calculate ERO

24. Ultimately, the patient received a CABG (SVG-RPDA SVG-RPL) and a 29-mm Carpentier-Edwards ThermaFix Bioprosthetic Mitral Valve Replacement. He recovered and he was discharged. According to the provided preoperative transesophageal images (VIDEO 28.10), which of the following segment(s) of the mitral valve leaflets appear to be flail?

A. A1 and P1
B. P1 and P2
C. A2 only
D. P2 only
E. P3 only
F. Not enough information

25. What are the wall motion abnormalities in this patient who suffered a myocardial infarction (VIDEO 28.11)?

A. Right ventricular free wall hypokinesis
B. Anterior and anteroseptal akinesis
C. Lateral and inferolateral wall akinesis
D. Apical akinesis
E. None of the options

26. A 45-year-old male with hypertension and significant family history of CAD presented with chest pain for several days. He underwent PCI to the LAD but had no reflow. An ACE inhibitor, beta-blocker, aspirin, and spironolactone were started. The assessment of left ventricular ejection fraction should be performed:

A. On admission prior to PCI.
B. 6 months after discharge.
C. Prior to discharge.
D. LVEF is not necessary at this time.
E. None of the options.

27. After obtaining the echocardiogram as shown in FIGURE 28.6 AND VIDEO 28.12, you decide:

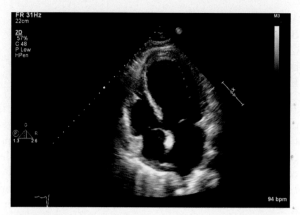

FIGURE 28.6

A. Start heparin as a bridge to Coumadin, keeping an INR of 2 to 3.
B. Keep aspirin at a dose of 325 mg.
C. Discharge the patient and have him return in 6 weeks.
D. Aspirin and Plavix should be sufficient.
E. None of the options.

28. He comes for follow-up at 6 weeks in your office, and you obtain an echocardiogram (FIG. 28.7). Which method is best to evaluate for ejection fraction?

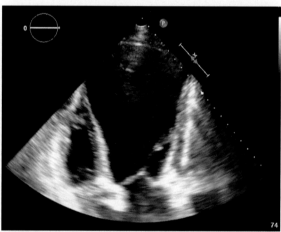

A

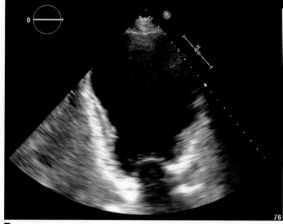

B

FIGURE 28.7

A. Fractional shortening
B. 2D echocardiography using biplane Simpson
C. 3D echocardiography
D. Speckle tracking
E. None of the options

29. This patient feels a little tired climbing stairs though he is doing most of his physical activities without much limitation. On a viability study, the left ventricular apex and apical cap are nonviable. He still has thrombus noted on the echocardiogram even after 6 months of anticoagulation, his LVEF is unchanged, and he has no evidence of mitral regurgitation. He had a syncopal episode and documented ventricular tachycardia on monitor even after VT ablation and antiarrhythmic therapy. What is your next course of action?

A. CABG
B. Aneurysmectomy
C. Aneurysmectomy, CABG, and mitral valve repair
D. AICD implantation only
E. None of the options

Answer 1: C. Segmental impairment of myocardial systolic thickening and motion precedes the clinical, electrocardiographic, and chemical manifestations of myocardial ischemia and acute coronary syndrome; ECG changes of myocardial ischemia usually follow chest pain with increase in troponin developing later (therefore, Options A, B, and D are incorrect). Echocardiography therefore can be used for the early detection of myocardial ischemia and/or infarction. A drop in systolic blood pressure during myocardial ischemia usually signifies extensive multivessel coronary artery disease or right ventricular infarction. Since this is not an early manifestation of myocardial ischemia, Option D is incorrect.

Answer 2: D. Normally, left ventricular wall thickness increases more than 50% during systole; *hypokinesis* is defined as an increase in systolic wall thickness of <40%. An increase of systolic left ventricular wall thickness of more than 70% implies a vigorous or hyperdynamic segment, while *akinesis* is defined as an increase of <10% (therefore, Options A, B, and E are incorrect). Visual assessment of systolic wall thickening by two-dimensional echocardiography may not distinguish a difference between 40% and 50% change in left ventricular wall thickness in systole; M-mode echocardiography can be useful in recording the temporal changes in wall thickness and allowing exact measurements of systolic and diastolic left ventricular wall thickness.

Answer 3: E. The left ventricular anterolateral papillary muscle usually has a dual supply from the right coronary and left circumflex coronary arteries, while the posteromedial papillary muscle has single coronary supply from the right or circumflex coronary artery; therefore, dysfunction, infarct, or rupture of the posteromedial papillary muscle with associated mitral regurgitation is 6 to 10 times more frequent than that of the anterolateral papillary muscle (which requires multivessel coronary artery disease). Left anterior descending coronary artery and ramus (intermediate)

coronary artery do not usually supply the papillary muscles (therefore, Options B, C, and D are incorrect).

Answer 4: C. Acute myocarditis can produce regional segmental wall motion abnormalities along with ST-segment–T-wave changes. For reasons not entirely clear, the inferolateral myocardial wall segment is commonly the involved region. This has been very well demonstrated on cardiac MRI late gadolinium enhancement studies, which frequently reveal "subepicardial enhancement" in this regional territory.

Stress-induced cardiomyopathy can produce clinical, electrocardiographic, and echocardiographic findings indistinguishable from acute coronary syndrome with segmental wall motion abnormalities involving any region of the LV; however, the distal LV myocardium and the entire LV apex ("apical ballooning syndrome" or "takotsubo cardiomyopathy") are most common. An isolated inferolateral regional wall motion would be much less common. The intimal flap during proximal aortic root dissection (type A) can involve the ostia of the left main and right coronary arteries and result in acute myocardial ischemia and infarct. A type B aortic dissection, which does not involve the ascending aorta, will not impact coronary flow.

Primary cardiac tumors like myxoma can embolize to the coronary arteries, and malignant metastatic cardiac tumors can infiltrate areas of the myocardium and produce segmental left ventricular wall motion abnormalities. Cardiac infiltration from primary or metastatic malignancy remains rare.

Apical hypertrophic cardiomyopathy represents <5% of all idiopathic hypertrophic cardiomyopathies and is localized exclusively to the apical area ("spade-like" appearance at end systole); it is associated with marked T-wave inversion on anterior ECG leads. It would not cause an inferolateral regional wall motion abnormality.

> *Editor's Note: The apical variant form of HCM may be misinterpreted as an apical aneurysm when the endocardial border definition is suboptimal and the apical LV cavity is filled with "myocardium." In this circumstance, the normal acoustic mismatch (necessary for image generation) created from the ventricular cavity/myocardial border interface is absent (there is cavity obliteration with myocardium replacing the LV cavity). At times, the apical myocardial wall may be so thick that the epicardial borders are displaced "outward" in systole, and therefore, the echo reader may be fooled into thinking this is an LV apical aneurysm. This can readily be discerned with LV contrast opacification or with cardiac MRI or CT scanning.*

Answer 5: A. In contrast with ST elevation or transmural myocardial infarcts, NSTEMI or subendocardial myocardial infarctions may have normal global and regional myocardial function or produce very limited and/or mild segmental wall motion abnormalities. Pericardial effusion, mitral regurgitation, and right ventricular dysfunction are usually associated with STEMI, and they are rarely seen with NSTEMI (therefore, Options B, C, and D are incorrect). Newer echocardiographic techniques including 2D strain with speckle tracking may provide more accurate and sensitive assessment of segmental wall motion abnormalities associated with NSTEMI.

Answer 6: E. The diagnosis can be established 90% of the time by transthoracic 2D echocardiography (TTE); TEE may be necessary in a small subgroup of patients with suboptimal transthoracic study. All other statements regarding post–myocardial infarction ventricular septal defect are correct (Options A, B, C, and D). The defect has a dyskinetic motion near the edge of the thinned myocardium and the border of the noninfarcted myocardium, and it is associated with left-to-right shunting by color-flow Doppler.

Answer 7: D. Although tricuspid regurgitation usually develops after right ventricular infarct, right ventricular systolic pressure is not elevated, and therefore, peak tricuspid regurgitation velocity is usually <2 m/s (with normal estimated right ventricular systolic pressure of 21 to 26 mm Hg, adding 5 to 10 mm Hg for right atrial pressure). However, the right ventricle and right atrium are dilated, and right atrial pressure may increase, thus causing right-to-left shunt through a patent foramen ovale and hypoxemia in some patients (therefore, Option E is correct as well as Options A, B, and C regarding the clinical manifestations of right ventricular infarction).

Answer 8: D. Although low-dose (5 to 20 µg/kg/min) dobutamine echo study can assess for viability of myocardial segments, it cannot distinguish between stunned and hibernating myocardium. Contrast echocardiography with myocardial perfusion has been shown to detect viable myocardium by demonstrating the extent of collateral blood flow within the infarct region (therefore, Option E as well as Options A, B, and C are correct statements); nonviable (fibrotic) myocardium may appear on resting 2D-echo as a thin, "echogenic," and akinetic segment.

Suggested Readings
Questions 1 to 8
Feigenbaum H. *Echocardiography.* 5th ed. Philadelphia, PA: Lea & Febiger, 1994.

Flachskampf FA, et al. Cardiac imaging after myocardial infarction. *Eur Heart J* 2011;32:272–283.

Mor-Avi V, et al. Current and evolving echocardiographic techniques for the quantitative evaluation of cardiac mechanics: ASE/EAE consensus statement on methodology and indications. *J Am Soc Echocardiogr* 2011;24(3):277–313.

Mulvagh SL, DeMaria AN, Feinstein SB, et al. Contrast echocardiography: current and future applications. *Am Soc Echocardiogr* 2000;13:331–342.

Oh J, Seward J, Tajik A. *The Echo Manual.* 1st ed. Boston, MA: Little Brown & Company, 1994.

Panidis J. *Cardiac Ultrasound.* 1st ed. Cambridge, MA: Blackwell Science, 1996.

Answer 9: B. Acute myocardial ischemia represents a mismatch of oxygen supply and demand. The subsequent series of events and provoked symptoms are termed "the ischemic cascade." Temporally, coronary ischemia impairs left ventricular compliance first (diastolic LV dysfunction),

myocardial contractility next (systolic LV dysfunction), induces ST-segment changes (ECG changes), and then produces angina.

Answer 10: C. Segmental LV wall motion scoring in echocardiography is based on the ACC/AHA 16-segment model. In order to calculate a wall motion score index (WMSI), ventricular wall motion is graded on a four-point scale. Normal or hyperkinesis, 1; hypokinesis, 2; akinesis, 3; dyskinesis or aneurysm, 4. The score of all 16 segments (the apical cap is not included) is added and divided by the total number of segments. The wall motion score index for stress echocardiography has been directly associated with the incidence of cardiac events during follow-up.

Answer 11: C. The video clip demonstrates a poorly opacified LV cavity with rapid destruction of ultrasound contrast. When imaging with ultrasound contrast, it is preferable to use the low mechanical index (MI) preset provided by the machine vendor. Ideally, the mechanical index (MI) should be 0.15 to 0.3. Suboptimal LV opacification can often be overcome by increasing the dose of contrast. A faster saline flush can increase the short-term effective contrast dose. Changing from harmonic imaging to fundamental would not provide an improvement in LV opacification.

Answer 12: D. All of the aforementioned are causes of mitral regurgitation. There is a wide clinical spectrum of involvement of the papillary muscle, from transient ischemia to frank infarction and papillary muscle rupture. The posteromedial papillary muscle is much more likely to become dysfunctional due to the usual single blood supply from the right coronary artery. The anterolateral papillary muscle is supplied by both the left circumflex and left anterior descending arteries.

Segmental wall motion abnormalities, often involving the inferior wall, can lead to significant mitral regurgitation. This may be a reflection of myocardial ischemia or frank infarction.

Over time, the left ventricle can dilate as a result of infarction or severe multivessel coronary artery disease. This will lead to mitral annular dilation and subsequent mitral regurgitation.

Answer 13: D. Although this large apical LV thrombus in association with extensive anterior myocardial infarction is pedunculated and somewhat mobile, thus having a higher chance of embolization, surgical removal is rarely indicated unless it is highly mobile and has already caused a systemic embolic event. Anticoagulation with warfarin for 3 to 6 months will likely cause a decrease in size or complete resolution of the thrombus; the benefit of continuous anticoagulation beyond that period is unclear.

Answer 14: C. Echocardiography is an excellent tool to help differentiate pseudoaneurysm from true ventricular aneurysms. The orifice of a pseudoaneurysm is usually seen as a distinct discontinuity in the ventricular wall. Typically, the ratio of orifice to cavity diameter for pseudoaneurysms is <0.5, while the ratio for true aneurysms is >0.9. Doppler color flow at the orifice of the cavity can also help differentiate pseudoaneurysms from true aneurysms. The presence of turbulent flow at the orifice of the cavity supports pseudoaneurysm. Ultrasound contrast can often be utilized to better delineate cavity anatomy and even superimposed thrombus.

Answer 15: D. Ventricular septal defects can be classified into four different subtypes:

1. Infundibular (including supracristal, subaortic, and subpulmonary)
2. Membranous (inferior to the crista and borders the septal tricuspid leaflet)
3. Inlet (deficient inlet septum leading to an AV canal)
4. Muscular (bordered only by trabecular septal muscle)

The images demonstrate a type 4 muscular VSD within the basal inferoseptum muscular septum.

Answer 16: C. The images demonstrate a successfully deployed Amplatzer atrial septal occluder device within the ventricular septal defect. There was no evidence of residual shunt.

Answer 17: D. This patient has an acute ascending aortic dissection complicated by extension into the left main coronary artery. Management of this condition requires emergent surgical repair.

Answer 18: A. Ascending aortic dissection extending into the right coronary artery is more common than involvement of the left main coronary artery. The remaining answer choices are all correct.

Answer 19: E. The image was acquired in the upper esophagus at the level of the aortic root and coronary arteries. A dissection flap is seen in the ascending aorta with involvement of the left main coronary artery.

Answer 20: C. The transthoracic echocardiogram images reveal hematoma in the pericardial space consistent with the probable diagnosis of myocardial rupture, complicating this patient's posterior myocardial infarction.

Answer 21: B. A site of rupture is not always visualized by echocardiography. Most commonly, only a pericardial effusion > 5 mm is seen containing pericardial hematoma. The remainder of the answer choices are true statements regarding myocardial rupture.

Answer 22: E. The two-chamber view demonstrates hypokinesis of the inferior wall with a flail posterior leaflet. Cardiac catheterization demonstrated a 100% mid-right coronary artery occlusion and a 100% third obtuse marginal occlusion. The result is ischemia and subsequent rupture of a chordae. Although the mitral valve may be described as somewhat thickened, this is not a typical myxomatous valve. There is no evidence of endocarditis.

Answer 23: E. Although the color-low Doppler suggests severe mitral regurgitation, the information provided for PISA calculation will probably not provide an accurate effective regurgitant orifice. Primarily, the Doppler signal for calculating the PISA radius is difficult to assess. Small changes in this assessment will significantly affect the calculate ERO.

In addition, there is a significant angle between the plane of the anterior and posterior leaflets. When the plane of the mitral leaflets is not nearly 180 degrees, the lack of correction for this angle will significantly affect the ERO.

Given this information, the ERO by the PISA method should not be calculated in order to avoid overestimation or underestimation of the mitral regurgitation.

Answer 24: E. The third scallop of the posterior leaflet appears to be flail. This is best seen in the two-chamber view at approximately 90 degrees.

A1 and P1 do not appear to be affected as seen in the four-chamber view at 0 degrees. A2 and A3 do not appear to be affected in multiple views. P2 does not appear to be flail at the 120-degree view.

Suggested Readings
Questions 9 to 24

Biaggi P, Jedrzkiewicz S, Gruner C, et al. Quantification of mitral valve anatomy by three-dimensional transesophageal echocardiography in mitral valve prolapse predicts surgical anatomy and the complexity of mitral valve repair. *J Am Soc Echocardiogr* 2012;25:758–765.

Brown SL, Gropler RJ, et al. Distinguishing left ventricular aneurysm from pseudoaneurysm. *Chest* 1997;111:1403–1409.

Flachskampf FA, Schmid M, Rost C, et al. Cardiac imaging after myocardial infarction. *Eur Heart J* 2011;32:272–283.

Mittle S, Makaryus AN, Mangion J. Role of contrast echocardiography in the assessment of myocardial rupture. *Echocardiography* 2003;20(1):77–81.

Mulvagh SL, Rakowski H, et al. American society of echocardiography consensus statement on the clinical applications of ultrasonic contrast agents in echocardiography. *J Am Soc Echocardigr* 2008;21:1179–1201.

Oh J, Seward J, Tajik A. *The Echo Manual.* 1st ed. Boston, MA: Little Brown & Company, 1994.

Panidis J. *Cardiac Ultrasound.* 1st ed. Cambridge, MA: Blackwell Science, 1996.

Pellikka PA, Nagueh, SF, et al. American society of echocardiography recommendations for performance, interpretation, and application of stress echocardiography. *J Am Soc Echocardigr* 2007;20:1021–1041.

Slater J, Brown RJ, Antonelli TAA, et al. Cardiogenic shock due to cardiac free wall rupture or tamponade after acute myocardial infarction: a report from the SHOCK Trial Registry. *J Am Coll Cardiol* 2000;36(3 suppl A):1117–1122.

Answer 25: C.

Option A is incorrect since the right ventricle appears normal in size and contracts normally.

Option B is incorrect.

Option C is correct. There is akinesis of the lateral and inferolateral wall when compared to the opposing walls, which appear hyperdynamic.

Option D is incorrect. There are more extensive abnormalities other than just the apex.

Option E is incorrect.

This patient suffered an acute myocardial infarction involving the lateral and inferolateral wall, which in this case was a circumflex obstruction, which was then successfully revascularized.

Suggested Reading

Lang RM, et al. Recommendations for cardiac chamber quantification by echocardiography in adults: an update from the American Society of Echocardiography and the European Association of Cardiovascular Imaging. *J Am Soc Echocardiogr* 2015;28(1):1–39.

Answer 26: C.

Option A is incorrect. There is no urgency in obtaining LVEF prior to PCI.

Option B is incorrect. After myocardial infarction, left ventricular assessment should be reassessed in patients with a large anterior wall myocardial infarction or LVEF < 40% approximately 6 weeks after MI.

Option C is correct. LVEF should be assessed in all patients after STEMI, which most accurately predicts future cardiac events.

Option D is incorrect. There should be an assessment of LVEF post–myocardial infarction to help determine treatment and aids in prognosis.

The assessment of LVEF is a Class I indication by the ACC/AHA guidelines in all patients after STEMI since.

Suggested Reading

Antman EM, Hand M, Armstrong PW, et al. 2007 Focused update of the ACC/AHA 2004 Guidelines for the Management of Patients with ST-Elevation Myocardial Infarction: a report of the American College of Cardiology/American Heart Association Task Force on Practice Guidelines: developed in collaboration with the Canadian Cardiovascular Society endorsed by the American Academy of Family Physicians: 2007 writing group to review new evidence and update the ACC/AHA 2004 Guidelines for the Management of Patients with ST-Elevation Myocardial Infarction, writing on behalf of the 2004 Writing Committee. *Circulation* 2008;117:296–329.

Answer 27: A.

Option A is correct. This patient has a laminated thrombus in the left ventricular apex. There is an extensive anteroapical myocardial infarction resulting in apical akinesis.

Option B is incorrect. Aspirin is insufficient to treat left ventricular thrombus.

Option C is incorrect. Even though the left ventricular thrombus is laminated, the apical akinesis leaves the patient at risk for development of further thrombus until there is improved left ventricular function.

Option D is incorrect. Though the patient will be on aspirin and Plavix post–myocardial infarction for secondary prevention and also for the prevention of stent thrombosis, it is insufficient to treat intracavitary thrombus.

Option E is incorrect.

Based on the guidelines for myocardial infarction, those after STEMI who have a large or anterior MI, atrial fibrillation,

previous embolus or known LV thrombus, or cardiogenic shock should receive IV unfractionated heparin or low molecular weight heparin. In addition to the treatment of left ventricular thrombus, the purpose of anticoagulation is to prevent stroke (0.75% to 1.2% of MIs).

Suggested Reading

Antman EM, Hand M, Armstrong PW, et al. 2007 Focused update of the ACC/AHA 2004 Guidelines for the Management of Patients with ST-Elevation Myocardial Infarction: a report of the American College of Cardiology/American Heart Association Task Force on Practice Guidelines: developed in collaboration with the Canadian Cardiovascular Society endorsed by the American Academy of Family Physicians: 2007 writing group to review new evidence and update the ACC/AHA 2004 Guidelines for the Management of Patients with ST-Elevation Myocardial Infarction, writing on behalf of the 2004 Writing Committee. *Circulation* 2008;117:296–329.

Answer 28: C.

Option A is incorrect. Fractional shortening is a one-dimensional method to calculate ejection fraction, which lends itself to inaccuracies due to assumptions that all the wall segments are equally contracting and it assumes a certain shape. Once the ventricle is irregularly shaped or has wall motion abnormalities beyond the septal and inferolateral wall, the method is not valid.

Option B is incorrect. Biplane Simpson is a better method than fractional shortening since there is more than one plane; however, this method is also based on a geometric assumption that the ventricle is bullet shaped. Volume estimation based on this method for dilated or aneurysmal ventricles is also inaccurate. There is usually foreshortening that occurs in the two-chamber view, which introduces inaccuracies.

Option C is correct. Three-dimensional echocardiography has been established as more accurate and reliable compared with M-mode or 2D echo methods since there is no geometric assumption and a common long axis is achieved with a 3D volumetric acquisition.

Option D is incorrect. Quantitation of volume and function has been investigated using speckle tracking; however, it is not well established.

Option E is incorrect.

The best method for volume estimation and ventricular function is three-dimensional echocardiography, which has been compared to MRI as a standard. The best method for volume estimation and ventricular function is three-dimensional echocardiography, which has been compared to cardiac MRI as a reference standard. Unlike 2D techniques, this method has no geometric assumptions; no errors in acquiring the correct, orthogonal, imaging plane along a common axis; and one-beat acquisitions with the capability of averaging multiple cardiac cycles is now possible.

Suggested Reading

Lang RM, Badano LP, Mor-Avi V, et al. Recommendations for Cardiac Chamber Quantification by Echocardiography in Adults: An Update from the American Society of Echocardiography and the European Association of Cardiovascular Imaging. *J Am Soc Echocardiogr* 2015;28(1):1–39.e14.

Answer 29: B.

Option A is incorrect. There is no evidence for CABG in this patient since there are nonviable segments in the previous area of infarct.

Option B is correct. An aneurysmectomy is indicated due to syncope and presence of ventricular tachycardia that is persistent even after antiarrhythmic and VT ablation. Persistent thrombus and congestive heart failure are also indications for aneurysmectomy.

Option C is incorrect. This patient does not have mitral regurgitation and nonviable myocardium; hence, there is no indication for mitral valve repair and bypass surgery.

Option D is incorrect. An AICD in this case may result in repetitive shocks since the patient has persistent VT despite antiarrhythmics and VT ablation.

Option E is incorrect.

Aneurysmectomy is a Class IIa recommendation in patients with intractable ventricular tachyarrhythmia and/or heart failure. The STICH trial (Surgical Treatment for Ischemic Heart Failure) sought to evaluate CABG versus intensive medical therapy and whether CABG along with surgical ventricular reconstruction would improve survival and rehospitalization in patients with decreased LVEF (≤35%) and coronary disease amenable for revascularization. From this trial, there was no difference in outcome between CABG and medical therapy.

Suggested Readings

Antman EM, Hand M, Armstrong PW, et al. 2007 Focused update of the ACC/AHA 2004 Guidelines for the Management of Patients with ST-Elevation Myocardial Infarction: a report of the American College of Cardiology/American Heart Association Task Force on Practice Guidelines: developed in collaboration with the Canadian Cardiovascular Society endorsed by the American Academy of Family Physicians: 2007 writing group to review new evidence and update the ACC/AHA 2004 Guidelines for the Management of Patients with ST-Elevation Myocardial Infarction, writing on behalf of the 2004 Writing Committee. *Circulation* 2008;117:296–329.

Velazquez EJ, Lee KL, Deja MA, et al. Coronary-artery bypass surgery in patients with left ventricular dysfunction. *N Engl J Med* 2011;364:1607–1616.

Chapter 29

Echo Features of Chronic CAD

Vincent L. Sorrell

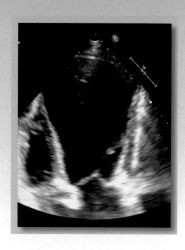

1. A 67-year-old hypertensive female presents with a neurologic deficit in the distribution of the right middle cerebral artery. Ten days prior to her presentation, she had a prolonged episode of mild chest discomfort lasting several hours, which resolved spontaneously and for which she did not seek any medical attention. Her ECG shows Q waves in anterior precordial leads along with mild ST elevation. Cardiac enzymes are within normal limits. A 2D echocardiogram is obtained (Videos 29.1 and 29.2). Which one of the following statements regarding the finding on her echocardiogram is *least* accurate?

A. The likelihood of an embolic event is highest in the first 2 weeks of an acute myocardial infarction.
B. The incidence of a left ventricular (LV) thrombus in anterior myocardial infarction has decreased since the advent of thrombolytic therapy.
C. Mobility and protrusion of LV thrombus have been associated with higher incidence of embolic events.
D. Left-sided contrast agents improve detection of LV apical thrombi.
E. Adult transducers are better designed than pediatric transducers to aid in resolving apical thrombi.

2. Which of the following statements regarding the abnormality shown in Videos 29.3 and 29.4 is *least* accurate?

A. Left ventricular aneurysms post myocardial infarction is associated with increased incidence of cardiac failure.
B. Left ventricular thrombi are frequently found in association with LV aneurysms and may result in systemic embolization.
C. Life-threatening arrhythmias may occur in these patients.
D. Left-sided contrast agents are helpful in detection and in defining aneurysms.
E. Transesophageal echo (TEE) may provide improved visualization of the LV apical aneurysm.

3. A 63-year-old female presented to the emergency room with her husband. The couple was out having dinner when the 67-year-old spouse started having chest pain. The restaurant owner called the EMT, and upon their arrival, an ECG was obtained that showed ST-segment elevation anteriorly.

The patient was immediately transferred to the nearest hospital. In the ER, the wife also started having chest pain, and her ECG showed ST-segment elevation of approximately 2 to 3 mm in the anterior leads. Cardiac troponin was ordered, but she was taken to the catheterization lab, which had just finished her husband's case. The wife is known to have hypertension and is a smoker. After the procedure, an echo was requested (shown in Videos 29.5 and 29.6). Cardiac troponin came back significantly elevated at four. Which of the following statements is correct?

A. Coronary angiography must be completely normal and cannot have nonobstructive CAD to make this diagnosis.
B. The clinical presentation is a manifestation of an aborted anterior MI with a long "wraparound" left anterior descending coronary artery.
C. It is estimated that one-third of cases may have right ventricular involvement.
D. Late gadolinium enhancement (LGE) on CMR is generally present in these cases.
E. The most common LV wall motion abnormality conforms to a single vascular territory, often confusing the 2D echocardiographic evaluation.

4. A 73-year-old male with a history of diabetes mellitus type 2, hypertension, and smoking presented to the ER with progressive shortness of breath. He had an acute MI about a week ago and had PCI and stent implantation. He had presented several hours after onset of his symptoms and did have a significant rise in his cardiac troponin. He has not felt better since he was discharged and has continued to have shortness of breath, now progressing to orthopnea and paroxysmal nocturnal dyspnea. On physical exam, he had difficulty breathing; vital signs were BP of 94/52 mm Hg, heart rate of 99/minute, and respiratory rate of 23/minute, and he was afebrile. Cardiovascular findings included JVD, bilateral rales, and an S3 gallop. The abdomen was nondistended and nontender. The lower extremities showed 1+ edema. The cardiologist who saw the patient on consultation decided to obtain an echocardiogram shown in Video 29.7. Regarding the diagnosis, which one of the following statements is most accurate?

A. A TTE is a reasonable first step and will make a definitive diagnosis in 75% of patients.

B. A TEE is rarely necessary and has a diagnostic accuracy only slightly higher than TTE compared to angiography.

C. Based upon the echo morphology, this is more likely a pseudoaneurysm than a true aneurysm.

D. TEE is the first test performed when the evaluation of the mitral valve is indicated.

E. Contrast echo is valuable in making the diagnosis and safe in this clinical setting, even with a suspected ventricular septal defect.

5. Which one of the following is the *least* likely mechanism of ischemic mitral regurgitation (MR)?

A. Dislocation of the papillary muscles

B. Septolateral dilation of the mitral valve annulus

C. Intraventricular dyssynchrony causing variable contraction of the papillary muscles

D. Increased tenting length and area

E. Increased zona coapta

6. Please review VIDEOS 29.8 AND 29.9. Which of the following is a direct morphologic echo feature of this type of MR (Type IIIb)?

A. Apical tethering with restriction of mitral valve leaflet motion especially involving the posterior leaflet

B. Decreased overlap of leaflet contact and decreased depth of coaptation

C. Dilated mitral annulus

D. Left ventricular wall motion abnormalities especially inferior or inferolateral

E. Posteriorly directed MR jet

7. Parameters that are used to assess LV remodeling include all of the following *except*:

A. Left ventricular end-systolic dimension and volume

B. Left ventricular end-diastolic dimension and volume

C. Left ventricular mass and ejection fraction (EF)

D. Left ventricular regional wall motion abnormalities

E. Myocardial strain

8. Which of the following parameters/statements regarding measures of LV remodeling has been proven in clinical studies to accurately identify the extent of disease in patients with heart failure?

A. LV end-diastolic volume is a reflection of the structural remodeling of the LV, and it is not influenced by the diastolic filling (end-diastolic myocyte fiber length).

B. Left ventricular end-systolic volume is influenced by both the end-diastolic volume and fiber shortening.

C. Left ventricular shape is not a useful parameter.

D. Left ventricular ejection fraction (LVEF) is derived from LV volume. Both heart rate and fiber shortening affect the LVEF to a greater extent than does the LV end-diastolic volume.

E. Fractional shortening provides a representative estimate of LV function, particularly when systolic impairment is regional.

9. Which of the following statements regarding the application of echocardiography in the diagnosis of Kawasaki disease (KD) is most accurate?

A. A coronary artery aneurysms are defined by an internal lumen diameter of >3 mm regardless of the age of the child.

B. Coronary artery aneurysms are defined by an internal diameter of an aneurysmal segment of at least three times the size of an adjacent coronary artery segment.

C. For optimal diagnosis of KD, one should adjust for patient size, which is an important determinant of the coronary artery dimension.

D. The coronary lumen should be smooth and without irregularities.

E. Echocardiography must also demonstrate other noncoronary artery abnormalities including depressed myocardial contractility, valvular lesions, and pericardial effusions to confirm the diagnosis.

10. Patients with Kawasaki disease (KD) are advised to undergo periodic testing to detect inducible ischemia and, if present, to quantify the degree of coronary insufficiency. All of the following statements regarding stress testing in KD are true *except*:

A. Exercise stress testing is preferred to pharmacologic stress testing because it is more physiologic.

B. Exercise testing for inducible ischemia with only electrocardiographic monitoring for ischemic changes has a relatively low mean sensitivity and specificity in adult series.

C. Stress testing is recommended in patients with KD with or without known coronary artery aneurysms.

D. Stress echocardiography, compared with SPECT perfusion imaging, has a higher success rate, has greater specificity, and avoids radiation exposure.

E. SPECT imaging has a higher sensitivity than stress echo.

11. Reliable techniques in the diagnosis of ischemic mitral regurgitation (MR) include both 2D and 3D echo. Which of the following statements regarding the diagnosis of ischemic MR is most accurate?

A. There is shortening of the mitral valve apparatus, resulting in failure of the leaflets to close completely and a resultant eccentric MR jet away from the diseased leaflet.

B. By 3D, the pattern of mitral valve deformation is asymmetric in ischemic MR and symmetric in functional MR.

C. By 3D, the LV chamber and mitral annulus are more enlarged in ischemic MR than in functional MR.

D. Exercise Doppler echocardiography may show a marked decrease in MR grade.

E. An ERO ≥ 0.4 cm^2 defines severe ischemic MR.

12. Which of the following statements regarding post-MI ventricular septal defect (VSD) is most accurate?

A. Due to the nature of the septal blood supply, patients with an MI due to occlusion of a "wraparound" left anterior descending artery (LAD) appear not to have an elevated risk of septal rupture.

B. Septal rupture is seen with higher frequency in anterior MI when compared to nonanterior infarctions.

C. With anterior MI, the defect is most commonly found in the apical septum, and with inferior MI, it most often occurs at the base.

D. Two-dimensional echocardiography alone visualizes the defect in only 10% to 20% of the patients, and therefore, a TEE as the initial imaging strategy is an appropriate consideration.

E. The septal perforation is rarely distinct and usually multiple with each defect ranging from one to several centimeters in size.

13. Which of the following statements on the assessment of regional LV function using strain rate imaging (SRI) from tissue Doppler echocardiography (TDE) during dobutamine stress echocardiography (DSE) is *least* accurate?

A. The increase in peak systolic strain during low-dose DSE allows accurate discrimination between different myocardial viability states.

B. The combination of SRI with wall motion scoring during DSE improves the sensitivity of viability assessment with DSE.

C. SRI has been shown to be superior to 2D DSE and TDE for the assessment of myocardial viability.

D. The specificity of wall motion scoring in assessment of myocardial viability has been shown to be superior to the SRI parameters.

E. After defining optimal cutoff for strain parameters, the sensitivity of low-dose SRI has been shown to be better though not significantly different from WMS.

14. The E-wave deceleration time (DT) on the mitral inflow spectral Doppler tracing may correlate with the extent of myocardial viability in patients with ischemic cardiomyopathy. Which of the following statements regarding the DT and low-dose dobutamine stress echocardiography (DSE) is most accurate?

A. A DT < 150 ms predicts an increase in LVEF after CABG of ≥5% with a sensitivity and specificity of about 80%.

B. At 1 year, the rate of death or heart transplantation is much lower in the patients with a DT <150 ms.

C. The higher number of viable segments on DSE correlates with a shorter DT on mitral inflow.

D. The presence of persistent restrictive pattern correlates with increased morbidity, but not mortality.

E. A DT of <130 ms in baseline echo correlates with decreased survival.

15. The following statements list nuclear SPECT, DSE, and FDG-PET imaging techniques in descending order for specificity, sensitivity, and predictive value. Please choose the correct descending order of the diagnostic test to predict functional recovery after revascularization:

A. Specificity, nuclear SPECT, DSE, and FDG-PET

B. Sensitivity, FDG-PET, nuclear SPECT, and DSE

C. Negative predictive value, DSE, FDG-PET, and nuclear SPECT

D. Positive predictive value, FDG-PET, DSE, and nuclear SPECT

16. Which of the following statements regarding stress echo is *least* accurate?

A. Exercise-induced ischemia has been shown to be an independent predictor of subsequent adverse cardiovascular outcomes.

B. Exercise-induced ischemia provides incremental predictive value beyond that provided by the clinical, resting 2D echo, and exercise data.

C. Patients referred for dobutamine stress echo (DSE) have an equal event rate when compared to those referred for exercise stress echo (ESE).

D. Adding data from coronary angiography to a positive pharmacologic stress echo is of little prognostic value.

E. Patients with resting LV wall motion abnormalities that have additional stress-induced myocardial ischemia have incrementally worse prognosis when compared to those who have either ischemia or resting abnormalities alone.

17. Which of the following stress echo parameters is *least* likely to identify patients at high risk for cardiovascular complications?

A. Postexercise wall motion score index (WMSI) > 2.0.

B. Increase in left ventricular end-systolic volume (ESV).

C. Exercise capacity and duration.

D. Postexercise LV ejection fraction (LVEF).

E. Postexercise EF is a more sensitive parameter than ESV and EDV changes.

18. Which one of the following responses best describes the biphasic response of the LV wall motion during dobutamine infusion?

A. Improvement at a low dose that improves further at a higher dose: This response indicates a viable myocardium.

B. Improvement at a low dose that deteriorates at a higher dose. This response indicates a viable myocardium with a high likelihood for functional recovery after coronary revascularization.

C. The response is seen in the setting of a stunned myocardium.

D. Worsening of resting LV wall motion abnormality in response to dobutamine infusion.

E. No response to either low or high dose of dobutamine infusion.

19. You are asked to evaluate a 63-year-old female with a past medical history significant for severe peripheral vascular disease (PVD), diabetes mellitus type 2, and hypertension. The patient is scheduled for kidney transplant. She has no history of CAD or CHF and currently is having no symptoms. Which of the following tests is most appropriate for the assessment of preoperative risk?

A. Exercise stress echocardiogram
B. Transthoracic 2D echo and, if LV function is normal, proceed with surgery
C. Dobutamine stress echo
D. Coronary angiogram
E. No further assessment

20. Which of the following statements regarding DSE in patients with end-stage renal disease (ESRD) is *least* accurate?

A. The percentage of ischemic segments by DSE is an independent predictor of mortality.
B. Dobutamine stress echo is a cost-effective approach in the cardiac evaluation of renal transplant patients because it poses no danger of nephrotoxicity.
C. Cardiac troponin does not predict significant CAD in this population.
D. Dobutamine has a short half-life of 30 minutes, which is not significantly increased in liver or kidney disease.
E. Atropine has a rapid-phase serum half-life of 2 hours and slow phase of 13 hours.

21. Both exercise myocardial perfusion imaging (MPI) and exercise echo have excellent negative predictive value for nonfatal MI and cardiac death, with an annual rate of <1% for a normal test. The prognostic value of the modalities has been shown to have greater accuracy in:

A. Male patients
B. Equal in both sexes
C. Female patients
D. Postmenopausal women

22. The correct numbers of LV regional myocardial wall segments as designated by the ASE and agreed upon by multiple other imaging societies in assessing regional wall motion abnormalities are:

A. 16 including the apex
B. 17 including the apex
C. 18 including the apex
D. 16 without the apex
E. 20 when considering both perfusion and function

23. Which of the following statements regarding LV wall motion score index (WMSI) is *least* accurate?

A. A score of 1 indicates normal wall motion.
B. The score ranges from 0 to 5, where 5 is the score of a normal segment.
C. It is a semiquantitative evaluation.
D. There is no geometric assumption.
E. WMSI is a real-time analysis.

24. Which of the following statements regarding the ischemic cascade is *least* accurate?

A. Angina is the last on the cascade.
B. Biochemical changes are the first to occur.
C. Electrocardiogram changes occur after LV wall motion abnormality and systolic dysfunction.
D. Elevated LV filling pressure occurs before systolic dysfunction and after diastolic dysfunction.
E. Diastolic dysfunction follows biochemical changes.

25. Which one of the following statements is true regarding the use of atropine in DSE?

A. The main effect of atropine on the heart is to induce tachycardia by blocking the vagal effects on the nicotinic receptors.
B. Atropine reduces GI motility and secretions, and therefore, it is not suitable for transesophageal stress testing.
C. Addition of atropine to dobutamine improves diagnostic specificity.
D. The risk for resistant ischemia decreases by adding atropine to dobutamine.
E. Atropine inhibits the acetylcholine action on the effectors innervated by postganglionic cholinergic nerves.

26. Which one of the following increases the sensitivity of stress echo?

A. Absence of variant angina
B. Presence of left circumflex disease versus left anterior descending disease
C. Absence of prior myocardial infarction
D. Intake of antianginal medications
E. Absence of hyperkinesia

Answer 1: E. This patient had an embolic complication from an apical thrombus she developed post myocardial infarction. History of prior chest discomfort, Q waves in ECG, and regional wall motion abnormality are supportive of this course of events. All choices except E are correct. The risk of embolization in patients with a documented LV thrombus who are not treated with anticoagulant therapy has been reported to be between 10% and 15%. Most embolic events occur within the first 3 to 4 months, although some occur later. The incidence of LV thrombi in the prereperfusion era was reported to be as high as 40% in patients with anterior infarction. Most thrombi developed within the first 2 weeks (median 5 to 6 days) after MI.

The incidence of LV thrombus in patients treated with fibrinolytic therapy was studied in 8,326 individuals in the GISSI-3 database; a predischarge transthoracic echocardiogram (TTE) was performed a mean of 9 days after symptom onset. LV thrombus was present in 5.1% of patients overall, 11.5% of those with an anterior wall infarction and 2.3% of those with infarctions at other sites.

Lower-frequency transducers have a decreased near-field resolution and do not enhance the detection of apical thrombi. Higher-frequency transducers (such as "pediatric" probes) with a shallow focal point are more effective in visualizing the near field due to higher spatial resolution (at a cost of lower penetration).

Suggested Readings

Cheesboro JH, Ezekowitz M, Badimon L, et al. Intracardiac thrombi and systemic thromboembolism: detection, incidence and treatment. *Annu Rev Med* 1985;36:576–605.

Chiarella F, Santoro E, Domenicucci S, et al. Predischarge two-dimensional echocardiographic evaluation of left ventricular thrombosis after acute myocardial infarction in the GISSI-3 study. *Am J Cardiol* 1998;81:822–827.

Natarajan D, Hotchandani RK, Nigam PD. Reduced incidence of left ventricular thrombi with intravenous streptokinase in acute myocardial infarction: prospective evaluation by cross sectional echo. *Int J Cardiol* 1988;20:201–207.

Visser CA, Kan G, Meltzer RS, et al. Embolic potential of left ventricular thrombus after myocardial infarction: a 2D echo study of 119 patients. *J Am Coll Cardiol* 1985;5:1276–1280.

Answer 2: E. All choices except E are correct. During systole, the paradoxical bulging of the aneurysmal segment results in "stealing" part of the LV stroke volume, thereby decreasing the effective cardiac output and inducing LV volume overload. The LV dilates, the wall stiffens, and the LV end-diastolic pressure rises. A mural thrombus is identified in 50% on autopsy or surgery in patients with LV aneurysm. The mechanism is stasis and contact of blood with potentially procoagulant fibrous tissue in the aneurysmal cavity. Ventricular arrhythmias that can lead to sudden cardiac death are common in patients with LV aneurysm. The potential mechanisms are ischemia and stretch of the myocardium, which can predispose to enhanced automaticity or triggered activity. The myocardium located at the border zone is heterogeneous and composed of fibrous tissue, inflammatory cells, and disorganized muscle fibers predisposing to reentrant activity. Contrast agents help to identify the aneurysmal cavity and the presence of thrombi. The LV aneurysm can grow and enlarge over time, but unlike pseudoaneurysm, it rarely ruptures due to its rich content in fibrous tissue. The LV apex is commonly foreshortened from the TEE approach, and the true apex may not be seen. Furthermore, the LV apex is in the far field and thus not well visualized using a high-frequency TEE transducer.

Suggested Reading

Visser CA, Kan G, Meltzer RS, et al. Incidence, timing and prognostic value of left ventricular aneurysm after myocardial infarction: a prospective serial echocardiographic study of 158 patients. *Am J Cardiol* 1986;57:729–732.

Answer 3: C. The diagnosis of stress-induced cardiomyopathy should be suspected in postmenopausal women who present with an acute coronary syndrome after intense psychological stress and in whom the clinical manifestations and ECG abnormalities are out of proportion to the degree of elevation in cardiac biomarkers. Coronary angiography typically demonstrates either normal vessels or mild to moderate coronary atherosclerosis. Therefore, Option A is incorrect. Some investigators have hypothesized that stress cardiomyopathy is not a distinct clinical entity but rather a manifestation of aborted anterior MI in patients with a long

"wraparound" left anterior descending artery. Transient occlusion in such a vessel, with subsequent spontaneous thrombolysis, could produce apical stunning and wall motion abnormalities that may improve over follow-up, but this hypothesis remains unproven. In one series of 256 patients, 82% were apical, 17% midventricular, and 1% basal, with 34% of cases demonstrating right ventricular involvement. Wall motion abnormalities are not necessarily confined to any one vascular territory. Therefore, Options B and E are incorrect. LGE on CMR is generally absent in stress-induced cardiomyopathy as compared to myocardial infarction in which intense subendocardial or transmural LGE is seen. Therefore, Option D is incorrect. A number of other syndromes in addition to stress-induced cardiomyopathy have been associated with ST-segment changes in the absence of significant coronary artery disease, including cardiac syndrome X, variant (Prinzmetal) angina, myocarditis, and cocaine abuse.

Suggested Readings

Dec GW. Recognition of the apical ballooning syndrome in the United States. *Circulation* 2005;111(4):388.

Eitel I, Knobelsdorff-Brekenhoff VF, Bernhardt P, et al. Clinical characteristics and cardiovascular magnetic resonance findings in stress (takotsubo) cardiomyopathy. *JAMA* 2011;306(3):277–286.

Hoyt J, Lerman A, Lennon RJ, et al. Left anterior descending artery length and coronary atherosclerosis in apical ballooning syndrome (Takotsubo/stress induced cardiomyopathy). *Int J Cardiol* 2010;145(1):112.

Answer 4: C. Video 29.7 shows a contrast-enhanced apical two-chamber view with a saccular aneurysm attached to the basal inferior wall by a narrow neck. The pseudoaneurysm neck is <40% of the maximal diameter of the aneurysm. True aneurysms have a wider neck, >40% of the maximal diameter of the aneurysm.

The incidence of LV aneurysm is 8% to 15% down from 35% due to the advances in therapy including thrombolytic therapy and PCI. Options A and B are incorrect since TTE is a reasonable first step, but a definitive diagnosis is made in only 26% of patients. TEE has a diagnostic accuracy of more than 75% compared to angiography, but data about its use are limited. We use TTE followed by contrast as initial studies. TEE is added when better assessment of the mitral valve is indicated. Option D is incorrect since a TTE study could still be performed initially or immediately prior to a TEE. Option E is incorrect since ultrasound contrast agents are contraindicated in cardiac shunts (based upon the package insert of Definity and Optison).

Suggested Readings

Glower DG, Lowe EL. Left ventricular aneurysm. In: Edmunds LH, ed. *Cardiac Surgery in the Adult*. New York: McGraw-Hill, 1997:677.

Yeo TC, Malouf JF, Oh JK, et al. Clinical profile and outcome in 52 patients with cardiac pseudoaneurysm. *Ann Intern Med* 1998;128(4):299.

Answer 5: E. Dislocation of the papillary muscle, septolateral dilation (simple annular dilation secondary to LV enlargement, which causes incomplete mitral valve coaptation associated with normal leaflet motion), intraventricular dyssynchrony (local LV remodeling with papillary muscle displacement causing apical tethering or tenting of the leaflets, with restricted systolic leaflet motion), and increased depth of tenting (secondary to LV remodeling and displacement of the papillary muscles) are all mechanisms of ischemic MR. It is decreased zona coapta (secondary to remodeling of the LV and tethering of the papillary muscles leading to tenting) rather than increased zona coapta that leads to ischemic MR.

Suggested Readings

Levine RA, Schwammenthal E. Ischemic mitral regurgitation on the threshold of a solution: from paradoxes to unifying concepts. *Circulation* 2005;112(5):745.

Timek TA, Lai DT, Liang D, et al. Effects of paracommissural septal-lateral annular cinching on acute ischemic mitral regurgitation. *Circulation* 2004;110(11 Suppl 1):1179–1184.

Uemura T, Otsuji Y, Nakashiki K, et al. Papillary muscle dysfunction attenuates ischemic mitral regurgitation in patients with localized basal inferior left ventricular remodeling: insights from tissue Doppler strain imaging. *J Am Coll Cardiol* 2005;46(1):113.

Answer 6: A. Mitral valve motion is used in Carpentier classifications of types I (normal motion), II (prolapse), and III (restriction). Type III is further classified into predominant diastolic impairment (IIIa) or systolic (IIIb). Most patients with ischemic MR have a type IIIb mitral valve pattern that results in apical tethering with restriction of mitral valve leaflet motion (especially involving the posterior leaflet and causing a posterior eccentric jet of MR).

Decreased overlap of leaflet contact and increased depth of coaptation leading to tenting is not an echocardiographic finding of ischemic MR, while all the other statements are applicable to a patient with ischemic MR.

Although these other features are indeed commonly found in patients with a type IIIb MV leaflet motion, the direct morphologic echo feature used for the Carpentier classification is the leaflet "motion." Therefore, Options B to E are not the single best answer.

Suggested Readings

Nagasaki M, Nishimura S, Ohtaki E, et al. The echocardiographic determinants of functional mitral regurgitation differ in ischemic and non-ischemic cardiomyopathy. *Int J Cardiol* 2006;108:171–176.

Otsuji Y, Handschumacher MD, Liel-Cohen N, et al. Mechanism of ischemic mitral regurgitation with segmental left ventricular dysfunction: three-dimensional echocardiographic studies in models of acute and chronic progressive regurgitation. *J Am Coll Cardiol* 2001;37:641–648.

Answer 7: D. Regional LV wall motion abnormalities are not a measure of remodeling. Option A, LV end-systolic volume, is influenced by both the LV end-diastolic volume and fiber shortening; however, asymmetric contraction may result in inaccurate estimates of LV end-systolic volume derived from M-mode or two-dimensional echocardiography. Option B, the LV end-diastolic volume, is a reflection of both structural remodeling and diastolic filling (end-diastolic myocyte fiber length). Option C, the LVEF, is derived from LV volume. Although heart rate and fiber shortening both affect LVEF, it is influenced to a far

greater extent by LV end-diastolic volume because changes in stroke volume tend to be much smaller than changes in LV end-diastolic volume. Option E, a refinement in the assessment of left ventricular function, has been strain rate imaging from tissue Doppler echocardiography (TDE). Strain rate imaging (SRI) measures regional thickening velocity using a transmural data set from color-coded TDE. The results are less subjective than wall motion scoring with traditional dobutamine echocardiography.

Suggested Readings

Abraham TP, Nishimura RA. Myocardial strain: can we finally measure contractility? *J Am Coll Cardiol* 2001;37(3):731.

Rumberger JA, Behrenbeck T, Breen JR, et al. Nonparallel changes in global left ventricular chamber volume and muscle mass during the first year after transmural myocardial infarction in humans. *J Am Coll Cardiol* 1993;21(3):673.

Answer 8: B. Option A is incorrect as the LV end-diastolic volume is a reflection of the structural remodeling of the LV and is influenced by the diastolic filling. Option B is correct as this statement is reflection of the Frank-Starling law. Option C is incorrect since the LV shape is an important determinant of the degree of LV remodeling. Option D is incorrect since heart rate will significantly affect LV diastolic volume. Option E is incorrect since fractional shortening is an echocardiographic measure of ventricular contractile function. However, since fractional shortening is derived from a single linear measurement of LV cavity at end diastole and end systole, it may not provide a representative estimate of LV function, particularly when systolic impairment is regional. The other listed measures are accurate.

Suggested Reading

Rumberger JA, Behrenbeck T, Breen JR, et al. Nonparallel changes in global left ventricular chamber volume and muscle mass during the first year after transmural myocardial infarction in humans. *J Am Coll Cardiol* 1993;21(3):673.

Answer 9: C. The criteria for diagnosis of coronary artery aneurysm as listed by the Japanese Ministry of Health are as follows: (1) internal lumen diameter is >3 mm for children <5 years of age and >4 mm in those older than 5 years; (2) the internal diameter is 1.5 times the size of an adjacent segment; and (3) there are clear luminal irregularities. These criteria do not adjust for patient size, an important determinant of coronary dimension. As a result, coronary arteries are often expressed as standard deviation units or Z-scores, adjusted for body surface area. It is likely that the most accurate system of classifying aneurysms relies on Z-scores rather than using absolute measurements. Interestingly, coronary dimensions in patients with KD at presentation are larger than normal. However, whether this is a reflection of the vasculitis or due to an associated factor such as fever is difficult to ascertain because there are no comparison Z-scores available for febrile children without KD.

Suggested Reading

Manlhiot C, Millar K, Golding F, et al. Improved classification of coronary artery abnormalities based only on coronary artery z-scores after Kawasaki disease. *Pediatr Cardiol* 2010;31(2):242.

Answer 10: C. Patients with aneurysms are advised to undergo periodic testing for inducible ischemia in order to detect and, if present, to quantify the degree of coronary insufficiency. Only small case series have reported the results of stress testing in children with KD and aneurysms. Thus, the choice of testing technique is based upon the larger adult literature, the ability of a child to cooperate, potential risks (such as radiation exposure or anesthesia), and the institutional experience. Because the risk of false-positive testing is highest when the probability of disease is low, we do not recommend stress testing in patients without a history of aneurysms.

In determining the most appropriate stress test to detect ischemia in children with coronary artery aneurysms, the following should be considered:

Exercise stress testing is preferred to pharmacologic stress testing because it is more physiologic. However, if children are unable to cooperate with the exercise protocol, pharmacologic stress test using dobutamine can be performed. Exercise stress ECG for detection of ischemia has relatively low sensitivity and specificity. The predictive value of exercise stress testing is enhanced using noninvasive imaging. Comparing stress echo (SE) versus SPECT, SE has higher success rate, has higher specificity, and avoids radiation. However, SE has lower sensitivity and greater interobserver variability. In patients with left main or triple-vessel disease leading to "balanced ischemia," the SPECT scan will have lower sensitivity than SE.

Suggested Reading

Kimball TR, Witt SA, Daniels SR. Dobutamine stress echocardiography in the assessment of suspected myocardial ischemia in children and young adults. *Am J Cardiol* 1997;79(3):380.

Answer 11: B. Option A is incorrect since with tethering and shortening, the leaflets will fail to close completely, and the resultant MR jet will be directed toward the diseased leaflet. Option B is correct since the pattern of deformation of the mitral valve is symmetric in functional cardiomyopathy and asymmetric in ischemic MR. Option C is incorrect since the LV chamber and mitral annulus are more enlarged in functional rather than ischemic MR. Exercise Doppler may show a marked increase in MR grade. Option E is incorrect as the ERO of more than 0.2 cm² defines severe ischemic MR.

Suggested Reading

Kwan J, Shiota T, Agler DA, et al. Geometric differences of the mitral apparatus between ischemic and dilated cardiomyopathy with significant mitral regurgitation: real-time three-dimensional echocardiography study. *Circulation* 2003;107(8):1135.

Answer 12: C. Option A is incorrect since due to the nature of the septal blood supply, patients with an MI due to occlusion of a "wraparound" LAD appear to have an elevated risk of septal rupture. Option B is incorrect since the frequency of VSD is equal in both anterior and nonanterior MI. Option D is incorrect since the sensitivity of 2D echo in diagnosing VSD post MI is only 40%, but the addition of color flow Doppler increases the sensitivity of the study. TEE is only occasionally required to delineate the defect. Option E is incorrect since the septal rupture occurs at the margin of necrotic and nonnecrotic tissue. The defect is usually single and extends from one to several centimeters. The defect is serpiginous in shape.

Suggested Readings

Batts KP, Ackermann DM, Edwards WD. Rupture of the left ventricular free wall: clinicopathologic correlates in 100 consecutive autopsy cases. *Hum Pathol* 1990;21(5):530.

Smyllie JH, Sutherland GR, Geuskens R. Doppler color flow mapping in the diagnosis of ventricular septal rupture and acute mitral regurgitation after myocardial infarction. *J Am Coll Cardiol* 1990;15(6):1449.

Answer 13: D.

A. In a study of 37 patients with ischemic LV dysfunction, Hoffman et al. have shown that an increase of peak systolic strain rate from rest to dobutamine stimulation by more than 0.23 1/S allowed accurate discrimination of viable from nonviable myocardium as determined by FDG-PET with a sensitivity of 83% and a specificity of 84%.

B. Hanekom et al. studied 55 patients with previous MI, wall motion scores and SRI parameters were measured, and the combination of WMS and SRI increased the sensitivity for prediction of functional recovery.

C. Hoffman showed the superiority of SRI over WMS in assessment of myocardial viability.

D. Is incorrect—the specificity of WMS (77%) was similar to SRI parameters.

E. This statement is correct.

Suggested Readings

Hanekom L, Jenkins C, Jeffries L, et al. Incremental value of strain rate analysis as an adjunct to wall-motion scoring for assessment of myocardial viability by dobutamine echocardiography: a follow-up study after revascularization. *Circulation* 2005;112(25):3892.

Hoffmann R, Altiok E, Nowak B, et al. Strain rate measurement by Doppler echocardiography allows improved assessment of myocardial viability in patients with depressed left ventricular function. *J Am Coll Cardiol* 2002;39(3):443.

Answer 14: E. Option A is incorrect since a DT >150 ms predicts an increase in LVEF after CABG of ≥5% with a sensitivity and specificity of about 80%. Option B is incorrect since, at 1 year, the rate of death or heart transplantation was much lower in patients with a DT >150 ms. Option C is incorrect since the higher number of viable segments on DSE correlates with a slower DT on mitral inflow. Option D is incorrect since the presence of persistent restrictive pattern correlates with increased mortality. A DT of <130 ms in baseline echo predicts decreased survival.

Suggested Reading

Yong Y, Nagueh SF, Shimoni S, et al. Deceleration time in ischemic cardiomyopathy: relation to echocardiographic and scintigraphic indices of myocardial viability and functional recovery after revascularization. *Circulation* 2001;103(9):1232.

Answer 15: *B.* PET has the highest sensitivity, and DSE has the highest specificity for detection of ischemia.

Review of the literature regarding the values for sensitivity and specificity of different modalities is as follows:

Exercise ECG (68% and 77%), planar thallium (both exercise and pharmacologic, 79% and 73%), thallium SPECT (both exercise and pharmacologic, 88% and 77%), stress echo (both exercise and pharmacologic, 76% and 88%), and PET (93% and 82%). SPECT (99 m)Tc has a slightly higher sensitivity and specificity than thallium (90% and 82%).

Suggested Readings

Bax JJ, Polderman D, Elhendy A, et al. Sensitivity, specificity, and predictive accuracies of various non-invasive techniques for detecting hibernating myocardium. *Curr Probl Cardiol* 2001;26:147–186.

Garber AM, Solomon NA. Cost effectiveness of alternative test strategies for the diagnosis of coronary artery disease. *Ann Intern Med* 1999;130(9):719.

Answer 16: *C.* Option C is incorrect. It is important to emphasize that an inability to exercise is in itself an ominous prognostic sign and patients referred for DSE have a higher event rate than those referred for ESE. The presence of ischemia on ESE can predict whether patients will experience an event independent of, and incremental to, clinical and exercise data. Otherwise, all other options are correct.

Suggested Readings

Chaowalit N, McCully RB. Outcomes after normal dobutamine stress echocardiography and predictors of adverse events: long-term follow-up of 3014 patients. *Eur Heart J* 2006;27:3039–3044.

Dhond MR, Nguyen TT, Sabapathy R, et al. Stress echo results predict mortality: a large scale multicenter prospective international study. *J Am Coll Cardiol* 2003;41:589–595.

Answer 17: *E.* Wall motion score index, LV end-systolic volume, exercise capacity, and postexercise LVEF are all predictors of high-risk stress test. Compared to EF, ESV may be a more sensitive indicator of ventricular function at the limits of contractile reserve when contractility is unable to match the normal physiologic increase in preload and afterload during exercise. LVEF during stress echocardiography is commonly used to risk stratify patients. However, EF is affected by loading conditions and heart rate, primarily through changes in EDV, and, therefore, may not adequately reflect contractile reserve.

Suggested Readings

Aranda-Olson AM, Juracan EM, Mahoney D, et al. Prognostic value of exercise echo. *J Am Coll Cardiol* 2002;39:625–631.

Burkhoff D, Mirsky I, Suga H. Assessment of systolic and diastolic ventricular properties via pressure-volume analysis: a guide for clinical, translational, and basic researchers. *Am J Physiol Heart Circ Physiol* 2005;289:H501–H512.

Answer 18: *B.* Low-dose viability dobutamine stress echo (DSE) is done to detect hibernating myocardium and predict recovery of a flow-limiting stenosis. No specific test is indicated in case of stunned myocardium, except for an echocardiogram to follow up on the recovery of LV myocardium following an MI.

A contractile response to dobutamine appears to require that at least 50% of the myocytes in a given segment are viable; the contractile response also correlates inversely with the extent of interstitial fibrosis on myocardial biopsy. In comparison, radionuclide myocardial perfusion imaging identifies segments with fewer viable myocytes. The predictive value of DSE appears to be highest when there is a biphasic response, improvement at low dose of dobutamine, and worsening at high dose. The initial improvement reflects the recruitment of the contractile reserve of the myocardium and hence viability. In comparison, higher dose is associated with deterioration due to onset of ischemia.

Suggested Readings

Barillà F, De Vincentis G, Mangieri E. Recovery of contractility of viable myocardium during inotropic stimulation is not dependent on an increase of myocardial blood flow in the absence of collateral filling. *J Am Coll Cardiol* 1999;33(3):697.

Cornel JH, Bax JJ, Elhendy A, et al. Biphasic response to dobutamine predicts improvement of global left ventricular function after surgical revascularization in patients with stable coronary artery disease: implications of time course of recovery on diagnostic accuracy. *J Am Coll Cardiol* 1998;31(5):1002.

Answer 19: *C.* Cardiovascular disease is the most common cause of death in patients with end-stage renal disease (ESRD). Therefore, preoperative risk assessment in these patients before renal transplant is very important. Current guidelines recommend noninvasive stress testing is performed based on the patient's estimated risk. The American Society of Nephrology (ASN) and the American Society of Transplantation (AST) recommend myocardial perfusion imaging or DSE as part of the preoperative evaluation. In comparison, the American College of Cardiology (ACC) and the American Heart Association (AHA) recommend no preoperative cardiac evaluation since kidney transplantation poses an intermediate risk if the patient has good functional status on perfusion imaging. Up to half of asymptomatic ESRD patients initiating renal replacement therapy with no known cardiac disease have significant coronary artery disease on angiography.

Suggested Readings

Kertai MD, Boersma E, Bax JJ, et al. A meta-analysis comparing the prognostic accuracy, of six diagnostic tests for predicting preoperative cardiac risk in patients undergoing major vascular surgery. *Heart* 2003;89:1327–1334.

Ohtake T, Kobayashi S, Moriya H, et al. Prevalence of occult coronary artery stenosis in patients with chronic kidney disease at the initiation of renal replacement therapy: an angiographic examination. *J Am Soc Nephrol* 2005;16(4):1141–1148.

Schouten O, Bax JJ, Polderman D. Assessment of cardiac risk prior to non-cardiac surgery. *Heart* 2006;S2:1866–1872.

Answer 20: *D.* All other options are correct. Troponin is chronically elevated in ESRD due to its decreased clearance. The half-life of dobutamine is 2 minutes (not 30 minutes as in Option D), and there is no need for renal or hepatic adjustments. The half-life of atropine is 2 hours.

Suggested Readings

Apple FS, Murakami MM, Pearce LA. et al. Dobutamine stress echo and cardiac troponin for detection of significant CAD and predicting outcomes in renal transplant candidates. *Eur J Echocardiogr* 2005;6:327–335.

De Lima JJ, Sabbaga E, Vieira ML. Prognostic value of dobutamine stress echo in patients with chronic kidney disease. *Am Heart J* 2007;153:385–391.

Answer 21: B. Equal in both sexes.

Suggested Readings

Bjork I, Asbjorn S, Stig A, et al. The prognostic value of normal exercise myocardial perfusion imaging and exercise echo: a meta-analysis. *J Am Coll Cardiol* 2007;49:227–237.

Buchthal SD, den Hollander JA, Merz CN. Prognostic value of exercise echocardiography in patients: Is there a gender difference? *J Am Coll Cardiol* 2002;39:625–631.

Answer 22: B. The 20-segment model would have provided smaller segments and a more complicated analysis. A reasonable trade-off between accuracy and feasibility is represented by the 16-segment model, which is recently modified to include the true apex, as the segment number 17. Each segment can be visualized from different echocardiographic views. The wall motion of each segment can be safely assessed if at least 50% of its entire length is visualized. The update to 17-segment model was especially important after the frequent use of contrast and identification of the apical cap. With the 17-segment model, all imaging modalities can share a standardized myocardial segmentation nomenclature.

Suggested Reading

Cerqueira MD, Weissman NJ, Dilsizian V, et al. Standardized myocardial segmentation and nomenclature for tomographic imaging of the heart: a statement for healthcare professionals from the Cardiac Imaging Committee of the Council on Clinical Cardiology of the American Heart Association. *Circulation* 2002;105:539–542.

Answer 23: B. This is based on 17 segments in which the normal segment is assigned a score of 1; mild or moderate hypokinesia, a score of 2; severe hypokinesia or akinesia, a score of 3; and dyskinesia, a score of 4. The WMSI is calculated by dividing the sum of the segmental score by the number of segments visualized. The normal WMSI is 1. A score between 1 and 1.9 suggests a smaller infarct, and a score >2.0 is suggestive of higher incidence of worse prognosis.

Suggested Reading

Bourdillon PD, Broderick TM, Swada S, et al. Regional wall motion index for infarct and noninfarct regions after reperfusion in acute myocardial infarction: comparison with global wall motion index. *J Am Soc Echocardiogr* 1989;2:398–407.

Answer 24: D. The ischemic cascade starts with perfusion abnormalities/biochemical changes, then diastolic dysfunction, followed by systolic dysfunction and ECG changes, and the last to occur is angina.

Suggested Reading

Hendryck CR, Baic H, Nelkins P, et al. Depression of regional blood flow and wall thickening after brief coronary occlusion. *Am J Physiology* 1978;234:H653–H660.

Answer 25: E. The main effect of atropine on the heart is to induce tachycardia by blocking the vagal effects on the muscarinic (M2) receptors in the sinoatrial node. Atropine inhibits the action of acetylcholine on anatomical effectors innervated by the postganglionic cholinergic nerves. Atrioventricular conduction is enhanced. Since atropine reduces GI motility and secretions, it can be administered before transesophageal stress. Atropine should not be given to patients with glaucoma or BPH. Addition of atropine to dobutamine or exercise improves the diagnostic sensitivity of the test, but there is no effect on specificity. Not surprisingly, however, the risk of resistant ischemia increases with atropine.

Suggested Readings

Attenhofer CH, Pellika PA, Roger VL, et al. Impact of atropine injection on heart rate response during treadmill exercise echocardiography: a double blind randomized study. *Echocardiography* 2000;17:221–227.

Erdogan O, Altun A, Akdemi O, et al. Unexpected occurrence of ST segment elevation during intravenous administration of atropine. *Cardiovasc Drugs Ther* 2001;15:367–368.

Mathias W Jr, Arruda A, Santos FC, et al. Safety of dobutamine-atropine stress echocardiography: a prospective experience of 4033 consecutive studies. *J Am Soc Echocardiogr* 1999;12:785–791.

Answer 26: E. All stresses yield better sensitivity results in populations with previous myocardial infarction and in patients off their antianginal medications. The evaluation of patients with variant angina inflates sensitivity since the stress agent, for example, dobutamine, may elicit coronary spasm and hence ischemia independent of organic stenosis. Submaximal stress test significantly reduces the sensitivity of the test. LAD disease will increase test sensitivity as compared to LCX disease. The lack of the expected LV regional hyperkinesis, when used as a marker of inducible myocardial ischemia (in the absence of a regional wall motion abnormality), will provide higher sensitivity at a cost of lowering specificity.

Suggested Readings

Bax JJ, Polderman D, Elhendy A, et al. Sensitivity, specificity, and predictive accuracies of various non-invasive techniques for detecting hibernating myocardium. *Curr Probl Cardiol* 2001;26:147–186.

Garber AM, Solomon NA. Cost effectiveness of alternative test strategies for the diagnosis of coronary artery disease. *Ann Intern Med* 1999;130(9):719.

Picano E. *Stress Echocardiography.* 5th ed. Springer-Verlag Berlin Heidelberg, 2009.

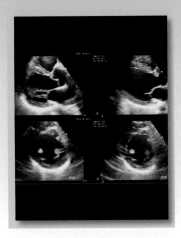

Chapter 30

Stress Echocardiography

Vincent L. Sorrell

1. A 65-year-old male with a history of type 2 diabetes mellitus and hypertension complains of chest tightness and shoulder and neck discomfort upon climbing stairs. The treating physician suspects coronary artery disease as the most likely explanation for this patient's symptoms. If the assumption is true, which of the following is the earliest abnormality to occur during graded, submaximal exercise?

A. Chest tightness
B. Impaired regional myocardial relaxation
C. Increased left ventricular filling pressures
D. Left ventricular wall motion abnormalities
E. ST-segment depression on EKG

2. A 56-year-old male with known coronary artery disease is evaluated for exertional shortness of breath. Transthoracic echocardiogram shows multiple resting regional wall motion abnormalities and left ventricular ejection fraction of 30%. He is scheduled for dobutamine echocardiography. Which of the response curves is most specific in predicting recovery of the regional and global systolic function after successful revascularization (Fig. 30.1)?

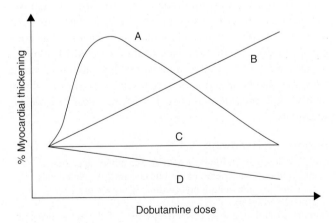

FIGURE 30.1

A. A
B. B
C. C
D. D

3. A 56-year-old overweight male with type 2 diabetes mellitus and hypertension complains of exertional shortness of breath and fatigue. He is referred for stress echocardiography for evaluation of his symptoms. He exercises on the Bruce protocol for 5:45 minutes reaching 6 METs. His heart rate increases to 148/minute, which is 90% of his maximal predicted heart rate. His blood pressure increases to 160/75 mm Hg from resting 116/56 mm Hg. Please review the images obtained during the study (Video 30.1).

The study results are most consistent with which of the following?

A. Normal response
B. Left anterior descending territory ischemia
C. Non–left anterior descending territory ischemia
D. Multivessel disease with transient ischemic dilation
E. Nonischemic cardiomyopathy

4. A 67-year-old male is evaluated for left-sided, sharp chest discomfort that happens occasionally with exertion and at rest. He has a history of hypertension, glucose intolerance, and hyperlipidemia. Stress echocardiography is performed. His baseline echocardiogram shows no regional wall motion abnormalities and normal left ventricular systolic function. He exercises following Bruce protocol for 8:40 minutes reaching 8.7 METs and stops because of fatigue. His peak heart rate is 151/minute, which corresponds to 99% of his maximally predicted heart rate. His blood pressure increases to 182/95 mm Hg from 145/90 mm Hg at rest. Postexercise images show normal enhancement of left ventricular contractility in all segments. In the next year, what is the expected probability of myocardial infarction or cardiac death in this patient?

A. 8%
B. 5%
C. 3%
D. 2%
E. <1%

5. A 62-year-old male with hypertension and hyperlipidemia complains of exertional chest discomfort. He describes the discomfort as tightness around his chest that is somewhat similar to asthma symptoms that he experiences occasionally. He is an exsmoker with a 20-pack-year smoking history. He has a strong family history of coronary artery disease. His electrocardiogram shows normal sinus rhythm and nonspecific T-wave changes. He is scheduled for an exercise echocardiogram. Which of the following would decrease the specificity of the test result in this patient?

A. Hypertensive response to exercise
B. Left circumflex artery disease
C. Mitral regurgitation
D. Suboptimal effort
E. Use of a beta-blocker prior to exercise

6. A 46-year-old man with known coronary artery disease complains of atypical chest discomfort. He also describes decreased exercise tolerance. Five years ago, he underwent a drug-eluting stent placement in his left anterior descending artery for resistant angina. His other past medical problems include hypertension and severe bilateral knee osteoarthritis. He is an exsmoker with a 20-pack-year smoking history. His BMI is 32 kg/m². He is scheduled for dobutamine echocardiography. Which of the following test findings is associated with benign prognosis in this patient?

A. Increase in left ventricular end-systolic volume at peak stress
B. Nonsustained ventricular tachycardia during dobutamine infusion
C. Stress-induced anterior wall hypokinesis
D. Resting hypokinesis of the posterior wall
E. A 1-mm ST-segment elevation in leads III and avF during the test

7. A 59-year-old male with hyperlipidemia and hypertension complains of chest discomfort and fatigue. He has no known history of coronary artery disease. He is referred for stress echocardiography for evaluation of his symptoms. He exercises on Bruce protocol for 6:00 minutes reaching 6.6 METs and stops because of fatigue. His heart rate increases to 153/minute, which is 95% of his maximal predicted heart rate. His blood pressure increases to 170/95 mm Hg from resting 136/80 mm Hg. Please review the images obtained (VIDEO 30.2).

The study results are most consistent with which of the following?

A. Normal response
B. Left anterior descending territory ischemia
C. Non–left anterior descending territory ischemia
D. Multivessel disease
E. Nonischemic cardiomyopathy

8. A 76-year-old male complains of left-sided chest and shoulder pain that is sometimes exacerbated by exertion. He has a history of hypertension treated with amlodipine and lisinopril. His father suffered from hypertension and died of a stroke. He is referred for stress echocardiography for evaluation of his symptoms. He exercises on Bruce protocol for 8:00 minutes reaching 8.2 METs and stops because of fatigue. His heart rate increases to 141/minute, which is 98% of his maximal predicted heart rate. His blood pressure increases to 165/85 mm Hg from resting 132/76 mm Hg. Please review the images obtained during the study (VIDEOS 30.3 AND 30.4).

Which of the following is the best next step in managing this patient?

A. Aspirin, beta-blocker, and atorvastatin
B. Cardiac catheterization
C. Further noninvasive cardiac testing
D. Reassurance and routine care

9. A 44-year-old male with no significant past medical history presents with progressive fatigue over the last 4 months. He denies any chest pain, palpitations, or syncope. His current exercise tolerance is about four blocks on a level ground. He has a strong family history of coronary artery disease with his father undergoing coronary artery grafting at the age of 48 years. Transthoracic echocardiogram shows a dilated left ventricle with global hypokinesis and ejection fraction of 30%. Electrocardiogram shows normal sinus rhythm with 1-mm lateral ST-segment depression and T-wave inversion. Which of the following is the best next step in managing this patient?

A. Treadmill exercise echocardiography using Bruce protocol
B. Treadmill exercise EKG using Bruce protocol
C. Dobutamine echocardiography using 2.5 to 40 μg/kg/min
D. Dobutamine echocardiography using 10 to 40 μg/kg/min
E. Dipyridamole echocardiography using 0.84 mg/kg

10. A 64-year-old male with type 2 diabetes mellitus and exertional chest discomfort undergoes dobutamine stress echocardiography. His resting left ventricular wall motion score index is 1.0, and ejection fraction is 65%. Right ventricle is normal in size and function. At 30 μg/kg/min of dobutamine infusion, he complains of chest discomfort. His heart rate is 115/minute, and his blood pressure is 155/90 mm Hg. Echocardiographic images show inferior wall hypokinesis. Additionally, the apical and midinferior wall of the right ventricle appears hypokinetic. The observed finding in the right ventricle is best described as which of the following?

A. It is a marker of worse prognosis.
B. It is associated with elevated left ventricular filling pressures.
C. It indicates right ventricular pressure overload.
D. Right ventricular wall motion cannot be reliably interpreted post stress.
E. The findings are consistent with pulmonary embolism.

11. A 44-year-old overweight female is evaluated for shortness of breath. Over the last year, she finds it progressively difficult to keep up with her daily activities due to exertional dyspnea. She denies any chest pain, palpitations, cough, or wheezing. Her past medical history is significant for hypertension treated with chlorthalidone. Her pulmonary function testing is unremarkable. Resting echocardiogram reveals mild concentric left ventricular hypertrophy, left ventricular ejection fraction of 65%, and normal right ventricular size and function. There are no major Doppler abnormalities. The estimated pulmonary artery systolic pressure is 35 mm Hg. Which of the following postexercise parameters are most likely to explain this patient's current symptoms?

A. Left ventricular ejection fraction
B. Left ventricular wall motion analysis
C. Right ventricular wall motion analysis
D. Transaortic and left ventricular outflow tract velocities
E. Transmitral flow velocities and tissue Doppler

12. A 43-year-old male presents to the hospital with palpitations. He had two similar episodes in the past that lasted several hours, but now, it seems to be persistent. He denies any chest pain, shortness of breath, or syncope. He was told 1 year ago that his blood pressure is "borderline" and his cholesterol is "fine." He does not smoke, exercises regularly, and tries to eat healthy. His father had a coronary artery bypass grafting at the age of 69 years. His blood pressure is 122/70 mm Hg, and his heart rate is 145/minute. His EKG shows atrial fibrillation with rapid ventricular response. Echocardiogram shows mild left atrial dilation, normal left ventricular wall motion, and left ventricular ejection fraction of 60%. There are no major Doppler abnormalities. He is admitted and started on a beta-blocker. Next morning, he is symptom-free and in normal sinus rhythm at the rate of 65/minute. Which of the following best describes appropriateness of exercise echocardiography in this patient before discharge?

A. Appropriate
B. Inappropriate
C. Uncertain

13. A 75-year-old male is scheduled for orthopedic surgery. The clinician considers dobutamine echocardiography after the preoperative assessment of clinical parameters. Based on the existing evidence, dobutamine echocardiography provides additional prognostic information in predicting perioperative adverse cardiac events due to which of the following?

A. High sensitivity in a high-risk patient
B. High specificity in a high-risk patient
C. High sensitivity in a low-risk patient
D. High specificity in a low-risk patient

Table 30.1	**Values Obtained at Baseline and During Intravenous Dobutamine Administration**	
	BASELINE	**WITH DOBUTAMINE**
LVOT PW VTI	11 cm	17 cm
LVOT PW velocity	0.6 m/s	0.8 m/s
Aortic valve CW VTI	56 cm	85 cm
Aortic valve CW velocity	3 m/s	4.1 m/s

CW, continuous wave; LVOT, left ventricular outflow tract; PW, pulsed wave; VTI, velocity time integral.

14. A 68-year-old male is evaluated for progressive exertional shortness of breath and poor exercise tolerance. Currently, he can walk less than one block on a level ground before getting dyspnea. Five years ago, he had cardiac catheterization for chest pain evaluation, and he was found to have normal coronary arteries. Baseline echocardiogram is performed showing left ventricular dilation and left ventricular ejection fraction of 20%. The aortic valve is thickened and has restricted opening. The following values were obtained at baseline and during intravenous dobutamine administration (20 µg/kg/min) (TABLE 30.1).

Which of the following is the best next step in managing this patient?

A. Aortic valve replacement
B. Beta-blocker and ACE inhibitor therapy
C. Evaluation for cardiac transplant
D. Treadmill exercise tolerance testing

15. A 57-year-old male presents to the stress echo laboratory with symptoms of worsening dyspnea on exertion. He is overweight at 5'10" and 227 pounds. He has a known cardiac murmur (diastolic) and ejection click. Resting HR 55 bpm; BP 139/74 mm Hg. ECG with sinus bradycardia, leftward axis, and nonspecific ST changes. He exercised for 7:43 Bruce protocol stopping with fatigue and dyspnea. HR increased to 151 bpm; BP 180/80 mm Hg. There was 1 mm upsloping ST depression V5, V6. Based upon the rest and stress echo images provided (FIGS. 30.2A–C and VIDEOS 30.5A–C), how would you interpret the results?

A. Normal stress echo
B. Abnormal stress echo, normal EF response, 1-vessel disease
C. Abnormal stress echo, abnormal EF response, 2-vessel disease (with LAD)
D. Abnormal stress echo, abnormal EF response, 2-vessel disease (without LAD)
E. Abnormal stress echo, abnormal EF response, nonischemic CM

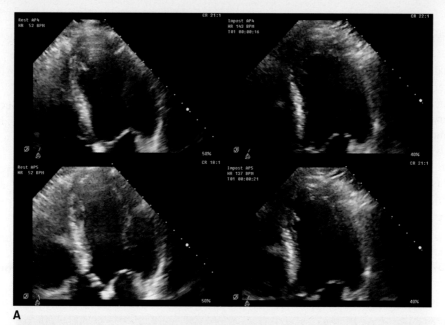

A

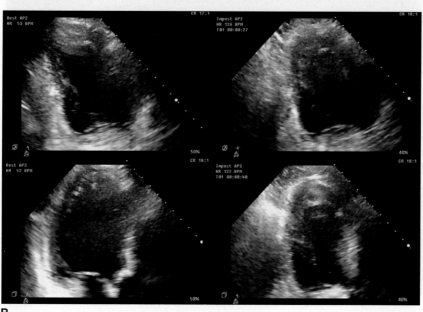

B

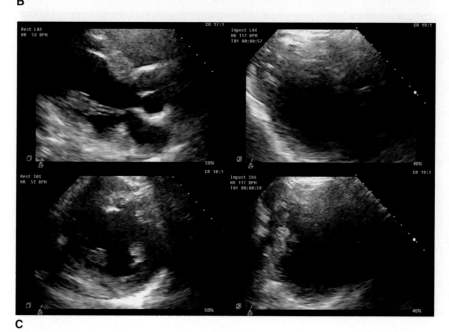

C

FIGURE 30.2

16. A 63-year-old female with new-onset chest pain 4 years after cardiac surgery (aortic aneurysm repair) is seen in the stress echocardiography laboratory. She has a long-standing history of hypertension, recently controlled, and continues to smoke 2 packs/day. She stands 5′3″ and weighs 148 pounds. She recently lost >60 pounds (by choice, through an exercise program). Her resting HR is 70 bpm and BP is 133/72 mm Hg. Resting ECG with normal sinus rhythm, RBBB and LAFB pattern.

She completes 3′24″ on a Bruce protocol stopping due to fatigue and dyspnea. She describes a mild chest pain similar (but not as severe) as her underlying complaint. Her maximal HR was 157 bpm and her BP at peak exercise (and 2 minutes in recovery) was 214/92 mm Hg. Her exercise ECG revealed sinus tachycardia without diagnostic ST changes or arrhythmias.

Based upon the rest and stress echo images provided (Figs. 30.3A–C and Videos 30.6A–C), how would you interpret the results?

A. Nondiagnostic stress echo

B. Abnormal stress echo, normal EF response, 1-vessel disease

C. Abnormal stress echo, abnormal EF response, 2-vessel disease (with LAD)

D. Abnormal stress echo, abnormal EF response, 2-vessel disease (without LAD)

E. Abnormal stress echo, abnormal EF response, nonischemic CM

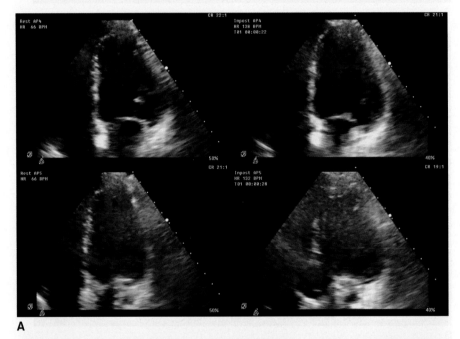

A

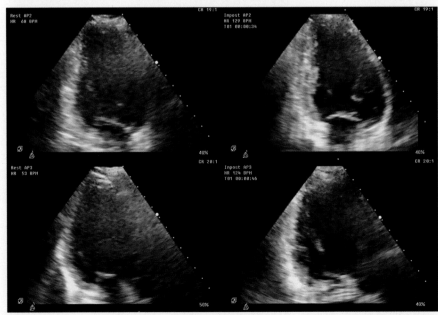

B

Figure 30.3

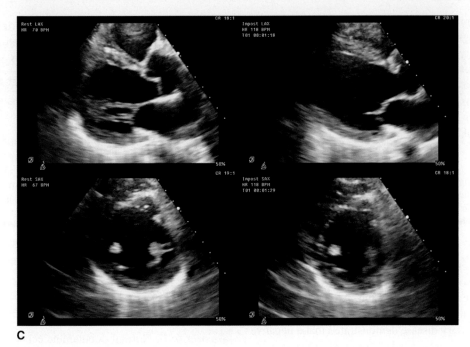

C

FIGURE 30.3 (*Continued*)

Answer 1: B. The ischemic cascade is the basic principle behind stress testing (1,2). It describes sequential pathophysiologic events that follow myocardial ischemia. Early after the onset of ischemia, myocardial perfusion heterogeneity is apparent that can be detected by myocardial perfusion imaging. Biochemical alterations in the myocardium due to ischemia result in impaired relaxation (regional diastolic dysfunction). The clinical utility of this finding has not been established, but it is a subject of active research. This is followed by systolic dysfunction (regional wall motion abnormalities), which is the basis of stress echocardiography. Depending on the extent of ischemia, left ventricular filling pressures may increase. EKG changes and anginal symptoms are late events in the ischemic cascade and may not be present depending on the extent and duration of ischemia (FIG. 30.4).

References

1. Nesto RW, Kowalchuk GJ. The ischemic cascade: temporal sequence of hemodynamic, electrocardiographic and symptomatic expressions of ischemia. *Am J Cardiol* 1987;59:23C–30C.
2. Kwong RY. Imaging the physiology of the ischemic cascade: are 2 tools better than 1? *Circ Cardiovasc Imaging* 2008;1:92–93.

Answer 2: A. Curve A demonstrates a biphasic response to dobutamine infusion: improvement in contractility (viability) at a low dose followed by worsening (ischemia) at a high dose. Biphasic response has the best positive predictive value for recovery of the regional systolic function of the segment after revascularization (1,2). Interestingly, sustained improvement response (monophasic, curve B) is much less specific for predicting functional recovery of the left ventricle. No significant change (curve C) and worsening (curve D) of segmental function with incremental dobutamine doses are usually associated with a low likelihood of the recovery of systolic function.

References

1. Cornel JH, Bax JJ, Elhendy A, et al. Biphasic response to dobutamine predicts improvement of global left ventricular function after surgical revascularization in patients with stable coronary artery disease: implications of time course of recovery on diagnostic accuracy. *J Am Coll Cardiol* 1998;31:1002–1010.
2. Afridi I, Kleiman NS, Raizner AE, et al. Dobutamine echocardiography in myocardial hibernation. Optimal dose and accuracy in predicting recovery of ventricular function after coronary angioplasty. *Circulation* 1995;91:663–670.

Answer 3: D. The stress echocardiogram shown demonstrates multiple wall motion abnormalities and left ventricular cavity dilation post exercise. In one study, abnormal transient ischemic dilation ratio values corresponded to left ventricular stress-to-rest volume ratios >1.17 and showed high sensitivity

Ischemic Cascade

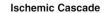

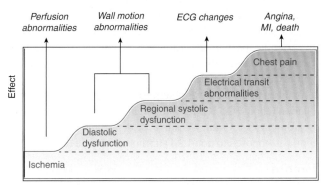

Increasing degree and duration of ischemia

FIGURE 30.4

(100%) and moderate specificity (54%) for detection of severe and extensive angiographic coronary artery disease (1). Also, left ventricular cavity dilation is a marker of poor prognosis. The presence of stress-induced marked regional wall motion abnormalities and postexercise transient cavity dilation makes other answer options such as single-vessel obstructive coronary disease (choices B and C) and nonischemic cardiomyopathy (choice E) less likely.

Reference

1. Yao SS, Shah A, Bangalore S, et al. Transient ischemic left ventricular cavity dilation is a significant predictor of severe and extensive coronary artery disease and adverse outcome in patients undergoing stress echocardiography. *J Am Soc Echocardiogr* 2007;20:352–358.

Answer 4: E. Studies consistently showed that the negative predictive value of normal exercise echocardiogram for short-term adverse cardiac events is very high. A meta-analysis of exercise imaging studies performed in patients with known or suspected coronary artery disease demonstrated that a negative stress echocardiogram is associated with a yearly adverse event rate (myocardial infarction or cardiac death) of 0.54% (1,2). Although stress-induced ischemia is a major determinant of prognosis, other exercise-related variables also contribute to prognosis, for example, poor exercise tolerance or inability to exercise and systolic blood pressure response (3).

References

1. Metz LD, Beattie M, Hom R, et al. The prognostic value of normal exercise myocardial perfusion imaging and exercise echocardiography: a meta-analysis. *J Am Coll Cardiol* 2007;49:227–237.
2. Yao SS, Qureshi E, Sherrid MV, et al. Practical applications in stress echocardiography: risk stratification and prognosis in patients with known or suspected ischemic heart disease. *J Am Coll Cardiol* 2003;42:1084–1090.
3. Myers J, Prakash M, Froelicher V, et al. Exercise capacity and mortality among men referred for exercise testing. *N Engl J Med* 2002;346:793–801.

Answer 5: A. The specificity of a test is determined by the false-positivity rate, whereas the sensitivity is determined by the false-negativity rate. Abnormal increase in blood pressure during stress can cause global or regional left ventricular dysfunction in the absence of epicardial coronary disease (1). This is due to increased myocardial oxygen demand exceeding the myocardial perfusion reserve (afterload mismatch). Other answer options list potential causes of a false-negative test (decreased sensitivity). The list of potential reasons for false-positive and false-negative stress echocardiography results is given in TABLE 30.2 (2).

References

1. Ha JW, Juracan EM, Mahoney DW, et al. Hypertensive response to exercise: a potential cause for new wall motion abnormality in the absence of coronary artery disease. *J Am Coll Cardiol* 2002;39:323–327.
2. Pellikka PA, Nagueh SF, Elhendy AA, et al. American Society of Echocardiography recommendations for performance, interpretation, and application of stress echocardiography. *J Am Soc Echocardiogr* 2007;20:1021–1041.

Table 30.2 **Potential Reasons for False-Positive and False-Negative Stress Echocardiography Results**

FALSE-POSITIVE RESULTS	FALSE-NEGATIVE RESULTS
Hypertensive response to stress	Inadequate level of stress
Hypertrophic cardiomyopathy	Delays in image acquisition postexercise
Microvascular disease (syndrome X)	Single-vessel disease, especially left circumflex
Nonischemic cardiomyopathy	Concentric left ventricular remodeling
Stress-induced cardiomyopathy	Hyperdynamic state in patients with mitral regurgitation or aortic regurgitation
Coronary spasm	
Abnormal septal motion due to pacing, conduction abnormalities, prior surgery, or right ventricular volume overload	Apical foreshortening

Answer 6: B. Normal dobutamine echocardiography carries a low short-term risk of adverse cardiac events. Stress-induced ischemia as described in option C is a major determinant of poor prognosis in patients undergoing stress echocardiography. At the same time, other test variables also carry prognostic significance. Resting wall motion abnormalities indicate a worse prognosis. Abnormal end-systolic volume response usually indicates severe ischemia. ST elevation during the test is uncommon, but it is a marker of severe coronary artery disease. Nonsustained ventricular tachycardia occurs in 3% to 5% of patients during dobutamine infusion and does not seem to have an independent prognostic significance (1,2).

References

1. Geleijnse ML, Krenning BJ, Nemes A, et al. Incidence, pathophysiology, and treatment of complications during dobutamine-atropine stress echocardiography. *Circulation* 2010;121:1756–1767.
2. De Sutter J, Poldermans D, Vourvouri E, et al. Long-term prognostic significance of complex ventricular arrhythmias induced during dobutamine stress echocardiography. *Am J Cardiol* 2003;91:242–244.

Answer 7: B. The stress echocardiogram shown demonstrates evidence of left anterior descending (LAD) territory ischemia. Normal response to exercise includes decrease in left ventricular cavity size and increase in myocardial contractility as evidenced by increased myocardial thickening and endocardial excursion (1). In this example, peak images show apical, anteroseptal, and anterior wall hypokinesis. Patients with multivessel obstructive coronary artery disease may demonstrate stress-induced wall motion abnormalities in different vascular territories and/or transient cavity dilation (choice D). It is also important to remember that stress echocardiography is more sensitive at identifying LAD territory ischemia as opposed to non-LAD territory ischemia (choice C).

Reference

1. Pellikka PA, Nagueh SF, Elhendy AA, et al. American Society of Echocardiography recommendations for performance, interpretation, and application of stress echocardiography. *J Am Soc Echocardiogr* 2007;20:1021–1041.

Answer 8: D. The echocardiographic images are obtained after administration of contrast. They show normal augmentation of wall motion with exercise in all visualized segments consistent with normal stress test. Therefore, reassurance and routine care including search for noncardiac causes of chest pain is warranted. Use of contrast agents during stress echocardiography is indicated when the image quality is suboptimal (≥2 contiguous segments are not seen on noncontrast images in any apical views), and it has been shown to be safe and well tolerated (1,2). It can increase the proportion of diagnostic studies and the reader's confidence in interpretation.

References

1. Mulvagh SL, Rakowski H, Vannan MA, et al. American Society of echocardiography consensus statement on the clinical applications of ultrasonic contrast agents in echocardiography. *J Am Soc Echocardiogr* 2008;21:1179–1201; quiz 1281.
2. Dolan MS, Gala SS, Dodla S, et al. Safety and efficacy of commercially available ultrasound contrast agents for rest and stress echocardiography a multicenter experience. *J Am Coll Cardiol* 2009;53:32–38.

Answer 9: C. In patients with systolic left ventricular dysfunction and significant resting wall motion abnormalities, dobutamine echocardiography allows assessment of both viability and ischemia. Inclusion of low-dose stages (2.5 and 5 μg/kg/min) facilitates identification of viability and ischemia in segments that are abnormal at rest (1–3). Treadmill exercise EKG, treadmill echocardiography, and vasodilator stress echocardiography have poor sensitivity in identifying both viable and ischemic myocardium.

References

1. Afridi I, Kleiman NS, Raizner AE, et al. Dobutamine echocardiography in myocardial hibernation. Optimal dose and accuracy in predicting recovery of ventricular function after coronary angioplasty. *Circulation* 1995;91:663–670.
2. Pellikka PA, Nagueh SF, Elhendy AA, et al. American Society of Echocardiography recommendations for performance, interpretation, and application of stress echocardiography. *J Am Soc Echocardiogr* 2007;20:1021–1041.
3. Chaudhry FA, Iskandrian AE. Assessing myocardial viability in ischemic cardiomyopathy. *Echocardiography* 2005;22:57.

Answer 10: A. Right ventricular wall motion should be interpreted during stress echocardiography since it has prognostic significance. In a study of 2,703 patients referred for stress echocardiography (both exercise and dobutamine), 112 (4%) patients had stress-induced right ventricular wall motion abnormalities. These abnormalities were more common in patients with a high number of cardiovascular risk factors and known coronary artery disease and congestive heart failure. Therefore, right ventricular wall motion abnormalities likely reflected a greater extent of coronary disease rather than other causes of right ventricular dysfunction (choices C and E). Abnormal right ventricle was a significant predictor of events (adjusted hazard ratio 2.7, *p* = 0.01) independent of left ventricular ischemia and ejection fraction (1). In the study, the assessment of the right ventricular wall motion was performed routinely in several echocardiographic views at rest and with stress, and it was feasible in 90% of patients (choice D).

Reference

1. Bangalore S, Yao SS, Chaudhry FA. Role of right ventricular wall motion abnormalities in risk stratification and prognosis of patients referred for stress echocardiography. *J Am Coll Cardiol* 2007;50:1981–1989.

Answer 11: E. Exertional dyspnea is a common reason for stress echocardiography referral. Although some patients with dyspnea without chest pain have postexercise wall motion abnormalities suggestive of coronary artery disease, a significant number has diastolic dysfunction. In recent years, it has been shown that postexercise transmitral flow velocities, tissue Doppler, and tricuspid regurgitation jet velocity can reliably identify stress-induced (latent) diastolic dysfunction. E/e′ ratio and estimated pulmonary artery systolic pressure often increase postexercise in patients with latent diastolic dysfunction indicating elevated left ventricular filling pressures (1). Although coronary heart disease is a possibility in this patient, she reports no anginal symptoms. A recent study showed that dyspnea is less likely to be angina equivalent in patients without known coronary artery disease (choices A, B, and C) (2).

References

1. Kane GC, Oh JK. Diastolic stress test for the evaluation of exertional dyspnea. *Curr Cardiol Rep* 2012;14:359–365.
2. Argulian E, Halpern DG, Agarwal V, et al. Predictors of ischemia in patients referred for evaluation of exertional dyspnea: a stress echocardiography study. *J Am Soc Echocardiogr* 2013;26:72–76.

Answer 12: B. Atrial fibrillation is an uncommon manifestation of coronary artery disease. In patients with newly diagnosed atrial fibrillation with no chest pain syndrome, no congestive heart failure, and normal left ventricular ejection fraction, exercise echocardiography should be considered as a part of evaluation only if the Framingham risk score is moderate to high. This patient seems to have lone atrial fibrillation, and he has a low risk for coronary artery disease. Therefore, exercise echocardiography before discharge will be considered inappropriate in this patient based on the appropriateness use criteria (1).

Reference

1. Douglas PS, Khandheria B, Stainback RF, et al. ACCF/ASE/ACEP/AHA/ASNC/SCAI/SCCT/SCMR 2008 appropriateness criteria for stress echocardiography: a report of the American College of Cardiology Foundation Appropriateness Criteria Task Force, American Society of Echocardiography, American College of Emergency Physicians, American Heart Association, American Society of Nuclear Cardiology, Society for Cardiovascular Angiography and Interventions, Society of Cardiovascular Computed Tomography, and Society for Cardiovascular Magnetic Resonance endorsed by the Heart Rhythm Society and the Society of Critical Care Medicine. *J Am Coll Cardiol* 2008;51:1127–1147.

Answer 13: A. Studies in patients undergoing vascular and nonvascular surgery have shown an excellent sensitivity and negative predictive value of dobutamine echocardiography in predicting adverse perioperative cardiac events (1,2). In the study by Das et al. (1), all patients who experienced adverse cardiac events had positive dobutamine echocardiogram (100% sensitivity). The specificity and positive predictive value of an abnormal dobutamine echocardiogram is modest meaning not all patients with stress-induced ischemia experience adverse events (choice B). Studies also showed that dobutamine echocardiography has limited prognostic information incremental to clinical parameters in low-risk patients (choices C and D) (3).

References

1. Das MK, Pellikka PA, Mahoney DW, et al. Assessment of cardiac risk before nonvascular surgery: dobutamine stress echocardiography in 530 patients. *J Am Coll Cardiol* 2000;35:1647–1653.
2. Poldermans D, Arnese M, Fioretti PM, et al. Improved cardiac risk stratification in major vascular surgery with dobutamine-atropine stress echocardiography. *J Am Coll Cardiol* 1995;26:648–653.
3. Boersma E, Poldermans D, Bax JJ, et al. Predictors of cardiac events after major vascular surgery: role of clinical characteristics, dobutamine echocardiography, and beta-blocker therapy. *JAMA* 2001;285:1865–1873.

Answer 14: *A.* Dobutamine echocardiography is proposed as a useful diagnostic tool in patients with suspected low-flow, low-gradient aortic stenosis (1,2). These patients typically have a depressed left ventricular ejection fraction, a low mean aortic gradient and peak transvalvular velocity, a calculated aortic valve area of <1.0 cm², and a dimensionless index of <0.25. True severe aortic stenosis in this setting should be differentiated from "pseudosevere" aortic stenosis created by a low-flow state and moderate or mild aortic stenosis. If the aortic stenosis is severe, the peak transvalvular velocity and the mean gradient augment during low-dose dobutamine infusion, while the calculated aortic valve area does not change compared to baseline. The dimensionless index (the ratio of LVOT VTI to aortic valve VTI) also stays unchanged in the severe range (<0.25). In our patient, the aortic valve VTI increased from 56 to 85 cm, the transvalvular velocity increased from 3 to 4.1 m/s, but the dimensionless index (11/56 cm = 0.20 at baseline) remained essentially unchanged (17/85 cm = 0.2) with dobutamine infusion. Therefore, the aortic stenosis is truly severe, and the patient will benefit from valve replacement. In patients with pseudosevere aortic stenosis, the augmentation in the mean gradient and the transvalvular velocity

during dobutamine infusion is accompanied by an increase in the calculated aortic valve area (>1.0 cm²) and the dimensionless index (>0.25). The primary problem in these patients is the cardiomyopathy, and the aortic stenosis is incidental. Appropriate treatment of cardiomyopathy is warranted (choice B). Some patients have little response to dobutamine infusion and do not augment their stroke volume due to poor contractile reserve. Prognosis in these patients is poor, and advanced therapies should be considered (choice C). Treadmill exercise tolerance testing may be considered in asymptomatic patients with severe aortic stenosis and normal left ventricular systolic function (choice D) (2).

References

1. Grayburn PA. Assessment of low-gradient aortic stenosis with dobutamine. *Circulation* 2006;113:604–606.
2. Bonow RO, Carabello BA, Chatterjee K, et al. 2008 focused update incorporated into the ACC/AHA 2006 guidelines for the management of patients with valvular heart disease: a report of the American College of Cardiology/American Heart Association Task Force on Practice Guidelines (Writing Committee to revise the 1998 guidelines for the management of patients with valvular heart disease). Endorsed by the Society of Cardiovascular Anesthesiologists, Society for Cardiovascular Angiography and Interventions, and Society of Thoracic Surgeons. *J Am Coll Cardiol* 2008;52:e1–e142.

Answer 15: *D.* This patient has a markedly abnormal stress echo with reduction in LV function immediately post exercise. There is significant apical foreshortening that could not be avoided by the sonographer performing the examination. Although this has a tendency of "falsely" improving the contractility in the LAD territory, the anteroseptal and anterior regional wall segments improved more than other regions. There is abnormal septal motion, but thickening is near-normal.

As shown on the coronary angiogram, the coronary artery anatomy was interpreted as normal (Fig. 30.5 and Videos 30.7A and B). As you recall from the history, this patient has a physical exam consistent with BAV and AR. It is important to perform a limited color-flow Doppler examination in these patients to understand other

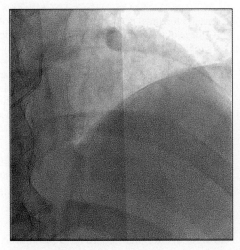
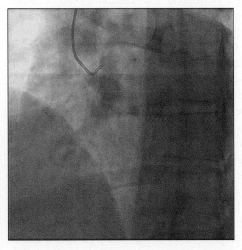

Figure 30.5

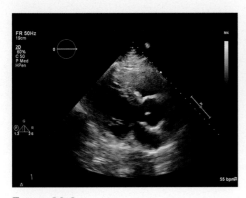

FIGURE 30.6

contributing factors to exercise cardiovascular physiology (see FIG. 30.6 and VIDEOS 30.8A AND B). In this case, it is likely that the regional dysfunction represents ischemia from coronary "mismatch" (myocardial perfusion impairment) despite normal epicardial coronary artery anatomy.

Answer 16: E. This patient has an abnormal stress echo result with reduced LV global systolic function. There are mild regional contraction variations coupled with slight variance in apical alignment (note: more foreshortening at rest), but no new regions of akinesis or severe hypokinesis. If you answered D (2-V CAD without LAD pattern), that would

not be entirely incorrect and likely many others would select this choice.

The coronary angiography is shown in FIGURE 30.7 and VIDEOS 30.9A AND B, and this was considered normal. In this clinical setting, where the BP markedly increases over a short period of time (>80 mm Hg increase in ~1 stage of exercise), this is known to result in impaired LV systolic contraction. Given her likely CAD (despite "normal" epicardial arteries) from years of smoking and hypertensive heart disease, she most likely has impaired coronary vasomotor tone and a component of microvascular CAD as well. This may cause the regional pattern to contraction that is demonstrated.

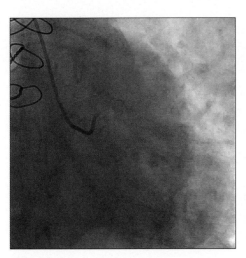
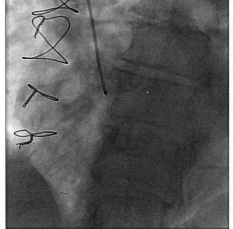

FIGURE 30.7

Chapter 31

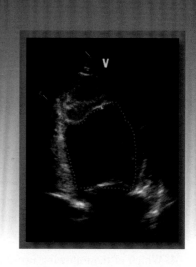

Dilated Cardiomyopathy

Maya E. Guglin

Questions 1 and 2

A 65-year-old female presents to the emergency department with complaints of shortness of breath and tightness across her chest after an argument with her husband. Her past medical history is significant for hypertension. An ECG in the ED is shown in FIGURE 31.1. Initial cardiac troponin T is elevated at 0.2 ng/mL. As the patient is preparing to go for emergent coronary angiography, a bedside echocardiogram is performed (VIDEOS 31.1 TO 31.3).

1. The most likely cause of the patient's presentation is:

   A. Severe multivessel coronary artery disease
   B. Acute thrombus within the left anterior descending coronary artery
   C. Acute thrombus within the right coronary artery
   D. Apical ballooning syndrome
   E. Acute myocarditis

2. Prior to the patient presenting in the catheterization laboratory, she becomes hypotensive (SBP 85 mm Hg). Dobutamine is initiated. The patient's systolic blood pressure is now 70 mm Hg, and she starts to show evidence of pulmonary edema. Dobutamine infusion is increased, but the patient remains unstable and is subsequently intubated. Exam reveals a systolic murmur that is difficult to hear because of the diffuse pulmonary crackles anteriorly and posteriorly. Repeat bedside echocardiogram is undertaken.

What is the most likely abnormality to be seen?

   A. Worsening systolic function with an LVEF now 10%
   B. Large pericardial effusion with tamponade physiology
   C. Ventricular septal defect
   D. LVOT gradient of 40 mm Hg and mitral regurgitation

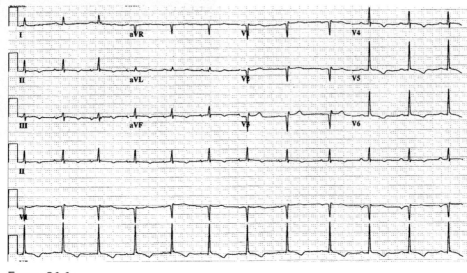

FIGURE 31.1

Questions 3 and 4

A 28-year-old female with a history of intravenous drug abuse comes to the emergency room complaining of shortness of breath. Initial evaluation in the emergency department reveals a thin anxious female with BP 100/50 mm Hg, HR 98 bpm, and a respiratory rate of 25/minute. Physical exam is remarkable for a jugular venous pressure of 10-cm H_2O. There are bibasilar crackles and an enlarged, displaced point of maximal impulse. An echocardiogram is performed (Video 31.4).

3. What is the most likely diagnosis?

   A. Systemic lupus erythematosus
   B. Infective endocarditis
   C. HIV/AIDS-related heart disease
   D. Amyloidosis-related cardiomyopathy
   E. Ischemic cardiomyopathy

4. Which of the following two-dimensional and Doppler profiles would not be indicative of hemodynamic compromise related to the pericardial effusion?

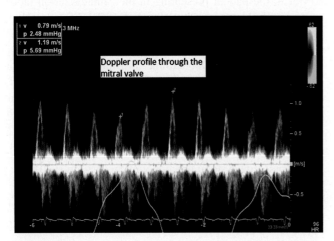

FIGURE 31.2

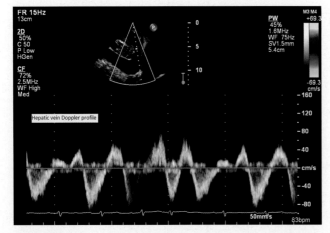

FIGURE 31.3

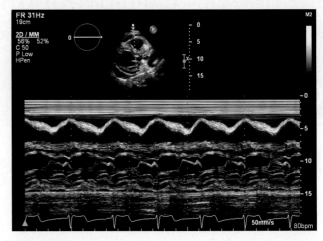

FIGURE 31.4

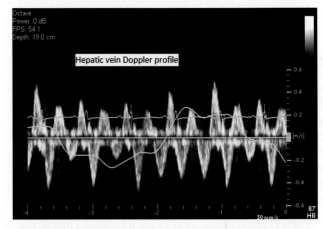

FIGURE 31.5

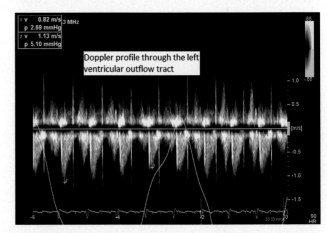

FIGURE 31.6

   A. FIGURE 31.2
   B. FIGURE 31.3
   C. FIGURE 31.4
   D. FIGURE 31.5
   E. FIGURE 31.6

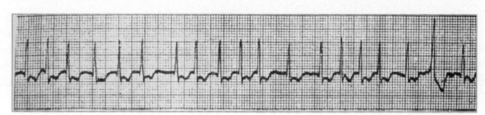

FIGURE 31.7

5. A 58-year-old female with weight loss, tremor, and palpitations undergoes an ECG (FIG. 31.7) and a transthoracic echocardiogram (VIDEO 31.5). Her systolic BP is 120/70 mm Hg, and her HR is 146 bpm at the time of evaluation.

The best *initial* treatment option for her after diagnosis is:

A. Methimazole and propranolol
B. Carvedilol and an ACE inhibitor
C. Immediate DC electrical cardioversion
D. Coronary angiography and PCI if indicated
E. Transesophageal echocardiogram–guided cardioversion

6. A 38-year-old female presents with an abnormal chest x-ray (FIG. 31.8) and syncope. An echocardiogram is performed (VIDEOS 31.6 TO 31.8).

What is the most likely diagnosis?

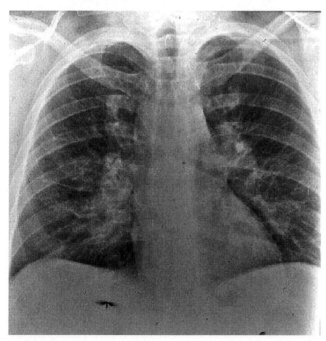

FIGURE 31.8

A. Multivessel coronary artery disease
B. Cardiac sarcoidosis
C. Left ventricular noncompaction
D. Familial dilated cardiomyopathy
E. Arrhythmogenic right ventricular cardiomyopathy (ARVC)

Questions 7 and 8

A 34-year-old female who is 37 weeks' pregnant reports to her obstetrician with complaints of shortness of breath and swelling of her lower extremities. Her past medical history is relatively unremarkable, yet she states she may have been told of a heart murmur in her teens. Blood pressure at the time of the visit is 90/55 mm Hg with a heart rate of 105 bpm. Physical exam reveals an elevated JVP (15 cm H_2O) with a V-wave, evidence of an S3 gallop, 2+ pitting lower extremity edema, and rales one-third of the way up bilaterally. An ECG performed reveals sinus tachycardia. A stat echocardiogram is ordered (FIG. 31.9, VIDEOS 31.9 TO 31.13).

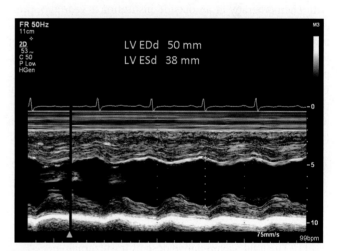

FIGURE 31.9

7. After the patient is admitted to the hospital, the next best step in the patient's management should be:

A. Intravenous ACE inhibitor
B. Immediate C-section
C. Intravenous nitroglycerin
D. Intravenous furosemide
E. Intravenous beta-blocker

8. Of the following, which is the best predictor of recovery of left ventricular systolic function?

A. Left ventricular end-diastolic diameter of 65 mm at the time of presentation
B. Normal troponin T level at the time of presentation
C. Fractional shortening <20% at the time of presentation
D. Left ventricular ejection fraction >20% at the time of presentation

Question 9.

A 59-year-old female presented with symptoms of heart failure 5 months ago to another institution where an echo was performed and demonstrated left ventricular global hypokinesis with an LVEF of 15%. She was started on lisinopril, carvedilol, and spironolactone with minimal symptom improvement. She is now being seen for a second opinion at your institution. Repeat echo is shown in VIDEOS 31.14A AND B.

After a procedure, she returns with marked improvement of symptoms and a 3-month follow-up video is shown (VIDEO 31.14C).

9. Which of the following procedures was most likely performed?

A. Placement of a left ventricular assist device
B. Cardioverter–defibrillator implantation
C. Cardiac resynchronization therapy
D. Stem cell therapy
E. Cardiac transplantation

Question 10

A 37-year-old female with a history of breast cancer, treated with chemotherapy at an outside institution 1 year ago, presents with symptoms of dyspnea on exertion, fatigue, and mild lower extremity edema. Physical exam reveals a heart rate of 98 bpm and BP 102/70. Cardiac exam is significant for a displaced PMI with a soft S3. The lungs reveal bibasilar crackles. Her records from the outside institution are limited but reveal that the patient received doxorubicin and trastuzumab (doses unknown). Echocardiogram is performed soon after admission (VIDEO 31.15).

10. Which of the following increases the patient's risk of chemotherapy-induced cardiomyopathy?

A. Her age <50
B. The use of trastuzumab with anthracycline
C. Use of birth control pills
D. The total accumulative dose of trastuzumab

11. A 25-year-old athlete has an echocardiogram performed to evaluate an episode of syncope (VIDEOS 31.16 AND 31.17). What is the most likely diagnosis?

A. Hypertrophic cardiomyopathy
B. Isolated left ventricular noncompaction
C. Dilated cardiomyopathy
D. Fabry disease
E. Arrhythmogenic right ventricular cardiomyopathy (ARVC)

12. A 68-year-old white male s/p myocardial infarction (MI) 1 month prior returns for follow-up echocardiography to assess left ventricular function (VIDEO 31.18).

What finding does the post-MI echocardiogram show?

A. Left ventricular pseudoaneurysm
B. Left ventricular aneurysm
C. Left ventricular apical thrombus
D. Finding associated with a high risk of myocardial rupture

13. A 50-year-old white male is referred for evaluation of palpitations and syncope. His physical exam is normal. A 24-hour Holter monitor reveals nonsustained monomorphic ventricular tachycardia. An echocardiogram is performed with images shown in VIDEOS 31.19 TO 31.22, and FIGURE 31.10.

What is the diagnosis shown?

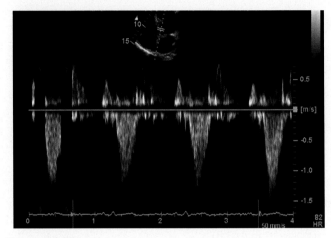

FIGURE 31.10

A. Hypertrophic obstructive cardiomyopathy
B. Apical hypertrophic cardiomyopathy
C. Arrhythmogenic right ventricular cardiomyopathy (ARVC)
D. Left ventricular noncompaction
E. Nonischemic dilated cardiomyopathy

Answer 1: D. The patient's clinical presentation is consistent with either an acute coronary event or apical ballooning. The argument with the spouse is a clue to stress-induced cardiomyopathy (apical ballooning syndrome or takotsubo cardiomyopathy). In addition, although the ECG does show evidence of slight ST elevation in the precordial leads, the findings are nonspecific and there are no reciprocal changes suggestive of an acute current of injury. The clinical case presented is fairly classic for stress-induced cardiomyopathy. Patients usually present after a stressor ("recent argument with husband" in this case) with an abnormal ECG (slight precordial ST elevation in the case). Coronary angiography revealed no significant epicardial coronary artery disease (VIDEOS 31.23 AND 31.24). The echocardiogram demonstrates regional wall motion abnormalities beyond the distribution of a single coronary artery territory. There is preserved to hyperdynamic basal function of the heart with significant hypokinesis to akinesis starting at the midwalls and continuing on to the apex. The LV cavity is dilated as well. It would be unusual for this to be due to multivessel disease given the well-preserved basal function of the heart. However, coronary angiography is frequently necessary to confirm the diagnosis. Complete recovery of function is typical as was true in this case and is seen on echocardiogram performed 5 days later (VIDEO 31.25). Multiple studies have now established no evidence of late gadolinium enhancement (LGE) on cardiac magnetic resonance imaging (CMR) and no evidence of acute pericarditis (epicardial or midmyocardial delayed hyperenhancement rather than endocardial). Troponins may be elevated in all of the choices, but the echo, ECG, and subsequent coronary angiogram are consistent with apical ballooning.

Answer 2: D. The recognition must be made that patients with apical ballooning are at risk for dynamic LVOT obstruction and systolic anterior motion of the mitral valve, causing mitral regurgitation (13% to 18% of cases) (VIDEO 31.26). Although pump failure is a potential issue with apical ballooning, the murmur and worsening hemodynamics should make alert you the LVOT obstruction with SAM and MR. Inotropes would make this condition worse, as this would worsen the hyperdynamic function at the base of the heart and thus increase the LVOT gradient. Treatment is volume and gentle beta blockade.

Suggested Readings

Bybee KA, Kara T, Prasad A, et al. Systematic review: transient left ventricular apical ballooning: a syndrome that mimics ST-segment elevation myocardial infarction. *Ann Intern Med* 2004;141:858.

Eitel I, von Knobelsdorff-Brenkenhoff F, Bernhardt P, et al. Clinical characteristics and cardiovascular magnetic resonance findings in stress (takotsubo) cardiomyopathy. *JAMA* 2011;306(3):277–286.

Sato H, Taiteishi H, Uchida T. Takotsubo-type cardiomyopathy due to multivessel spasm. In: Kodama K, Haze K, Hon M, eds. *Clinical Aspect of Myocardial Injury: From Ischemia to Heart Failure*. Tokyo, Japan: Kagakuhyouronsha, 1990:56.

Sharkey SW, Lesser JR, Zenovich AG, et al. Acute and reversible cardiomyopathy provoked by stress in women from the United States. *Circulation* 2005;111:472.

Syed IS, Prasad A, Oh JK, et al. Apical ballooning syndrome or aborted acute myocardial infarction? Insights from cardiovascular magnetic resonance imaging. *Int J Cardiovasc Imaging* 2008;24(8):875–882.

Villareal RP, Achari A, Wilansky S, et al. Anteroapical stunning and left ventricular outflow tract obstruction. *Mayo Clin Proc* 2001;76:79–83.

Answer 3: C; Answer 4: B. The patient most likely has HIV/AIDS given her intravenous drug use and echocardiographic findings. There is no evidence of valvular pathology to suggest endocarditis. Clinical cardiac involvement occurs in 10% of patients with AIDS. The most common cardiac involvement is pericardial effusion/pericarditis. However, on autopsy, myocarditis is seen 50% of the time. Clinical manifestations of myocarditis, however, occur more rarely (10%) but can result in a dilated cardiomyopathy. The echocardiogram demonstrates a circumferential pericardial effusion without evidence of chamber collapse. The LV systolic function appears normal on this limited view with normal wall thickness. The myocardial acoustic characteristics and wall thickness do not suggest an infiltrative cardiomyopathy as would be present in amyloidosis. There is no evidence of any regional wall motion abnormalities on limited imaging but clinically would be highly unlikely. Although a pericardial effusion may be seen with systemic lupus erythematosus, the history is more consistent with HIV-related cardiomyopathy.

It is very important when assessing pericardial effusion to identify if there is hemodynamic compromise related to the effusion. The diagnosis of tamponade is a clinical one, but

two-dimensional and Doppler echocardiography play major roles in identifying the location and characteristics of effusions as well as their hemodynamic significance. Certain echocardiographic findings can be indicative of increased intrapericardial pressure, leading to tamponade physiology. FIGURE 31.11 shows the mitral inflow Doppler signal. Respirometer tracing is seen on the bottom of the view. Mitral inflow E velocity decreases >25% during inspiration (point 1). During inspiration, the flow to the right ventricle increases. In tamponade, this increased RV flow causes a decrease of flow through the left side due to the shift of the ventricular septum leftward (a process called ventricular interdependence). Thus, a decrease in early mitral inflow is seen by a reduction in the E velocity. Accordingly, the flow out of the aortic valve will show a decrease during inspiration as well which is illustrated in FIGURE 31.12. These changes play a primary role in the finding of pulsus paradoxus seen in clinical tamponade. FIGURE 31.4 reveals an M-Mode tracing through the heart from the parasternal long-axis view. The still picture shows the pericardial effusion anterior to the right ventricle. The M-mode tracing reveals early right ventricular diastolic collapse (FIG. 31.13 and seen in 2D here in VIDEO 31.27). The hepatic vein Doppler tracing in FIGURE 31.4 shows evidence of end-expiratory diastolic flow reversal (FIG. 31.14). This is seen in constrictive pericarditis as well and reflects the ventricular interdependence and the dissociation between intracardiac and

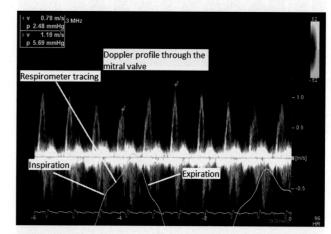

FIGURE 31.11

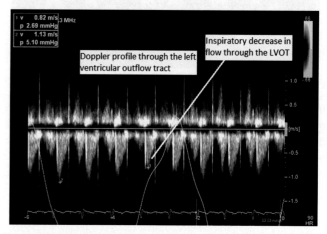

FIGURE 31.12

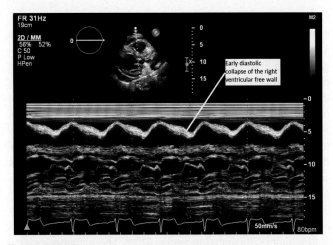

FIGURE 31.13

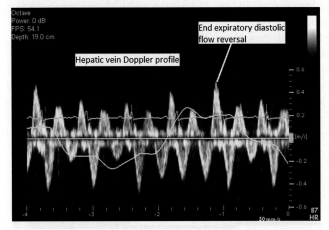

FIGURE 31.14

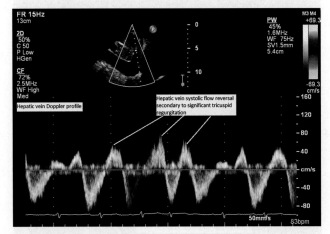

FIGURE 31.15

intrathoracic pressures. FIGURE 31.3 is a hepatic vein Doppler tracing in a patient with severe tricuspid regurgitation. Systolic flow reversal within the hepatic vein is seen with each cardiac beat (FIG. 31.15). This pattern is the least likely to be seen in a patient with a hemodynamically significant pericardial effusion.

Suggested Readings

Anderson DW, Virmani R, Reilly JM, et al. Prevalent myocarditis at necropsy in the acquired immunodeficiency syndrome. *J Am Coll Cardiol* 1988;11:792.

Cammarosano C, Lewis W. Cardiac lesions in acquired immune deficiency syndrome (AIDS). *J Am Coll Cardiol* 1985;5:703.
De Castro S, d'Amati G, Gallo P, et al. Frequency of development of acute global left ventricular dysfunction in human immunodeficiency virus infection. *J Am Coll Cardiol* 1994;24:1018.
De Castro S, Migliau G, Silvestri A, et al. Heart involvement in AIDS: a prospective study during various stages of the disease. *Eur Heart J* 1992;13:1452.
Eisenberg MJ, Gordon AS, Schiller NB. HIV-associated pericardial effusions. *Chest* 1992;102:956.
Shannon RP, Simon MA, Mathier MA, et al. Dilated cardiomyopathy associated with simian AIDS in nonhuman primates. *Circulation* 2000;101(2):185–193.
Sudano I, Spieker LE, Noll G, et al. Cardiovascular disease in HIV infection. *Am Heart J* 2006;151:1147.

Answer 5: A. The patient's clinical presentation is that of hyperthyroidism, which has resulted in atrial fibrillation. The rapid atrial fibrillation has subsequently led to a tachycardia-induced dilated cardiomyopathy. The four-chamber and two-chamber views reveal a dilated LV with a reduced ejection fraction and global hypokinesis. The best initial treatment option *is to treat the underlying hyperthyroid state and add beta-blockers to control the heart rate.* Typically, these patients do not need traditional heart failure treatment regimens as the left ventricular systolic function returns to normal with treatment of the tachyarrhythmia. Cardioversion should be performed if the atrial fibrillation is persistent after reaching a euthyroid state or if the patient is clinically unstable. Sinus rhythm will be unlikely to be maintained, however, unless the patient is euthyroid. Anticoagulation is also more problematic in patients with hyperthyroidism.

Suggested Readings

Kellett HA, Sawers JS, Boulton FE, et al. Problems of anticoagulation with warfarin in hyperthyroidism. *Q J Med* 1986;58:43.
Klein I, Danzi S. Thyroid disease and the heart. *Circulation* 2007;116:1725.
Klein I, Ojamaa K. Thyroid hormone and the cardiovascular system. *N Engl J Med* 2001;344:501.
Mercé J, Ferrás S, Oltra C, et al. Cardiovascular abnormalities in hyperthyroidism: a prospective Doppler echocardiographic study. *Am J Med* 2005;118:126.
Osman F, Franklyn JA, Holder RL, et al. Cardiovascular manifestations of hyperthyroidism before and after antithyroid therapy: a matched case–control study. *J Am Coll Cardiol* 2007;49:71.

Answer 6: B. Clinical manifestations of cardiac sarcoidosis depend upon the location and extent of the granulomatous inflammation. Unusual wall motion abnormalities that do not clearly follow a coronary artery distribution can be seen and, in addition, left ventricular aneurysms are sometimes present. The depositions of granulomas can be anywhere throughout the myocardium but are most common within the intraventricular septum and left ventricular free wall. The clinical scenario is very helpful in making the diagnosis. The diagnosis of cardiac sarcoid should be entertained in young individuals who present with syncope in the setting of an abnormal chest x-ray. Echocardiographic abnormalities in sarcoid are frequently found after the diagnosis has already been established. The myocardium has scar related to infiltrating noncaseating granulomas. The scar tissue may lead to heart block, syncope, or sudden cardiac death. In the echo images shown, there is a dilated cardiomyopathy with a superimposed basal septal aneurysm (this would be very unusual to be caused by coronary artery disease, given the lack of abnormality specifically in the anterior wall). Given the patient's abnormal chest x-ray, revealing bilateral hilar adenopathy and reticular opacities, and syncope, most likely from heart block, the likely etiology of the cardiomyopathy of the choices shown is cardiac sarcoidosis, although this is a difficult diagnosis to make unless there is a biopsy from the heart or other tissue showing the characteristic noncaseating granulomas.

Familial dilated cardiomyopathy is less likely because of the definite regional wall motion abnormality (aneurysm) in the basal septum. The patient's history also is a clue to a systemic disease. Arrhythmogenic right ventricular cardiomyopathy is incorrect. The right ventricle does have an unusual contour, likely related to the dilated left ventricle. Although it is not unusual to also have right ventricular involvement with cardiac sarcoidosis, the primary abnormality shown is a left ventricular problem. Right ventricular function is relatively preserved. Cardiovascular magnetic resonance (CMR) imaging has become a very useful tool to help establish the diagnosis of cardiac sarcoid. Edema from inflammation, wall motion abnormalities, and delayed enhancement secondary to fibrosis and scar can be assessed by CMR and help guide in the diagnosis and possible treatment response.

Suggested Readings

Chapelon-Abric C, de Zuttere D, Duhaut P, et al. Cardiac sarcoidosis: a retrospective study of 41 cases. *Medicine (Baltimore)* 2004;83:315.

Kim JS, Judson MA, Donnino R, et al. Cardiac sarcoidosis. *Am Heart J* 2009;157:9.

Schulte W, Kirsten D, Drent M, et al. Cardiac involvement in sarcoidosis. *Eur Respir Mon* 2005;32:130.

Smedema JP, Snoep G, van Kroonenburgh MP, et al. Cardiac involvement in patients with pulmonary sarcoidosis assessed at two university medical centers in the Netherlands. *Chest* 2005;128:30.

Smedema JP, Snoep G, van Kroonenburgh MP, et al. Evaluation of the accuracy of gadolinium-enhanced cardiovascular magnetic resonance in the diagnosis of cardiac sarcoidosis. *J Am Coll Cardiol* 2005;45(10):1683.

Answer 7: D; Answer 8: B. The patient presents with severe heart failure related to peripartum cardiomyopathy. The acute heart failure must be addressed first. The patient shows evidence of volume overload primarily. Intravenous nitroglycerin or ACE inhibition would not be indicated in a relatively hypotensive patient. Furthermore, because ACE inhibitors and ARBs are contraindicated in pregnancy, hydralazine would be the drug of choice when antepartum oral vasodilator therapy is necessary. It has been used for many years in the treatment of hypertension during pregnancy and appears to be safe for both the mother and fetus, but probably not in this patient given the relative hypotension. Intravenous beta-blocker would not be used initially given the volume overload that is present. Although removal of the fetus may be necessary, it is not the first step, given the patient's overall clinical status. If the patient was more acutely decompensating, immediate delivery may be warranted. Recently, a potentially pathophysiologic

role of a defective antioxidant defense mechanism triggering pathogenic prolactin fragments has been implicated in peripartum cardiomyopathy; hence, suppression of prolactin production with bromocriptine may also be indicated.

There are certain conditions that increase the risk of peripartum cardiomyopathy. These include African American race, multiparity, age > 30 years, maternal cocaine use, and a history of preeclampsia or eclampsia. There are certain features that predict persistent LV dysfunction. These include LVEF < 30%, fractional shortening <20%, LVEDD ≥ 60 mm, and an elevated troponin.

Suggested Readings

Chapa JB, Heiberger HB, Weinert L, et al. Prognostic value of echocardiography in peripartum cardiomyopathy. *Obstet Gynecol* 2005;105:1303.

Elkayam U, Akhter MW, Singh H, et al. Pregnancy-associated cardiomyopathy: clinical characteristics and a comparison between early and late presentation. *Circulation* 2005;111:2050.

Elkayam U, Goland S. Bromocriptine for the treatment of peripartum cardiomyopathy. *Circulation* 2010;121:1463.

Goland S, Bitar F, Modi K, et al. Evaluation of the clinical relevance of baseline left ventricular ejection fraction as a predictor of recovery or persistence of severe dysfunction in women in the United States with peripartum cardiomyopathy. *J Card Fail* 2011;17:426.

Hu CL, Li YB, Zou YG, et al. Troponin T measurement can predict persistent left ventricular dysfunction in peripartum cardiomyopathy. *Heart* 2007;93:488.

Lampert MB, Lang RM. Peripartum cardiomyopathy. *Am Heart J* 1995;130:860.

Lee W. Clinical management of gravid women with peripartum cardiomyopathy. *Obstet Gynecol Clin North Am* 1991;18:257.

Sliwa K, Blauwet L, Tibazarwa K, et al. Evaluation of bromocriptine in the treatment of acute severe peripartum cardiomyopathy: a proof-of-concept pilot study. *Circulation* 2010;121:1465.

Sliwa K, Fett J, Elkayam U. Peripartum cardiomyopathy. *Lancet* 2006;368:687.

Answer 9: C. On baseline echocardiography (Videos 31.28 and 31.29), severe global hypokinesis and marked intraventricular dyssynchrony is noted. The septum moves away from the left ventricular free wall. In addition, the running ECG on the bottom of the screen, although not precise to allow adequate analysis of the morphology of the QRS, demonstrates a wide complex QRS. After 3 months of guidelines-recommended medical therapy, the next step is the implantation of BiV/AICD. Neither LVAD nor heart transplantation should be performed until all potentially reversible conditions are addressed.

Women with nonischemic cardiomyopathy and recent onset of symptoms, like the patient in our question, have the best chances of being superresponders to CRT, with almost complete resolution of left ventricular dyssynchrony and dysfunction. Stem cells were never shown to provide such a marked improvement in left ventricular geometry and function. Implantable cardioverter–defibrillators, although important for sudden cardiac death prevention, do not have any impact on cardiac function.

Suggested Readings

Gho JM, Kummeling GJ, Koudstaal S, et al. Cell therapy, a novel remedy for dilated cardiomyopathy? A systematic review. *J Card Fail* 2013;19(7):494–502.

Miller LW, Guglin M. Patient selection for ventricular assist devices: a moving target. *J Am Coll Cardiol* 2013;61(12):1209–1221.

Steffel J, Ruschitzka F. Superresponse to cardiac resynchronization therapy. *Circulation* 2014;130(1):87–90.

Yancy CW, Jessup M, Bozkurt B, et al. 2013 ACCF/AHA guideline for the management of heart failure: a report of the American College of Cardiology Foundation/American Heart Association Task Force on Practice Guidelines. *J Am Coll Cardiol* 2013;62(16):e147–e239.

Answer 10: B. Because the patient has received chemotherapy, there are important considerations with regard to her risk of developing a DCM. Anthracycline-based regimens are well established as a potential cause for a dilated cardiomyopathy. Total accumulative dose closely correlates with the risk. A recently published study on a cohort of 607 children with long-term follow-up (mean 6.3 years) has shown that the only independent risk factor is a cumulative dose of >300 mg/m^2. Present recommendations are not to exceed lifetime total doses of >450 to 500 g/m^2 in adults. Trastuzumab use in conjunction with an anthracycline increases the risk further. Unlike anthracyclines, the total accumulative dose of trastuzumab does not appear to be related to the risk of cardiotoxicity. The biggest risk for trastuzumab for causing cardiotoxicity is previous or concurrent use of an anthracycline and the patient's age > 50 years. Trastuzumab cardiotoxicity differs substantially from anthracycline cardiotoxicity in that it occurs much more frequently but is also more reversible. The incidence of cardiotoxicity is increased when trastuzumab is used in combination with anthracyclines. A prior history of chest irradiation increases the risk of cardiotoxicity related to the doxorubicin (but does not seem to increase the risk in a trastuzumab-alone regimen). In addition, the presence of traditional risk factors, such as hypertension, hyperlipidemia, and diabetes, increases the risk of an anthracycline-induced cardiomyopathy (less so with trastuzumab alone).

Suggested Readings

Bowles EJ, Wellman R, Feigelson HS, et al.; Pharmacovigilance Study Team. Risk of heart failure in breast cancer patients after anthracycline and trastuzumab treatment: a retrospective cohort study. *J Natl Cancer Inst* 2012;104(17):1293–1305.

Ewer MS, Vooletich MT, Durand JB, et al. Reversibility of trastuzumab-related cardiotoxicity: new insights based on clinical course and response to medical treatment. *J Clin Oncol* 2005;23(31):7820–7826.

Gharib MI, Burnett AK. Chemotherapy-induced cardiotoxicity: current practice and prospects of prophylaxis. *Eur J Heart Fail* 2002;4(3):235–242.

Plana JC, Galderisi M, Barac A, et al. Expert consensus for multimodality imaging evaluation of adult patients during and after cancer therapy: a report from the American Society of Echocardiography and the European Association of Cardiovascular Imaging. *J Am Soc Echocardiogr* 2014;27:911–939.

Answer 11: E. ARVC is a rare inherited heart–muscle disease that can lead to sudden cardiac death from arrhythmia. First described in 1736 by Giovanni Maria Lancisi, it results from an abnormality in desmosomal proteins. The original task force recommendations identified the following as major criteria for the diagnosis of ARVC: (1) severe dilation and reduction of right ventricular ejection fraction with no (or only mild) left ventricular impairment, (2) localized right ventricular aneurysms (akinetic or dyskinetic areas with diastolic bulging), (3) severe segmental dilation of the right ventricle, (4) fibrofatty replacement of myocardium on endomyocardial biopsy, (5) epsilon-wave or localized prolongation (>110 ms) of the QRS complex in right precordial leads (V1 to V3), (6) familial disease confirmed at necropsy or surgery, and (7) ventricular arrhythmias. These criteria were later modified to include ARVC in a first-degree relative plus one of the following: (1) ECG T-wave inversion in right precordial leads (V2 and V3); (2) late potentials on signal-averaged ECG; (3) left bundle-branch block–type VT on ECG, on Holter monitoring, or during exercise testing; (4) extrasystoles of more than 200 over a 24-hour period; (5) mild global right ventricular dilation or ejection fraction reduction with normal left ventricle; (6) mild segmental dilation of the right ventricle; and (7) regional right ventricular hypokinesia.

The echocardiographic features of ARVC have also been described and include (1) dilation of the right ventricle (RV)—RV outflow tract ≥30 mm in parasternal long-axis view or RV outflow tract ≥32 mm in parasternal short axis view, (2) RV apical pouching, (3) prominent RV trabeculation, and (4) prominent RV moderator band.

Hypertrophic cardiomyopathy is incorrect. Although probably the most common cause of sudden cardiac death in athletes, the echocardiographic findings do not suggest this diagnosis. The abnormalities of a prominent RV moderator band and prominent RV trabeculation are more consistent with ARVC. Isolated LV noncompaction is incorrect because the LV looks unremarkable on echocardiography. Although the RV can be involved in noncompaction, this diagnosis is unlikely given the isolated RV abnormalities shown. Dilated cardiomyopathy is unlikely because the LV is not dilated and has a normal ejection fraction. Fabry disease is an inherited X-linked recessive disorder due to a lysosomal storage disease secondary to α-galactosidase A enzyme deficiency and leads to intralysosomal accumulation of the glycosphingolipid globotriaosylceramide. It is manifest on echocardiography as an infiltrative cardiomyopathy of the left ventricle and often mistaken for hypertrophic cardiomyopathy or amyloidosis. The myocardium has been described as having a binary appearance with echo brightness in the endocardium and epicardium (and darker appearance in the midmyocardium).

Suggested Readings

Hamid MS, Norman M, Quraishi A, et al. Prospective evaluation of relatives for familial arrhythmogenic right ventricular cardiomyopathy/dysplasia reveals a need to broaden diagnostic criteria. *J Am Coll Cardiol* 2002;40(8):1445–1450.

McKenna WJ, Thiene G, Nava A, et al. Diagnosis of arrhythmogenic right ventricular dysplasia/cardiomyopathy. Task Force of the Working Group Myocardial and Pericardial Disease of the European Society of Cardiology and of the Scientific Council on Cardiomyopathies of the International Society and Federation of Cardiology. *Br Heart J* 1994;71(3):215–218.

Pieroni M. Echocardiographic assessment of Fabry cardiomyopathy: early diagnosis and follow-up. *J Am Soc Echocardiogr* 2011;24(9):1033–1036.

Pieroni M, Chimenti C, De Cobelli F, et al. Fabry's disease cardiomyopathy: echocardiographic detection of endomyocardial glycosphingolipid compartmentalization. *J Am Coll Cardiol* 2006;47(8):1663–1671.

Yoerger DM, Marcus F, Sherrill D, et al.; Multidisciplinary Study of Right Ventricular Dysplasia Investigators. Echocardiographic findings in patients meeting task force criteria for arrhythmogenic

Table 31.1	Echocardiographic Criteria for IVNC Diagnosis	

CHIN CRITERIA (1990)	JENNI CRITERIA (1999)
Absence of any other coexisting cardiac structural abnormality	Absence of any other coexisting cardiac structural abnormality
Numerous, excessively prominent trabeculations and deep intertrabecular recesses	Numerous, excessively prominent trabeculations and deep intertrabecular recesses
Views: parasternal long axis, subxiphoid, and apical	Views: parasternal short axis and apical
Focus on depth of recesses	Focus on a two-layer structure
Measured in end diastole	Measured in end systole
Ratio of distance from the epicardial surface to the trough of the trabecular recesses and distance from the epicardial surface to peak of trabeculation ≤0.5	Ratio of thick noncompacted layer to thin compacted ≥2 perfused intertrabecular recesses supplied by intraventricular blood on color Doppler analysis

Adapted from Song Z. Echocardiography in the diagnosis left ventricular noncompaction. *Cardiovasc Ultrasound* 2008;6:64.

right ventricular dysplasia: new insights from the multidisciplinary study of right ventricular dysplasia. *J Am Coll Cardiol* 2005;45(6):860–865.

Answer 12: B. The image shown demonstrates a classic post-MI LV apical aneurysm. There is thinning and expansion of the apical myocardium, and the usual treatment is conservative unless there is refractory angina, heart failure, or ventricular arrhythmia. There is relatively low risk of rupture because of the fibrous scar forming the wall of the aneurysm.

LV pseudoaneurysm is incorrect. The echo image shown demonstrates thinning and expansion of the LV apex characteristic of an LV apical aneurysm. Post-MI LV pseudoaneurysm occurs when a rupture of the LV free wall is contained by an overlying, adherent pericardium, and the usual treatment is urgent surgical repair because there is high risk of rupture of the overlying pericardium. An example of a post-MI LV pseudoaneurysm is shown (VIDEOS 31.30 AND 31.31).

LV aneurysm demonstrates a wide neck-to-base ratio while LV pseudoaneurysm demonstrates a narrow (<0.4 to 0.5) ratio of diameter of entry to maximum cavity.

LV apical thrombus is incorrect. There is no mass seen at the LV apex. Findings consistent with a high risk of rupture are not correct because there is a relatively low risk of aneurysm rupture due to the fibrous scar representing all three layers of myocardium that is present. Although rupture may occur, the risk appears relatively low.

Suggested Reading

Brown SL, Gropler RJ, Harris KM. Distinguishing left ventricular aneurysm from pseudoaneurysm. A review of the literature. *Chest* 1997;111(5):1403–1409.

Answer 13: D. The image shown demonstrates classic findings of left ventricular (LV) noncompaction. The myocardium is noncompacted or "spongy myocardium." This disorder results from an arrest in normal endomyocardial embryogenesis. Both isolated noncompaction and types associated with other complex congenital diseases may be seen. The right ventricle is involved in less than half of cases.

Echocardiography is pivotal to the diagnosis. 2D echocardiography demonstrates the classic deep sinusoids with multiple prominent trabeculations. Color Doppler echocardiography as well as contrast echocardiography can be very helpful for the

diagnosis. The characteristic deep intertrabecular recesses communicating with the ventricular cavity can be better demonstrated using these modalities. Cardiac MRI is another useful imaging modality to diagnose LV noncompaction and does so by assessing the ratio of noncompacted to compacted myocardium.

In a recent series, isolated LV noncompaction was present in 0.045% of adult transthoracic echocardiograms. There are two sets of echocardiographic criteria for LV noncompaction diagnosis: the Jenni criteria, which stress the presence of a two-layered structure, and the Chin criteria, which focus on the depth of the recess compared with the height of the trabecular (TABLE 31.1).

In addition, 3D echocardiography may be helpful to establish the diagnosis (VIDEO 31.32) and can also help demonstrate one of the feared complications that can be seen when LV systolic dysfunction is present: LV thrombus (VIDEO 31.33).

Suggested Readings

Baker GH, Pereira NL, Hlavacek AM, et al. Transthoracic real-time three-dimensional echocardiography in the diagnosis and description of noncompaction of ventricular myocardium. *Echocardiography* 2006;23:490–494.

Chin TK, Perloff JK, Williams RG, et al. Isolated noncompaction of left ventricular myocardium: a study of eight cases. *Circulation* 1990;82:507–513.

Ichida F, Hamamichi Y, Miyawaki T, et al. Clinical features of isolated noncompaction of the ventricular myocardium. *J Am Coll Cardiol* 1999;34:233–240.

Jenni R, Oechslin E, Schneider J, et al. Echocardiographic and pathoanatomical characteristics of isolated left ventricular non-compaction: a step towards classification as a distinct cardiomyopathy. *Heart* 2001;86:666–671.

Koo BK, Choi D, Ha JW, et al. Isolated Noncompaction of the ventricular myocardium: contrast echocardiographic findings and review of the literature. *Echocardiography* 2002;19:153–156.

Lowery MH, Martel JA, Zambrano JP, et al. Noncompaction of the ventricular myocardium: the use of contrast-enhanced echocardiography in diagnosis. *J Am Soc Echocardiogr* 2003;16:94–96.

Oechslin E, Attenhofer Jost CH, Rojas JR, et al. Long-term follow-up of 34 adults with isolated left ventricular non-compaction: a distinct cardiomyopathy with poor prognosis. *J Am Coll Cardiol* 2000;36:493–497.

Ritter M, Oechslin E, Sütsch G, et al. Isolated noncompaction of the myocardium in adults. *Mayo Clin Proc* 1997;72(1):26–31.

Song, ZZ. Echocardiography in the diagnosis of left ventricular non-compaction. *Cardiovasc Ultrasound* 2008;6:64.

Stöllberger C, Finsterer J. Left ventricular hypertrabeculation/ non-compaction. *J Am Soc Echocardiogr* 2004;17(1):91–100.

Weiford BC, Subbarao VD, Mulhern KM. Noncompaction of the ventricular myocardium. *Circulation* 2004;109:2965–2971.

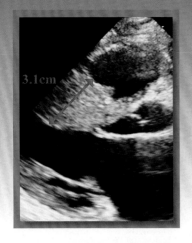

Chapter 32

Hypertrophic Cardiomyopathy

Maya E. Guglin

1. Which of the following statements regarding the 2D echo-cardiographic features of hypertrophic cardiomyopathy (HCM) is most accurate?

A. Asymmetric septal hypertrophy is the most common type.

B. Isolated posterior wall hypertrophy should raise suspicion for another etiology.

C. Apical hypertrophy is best seen in the parasternal long-axis orientation.

D. Right ventricular hypertrophy would only be present with concomitant pulmonary hypertension.

E. Diffuse concentric hypertrophy (>50% of the myocardium) is more common than discreet focal hypertrophy (less than two segments).

2. Which of the following statements regarding conditions of increased left ventricular (LV) wall thickness is true?

A. It is common for increased LV wall thickness due to athlete's heart to have an increased wall thickness of >13 mm.

B. In patients with increased LV wall thickness due to cardiac amyloidosis, the basal wall function is better preserved than apical wall function (as assessed by strain imaging).

C. In patients with increased LV wall thickness due to cardiac amyloidosis, basal longitudinal LV strain predicts mortality.

D. It is common for increased LV wall thickness due to athlete's heart to also have severe left atrial enlargement.

E. It is common for increased LV wall thickness due to athlete's heart to also have relatively small LV cavity size.

3. The images in Video 32.1 were obtained at baseline, and following echo contrast enhancement images in Video 32.2 were obtained. What is the diagnosis?

A. Hypertrophic cardiomyopathy

B. Ischemic heart disease

C. Chagas

D. Takotsubo

E. LV apical thrombus

4. Among family members of an HCM patient, which of the following Doppler echocardiographic findings would best predict the HCM genotype, in the absence of overt hypertrophy?

A. Figure 32.1A: Tissue Doppler imaging signal obtained by interrogation of the medial mitral annulus

B. Figure 32.1B: Pulsed-wave Doppler recording obtained with sample volume at the tips of the mitral leaflets

C. Figure 32.1C: Tissue Doppler imaging signal obtained by interrogation of the medial mitral annulus

D. Figure 32.1D: Pulsed-wave Doppler recording obtained with sample volume at the tips of the mitral leaflets

5. Which of the following best describes the mitral regurgitation color Doppler jet that results from systolic anterior motion of the mitral valve in the absence of other valvular pathology?

A. Eccentric anteriorly directed jet from the systolic anterior motion in the LV outflow tract

B. Eccentric posterolaterally directed jet due to misalignment of the MV leaflets with resultant reduced coaptation

C. Eccentric posterolaterally directed jet that is holosystolic and unrelated to the systolic anterior motion of the mitral valve

D. Central jet due to annular dilation from the chronic diastolic dysfunction and LA dilation

6. Which of the following transesophageal echocardiographic video clips would *most* likely accompany the transthoracic M-mode tracing in Figure 32.2?

A. Video 32.3

B. Video 32.4

C. Video 32.5

D. Video 32.6

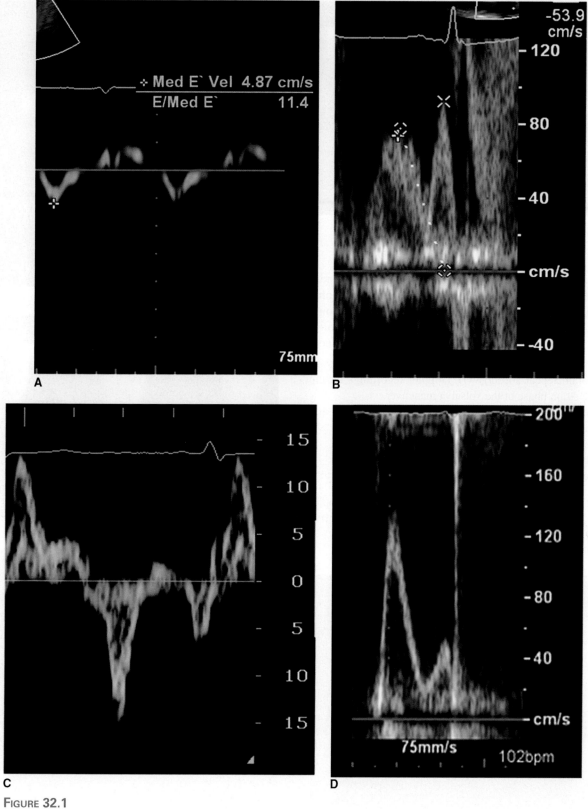

FIGURE 32.1

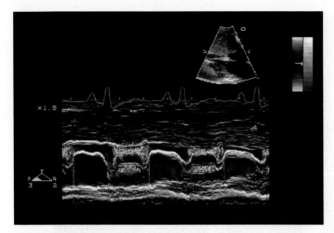

FIGURE 32.2

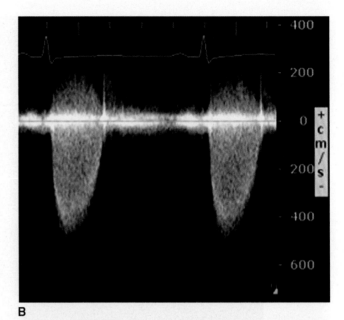

B

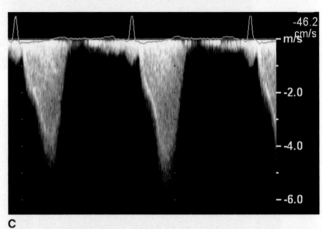

C

7. A 48-year-old male with significant light-headedness and dyspnea on exertion undergoes echocardiography, and the images in VIDEO 32.7 are obtained. Continuous-wave Doppler recordings across the LVOT and aortic valve are <1.5 m/s. What would be the appropriate next intervention?

A. Obtain repeat aortic/LVOT Doppler recordings during the strain phase of the Valsalva maneuver.
B. Refer the patient for cardiac catheterization and endomyocardial biopsy.
C. Perform a transesophageal echocardiogram.
D. Refer the patient for surgical myectomy.
E. Refer the patient for alcohol septal ablation.

8. Which of the following continuous-wave (CW) Doppler signals is most closely associated with obstructive HCM?

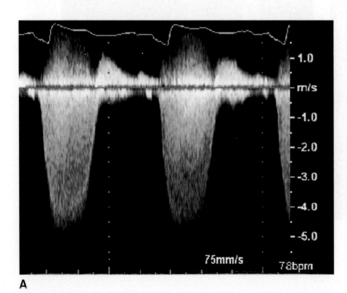

A

FIGURE 32.3

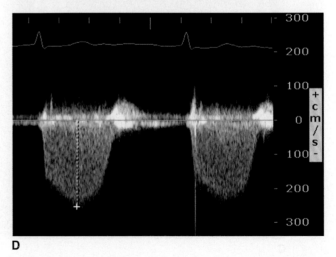

D

FIGURE 32.3 (Continued)

A. FIGURE 32.3A
B. FIGURE 32.3B
C. FIGURE 32.3C
D. FIGURE 32.3D

9. Which of the following risks is *least* commonly associated with hypertrophic cardiomyopathy?

A. Sudden cardiac death
B. Diastolic left ventricular heart failure
C. Aortic root dilation
D. Systolic left ventricular heart failure
E. Atrial fibrillation

10. A 45-year-old sedentary man presents with palpitations and shortness of breath first noted during a recreational football game he played while on vacation. He is now back to his usual lifestyle but has noticed mild dyspnea on exertion and is now being seen in your ambulatory consultation clinic. He describes a single syncopal event after exertion and blamed this on dehydration. He has no siblings and his parents died in a car crush when he was little. Echocardiograph is shown in Video 32.1.

What is the most appropriate next step in management of this patient?

A. Surgical myectomy
B. Cardiovascular MRI
C. Ambulatory rhythm monitor
D. AICD implantation
E. Electrophysiology study

11. A 42-year-old male with exertional chest pain and dyspnea is diagnosed with HCM. Which of the following recommendations, alone or in combination, would be appropriate for his first-degree family members?

a. Yearly screening echocardiograms
b. Yearly screening echocardiograms for adolescents
c. Screening echocardiograms every 5 years for adults
d. Echocardiogram if symptoms of HCM develop

A. a
B. b and d
C. b and c
D. b, c, and d
E. d

12. Which of the following echocardiographic findings is *least* associated with increased risk of sudden death in HCM?

A. Figure 32.4A: End-diastolic 2D image with measurement of anteroseptal thickness.
B. Figure 32.4B: Continuous-wave Doppler recording obtained by interrogation across the aortic valve and LV outflow tract.
C. Figure 32.4C: End-diastolic and end-systolic 2D images with corresponding LV ejection fraction.
D. Figure 32.4D: End-systolic 2D and color Doppler image obtained from the apical four-chamber view.
E. None of these echo findings have been associated with increased mortality.

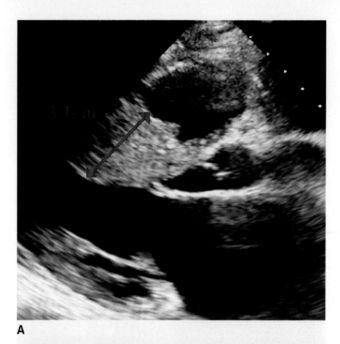

A

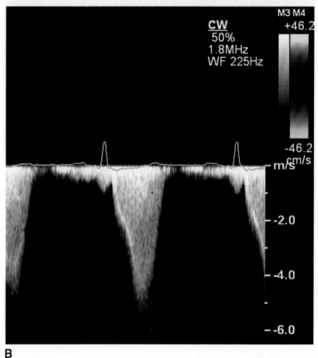

B

FIGURE 32.4

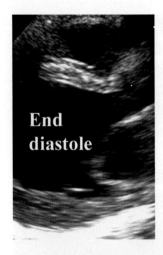
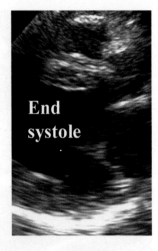

LV ejection fraction = 40%

C

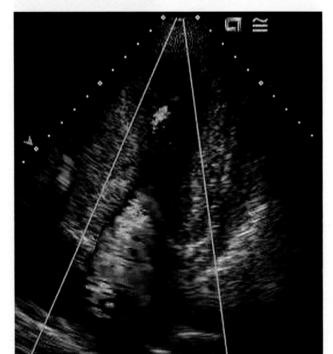

D

FIGURE 32.4 (Continued)

13. The decision has been made to proceed with alcohol septal ablation in a symptomatic 45-year-old female with obstructive HCM. What imaging modality would be most appropriate during the procedure?

A. 3D echocardiography to define the extent of septal hypertrophy

B. Transesophageal echo to better image systolic anterior motion of the mitral valve

C. Myocardial contrast echocardiography to guide the coronary intervention

D. Echocardiographic imaging during dobutamine administration to define magnitude of provocable gradient after the ablation

14. Which of the following reasons for considering an intraoperative transesophageal echocardiography essential during surgical septal myectomy is *least* accurate?

A. Direct insertion of the anterolateral papillary muscle into the mitral valve may be identified and surgically corrected.

B. The surgeon can use transesophageal echo measurements of maximal septal thickness and distance of maximum septal thickness from the aortic annulus to guide the location and extent of the myectomy.

C. Postprocedure complications such as residual LV outflow tract obstruction, mitral regurgitation, and iatrogenic ventricular septal defects and aortic regurgitation can be identified.

D. TEE imaging may assist the anesthesiologist with monitoring fluid status but has *not* been shown to improve outcomes in this operation.

E. Myectomy is performed via a retrograde aortic approach, and without TEE, the surgeon has difficulty visualizing the septal hypertrophy.

Answer 1: E. Hypertrophy involving the left ventricle is most common in HCM; however, right ventricular hypertrophy can also be observed. Therefore, Option D is incorrect. The most common location of left ventricular hypertrophy has been reported to be the anterior free wall and contiguous anterior ventricular septum. Diffuse LV hypertrophy (involving >50% of the LV) is more common than focal (≤2 myocardial segments). Therefore, Option E is correct. Although less common, cases of isolated hypertrophy involving the LV posterior wall or of the LV apex (apical variant of HCM) have been reported. Option B is incorrect. The best echo window to visualize apical variant HCM is the apical views and may require the administration of a contrast agent to confirm this finding and to rule out other apical pathologies (such as LV noncompaction). Option A is incorrect.

Suggested Readings

Klues HG, Schiffers A, Maron BJ. Phenotypic spectrum and patterns of left ventricular hypertrophy in hypertrophic cardiomyopathy: morphologic observations and significance as assessed by two-dimensional echocardiography in 600 patients. *J Am Coll Cardiol* 1995;26:1699–1708.

Maron MS, Maron BJ, Harrigan C, et al. Hypertrophic cardiomyopathy phenotype revisited after 50 years with cardiovascular magnetic resonance. *J Am Coll Cardiol* 2009;54:220–228.

Nagueh SF, Bierig SM, Budoff MJ, et al. American Society of echocardiography clinical recommendations for the multimodal cardiovascular imaging of patients with hypertrophic cardiomyopathy. *J Am Soc Echocardiogr* 2011;24:473–498.

Answer 2: D. Marfan syndrome is an autosomal dominant disorder of the connective tissue that is characterized by mitral and/or aortic valve prolapse and aortic dilation; LV hypertrophy, as in HCM, is not a typical feature. Therefore, Option D is an inaccurate statement and the single best answer. Because left ventricular hypertrophy can be seen in a wide array of conditions and diseases other than HCM, it can easily be mimicked. Infiltrative myopathies such as glycogen storage diseases like

Pompe disease can mimic HCM. Friedreich ataxia is associated with concentric LV hypertrophy or asymmetric septal hypertrophy and can resemble HCM. Fabry disease, an X-linked recessive disorder of glycosphingolipid metabolism caused by the lysosomal enzyme alpha-galactosidase A mutation, can be mistaken for HCM. LV hypertrophy can occur in multisystem disorders like Noonan syndrome characterized by craniofacial and congenital heart malformations (pulmonic valve stenosis and septal defects). Physiologic hypertrophy resulting from athletes' heart can also mimic HCM.

Suggested Readings

Burch M, Sharland M, Shinebourne E, et al. Cardiologic abnormalities in Noonan syndrome: phenotypic diagnosis and echocardiographic assessment of 118 patients. *J Am Coll Cardiol* 1993;22(4):1189–1192.

Child JS, Perloff JK, Bach PM, et al. Cardiac involvement in Friedreich's ataxia: a clinical study of 75 patients. *J Am Coll Cardiol* 1986;7(6):1370–1378.

Maron BJ, Seidman CE, Ackerman MJ, et al. How should hypertrophic cardiomyopathy be classified? *Circ Cardiovasc Genet* 2009;2:81–86.

Monserrat L, Gimeno-Blanes JR, Marin F, et al. Prevalence of Fabry disease in a cohort of 508 untreated patients with hypertrophic cardiomyopathy. *J Am Coll Cardiol* 2007;50:2399–2403.

Answer 3: *A.* The baseline apical four-chamber view demonstrates poor endocardial definition of the LV apex; following contrast enhancement, the presence of significant hypertrophy of the apical myocardium becomes apparent consistent with the diagnosis of apical HCM. Contrast has been shown to be of incremental value in identifying apical HCM in the setting of nondiagnostic transthoracic echocardiograms. Apical HCM can be misdiagnosed as apical thrombus or apical akinesis. Other listed answers are associated with abnormalities of the LV apex but do not cause hypertrophy of the apical myocardium as in this case.

Ischemic heart disease can manifest with apical wall motion abnormalities and aneurysm but not increased apical wall thickness. In takotsubo, there is a ballooning appearance of the LV apex in systole with sparing of the LV base and, in some cases, associated wall motion abnormality involving the right ventricular apex. Unlike ischemic heart disease, however, the apical wall motion abnormalities seen with takotsubo do not respect coronary artery blood flow territories. Apical wall motion abnormalities can be observed in both the acute and chronic phases of Chagas heart disease. In the chronic phase, apical aneurysms of varying sizes can be observed. Apical thrombus can be mural or protruding and is typically attached to akinetic or severely hypokinetic myocardium. The increased myocardial wall thickness in apical HCM can be distinguished from extensive thrombus within the apex by observing the presence of systolic wall thickening, which is not present with thrombus.

Suggested Readings

Acquatella H. Echocardiography in Chagas heart disease. *Circulation* 2007;115:1124–1131.

Donohue D, Ahsan C, Sanaei-Ardekani M, et al. Early diagnosis of stress-induced apical ballooning syndrome based on classic echocardiographic findings and correlation with cardiac catheterization. *J Am Soc Echocardiogr* 2005;18(12):1423.

Soman P, Swinburn J, Callister M, et al. Apical hypertrophic cardiomyopathy: bedside diagnosis by intravenous contrast echocardiography. *J Am Soc Echocardiogr* 2001;14(4):311–313.

Thanigaraj S, Perez JE. Apical hypertrophic cardiomyopathy: echocardiographic diagnosis with the use of intravenous contrast image enhancement. *J Am Soc Echocardiogr* 2000;13(2):146–149.

Ward RP, Weinert L, Spencer KT, et al. Quantitative diagnosis of apical cardiomyopathy using contrast echocardiography. *J Am Soc Echocardiogr* 2002;15(4):316–322.

Answer 4: *A.* In studies attempting to distinguish preclinical HCM in genotype-positive individuals from genotype-negative controls, transmitral parameters have not proven to be useful and neither have sensitive markers of systolic function such as tissue Doppler systolic annular velocity (Sa) or speckle tracking–derived global longitudinal strain. Tissue Doppler early diastolic annular velocity (Ea), however, has been found to be useful in this regard with good positive predictive value (86% for Ea ≤12) albeit poor negative predictive value (22%).

Suggested Reading

Ho CY, Carlsen C, Thune JJ, et al. Echocardiographic strain imaging to assess early and late consequences of sarcomere mutations in hypertrophic cardiomyopathy. *Circ Cardiovasc Genet* 2009;2(4):314–321.

Answer 5: *B.* Mitral regurgitation caused by systolic anterior motion of the mitral valve in HCM is eccentric and posterolaterally directed in the absence of other valvular pathology. Mitral valve leaflet pathology in addition to systolic anterior motion may alter posterolateral direction of regurgitation in obstructive HCM. Identification of an anteriorly directed jet in this condition warrants further investigation regarding its cause. Although rare, cases of flail posterior leaflet have been reported in obstructive HCM with an anteriorly directed mitral regurgitation jet.

Suggested Reading

Yeo TC, Miller FA, Oh JK, et al. Hypertrophic cardiomyopathy with obstruction: important diagnostic clue provided by the direction of the mitral regurgitation jet. *J Am Soc Echocardiogr* 1998;11(1):61–65.

Answer 6: *B.* The color M-mode tracing demonstrates systolic anterior motion of the mitral valve resulting in flow acceleration in the left ventricular outflow tract and mitral regurgitation; findings are consistent with obstructive HCM. Of the transesophageal echo video clips, (B) is the correct choice as it demonstrates posterolaterally directed mitral regurgitation and increased velocity of flow in the LV outflow tract (as evidenced by the mosaic and aliased color Doppler signal). On careful review, the anterior mitral valve leaflet can also be seen to obstruct the LV outflow tract in systole. Video (A) is incorrect; it demonstrates highly eccentric and anteriorly directed mitral regurgitation that was the result of a partially flail middle scallop of the posterior mitral valve leaflet. Video (C) demonstrates two mitral regurgitation jets, one highly eccentric and anterior and the other more central; in this case, regurgitation was the result of vegetation on the posterior mitral valve leaflet, and the mitral regurgitation jets are not characteristic of obstructive

HCM in the absence of other valvular pathology. Video (D) is also incorrect as it demonstrates functional and central mitral regurgitation resulting from mitral annular dilation in the setting of dilated cardiomyopathy.

Suggested Reading

Nagueh SF, Bierig SM, Budoff MJ, et al. American Society of echocardiography clinical recommendations for the multimodal cardiovascular imaging of patients with hypertrophic cardiomyopathy. *J Am Soc Echocardiogr* 2011;24:473–498.

Answer 7: A. The video demonstrates findings of asymmetric septal hypertrophy with systolic anterior motion of the mitral valve and chordae tendineae, consistent with HCM. In the absence of a resting LV outflow tract gradient, imaging during the strain phase of the Valsalva maneuver, during exercise, or following administration of amyl nitrite is indicated to determine whether a provocable gradient is present. Demonstrating LV outflow tract obstruction is important as it has been shown to contribute to debilitating heart failure symptoms in HCM. The magnitude of rest or provocable peak instantaneous pressure gradient also serves as the basis to consider surgical or percutaneous interventions with a conventional threshold of 50 mm Hg in the setting of medication refractory symptoms.

Suggested Readings

Gersh BJ, Maron BJ, Bonow RO, et al. 2011 ACCF/AHA guideline for the diagnosis and treatment of hypertrophic cardiomyopathy: a report of the American College of cardiology Foundation/American Heart Association task force on practice guidelines. *Circulation* 2011;124:E783–E831.

Maron MS, Olivotto I, Zenovich AG, et al. Hypertrophic cardiomyopathy is predominantly a disease of the left ventricular outflow tract obstruction. *Circulation* 2006;114:2232–2239.

Wigle ED, Rakowski H, Kimball BP, et al. Hypertrophic cardiomyopathy: clinical spectrum and treatment. *Circulation* 1995;92:1680–1692.

Answer 8: C. Continuous-wave (CW) Doppler signal contour can differentiate left ventricular outflow tract obstruction from other systolic high-velocity signals such as mitral regurgitation or aortic stenosis. The CW Doppler signal of obstruction in HCM is late peaking and "dagger" shaped as in the tracing seen in answer (C). Answer (A) is a CW Doppler signal of mitral regurgitation; note the symmetric and holosystolic envelope and typical mitral inflow pattern above the baseline. The CW Doppler signal of aortic stenosis is early peaking as in answer (B). Answer (D) is a CW Doppler signal of tricuspid regurgitation, which is similar in appearance to mitral regurgitation although lower in velocity in the absence of pulmonary hypertension and with lower E-wave velocity above the baseline.

Suggested Reading

Oh JK, Seward JB, Tajik AJ. Valvular heart disease. In: Oh JK, Seward JB, Tajik AJ, eds. *The Echo Manual*. 3rd ed. Rochester, NY: Lippincott Williams & Wilkins, 2006:189–225.

Answer 9: C. Aortic root dilation is not a feature of all HCM. However, this is not an uncommon finding in patients with LVH from poorly controlled hypertension. Sudden cardiac death resulting from unpredictable ventricular tachyarrhythmias occurs most commonly in patients under 35 years of age and in those involved with competitive athletics. Heart failure symptoms are common in HCM mostly with preserved systolic function and diastolic dysfunction. However, heart failure may progress to an end stage with myocardial scarring and systolic dysfunction. Atrial fibrillation is associated with HCM and portends a poor prognosis due to excessive heart failure mortality, functional disability, and stroke. For this reason, individuals with apical variant HCM are best followed by serial LAVI measurements.

Suggested Readings

Harris KM, Spirito P, Maron MS, et al. Prevalence, clinical profile, and significance of left ventricular remodeling in the end-stage phase of hypertrophic cardiomyopathy. *Circulation* 2006;114:216–225.

Moon J, Shim CY, Ha JW, et al. Clinical and echocardiographic predictors of outcomes in patients with apical hypertrophic cardiomyopathy. *Am J Cardiol* 2011;108(11):1614–1619.

Olivotto I, Cecchi F, Casey SA, et al. Impact of atrial fibrillation on the clinical course of hypertrophic cardiomyopathy. *Circulation* 2001;104(21):2517–2524.

Wigle ED, Rakowski H, Kimball BP, et al. Hypertrophic cardiomyopathy: clinical spectrum and treatment. *Circulation* 1995;92:1680–1692.

Answer 10: D. Several factors have been identified as predictors of sudden cardiac death in hypertrophic cardiomyopathy. They include history of cardiac arrest, history of sudden death in the family, *unexplained syncope*, nonsustained ventricular tachycardia on ambulatory monitor, decrease in systolic blood pressure on physical exercise such as treadmill stress test, and focal myocardial wall thickness of the ventricular septum greater than 3.0 cm. This patient meets two of these criteria with the severely thickened septal thickness noted on echo and the history of a syncopal episode. AICD is therefore indicated. Electrophysiology study was never demonstrated to add to risk stratification in the setting of hypertrophic cardiomyopathy.

Surgical myectomy or alcohol septal ablation may be indicated in symptomatic patients with a significant resting or induced gradient (>50 mm Hg), but medical treatment should be tried first. The other options are less satisfactory. EP study, rhythm monitor, and CMR are all techniques for additional risk stratification but would not be adequate to lower the risk enough to exclude the ICD placement recommendation.

Suggested Readings

Gersh BJ, Maron BJ, Bonow RO, et al. 2011 ACCF/AHA guideline for the diagnosis and treatment of hypertrophic cardiomyopathy: executive summary: a report of the American College of Cardiology Foundation/American Heart Association Task Force on Practice Guidelines. *J Thorac Cardiovasc Surg* 2011;142(6):1303–1338.

Maron BJ, Ommen SR, Semsarian C, et al. Hypertrophic cardiomyopathy: present and future, with translation into contemporary cardiovascular medicine. *J Am Coll Cardiol* 2014;64(1):83–99.

Answer 11: D. In HCM, hypertrophy most commonly develops during adolescence but may also develop into the fifth and sixth decades of life. As such, screening echocardiograms for asymptomatic first-degree relatives are recommended yearly for adolescents and every 5 years for adults. Echocardiography is also indicated if symptoms of HCM develop.

Suggested Readings

Gersh BJ, Maron BJ, Bonow RO, et al. 2011 ACCF/AHA Guideline for the diagnosis and treatment of hypertrophic cardiomyopathy: a report of the American College of Cardiology foundation/ American Heart Association task force on practice guidelines. *Circulation* 2011;124:e783–e831.

Nagueh SF, Bierig SM, Budoff MJ, et al. American society of echocardiography clinical recommendations for multimodality cardiovascular imaging of patients with hypertrophic cardiomyopathy. *J Am Soc Echocardiogr* 2011;24:473–498.

Answer 12: D. Maximal wall thickness ≥3.0 cm has been shown to be an independent predictor of sudden cardiac death and is considered a class IIa indication for primary prevention implantable cardioverter–defibrillator. LV outflow tract obstruction severity has been shown to positively correlate with the risk of sudden cardiac death. A resting gradient ≥30 mm Hg has been associated with increased risk of sudden cardiac death. HCM can progress to an end-stage cardiomyopathy characterized by reduced systolic function and the risk of sudden cardiac increases when LV ejection fraction is <50%. Apical aneurysms with thinned wall and scarring have also been reported to be associated with increased risk of sudden cardiac death. The image in (D) demonstrates mid-LV cavity obstruction; however, there is no evidence of wall thinning of the apex, and as such, it is not consistent with apical aneurysm. Mid-LV cavity obstruction as in this case, however, may over time progress to aneurysm formation. Other important clinical risk factors would include family history of sudden death in first-degree relatives, recent unexplained syncope, nonsustained ventricular tachycardia, and abnormal systolic BP response to exercise (drop or failure to appropriately increase).

Suggested Readings

Gersh BJ, Maron BJ, Bonow RO, et al. 2011 ACCF/AHA guideline for the diagnosis and treatment of hypertrophic cardiomyopathy: a report of the American College of cardiology Foundation/ American Heart Association task force on practice guidelines. *Circulation* 2011;124:E783–E831.

Answer 13: Question 14 is an example of a transthoracic echocardiogram, apical four-chamber view, performed during an ETOH septal ablation procedure. Contrast has been injected directly into the isolated septal perforator being considered for ETOH administration. Note the very bright, focal proximal IVS that extends toward the mid septum. This region of contrast enhancement can be compared with the location of the systolic anterior motion of the mitral valve to insure that the contact point (location of obstruction) is the same location as the impending infarct prior to ablation in VIDEO 32.8.

Answer 14: D. Transesophageal echo has been shown to improve the surgical outcomes of myectomy in obstructive HCM. Abnormalities of the mitral valve including leaflet elongation/redundancy or direct insertion of the papillary muscle into the mitral valve can occur in HCM, and such findings guide the surgical procedure. Myectomy is performed via a retrograde aortic approach that limits the surgeons' view of the full extent of septal hypertrophy. Transesophageal echo measures of septal thickness and location of maximal thickness can guide the extent of the myectomy. Following cardiopulmonary bypass, intraoperative transesophageal echo imaging can determine the outcome of the myectomy and identify potential complications as listed in option (C) that may need to be surgically treated before leaving the operating room.

Suggested Readings

Grigg LE, Wigle ED, Williams WG, et al. Transesophageal Doppler echocardiography in obstructive hypertrophic cardiomyopathy: clarification of pathophysiology and importance in intraoperative decision making. *J Am Coll Cardiol* 1992;20:42–52.

Maron BJ, Nishimura RA, Danielson GK. Pitfalls in clinical recognition and a novel operative approach for hypertrophic cardiomyopathy with severe outflow obstruction due to anomalous papillary muscle. *Circulation* 1998;98:2505–2508.

Ommen SR, Park SH, Click RL, et al. Impact of intraoperative transesophageal echocardiography in the surgical management of hypertrophic cardiomyopathy. *Am J Cardiol* 2002;90:1022–1024.

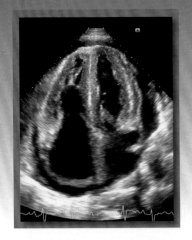
Echo Features of Restrictive Cardiomyopathy

Vincent L. Sorrell

1. *Which of the following statements is most accurate* regarding restrictive cardiomyopathies:

A. It is not uncommon, even early in the disease process, that the left ventricle is dilated with increased wall thickness and decreased systolic function.

B. Grade III (restrictive pattern) diastolic dysfunction is always found.

C. The peak early diastolic mitral annular velocity is normal or increased.

D. The pulmonary artery pressure is typically normal or mildly increased.

E. Biatrial dilatation is expected.

2. Which of the following statements is most accurate regarding the M-mode echocardiogram (FIG. 33.1) and electrocardiogram (FIG. 33.2) shown?

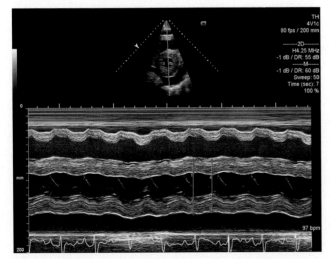

FIGURE 33.1

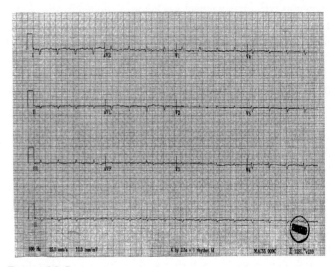

FIGURE 33.2

A. This patient likely has a sarcomeric gene mutation.

B. Reduced basal relative to apical longitudinal strain ratio.

C. Additional imaging would likely confirm pericardial thickening.

D. Severe pulmonary artery hypertension is present.

E. Urgent pericardiocentesis is warranted.

3. Which statement is most accurate regarding cardiac hemochromatosis?

A. The triad of cirrhosis, diabetes, and tanned skin is commonly seen on presentation.

B. The classic hereditary form of the disease is an autosomal dominant genetic disorder resulting in iron overload whose chromosomal mutation is not well characterized.

C. The left ventricle on echocardiography is normal sized and thick walled with normal systolic function.

D. Phlebotomy and chelation therapy have been shown to reduce abnormal echocardiographic findings and reverse the cardiomyopathy.

4. Match the disease entities (1 to 5) with the single best description or comment (A to E):

1. Fabry disease
2. Endomyocardial fibrosis
3. Radiation cardiotoxicity
4. Idiopathic restrictive cardiomyopathy
5. Cardiac sarcoidosis

A. Superimposed apical thrombus formation in either the LV or RV is common.
B. May present either as a restrictive cardiomyopathy or as a constrictive pericarditis.
C. Endomyocardial biopsy is necessary for the diagnosis.
D. It may be confused with hypertrophic cardiomyopathy in adults.
E. It may be confused with an old myocardial infarction in adults.

5. Match the transthoracic echocardiogram in Figure 33.3 and Video 33.1 with the single most likely pathologic entity:

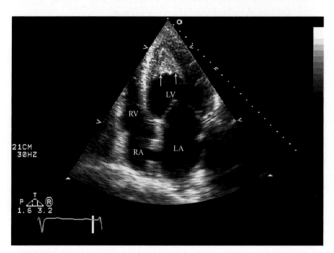

Figure 33.3 Reproduced from Armstrong WF, Ryan T. *Feigenbaum's Echocardiography.* 7th ed. Philadelphia, PA: Lippincott Williams & Wilkins, 2010, with permission.

A. Fabry disease
B. Endomyocardial fibrosis
C. Radiation cardiotoxicity
D. Idiopathic restrictive cardiomyopathy
E. Cardiac sarcoidosis

6. Which of the following statements regarding the differentiation of restrictive cardiomyopathy versus constrictive pericarditis is most accurate?

A. The systolic area index is a highly accurate cath finding in restrictive cardiomyopathy.
B. Equalization of end-diastolic pressures is the single most accurate hemodynamic measurement to differentiate these entities.
C. Mitral annular tissue Doppler findings are impaired in both of these entities.

D. Respiratory variation in early diastolic mitral inflow velocity (E wave) demonstrated by pulsed-wave Doppler echo occurs in both constrictive pericarditis and restrictive cardiomyopathy.
E. Pericardial thickening and/or calcification is pathognomonic of constrictive pericarditis, and its absence excludes the diagnosis.

7. A patient with eosinophilia is referred to you from a colleague in the hematology department with a new diagnosis of heart failure. Echocardiography confirms HFnEF with an LVEF of 55%. Which of the following statements is most accurate?

A. The diagnosis of this condition requires an eosinophil count that is elevated above the upper limits of normal for a standard reference population on at least one occasion.
B. Echocardiography reveals typical features consistent with a restrictive cardiomyopathy without distinguishing or unique features.
C. Eosinophils are felt to be incidental and not causative of the cardiac damage.
D. Parasitic infections or allergic conditions may play a role in the etiology of this condition.
E. Specific chromosomal mutations may help in the selection of treatment.

Questions 8 and 9

A 64-year-old male with a history of multiple myeloma being treated with Velcade and Adriamycin is referred from oncology for increased shortness of breath, orthopnea, paroxysmal nocturnal dyspnea, and peripheral edema. Transthoracic echocardiography is ordered and shown in Figure 33.4 and Video 33.2.

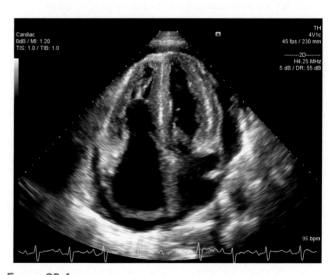

Figure 33.4

8. Which of the following statements is most accurate?

A. Endomyocardial biopsy is necessary to confirm the diagnosis before treating.

B. If the E/a ratio is high and deceleration time is short, the chemotherapy should be stopped.

C. Global longitudinal strain bull's-eye will demonstrate a normal LV apex.

D. Pericardiocentesis needs to be performed urgently.

E. The cardiomyopathy is likely an incidental finding and unrelated to the patient's history.

9. Which of the following statements is most accurate regarding the echocardiographic diagnosis of this condition and the video provided?

A. The global longitudinal strain pattern is able to distinguish this from LVH and HCM.

B. Granular sparkling appearance of the myocardium is a highly specific finding.

C. Increased atrial septal thickness is a sensitive but not specific finding.

D. Pericardial effusions are present in 10% to 20% of cases.

E. LA thrombi are common (see the echo-bright mass in the LA).

10. A 58-year-old male with a history of Hodgkin lymphoma treatment 20 years earlier presents with severe fatigue, lower extremity edema, and ascites. He has gained more than 40 pounds in the past 6 months.

Which of the following would be consistent with radiation cardiotoxicity causing this presentation?

A. Dilated LV and RV cavities with restrictive filling pattern on mitral inflow.

B. Coronary artery calcium Agatston score = 0.

C. Lower likelihood if concomitant Adriamycin chemotherapy was given.

D. RV involvement is greater than LV involvement.

E. It would be rare to have features of both constriction and restriction together.

11A. A 55-year-old male presents with severe heart failure symptoms despite maximal medical therapy to your ambulatory clinic. He has been treated for the past 15 years by a cardiologist in the community who is now referring him to you for consideration of possible cardiac transplantation. His past history is significant for LVEF < 25% for the past 5 years with a restrictive MV filling pattern and persistently increased E/e' ratio > 15. His very initial presentation 15 years ago was syncope and third-degree heart block at which time he received a PPMI. Coronary angiography has been normal (most recent cath 1 year ago). He has frequent PVCs and non-sustained VT. Because of severe RV dysfunction (and PVCs with RV origin), he recently underwent a cardiac MRI (with compatible pacemaker sequences) to exclude arrhythmogenic RV cardiomyopathy and this revealed the following findings:

LVVd= 260 mL
LVVs = 200 mL
RVVd = 290 mL
RVVs = 220 mL
Qs = 60
Qp = 60
No focal RV aneurysms
Contrast enhancement: focal, midseptal transmural infarct and papillary muscle fibrosis

Given this clinical presentation and the findings on echo and CMR, which of the following statements is most accurate?

A. Noncaseating granulomas will be found at the time of cardiac transplantation.

B. Extensive 3V CAD is likely present if coronary angiography is repeated.

C. Viral myocarditis causing an idiopathic CM presentation is expected.

D. The LV dysfunction may be explained by the pacemaker-induced dyssynchrony.

E. Genetics may demonstrate a gap junction mutation.

11B. Based upon the reported quantitative CMR findings, which of the following is correct?

A. There is moderate MR.

B. There is mild TR.

C. There is a small intracardiac shunt.

D. The LVEF is 30%.

E. The RVEF is 21%.

Answer 1: *E.* The 1995 World Health Organization/International Federation of Cardiology Task Force on the Definition and Classification of Cardiomyopathies defined cardiomyopathies as "diseases of the myocardium associated with cardiac dysfunction" and "classified as dilated cardiomyopathy, hypertrophic cardiomyopathy, restrictive cardiomyopathy, and arrhythmogenic right ventricular cardiomyopathy" (1). Restrictive cardiomyopathy is the least common of the cardiomyopathies and is "characterized by restrictive filling and reduced diastolic volume of either or both ventricles with normal or near-normal systolic function and wall thickness" (1). It is notable that the cardiomyopathies in general are categorized using morphologic criteria, whereas restrictive cardiomyopathy is a physiologic or functional classification (2). The category, therefore, contains a variety of diseases with a degree of anatomic variability all sharing an impairment in diastolic filling.

The restrictive cardiomyopathies can be subcategorized in a number of ways. One attempted subcategorization with the most common or prototypical examples in parentheses is non-infiltrative (idiopathic restrictive cardiomyopathy), infiltrative (amyloidosis, sarcoidosis), storage diseases (hemochromatosis, Fabry disease, glycogen storage disease), and endomyocardial (endomyocardial fibrosis, hypereosinophilic or Loeffler endomyocardial fibrosis, radiation) (3).

There are no specific individual echocardiographic findings that make the diagnosis of restrictive cardiomyopathy but rather a combination of features, which together make the diagnosis. The classic echocardiogram includes normal-sized ventricles with normal to thickened walls and preserved systolic function combined with biatrial enlargement (3,4). Classic Doppler echo findings include grade III (restrictive) diastolic dysfunction and moderate to severe pulmonary hypertension. Therefore, **Option D** is incorrect.

There are, of course, variations on this classic echocardiographic picture. Toward the end stage of disease, left ventricular function may be mildly reduced, and it may be difficult to distinguish from a dilated cardiomyopathy. Therefore, **Option A** is incorrect. Impaired diastolic function is, by definition, required for the diagnosis of a restrictive cardiomyopathy and, typically when a patient with this diagnosis becomes symptomatic and is finally diagnosed, grade III (restrictive) diastolic dysfunction is usually present. Advanced diastolic dysfunction is, however, not a requirement; and during the early stages of disease, milder degrees of diastolic dysfunction such as grade I (abnormal relaxation) or grade II (pseudonormal) diastolic dysfunction may be found (4,5). Therefore, **Option B** is incorrect.

In recent years, the development of newer tissue Doppler modalities has further refined the diagnosis of restrictive cardiomyopathy. As milder forms of the disease give way to more advanced stages, advanced diastolic dysfunction becomes inevitable, and LA pressure increases as the stiff left ventricle results in poor diastolic compliance and high LV diastolic pressures. At this point, there is impairment in left ventricular expansion measured at the mitral annulus during diastole on the longitudinal axis. This is measured by tissue Doppler and is represented by a reduced e′ velocity typically much <8 cm/s (often <5 cm/s) that is supportive of the diagnosis of a restrictive cardiomyopathy. Therefore, **Option C** is incorrect. If, on the other hand, the e′ velocity is equal to or >8 cm/s, then this may be a clue that constrictive pericarditis, often confused clinically with this entity, should be considered as an alternative diagnosis (6–8).

References

1. Richardson P, McKenna W, Bristow M, et al. Report of the 1995 World Health Organization/International Society and Federation of Cardiology Task Force on the Definition and Classification of cardiomyopathies. *Circulation* 1996;93:841.
2. Nihoyannopoulos P, Dawson D. Restrictive cardiomyopathies. *Eur J Echocardiogr* 2009;10:iii23.
3. Kushwaha SS, Fallon JT, Fuster V. Restrictive cardiomyopathy. *N Engl J Med* 1997;336(4):267.
4. Tam JW, Shaikh N, Sutherland E. Echocardiographic assessment of patients with hypertrophic and restrictive cardiomyopathy: imaging and echocardiography. *Curr Opin Cardiol* 2001;17:470–477.
5. Asher CR, Klein AL. Diastolic heart failure: restrictive cardiomyopathy, constrictive pericarditis, and cardiac tamponade: clinical and echocardiographic evaluation. *Cardiol Rev* 2002;10(4):218–229.
6. Garcia MJ, Rodriguez L, Ares M, et al. Differentiation of constrictive pericarditis from restrictive cardiomyopathy: assessment of left ventricular diastolic velocities in longitudinal axis by Doppler tissue imaging. *J Am Coll Cardiol* 1996;27(1):108–114.
7. Rajagopalan N, Garcia MJ, Rodriguez L, et al. Comparison of new Doppler echocardiographic methods to differentiate constrictive pericardial heart disease and restrictive cardiomyopathy. *Am J Cardiol* 2001;87:86–94.
8. Ha JW, Ommen SR, Tajik AJ, et al. Differentiation of constrictive pericarditis from restrictive cardiomyopathy using mitral annular velocity by tissue Doppler echocardiography. *Am J Cardiol* 2004;94:316–319.

Answer 2: *B.* True. See discussion. This is the classic method to diagnose amyloidosis. Please add here:

Recently, it has been demonstrated that the global longitudinal strain assessment of the LV in patients with amyloidosis have an "apical-sparing," bull's-eye pattern. This results from higher strain values (normal or supranormal) in the apical segments with markedly "reduced" strain values (less negative; "reduced" from their distance from a zero value) in the basal and mid-LV segments.

Answer 3: *D.* Hemochromatosis is an iron storage disease that occurs in two forms: primary or hereditary hemochromatosis that is an autosomal recessive disease that affects the absorption of iron and secondary hemochromatosis due to repetitive blood transfusions for chronic hematologic disorders such as thalassemia, hemolytic anemia, or sickle cell anemia. The excessive iron overload then deposits to varying degrees in the liver, heart, pancreas, and testicles, potentially resulting in cirrhosis, cardiomyopathy, diabetes, and hypogonadism, respectively (1). The classic triad of cirrhosis, diabetes, and tanned skin was first described in the 19th century and is not commonly seen in modern practice possibly due to earlier diagnosis with the advent of serologic and genetic testing. The most common symptoms/findings are fatigue, arthralgias, and hepatomegaly (with mild elevation of the transaminases) (2).

Primary or hereditary hemochromatosis is classically due to a single mutation in the HFE gene located on chromosome 6 at position 282 of the HFE protein (2). Homozygosity for this mutation is present in 0.5% of persons of Northern European ancestry. However, there is a wide degree of phenotypic expression or penetrance due to the complexity of iron metabolism, the effect of other gene mutations on iron metabolism, and a number of other variables. There are other known genetic mutations associated with other forms of hemochromatosis such as the juvenile-onset form of the disease.

Cardiac involvement may be present in up to 15% of hemochromatosis cases. When heart failure occurs, it is commonly more right sided than left sided and manifested by ascites and peripheral edema. Electrocardiographic changes are common but nonspecific. Low voltage can be seen but not uniformly. **Echocardiographic features commonly show LV dilatation with decreased systolic function but with normal wall thickness. This latter point is consistent with its status as a storage disease rather than an infiltrative disease** (3). **Less frequently, findings more consistent with a restrictive cardiomyopathy may be observed** (4). This, however, remains an important distinction since it is one of the few restrictive cardiomyopathies that are reversible with treatment.

When suspecting hemochromatosis, the first serologic tests performed are usually a transferrin saturation and serum ferritin. There are different guidelines for cutoff points, but one proposed by the American College of Physicians suggests that a transferrin saturation of >55% and a serum ferritin level of >200 μg/L in women and >300 μg/L in men are sufficient to warrant additional investigation (5). Genetic testing is now available and can be used to detect mutations of the HFE gene. In addition, cardiac MRI (CMR) can now be used to assess hepatic and cardiac iron concentrations. CMR is now considered the most important noninvasive diagnostic tool and is used to predict patient outcomes. These new diagnostic tests are very helpful, but liver biopsy remains the gold standard in assessing the degree of iron overload and liver damage. Endomyocardial biopsy is not commonly needed unless clinical, serologic, and genetic testing is equivocal. If endomyocardial biopsy is needed, it should be noted that iron deposition in the heart is concentrated in the subepicardium, and therefore, false-negative biopsies are possible.

Phlebotomy and iron chelation treatments using desferrioxamine have been shown to improve abnormal echocardiographic findings and left ventricular function (6). Those patients with cirrhosis have a poor prognosis despite treatment, whereas those patients without cirrhosis have a life expectancy comparable to the normal population with phlebotomy (7).

References

1. Pereira NL, Dec GW. Restrictive and infiltrative cardiomyopathies. In: Crawford MH, DiMarco JP, Paulus WJ, eds. *Cardiology*. 3rd ed. Philadelphia, PA: Elsevier, 2010.
2. Piertrangelo A. Hereditary hemochromatosis—a new look at an old disease. *N Engl J Med* 2004;350:2383–2397.
3. Olson LJ, Baldus WP, Tajik AJ. Echocardiographic features of idiopathic hemochromatosis. *Am J Cardiol* 1987;60:885–889.
4. Cutler DJ, Isner JM, Bracey AW, et al. Hemochromatosis heart disease: an unemphasized cause of potentially reversible restrictive cardiomyopathy. *Am J Med* 1980;69:923–928.
5. Qaseem A, Aronson M, Fitterman N, et al. Screening for hereditary hemochromatosis: a clinical practice guideline from the American College of Physicians. *Ann Int Med* 2005;143:517–521.
6. Candell-Riera J, Lu L, Seres L, et al. Cardiac Hemochromatosis: beneficial effects of iron removal therapy. *Am J Cardiol* 1983;52:824–829.
7. Niederau C, Fischer R, Sonnenberg A, et al. Survival and causes of death in cirrhotic and in non-cirrhotic patients with primary hemochromatosis. *N Engl J Med* 1985;313:1256–1262.
8. Kirk P, Roughton M, Porter JB, et al. Cardiac T2* magnetic resonance for prediction of cardiac complications in thalassemia major. *Circulation* 2009;120:1961–1968.

Answer 4: **1 = D, 2 = A, 3 = B, 4 = C, and 5 = E**

Fabry disease = Endocardium with a two-layered or binary appearance on echo (FIG. 33.5)

Fabry disease is a rare X-linked recessive genetic disorder that results in the lack of an enzyme, alpha-galactosidase A, which is involved in glycosphingolipid metabolism and results in deposition of glycosphingolipids in various organs. Symptoms often start in childhood and include severe pain and numbness in the limbs and skin manifestations, including telangiectasias and angiokeratomas. As the patient ages,

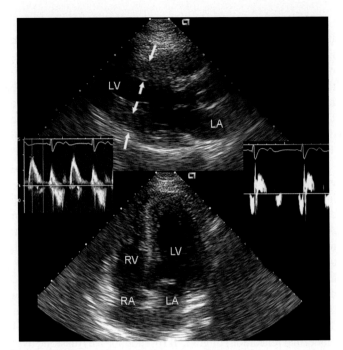

FIGURE 33.5 Reproduced from Armstrong WF, Ryan T. *Feigenbaum's Echocardiography.* 7th ed. Philadelphia, PA: Lippincott Williams & Wilkins, 2010, with permission.

renal manifestations develop with a significant number of the patient's developing end-stage renal disease and requiring dialysis. Cerebral involvement can occur in young adulthood leading to TIAs and strokes. Cardiac involvement is frequent and commonly seen in midlife. Left ventricular hypertrophy is the most prominent cardiac finding and is usually concentric. Cardiac manifestations include congestive heart failure, valvular abnormalities, and conduction system disease. There is also an atypical cardiac variant of the disease that presents later in life and is devoid of the classic noncardiac manifestations of the disease. One study of men diagnosed with a hypertrophic cardiomyopathy later in life found 6% to have Fabry disease (1). Another study of males with unexplained left ventricular hypertrophy showed 10% to have Fabry disease (2). Therefore, Fabry disease may be more frequent than previously thought.

The echocardiogram has been described as having a two-layered or binary appearance in the endocardium of the left ventricle likely due to deposits of glycosphingolipid in the endocardium (3). This finding has been arguably felt to be a fairly sensitive and specific indicator of Fabry disease although others feel it is not as sensitive and specific as originally hoped and poor at differentiating Fabry disease from hypertrophic cardiomyopathy (4). Late gadolinium enhancement of cardiac MRI shows a characteristic involvement of the basilar inferolateral wall (5). Once the correct diagnosis is made, enzyme replacement therapy is now available and has been shown to result in reduction of LV hypertrophy and improvement in cardiac function (6). Enzyme replacement therapy may not be as effective once Fabry disease has progressed and myocardial fibrosis has become more extensive, but predictors to therapeutic response are not well established.

References

1. Sachdev B, Takenaka T, Teraguchi H, et al. Prevalence of Anderson-Fabry disease in male patients with late onset hypertrophic cardiomyopathy. *Circulation* 2002;105:1407–1411.
2. Nakao S, Takenaka T, Maeda M, et al. An atypical variant of Fabry's disease in men with left ventricular hypertrophy. *N Engl J Med* 1995;333:288–293.
3. Pieroni M, Chimenti C, De Cobelli F, et al. Fabry's disease cardiomyopathy: echocardiographic detection of endomyocardial glycosphingolipid compartmentalization. *J Am Coll Cardiol* 2006;47:1663–1671.
4. Kounas S, Demetrescu C, Pantazis AA, et al. The binary endocardial appearance is a poor discriminator of Anderson-Fabry disease from familial hypertrophic cardiomyopathy. *J Am Coll Cardiol* 2008;51:2058–2061.
5. Moon JCC, Sachdev B, Elkington AG, et al. Gadolinium enhanced cardiovascular magnetic resonance in Anderson-Fabry disease 1: evidence for a disease specific abnormality of the myocardial interstitium. *Eur Heart J* 2003;24:2151–2155.
6. Weidemann F, Breunig F, Beer M, et al. Improvement of cardiac function during enzyme replacement therapy in patients with Fabry's disease: a Prospective Strain Rate Imaging Study. *Circulation* 2003;108:1299–1301.

Endomyocardial fibrosis = Left ventricular and/or right ventricular apical fibrosis often with superimposed thrombus formation

This is also shown in FIGURE 33.3 and VIDEO 33.1 (see question 5). Although the other options are difficult to distinguish with echo imaging alone as they mimic other diseases (Fabry with HCM; radiation CM with infiltrative CM and constriction) or are a diagnosis of exclusion (idiopathic CM), this is one of the rare instances where echo can make the diagnosis due to the very distinct 2D appearance.

Endomyocardial fibrosis is a restrictive cardiomyopathy featuring fibrosis of the endocardium especially at the apices of the left and/or right ventricles. This results in impairment in ventricular filling and subsequent congestive heart failure. It was first diagnosed in Uganda and is endemic to tropical areas worldwide, including other central African countries such as Nigeria as well as portions of India and Brazil. It is felt to be the most prevalent restrictive cardiomyopathy in the world. Etiology is not certain although it resembles Loeffler endocarditis (eosinophilic myocarditis) that is linked with eosinophilia. Infectious and environmental etiologies have also been considered. Onset is usually from childhood to young adulthood. In addition to the usual physical findings of congestive heart failure, an exudative ascites without peripheral edema is characteristic, and an exudative pericardial effusion is common (1). Echocardiographic findings are typical of a restrictive cardiomyopathy but also have characteristic findings of apical obliteration of the left and/or right ventricles due to fibrosis and underlying thrombus (2,3). In contradistinction to apical thrombus formation due to hypokinesis or akinesis, the underlying apical myocardium in endomyocardial fibrosis has preserved contractility (2). Endomyocardial fibrosis also results in papillary muscle dysfunction and commonly some degree of mitral and tricuspid regurgitation. Prognosis is generally poor due to the presentation usually occurring in the end stages of

the disease. Symptomatic medical treatment as is common in most restrictive cardiomyopathies is indicated. Surgical treatment with myocardial resection and valvular replacement, if indicated, has been performed and may improve survival in selected cases (4).

References

1. Sliwa K, Damasceno A, Mayosi BM. Epidemiology and etiology of cardiomyopathy in Africa. *Circulation* 2005;112:3577–3583.
2. Acquatella H, Schiller NB, Puigbo JJ, et al. Value of two-dimensional echocardiography in endomyocardial disease with and without eosinophilia. *Circulation* 1983;67(6):1219–1226.
3. Berensztein CS, Pineiro D, Marcotegui M, et al. Usefulness of echocardiography and Doppler echocardiography in endomyocardial fibrosis. *J Am Soc Echocardiogr* 2000;13:385–392.
4. Schneider U, Jenni R, Turina J, et al. Long term follow up of patients with endomyocardial fibrosis: effects of surgery. *Heart* 1998;79:362–367.

Radiation cardiotoxicity = May present as restrictive cardiomyopathy or constrictive pericarditis (FIG. 33.6)

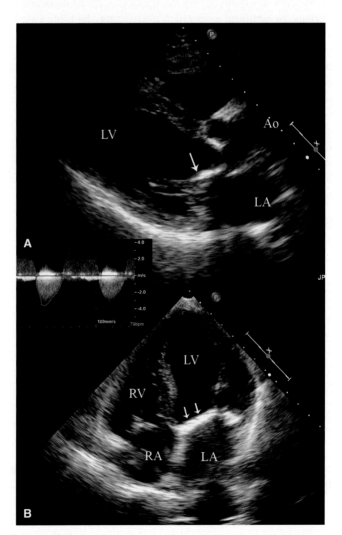

FIGURE 33.6 Reproduced from Armstrong WF, Ryan T. *Feigenbaum's Echocardiography.* 7th ed. Philadelphia, PA: Lippincott Williams & Wilkins, 2010, with permission.

Radiation therapy has been a long-established and effective method of treatment for thoracic malignancies, most notably breast cancer and Hodgkin lymphoma. The anatomic location of these malignancies commonly results in the heart being in the field of irradiation. Cardiac irradiation may result in coronary artery disease, valvular heart disease, heart conduction abnormalities, cardiomyopathy, heart failure, and pericardial disease. Studies have established the increased incidence of death from cardiovascular causes in patients receiving radiation therapy for these malignancies (1,2). Contemporary radiation techniques focused on limiting the radiation dose, and radiation field is likely to have reduced the incidence of cardiotoxicity in breast cancer but probably has not eliminated it altogether (3). Risk factors for developing cardiotoxicity include not only radiation dose and field but also concomitant cardiotoxic chemotherapy such as anthracycline (2). Diastolic function has been found to be impaired after mediastinal radiation for Hodgkin disease even in asymptomatic patients (4). Ultimately, this may progress to a restrictive cardiomyopathy through a process of myocardial fibrosis. In addition, myocardial fibrosis may be more extensive and frequent in the right ventricle than the left ventricle, presumably due to greater radiation exposure to this part of the heart (5). Radiation is one of the few causes of restrictive cardiomyopathy that may also cause constrictive pericarditis through fibrosis of the pericardium. Pericardial effusion is more likely to occur early after irradiation, whereas pericardial constriction is a late manifestation of irradiation. Restrictive cardiomyopathy is normally difficult to distinguish from constrictive pericarditis but may be particularly hard in cases of radiation cardiotoxicity since both entities may coexist in any one patient.

References

1. Jones JM, Ribeiro GG. Mortality patterns over 34 years of breast cancer patients in a clinical trial of post-operative radiotherapy. *Clin Radiol* 1989;40:204–208.
2. Aleman BMP, van den Belt-Duselbout AW, De Bruin ML, et al. Late cardiotoxicity after treatment for Hodgkin lymphoma. *Blood* 2007;109:1878–1886.
3. Demirci S, Nam J, Hubbs JL, et al. Radiation-induced cardiac toxicity after therapy for breast cancer: interaction between treatment era and follow-up duration. *Int J Radiat Oncol Biol Phys* 2009;73(4):980–987.
4. Heidenreich PA, Hancock SL, Vagelos RH, et al. Diastolic dysfunction after mediastinal irradiation. *Am Heart J* 2005;150:977–982.
5. Brosium FC III, Waller BF, Roberts WC. Radiation heart disease: analysis of 16 young (aged 15 to 33 years) necropsy patients who received over 3,500 rads to the heart. *Am J Med* 1981;70:519–530.

Idiopathic restrictive cardiomyopathy = Endomyocardial biopsy is necessary for the diagnosis

Idiopathic restrictive cardiomyopathy is a myocardial disorder that has all the features characteristic of restrictive cardiomyopathy, including a nondilated left ventricle with preserved systolic function, impaired diastolic function, and biatrial enlargement. There is no obvious underlying etiology (1,2). It is a diagnosis of exclusion, and, therefore, known etiologies of restrictive cardiomyopathy need to be investigated and excluded such as amyloidosis, sarcoidosis, hemochromatosis, familial restrictive cardiomyopathy, endomyocardial fibrosis, Loeffler endocarditis(eosinophilic myocarditis), and radiation-induced cardiotoxicity. Constrictive pericarditis can have a similar clinical presentation and also needs to be excluded. As part of the workup, the above conditions cannot effectively be excluded without an endomyocardial biopsy. Prognosis is limited with one cohort demonstrating a 5-year survival of 64% (3). Survival is adversely affected by male gender, age > 70 years, worse NYHA functional class, and left atrial diameter > 60 mm (3). There is no specific treatment for idiopathic restrictive cardiomyopathy. Treatment is focused on symptomatic management of congestion. Cardiac transplantation is an option in patients who are eligible.

References

1. Benotti JR, Grossman W, Cohn PF. Clinical profile of restrictive cardiomyopathy. *Circulation* 1980;61(6):1206–1212.
2. Siegel RJ, Shah PK, Fishbein MC. Idiopathic restrictive cardiomyopathy. *Circulation* 1984;70(2):165–169.
3. Ammash NM, Seward JB, Bailey KR, et al. Clinical profile and outcome of idiopathic restrictive cardiomyopathy. *Circulation* 2000;101:2490–2496.

Cardiac sarcoidosis = Frequently associated with focal wall motion abnormalities out of distribution to classic myocardial perfusion coronary anatomy (Fig. 33.7)

The American Thoracic Society in its 1999 statement on sarcoidosis defined sarcoidosis as "a multisystem disorder of unknown causes. It commonly affects young and middle-aged adults and frequently presents with bilateral hilar lymphadenopathy, pulmonary infiltration, and ocular and skin lesions. The liver, spleen, lymph nodes, salivary glands, heart, nervous system, muscles, bones, and other organs may be involved (1)." The characteristic histologic lesion is a noncaseating epithelioid cell granuloma.

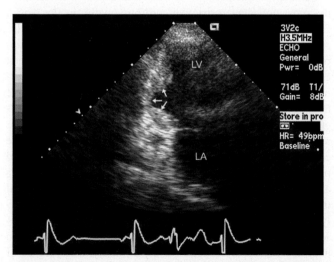

FIGURE 33.7 Reproduced from Armstrong WF, Ryan T. *Feigenbaum's Echocardiography.* 7th ed. Philadelphia, PA: Lippincott Williams & Wilkins, 2010, with permission.

Clinically evident cardiac sarcoidosis is present in only 5% of cases, but autopsy studies suggest that the incidence is likely much higher (1). The clinical course of the disease is highly variable. Granulomatous involvement of the myocardium results in inflammation and scarring, which lead to diastolic dysfunction and, in advanced cases, global systolic dysfunction. Involvement of the AV node can result in heart block and, the most common presentation of cardiac sarcoidosis, complete heart block. Myocardial scarring may result in abnormal automaticity leading to ventricular arrhythmias. Sudden cardiac death is, therefore, a common cause of death in those with cardiac sarcoidosis. Mitral regurgitation may occur due to annular dilatation from the development of a cardiomyopathy or due to papillary muscle infiltration. Coronary artery involvement is found on occasion and may result in symptoms, electrocardiographic findings, and echocardiographic findings suggestive of a myocardial infarction. It is also common for focal wall motion abnormalities to occur that do not correspond to perfusion patterns of classic coronary anatomy (2). This is likely due to the variable pattern of granulomatous involvement in the myocardium that results in the focal wall motion abnormalities. Left ventricular wall thickening may occur due to granulomatous involvement and later wall thinning due to fibrosis and scarring. Therefore, the echocardiogram may sometimes mimic concentric left ventricular hypertrophy or asymmetric septal hypertrophy and be confused with a hypertrophic cardiomyopathy.

Cardiac sarcoidosis should be considered in young adults with unexplained heart block or unexplained ventricular arrhythmias or when there is a diagnosis of extracardiac sarcoidosis even without cardiac symptoms. The first diagnostic tests should include echocardiography and Holter monitoring. If the Holter and/or the echocardiogram is abnormal, cardiac magnetic resonance (CMR) is indicated since it is more sensitive than radionuclide techniques and may have prognostic importance (3,4). Endomyocardial biopsy may be helpful in diagnosing cardiac sarcoidosis especially when there is no histologic proof of noncaseating granulomas from extracardiac sources, but is limited due to its low sensitivity of 20%. This is due to the patchy distribution of granulomas in the myocardium (5).

References

1. Statement on Sarcoidosis. Joint Statement of the American Thoracic Society (ATS), the European Respiratory Society (ERS) and the World Association of Sarcoidosis and Other Granulomatous Disorders (WASOG) adopted by the ATS Board of Directors and by the ERS Executive Committee, February 1999. *Am J Respir Crit Care Med* 1999;160:736–755.
2. Seward JB, Casaclang-Verzosa G. Infiltrative cardiovascular diseases. *J Am Coll Cardiol* 2010;55:1769–79.
3. Smedema JP, Snoep G, van Kroonenburg MPG, et al. Evaluation of the accuracy of gadolinium-enhanced cardiovascular magnetic resonance in the diagnosis of cardiac sarcoidosis. *J Am Coll Cardiol* 2005;45:1683–90.
4. Vignaux O, Dhote R, Duboc D, et al. Clinical significance of myocardial resonance abnormalities in patients with sarcoidosis: a 1-year follow-up study. *Chest* 2002;122(6):1895–1901.
5. Uemura A, Morimoto SI, Hiramitsu S, et al. Histologic diagnostic rate of cardiac sarcoidosis: evaluation of endomyocardial biopsies. *Am Heart J* 1999;138:299–302.

Answer 5: *B.* See answer 4 for additional details on endomyocardial fibrosis.

Answer 6: *E.* Hypereosinophilic syndrome is a disorder of increased eosinophils whose infiltration causes damage to several organs including the heart. By definition, eosinophilia must be >1,500/μL on at least two separate occasions and without obvious etiologies such as parasites or allergies (1). Endomyocardial fibrosis is typically the end result of the cardiac damage sustained as a result of hypereosinophilic syndrome. This was first described by Loeffler in 1936 and is, therefore, called Loeffler endocarditis (also eosinophilic endomyocardial disease, eosinophilic myocarditis, eosinophilic cardiomyopathy). Eosinophil granule proteins have been found in the necrotic tissue in the areas of endocardial and blood vessel damage and are hypothesized to be involved in the cardiac damage, leading to the endomyocardial fibrosis (2). This type of endomyocardial fibrosis is often linked to tropical endomyocardial fibrosis seen in equatorial countries like Africa because of their similarities with both conditions showing **fibrosis of the apices of the left and/or right ventricle, obliteration of these apices on echo with overlying thrombus formation, endocardial thickening, and thickening of the posterior mitral valve leaflet or posterior wall. Otherwise, echocardiographic findings are typical of a restrictive cardiomyopathy** (3–5). Cardiac MRI has become an increasingly valuable tool with its ability to detect and quantify myocardial fibrosis and inflammation. Cardiac involvement is somewhat unpredictable and does not necessarily correlate with the severity of eosinophilia. In recent years, it has been found that there are several hypereosinophilic syndrome variants, one of which is a myeloproliferative variant that has a high incidence of cardiac involvement. This variant has been associated with a chromosomal mutation resulting in a fusion of two genes (FIP1L1 and PDGFRA). Patients with this specific chromosomal alteration are less likely to respond to corticosteroid therapy and more likely to respond to imatinib, a tyrosine kinase inhibitor that has been shown to result in regression in clinical symptoms, eosinophilia, and arguably the cardiomyopathy (5–7).

References

1. Klion AD, Bochner BS, Gleich GJ, et al. Approaches to the treatment of hypereosinophilic syndromes: a workshop summary report. *J Allergy Clin Immunol* 2006;117:1292.
2. Tai PC, Spry CJF, Olsen EGJ, et al. Deposits of eosinophil granule proteins in cardiac tissues of patients with eosinophilic endomyocardial disease. *Lancet* 1987;329:643–647.
3. Gottdiener JS, Maron BJ, Schooley RT, et al. Two-dimensional echocardiographic assessment of the idiopathic hypereosinophilic syndrome: anatomic basis of mitral regurgitation and peripheral embolization. *Circulation* 1983;67(3):572–578.
4. Ommen SR, Seward JB, Tajik AJ. Clinical and echocardiographic features of hypereosinophilic syndromes. *Am J Cardiol* 2000;86:110–113.
5. Ogbogu P, Rosing DR, Home MK III. Cardiovascular manifestations of hypereosinophilic syndromes. *Immunol Allergy Clin North Am* 2007;27(3):457–475.
6. Cools J, DeAngelo DJ, Gotlib J, et al. A tyrosine kinase created by fusion of the PDGFRA and FIP1L1 genes as a therapeutic target of imatinib in idiopathic hypereosinophilic syndrome. *N Engl J Med* 2003;348(13):1201–1214.

7. Rotoli B, Catalano L, Galderisi M, et al. Rapid reversion of Loeffler's endocarditis by imatinib in early stage clonal hypereosinophilic syndrome. *Leuk Lymphoma* 2004;45(12):2503–2507.

Answer 7: *C.* The mitral annular TDE findings are altered in both diseases, but importantly for the echocardiographer, their impairments are in "opposite" directions. The lateral wall e' velocity is ***reduced*** in restriction and ***increased*** in constriction.

Answer 8: *C.* Figure 33.4 shows a transthoracic echocardiogram in the apical four-chamber plane. The LV is normal in size with concentric hypertrophy, and the video demonstrates normal systolic function. The myocardium has a somewhat granular appearance of unclear significance. The RV is somewhat borderline in size in this frame and is notable for hypertrophy of the RV free wall. The atria appear enlarged, and the septum separating the atria is thick. A small pericardial effusion is present.

There has been much recent work with strain imaging in patients with cardiac amyloidosis (CA), and our understanding of the incremental value of this continues to grow. At this time, apical sparing with GLS is a unique finding in CA and relatively simple to obtain. Continued investigation into the prognostic implications, the subclassification of CA types, and the unique findings in the atria (atrial strain) may soon offer new insights.

Suggested Readings

Koyama J, Falk RH. Prognostic significance of strain Doppler imaging in light-chain amyloidosis. *JACC Cardiovasc Imaging* 2010;3:333–342.
Phelan D, Collier P, Thavendiranathan P, et al. Relative apical sparing of longitudinal strain using two-dimensional speckle-tracking echocardiography is both sensitive and specific for the diagnosis of cardiac amyloidosis. *Heart* 2012;98:1442–1448.

Answer 9: *A.* The echocardiographic diagnosis of cardiac amyloidosis includes all of the features previously discussed for restrictive cardiomyopathy in general. There are features on echocardiography that are more typical for infiltrative cardiomyopathies and cardiac amyloidosis in particular. These include the classic granular sparkling myocardium described in 1981 by Siqueira-Filho et al. (1), and although this finding is typical for cardiac amyloidosis and has had studies suggesting its high specificity, the advent of harmonic imaging and modern-day processing techniques have rendered this finding less specific and less useful. Therefore, **Option B** is incorrect. Hypertensive heart disease, especially associated with end-stage renal disease, will often have this appearance as well. If one suspects that a myocardium has increased echogenicity, turning off harmonic imaging may be of some help. Increased atrial septal thickness is only moderately sensitive at 60% but highly specific at up to 100% for cardiac amyloidosis (2) although the echocardiographer must be careful to make sure it is not lipomatous hypertrophy of the septum. Therefore, **Option C** is incorrect. Pericardial effusions are found in cardiac amyloidosis >50% of the time but are usually not

severe enough to cause cardiac tamponade (1). Its presence, therefore, should not be surprising and should not point the physician in a different direction as long as all the other echocardiographic findings point toward cardiac amyloidosis and there are no findings suggesting alternatives such as constrictive pericarditis or cardiac tamponade. Therefore, **Option D** is incorrect.

The classic findings described such as grade III diastolic dysfunction and significant hypertrophy of both ventricular walls and the atrial septum are typical in advanced cases. By the time of diagnosis, however, prognosis is often poor. Strain and strain rate have evolved as a method that can detect myocardial involvement despite normal standard echo features. Studies reveal that longitudinal myocardial function is reduced or impaired as evidenced by abnormal systolic strain and strain rate in patients with cardiac amyloidosis despite normal standard echo and tissue Doppler findings (3,4). At least one study suggests that this may have prognostic significance regarding cardiac and total mortality (5).

The echo-bright LA structure is located at the junction of the LA appendage and the left superior pulmonary vein. This "tissue infolding" is sometimes referred to as the Coumadin ridge and is more commonly noted on TEE exams. Since the LA is in the far field on TTE orientation, LA thrombi are not commonly found, and TEE is frequently beneficial for this diagnosis. Therefore, **Option E** is incorrect.

References

1. Siqueira-Filho AG, Cunha CLP, Tajik AJ, et al. M-mode and two-dimensional echocardiographic features of cardiac amyloidosis. *Circulation* 1981;63(1):188–196.
2. Falk RH, Plehn JF, Deering T, et al. Sensitivity and specificity of the echocardiographic features of cardiac amyloidosis. *Am J Cardiol* 1987;59:418–422.
3. Koyama J, Ray-Sequin PA, Falk RH. Longitudinal myocardial function assessed by tissue velocity, strain, strain rate tissue Doppler echocardiography in patients with al (primary) cardiac amyloidosis. *Circulation* 2003;107:2446–2452.
4. Bellavia D, Pellikka PA, Abraham TP, et al. Evidence of impaired left ventricular systolic function by Doppler myocardial imaging in patients with systemic amyloidosis and no evidence of cardiac involvement by standard two-dimensional and Doppler echocardiography. *Am J Cariol* 2008;101:1039–1045.
5. Koyama J, Falk RH, Prognostic significance of strain Doppler imaging in light-chain amyloidosis. *J Am Coll Cardiol Imaging* 2010;3:333–342.

Answer 10: *D.* See discussion in question 4 for a detailed explanation.

Answer 11A: See question 4 for additional discussion on cardiac sarcoidosis.

Option B. It is incorrect since it would be unlikely that CAD caused this degree of LV dysfunction given the recently normal cath findings as well as the atypical (noncoronary) septal infarct on CMR.

Option C. Although there are no absolute criteria and dilated CM from a remote history of myocarditis is always a consideration, the presence of third-degree heart block, septal scar, and RV involvement lowers this likelihood.

Option D. It is true that persistent RV pacing can result in LV systolic dysfunction. It would not explain the other findings.

Option E. ARVD/C is a real consideration and is known to cause biventricular dysfunction in 10% to 15% of cases. However, ARVD/C, due to gap junction mutations, does not usually cause third-degree heart block (although this is common in cardiac sarcoidosis).

Answer 11B:

Option A is incorrect. The anatomic (total ventricular) stroke volume (LVVd–LVVs) is the same as the physiologic (forward) stroke volume (Qs). As MR increases, this difference becomes greater.

Option B is correct and assumes that there is 10 mL of TR.

Option C is incorrect as the Qp/Qs ratio is equal.

Options D and E are both incorrect. The LVEF is 23% and the RVEF is 24% (volumetric stroke volume/diastolic volume).

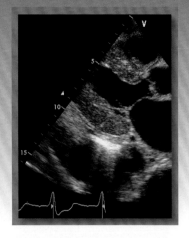

Chapter 34

Echo Features of Other Cardiomyopathies

Maya E. Guglin

1. A 40-year-old female is referred to you for evaluation of exertional dyspnea. A transthoracic echocardiogram is performed. Selected images are shown in FIGURE 34.1 and VIDEO 34.1.

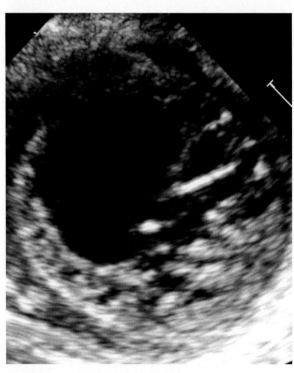

FIGURE 34.1

Which of the following statements best describes the condition shown?

A. A ratio of compacted to noncompacted myocardium >3:1 is a characteristic diagnostic criterion that balances the sensitivity and specificity of 2D echocardiography.

B. Since familial occurrence is rare, screening echocardiography is not recommended for first-degree relatives.

C. Prominent trabecular meshwork is seen primarily in the anterior wall.

D. Left ventricular systolic function remains normal with increasing age.

E. This condition may at times be confused with both a dilated cardiomyopathy and an apical-variant hypertrophic cardiomyopathy.

2. A 33-year-old male is admitted to the hospital with complaints of dizziness and a syncopal event. Telemetry monitoring is significant for recurrent episodes of nonsustained ventricular tachycardia. A transthoracic echocardiogram is performed. Selected images are shown in FIGURES 34.2 AND 34.3 and VIDEOS 34.2 AND 34.3.

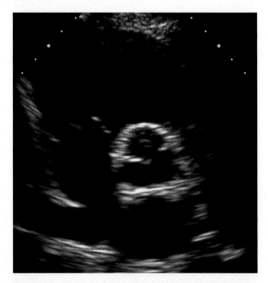

FIGURE 34.2

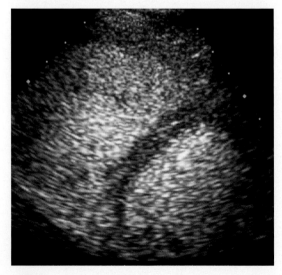

FIGURE 34.3

Based on this information, what is the next best step in establishing a primary diagnosis?

A. Left heart catheterization
B. Endomyocardial biopsy
C. Electrophysiologic study
D. Nuclear myocardial perfusion study
E. Cardiac MRI

3. You are asked to see a 51-year-old female in the emergency department. She complains of several hours of moderate-intensity, persistent midsternal chest pressure. Past medical history is significant for hypertension that is well controlled with chlorthalidone and lisinopril. She is recently divorced, lives with her 16-year-old daughter, and reports ongoing child custody problems with her ex-spouse. Social history is significant for smoking and occasional use of marijuana in the past; she denies any current illicit drug use.

An electrocardiogram is performed, which is significant for precordial (V1 to V4) ST-segment elevations, and the patient is brought urgently to the cardiac catheterization lab for coronary angiography. Coronary angiography is completed and reveals normal coronary arteries. Provocative testing performed with intracoronary acetylcholine injection is unremarkable. A transthoracic echocardiogram is performed following the cardiac catheterization (Figs.34.4 and 34.5; Videos 34.4 and 34.5).

Which of the following statements is most accurate given the most likely diagnosis?

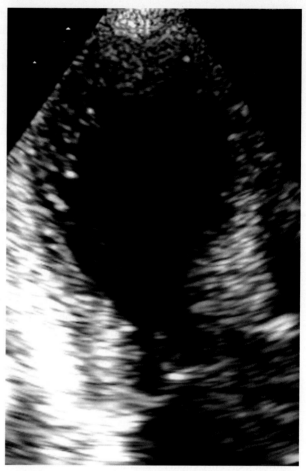

Figure 34.5

A. The normal coronary angiogram confirms the diagnosis of Prinzmetal variant angina.
B. This disease is much more common in women than in men.
C. An exercise echocardiogram would be valuable early in the diagnostic algorithm of this patient.
D. A 24-hour Holter monitor is necessary to confirm the suspected diagnosis.
E. Obtaining a urine drug screen would be necessary to confirm the most likely etiology.

4. Which of the following statements is true regarding anthracycline-related cardiomyopathy?

A. Cumulative dose of anthracycline therapy is the highest risk factor for cardiotoxicity.
B. Cumulative doxorubicin dose up to 900 mg/m^2 is considered safe.
C. Current guidelines recommend baseline-only assessment of LVEF, without the need for follow-up evaluation.
D. Global longitudinal strain value of −5% in a patient undergoing anthracycline therapy is associated with a low risk of cardiotoxicity.
E. In patients with anthracycline-related cardiotoxicity, 90% will show LVEF improvement following anthracycline cessation and initiation of a heart failure regimen.

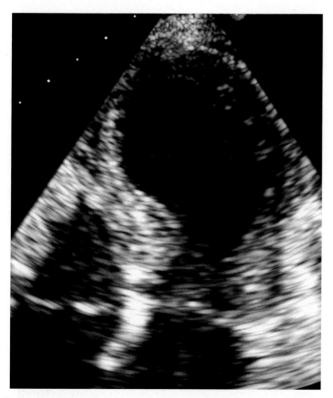

Figure 34.4

5. Distinguishing hypertrophic cardiomyopathy from athlete's heart can be challenging. Which of the following statements is least correct?

A. In athlete's heart, left ventricular wall thickness will decrease with deconditioning.

B. Left ventricular end-diastolic dimensions (LVEDD) commonly differ as follows: hypertrophic cardiomyopathy LVEDD < 45 mm and athlete's heart LVEDD >55 mm.

C. First-degree relatives of patients with hypertrophic cardiomyopathy should receive screening evaluation.

D. Strength training, compared to endurance training, results in thicker myocardial walls but less LV dilation.

E. Normal values for LV mass and wall thickness vary with gender and type of sport, but a septal wall thickness >13 mm in a male is pathognomonic of hypertrophic cardiomyopathy and not achieved in an athlete's heart.

6. A 30-year-old African American female is referred to you from the obstetrics clinic for evaluation. She has no past medical history, and she is currently 36 weeks' pregnant (first pregnancy). She reports several weeks of worsening dyspnea, which she primarily attributes to her pregnancy. Relevant exam findings are as follows:

BP 100/55; HR 110; RR 18; Temp 36.8
Jugular venous pulsation 12 cm
S3 gallop
Bibasilar crackles
1+ lower extremity edema bilaterally

A transthoracic echocardiogram is performed, which is significant for left ventricular systolic dysfunction with EF = 35%. Which of the following statements is least accurate given the listed findings?

A. Angiotensin-converting enzyme inhibitors should be avoided during the third trimester of pregnancy.

B. Peripartum cardiomyopathy is defined by the development of heart failure in the last month of pregnancy or within 5 months of delivery.

C. Peripartum cardiomyopathy occurs most commonly in women >30 years old.

D. Women with a history of peripartum cardiomyopathy and persistent left ventricular dysfunction should be counseled against repeat pregnancy.

E. Seventy-five percent of all peripartum cardiomyopathy patients will have recovery of left ventricular systolic function to EF > 50%.

7. You are asked to a see a 35-year-old male in the emergency department who presents to the hospital with several weeks of light-headedness and dizziness. His past medical history and family history are unremarkable. He smokes about one pack of cigarettes per week. He consumes 4 to 5 servings of alcohol per week, and he denies illicit drug use. He is originally from South America, and he travels there frequently on business.

A transthoracic echocardiogram is performed (FIGS. 34.6 AND 34.7; VIDEOS 34.6 AND 34.7). Based upon the clinical history and the findings on echocardiography, which of the following is most accurate?

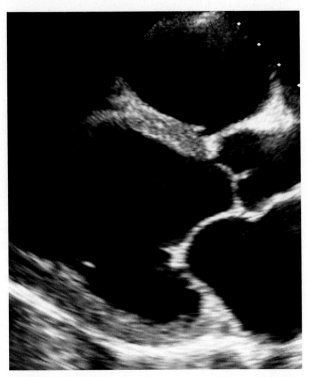

FIGURE 34.6

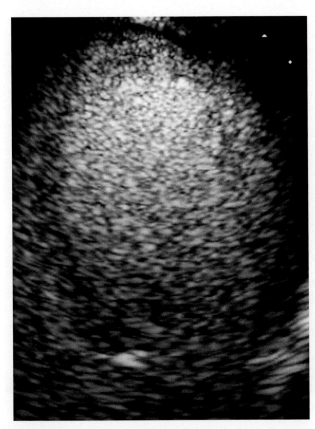

FIGURE 34.7

A. Urgent coronary revascularization will likely result in complete recovery of LV function.

B. Serial evaluation of coxsackievirus B or echovirus titers will confirm the diagnosis.

C. Intravenous injection of contrast microbubbles will show prominent recesses and extensive trabeculation.

D. He likely has a parasitic infection from his travels.

E. An abdominal fat biopsy may be diagnostic.

8. Which of the following statements describing the features of cardiac sarcoidosis is true?

A. Cardiac and pulmonary involvement occurs with similar frequency.

B. Granulomatous involvement typically spares the cardiac conduction system.

C. Echocardiography may show regional wall motion abnormalities that occur in a noncoronary distribution.

D. Granulomatous myocardial involvement will result in diastolic dysfunction; systolic function is usually unaffected.

E. Contrast echocardiography can be used to enhance areas of myocardial granulomatous infiltration.

9. A 56-year-old male is referred to your office for evaluation of progressive dyspnea and lower extremity edema. He has a past medical history of hyperlipidemia that is well controlled with atorvastatin. Laboratory data provided by the patient's primary care provider are significant for borderline normal creatinine and increased urine protein. Vital signs are normal. Physical exam is significant for increased jugular venous pulsation, bilateral lower extremity edema, and mild hepatomegaly. A transthoracic echocardiogram is performed (Fig. 34.8 and Video 34.8).

Which of the following statements about this patient's condition is true?

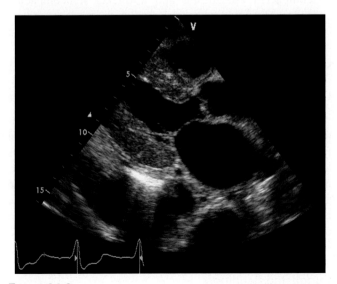

Figure 34.8

A. Electrocardiogram shows left ventricular hypertrophy.

B. The conduction system is usually unaffected.

C. The mitral inflow Doppler pattern is typically normal.

D. Cardiac valves are thickened.

E. Increased wall thickness is limited to the left ventricle.

10. Which of the following conditions best describes the images shown in Figures 34.9 and 34.10 and Video 34.9?

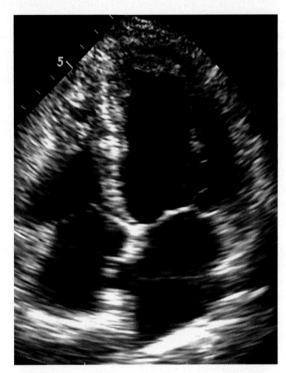

Figure 34.9

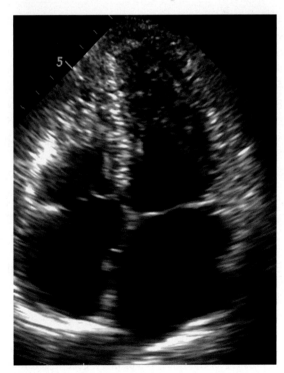

Figure 34.10

A. Apical-variant hypertrophic cardiomyopathy
B. Amyloid cardiomyopathy
C. Cardiac sarcoidosis
D. Hypereosinophilic syndrome
E. Hemochromatosis

11. A 66-year-old male who lives alone called EMS for weakness and severe dyspnea increasing over the past 10 days. They arrived within 5 minutes and found a profoundly dyspneic patient in acute respiratory distress requiring urgent intubation prior to transport to the emergency room. Upon exam in the ER, he was cold and clammy with blood pressure measured at 67/49 mm Hg, HR 115 bpm, and diffuse bilateral infiltrates on chest X-ray.

Echocardiographic findings are shown in Video 34.10.

Which of the following would most likely explain the echo findings?

A. Past history of infection from *Trypanosoma cruzi*
B. Peripheral eosinophil count >1,500/µL
C. Remote viral myocarditis
D. Severe CAD
E. Recent stressful event

12. The patient in question 11 had persistent hemodynamic instability and worsening renal and liver function and was evaluated for mechanical circulatory support.

Which device would you choose?

A. HeartMate 2
B. HeartWare
C. VV ECMO
D. TandemHeart
E. VA ECMO

13. 40-year-old female underwent heart transplantation 5 years ago. She is admitted with gradual onset of shortness of breath and peripheral edema. A transthoracic echocardiogram is shown in Videos 34.11A–C and Figures 34.11A and B.

Based upon the available images, which of the following statements is most accurate?

A. These are expected findings on a posttransplant echocardiogram.
B. This echocardiogram strongly suggests acute allograft rejection.
C. The TV leaflets are flail and likely iatrogenic from recent biopsy.
D. These findings are consistent with constrictive pericarditis.
E. This patient likely has severe coronary vasculopathy.

Answer 1: E. The echocardiogram is significant for prominent lateral wall trabeculations with deep recesses and increased ratio of noncompacted to compacted myocardium. These findings are most consistent with left ventricular noncompaction (LVNC). LVNC is classified as a primary, genetic cardiomyopathy. It is characterized by first-trimester failure of intrauterine compaction. Familial occurrence is frequent (18% to 50% in

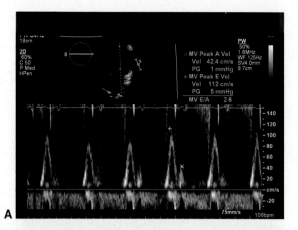

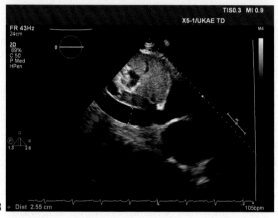

FIGURE 34.11

different series), and screening ECGs and echocardiograms should be performed on all first-degree relatives. The most commonly used echocardiographic criteria are those by Jenni et al., which describe LVNC as follows:

A. No coexistent cardiac abnormalities
B. Thick left ventricular wall with two layers—a thin compacted epicardium and a thicker noncompacted endocardium with trabecular meshwork and deep recesses (2:1 ratio of noncompacted to compacted myocardium at end systole in the parasternal short-axis view)
C. Prominent "trabecular" infoldings in left ventricular apex or midleft ventricular segments of inferior and lateral wall
D. Color Doppler evidence of flow within intertrabecular recesses

The use of color Doppler or a contrast agent may help to identify the presence of intertrabecular recesses. Although the clinical features of LVNC may vary, the natural history usually includes left ventricular systolic dysfunction and heart failure. LVNC may be misinterpreted as either a dilated cardiomyopathy or an apical-variant hypertrophic cardiomyopathy. Thromboembolic complications are an important concern; however, current expert consensus does not recommend use of anticoagulation in LVNC patients with sinus rhythm and preserved LVEF.

Suggested Readings

Murphy RT, Thaman R, Blanes JG, et al. Natural history and familial characteristics of isolated left ventricular non-compaction. *Eur Heart J* 2005;26(2):187–192.

Oechslin E, Jenni R. Left ventricular non-compaction revisited: a distinct phenotype with genetic heterogeneity? *Eur Heart J* 2011;32(12):1446–1456.

Answer 2: E. This patient's presentation and images are most consistent with arrhythmogenic right ventricular cardio-myopathy/dysplasia (ARVC/ARVD). The echocardiogram shows severe RV dilation and systolic dysfunction. Contrast-enhanced images are significant for the presence of localized RV free wall aneurysms. ARVC is typically characterized by a scarred right ventricular appearance with fibrofatty replacement of the myocardium. Regional RV involvement is most common initially; however, ARVC can progress to diffuse RV disease and LV involvement. ARVC is an important cause of sudden cardiac death in young adults, and familial inheritance is common. Increased ARVC incidence has been observed in the Mediterranean population.

Clinically, ARVC may be characterized by symptoms such as dizziness, palpitations, syncope, or sudden death. Ventricular tachyarrhythmias in the absence of coronary disease (typically right heart origin/left bundle branch block ECG pattern) may also occur. Echocardiographic features of ARVC may include RV dilation (particularly right ventricular outflow tract), RV systolic dysfunction, RV regional wall motion abnormalities, localized RV free wall aneurysms, echogenic appearance of affected RV myocardium, RV trabecular derangement, and a hyperreflective moderator band. Cardiac MRI and echocardiography are typically the most useful diagnostic tests to assess right heart morphology and function.

Left heart catheterization or nuclear myocardial perfusion imaging is most helpful if there is a strong clinical suspicion of ischemic heart disease. Although lacking in sensitivity and specificity, in selected patients with contraindications to MRI being evaluated at experienced centers, endomyocardial biopsy may be performed to assist with ARVC diagnosis. While electrophysiologic testing may indicate ventricular tachyarrhythmias of RV origin, these findings are not diagnostic of ARVC.

Suggested Readings

Marcus FI, McKenna WJ, Sherrill D, et al. Diagnosis of arrhythmogenic right ventricular cardiomyopathy/dysplasia. *Circulation* 2010;121(13):1533–1541.
Yoerger DM, Marcus F, Sherrill D, et al. Echocardiographic findings in patients meeting task force criteria for arrhythmogenic right ventricular dysplasia: new insights from the multidisciplinary study of right ventricular dysplasia. *J Am Coll Cardiol* 2005;45(6):860–865.

Answer 3: B. This patient's presentation is most consistent with stress-induced cardiomyopathy (also known as Takotsubo syndrome or transient apical ballooning). The echocardiogram is remarkable for mid to distal LV akinesis/dyskinesis with aneurysm and sparing of basal segment systolic function. This cardiomyopathy is far more common in women and may be triggered by an emotional or physical stressor or acute medical illness. Stress-induced cardiomyopathy is typically characterized by transient systolic dysfunction of the apical and mid LV segments with basal wall hyperkinesis. Its presentation may mimic a myocardial infarction; however, there is usually an absence of obstructive coronary disease. Clinical presentation may involve a trigger and may include symptoms of chest pain, dyspnea, or even cardiogenic shock. ST-segment elevations and T-wave inversions are common on ECG, and cardiac biomarkers are often mildly elevated. Clinical, ECG, and echocardiographic presentation may often resemble that of an anterior wall myocardial infarction. The diagnosis of stress-induced cardiomyopathy is usually made only once obstructive or occlusive coronary artery disease has been excluded. Similar to extensive anterior and apical wall myocardial infarction, stress-induced cardiomyopathy may be complicated by left ventricular outflow tract obstruction, systolic anterior motion (SAM) of the mitral valve, and mitral regurgitation. In the presence of shock, echocardiography is important in order to evaluate LV systolic function and to assess for the presence of dynamic LVOT obstruction.

There is no optimal therapeutic regimen for the treatment of stress-induced cardiomyopathy. Medical therapy usually entails a standard heart failure regimen (beta-blockers, angiotensin-converting enzyme inhibitors). The majority of patients have complete recovery of LV systolic function within weeks.

Prinzmetal variant angina is much less likely given the clinical history of emotional stressors with normal provocative testing in the catheterization lab. The patient's clinical presentation and workup thus far are sufficient to make a diagnosis; further cardiac testing (Holter monitor, exercise echocardiogram) is unnecessary. A urine drug screen should be performed to exclude the possibility of cocaine-related vasospasm; however, in the current scenario, this diagnosis is less likely.

Suggested Readings

Prasad A, Lerman A, Rihal CS. Apical ballooning syndrome (Tako-Tsubo or stress cardiomyopathy): a mimic of acute myocardial infarction. *Am Heart J* 2008;155(3):408–447.
Sharkey SW, Windenburg DC, Lesser JR, et al. Natural history and expansive clinical profile of stress (Tako-Tsubo) cardiomyopathy. *J Am Coll Cardiol* 2010;55(4):333–341.

Answer 4: A. Cardiotoxicity may occur at any dose level of anthracycline therapy. The most significant risk factor for irreversible myocardial toxicity is cumulative dose of therapy; lifetime doxorubicin dosage >450 to 500 mg/m^2 is associated with significantly increased risk. Some patients develop LV dysfunction prior to this dose, and therefore, serial screening surveillance is required. Current recommendations state that LVEF should be evaluated at baseline by either echocardiography or multigated radionuclide angiography and periodically thereafter. FDA labeling for doxorubicin defines deterioration in cardiac function as a 10% decline in LVEF below the lower limit of normal or an absolute LVEF below 45% or a 20% decline in LVEF to any level. In studies involving patients receiving chemotherapeutic agents with potential for cardiotoxicity, echocardiographic techniques such as strain, strain rate imaging, tissue Doppler, and 3D echocardiographic LVEF assessment have shown promise as a means to evaluate for early signs of cardiomyopathy. In one study of breast cancer patients treated with anthracyclines, LV global longitudinal strain less negative than −19% was predictive of subsequent cardiotoxicity and preceded changes in LVEF. In patients undergoing chemotherapy, noncontrast 3D echocardiographic assessment of LVEF was found to be the most reproducible technique for serial evaluation of LV function. The incidence of LV recovery is greatest in patients with the shortest time between the end of anthracycline chemotherapy and the initiation of heart failure treatment (beta-blockers and angiotensin-converting enzyme inhibitors). In one series of 201 patients, there was an approximately 50% incidence of LVEF response/improvement following chemotherapy cessation and HF treatment.

Suggested Readings

Cardinale D, Colombo A, Lamantia G, et al. Anthracycline-induced cardiomyopathy: clinical relevance and response to pharmacologic therapy. *J Am Coll Cardiol* 2010;55(3):213–220.

Feenstra J, Grobbee DE, Remme WJ, et al. Drug-induced heart failure. *J Am Coll Cardiol* 1999;33(5):1152–1162.

Sawaya H, Sebag IA, Plana JC, et al. Assessment of echocardiography and biomarkers for the extended prediction of cardiotoxicity in patients treated with anthracyclines, taxanes, and trastuzumab/clinical perspective. *Circ Cardiovasc Imaging* 2012;5(5):596–603.

Thavendiranathan P, Grant AD, Negishi T, et al. Reproducibility of echocardiographic techniques for sequential assessment of left ventricular ejection fraction and volumes application to patients undergoing cancer chemotherapy. *J Am Coll Cardiol* 2013;61(1):77–84.

Answer 5: E. The cardiac morphology of trained athletes may often be different from that of other "normal" patients and can be mistaken for conditions such as hypertrophic cardiomyopathy (HCM). Family history, ECG findings, and echocardiographic evaluation are often helpful in making this distinction.

Patients with cardiac morphologic changes due to athlete's heart will usually display a homogeneous pattern of wall thickening that involves all of the left ventricle rather than the septum alone. As opposed to HCM, the LV wall thickness seen in athlete's heart will reliably regress following a period of deconditioning. Trained athletes will often have enlarged left ventricular internal dimensions and normal or mildly increased left atrial size indices. Diastolic flow patterns are normal and are significant for increased early diastolic flow velocity (E wave) and increased LV tissue Doppler E-wave velocities (up to 16 and 19 cm/s for septal and lateral walls, respectively, in one series of endurance athletes).

In patients with HCM, maximal wall thickening most commonly occurs in a heterogeneous manner (septal wall), resulting in an asymmetric pattern. Compared to endurance training, strength training results in increased wall thickness but less LV dilation (concentric rather than eccentric hypertrophy). The maximal wall thickness generally associated with HCM is greater than that of athlete's heart. Although 13 mm is an important echocardiographic "cutoff" that helps to distinguish between these two entities in males, it is not pathognomonic for HCM. A small number of elite athletes may show septal wall thicknesses in the 13- to 15-mm range, potentially overlapping with the wall thicknesses seen in HCM patients. Therefore, Option E is least correct and the single best answer for this question. Compared to athlete's heart, HCM patients will have smaller left ventricular internal dimensions, enlarged

left atrial size indices, and abnormal diastolic flow parameters (E/A reversal, prolonged E-wave deceleration time, decreased LV tissue Doppler velocities).

Normative values for LV mass and wall thickness vary with gender.

Suggested Readings

D'Andrea A, Cocchia R, Riegler L, et al. Left ventricular myocardial velocities and deformation indexes in top-level athletes. *J Am Soc Echocardiogr* 2010;23(12):1281–1288.

Maron BJ. Distinguishing hypertrophic cardiomyopathy from athlete's heart: a clinical problem of increasing magnitude and significance. *Heart* 2005;91(11):1380–1382.

Maron BJ, Pelliccia A, Spirito P. Cardiac disease in young trained athletes. *Circulation* 1995;91(5):1596–601.

Weiner RB, Baggish AL. Exercise-induced cardiac remodeling. *Prog Cardiovasc Dis* 2012;54(5):380–386.

Answer 6: E. Peripartum cardiomyopathy is defined as the development of heart failure with left ventricular ejection fraction <45% in the last month of pregnancy or within 5 months of delivery, along with an absence of recognizable heart disease prior to the last month of pregnancy and absence of other identifiable causes of heart failure. Peripartum cardiomyopathy is a rare cause of heart failure in the United States; however, worldwide incidence is variable. Risk factors associated with peripartum cardiomyopathy include age >30 years, multiparity, multifetal pregnancy, African descent, history of preeclampsia, eclampsia, or postpartum hypertension. Prognosis is variable. Case series from South Africa report a 6-month and 2-year mortality rate of 10% and 28%, respectively. The percentage of patients who demonstrate normalization of left ventricular function is also variable with estimates ranging from 20% to 50%. Therefore, Option E is an incorrect statement and the single best answer to this question. Women with a history of peripartum cardiomyopathy with severe left ventricular dysfunction at diagnosis (EF <25%) or those who have persistent left ventricular dysfunction should be counseled against repeat pregnancy. Angiotensin-converting enzyme inhibitors are associated with an increased risk of fetal malformations, and their use is contraindicated during all three trimesters of pregnancy.

Suggested Readings

Ramaraj R, Sorrell VL. Peripartum cardiomyopathy: causes, diagnosis, and treatment. *Cleve Clin J Med* 2009;76(5):289–296.

Sliwa K, Hilfiker-Kleiner D, Petrie MC, et al. Current state of knowledge on aetiology, diagnosis, management, and therapy of peripartum cardiomyopathy: a position statement from the Heart Failure Association of the European Society of Cardiology Working Group on peripartum cardiomyopathy. *Eur J Heart Fail* 2010;12(8):767–778.

Answer 7: D. Chagas disease is caused by ***Trypanosoma cruzi*** parasitic infection and is endemic to many South American regions. Worldwide, it is a common cause of significant cardiac morbidity (heart failure, stroke) and mortality. Acute Chagas disease is commonly associated with pericardial effusion. Chronic Chagas cardiac disease may present as severe biventricular systolic dysfunction, and it can be associated with ventricular wall aneurysms (predominantly apical) and thromboembolism. Ventricular tachyarrhythmias and significant conduction disease are also common and are the likely causes for this patient's symptoms. The echocardiogram is significant for severe LV dilation and severe global LV systolic dysfunction. The patient's travel history and clinical presentation make Option D the most likely answer.

Coronary revascularization would be most helpful in a patient with ischemic cardiomyopathy. Coxsackie B virus and echovirus are commonly associated with viral myocarditis. Left ventricular noncompaction cardiomyopathy is characterized by prominent LV recesses and trabeculations. Abdominal fat pad biopsy is useful in the diagnostic workup of cardiac amyloidosis.

Suggested Readings

Acquatella H. Echocardiography in Chagas heart disease. *Circulation* 2007;115(9):1124–1131.
Bern C. Evaluation and treatment of Chagas disease in the United States: a systematic review. *JAMA* 2007;298(18):2171–2181.

Answer 8: C. Sarcoidosis is a multisystem disease that is characterized by the presence of noncaseating granulomas. It most commonly involves the lungs and usually results in hilar adenopathy and reticular opacities, although its appearance can vary considerably by stage. Cardiac sarcoidosis is less common and usually manifests itself clinically as conduction abnormalities, ventricular arrhythmias, and heart failure. Granulomatous involvement can occur in any area of the heart, including the pericardium and the myocardium. The patchy nature of granuloma distribution can cause regional wall motion abnormalities that occur in a noncoronary distribution. Extensive granulomatous infiltration may result in both systolic and diastolic dysfunction. Gadolinium-enhanced cardiac magnetic resonance imaging has been shown to be helpful in the evaluation of cardiac sarcoidosis. At present, there is no accepted role for the use of contrast echocardiography in the assessment of myocardial sarcoid involvement.

Suggested Readings

Ayyala US, Nair AP, Padilla ML. Cardiac sarcoidosis. *Clin Chest Med* 2008;29(3):493–508.
Kim JS, Judson MA, Donnino R, et al. Cardiac sarcoidosis. *Am Heart J* 2009;157(1):9–21.
Youssef G, Beanlands RSB, Birnie DH, et al. Cardiac sarcoidosis: applications of imaging in diagnosis and directing treatment. *Heart* 2011;97(24):2078–2087.

Answer 9: D. This patient's presentation and echocardiogram are most consistent with a diagnosis of cardiac amyloidosis. The echocardiogram is significant for increased myocardial echogenicity, LV systolic dysfunction, and concentric LV thickening. The mitral and aortic valves are mildly thickened, and the left atrium is enlarged.

There are several different types of amyloidosis that can result in heart disease: primary (AL), secondary, familial, and senile. Cardiac amyloidosis is characterized by immunoglobulin deposition in the myocardium, cardiac valves, and pericardium. On echocardiography, it is commonly associated with

ventricular wall thickening due to amyloid deposition; however, the electrocardiogram will usually show low-voltage or a pseudoinfarct pattern, without evidence of left ventricular hypertrophy. The myocardium is classically described as having a granular, speckled appearance; however, in the current era of harmonic imaging, this is not a very specific finding. Amyloid deposits may also be found in the conduction system and can result in the need for pacemaker implantation. The cardiac valves are also involved and will commonly appear thickened. Symptomatic individuals with advanced disease will usually have mitral inflow Doppler spectra that are consistent with a restrictive filling pattern: tall E wave, increased E/A ratio, short deceleration time, and decreased isovolumic relaxation time. Tissue Doppler, strain, and strain rate imaging are typically abnormal prior to a decrease in ejection fraction and may be of diagnostic and prognostic value. In addition to increased LV wall thickness, amyloid cardiomyopathy is also commonly associated with RV wall thickening and biatrial dilation.

Suggested Reading

Falk RH. Diagnosis and management of the cardiac amyloidoses. *Circulation* 2005;112(13):2047–2060.

Answer 10: D. The hypereosinophilic syndrome (HES) consists of a group of disease states that are characterized by eosinophil deposition. Myocardial, pericardial, and coronary vascular inflammation may occur. Clinical and pathologic changes are similar irrespective of etiology; early diagnosis and treatment can improve patient outcomes. The natural history of the condition is characterized by three stages: an acute necrotic stage, an intermediate thrombotic stage, and a late fibrotic stage. On echocardiography, HES is most commonly characterized by LV and RV apical thrombi and scarring (as in the figure and video). Endomyocardial thickening is also common and may result in leaflet tethering and regurgitation in both the mitral and tricuspid valves. Advanced diastolic dysfunction with restrictive physiology may also be seen. Left ventricular systolic function is usually preserved.

Apical HCM is associated with myocardial hypertrophy in the distal/apical LV segments with abnormalities limited to the LV. The left ventriculogram classically shows a "spade-like" LV pattern similar to that seen here. Contrast echocardiography and cardiac MRI are useful modalities in making this diagnosis. Amyloid cardiomyopathy is typically associated with diffuse myocardial wall thickening, valve thickening, and abnormal diastolic function. Cardiac sarcoidosis may result in many nonspecific echocardiographic findings and can involve the pericardium and the myocardium and may result in both systolic and diastolic dysfunctions. Patchy granulomatous infiltration of the heart may cause regional wall motion abnormalities that occur in a noncoronary distribution. Hereditary hemochromatosis is associated with myocardial iron deposition and subsequent systolic heart failure; cardiac MRI is a useful diagnostic modality to assess for cardiac infiltration.

Suggested Readings

Hunt SA, Abraham WT, Chin MH, et al. 2009 focused update incorporated into the ACC/AHA 2005 guidelines for the diagnosis and management of heart failure in adults. *Circulation* 2009;119(14):e391–e479.

Ogbogu PU, Rosing DR, Horne MK III. Cardiovascular manifestations of hypereosinophilic syndromes. *Immunol Allergy Clin North Am* 2007;27(3):457–475.

Answer 11: D. This echo is most consistent with an "ischemic cardiomyopathy" (probable proximal left anterior descending artery-related myocardial infarction chronic and/or subacute). This was complicated by true left ventricular aneurysm (chronic) and an LV pseudoaneurysm (probably more recent). VIDEO 34.12A shows severe global hypokinesis to akinesis of the left ventricle with only very proximal part of septum moving. The ventricle is dilated with dense spontaneous echo contrast consistent with low flow. You can see small thrombus on VIDEO 34.12B. VIDEO 34.12C demonstrates the adjacent echo-free space consistent with the LV pseudoaneurysm.

Both left ventricular aneurysms and pseudoaneurysms are typical complications of myocardial infarction. The true LV aneurysm has a wide neck (and is confirmed by the "diastolic deformation" and outpouching). Pathologically, the wall of the aneurysm is composed of the all "three" layers of the normal ventricular myocardium. A pseudoaneurysm (PA), or false aneurysm, develops after a ventricular free wall rupture that is contained by pericardium. Unlike the true aneurysm, the neck is relatively narrow compared to the full extent of the body of the PA (not shown on the video). Pseudoaneurysms can rupture and surgical repair should be considered. In this case, the patient was fortunate to receive heart transplant.

Although apical aneurysm is typical for Chagas disease (chagasic cardiomyopathy), neither the clinical history nor the left ventricular pseudoaneurysm is consistent. Takotsubo, or stress-induced cardiomyopathy, typically has apical ballooning and akinesis on echo, but would not result in partial rupture of the free wall and PA. The low-flow state and clinical presentation with cardiogenic shock and pulmonary edema in a 66-year-old man are much more consistent with a cardiomyopathy from CAD.

Suggested Readings

Acquatella H. Echocardiography in Chagas heart disease. *Circulation* 2007;115(9):1124–1131.

Acquatella H, et al. Recommendations for multimodality cardiac imaging in patients with chagas disease: a report from the American Society of Echocardiography in Collaboration with the InterAmerican Association of Echocardiography (ECOSIAC) and the Cardiovascular Imaging Department of the Brazilian Society of Cardiology (DIC-SBC). *J Am Soc Echocardiogr* 2018;31(1):3–25.

Vlodaver Z, Coe JI, Edwards JE. True and false left ventricular aneurysms. Propensity for the latter to rupture. *Circulation* 1975;51:567.

Answer 12: D. The TandemHeart is the only device which may be feasible in this patient.

HeartMate 2 and HeartWare are both long-term ventricular assist devices. The patient is a typical INTERMACS 1, or "crash and burn" profile, which has the worst outcomes of all LVAD candidates. Preferably, patients should be stabilized first, with optimization of end-organ function, including renal and hepatic impairment.

Also, since this patient is intubated, sedated, and on a ventilator, he is currently unable to understand, discuss, and make informed decisions about long-term options or agree with all of the necessary lifestyle changes resulting from the implantation of a long-term assist device.

Importantly, the left ventricular wall in the apical region is compromised by the pseudoaneurysm and apical thrombus and placement of the inflow cannula may present technical difficulties.

A venovenous ECMO (extracorporeal membrane oxygenation) will oxygenate the blood and can support the lungs, but this will not treat shock or provide circulatory support.

VA ECMO would provide the required support, but since this pumps blood in a retrograde manner into the artery and increases the left ventricular end-diastolic pressure, it may result in further ventricular distension. Because the left ventricular end-diastolic pressure is already elevated (low ejection fraction, low flow) and pulmonary edema is present, VA ECMO would cause further flooding of the lungs.

To the contrary, TandemHeart, which is inserted transseptally into the left atrium, does not only support circulation but it drains the left side of the heart.

Answer 13: B. This echocardiogram indicates that both the left-sided and right-sided intracardiac filling pressures are elevated. This may indicate acute or chronic rejection.

Tricuspid regurgitation is nearly universal after heart transplantation. There are many reasons for this, including the "normal" donor heart is placed into an "abnormal" environment with some degree of elevated pulmonary arterial resistance; the heart undergoes some degree of stress at the time of procurement which is often felt by the lower pressure RV and delicate TV apparatus; and because the patient undergoes frequent endomyocardial biopsies, which may damage the tricuspid valve further. However, right ventricular failure with dilated inferior vena cava is unusual.

Moderate or severe mitral regurgitation with a restrictive filling pattern is not common.

Another prominent feature of this echo is biatrial enlargement. The heart was transplanted using the "bicaval" technique. In essence, the procedure uses resection of the superior and inferior vena cava, preserving the integrity of the right atrium, which results in preservation of atrial contractility and sinus node function and greater tricuspid valve competence. Although this procedure decreases the burden of atrial arrhythmias and tricuspid regurgitation, some degree of TR still usually develops. In the first month after the transplantation, biopsies are done weekly and then monthly, with 5 to 6 pieces of endomyocardium taken during each procedure.

Suggested Readings

Aziz T, Burgess M, Khafagy R, et al. Bicaval and standard techniques in orthotopic heart transplantation: medium-term experience in cardiac performance and survival. *J Thorac Cardiovasc Surg* 1999;118:115–122.

Thorn EM, de Filippi CR. Echocardiography in the cardiac transplant recipient. *Heart Fail Clin* 2007;3(1):51–67.

Chapter 35

Normal and Abnormal Appearance of Cardiac Devices

Maya E. Guglin

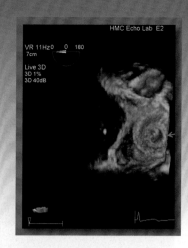

1A. A 71-year-old male is brought by EMS with altered mental status and new weakness on his right side. He has a normally functioning left ventricular assist device. CT scan of the brain is consistent with two old infarcts and a small subarachnoid hemorrhage. He has a very weak pulse; blood pressure cannot be obtained.

A transthoracic echocardiogram is obtained (VIDEO 35.1).

Which of the following statements is most accurate?

A. There is thrombosis of the inflow cannula.
B. This is a normal inflow cannula.
C. This is a normal outflow cannula.
D. There is an LV thrombosis not involving the cannula.

1B. In the same patient, additional images are obtained (VIDEO 35.2). The color flow Doppler pattern demonstrated on this echo increases the risk of:

A. Ischemic stroke
B. Hemorrhagic stroke
C. Gastrointestinal bleeding
D. Worsened heart failure

2. A 46-year-old man on LVAD support for the last 3 years complains of fatigue and generally not feeling well in the emergency room. He looks tired but not in acute distress. The LVAD coordinator cannot find anything wrong with the function of the LVAD.

A bedside echo is performed (FIG. 35.1A) and compared with a prior outpatient echo study performed 1 month earlier when he was feeling well (FIG. 35.1B).

Which of the following is the most important next step in the management of this patient?

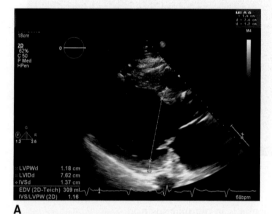

A

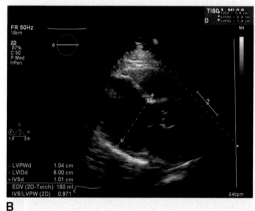

B

FIGURE 35.1

A. Routine care and observation
B. Replace the battery
C. Obtain hemoglobin and hematocrit
D. Obtain lactate dehydrogenase
E. Urgent pericardiocentesis

3. A 57-year-old male had unsuccessful attempt of a stent placement in an ostial left anterior descending coronary artery. There is now total occlusion, and the patient is hemodynamically unstable. An Impella 2.5 is placed prior to transporting to the CV ICU, and the patient's hemodynamic status was improved.

Hours later, his hemodynamic status deteriorated requiring norepinephrine therapy for stabilization, and a portable echocardiogram was performed (FIG. 35.2). Subsequently, his urine output became scant and you reevaluated the patient. Hemodynamics remained stable. Repeat echo is shown in VIDEO 35.3.

Which of the following options is most correct?

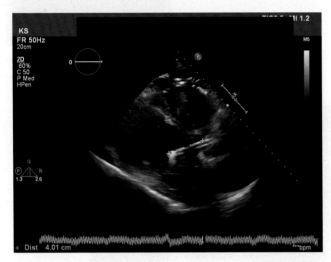

FIGURE 35.2

A. The Impella is in optimal position.
B. The Impella needs to be withdrawn into the aorta.
C. The Impella needs to be inserted into the LV.
D. The Impella requires urgent surgical removal.

4. A 65-year-old male with idiopathic cardiomyopathy and is pacemaker dependent with an EF of 30% presents with fever and chills and 2/2 blood cultures positive for *Staphylococcus aureus*. The TEE image in FIGURE 35.3 and VIDEO 35.4 is obtained. What is the most appropriate therapeutic strategy?

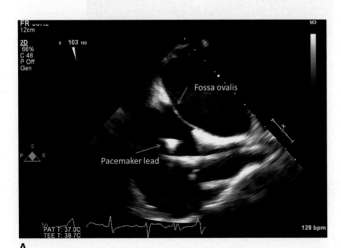

A

FIGURE 35.3

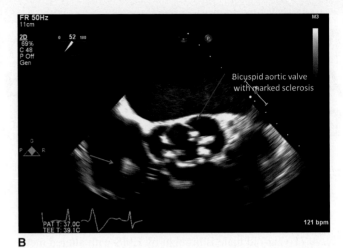

B

FIGURE 35.3 *(Continued)*

A. Complete 6 weeks of IV antibiotics, and repeat TEE after treatment.
B. Extract pacemaker/ICD leads, and place temporary transvenous pacemaker.
C. Start heparin therapy.
D. Extract pacemaker/ICD leads, and place subcutaneous pacemaker.

5. Pacemakers in the right ventricle have been noted to cause tricuspid regurgitation (FIG. 35.4 and VIDEO 35.5). All of the below answers are known mechanisms of causing tricuspid regurgitation, but which mechanism is the most common?

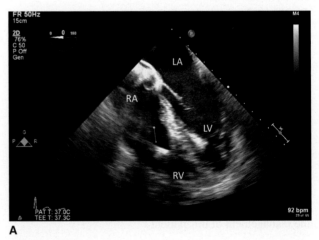

A

FIGURE 35.4

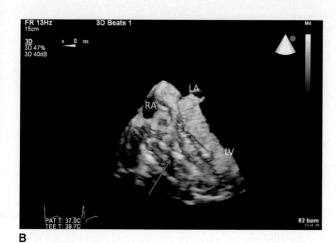

B

FIGURE 35.4 (*Continued*)

A. Interference with complete closure of the TV leaflet
B. "Spearing" of a tricuspid leaflet
C. Atrioventricular dyssynchrony caused by single-chamber pacing
D. Right ventricular dyssynchrony leading to right ventricular enlargement

Questions 6 to 12

Refer to FIGURE 35.5 and VIDEO 35.6.

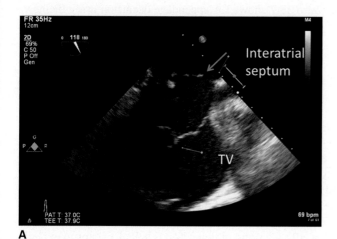

A

FIGURE 35.5

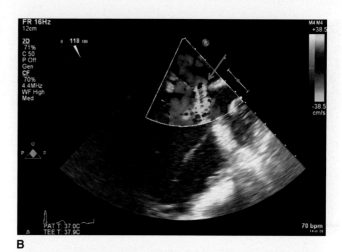

B

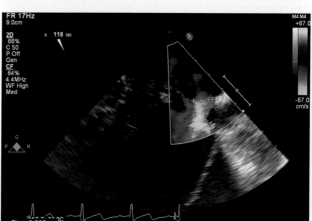

C

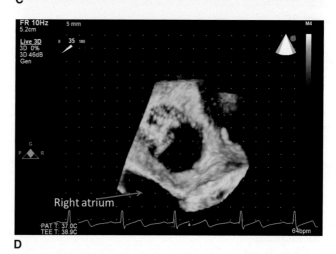

D

FIGURE 35.5 (*Continued*)

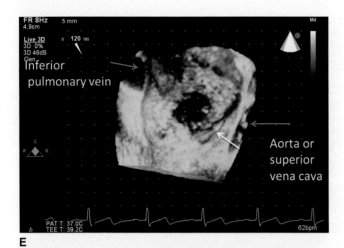

E

F

FIGURE 35.5 (*Continued*)

6. The images show a patient with a congenital heart defect. On ECG, the defect should have:

    A. Left axis deviation
    B. Normal axis
    C. Right axis deviation
    D. Left bundle branch block

7. Three-dimensional echocardiography is not helpful for evaluating percutaneous closure in atrial septal defects that are:

    A. Circular
    B. Elliptical
    C. Fenestrated
    D. Sinus venosus type
    E. None of the above

8. The largest-sized defect that can be closed percutaneously is:

    A. 25 mm
    B. 38 mm
    C. 15 mm
    D. 45 mm

9. Other than the overall size of the defect, what is the other most important factor that is important for determining whether this defect can be closed percutaneously?

    A. Presence of Chiari network
    B. Right ventricular systolic function
    C. Size of the aorta
    D. Size of the surrounding rim of tissue
    E. Pulmonary artery pressure

10. In FIGURE 35.5E, the structure depicted by the *white arrow* is:

    A. Gandalf staff
    B. A wire
    C. A catheter
    D. Part of the nitinol that holds the two sides of the closure device together

11. In the PROTECT AF trial, the WATCHMAN device group was found to have higher safety events (i.e., adverse events) in the device versus the control group (7.4% versus 4.4%), odds ratio 1.69 with confidence interval 1.1 to 3.19. Most of these adverse events occurred early, and 50% were:

    A. MI
    B. Stroke
    C. Catheter migration
    D. Pericardial effusion

12. VIDEO 35.7 shows LA appendage occlusion using the newest type of device. The device used here is:

    A. WATCHMAN
    B. Amplatz
    C. PLAATO
    D. LARIAT

Answer 1A: B. This is a normal appearance of the inflow cannula of left ventricular assist device. The outflow cannula drains the blood into the ascending aorta. It requires special effort to demonstrate the outflow cannula on echo, and it is rarely visible on standard views. There is no visible thrombus either in the cannula or in the left ventricular cavity on the images shown (although it is important to review all views and obtain off-axis apical sweeps to exclude thrombus).

Stroke, both hemorrhagic and ischemic, is a relatively common complication of left ventricular assist device. Subarachnoid hemorrhage is usually secondary to supratherapeutic anticoagulation with warfarin. Old ischemic strokes may be unrelated to left ventricular assist device. If strokes have minimal or no residual deficits, they are not necessarily a contraindication for LVAD implantation. Because all currently used LVADs have continuous flow, pulse is barely palpable or not palpable at all and blood pressure measurement usually requires peripheral Doppler interrogation.

Suggested Readings

Boyle AJ, Russell SD, Teuteberg JJ, et al. Low thromboembolism and pump thrombosis with the HeartMate II left ventricular assist device: analysis of outpatient anti-coagulation. *J Heart Lung Transplantation* 2009;28:881–887.

Estep JD, Stainback RF, Little SH, et al. The role of echocardiography and other imaging modalities in patients with left ventricular assist devices. *JACC Cardiovasc Imaging* 2010;3(10):1049–1064.

Answer 1B: *D.* Aortic regurgitation develops or progresses on continuous flow LVAD support. LVAD alters blood flow dynamics and kinetics. Part of the alterations is dilation of the aortic root, which is mild but still enough to promote valve malcoaptation and aortic regurgitation development. Significant aortic regurgitation creates a closed loop in the flow cannula–LVAD–outflow cannula–ascending aorta–left ventricle with decreased forward flow. This presents clinically as heart failure. Aortic regurgitation is not linked to increased stroke risk or gastrointestinal bleeding.

Suggested Readings

Cowger J, Pagani FD, Haft JW, et al. The development of aortic insufficiency in left ventricular assist device-supported patients. *Circ Heart Fail* 2010;3(6):668–674.

Topilsky Y, Hasin T, Oh JK, et al. Echocardiographic variables after left ventricular assist device implantation associated with adverse outcome. *Circ Cardiovasc Imaging* 2011;4(6):648–661.

Answer 2: *D.* The most important finding on the new echocardiogram is a bigger left ventricular end-diastolic dimension than 2 months ago. This means that the ventricle is less unloaded than before. Pump stoppage due to lack of power/discharged batteries can result in such dilation, but this would be inconsistent with normal interrogation of the LVAD by the coordinator. Inconsistency in measurements is always a possibility, but new symptom of fatigue makes it a diagnosis of exclusion. Bleeding does not cause left ventricular dilation.

Pump thrombosis occurs, by different sources, in 2% to 12% of patients on LVAD support and presents as new symptoms of heart failure, new or more severe mitral regurgitation, and signs of hemolysis such as elevated lactate dehydrogenase, free hemoglobin, and low haptoglobin. CT of the LVAD may confirm the diagnosis. In this case, CT showed thrombus in the outflow cannula.

While the thrombus is nonocclusive, LVAD interrogation may be normal, but in more severe cases, power spikes are common.

Suggested Reading:

Estep JD, Stainback RF, Little SH, et al. The role of echocardiography and other imaging modalities in patients with left ventricular assist devices. *JACC Cardiovasc Imaging* 2010;3(10):1049–1064.

Kirklin JK, Naftel DC, Kormos RL, et al. Interagency Registry for Mechanically Assisted Circulatory Support (INTERMACS) analysis of pump thrombosis in the HeartMate II left ventricular assist device. *J Heart Lung Transplantation* 2014;33:12–22.

Starling RC, Moazami N, Silvestry SC, et al. Unexpected abrupt increase in left ventricular assist device thrombosis. *N Engl J Med* 2014;370:33–40.

Answer 3: *C.* With optimal positioning of the Impella, the inlet should be about 4 cm below the aortic valve. The original position of the pump was correct. With such position, the outflow is well above the aortic valve, and hemolysis does not occur. On the second echocardiogram, the tip of the device appears to be entangled in the subvalvular apparatus of the mitral valve. Surgery should not be necessary, at least not as a next step—adjustment of the position of the inflow cannula can be done by gently manipulating the pump.

Suggested Reading

Mehrotra AK, Shah D, Sugeng L, et al. Echocardiography for percutaneous heart pumps. *JACC Cardiovasc Imaging* 2009;2(11):1332–1333.

Answer 4: *B.* Other options are not as aggressive. Option D is incorrect because subcutaneous pacemaker would be, in theory, an intolerable level of infection risk.

Recommendations for removal of infected CIED

Class I

Complete device and lead removal is recommended for all patients with definite CIED infection, as evidenced by valvular and/or lead endocarditis or sepsis (level of evidence A).

Complete device and lead removal is recommended for all patients with CIED pocket infection as evidenced by abscess formation, device erosion, skin adherence, or chronic draining sinus without clinically evident involvement of the transvenous portion of the lead system (level of evidence B).

Complete device and lead removal is recommended for all patients with valvular endocarditis without definite involvement of the lead(s) and/or device (level of evidence B).

Complete device and lead removal is recommended for patients with occult staphylococcal bacteremia (level of evidence B).

Class IIa

Complete device and lead removal is reasonable in patients with persistent occult gram-negative bacteremia despite appropriate antibiotic therapy (level of evidence B).

Class III

CIED removal is not indicated for a superficial or incisional infection without involvement of the device and/or leads (level of evidence C).

CIED removal is not indicated for relapsing bloodstream infection due to a source other than a CIED and for which long-term suppressive antimicrobials are required (level of evidence C).

Recommendations for New CIED Implantation after Removal of an Infected CIED

Class I

Each patient should be evaluated carefully to determine whether there is a continued need for a new CIED (level of evidence C).

The replacement device implantation should not be ipsilateral to the extraction site. Preferred alternative locations include the contralateral side, the iliac vein, and epicardial implantation (level of evidence C).

Class IIa

When positive before extraction, blood cultures should be drawn after device removal and should be negative for at least 72 hours before new device placement is performed (level of evidence C).

New transvenous lead placement should be delayed for at least 14 days after CIED system removal when there is evidence of valvular infection (level of evidence C).

Suggested Reading

Baddour LM, Epstein AE, Erickson CC, et al. Update on cardiovascular implantable electronic device infections and their management: a scientific statement from the American Heart Association. *Circulation* 2010;121(3):458.

Answer 5: A. In an echo/surgery series by Lin et al., the most common mechanism was interfering with closure of the leaflet. Pacing dyssynchrony may play a role in the interference as well and as such may be a complimentary mechanism. Entanglement with subvalvular mechanism, including the chordae and papillary muscles, is another cause not listed here. Spearing of the tricuspid leaflet is quite uncommon.

Suggested Reading

Lin G, Nishimura RA, Connolly HM, et al. Severe symptomatic tricuspid valve regurgitation due to permanent pacemaker or implantable cardioverter-defibrillator leads. *J Am Coll Cardiol* 2005;45(10):1672–1675.

Answer 6: C. The congenital defect is a secundum-type atrial septal defect. The ECG findings in atrial septal defects include left axis deviation in septum primum defects, no particular axis in sinus venosus defects, and right axis deviation in secundum defects. Secundum-type atrial septal defects are also associated with incomplete right bundle branch block. No ASD is associated with left bundle branch block (Answer D). Sinus venosus defects are associated with crochetage sign, a notch toward the apex of the QRS in the inferior leads.

Suggested Reading

Stouffer G. *Practical ECG Interpretation: Clues to Heart Disease in Young Adults.* John Wiley & Sons, 2009:32.

Answer 7: D. The superior form of the sinus venosus ASD constitutes 5% to 10% of all ASDs. Its posterior aspect is the right atrial free wall, and its superior border is often absent because of an overriding superior vena cava (SVC). Anomalous connection of some or all of the right pulmonary veins to the SVC or the right atrium is very common. Diagnosis is often more difficult than for other forms of ASD and may require special imaging, such as transesophageal echocardiography, magnetic resonance imaging (MRI), and computed tomographic scanning, and the possibility of a sinus venosus ASD should be considered for any patient with unexplained right atrial and right ventricular dilation. Catheter closure is not possible, and the treatment is surgical.

Three-dimensional echocardiography is helpful in all atrial septal defects that can be closed percutaneously. Of note is that sinus venosus–type ASDs cannot be closed percutaneously because of the frequent association with the anomalous pulmonary vein and the close approximation of the anomalous pulmonary vein to the actual defect. Also, it should be noted that 3D echo is useful to appreciate the variation in size of the defect that occurs during the cardiac cycle.

Suggested Reading

Webb G, Gatzoulis MA. Atrial septal defects in the adult recent progress and overview. *Circulation* 2006;114:1645–1653.

Answer 8: B. Transcatheter atrial septal defect (ASD) closure is now a widely recognized alternative to surgical closure for suitable secundum ASDs. We report closure of a large ostium secundum ASD (OS-ASD) that measured 40 mm on transesophageal echo (TEE) and was closed with a 46-mm device (Lifetech Scientific, Inc., China). To the best of our knowledge, this is the largest size of the device used for closure of ASD to date.

This is the largest-size closure device that is available. In some cases, operators have gone as high as 40 mm, but not 45.

Suggested Reading

Sugaonkar P, et al. Largest ASD device closure. *Ann Pediatr Cardiol* 2011;4(2):218–219.

Answer 9: D. There must be 5 mm of a rim of tissue around the entire defect to be certain that there will not be embolization of the device and also that the device will not cause aortic perforation. Aortic erosion with perforation has been associated with a small rim of tissue next to the aortic knob. Probably, this has resulted from operators trying to oversize the device and having it press on the aortic knob for support. Chiari network is a congenital remnant of the right valve of the sinus venosus. It has been found in 1.3% to 4% of autopsy studies and is believed to be of little clinical consequence.

Suggested Reading

Warnes CA, Williams RG, Bashore TM, et al. Atrial septal defect: ACC/AHA 2008 guidelines for the management of adults with congenital heart disease. A report of the American College of Cardiology/American Heart Association Task Force on Practice Guidelines (Writing Committee to Develop Guidelines on the Management of Adults With Congenital Heart Disease). Developed in Collaboration With the American Society of Echocardiography, Heart Rhythm Society, International Society for Adult Congenital Heart Disease, Society for Cardiovascular Angiography and Interventions, and Society of Thoracic Surgeons. *J Am Coll Cardiol* 2008;52:e1–e121.

Answer 10: B.

Option A: A joke albeit a bad one.

Option B: The correct answer—this is a wire for placement of the Amplatz device.

Option C: The wire has been placed up through a catheter.

Option D: Nitinol is the material that the Amplatz device is made of. It is uniquely suited to these procedures because it has a memory of its shape, and so after shrinking it within a catheter for delivery, it expands to its original shape after deployment.

Answer 11: D. Most of the events were pericardial effusion. Other events were quite equivalent, particularly stroke.

Suggested Reading

Holmes DR, Reddy VY, Turi ZG, et al. Percutaneous closure of the left atrial appendage versus warfarin therapy for prevention of stroke in patients with atrial fibrillation: a randomised non-inferiority trial. *Lancet* 2009;374:534.

Answer 12: D. The device used is LARIAT. The other three choices are not correct because a device is seen postprocedure with those. In the LARIAT, the LA appendage is snared from exterior to the heart and tied off. Hence, no device remains postprocedure.

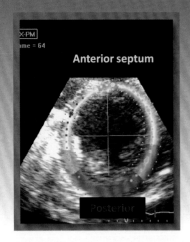

Anterior septum

Posterior

Chapter 36

LV Dyssynchrony and Resynchronization Therapy

Vincent L. Sorrell

Author's Note: *Determination of echocardiographic dyssynchrony is currently considered an adjunct to patient selection for cardiac resynchronization therapy. Guidelines have suggested electrocardiographic criteria as a surrogate for mechanical dyssynchrony, so echocardiographic dyssynchrony is presently not part of routine selection criteria. However, recent data continue to emerge that support the importance of echocardiographic dyssynchrony to potentially assist with patient selection, in borderline situations, for example, as in intermediate QRS width or non–left bundle branch morphology.*

1. Heart failure patients with depressed ejection fractions and with which of the following have the greatest level of evidence of response to cardiac resynchronization therapy (CRT)?

    A. QRS width ≥ 150 ms regardless of QRS morphology
    B. QRS width ≥ 120 ms and left bundle branch block
    C. QRS width ≥ 150 ms and right bundle branch block
    D. QRS width ≥ 150 ms and left bundle branch block

2. Which echocardiographic technique to determine dyssynchrony is the most reproducible and most widely available on all echocardiographic equipment?

    A. Tissue Doppler velocity Yu index
    B. Tissue Doppler longitudinal strain delay
    C. Speckle tracking radial strain delay
    D. Interventricular mechanical delay

3. Intraventricular dyssynchrony can be assessed by the time to peak tissue Doppler longitudinal velocity curve. Which technical approach will give the most reproducible velocity signal?

    A. Pulsed tissue Doppler in the midseptum and midlateral wall
    B. Color-coded tissue Doppler with a 3-mm circular region of interest at base or midlevels
    C. Color-coded tissue Doppler with a 5-mm × 7-mm region of interest at base or midlevels
    D. Color-coded tissue Doppler with a 5-mm circular region of interest at the apical level

4. The 12-site standard deviation in time to peak tissue Doppler velocities, also known as the Yu index shown in FIGURE 36.1, has been shown to be an important measure of dyssynchrony associated with cardiac resynchronization therapy. Which of the following statements is true?

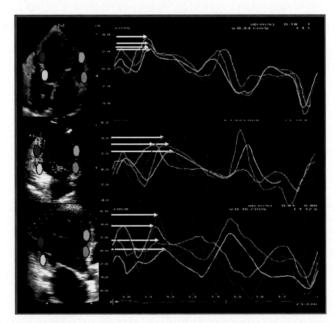

FIGURE 36.1

A. Velocity cannot differentiate between active contraction and passive motion.
B. Tissue Doppler has a stronger signal-to-noise ratio than speckle tracking.
C. Determination of peak velocities used for the Yu index requires training and experience.
D. The Yu index was shown to have low yield in the PROSPECT study.
E. All of the above.

5. Baseline dyssynchrony detected by which of the following methods has been associated with long-term survival after cardiac resynchronization therapy?

A. Tissue Doppler longitudinal strain
B. Tissue Doppler longitudinal tissue tracking
C. Speckle tracking longitudinal strain rate
D. Speckle tracking radial strain

6. Of the following technical tips associated with speckle tracking radial strain acquisition and analysis, which is *the least correct*?

A. Image gain and contrast should be set to optimize visualization of wall motion.
B. Frame rates should be set at least 120 Hz.
C. The region of interest needs to be adjusted to track the endocardium.
D. Because of beat-to-beat variability, three or more beats should be analyzed, even in normal sinus rhythm.

7. A 63-year-old male undergoes cardiac resynchronization therapy and returns to the echocardiography laboratory after 3 months for atrioventricular (AV) optimization because of continued dyspnea. His AV delay was set at 120 ms at the time of implantation, and his baseline mitral inflow pulsed Doppler pattern appears in FIGURE 36.2A.

Using the iterative technique, AV delay was increased from 120 to 160 ms, then to 200 ms, as shown in FIGURE 36.2B.

The most likely explanation for these findings is:

A. Intra-atrial conduction delay
B. Dislodged right atrial lead
C. Loss of biventricular pacing capture
D. Persistent atrial fibrillation

8. In addition to nonresponders to cardiac resynchronization implantation, which of the following patient subgroups appears to derive the most benefit from atrioventricular optimization?

A. Patients with echo-guided lead positioning
B. Women with nonischemic cardiomyopathy
C. Men with ischemic cardiomyopathy
D. Patients on beta-blocker therapy

9. A 58-year-old female has marked improvement in her symptoms of heart failure after cardiac resynchronization therapy (CRT). In addition to an improvement in ejection fraction, a decrease in her mitral regurgitation was observed, as shown in FIGURE 36.3. Which of the following has been mechanistically associated with reduction in mitral regurgitation after CRT?

A. Increases in mitral leaflet tenting angle
B. Decreases in the degree of mitral valve prolapse
C. Increases in reverse remodeling of papillary muscle scar
D. Decreases in the timing of papillary muscle closing forces

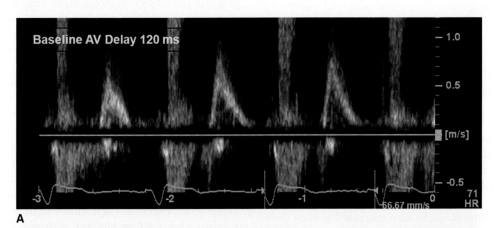

A

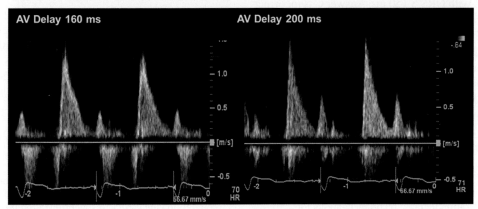

B

FIGURE 36.2

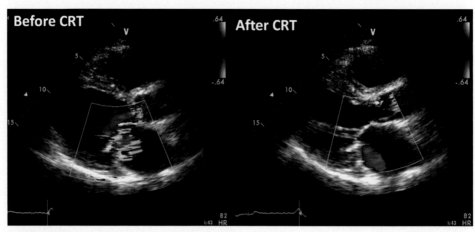

FIGURE 36.3

10. When considering factors other than mechanical dyssynchrony that may influence patient response to cardiac resynchronization therapy (CRT), which of the following has been shown to be associated with a favorable response among heart failure patients with widened QRS and low ejection fractions?

A. Biventricular pacing of ischemic cardiomyopathy patients with large scar burdens
B. Pacing with the left ventricular lead at the site of latest mechanical activation
C. Pacing using only the right ventricular lead from an apical position
D. Pacing with the left ventricular lead carefully positioned in the great cardiac vein

Answer 1: D. Cardiac resynchronization therapy (CRT), also known as biventricular pacing, has been a major therapeutic advance for heart failure patients with depressed ejection fraction. Current guidelines focus on the electrocardiographic QRS width *and morphology* for selection of patients for CRT. Answer A is partially correct, but not the single best option, since both the morphology and the QRS width are important. Answer B is partially correct. Previous guidelines were revised in 2012 for patients with QRS width 120 to 149 ms as a class II indication, because the strongest response rate has been demonstrated in patients with QRS > 150 ms. Answer C is incorrect because patients with right bundle branch block have a variable response to CRT, with more than half as nonresponders. Note that many studies have demonstrated that QRS width and QRS morphology are surrogates for mechanical dyssynchrony, which is the uncoordinated timing of regional contraction improved by CRT. Echocardiography may play a role in measuring dyssynchrony, which may refine patient selection for those patients who are borderline to meet criteria or for future patient selection for CRT.

Suggested Readings

Gorcsan J, Abraham T, Agler DA, et al. Echocardiography for cardiac resynchronization therapy: recommendations for performance and reporting—a report from the American Society of Echocardiography dyssynchrony writing group endorsed by the Heart Rhythm Society. *J Am Soc Echocardiogr* 2008;21:191–213.
Tracy CM, Epstein AE, Darbar D, et al. 2012 ACCF/AHA/HRS focused update of the 2008 guidelines for device-based therapy of cardiac rhythm abnormalities: a report of the American College of Cardiology Foundation/American Heart Association Task Force on practice guidelines. *Circulation* 2012;126:1784–1800.

Answer 2: D. Answer D, interventricular mechanical delay (IVMD), is the most correct because it is the simplest of the dyssynchrony indices listed above. IVMD requires pulsed Doppler recordings from the right ventricular (RV) outflow tract and left ventricular (LV) outflow tract and is the time difference between the onset of QRS complex and the onset of flow at each site (FIG. 36.4). Pulsed Doppler of blood flow has a strong signal-to-noise ratio, is readily available on virtually all echo–Doppler systems, and has a high yield. A cutoff IVMD delay from onset of RV to LV flow ≥40 ms is typically considered a significant dyssynchrony. Tips to be aware of include recording RV and LV outflow tract pulsed Doppler velocities at similar heart rates and placing the sample volume and filters so that an abrupt onset of Doppler flow can be easily measured. A limitation of IVMD is that it reflects major global dyssynchrony and may be insensitive to subtle intraventricular dyssynchrony. IVMD has been shown to be predictive of patient survival after CRT in patients with non–left bundle branch morphology and has potential to play a role in patient selection. Answers A, B, and C are all incorrect. Tissue Doppler Yu index, tissue Doppler longitudinal strain delay, and speckle tracking radial strain delay all require special equipment and software for analysis and a much higher level of training and experience.

Suggested Readings

Chung ES, Leon AR, Tavazzi L, et al. Results of the predictors of response to cardiac resynchronization therapy (PROSPECT) trial. *Circulation* 2008;117:2608–2616.
Hara H, Oyenuga OA, Tanaka H, et al. The relationship of QRS morphology and mechanical dyssynchrony to long-term outcome following cardiac resynchronization therapy. *Eur Heart J* 2012;33(21):2680–2691.

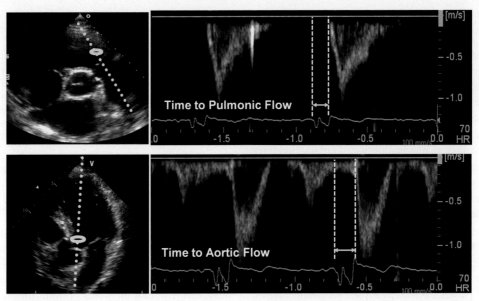

FIGURE 36.4

Answer 3: C. Answer C is the single best answer because the majority of literature supports using color-coded tissue Doppler because it can sample different regions of the left ventricle from the same beat and a larger region of interest to achieve more spatial averaging, which can improve reproducibility (FIG. 36.5A). Answer A is partially correct, but not the single best answer, because there was one study using simple pulsed tissue Doppler timing from the apical views to assess dyssynchrony. Answer B is incorrect because there is known variability in tissue Doppler time velocity curves and a 3-mm circular region of interest is small and usually is noisy (FIG. 36.5B). Answer D is incorrect because apical regions should be avoided because of an unfavorable Doppler angle of incidence and near-field noise.

Suggested Reading

Gorcsan J, Abraham T, Agler DA, et al. Echocardiography for cardiac resynchronization therapy: recommendations for performance and reporting—a report from the American Society of Echocardiography dyssynchrony writing group endorsed by the Heart Rhythm Society. *J Am Soc Echocardiogr* 2008;21:191–213.

Answer 4: E. All of the above answers A to D are correct. C.M. Yu was one of the first people to use echo–Doppler to assess cardiac dyssynchrony associated with response to CRT and proposed the 12-site standard deviation from basal and midlevels using the three standard apical views: apical four-chamber view, apical two-chamber view, and apical long-axis views (see FIG. 36.1). The most cited cutoff for the Yu index has been ≥32 ms. Answer B is correct because one of the advantages of the Yu index is that tissue Doppler has a favorable signal-to-noise ratio (more than speckle tracking). Answer A is correct because a disadvantage of tissue Doppler velocity is that it cannot differentiate between active contraction and passive motion seen with scarred regions. Another disadvantage is that one needs to calculate standard deviation. Answers C and D are also correct because without proper training and experience, a low yield of Yu index could be anticipated, as was shown in the multicenter PROSPECT study.

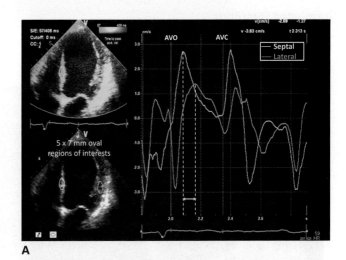

A

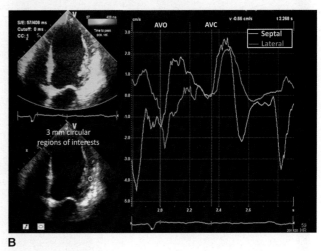

B

FIGURE 36.5 AVO, aortic valve opening; AVC, aortic valve closure.

Suggested Readings

Chung ES, Leon AR, Tavazzi L, et al. Results of the predictors of response to cardiac resynchronization therapy (PROSPECT) trial. *Circulation* 2008;117:2608–2616.

Yu CM, Gorcsan J, Bleeker GB, et al. Usefulness of tissue Doppler velocity and strain dyssynchrony for predicting left ventricular reverse remodeling response after cardiac resynchronization therapy. *Am J Cardiol* 2007;100:1263–1270.

Answer 5: D. Baseline mechanical dyssynchrony by echocardiography has been linked to patient response after CRT. Specifically, patients who have QRS widening but do not have mechanical dyssynchrony have a less favorable response. A variety of v methods to measure regional timing of contraction have been associated with CRT response defined by clinical variables or ventricular reverse remodeling. Answers A, B, and C may be considered partially correct because tissue Doppler longitudinal strain, tissue Doppler tissue tracking, and speckle tracking longitudinal strain rate have been associated with CRT response. Of the methods listed, Answer D, speckle tracking radial strain (septal to posterior wall delay of ≥130 ms) (Fig. 36.6), is the single best option because this has been associated with the important outcome variable of patient survival by several long-term studies.

Suggested Readings

Delgado V, van Bommel RJ, Bertini M, et al. Relative merits of left ventricular dyssynchrony, left ventricular lead position, and myocardial scar to predict long-term survival of ischemic heart failure patients undergoing cardiac resynchronization therapy. *Circulation* 2011;123:70–78.

Gorcsan J III, Oyenuga O, Habib PJ, et al. Relationship of echocardiographic dyssynchrony to long-term survival after cardiac resynchronization therapy. *Circulation* 2010;122:1910–1918.

Tanaka H, Nesser HJ, Buck T, et al. Dyssynchrony by speckle-tracking echocardiography and response to cardiac resynchronization therapy: results of the speckle tracking and resynchronization (STAR) study. *Eur Heart J* 2010;31:1690–1700.

Answer 6: B. Speckle tracking echocardiography is an important new advance that can derive strain data used for dyssynchrony analysis from routine black and white digital images. The ideal frame rate for current speckle tracking software appears to be between 30 and 90 Hz. Answer B is the single best answer as *an incorrect* option because high frame rates over 120 Hz may be associated with a high level of signal noise ratio with speckle tracking. Answer A is a correct statement and, therefore, an incorrect option. Speckle tracking analysis uses raw digital data and performs best when the routine image is optimized for wall motion. Answer C is a correct statement and, therefore, an incorrect option. The region of interest needs to be carefully adjusted and anchored to the motion of the LV.

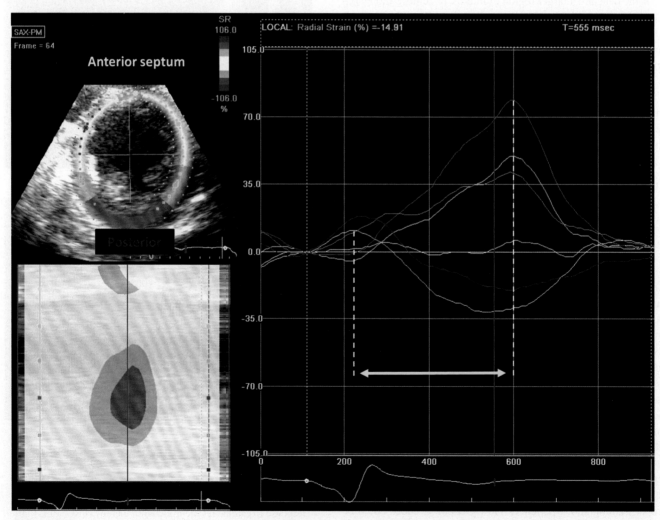

Figure 36.6

Answer D is a correct statement and, therefore, an incorrect option. Analyzing three or more beats is recommended because of beat-to-beat variability with speckle tracking radial strain, even in regular sinus rhythm.

Suggested Readings

Gorcsan J, Tanabe M, Bleeker GB. Combined longitudinal and radial dyssynchrony predicts ventricular response after resynchronization therapy. *J Am Coll Cardiol* 2007;50:1476–1483.

Suffoletto MS, Dohi K, Cannesson M. Novel speckle-tracking radial strain from routine black-and-white echocardiographic images to quantify dyssynchrony and predict response to cardiac resynchronization therapy. *Circulation* 2006;113:960–968.

Answer 7: *A.* Answer A is correct. The out-of-the-box AV delay of 120 ms was too short for this patient whose mitral inflow A wave could not be seen at baseline. The A wave appeared at an AV delay of 160 ms and was optimal with an AV delay of 200 ms. This patient most likely has an intra-atrial conduction delay and needs a longer programmed AV delay to include the atrial kick to ventricular filling. Patients with AV delays set too short may suffer from pacemaker syndrome where the left atrium contracts against a closed mitral valve and increases left atrial pressure. Answer B is incorrect because the above Doppler tracings would not change as they do with a dislodged atrial lead, used for sensing in this case. Answer C is incorrect because the baseline mitral inflow would show both E and A waves in normal sinus rhythm. Answer D is incorrect because A waves are seen with AV delays of 160 and 200 ms. These would not appear with persistent atrial fibrillation. A subgroup of patients who appear to be nonresponders to CRT may benefit from AV optimization, including patients with intra-atrial conduction delays.

Suggested Reading

Mullens W, Grimm RA, Verga T, et al. Insights from a cardiac resynchronization optimization clinic as part of a heart failure disease management program. *J Am Coll Cardiol* 2009;53:765–773.

Answer 8: *B.* Answer B is the single best answer. Although atrioventricular (AV) and ventricular–ventricular (VV) optimization may not play a critical role in all routine CRT patients, the SMART-AV randomized trail observed that women with nonischemic cardiomyopathy were the subgroup that appeared to benefit the most from AV optimization. Answer C is incorrect (men with ischemic cardiomyopathy) because the SMART-AV trial showed that CRT patients randomized to a routine "out-of-the-box" AV interval setting of 120 ms and VV interval setting of 0 had a similar response to CRT as those who underwent AV and VV optimization procedures. Answer A is incorrect, because, to date, there are little data known about AV optimization and echo-guided lead positioning. Answer D is incorrect because lack of beta-blocker therapy may result in tachycardia, which makes AV optimization very difficult secondary to the common mitral inflow finding of E and A wave fusion.

Suggested Readings

Cheng A, Gold MR, Waggoner AD, et al. Potential mechanisms underlying the effect of gender on response to cardiac resynchronization therapy: insights from the SMART-AV multicenter trial. *Heart Rhythm* 2012;9:736–741.

Ellenbogen KA, Gold MR, Meyer TE, et al. Primary results from the SmartDelay determined AV optimization: a comparison to other AV delay methods used in cardiac resynchronization therapy (SMART-AV) trial: a randomized trial comparing empirical, echocardiography-guided, and algorithmic atrioventricular delay programming in cardiac resynchronization therapy. *Circulation* 2010;122:2660–2668.

Answer 9: *D.* Improvements in mitral regurgitation (MR) have been associated with favorable outcomes after CRT. Reasons for improvement in MR after are complex. Resynchronization of papillary muscle closing forces has been associated with reductions in MR. Answer A is incorrect because reductions in MR have been associated with *decreases* in mitral leaflet tenting angle from left ventricular reverse remodeling. Answer B is incorrect because structural mitral valve disease, such as prolapsed or flail leaflets, is not improved by CRT. Answer C is incorrect because although there is ventricular myocardial reverse remodeling, myocardial infarction and scar involving the papillary muscle are usually not thought to be directly improved by CRT.

Suggested Reading

Kanzaki H, Bazaz R, Schwartzman D, et al. A mechanism for immediate reduction in mitral regurgitation after cardiac resynchronization therapy: insights from mechanical activation strain mapping. *J Am Coll Cardiol* 2004;44:1619–1625.

Answer 10: *B.* Two recent randomized trials have independently shown a clinical benefit of CRT with the left ventricular (LV) lead at the site of latest mechanical activation using speckle tracking radial strain. The TARGET trial showed a greater improvement in the primary end point of left ventricular reverse remodeling and secondary end point of heart failure hospitalizations or death. The STARTER trial demonstrated a significant reduction of the primary end point of heart failure hospitalizations or deaths in patients randomized to the echo-guided LV lead strategy. Answer A is incorrect because patients with ischemic cardiomyopathy, especially with proven large scar burdens, have a less favorable response to CRT. Answer C is incorrect. Patients who are paced only from the right ventricle do not derive the clinical benefits of CRT. Furthermore, RV pacing alone may create or exacerbate LV dyssynchrony. Answer D is incorrect. The great cardiac vein is in the anterior interventricular groove and has been shown to be an unfavorable LV lead position. The most favorable LV lead positions are typically posterior or lateral.

Suggested Readings

Khan FZ, Virdee MS, Palmer CR, et al. Targeted left ventricular lead placement to guide cardiac resynchronization therapy: the TARGET study: a randomized, controlled trial. *J Am Coll Cardiol* 2012;59:1509–1518.

Saba S, Marek J, Schwartzman D, et al. Echocardiography-guided left ventricular lead placement for cardiac resynchronization therapy: results of the speckle tracking assisted resynchronization therapy for electrode region (STARTER) trial. *Circ Heart Fail* 2013;6(3):427–434.

Chapter 37

Echo in Cardiac Shunt Lesions

Majd Makhoul

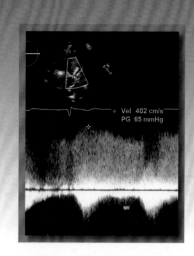

1. Which of the following statements is most accurate?

A. Secundum ASD is a defect of the superior caval vein.

B. Secundum ASD is commonly associated with a biatrial SVC connection.

C. Primum ASD is commonly associated with a biatrial SVC connection.

D. Superior sinus venosus ASD is commonly associated with an anomalous right pulmonary vein.

E. Inferior sinus venosus ASD overriding the IVC is more common than is its superior counterpart.

2. Which of the following echocardiographic findings is most suggestive of a hemodynamically significant ASD in an adult with poor-quality transthoracic images?

A. Color flow Doppler disturbance at the atrial septum in the four-chamber or subcostal view.

B. 2D image in the parasternal short-axis image to look for atrial septal tissue dropout.

C. A dilated RA and RV on apical four-chamber view.

D. A high-velocity CW Doppler at the tricuspid or pulmonic valve.

E. A normal bubble study excludes the possibility of a hemodynamically significant ASD.

3. Which of the following statements is most accurate regarding the 2D echo investigation of a secundum ASD?

A. Despite the common echo "dropout" associated with imaging the atrial septum from the apical four-chamber view, this window can *rule out* an ASD if the septum is seen to be intact.

B. The absence of right atrial and ventricular dilation excludes a hemodynamically significant ASD.

C. Most ASDs are round, permitting a relatively simple geometric approach to their investigation.

D. It would be rare for an individual to have more than one ASD.

E. With the use of an agitated saline bubble study, injected in the lower extremity, a superior sinus venosus ASD can be confirmed by the presence of a filling defect seen in the right atrium next to an intact-looking atrial septum adjacent to where a right upper pulmonary vein would drain into the LA.

4. Which of the following is considered the least important parameter in determining the degree of shunt across an ASD?

A. The blood viscosity, as estimated by the hematocrit

B. The size of the defect

C. The pressure gradient across the defect

D. The difference in compliance of both ventricles

E. The heart rate

5. A 24-year-old obese female patient presented for routine checkup to the primary care physician's office prior to starting an exercise weight loss program. She was found to have a systolic ejection murmur at the base of the heart and a fixed split S2. Vital signs were normal. An ECG was obtained and showed no conduction abnormalities. She was sent for cardiology consultation and an echocardiogram. The TTE was limited due to poor acoustic transmission, but the sonographer thought the right heart was dilated. As the reading cardiologist in the echo lab, which of the following would be the most appropriate next step?

A. Perform an urgent TEE.

B. Calculate the Qp/Qs, and if this is normal, perform a contrast echocardiogram to improve the quality of the study.

C. Perform an agitated saline bubble study.

D. Perform a carefully mapped pulsed-wave Doppler examination of the right side of the ventricular septum since you suspect a ventricular septal defect.

E. Obtain ductal view from the suprasternal window to search for PDA.

Questions 6 and 7

6. Assign the correct ultrasound window and transducer location with the optimal pulsed-wave Doppler sample volume position to obtain the most accurate Qp/Qs (Fig. 37.1).

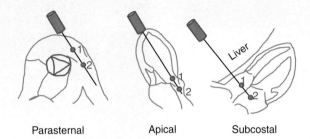

Parasternal   Apical   Subcostal

Figure 37.1

   A. Position 1 parasternal with position 2 apical
   B. Position 2 parasternal with position 2 apical
   C. Position 1 parasternal with position 1 subcostal
   D. Position 2 parasternal with position 1 apical
   E. Position 1 parasternal with position 2 subcostal

7. What is the Qp/Qs using the measurements obtained from the correct location in Question 6?

LVOT diameter = 20 mm	Aortic root = 34 mm	Atrial septum = 42 mm
RVOT diameter = 22 mm	Main PA = 25 mm	IVC = 18 mm
LVOT VTI = 24 cm	Aortic VTI = 60 cm	ASD flow VTI = 10 cm
RVOT VTI = 30 cm	Main PA VTI = 26 cm	LA flow VTI = 8 cm

   A. Small ASD with Qp/Qs = 1.7
   B. Small ASD with Qp/Qs = 1.5
   C. Moderate ASD with Qp/Qs = 2.0
   D. Large ASD with Qp/Qs >2.5
   E. Large ASD with cyanosis and a (−) Qp/Qs = (−) 2.0

8. Which of the following is the most accurate statement regarding the echocardiographic finding(s) in a patient with a ventricular septal defect (VSD)? Consider Figure 37.2.

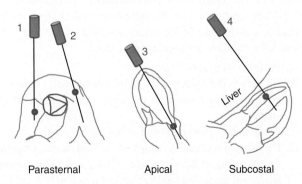

Parasternal   Apical   Subcostal

Figure 37.2

   A. The most common type of VSD is the membranous VSD. These may close before adulthood, and a residual septal aneurysm may remain. These are commonly seen in position C below.
   B. Inlet VSD is often associated with other congenital anomalies such as primum ASD, AV valve pathology, or complete heart block. This defect is most commonly seen in position D below.
   C. A supracristal (or subarterial) VSD is rarely first found in adulthood. These defects are best seen in the apical four-chamber view and would not be seen on the figure below.
   D. A muscular VSD may occur anywhere in the ventricular septum and may be small, multiple, and difficult to image with 2D echo alone. It would not be seen on the figure below. Basal to apical short-axis sweep is helpful.
   E. Continuous-wave Doppler is necessary for diagnosis of a VSD. It will show a spectral pattern similar to MR. It is only noted in systole unless Eisenmenger physiology is present.

Questions 9 to 11

A 50-year-old female with a known secundum ASD followed since childhood has been asymptomatic. She now presents to the emergency department with a dilated cardiac silhouette on chest x-ray and hypotension. Her recent history is significant for low-grade fever, malaise, and "cold-like" symptoms. Slight pleuritic, nonexertional chest pain became more prolonged and more severe, resulting in her presenting to the local emergency department. On examination, O_2 Sat is 89%, BP is 86/60 mm Hg, and HR is 120 bpm, and she is cool and clammy. Her JVP is elevated. There was no noticeable pulsus paradoxus on exam. An arterial line was placed and confirmed the BP and the lack of respiratory variation. ECG demonstrates sinus tachycardia and nonspecific ST changes. Bedside echocardiography demonstrated a large pericardial effusion with a dilated IVC, diastolic RV, and RA collapse. The LV is small and hyperdynamic. The estimated RVSP is 40 mm Hg using the TR gradient. The cardiac output was >4.0 L/min using the RVOT VTI × CSA method.

9. The most likely reason for shock is:

   A. The patient has sepsis and high-output cardiac failure.
   B. The patient has myocarditis with severe LV systolic dysfunction.
   C. The patient is having an acute myocardial infarction.
   D. The patient likely has cardiac tamponade despite the absence of a pulsus paradoxus.
   E. The patient most probably had acute pulmonary emboli.

10. The patient's desaturation is most accurately described by which of the following statements?

   A. Incomplete patient follow-up has resulted in Eisenmenger physiology and right-to-left atrial level shunting.
   B. Cardiogenic shock has led to severe tissue hypoperfusion and desaturation.
   C. Transient right-to-left flow across the ASD that is acute and transient due to comorbidities.
   D. Massive pulmonary embolism.
   E. Acute myocardial infarction with an acute ventricular septal rupture.

11. Why is the estimated cardiac output normal despite the clinical shock state?

   A. Sepsis
   B. VSD with left-to-right shunting
   C. ASD with left-to-right shunting
   D. ASD with right-to-left shunting
   E. Incorrect CO estimate in the setting of RV dysfunction from acute PE

Questions 12 and 13

An 18-year-old female, who is a refugee from Africa, presented with SOB and history of "hole in the heart" with no interventions. On exam, her precordium is hyperactive. She has loud S2 in addition to a harsh 3/6 holosystolic murmur with some extension into diastole. She has always been thin and short as per her family. Her BP is 127/75, and her O_2 saturation is 95% in room air at rest.

12. Based on VIDEOS 37.1 AND 37.2 what are her likely diagnoses?

   A. Inlet VSD and large PDA
   B. Subarterial/supracristal VSD and small PDA
   C. Inlet VSD with AP window
   D. VSD and coarctation of the aorta
   E. Large perimembranous VSD and large PDA

13. Based on FIGURES 37.3 AND 37.4, which of the following actions is the best next step in her management, knowing

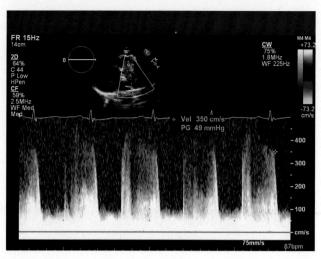

FIGURE 37.4

that there is no tricuspid or pulmonary valve stenosis and her IVC collapses normally with breathing?

   A. Perform right heart catheterization with pulmonary vasoreactivity testing.
   B. Refer for cardiac transplantation evaluation.
   C. Cardiac catheterization with aortic arch angioplasty.
   D. Start sildenafil and see her back in 3 months.
   E. Refer for immediate surgical intervention.

Questions 14 and 15

A 20-year-old healthy and athletic woman was seen by her PCP for routine checkup. Upon exam, she was found to have a murmur heard only over the back (interscapular area). Her BP was 100/70 in right arm. EKG was normal, and she was sent to have an echocardiogram. See VIDEO 37.3 of shunt small PDA ductal view.

14. Knowing that her echo was normal except for what is seen in the video above, what is her diagnosis?

   A. Left pulmonary artery sling
   B. Coronary artery fistula
   C. Anomalous origin of left coronary artery from pulmonary artery (ALCAPA)
   D. Patent ductus arteriosus

15. Based on the spectral Doppler signal seen in FIGURE 37.5 of the structure seen in previous question's video, what additional diagnosis can be made in this patient?

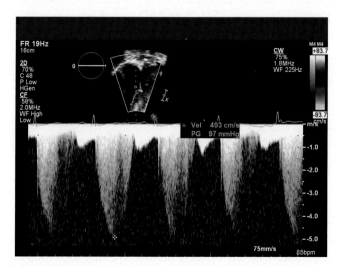

FIGURE 37.3

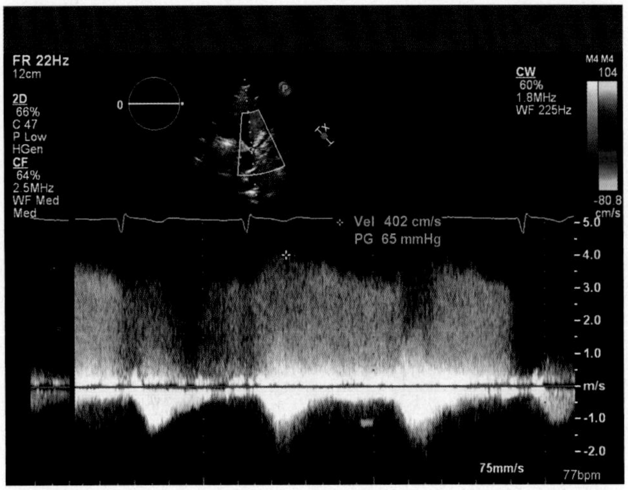

FIGURE 37.5

A. LPA stenosis
B. Narrowing of the coronary artery fistula
C. Narrowing of the anomalous coronary artery at its connection with pulmonary arteries
D. Normal pulmonary artery pressures

Answer 1: *D.* Options A, B, and C are incorrect since these describe common features of a superior sinus venosus ASD, which is a more common sinus venosus defect than its inferiorly located counterpart (therefore, Option E is also incorrect).

ASD and bicuspid aortic valve are the two most common types of congenital heart lesions presenting in adulthood. ASDs occur in 6% to 10% of all cardiac malformations and are more common in females (2:1). Secundum ASD is a defect of the fossa ovalis and is by far the most common type of ASD (60%). Primum ASD accounts for 20% and is considered an endocardial cushion defect (atrioventricular canal defect). This can be part of complete AV canal defect (along with inlet-type VSD and common atrioventricular valve) or part of partial AV canal defect (along with cleft in mitral valve).

Sinus venosus ASD accounts for about 15% of all ASDs. It can be superior or inferior in location. Superior type is more common and often called SVC-type sinus venosus defect and is commonly associated with anomalous drainage of right upper and middle pulmonary veins to SVC/right atrium. This is best imaged from subcostal or right parasternal window. The inferior type is called IVC sinus venosus defect and is quiet rare.

The rarest type of ASD is the coronary sinus defect, which is associated with unroofed coronary sinus and often a left-sided SVC draining to the roof of the left atrium. These echo findings are easily seen from parasternal long-axis view, which shows the dilated coronary sinus (CS) in the back of the left atrium with defect in the tissue separating the CS from LA (unroofed CS).

Suggested Readings

Ettedgui JA, Siewers RD, Anderson RH, et al. Diagnostic echocardiographic features of the sinus venosus defect. *Br Heart J* 1990; 64:329–331.

Mehta RH, Helmcke F, Nanda NC, et al. Uses and limitations of transthoracic echocardiography in the assessment of atrial septal defect in the adult. *Am J Cardiol* 1991;67:288–294.
Pascoe RD, Oh JK, Warnes CA, et al. Diagnosis of sinus venosus atrial septal defect with transesophageal echocardiography. *Circulation* 1996;94:1049–1055.

Answer 2: *C.* Option A is incorrect since there are many causes of CFD "disturbances" near the atrial septum, since vena cava inflow is directed along the septum and many patients have blood flow redirected by a residual eustachian valve.

Option B is incorrect since the atrial septum is parallel to the 2D image in this view and "dropout" of tissues is relatively common given the very thin tissue (especially near the fossa) combined with septal motion and limits in temporal resolution. This is less likely with subcostal window since the atrial septum is perpendicular to the 2D ultrasound beam.

Option D is incorrect. Although a significant ASD will increase flow across the TV and PV, many pathologies cause increased flow velocities at the TV and PV.

Option E is incorrect. Most significant, uncomplicated left-to-right ASD shunts can indeed be associated with some microbubbles shunting to the left side transiently. This R-to-L relative pressure gradient occurs at onset of LV contraction, but this is not 100% specific and cannot exclude an ASD. This can be augmented with a carefully timed Valsalva (release) maneuver.

With a hemodynamically significant ASD and absence of RV pathology or RV outflow obstruction, a left-to-right shunt occurs because the RV fills more easily than does the LV (higher RV compliance). This leads to volume load on the RA and RV in addition to increased pulmonary blood flow. Typically, the atrial pressures are low, so a large ASD will not lead to RV and pulmonary artery pressure overload in the short and mid-term. However, in some cases, the increased pulmonary blood flow can over several decades lead to irreversible changes in the pulmonary arterial bed and pulmonary hypertension. If this occurs, the atrial level shunting can reverse (becomes right to left) leading to Eisenmenger syndrome.

A contrast study is routine in patients with a dilated right side since color flow Doppler is not very sensitive at detecting ASDs in adults.

Many times, the dilated RA and RV are the first echocardiographic signs of an ASD. If an ASD cannot be confirmed on TTE, and other causes of right heart dilation are not seen (such as TR), then a TEE (or cardiac MRI) is indicated to exclude a sinus venosus–type ASD or partial anomalous pulmonary venous return (or both).

Suggested Readings

Mulvagh S, et al. American Society of echocardiography consensus statement on the clinical applications of ultrasonic contrast agents in echocardiography. *J Am Soc Echocardiogr* 2008;21(11):1179–1201.
Solimana O II, Geleijnsea ML, Meijbooma FJ, et al. The use of contrast echocardiography for the detection of cardiac shunts. *Eur J Echocardiogr* 2007;8(3):S2–S12.

Answer 3: *B.* Option A is incorrect since the apical four-chamber view has a scan plane that aligns the atrial septum in parallel with the thinnest portion, creating this common "dropout" artifact. Furthermore, even an intact-appearing atrial septum may have a small ASD out of the imaging plane that could readily be missed if only one view is used for diagnosis.

Option B is correct. The right atrium and ventricle respond to the increased volume by compensatory dilation. If the RA and RV sizes are normal, then the increased flow is not likely to be hemodynamically significant (often defined as Qp/Qs >2:1).

Option C is incorrect since most ASDs are actually oblong or elliptical. This is an important concept learned primarily via the increased use of 3D echo. It is important to image the septum in multiple orientations and many windows to obtain the maximal dimension of the defect.

Option D is incorrect since it is relatively common that multiple ASDs are often present in the same patient.

Option E is incorrect since that description is a common normal finding that occurs from the nonopacified blood entering the RA from the SVC and creating a "filling defect" from mixing with the agitated saline entering via the IVC (lower extremity injection). A sinus venosus ASD should be considered whenever marked bubble contrast shunts to the left side across an "intact-appearing" atrial septum and is likely significant if the right heart is dilated. This is commonly associated with a partial anomalous pulmonary venous return (usually the right superior pulmonary vein).

Suggested Reading
Staffen RN, Davidson WR Jr. Echocardiographic assessment of atrial septal defects. *Echocardiography* 1993;10:545–552.

Answer 4: **A.** The viscosity of the blood has little impact on the degree of cardiac shunting. However, the other parameters above directly or indirectly influence the direction and degree of shunting.

Option B is a significant anatomic feature that impacts the amount of shunting. However, the size alone is not enough to predict the degree of shunt.

Option C is a very important parameter that contributes to the degree and direction of shunting. An ASD will usually shunt left-to-right since the LA pressure is greater than the RA pressure. Sometimes, RA pressure can surpass LA pressure transiently and an R-to-L shunting may occur for short period of time during cardiac cycle.

Option D is the major reason that ASD will shunt from left to right. The normally low pulmonary vascular resistance makes the RV more compliant than the LV, and this is the major contributor to the direction of shunting.

Option E is an indirect contributor to the degree of shunting. Very fast HR will lead to less shunting across an ASD. This hemodynamic alteration is attributed to the difference in diastolic distensibility (compliance) between the left and right ventricles.

Suggested Reading
Dittmann H, Jacksch R, Voelker W, et al. Accuracy of Doppler echocardiography in quantification of left to right shunts in adult patients with atrial septal defect. *J Am Coll Cardiol* 1988;11:338.

Answer 5: C. Option A is incorrect since there is no indication for an urgent or emergent TEE. Although a TEE would likely be a valuable diagnostic test to search for a suspected ASD, it is not urgent and not the single best answer.

Option B is incorrect since there are limitations to measuring the Qp/Qs, and this would not be adequate evidence for the lack of a shunt prior to administering a manufactured contrast agent that lists "known or suspected cardiac shunt" as a contraindication in the package insert.

Option C is correct. This is always an appropriate next step when the right heart is dilated and demonstration of marked shunting (microbubbles in the left heart) warrants additional diagnostic investigations (and excludes the routine use of a manufactured contrast agent).

Option D is incorrect since the right ventricle does not become dilated from a VSD. Also, a color Doppler sweep of the ventricular septum is more helpful than PW Doppler assessment to diagnose VSDs.

Option E is incorrect since the right heart does not become dilated from a PDA. Ductal view is obtained with the probe in suprasternal notch and marker around 11 o'clock, which will show proximal descending aorta parallel to main pulmonary artery. Any PDA even small one will usually show in this view with color Doppler.

Whenever the right heart is dilated, one should rule out an atrial level shunt. In this patient, she was reported to have a fixed split S2, and this is consistent with an ASD, especially that her EKG did not show an RBBB. This can be most simply and accurately evaluated with an agitated saline bubble study. Significant shunting can be seen at rest or after maneuvers to transiently elevate the right atrial pressure such as Valsalva (or Valsalva release). Coughing or abdominal thrust may be more successful for some patients. Since there are many other causes for a dilated right heart, the presence of this finding alone does not preclude the use of the manufactured ultrasound contrast agent (UCA) microbubbles to improve the quality of the TTE. However, agitated saline should be used first until intracardiac shunt is ruled out (a shunt will be a contraindication to use UCA).

A systolic murmur, dilated right heart, and recognition first in adulthood make ASD likely. PDA flow results in volume overload on the LA and LV and not the right heart. A VSD is usually associated with a normal-sized right ventricle since the RV directs the "extra" blood flow directly into the pulmonary artery, which eventually comes back to the left heart as extra volume. Therefore, it is the left-sided chambers that "see" the extra flow and dilate in response.

Suggested Readings
Attaran RR, Ata I, Kudithipudi V, et al. Protocol for optimal detection and exclusion of a patent foramen ovale using transthoracic echocardiography with agitated saline microbubbles. *Echocardiography* 2006;23:616–622.

Solimana O II, Geleijnsea ML, Meijbooma FJ, et al. The use of contrast echocardiography for the detection of cardiac shunts. *Eur J Echocardiogr* 2007;8(3):S2–S12.

Answer 6: D. The stroke volume is readily obtained using the velocity time integral (VTI) × the cross-sectional area (CSA).

The CSA must be measured at the site of the sample volume placement for optimal accuracy. Many times, a major source of error for stroke volume calculation is the incorrect matching of these two. Since the RVOT diameter (d × d × 0.785 = CSA) is difficult to measure (parasternal position 1), the main pulmonary artery is measured instead. This is also more circular and adheres to a potentially more accurate CSA than the RVOT (assumed to be circular, but rarely ever is this the case). When the PA is used to measure the CSA, the sample volume must be placed at this site to calculate the stroke volume (Qp). This is parasternal position 2.

The systemic stroke volume (Qs) is measured in the LVOT using either the apical five-chamber view or the apical long-axis (three-chamber) view. This latter window is often better aligned to the Doppler cursor. As with the Qp measurement, it is imperative that the CSA and pulsed-wave Doppler sample volume be at the same location to optimally obtain the stroke volume. The LVOT diameter is usually measured in the parasternal long axis at the site of aortic valve leaflet attachment. This is the aortic annulus. If the LVOT flow is increased, then the PWD sample volume is often lowered into the LV, but this is no longer at the site of the CSA and invokes an incorrect systemic stroke volume estimate (Qs). The optimal location is demonstrated on apical position 1 in the schematic. Moving the sample volume further into the aorta (apical position 2), unlike the pulmonary artery, is not accurate for the systemic stroke volume since the diameter is difficult to measure at this location and it is not circular (due to the sinuses of Valsalva).

The subcostal window and PWD sample volume position 1 is sometimes used to measure the flow across the atrial septal defect but is not used to calculate the Qp/Qs. Subcostal position 2 would seldom be obtained and is not useful for Qp/Qs calculations.

Suggested Readings

Lopez L, et al. Recommendations for quantification methods during the performance of a pediatric echocardiogram: a report from the Pediatric Measurements Writing Group of the American Society of Echocardiography Pediatric and Congenital Heart Disease Council. *J Am Soc Echocardiogr* 2010;23:465–495.

Staffen RN, Davidson WR Jr. Echocardiographic assessment of atrial septal defects. *Echocardiography* 1993;10:545–552.

Answer 7: *A.* Option A is obtained using the parasternal position 2 and the apical position 1 in Figure 37.1.

Option B is incorrect and is obtained using the data for parasternal position 1 and apical position 1, which is commonly used, but not one of the choices above for this example.

Options C, D, and E are incorrect, and the answers did not use any of the provided Doppler measures.

LVOT diameter of 20 mm provides an SCA of 3.14 cm² × VTI 24 = 75 mL (Qs).

The MPA CSA = 4.9 cm². This area × the MPA VTI = 128 mL (Qp).

If you used the RVOT diameter (CSA = 3.8 cm²) × the RVOT VTI, then the Qp was estimated at 114 mL.

The aortic root, atrial septum, and LA flow should not be used to measure the Qp/Qs.

Answer 8: *D.* Option D is the most accurate option. Each of the other options is partially correct.

Option A is incorrect since these membranous/perimembranous VSDs are most commonly seen in this view at the 10 o'clock position (position B on figure). Option B is incorrect since these inlet VSDs are best seen in the apical view, although depending on the extent of the inferior angulation (below the aortic valve), these may be seen at position A in the figure. Option C is incorrect since the basal SAX view is a commonly used view to image these defects. Position D (2 o'clock) is the common location for the supracristal/subarterial VSDs. Option E is incorrect since the CW Doppler will demonstrate both systolic (high-velocity jet, when restricted) and diastolic (low-velocity jet) left-to-right shunting.

Eisenmenger physiology may occur if the VSD is large and unrepaired in the adult, leading to equalization of ventricular pressures and later to pulmonary vascular resistance surpassing systemic vascular resistance. The shunt will be either bidirectional or all right to left in that case and can be assessed using color Doppler.

The basal parasternal short-axis view is an important tomographic 2D image for patients with cardiac shunting. The image should be swept superiorly to inferiorly while color flow Doppler is being recorded. The location of the shunt in this view helps to determine the type and etiology of the defect.

Suggested Reading

Hagler DJ, et al. Standardized nomenclature of the ventricular septum and ventricular septal defects, with applications for 2D echocardiography. *Mayo Clin Proc* 1985;60:741–752.

Answer 9: *D.* Option A is incorrect since the calculated CO was not obtained in the left heart (is not the systemic CO).

Option B is incorrect since it is unlikely that the patient has severe LV systolic dysfunction given the "small, hyperdynamic" LV seen on bedside echo. Myocarditis is possible given the clinical presentation and abnormal ECG.

Option C is incorrect. Although the patient is female, has an abnormal ECG, and has a chest pain syndrome, and therefore, an acute myocardial infarction should be considered, it would not be the cause for the shock state given the small, hyperdynamic LV.

Option D is correct.

Option E is incorrect since it is not the single best answer. Although a patient with hypotension, chest pain, nonspecific ECG changes, tachycardia, and desaturation should be assessed for possible acute pulmonary emboli, it would not account for the pericardial effusion and tamponade findings. There is no reason to investigate this etiology since the presentation can be entirely accounted for.

Answer 10: *C.* Option A is incorrect since there appears to have been good patient follow-up and she has been asymptomatic until this presentation. Eisenmenger physiology would not occur this rapidly. However, right-to-left atrial level shunting is indeed present here, but due to other reasons.

Option B is incorrect since cardiogenic shock resulting in severe tissue hypoperfusion does not take into consideration the ASD and would be unlikely given the small, hyperdynamic LV seen on echo.

Option C is correct. There is transient right-to-left flow across the ASD that is acute and transient due to the hemodynamically significant pericardial effusion.

Option D is not the single best answer and does not account for the pericardial effusion and tamponade findings. Providing an additional etiology for this patient's presentation is not necessary.

Option E is unlikely since an acute ventricular septal rupture would cause left-to-right shunting, which would not cause desaturation.

Answer 11: C. Option A is incorrect since the cardiac output is pseudo-elevated.

Option B is incorrect and not the single best answer since another cause for left-to-right shunting is not necessary to account for the increased CO measured from the RVOT.

Option C is the correct answer.

Option D is incorrect since an ASD with right-to-left shunting would NOT increase the Qp.

Option E is incorrect. It is possible to estimate the CO from the RVOT in the setting of RV dysfunction from acute PE, and this information is clinically valuable to assist in the determination of the pulmonary vascular resistance (PVR [Wood u] = TR velocity/RVOT VTI + 0.16).

It is important to understand the physiology of atrial level shunting and how this is likely to influence hemodynamic parameters. This patient has been followed since childhood. Although many patients with congenital heart diseases are lost to follow-up after adolescence, this patient appears to have had careful follow-up, so there is no reason to suspect that she has developed Eisenmenger physiology and pulmonary hypertension.

Her current presentation is consistent with a viral illness and development of a hemodynamically significant pericardial effusion. Her vital signs support this diagnosis with hypotension, narrow pulse pressure, tachycardia, poor peripheral perfusion, and an elevated JVP. The echo findings are also supportive of this diagnosis as demonstrated by the large pericardial effusion, dilated IVC, and right heart diastolic collapse. Other echocardiographic signs of tamponade that are not mentioned in this scenario are significant respiratory variation in MV inflow Doppler velocity (>25% difference) and TV inflow Doppler velocity (>50%).

Major clinical, echo, and hemodynamic confusion arises because of the new, acute desaturation, the absence of pulsus paradoxus despite tamponade, and the measured high cardiac output. These features can be accounted for when one understands the impact of elevated pericardial pressures in patients with intracardiac shunting. The lack of a pulsus paradoxus in patients with atrial level shunting should not be unexpected. The atrial and ventricular volumes remain fixed during respiration in patients with ASD since the increased venous return associated with inspiration results in an equal decrease in left-to-right atrial shunting.

Clinical desaturation is present because of right-to-left shunting that occurs during the transient atrial collapse from tamponade. During these periods, the shunting reverses, and desaturated blood is shunted into the left atrium and then become systemic.

Finally, the high cardiac output is a reflection of the Qp. Since the sonographer measured the cardiac output using the RVOT, this stroke volume is not the true systemic CO (Qs) and includes the Qs as well as the shunt flow (which is mostly left to right).

Suggested Readings

Hausmann D, et al. Value of TEE color Doppler echo for detection of different types of ASD in adults. *J Am Soc Echocardiogr* 1992;5:481–488.

Kronzon I, Tunick PA. *Challenging Cases in Echocardiography.* Philadelphia, PA: Lippincott Williams & Wilkins, 2005.

McNamara DG. The adult with congenital heart disease. *Curr Probl Cardiol* 1998;14:63–114.

Perloff JK, et al. 22nd Bethesda Conference. Congenital heart disease after childhood: an expanding patient population. *J Am Coll Cardiol* 1991;18:311–342.

Relier MD, et al. Cardiac embryology: basic review and clinical correlations. *J Am Soc Echocardiogr* 1991;4:519–531.

Answer 12: E. Correct answer is E. VIDEO 37.1 is a parasternal long-axis view at the LVOT/aortic annulus level showing a large VSD in the membranous area with left-to-right shunting by color Doppler. VIDEO 37.2 is a ductal view from suprasternal window showing proximal descending aorta (blue flow) with large PDA (red flow) heading toward the main pulmonary artery.

Option A is incorrect as inlet VSD is usually not well seen in this view but at around 7 to 8 o'clock from parasternal short-axis view (base of the heart) or 4-chamber apical view (atrioventricular valves level). It is typically part of endocardial cushion defect.

Option B is incorrect as the PDA is large in this patient. Supracristal/subarterial VSD can be hard to differentiate from membranous one in parasternal long-axis view but is usually seen at 2 o'clock on parasternal short-axis view (base of the heart).

Option C is incorrect as the VSD is perimembranous in location and there is no indication of aortopulmonary (AP) window from the videos seen. AP window is a communication between the ascending aorta and pulmonary artery distal to the semilunar valve level. This is best imaged from parasternal short-axis view with anterosuperior angulation (FIG. 37.6).

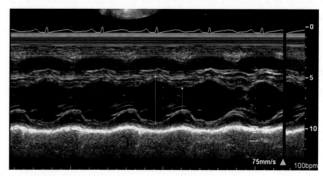

FIGURE 37.6

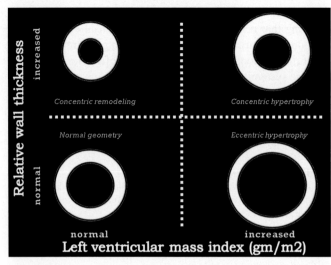

FIGURE 37.7

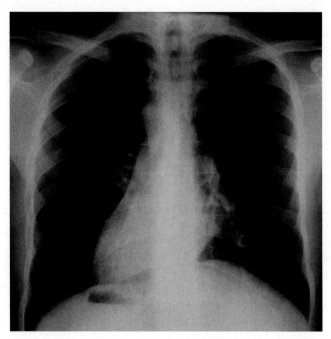

FIGURE 37.8

It cannot be seen from parasternal long-axis view. PW Doppler sampling in the branch pulmonary arteries is a good screening test for AP window as it shows abnormal continuous antegrade flow secondary to the left-to-right shunt during systole and diastole from the aorta into the pulmonary arteries (Fig. 37.7). Option D is incorrect as the aortic arch looks widely patent from Video 37.2 although large PDA makes it difficult to completely rule out aortic coarctation in infants but that is not usually the case in adults.

It is quite uncommon nowadays in the developed world to see large PDA and/or VSD that are not repaired in teens or young adults. This case presents a rare natural history example of unrepaired large left-to-right shunts. Her failure to thrive as a child can be well explained by her increased pulmonary blood flow. After several years, pulmonary vascular bed starts developing changes that lead to increase in pulmonary vascular resistance (PVR) and limits the amount of left-to-right shunting. This is why such patients are not that symptomatic at rest later in childhood. If this goes unrepaired longer, the PVR can become higher than systemic vascular resistance (SVR) and the shunts reverse to right to left. This is called Eisenmenger physiology and is associated with cyanosis at rest and/or with activity. Our patient underwent a cardiac catheterization to evaluate her shunt and PVR. Her Qp:Qs was estimated at 3:1, and her PVR was elevated but partially responsive to pulmonary vasodilators. After that, she had VSD closure and PDA ligation in addition to creation of atrial septal fenestration. The atrial fenestration works as a pop-off valve that allows right-to-left shunting in case of pulmonary hypertension crisis, which leads to cyanosis but maintains some cardiac output.

Suggested Reading

Eidem BW, et al. Echocardiography in pediatric and adult congenital heart disease. *Chapter 19: Patent Ducts Arteriosus and Aortopulmonary Window*. 364–373.

Answer 13: A. Option A is correct as we need to evaluate her Qp:Qs ratio in addition to her pulmonary vascular resistance (see below explanation of how to estimate her pulmonary

arterial pressures) and, if elevated, do pulmonary vasoreactivity testing to determine her surgical candidacy.

Figure 37.8 shows CW Doppler across TV with TR peak velocity of 4.9 m/s. Using the modified Bernoulli equation ($P2-P1 = 4\,[V2]^2$),

P2 represents RV systolic pressure.

P1 represents RA pressure (same as CVP = 10 mm Hg as no tricuspid valve stenosis).

V2 represents tricuspid regurgitation peak velocity (4.9 m/s).

Using the above numbers, RV systolic pressure = CVP + 4 $(4.9)^2$ = 10 + 96 = 97 mm Hg.

This is equal to pulmonary artery systolic pressure as the case mentioned no pulmonary valve stenosis.

Figure 37.9 shows CW Doppler across PV with pulmonary insufficiency end-diastolic (PIED) velocity of 3.5 m/s. Using the Bernoulli equation ($P2-P1 = 4\,[V2]^2$),

P2 represents PA diastolic pressure.

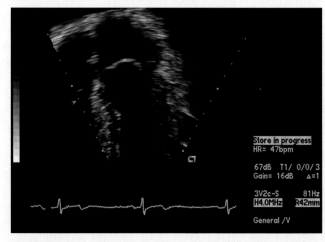

FIGURE 37.9

P1 represents RV diastolic pressure (same as RA pressure and CVP = 10 mm Hg as no tricuspid valve stenosis).

V2 represents PIED velocity (3.5 m/s).

Using the above numbers, PA diastolic pressure = CVP + 4 $(3.5)^2$ = 10 + 49 = 59 mm Hg.

Option B is incorrect. This patient deserves further hemodynamic evaluation to determine her surgical candidacy. If her PVR is very elevated and fixed with no response to pulmonary vasodilators, she can still have pretty functional lifestyle with the newer pulmonary hypertension treatment options and transplant will not be needed at this point.

Option C is incorrect. There is no coarctation of the aorta here so no angioplasty is needed.

Option D is incorrect. This patient will likely need pulmonary vasodilators like sildenafil, but that should be done after getting accurate evaluation of her PVR and the left-to-right shunting degree. Delaying her next step of action for 3 months is definitely not the best action for her either.

Option E is incorrect. Patients with obvious elevation in pulmonary arterial pressures need hemodynamic evaluation to determine how elevated the PVR is and if it changes at all with pulmonary vasodilators. Patients with fixed and elevated PVR have higher risk of death and clinical problems if their septal defects are closed compared to managing them medically with pulmonary vasodilators.

Suggested Reading

Eidem BW, et al. Echocardiography in pediatric and adult congenital heart disease. *Chapter 29: Pulmonary Hypertension*: 507–510.

Answer 14: D. The video here is a parasternal short-axis view at level of pulmonary arteries and ascending aorta showing small PDA with shunt from proximal descending aorta to MPA (left to right). This view can be best obtained from high left parasternal window in kids and young adults with slight anterior tilting of probe. It is great for showing pulmonary artery branching pattern and PDA. Best PDA view though is from suprasternal notch with marker around 11 o'clock, which shows proximal descending aorta and MPA in parallel way with PDA as a connecting vessel between them.

Option A is incorrect. LPA sling occurs when LPA originates from RPA instead of MPA and courses posteriorly between trachea and esophagus. The video here shows no indication of abnormal branching of pulmonary arteries.

Option B is incorrect. Coronary artery fistula will show as a diastolic Doppler signal ending in pulmonary artery and not continuous signal as in this video. It will also be better seen from lower parasternal views coming from aortic root (coronaries) and not proximal descending as in this video.

Option C is incorrect. ALCAPA will also show as diastolic flow signal that ends in MPA. The difference from coronary fistula is the direction of blood flow in LAD by color Doppler. In ALCAPA, blood flow will be reversed (toward aorta) compared to forward flow in fistula (away from aorta). Showing normal origin of LCA from aorta also helps differentiate these two conditions.

Suggested Reading

Schneider DJ, Moore JW. Patent ductus arteriosus. *Circulation* 2006; 114:1873–1882.

Answer 15: D. Option A is incorrect. LPA stenosis (commonly seen in LPA sling) Doppler signal is systolic one with early systolic peak velocity and not continuous as seen in the figure in this question.

Option B is incorrect. Coronary artery fistula can be narrowed, but its Doppler signal will never show high velocity as seen in the figure in this question.

Option C is incorrect. ALCAPA is rarely associated with narrowing of the actual coronary artery. It is not unusual for coronary collateral vessels between left and right systems to have some narrowing though (seen by cath), which can affect myocardial supply and ventricular function.

Option D is correct. PDA in this patient is small with minimal amount of shunting. This is evident from the small diameter and normal LA and LV dimensions. It has likely been this small for most of this patient's life as evident by the high velocity seen in the figure in this question.

The peak gradient estimated from this PDA peak velocity of 4 m/s is 65 mm Hg and represents the difference between aortic and pulmonary systolic pressures. This means that pulmonary artery systolic pressure is 100–65 = 35 mm Hg, which is normal.

Suggested Reading

Schneider DJ, Moore JW. Patent ductus arteriosus. *Circulation* 2006;114:1873–1882.

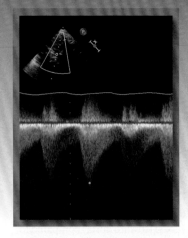

Chapter 38

Congenital Valve Lesions

Kristopher M. Cumbermack

1. Based upon the demonstrated findings on the echo shown (Video 38.1 and Fig. 38.1), what additional congenital lesions should be sought in an asymptomatic 24-year-old female with a blood pressure of 152/84?

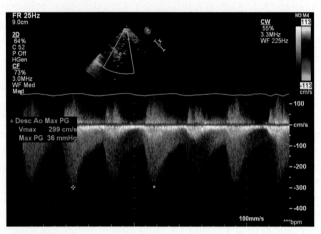

FIGURE 38.1

A. Bicuspid aortic valve and subaortic membrane
B. Bicuspid aortic valve and bicuspid pulmonary valve
C. Cor triatriatum dexter
D. Parachute tricuspid valve with stenosis
E. Hypoplastic left heart syndrome (HLHS)

2. When would it be reasonable to refer the patient with the congenital heart lesion shown in Video 38.2 for surgical repair?

A. LVOT peak Doppler gradient is 40 mm Hg; the patient is asymptomatic.
B. Pregnancy is being planned; LVOT mean Doppler gradient is <30 mm Hg.
C. The patient plans to join a recreational curling team; LVOT mean Doppler gradient is <30 mm Hg.
D. Echo demonstrates mild aortic regurgitation.
E. Chordal systolic anterior motion of the mitral apparatus is noted with no mitral regurgitation.

3. What would be the most appropriate recommendation for a 30-year-old with dyspnea on exertion and echo findings

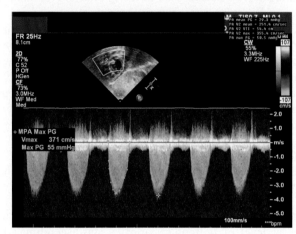

FIGURE 38.2

similar to those shown in Video 38.3 and Figure 38.2? Assume significant valvular regurgitation is absent.

A. Exercise stress test and Holter.
B. Clinical follow-up in 1 to 2 years.
C. Schedule balloon valvuloplasty.
D. Refer to pulmonary hypertension service.
E. Refer for Melody valve/percutaneous pulmonary valve implant.

4. What additional findings would lead to recommend surgery for the asymptomatic patient with repaired tetralogy of Fallot and the echocardiographic finding shown in Video 38.4?

A. Right ventricular enlargement (RVEDVi > 170 mL/m^2) on cardiac MRI
B. Mild right ventricular dysfunction
C. Asymptomatic nonsustained arrhythmias noted on Holter monitor
D. Systemic hypertension
E. Mild tricuspid regurgitation predicting RVSP of 30 mm Hg + CVP

5. What is the underlying congenital heart defect in this 21-year-old who has undergone an extracardiac Fontan procedure (VIDEO 38.5)?

A. Ebstein malformation

B. Hypoplastic left heart syndrome

C. Tricuspid atresia

D. Uhl anomaly

E. D-Transposition of the great vessels

6. What is the likely underling cardiac malformation (VIDEO 38.6) affecting a 44-year-old with no prior cardiac history who presents with pulmonary edema and CHF symptoms?

Note: Apical echo image is inverted upright (apex down) as preferred by congenital cardiologist.

A. D-Transposition of the great vessels

B. Double outlet right ventricle

C. Shone-like complex

D. L-Transposition of the great vessels

E. Tricuspid atresia

7. Which of the following repairs for congenital heart disease does *not* include placement of a right ventricular to pulmonary artery conduit?

A. Ross procedure

B. Konno procedure

C. Complete truncus arteriosus repair

D. Rastelli procedure

8. A 50-year-old obese female with trisomy 21 presents to outreach clinic to establish care. She has had heart surgery in the remote past, but family is unable to provide details and no records are available. She has had a recent decrease in her activity level and has difficulty breathing after walking out to her mailbox. Her examination reveals a holosystolic murmur most prominent at the apex. What is her most likely form of congenital heart disease and residual defect?

A. Tetralogy of Fallot with residual VSD

B. Tetralogy of Fallot with free pulmonary insufficiency

C. Perimembranous VSD with subsequent subaortic membrane

D. Complete atrioventricular canal defect with residual ASD

E. Complete atrioventricular canal defect with left atrioventricular valve regurgitation

9. A 21-year-old female college athlete with a history of bicuspid aortic valve (BAV) presents for cardiac clearance for sports participation. Her prior echos have not demonstrated aortic stenosis, insufficiency, or other forms of congenital heart disease. Of the following options, what should be the focus of her echocardiogram evaluation?

A. Coarctation of the aorta

B. Hypertrophic cardiomyopathy

C. Parachute mitral valve

D. Ascending aorta

E. Ruptured berry aneurysms

10. A 30-year-old female with a history of Marfan syndrome and abdominal aortic aneurysm s/p graft repair presents for routine follow-up. What should be the primary focus of her annual echocardiogram?

A. Atrial and ventricular septum

B. Pericardial space

C. Mitral valve and aortic root

D. Aortic and pulmonary valves

E. Assessment for pulmonary hypertension

11. A 19-year-old male is seen in adult congenital heart clinic after being lost to follow-up. He has been reporting new exercise intolerance. A sternotomy scar is present and a loud systolic murmur is appreciated on auscultation. Records are unavailable, but he reports being a blue baby that required heart surgery. Which of the following forms of congenital heart disease is most consistent with the spectral Doppler pattern shown in FIGURE 38.3?

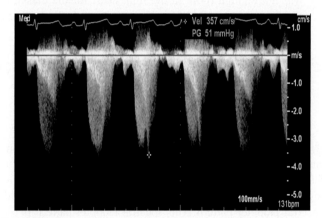

FIGURE 38.3

A. Aortic valve stenosis

B. Isolated intracavitary obstruction in hypertrophic cardiomyopathy

C. Tetralogy of Fallot

D. Pulmonary valvular stenosis

E. Discrete subaortic membrane

12. A 27-year-old female with a history of unrepaired pulmonary atresia with VSD has an oxygen saturation level of 79% and a continuous murmur heard both anteriorly and posteriorly. What is the most likely cause of this murmur?

A. Ventricular septal defect

B. RV to PA conduit stenosis and insufficiency

C. Coronary artery fistulas

D. Multiple aortopulmonary collateral arteries

E. Patent ductus arteriosus

13. A 24-year-old male presents to the ER with fractured arm requiring surgical intervention. They have an unclear cardiac history. His mother sends an image of an old echo report describing cardiac anatomy of dextrocardia, DORV with malposed great vessels, subpulmonary VSD, and pulmonary stenosis. This however was a preoperative report and surgical records are unavailable. The patient never understood his heart diagnosis. An echocardiogram is performed prior to anesthesia and surgery. Based upon the described anatomy and images (Videos 38.7 and 38.8), what surgical repair was most likely?

A. Rastelli repair
B. REV (réparation à l'étage ventriculaire) repair
C. Nikaidoh repair
D. Ross repair
E. Arterial switch operation

14. An adult patient with D-TGA states to you that their heart surgeon told them "their aorta was too far away and there was not enough room in the right heart for the classical switch procedure." What alternative surgical approach might the surgeon have performed instead?

A. Rastelli repair
B. REV repair
C. Nikaidoh repair
D. Ross repair
E. Arterial switch operation

Answer 1: A. The images of this hypertensive adult demonstrate a coarctation of the aorta at the aortic isthmus (distal to left subclavian artery and typical site of ductal insertion) resulting in flow acceleration by color Doppler and a "sawtooth" spectral Doppler pattern. This spectral Doppler pattern is the result of aortic pressures proximal to the obstruction being significantly higher than distal to the obstruction in both systole and diastole (Fig. 38.4). Persistence of antegrade diastolic flow is normal but should be <30 cm/s. A similar spectral Doppler pattern is seen in any discrete stenosis of an arterial vessel, including significant branch pulmonary artery stenosis and restrictive ductus arteriosus. Cardiovascular lesions associated with coarctation of the aorta can occur at the aortic valve and mitral valve levels as abnormalities in flow impair downstream cardiac development. Lesions include bicuspid aortic valve (BAV), subaortic membrane/stenosis, and mitral valve abnormalities. Shone complex, consisting of a supramitral valve ring, parachute mitral valve, subaortic stenosis, and coarctation of the aorta, is a rare form of congenital heart disease (CHD), though Shone-like complex is a term often used to describe any subset of multiple left-sided obstructive lesions.

Answer B is incorrect as though bicuspid pulmonary valves exist, they are not associated with aortic coarctation or BAV.

Answer C is incorrect as cor triatriatum *dexter* is a potentially obstructive membrane that can develop in the right atrium and is not associated with coarctation of the aorta. Cor triatriatum *sinister* occurs in the left atrium above the left atrial appendage (in contrast to supramitral valve ring, which is located below the left atrial appendage) and could theoretically

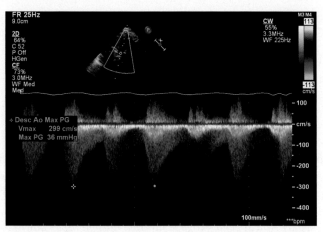

Figure 38.4 Continuous-wave Doppler through the aortic isthmus creates a "sawtooth" pattern with high-velocity, antegrade flow persisting through diastole seen in aortic coarctation.

impair growth of downstream structures including aortic arch, but is not a typical association, nor would remain asymptomatic in our scenario.

Answer D is incorrect since tricuspid valve abnormalities are not generally associated with aortic coarctation or other forms of left heart disease. Parachute *mitral* valve, the result of chordal attachments to a solitary papillary muscle, can be associated with a coarctation of the aorta in the setting of Shone complex as described above.

Answer E is also incorrect. Though HLHS is felt to have a genetic link to BAV and coarctation of the aorta is typically a component, HLHS is a ductal-dependent lesion for systemic flow and patients with HLHS would not remain asymptomatic, yet alone survive, until adulthood without palliative surgery.

Suggested Readings

Barron DJ, et al. Hypoplastic left heart syndrome. *Lancet* 2009;374:551–564.

Goudar SP, et al. Echocardiography of coarctation of the aorta, aortic arch hypoplasia, and arch interruption. *Cardiol Young* 2016;26(8):1553–1562.

Kiefer TL, Wang A, Hughes GC, et al. Management of patients with bicuspid aortic valve disease. *Curr Treat Options Cardiovasc Med* 2011;13(6):489–505.

Moral S, et al. Differential diagnosis and clinical implications of remnants of the right valve of the sinus venosus. *J Am Soc Echocardiogr* 2016;29:183–194.

Siu SC, Silversides CK. Bicuspid aortic valve disease. *J Am Coll Cardiol* 2010;55(25):2789–2800. doi:10.1016/j.jacc.2009.12.068.

Answer 2: B. Echo demonstrates a discrete subaortic membrane without left ventricular hypertrophy. Subaortic membrane resection can be considered for female patients with lesser degrees of subaortic obstruction who desire to become pregnant. Subaortic membrane can develop in isolation, in association with left-sided cardiac lesions, and late in the natural history of patients with a perimembranous VSD.

Answer A is incorrect because surgical resection of subaortic membrane should be recommended for asymptomatic patients with peak gradients >50 mm Hg.

Answer C is incorrect because while subaortic membrane resection can be considered for patients with mean subaortic stenosis gradients <30 mm Hg considering engaging in strenuous sports, curling is not considered a strenuous sport (class 1A).

Answer D is incorrect because mild aortic regurgitation is common in subaortic membrane patients and resection is not recommended to prevent progressive AR in patients with trivial or mild AR.

Answer E is not correct. Isolated chordal systolic anterior motion of the mitral apparatus without mitral regurgitation is not an indication for subaortic membrane resection.

Suggested Readings

Mitchell JH, Haskell W, Snell P, et al. Task force 8: classification of sports. *J Am Coll Cardiol* 2005;45(8):1364–1367.

van der Linde D, Takkenberg JJ, Rizopoulos D, et al. Natural history of discrete subaortic stenosis in adults: a multicentre study. *Eur Heart J* 2013;34(21):1548–1556.

Warnes CA, et al. ACC/AHA 2008 guidelines for the management of adults with congenital heart disease: executive summary. *J Am Coll Cardiol* 2008;52(23):1890–1947.

Answer 3: C. Images show a doming pulmonary valve with pulmonary stenosis (peak gradient >50 mm Hg). In symptomatic patients with pulmonary valve stenosis with less than moderate pulmonary regurgitation, balloon valvuloplasty is recommended.

Answers A and B are not adequate recommendations for a *symptomatic* patient with pulmonary valve stenosis.

Answer D is not correct, as isolated pulmonary valve stenosis does not result in pulmonary vascular occlusive disease.

Answer E is incorrect as percutaneous pulmonary valve placement is not indicated for native right ventricular/pulmonary valve anatomy; rather, transcatheter PVR is currently only FDA approved for patients with severe stenosis/regurgitation due to existing RV–PA conduit or bioprosthetic PVR dysfunction, though this is expected to see approval for broader use in the near future.

Suggested Readings

Cheatham JP, et al. Clinical and hemodynamic outcomes up to 7 years after transcatheter pulmonary valve replacement in the US melody valve investigational device exemption trial. *Circulation* 2015;131(22):1960–1970.

Fitzgerald KP, Lim MJ. The pulmonary valve. *Cardiol Clin* 2011;29(2):223–227.

McElhinney DB, Hellenbrand WE, Zahn EM, et al. Short-and medium-term outcomes after transcatheter pulmonary valve placement in the expanded multicenter US melody valve trial. *Circulation* 2010;122(5):507–516.

Warnes CA, et al. ACC/AHA 2008 guidelines for the management of adults with congenital heart disease: executive summary. *J Am Coll Cardiol* 2008;52(23):1890–1947.

Answer 4: A. The echocardiographic image demonstrates pulmonary valve stenosis and severe pulmonary valve regurgitation. In the postop tetralogy of Fallot patient with severe pulmonary regurgitation, pulmonary valve replacement is reasonable in adults with any of the following:

A. Moderate to severe RV dysfunction
B. Moderate to severe RV enlargement (RVEDVi > 150 to 170 mL/m^2)
C. Development of symptomatic or sustained atrial and/or ventricular arrhythmias
D. Moderate to severe tricuspid regurgitation

Editor's Note: *Much has been written on this topic regarding optimal timing of PVR in relation to RV size. The volumes used to refer patients are decreasing in deference to improved percutaneous and surgical repairs as well as a goal to preserve RV systolic function. At the time of this review, the above RVEDVi guidelines were valid, but may soon be smaller still.*

Suggested Readings

Burchill LJ, Wald RM, Harris L, et al. Pulmonary valve replacement in adults with repaired tetralogy of Fallot. *Semin Thorac Cardiovasc Surg Pediatr Card Surg Annu* 2011;14(1):92–97.

Graham TP Jr, Bernard Y, Arbogast P, et al. Outcome of pulmonary valve replacements in adults after tetralogy repair: a multi-institutional study. *Congenit Heart Dis* 2008;3(3):162–167.

Warnes CA, et al. ACC/AHA 2008 guidelines for the management of adults with congenital heart disease: executive summary. *J Am Coll Cardiol* 2008;52(23):1890–1947.

Answer 5: C. Image shows tricuspid atresia (TA), with a lack of a direct connection between the right atrium and a hypoplastic right ventricle. Patients with tricuspid atresia may have a wide variety of morphologic subtypes. When the ventricular septum is *intact* or a small, *restrictive* VSD is present, the RV and pulmonary valve are more likely to be hypoplastic given impact on downstream blood flow. This represents a ductal-dependent lesion at birth. In utero, retrograde flow from ductus arteriosus can allow normal branch pulmonary artery growth. When TA is associated with an *unrestrictive* VSD, the right ventricle can be larger with minimal impact on development of the outflow tract and associated semilunar valve to the right ventricle. This form of CHD is not ductal dependent and need for surgery to provide pulmonary blood flow as neonate is not needed. In fact, pulmonary artery banding may be required to limit pulmonary overcirculation and development of congestive heart failure. Up to 30% of cases of tricuspid atresia are associated with transposition of the great arteries, which can lead to aortic valve and arch abnormalities, particularly when intact ventricular septum or small VSD. Single ventricle surgical pathway is uniformly followed. If ductal dependent, a modified Blalock-Taussig (BT) shunt (Gore-Tex tube connecting right subclavian artery to right pulmonary artery) is performed in the first 7 to 10 days of life to maintain pulmonary blood flow, followed by bidirectional Glenn (SVC connected to right pulmonary artery with BT shunt takedown) at 3 to 6 months, and completion of the cavopulmonary anastomosis with the Fontan procedure (IVC connect to pulmonary artery) between 2 and 5 years depending on surgical center.

The atrioventricular valves develop from the ventricles themselves and cannot be incongruous to the associated ventricle. If present, the mitral valve is always associated with the morphologic left ventricle, and the tricuspid valve is always connected with the morphologic right ventricle regardless of ventricular relationship (D- or L-looped ventricles). Ebstein malformation results from abnormal delamination (process of separation from ventricular walls) of the tricuspid valve leaflets that leads to apical displacement of the effective tricuspid valve annulus. Limitations on excursion of the leaflets can lead to varying degrees, from mild to severe, tricuspid regurgitation. Severe right atrial dilation and atrialization of portions of the ventricle above the apically displaced tricuspid valve can occur. Repair of Ebstein malformations does not typically include the Fontan repair, and in milder forms, no surgical intervention is needed. Severe in utero cases often lead to fetal or neonatal demise; if survive, neonatal surgery can include fenestrated right ventricular exclusion, or Starnes procedure, and subsequent single ventricle pathway.

Hypoplastic left heart syndrome has a spectrum of morphologic subtypes including combinations of mitral and aortic valve stenosis and atresia. The obligatory feature is inadequate systemic blood flow. While the Fontan repair is part of HLHS palliation, the images shown here demonstrate normal left ventricular size with hypoplastic right ventricle.

Uhl anomaly is an extremely rare congenital heart defect that is caused by a lack of right ventricular muscle that results in a significantly enlarged right ventricular cavity with poor function. The image shown here shows a diminutive right ventricular cavity.

D-transposition of the great vessels is a conotruncal defect resulting in discordance of ventricular–arterial connections. By definition, the aorta connects to a morphologic right ventricle and the pulmonary artery connects to a morphologic left ventricle regardless of ventricular position. Though D-TGA can occur in tricuspid atresia, one cannot make that diagnosis from images provided. In isolated forms of D-TGA without semilunar valve stenosis or hypoplasia, both ventricles are typically normal in size. Cardiac repair of D-TGA involves either an atrial or arterial switch to separate the pulmonary and systemic circulations and return blood flow to series instead of flowing in parallel.

Suggested Readings
Allen HD, et al, ed. *Moss and Adams' Heart Disease in Infants, Children, and Adolescents, Including the Fetus and Young Adult.* 9th ed. Baltimore, MD: Lippincott Williams & Wilkins, 2016.
Booker OJ, Nanda NC. Echocardiographic assessment of Ebstein's anomaly. *Echocardiography* 2015;32(suppl 2):S177–S188.

Answer 6: *D.* Image shows that the left-sided ventricle has a moderator band and the left-sided AV valve is apically displaced, findings consistent with a morphologic right ventricle and associated tricuspid valve on the left side of the heart. In an adult with no history of congenital heart surgeries, the patient's presenting symptoms and echo findings are consistent with congenitally corrected TGA (CCTGA) or L-TGA. The term "corrected" refers to physiologically normal blood flow caused by the "double discordance" of both the atrioventricular connection and the ventricular–arterial connection. Symptoms

develop in young adulthood related to failure of the systemic morphologic right ventricle.

D-transposition of the great vessels is a cyanotic heart defect with discordance of only ventricular–arterial connections that requires surgical intervention (atrial or arterial switch repair) and therefore a significant cardiac history for survival into adulthood.

Double outlet right ventricle (DORV) heart defects consist of both the aortic and pulmonary valves being committed to the right ventricle usually associated with a VSD. DORV can be defined by >50% of second semilunar valve being committed to the right ventricle and more stringently by mitral–aortic fibrous discontinuity. Most individuals with DORV present and undergo surgical repair during childhood.

Shone complex refers to obstructive left heart disease at the mitral, aortic, and aortic arch levels. There is no atrial, ventricular, or arterial discordance in Shone patients like the images shown here.

Tricuspid atresia is a congenital heart defect with three functional cardiac chambers and a lack of a direct connection between the right atrium and a hypoplastic right ventricle. A patient with tricuspid atresia would have a significant cardiac history including surgical interventions (up to and including a Fontan palliation) to survive into adulthood.

Suggested Readings
Allen HD, et al, ed. *Moss and Adams' Heart Disease in Infants, Children, and Adolescents, Including the Fetus and Young Adult.* 6th ed. Baltimore, MD: Lippincott Williams & Wilkins, 2000.
De León LE, et al. Mid-term outcomes in patients with congenitally corrected transposition of the great arteries: a single center experience. *J Am Coll Surg* 2017;224:707–715. doi:10.1016/j.jamcollsurg.2016.12.029.

Answer 7: *B.* The Konno procedure is a cardiac repair to address a small left ventricular outflow tract (typically long-segment tunnel-like) and concomitant aortic stenosis. The original description by Konno consisted of an aortoventriculoplasty and aortic valve replacement. More recent advances have focused on valve-sparing enlargement of the left ventricular outflow tract termed modified or valve-sparing Konno procedure. The Konno procedure does not require an RV–PA conduit.

The Ross procedure is an approach for aortic valve disease in children and young adults that replaces the diseased aortic valve with an autograft using the patient's pulmonary valve. This approach has the obligate requirement of inserting an RV–PA conduit to replace the translocated pulmonary valve. This approach results in growth of the aortic autograft and relatively low reoperation risks to replace the RV–PA conduit.

Truncus arteriosus is a significant congenital heart defect where a single "truncal" semilunar valve overrides a VSD. This single outflow provides systemic, pulmonary, and coronary circulation. A main PA trunk or separate branch pulmonary arteries can connect directly to the truncal vessel. The truncal valve can have one to four leaflets and can have significant stenosis or insufficiency, which significantly impacts survival. To achieve a complete truncus repair, VSD closure incorporates the truncal valve into the systemic circulation and separates from the pulmonary circulation. An RV–PA conduit connects the RV to the surgically isolated pulmonary arteries. Coronary arteries remain attached to the truncal or neo-aortic root.

The Rastelli procedure involves placement of an RV–PA conduit as a core feature of the repair (see answer to question 13).

Suggested Readings

Erentug V, Bozbuga N, Kirali K, et al. Surgical treatment of subaortic obstruction in adolescent and adults: long-term follow-up. *J Card Surg* 2005;20(1):16–21.

Gonzalez-Lavin L, Geens M, Ross D. Aortic valve replacement with a pulmonary valve autograft: indications and surgical technique. *Surgery* 1970;68(3):450–455.

Konno S, Imai Y, Iida Y, et al. A new method for prosthetic valve replacement in congenital aortic stenosis associated with hypoplasia of the aortic valve ring. *J Thorac Cardiovasc Surg* 1975;70(5):909–917.

McGoon DC, Wallace RB, Danielson GK. The Rastelli operation. Its indications and results. *J Thorac Cardiovasc Surg* 1973;65(1):65–75.

Answer 8: E. Complete atrioventricular canal defect (CAVC), also known as atrioventricular septal defect, is the result of abnormal development of the endocardial cushions resulting in a common atrioventricular valve, a primum ASD, and an inlet VSD. Various subtypes can include a partial AVC consisting of a primary ASD with a cleft in the left atrioventricular valve (a true mitral valve is not present in atrioventricular canal defects) and transitional AVC with small inlet VSD component. These defects can also develop an imbalance with the degree of atrioventricular valve tissue associated with each ventricular leading to impairments of blood flow, subsequent growth of ventricles, and ultimately hypoplastic left or right ventricles.

AVC defects are associated with trisomy 21. The goals of surgical repair are to patch close the primum ASD and inlet VSD and create too functional inflow valves, typically tolerating more insufficiency than stenosis. The holosystolic murmur in this case is caused by the severe left AV valve regurgitation demonstrated in VIDEO 38.9 matching the most prominent location at the apex resulting in left atrial dilation.

Answers A and B are incorrect. Despite TOF being seen in trisomy 21 patients with and without AVC defects, murmurs in patients with repaired TOF are typically systolic ejection type due to residual RV outflow tract, valvular or supravalvar obstruction with possible diastolic murmur from pulmonary insufficiency. A residual VSD after repair can cause a holosystolic murmur but is typically most prominent at left sternal border not apex. AVC defects are also significantly more common than TOF in patients with trisomy 21.

Answer C is incorrect as subaortic membrane classically causes a systolic ejection murmur at the upper right sternal border.

Answer D is incorrect. A residual ASD after AVC repair could potentially cause a systolic ejection murmur at upper left sternal border from increased flow across the pulmonary valve due to atrial left-to-right shunt, but not a holosystolic murmur at the apex.

Suggested Readings

Hazekamp MG, et al. Long-term results of reoperation for left atrioventricular valve regurgitation after correction of atrioventricular septal defects. *Ann Thorac Surg* 2012;93(3):849–855.

Valente AM, et al. Multimodality imaging guidelines for patients with repaired tetralogy of Fallot: a report from the American Society of Echocardiography: developed in collaboration with the Society for Cardiovascular Magnetic Resonance and the Society for Pediatric Radiology. *J Am Soc Echocardiogr* 2014;27(2):111–141.

Answer 9: D. BAV is associated with an aortopathy of the ascending aorta (the portion of the aorta extending from the sinotubular junction to the innominate/brachiocephalic artery) that can result in dilation and rupture. VIDEO 38.10 provides an example of a significantly dilated ascending aorta in a modified parasternal long axis (rock probe to patient's right without rotation or slight slide of probe cephalad and rightward along probe marker line). In addition, patients with BAV can develop aortic insufficiency and stenosis overtime. Of note, ascending aorta dilation can occur in absence of significant stenosis and insufficiency. Over time, sinuses of Valsalva can also become dilated in patients with BAV.

Answer A is incorrect as coarctation of the aorta would not develop over time if not present on initial evaluation in an adult with BAV despite the known association.

Answer B is incorrect as the diagnosis of hypertrophic cardiomyopathy requires absence of secondary causes such as significant aortic stenosis or coarctation that would cause a pressure overload on the left ventricle resulting in ventricular hypertrophy to reduce wall stress.

Answer C is incorrect as parachute mitral valve is a congenital abnormality consisting of mitral valve chordae attaching to a solitary papillary muscle creating the appearance of a parachute. Though can be seen in BAV and coarctation, this anomaly is either present or absent at birth and does not develop over time.

Answer D is incorrect as berry aneurysms, saccular cerebral aneurysms with a stem resembling a berry that typically form at bifurcation points within the circle of Willis, are associated with coarctation and hypertension but not associated with isolated bicuspid aortic valve.

Suggested Readings

Cook SC, Hickey J, Maul TM, et al. Assessment of the cerebral circulation in adults with coarctation of the aorta. *Congenit Heart Dis* 2013;8(4):289–295.

Hakim FA, Kendall CB, Alharthi M, et al. Parachute mitral valve in adults—a systematic overview. *Echocardiogr* 2010;27(5):581–586.

Hiratzka LF, Creager MA, Isselbacher EM, et al. Surgery for aortic dilatation in patients with bicuspid aortic valves: a statement of clarification from the American College of Cardiology/American Heart Association Task Force on Clinical Practice Guidelines. *J Am Card Cardiol* 2016;67(6):724–731.

Answer 10: C. Patients with Marfan syndrome are at risk for developing cardiovascular abnormalities including mitral valve prolapse (MVP), tricuspid valve prolapse, dilation of the sinuses of Valsalva, and dilation of the main pulmonary artery (VIDEOS 38.11A AND B). From an echocardiographic standpoint, mitral valve prolapse is defined by buckling of a leaflet, typically the anterior leaflet, more than 2 mm past the annulus into the left atrium. Leaflet thickening and mitral regurgitation can also be seen. Though pulmonary hypertension and abnormalities of the atrial septum, ventricular septum, and pulmonary valve can occur in Marfan syndrome as in the general population, they are not typical associated cardiovascular abnormalities and would not be the primary focus of her follow-up echocardiogram.

Suggested Readings

Loeys BL, et al. The revised Ghent nosology for the Marfan syndrome. *J Med Genet* 2010;47(70):476–485.

Stout M. The Marfan syndrome: implications for athletes and their echocardiographic assessment. *Echocardiography* 2009;26(9):1075–1081.

Answer 11: *C.* The spectral Doppler signal in Figure 38.3 consists of two different overlapping waveforms highlighted in Figure 38.5. One is a static waveform with a convex shape peaking early in systole; a later peak and more rounded shape occur with increasing severity (blue). The second pattern is consistent with dynamic obstruction with an initial concave shape and a peak later in systole caused by changing degree of obstruction (yellow). The spectral Doppler pattern shown was obtained in a patient with tetralogy of Fallot s/p repair with both residual infundibular (dynamic) and valvular (static) stenosis.

Subaortic membrane, semilunar valve stenosis, and supravalvar stenosis (Fig. 38.6) create fixed or static patterns of obstruction. Intracavitary obstruction seen in hypertrophic cardiomyopathy causes a dynamic spectral Doppler pattern (Fig. 38.7). Only Answer C would create an overlap of both spectral Doppler patterns.

Suggested Reading

Apitz C, et al. Tetralogy of fallot. *Lancet* 2009;374(9699):1462–1471.

Answer 12: *D.* Pulmonary atresia with VSD is typically associated with multiple aortopulmonary collateral arteries (MAPCAs), which are abnormal arterial connections between the aorta and the pulmonary arterial system of lobes of the

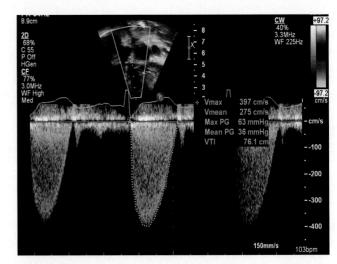

FIGURE 38.6 Fixed obstructive spectral Doppler pattern seen in subaortic membrane.

lungs (Videos 38.12A and B). These vessels form in a haphazard fashion of variable sizes typically with small or even absent branch pulmonary arteries. Continuous high-velocity flow from aorta to pulmonary artery causes a continuous murmur radiating to the back. This lesions can be surgically repaired by closure of VSD, unifocalization of MAPCAs to main pulmonary arteries (if present), and an RV–PA conduit. However, based on the challenging anatomy and suboptimal surgical outcomes, some congenital cardiologists believe that no surgery should be pursued as decades of survival with decent quality of life can ensue. As a mixing lesion at the ventricular level, O2 saturations are in the midseventies if Qp:Qs is near 1:1, which can occur when pulmonary vascular resistance is elevated.

Answer A is incorrect as VSD does not cause a continuous murmur, and in PA/VSD, the VSD often causes no murmur at all given its large, unrestrictive nature and equalization of RV and LV pressure.

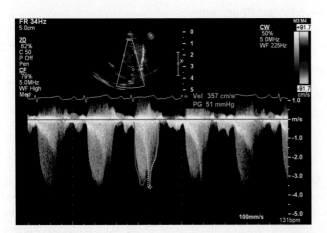

FIGURE 38.5 Spectral Doppler pattern in patient status post tetralogy of Fallot repair. There is overlap of two distinct patterns, fixed (convex outlined in *blue*) and dynamic (concave outlined in *yellow*).

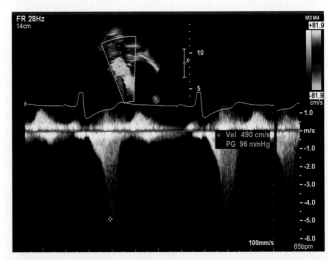

FIGURE 38.7 Dynamic obstructive spectral Doppler pattern seen intracavitary LV obstruction in hypertrophic cardiomyopathy.

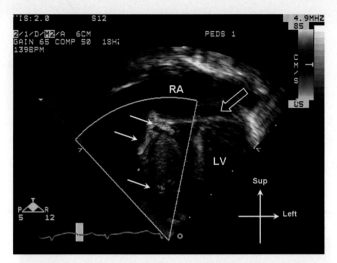

FIGURE **38.8**

Answer B is incorrect. RV–PA conduits can develop significant stenosis and insufficiency, but this results in distinct systolic ejection and diastolic murmurs ("to and fro") as opposed to continuous murmur.

Answer C is incorrect. Though coronary artery fistulas can cause continuous murmurs, they are seen in pulmonary atresia with intact ventricular septum (PA/IVS), not PA/VSD (Fig. 38.8; Videos 38.13A and B).

Answer E is incorrect. Patent ductus arteriosus does cause a continuous murmur but is typically absent in pulmonary atresia with VSD.

Suggested Readings

Malhotra SP, Hanley FL. Surgical management of pulmonary atresia with ventricular septal defect and major aortopulmonary collaterals: a protocol-based approach. *Semin Thorac Cardiovasc Surg Pediatr Card Surg Annu* 2009:145–151.

Schneider AW, et al. More than 25 years of experience in managing pulmonary atresia with intact ventricular septum. *Ann Thorac Surg* 2014;98(5):1680–1686.

***Answer 13:** A.* Video 38.7 is an anterior parasternal long-axis view demonstrating an RV to PA conduit with no more than mild stenosis and insufficiency. Video 38.8 shows an LV baffle tunnel to the aortic valve from a subcostal view.

Both of these findings comprise the core components of the Rastelli repair. Creation of a large intraventricular baffle simultaneously closes the VSD, separates the right and left ventricles, and redirects systemic blood flow to the aorta. Pulmonary blood flow is established by placement of a valved homograft conduit connecting the right ventricle and main pulmonary

artery. Forms of complex congenital heart defects that require Rastelli procedure include D-transposition of the great arteries with VSD and pulmonary stenosis, pulmonary valve atresia with VSD, and double outlet right ventricle (DORV) with pulmonary stenosis or atresia.

Complications of the Rastelli repair include conduit stenosis and regurgitation, branch pulmonary artery stenosis, baffle/tunnel obstruction, residual VSD, RV volume loss impairing RV cardiac output, RV and LV dysfunction. Typically, this surgery is pursued in early childhood and obviates replacement of conduit in the future due to becoming inadequate in size over time. Once adult-sized conduit is in place, transcatheter pulmonary valve placement can be pursued in appropriate cases instead of open heart surgery.

Answer B is incorrect as the REV (Réparation à l'Etage Ventriculaire) repair creates a direct connection from RV to PA without conduit.

Answer C is incorrect as Nikaidoh repair does not involve baffle tunnel of LV outflow to aortic valve aligned with RV (see question 14).

Answer D is incorrect as a Ross repair is used in cases of aortic valve stenosis, not pulmonary valve stenosis (see question 7).

Answer E is incorrect as arterial switch is not used in isolation in cases of significant pulmonary stenosis as the pulmonary valve becomes the aortic valve. This is a surgery used in D-TGA without significant valvular stenosis.

Suggested Readings

Di Carlo D, et al. Long-term results of the REV (réparation à l'ètage ventriculaire) operation. *J Thorac Cardiovasc Surg* 2011;142(2):336–343.

Mahle WT, et al. Anatomy, echocardiography, and surgical approach to double outlet right ventricle. *Cardiol Young* 2008;18(suppl 3):39–51.

***Answer 14:** C.* Nikaidoh repair, also known as aortic translocation, involves resecting the stenotic pulmonary valve and root and moving the aortic valve and root to that location. This results in a closer to normal LV outflow contour without tunnel across to an aortic valve aligned with a right ventricle. Blood flow dynamics are felt to be closer to normal and RV volume loss due to tunnel through ventricular septum and RV does not occur. Risk of tunnel stenosis is also removed. An RV–PA conduit is then used to establish pulmonary blood flow.

Suggested Reading

Yeh T Jr, et al. The aortic translocation (Nikaidoh) procedure: midterm results superior to the Rastelli procedure. *J Thorac Cardiovasc Surg* 2007;133(2):461–469.

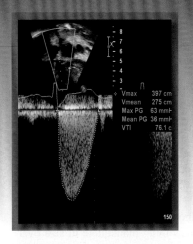

Chapter 39

Arterial Anomalies

Majd Makhoul

1. An asymptomatic 25-year-old with D-transposition of great arteries, who is s/p Mustard repair at 6 months of age, has the following findings on a routine transthoracic echocardiogram: a dilated right ventricle with moderate tricuspid regurgitation and peak velocity of 4.5 m/s. What is the most likely interpretation of this finding?

   A. Severe pulmonary arterial hypertension
   B. Severe aortic stenosis
   C. Expected finding in patients after Mustard operation
   D. Congenitally abnormal tricuspid valve

2. Which of the following clinical or echo findings would be unexpected after Mustard or Senning repair of D-transposition of great arteries?

   A. Sinus node dysfunction
   B. Atrial flutter
   C. Atrial baffle leak
   D. Pulmonary stenosis
   E. Systemic ventricular dysfunction

Questions 3 and 4

A 23-year-old asymptomatic male with uncontrolled hypertension is referred for an echocardiogram. Vital signs show right upper extremity blood pressure of 150/90 mm Hg. His heart rate is 88 bpm; cardiac exam is significant for grade 2/6 systolic ejection murmur loudest at the upper left sternal border. Femoral pulses are poorly palpable. He has been tried on thiazide with no significant response.

3. Which of the following conditions is not a common associated finding with the patient's condition, demonstrated in VIDEO 39.1 and FIGURE 39.1?

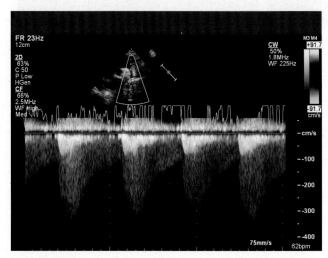

FIGURE 39.1

   A. Bicuspid aortic valve
   B. Systemic hypertension
   C. Cerebral aneurysms
   D. Supraventricular tachycardia
   E. Rib notching

4. What is the best next step for this patient?

   A. Add a beta-blocker as a second agent and see him back in 3 months.
   B. EP study for further stratification.
   C. Aortic arch repair with either surgery or percutaneously.
   D. Balloon aortic valvuloplasty of the bicuspid aortic valve.
   E. Chest CT scan to further evaluate the rib lesions.

Questions 5 and 6

A 20-year-old female college student was referred for evaluation of a murmur. She reports she has never had menstrual periods. On physical examination, you find the following: short stature, hypertelorism, lower extremity nonpitting edema, and neck webbing. Her murmur is grade III/VI systolic ejection murmur heard best at right upper sternal border in sitting position and radiates to the neck. An echocardiogram was performed (VIDEO 39.2 and FIGS. 39.2 AND 39.3).

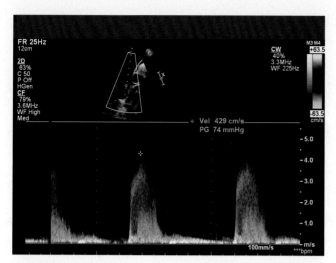

FIGURE 39.2

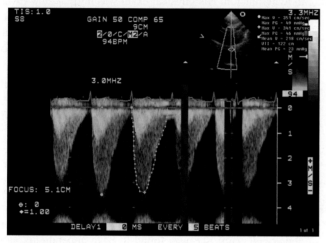

FIGURE 39.3

5. Which of the following best explains the etiology of her murmur?

A. Bicuspid aortic valve with aortic regurgitation.
B. Bicuspid aortic valve with aortic stenosis.
C. Tricuspid aortic valve with aortic stenosis.
D. Still heart murmur.

6. Which of the following associated conditions is least likely to be present?

A. Coarctation of the aorta
B. Bicuspid aortic valve
C. Increased risk for aortic dissection
D. Pulmonary valve stenosis
E. Renal abnormalities

7. All of the following conditions are commonly associated with the diagnosis demonstrated in Videos 39.3 and 39.4 except:

A. Ventricular septal defect
B. Pulmonary stenosis
C. Atrioventricular discordance
D. Coarctation of the aorta
E. Complete heart block

8. A 20-year-old pregnant female presents for evaluation of a murmur. The following flow signal is recorded on her echo (Fig. 39.4). The most likely diagnosis is:

A. Normal flow murmur of pregnancy
B. Ventricular septal defect
C. Anomalous pulmonary venous connection
D. Patent ductus arteriosus
E. Atrial septal defect

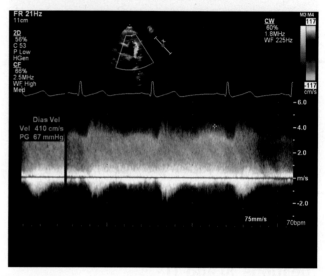

FIGURE 39.4

9. A 22-year-old female college student athlete is referred for evaluation of exertional chest pain. A 12-lead EKG showed no abnormalities, and echocardiogram was performed (Figs. 39.5 and 39.6 and Video 39.5). What is the most likely diagnosis?

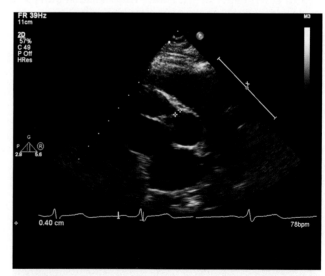

FIGURE 39.5

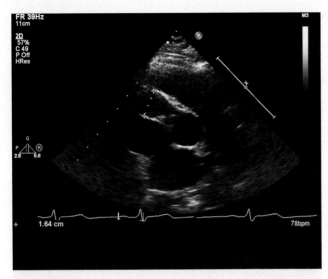

FIGURE 39.6

A. Aortopulmonary window
B. Coronary artery aneurysm
C. Sinus of Valsalva aneurysm
D. Pericardial cyst
E. Coronary artery thrombus

Questions 10 and 11

An 18-year-old young lady presented to cardiology office due to remote history of muscular VSD and family history of sudden cardiac death in her uncle at age 28. Autopsy showed no structural cardiac causes, so arrhythmia was the proposed cause. She is asymptomatic and last echo at age 6 months showed small muscular VSD with trivial left-to-right shunting. Today, her EKG is normal; her cardiac exam reveals grade II/VI SEM at left upper sternal border with radiation toward the left side of her back. Her BP was normal too. An echocardiogram was obtained (Video 39.6 and Fig. 39.7).

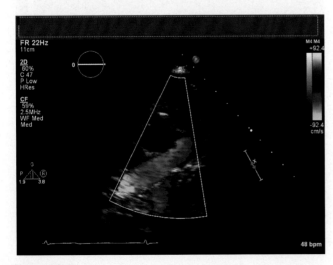

FIGURE 39.7

10. Based on the figure and video attached, what is the likely diagnosis and cause of her murmur?

A. Severe coarctation of the aorta
B. Abnormal origin of left pulmonary artery
C. Aortopulmonary window
D. L-transposition of the great arteries

11. What is the best next step of action in her management plan?

A. Referral for repair of coarctation of the aorta.
B. Cardiac MRI to better evaluate her pulmonary artery branching pattern.
C. Right heart catheterization to evaluate her pulmonary vascular resistance due to unrepaired AP window.
D. Repeat echo in 1 year to follow her ventricular function.

12. A 20-year-old young man presented for an evaluation due to hypertension. His physical exam was normal, and EKG showed no abnormalities. An echocardiogram was done and showed normal ventricular wall thickness and a patent aortic arch (Video 39.7). Based upon the clinical and echo findings, what is the most likely diagnosis?

A. Anomalous origin of left main coronary artery from pulmonary artery (ALCAPA)
B. Anomalous origin of right coronary artery from left sinus of Valsalva
C. Coronary artery aneurysm
D. Anomalous origin of left main coronary artery form right sinus of Valsalva

13. A 20-year-old young lady, who had arterial switch operation for D-TGA at 1 month of age, presented to the ER for abdominal pain. She was found to have appendicitis and needed clearance for appendectomy. EKG was normal and an echocardiogram was done. Based on Figure 39.8 and Video 39.8 that were obtained from her parasternal short-axis views, what is the best explanation of the finding you see?

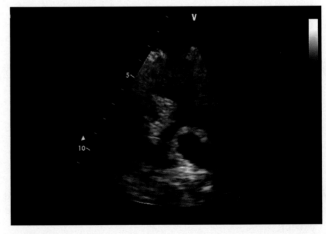

FIGURE 39.8

A. Retroaortic course of innominate vein.
B. Moving pulmonary arteries anteriorly is a common maneuver in arterial switch operation.
C. Aneurysmal dilation of the ascending aorta.
D. Arteriovenous connection between innominate vein and pulmonary arteries.

Answer 1: C.

A. False: No information is given regarding pulmonary arterial pressure or subpulmonary ventricular (left ventricle) pressure that would suggest increased pulmonary arterial pressure. If there was mitral regurgitation with elevated peak velocity instead, one could conclude that pulmonary hypertension is present as long as no obstruction at the LV outflow tract/pulmonary valve level.
B. False: From the tricuspid regurgitation jet, one could estimate that the systemic right ventricular pressure is 81 mm Hg + the left atrial pressure. One cannot conclude from this that there is severe aortic stenosis.
C. True: See discussion below.
D. False: D-transposition of great arteries is not typically associated with congenital tricuspid valve abnormalities. Such abnormalities are common in L-transposition of great arteries where aorta is typically anterior and to the left of pulmonary artery and there is L-looped ventricles (atrioventricular and ventricular–arterial discordance).

In D-transposition of great arteries, there is atrioventricular concordance and ventricular–arterial discordance. The systemic venous return is into a right atrium that connects with a morphologic right ventricle, which in turn gives rise to an aorta. The left atrium is connected to a morphologic left ventricle, which gives rise to a pulmonary artery. Mustard or Senning repair consists of redirecting blood return at the atrial level using a baffle made of Dacron or pericardium (Mustard operation) or atrial flaps (Senning operation). Thus, systemic venous return is redirected to the morphologic LV and into a pulmonary artery, and the pulmonary venous return is redirected into the morphologic RV and into the aorta. The morphologic RV is the systemic ventricle. Systemic ventricular dysfunction and systemic atrioventricular valve regurgitation (tricuspid regurgitation) are common complications of this procedure and occur in approximately 40% of patients. Therefore, moderate TR with a dilated RV would be a common finding in this type of a patient. Also, the systemic right ventricle is expected to have elevated systolic pressure (estimated by TR peak gradient) as it is connected to the aorta.

Suggested Readings

Child JS. Echocardiographic evaluation of the adult with postoperative congenital heart disease. In: Otto CM, ed. *Chapter 44: The Practice of Clinical Echocardiography*. 3rd ed. Philadelphia, PA: Saunders Elsevier, 2009.

Mertens LL, Vogt MO, Marek J, et al. Transposition of the great arteries. In: Lai WW, Mertens LL, Cohen MS, et al., eds. *Chapter 24: Echocardiography in Pediatric and Congenital Heart Disease: From Fetus to Adult*. Chichester, West Sussex, UK: Wiley-Blackwell Publishers, 2009.

Wernovsky G. Transposition of the great arteries. In: Allen HD, Driscoll DJ, Shaddy RE, et al., eds. *Chapter 51: Moss and Adams' Heart Disease in Infants, Children and Adolescents*. 7th ed. Philadelphia, PA: Lippincott Williams & Wilkins, 2008.

Answer 2: D.

A. Common complication; see discussion below.
B. Common complication; see discussion below.
C. Common complication; see discussion below.
D. False. Pulmonary stenosis is not usually a complication of Mustard or Senning procedures. Supravalvar pulmonary stenosis is, however, a complication following arterial switch repair of D-TGA, during which the pulmonary artery is brought anteriorly and connected to the morphologic right ventricle. This occurs in at least 5% of patients.
E. Common complication; see discussion below.

Mustard or Senning operations for correcting D-transposition of great arteries consist of redirecting blood from the systemic venous return via a baffle into the morphologic left ventricle and into the pulmonary artery and from the pulmonary veins into the morphologic right ventricle and into the aorta. Common complications include sinus bradycardia with junctional escape beats, sinus node dysfunction, and atrial flutter and fibrillation. The probability of being in sinus rhythm is only 50% at 10 years after atrial switch. Nearly half (48%) of patients followed for 23 years after Mustard had at least one episode of supraventricular tachycardia; of these, 73% had atrial flutter. Other complications include systemic venous baffle obstruction and baffle leaks in up to 10% of patients. Pulmonary venous baffle obstruction is less common, in only approximately 2% of patients. The right ventricle assumes the role of systemic ventricle and commonly shows signs of systolic dysfunction after several years of the procedure.

Suggested Readings

Gatzoulis MA, Walters J, McLaughlin PR, et al. Late arrhythmia in adults with the Mustard procedure for transposition of great arteries: a surrogate marker for right ventricular dysfunction? *Heart* 2000;84:409–415.

Hornung T. Transposition of the great arteries. In: Gatzoulis MA, Webb GD, Daubeney PEF, eds. *Chapter 41: Diagnosis and Management of Adult Congenital Heart Disease*. London, UK: Churchill Livingstone, 2004.

Puley G, Siu S, Connelly M, et al. Arrhythmia and survival in patients >18 years of age after the Mustard procedure for complete transposition of the great arteries. *Am J Cardiol* 1999;83:1080–1084.

Answer 3: D. Arrhythmias are rare in patients with coarctation of the aorta. VIDEO 39.1 shows a suprasternal notch view of the aortic arch with a tight narrowing at the aortic isthmus level, just distal to the left subclavian artery origin, consistent with coarctation of the aorta. Color Doppler interrogation shows turbulent flow pattern in this area consistent with obstruction. FIGURE 39.1 shows a characteristic "serrated" or "shark-tooth" Doppler pattern with early high-velocity systolic peak, followed by gradual deceleration throughout diastole (diastolic tailing). Peak flow velocity is elevated at 3.5 m/s and end-diastolic velocity is also abnormally elevated at 1 m/s (normal <0.5 m/s), both of which are consistent with severe coarctation of the aorta.

A. Bicuspid aortic valve occurs in up to 85% of patients with coarctation of the aorta.

B. Arterial hypertension is a common complication in such patients even after successful repair of coarctation of the aorta. Patients repaired at an older age are at greater risk than those operated in infancy or early childhood. Several factors that contribute to hypertension in these patients include residual coarctation or unrepaired hypoplastic aortic arch, alterations in renin–angiotensin receptors, structural changes in the vessel walls, and/or increased plasma epinephrine and norepinephrine concentrations.

C. Aneurysms of the circle of Willis (Berry aneurysms) occur in approximately 5% of adult patients with aortic coarctation.

D. Rib notching on the underside of ribs on a chest radiograph can be seen in patients with unrepaired coarctation of the aorta who are older than 5 years of age. It is caused by erosion of the underside of ribs by dilated collateral vessels.

Suggested Readings

Kaemmerer H. Aortic coarctation and interrupted aortic arch. In: Gatzoulis MA, Webb GD, Daubeney PEF, eds. *Chapter 30: Diagnosis and Management of Adult Congenital Heart Disease.* London, UK: Churchill Livingstone, 2004.

Marek J, Fenton M, Khambadkone S. Aortic arch anomalies: coarctation of the aorta and interrupted aortic arch. In: Lai WW, Mertens LL, Cohen MS, et al., eds. *Chapter 21: Echocardiography in Pediatric and Congenital Heart Disease: From Fetus to Adult.* Chichester, West Sussex, UK: Wiley-Blackwell Publishers, 2009.

Warnes CA. The adult with congenital heart disease: born to be bad? *J Am Coll Cardiol* 2005;46:1–8.

Answer 4: C.

A. False: Hypertension should be controlled with beta-blockers, ACE inhibitors, or angiotensin receptor blockers; however, the patient should undergo definite repair (see below) soon after diagnosis. Waiting for 3 months to reevaluate is not the correct action.

B. False: Arrhythmias are not a usual complication of this condition.

D. False: Bicuspid aortic valve is commonly associated with coarctation of the aorta; however, no information is given in this question on whether or not this patient has significant aortic stenosis to require valvuloplasty.

E. False: Rib notching is common long-term feature on CXR in patients with unrepaired coarctation of the aorta. No further imaging is needed for that.

Class I indications for surgical or interventional treatment of coarctation of the aorta include:

a. Peak-to-peak coarctation gradient ≥20 mm Hg (Level of Evidence C)

b. Peak-to-peak gradient <20 mm Hg, in the presence of anatomic imaging evidence of significant coarctation with radiologic evidence for significant collateral flow (significant collateral flow may underestimate the degree of obstruction) (Level of Evidence C)

The appropriate type of treatment for native coarctation of the aorta in adults, whether surgery or catheter interventional therapy, remains controversial at this time. Percutaneous catheter intervention is indicated for recurrent discrete coarctation and a peak-to-peak gradient of at least 20 mm Hg.

Suggested Reading

Warnes CA, Williams RG, Bashore TM, et al. ACC/AHA 2008 guidelines for the management of adults with congenital heart disease. *J Am Coll Cardiol* 2008;52:e143–e126.

Answer 5: B.

This patient has Turner syndrome, which is a clinical syndrome due to 45XO karyotype. Most common characteristics seen in patients with Turner syndrome are short stature and ovarian failure. BAV is a common problem in such patients (see next question discussion).

Answer A is incorrect as aortic regurgitation is associated with diastolic murmur.

Answer C is incorrect as the video clearly shows fusion of right and noncoronary aortic cusps causing bicuspid aortic valve.

Answer D is incorrect as this is a pathologic and not innocent murmur. Still murmur is the most common innocent heart murmur in children and young adults. It is seen in as many as 60% of children and typically heard the best at left sternal border and has characteristic vibratory quality. It is louder in supine position and does not radiate.

Answer B is correct, as Video 39.2 shows bicuspid aortic valve. Figure 39.2 shows a spectral Doppler evaluation across the aortic valve with peak gradient of 74 mm Hg, suggestive of aortic stenosis.

Suggested Readings

Goldmuntz E, Lin AE. Genetics of congenital heart defects. In: Allen HD, Driscoll DJ, Shaddy RE, et al., eds. *Chapter 23: Moss and Adams' Heart Disease in Infants, Children and Adolescents.* 7th ed. Philadelphia, PA: Lippincott Williams & Wilkins, 2008.

Goldmuntz E, Lin AE. Genetics of congenital heart defects. In: Allen HD, Driscoll DJ, Shaddy RE, et al., eds. *Chapter 26: Moss and Adams' Heart Disease in Infants, Children and Adolescents.* 7th ed. Philadelphia, PA: Lippincott Williams & Wilkins, 2008.

Answer 6: D.

Associated cardiac findings in Turner syndrome include bicuspid aortic valve in 10% to 20% and aortic coarctation (8%). These patients are at increased risk for aortic dissection and require periodic screening for this.

Renal abnormalities are commonly seen in patients with Turner syndrome and include horseshoe kidney and abnormal vascular supply. Patients should undergo renal ultrasound to screen for these problems at the time of diagnosis.

Pulmonary valve stenosis is an associated cardiac finding in patients with Noonan syndrome; it is not typically associated with Turner syndrome.

Suggested Readings

Bondy CA; Turner Syndrome Study Group. Care of girls and women with Turner syndrome: a guideline of the Turner syndrome study group. *J Clin Endocrinol Metab* 2007;92(1):10–25.

Hiratzka LF, Bakris GL, Beckman JA, et al. 2010 ACCF/AHA/AATS/ACR/ASA/SCA/SCAI/SIR/STS/SVM guidelines for the diagnosis and management of patients with thoracic aortic disease. *Circulation* 2010;121:e266–e369.

Answer 7: D. Echocardiographs cannot make assumptions regarding identification of great vessels and ventricles based upon location and typical views in congenital heart diseases. MUST PROVE IT through the segmental approach to echocardiography confirming morphologic features and connections.

Video 39.3 is that of an apical four-chamber view demonstrating more apical displacement of the left-sided atrioventricular valve insertion at the crux with faintly visible septal attachments indicating that this is the tricuspid valve. Therefore, the left-sided ventricle is the morphologic right ventricle. Moderator band is also seen. These structures are labeled on Figure 39.9. Video 39.4 shows that the posterior great artery divides, therefore making it the pulmonary artery. The anterior great artery, shown as a round circular structure, is slightly to the left of the posterior pulmonary artery. These findings are characteristic of congenitally corrected transposition of great arteries (synonyms include L-transposition of great arteries, ventricular inversion).

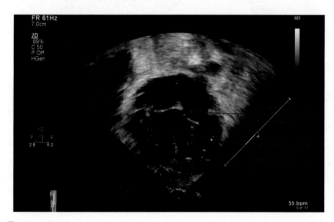

Figure 39.9

Systemic venous return is into the right-sided, morphologic right, atrium, through a morphologic mitral valve into a right-sided, morphologic left, ventricle, giving rise to the pulmonary artery. Pulmonary venous return is into the left-sided, morphologic left, atrium, through a morphologic tricuspid valve into a left-sided, morphologic right, ventricle and out into the aorta. The left-sided, morphologic right, ventricle is thus the systemic pumping chamber.

Common associated lesions include pulmonary valve stenosis, ventricular septal defect, and complete heart block. Using the segmental nomenclature, this condition is described as atrioventricular discordance and ventricular–arterial discordance. These patients are at risk for systemic, right ventricular failure with congestive heart failure at any point of life but commonly by fourth and fifth decades.

Coarctation of the aorta is not a common lesion in patients with L-TGA.

Suggested Readings

Graham TP Jr. Congenitally corrected transposition. In: Gatzoulis MA, Webb GD, Daubeney PEF, eds. *Chapter 43: Diagnosis and Management of Adult Congenital Heart Disease*. London, UK: Churchill Livingstone, 2004.

Hornung TS, Calder L. Congenitally corrected transposition of the great arteries. *Heart* 2010;96:1154–1161.

Answer 8: D. The accompanying still frame shows a continuous-wave Doppler signal with a high peak velocity of 4.1 m/s, characteristic of a pressure restrictive patent ductus arteriosus with a left-to-right shunt and a high peak instantaneous gradient of 67 mm Hg between the aorta and pulmonary artery.

Answer A is false as a normal flow murmur of pregnancy would not be expected to be associated with a high-velocity Doppler signal. During pregnancy, especially in third trimester, there is significant increase in maternal blood volume, which can cause flow-type murmurs across pulmonary valve. This is typically associated with peak velocity <2 m/s.

Answer B is incorrect as a typical Doppler pattern for a ventricular septal defect is a holosystolic signal, not a continuous signal throughout the cardiac cycle.

Answer C is false as Doppler signal associated with anomalous, possibly obstructed pulmonary venous connection would be continuous but velocities will be in the range as high as 2 m/s but not >4 m/s as demonstrated in this example. We typically report the mean gradient in cases of venous obstruction as they are more likely to correlate with cath data.

Answer E is false as atrial level shunts associated with atrial septal defects are not high velocity.

Suggested Readings

Moore P, Brook MM, Heymann MA. Patent ductus arteriosus and aortopulmonary window. In: Allen HD, Driscoll DJ, Shaddy RE, et al., eds. *Chapter 33: Moss and Adams' Heart Disease in Infants, Children and Adolescents*. 7th ed. Philadelphia, PA: Lippincott Williams & Wilkins, 2008.

Tacy TA. Abnormalities of ductus arteriosus and pulmonary arteries. In: Lai WW, Mertens LL, Cohen MS, et al., eds. *Chapter 18: Echocardiography in Pediatric and Congenital Heart Disease: From Fetus to Adult*. Chichester, West Sussex, UK: Wiley-Blackwell Publishers, 2009.

Answer 9: B. The accompanying video and still frames show a parasternal short-axis view, demonstrating a giant coronary artery aneurysm of the proximal right coronary artery. The origin of the right coronary artery is shown and measures 4 mm; the giant aneurysm measures 16.4 mm. See below for additional information on Kawasaki disease.

Answer A is false as aortopulmonary window consists of a defect in the proximal portion of the aortopulmonary septum between the semilunar valves and the pulmonary bifurcation. The defects are usually large and located between the main pulmonary artery and adjacent aorta.

Answer C is false because the origin of the right coronary artery is shown from the right sinus of Valsalva with no dilation of the sinus itself. There is severe dilation of the proximal coronary artery though.

Answer D is false as the aneurysm is located in the right coronary artery. A pericardial cyst will have echo-lucent appearance but in different location.

Answer E is false because a thrombus would appear echo-dense, not echo-lucent as shown in Figures 39.5 and 39.6.

Kawasaki disease was first reported by Tomisaku Kawasaki in 1967. It is an acute systemic vasculitis of unknown etiology. It is characterized by fever, bilateral nonexudative conjunctivitis, erythema of the lips and oral mucosa, changes in extremities, rash, and cervical lymphadenopathy. It occurs predominantly in infants and young children. Coronary artery aneurysms or ectasia develops in 15% to 25% of patients who do not receive treatment with intravenous gamma globulin (IVIG). Late cardiovascular complications include coronary artery aneurysms, coronary artery stenosis after aneurysmal healing, ischemic heart disease, acute myocardial infarction, sudden death, arrhythmia, congestive heart failure, systemic artery aneurysms, valvulopathy (mitral regurgitation), and early-onset atherosclerosis. Coronary aneurysms present abnormal blood flow and predispose to thrombus formation.

Suggested Readings

Daniels LB, Tjajadi MS, Walford HH, et al. Prevalence of Kawasaki disease in young adults with suspected myocardial ischemia. *Circulation* 2012;125:2447–2453.

Niwa K, Tateno S. Kawasaki's disease. In: Gatzoulis MA, Webb GD, Daubeney PEF, eds. *Chapter 49: Diagnosis and Management of Adult Congenital Heart Disease*. London, UK: Churchill Livingstone, 2004.

Newburger JW, Takahashi M, Beiser AS, et al. A single intravenous infusion of gamma globulin as compared with four infusions in the treatment of acute Kawasaki syndrome. *N Engl J Med* 1991;324:1633–1639.

Newburger JW, Takahashi M, Gerber MA, et al. Diagnosis, treatment and long-term management of Kawasaki disease: a statement for health professionals from the committee on rheumatic fever, endocarditis, and Kawasaki disease, council on cardiovascular disease in the young, American Heart Association. *Pediatrics* 2004;114:1708–1733.

Answer 10: B. Option A is incorrect. Figure 39.7 and Video 39.6 do not show the aortic arch well, but a normal BP in upper extremities makes it very unlikely for this case to be a severe coarctation of the aorta. Also, coarctation murmur will typically radiate to interscapular area over the back and not to one side. The best window to evaluate aortic arch is suprasternal window with marker around 1 o'clock, which delineated the arch in long axis.

Option C is incorrect. Aortopulmonary window consists of a defect in the proximal portion of the aortopulmonary septum between the semilunar valves and the pulmonary bifurcation. The defects are usually large and located between the main pulmonary artery and adjacent aorta. It is not that common to be seen first in later childhood or adulthood as unrepaired defects will lead to significant increase in pulmonary blood flow and congestive heart failure early followed by development of pulmonary hypertension. This is best imaged from parasternal short axis but can be hard to completely be ruled out based on 2D and color Doppler images only. Spectral Doppler evaluation of branch pulmonary arteries is key part of any congenital TTE, especially in AP window cases, where this will show abnormal continuous forward flow in branch PAs due to the abnormal connection between aorta and pulmonary artery, unlike the normal pattern with systolic flow only.

Option D is incorrect. We do not have enough echo images to evaluate all aspects of L-TGA in this patient, but the short-axis video (Video 39.6) and figure (Figure 39.7) provided in this case show the aorta rightward and posterior to the main PA, which is the normal relationship of great arteries. In L-TGA

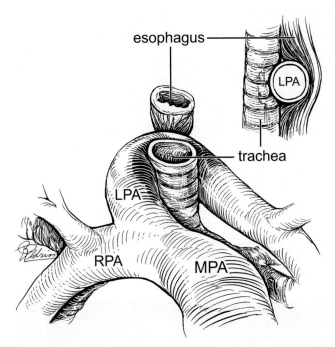

Figure 39.10

cases, the aorta and PA will be both seen as circles in a parasternal short-axis view with aorta anterior and leftward to the branching vessel (PA).

Option B is correct. Video 39.6 shows clearly the main PA giving rise to the RPA but does not show the LPA very clearly where it typically comes off (see Video 39.9 for normal origin of branch PAs). This should be a red flag for abnormal origin of LPA. One possible scenario here is LPA coming off the aorta, which puts the left lung vasculature under systemic pressure and leads to unilateral and sometimes bilateral pulmonary hypertension. The other possibility is LPA sling, which means LPA coming off the RPA instead of MPA with abnormal course between the trachea and esophagus (see Fig. 39.10). This is a rare congenital vascular abnormality that is usually diagnosed in infants and young children but can go undiagnosed into adulthood. This condition is often associated with complete tracheal rings in the area in touch with abnormal LPA vessel. Complete tracheal rings usually causes tracheal stenosis and can be devastating if undiagnosed before any endotracheal intubation as patient might be very hard to extubate after that. Due to the abnormal course of LPA, children with this issue might have swallowing difficulties of solids (esophageal compression) and sometimes airway issues with asthma like symptoms (tracheal compression). Barium swallow in such case would demonstrate anterior indentation of the esophagus, which can confirm diagnosis.

Suggested Reading

Eidem BW, et al. Chapter 20: Abnormalities of the aortic arch. In: O'Leary PW, Cetta F, eds. *Echocardiography in Pediatric and Adult Congenital Heart Disease*. 2nd ed. Philadelphia, PA: Wolters Kluwer, 2015:378–379.

Answer 11: B. Answer A will be correct if patient has severe coarctation of the aorta.

Answer C will be correct if patient has unrepaired AP window.

Answer D will be correct if patient has L-TGA.

As explained in previous question answers, this patient did not have normal-looking pulmonary artery branching, which is an indication to investigate more with another imaging modality. CMR is radiation free imaging and is the best option in this patient who is old enough to cooperate with instruction about breath holding and does not have any contraindication for the test. CT angiography is another possible modality that sometimes is used in younger patient to avoid sedation or if there is a contraindication for CMR. It does expose to ionizing radiation though.

This patient had CMR that showed LPA sling with LPA coming off the RPA and coursing posteriorly, posterior to trachea and anterior to esophagus. The LPA was mildly stenotic compared to RPA as expected in such case. Another advantage of CMR is ability to evaluate relative pulmonary blood flow between left and right lungs without need to do lung perfusion scan. In this case, the patient had 65% of her pulmonary blood flow directed to right lung and 35% to her left one. Normal range is about 55% to right lung and 45% to left one, but most experts agree that in asymptomatic patients, intervention is not needed unless the values are more in 75%, 25% range.

Most cases are quiet symptomatic in early childhood with swallowing difficulties and/or airway-related problems. Those are usually repaired with LPA reimplantation into MPA in addition to tracheoplasty to repair the complete tracheal rings and stenosis. This patient is being monitored with PFTs and CMRs every few years as an intervention may be required in the future.

Suggested Readings

Odell DD, et al. Pulmonary artery sling: a rare cause of tracheomalacia in the adult. *J Bronchology Interv Pulmonol* 2011;18:278–280.
Zabad A, et al. Anomalous origin of the left pulmonary artery from the right pulmonary artery (pulmonary artery sling). *Anesthesiology* 2013;119:1470.

Answer 12: D. The best view to evaluate coronary artery origin and proximal courses is a short-axis clip at the base of the heart just above the level of the aortic cusps (see Video 39.10). One should always try to confirm the 2D findings with color Doppler as artifacts are common in this view. Diastolic low-velocity flow in LAD and left main, away from the aorta, is important to confirm normal flow. The video provided shows the left main coronary artery originating right next to the right main coronary artery origin from the right sinus of Valsalva. The left main then courses anteriorly and leftward between the aorta and main PA (interarterial course). This anomaly is quite rare and seen in about 0.03% to 0.05% but has been clearly linked to increased risk of sudden cardiac death, usually during or shortly after vigorous exercise. The reported cases of sudden cardiac death are usually reported in teens or young adults and rarely in older adults (less likely to participate in high-intensity sports after certain age). In some cases, the left main coronary artery has an abnormal, slit-like, ostium and a short segment of it runs inside the anterior aortic wall (intramural course) before it exits and continues its course leftward. The definite diagnosis sometimes is not made until a different imaging modality is used (most commonly a CT angiography). This usually confirms the anatomy of coronary arteries, shows the course (intramural course increases the risk), and helps with surgical planning (3D visualization).

Answer A is incorrect. ALCAPA is a rare anomaly seen in 1:300,000 people. The left main coronary artery originates usually from the leftward and posterior aspect of the main pulmonary artery. This has variable presentations from significant ischemia and LV failure in early infancy due to pulmonary artery stealing blood from LCA system after the normal decrease in pulmonary vascular resistance (poorly developed collaterals from RCA) to accidental finding on autopsy in an adult who passed from different reason (collaterals from RCA perfuse LV myocardium well and preserve LV function). This is best visualized in parasternal long- and short-axis views. Color Doppler is very important in some cases as the left main CA sometimes gets very close to the left sinus of Valsalva before it turns anteriorly and inserts into the MPA (see Fig. 39.11). The color Doppler shows retrograde diastolic flow in LAD instead of the normal direction away from the aorta (see Fig. 39.12). One can sometimes show diastolic flow into the posterior

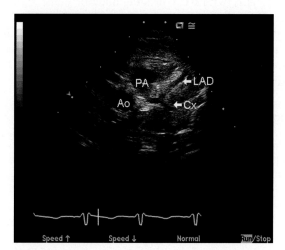

Figure 39.11

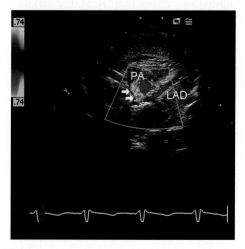

Figure 39.12

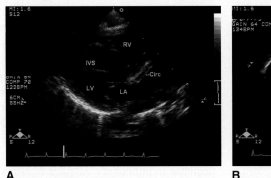
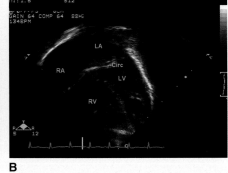

A   **B**

FIGURE 39.13

aspect of MPA. Treatment is usually surgical reimplantation into left sinus of Valsalva and, if done early in infancy, can be associated with excellent outcome.

Answer B is incorrect. The right coronary arises normally from the right sinus in this patient. Anomalous origin of right main coronary from left sinus of Valsalva is also rare and its association with sudden cardiac death is less clear than the one in answer E. The course is also interarterial usually with RCA heading anteriorly and rightward (VIDEO 39.11).

Answer C is incorrect. There are no signs of coronary artery dilation in the clip provided. Coronary artery aneurysms are often seen in the settings of Kawasaki disease and increase risk of thrombosis and ischemia.

Suggested Readings

Eidem BW, et al. Chapter 26: Vascular abnormalities. In: *Echocardiography in Pediatric and Adult Congenital Heart Disease.* 472–485.

Angelini P. Coronary artery anomalies: an entity in search of an identity. *Circulation* 2007;115:1296–1305.

Answer 13: *B.* In arterial switch operation and after aortic cross clamping, the ascending aorta and main pulmonary artery are transected. The left and right coronary artery ostia are visualized and excised from the aortic root with adjacent aortic wall as "buttons." The coronary artery buttons are then shifted posteriorly and implanted into the facing sinuses of the main pulmonary artery root. Next, the distal pulmonary artery and its branches are brought forward (**LeCompte maneuver**), and the distal aorta is moved posteriorly. The distal aorta is now anastomosed to the "new" aortic root. Reconstruction of the pulmonary artery is undertaken next, utilizing a patch of cryopreserved pulmonary artery homograft (see FIG. 39.13). Due to the LeCompte maneuver the branch pulmonary arteries straddle the ascending aorta as seen in the video in this patient. This increases the risk of stretching of the vessels and developing of branch pulmonary artery stenosis.

Answer A is incorrect. Retroaortic course of innominate vein is a normal and rare variant that shows a venous structure posterior to the aortic arch in suprasternal views, just superior to the normal right pulmonary artery.

Answer C is incorrect. There is clear separation between the branch pulmonary arteries and ascending aorta so this is not a dilation of the aorta.

Answer D is incorrect. This is not a true entity. Arteriovenous malformation can form at various locations but not between the innominate vein and pulmonary artery.

Suggested Readings

Delmo Walter EM, et al. Onset of pulmonary stenosis after arterial switch operation for transposition of great arteries with intact ventricular septum. *HSR Proc Intensive Care Cardiovasc Anesth* 2011;3(3):177–187.

Eidem BW, et al. Chapter 16: D-Transposition of the great arteries. *Echocardiography in Pediatric and Adult Congenital Heart Disease.*

Chapter 40

Venous Anomalies

Kristopher M. Cumbermack

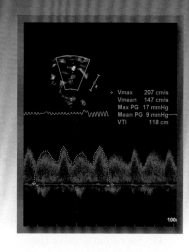

1. A 20-year-old female is referred for cardiac consultation due to murmur after recent post streptococcal arthralgia. What is the most likely cardiac diagnosis based upon the images provided in Videos 40.1 to 40.3?

   A. Partial anomalous pulmonary venous return (PAPVR)
   B. Total anomalous pulmonary venous return (TAPVR)
   C. Large sinus venosus ASD
   D. Large cerebral arteriovenous malformation
   E. Left SVC to coronary sinus

2. A 30-year-old male with a history of Tetralogy of Fallot (TOF) repair performed in Hungary presents to establish care. Records are unavailable. He works in construction and has been experiencing progressive shortness of air and fatigue at work over the last 6 months. What venous anomaly should be evaluated for via echocardiography prior to potential surgical intervention if indicated?

   A. Retroaortic innominate vein
   B. Pulmonary arteriovenous malformation
   C. Venovenous collaterals
   D. TAPVR
   E. Persistent left SVC to coronary sinus

3. A 37-year-old female presents with dyspnea on exertion. Pulse oximetry reveals normal O_2 saturation. A chest x-ray reveals mesocardia, a hazy right lung field with probable right lung hypoplasia, and a vertical density noted from the right heart border to just below the right diaphragm. An echocardiogram with limited imaging is performed (see Videos 40.4 and 40.5).

   The most likely diagnosis is:

   A. Pulmonary hypertension
   B. Eventration of right diaphragm
   C. Pulmonary arteriovenous malformations of the right lung
   D. Scimitar syndrome
   E. Tracheoesophageal fistula with chronic aspiration

4. Videos 40.6 to 40.8 are obtained on an outpatient 18-year-old referred secondary to a heart murmur. Based on your interpretation of the following images, this patient is most at risk for which of the following?

   A. Intracranial berry aneurysms
   B. Fulminant sepsis secondary to *Streptococcus pneumoniae*
   C. Cirrhosis
   D. Early-onset atherosclerosis
   E. Pulmonary embolism

5. A 27-year-old female without prior cardiac history presents to ER with 2-week history of worsening cough and fever. Her chest x-ray is shown in Figure 40.1. Based on this image and Videos 40.9 and 40.10, for what medical problem is she at increased risk assuming no outflow tract or conotruncal abnormalities?

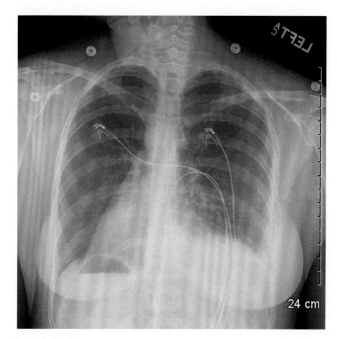

Figure 40.1

   A. Recurrent respiratory infections
   B. Intestinal malrotation
   C. Congenital heart disease
   D. Infections from encapsulated bacteria
   E. Cardiac dysrhythmia

6. An 18-year-old male with developmental delay presents to the ER from an assisted living facility with tachypnea and

respiratory distress. He has a sternotomy scar, but records are currently unavailable. A chest x-ray demonstrates pulmonary edema. What is the most likely original form of congenital heart disease based upon this history and the postoperative complication shown in Video 40.11?

A. Sinus venosus ASD with partial anomalous pulmonary venous return (PAPVR)
B. Supracardiac type of total anomalous pulmonary venous return (TAPVR)
C. Transposition of great arteries
D. Supramitral valve ring
E. TAPVR to coronary sinus

7. A 37-year-old female with a history of D-transposition of the great arteries (D-TGA) status post Mustard procedure presents with swelling of her neck and left arm in addition to a noticeable decrease in her energy level. What should be the focus of her echocardiogram?

A. Branch pulmonary arteries
B. Coronary arteries
C. Superior limb of the systemic venous baffle
D. Inferior limb of the systemic venous baffle
E. Pulmonary venous baffle

8. A 23-year-old male with a history of double-inlet left ventricle s/p bidirectional Glenn and extracardiac, fenestrated Fontan procedure presents to the clinic for annual evaluation. Family members report increasing episodes of blue lips especially with exercise. In the office, O_2 saturations are 80% compared to 90% 1 year prior. An exercise stress test is performed and O_2 saturations drop to the 70s without dysrhythmias or signs of ischemia. Patient is taken to cardiac cath lab for hemodynamic study and intervention. What intervention is undertaken as shown in attached video clips (Videos 40.12 to 40.15) to address his desaturation?

A. Device closure of ASD
B. Balloon dilation of Fontan circuit stenosis
C. Device closure of fenestration
D. Device closure of venovenous collateral
E. Device closure of coronary fistula to right atrium

Answer 1: A. PAPVR is the term used when one or more pulmonary veins, but not all pulmonary veins, return anomalously to the right atrium via a variety of potential routes. They can connect superiorly to the innominate vein or SVC, to the right atrium directly or via the coronary sinus, or inferiorly to the IVC, hepatic veins, ductus venosus, or portal veins. Physiology of this left-to-right shunt (oxygenated pulmonary venous return to right atrium) is similar to that of a secundum ASD with a volume load to and subsequent dilation of the right atrium and right ventricle (Video 40.1). PAPVR is often seen in cases of superior and inferior sinus venosus ASDs though can occur in isolation. Risk of upper respiratory infection is increased and exercise tolerance can be impaired though patients can be relatively asymptomatic for decades.

B is incorrect as TAPVR causes critical illness as a neonate if obstructed and presents in infancy if unobstructed. Diagnosis or death would occur prior to 20 years of age.

C is incorrect as the subcostal bicaval view (Video 40.3) demonstrates absence of sinus venosus defects both inferiorly and superiorly.

D is incorrect as a large cerebral arteriovenous malformation would cause an increase in flow from the cerebral arterial to venous circulation causing dilation and prominence of flow in the SVC not seen in Video 40.3. Significant diastolic reversal of flow in the aortic arch can also be seen if shunt is large. In congenital forms, this can be detected in infancy via a cranial bruit through anterior fontanelle or from associated symptoms.

E is incorrect as a left coronary sinus causes dilation of the coronary sinus but would not cause dilation of the right atrium or ventricle as volume of blood flow to right-sided heart structures is normal.

Suggested Readings

Allen HD, et al, ed. *Moss and Adams' Heart Disease in Infants, Children, and Adolescents, Including the Fetus and Young Adult.* 9th ed. Baltimore, MD: Lippincott Williams & Wilkins, 2016.

Crystal MA, Al Najashi K, Williams WG, et al. Inferior sinus venosus defect: echocardiographic diagnosis and surgical approach. *J Thorac Cardiovasc Surg* 2009;137(6):1349–1355.

Oliver JM, Gallego P, Gonzalez A, et al. Sinus venosus syndrome: atrial septal defect or anomalous venous connection? A multiplane transesophageal approach. *Heart* 2002;88(6):634–638.

Snarr BS, et al. The parasternal short-axis view improves diagnostic accuracy for inferior sinus venosus type of atrial septal defects by transthoracic echocardiography. *J Am Soc Echocardiogr* 2017. pii: S0894-7317(16)30755-6.

Answer 2: E. Persistent LSVC to coronary sinus can be seen in isolation but also is associated with congenital heart disease including TOF. This benign variant does not require intervention. However, congenital heart surgeons need to know of its presence for cannulation purposes to avoid blood flowing into their surgical field. First sign is often a dilated coronary sinus seen in the parasternal long axis or apical view (Figs. 40.2 and 40.3). Subsequent imaging is focused on identifying the cause

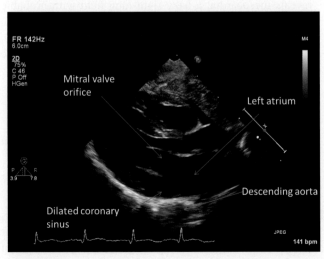

Figure 40.2

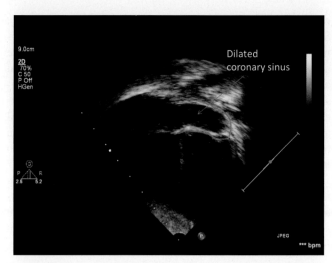

FIGURE 40.3

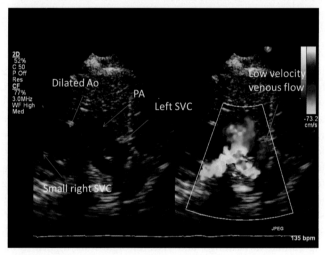

FIGURE 40.4

of dilated coronary sinus, which is most commonly persistent LSVC (Fig. 40.4, Video 40.16).

A is incorrect as a retroaortic innominate vein is a benign finding without surgical significance. In suprasternal sagittal imaging of the aortic arch, the innominate vein is seen passing caudal to the aortic arch as an additional lumen to the usually solitary right pulmonary artery seen in short axis. The innominate vein typically passes cephalad to the aortic arch as it traverses toward the right SVC (Video 40.17).

B is incorrect as pulmonary arteriovenous malformations are abnormal connections between the pulmonary artery and pulmonary veins typically seen in single ventricle patients having undergone Glenn operation, typically prior to Fontan procedure as felt to be related to lack of yet to be identified hepatic factor flowing to the pulmonary vasculature. These can be identified via a microcavitation or agitated saline study with injection into an upper extremity leading to microcavitations seen in the left atrium (from pulmonary artery to pulmonary vein to left atrium), whereas if pulmonary AVMs were absent, microcavitations would be filtered out by the pulmonary microvasculature (Video 40.18).

C is incorrect. Venovenous collaterals are not associated with Tetralogy of Fallot and are most commonly seen in single ventricle patients that have undergone Fontan procedure. When Fontan circuit pressures rise, venovenous collaterals can develop serving as a pressure pop-off. A common example is innominate vein to left atrium. These are typically diagnosed by cardiac catheterization and not by echocardiography.

D is incorrect as though TAPVR can be seen in patients with TOF, this would have required surgical intervention in infancy.

Suggested Readings

Geva T, Van Praagh S. Abnormal systemic venous connections. In: Allen HD, et al, eds. *Chapter 38: Moss and Adams' Heart Disease in Infants, Children and Adolescents.* 7th ed. Philadelphia, PA: Lippincott Williams & Wilkins, 2008:792–817.

Goyal SK, Punnam SR, Verma G, et al. Persistent left superior vena cava: a case report and review of literature. *Cardiovasc Ultrasound* 2008;6:50.

Kavarana MN, et al. Pulmonary arteriovenous malformations after the superior cavopulmonary shunt: mechanisms and clinical implications. *Expert Rev Cardiovasc Ther* 2014;12(6):703–713. doi:10. 1586/14779072.2014.912132.

Answer 3: D.

Option A: False. Possible with scimitar syndrome if anomalous veins are obstructed but not seen here.

Option B: False. In differential of abnormal shadow on chest x-ray and occasionally associated with congenital heart anomalies but not classically with those presented here.

Option C: False. Pulmonary AVMs are associated with desaturation.

Option D: *Correct. See discussion below.*

Option E: False. The majority of patients with TE fistula are symptomatic in the neonatal period and the patient in this scenario is 37 years old. Rarely, H-type fistulae may present later but are not a common association with scimitar syndrome.

Scimitar syndrome is a type of partial anomalous pulmonary venous return in which some or occasionally all of the right pulmonary veins drain anomalously to the IVC. The name scimitar derives from the abnormal chest x-ray finding of a curved linear shadow along the right heart border (resembling a Turkish sword) of the anomalous right pulmonary veins coalescing and draining inferiorly to the IVC. The right lung and right pulmonary artery are typically hypoplastic. The echocardiogram images presented in this case reveal severe RPA hypoplasia and an abnormal flow pattern in the IVC near insertion into the right atrium, which in the setting of mesocardia or dextrocardia (secondary to right lung hypoplasia) should lead to the suspicion of scimitar syndrome. Frequently, additional imaging (cardiac CT, MRI, and/or catheterization) is required to confirm the diagnosis. Additionally, sequestration of a right pulmonary lobe may occur with the only source of blood flow to the affected area originating from collaterals off the descending or abdominal aorta. There is significant clinical variation with scimitar as some children present in infancy with severe symptoms and pulmonary hypertension, whereas adults may be discovered incidentally based on an abnormal chest x-ray.

Suggested Readings

Gudjonsson U, Brown JW. Scimitar syndrome. *Semin Thorac Cardiovasc Surg Pediatr Card Surg Annu* 2006:56–62.

Najm HK, Williams WG, Coles JG, et al. Scimitar syndrome: twenty years' experience and results of repair. *J Thorac Cardiovasc Surg* 1996;112(5):1161.

Answer 4: B.

Option A: False. Berry aneurysms are seen in approximately 5% to 10% of patients with coarctation of the aorta.

Option B: *Correct. See discussion.*

Option C: False. Cirrhosis is not typically associated with heterotaxy syndromes.

Option D: False. Atherosclerosis is not a common complication of heterotaxy syndromes.

Option E: False. Pulmonary hypertension occurs commonly in heterotaxy secondary to complex congenital heart disease, but pulmonary embolism is infrequent.

The subcostal transverse image in VIDEO 40.6 shows a midline liver with a small, low-velocity venous structure posterior and rightward of the pulsatile, abdominal aorta. As opposed to the normal relationship, situs solitus (VIDEO 40.7), where the liver is located on the right and the IVC is anterior and rightward of the abdominal aorta, VIDEO 40.6 demonstrates one of several forms of situs ambiguous where the liver is midline and the IVC is interrupted with azygous continuation (the posterior venous structure is termed "hemiazygous" if located leftward of the abdominal aorta). Situs ambiguous is a feature of heterotaxy syndrome, which is the result of failed signaling pathways that differentiate right- and left-sided organ development.

The two primary forms of heterotaxy syndrome are left and right atrial isomerism meaning "double left" or "double right" respectively with cardiac atria, lung morphology (including lobes and pulmonary and bronchial branching patterns), and abdominal viscera matching in the vast majority of cases (FIG. 40.5). The term left atrial isomerism is used when two morphologic left atria, two bilobed left lungs and multiple spleens ("polysplenia") form as in the case described here. In right atrial isomerism, two morphologic right atria develop; two trilobed, morphologic

right lungs form; and the spleen never develops ("asplenia"). Subcostal transverse imaging is a critical component of the segmental approach to echocardiography in congenital heart disease as it confirms situs solitus or identifies cases of situs inversus and ambiguous. VIDEO 40.8 shows an example of juxtaposed relationship of the abdominal aorta and IVC as seen in right atrial isomerism. Systemic and pulmonary venous abnormalities, as well as, a variety of complex congenital heart disease are common in heterotaxy syndrome, though venous abnormalities can occur in isolation without diagnosis of heterotaxy in rare cases.

Important noncardiac abnormalities to consider in heterotaxy syndrome are intestinal malrotation with risk of volvulus and susceptibility to infections from encapsulated organisms, such as *Streptococcus pneumoniae*, due to asplenia or functional asplenia in the case of polysplenia.

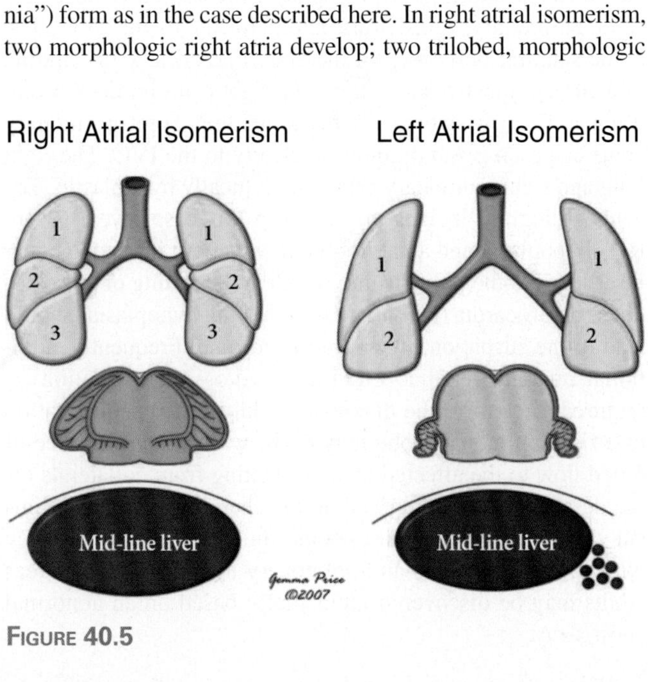

Suggested Reading

Jacobs JP, et al. The nomenclature, definition and classification of cardiac structures in the setting of heterotaxy. *Cardiol Young* 2007;17(suppl 2):1–28. doi:10.1017/S1047951107001138

Answer 5: A. The chest x-ray demonstrates dextrocardia. Situs inversus is demonstrated in VIDEO 40.9 with liver on the left, aorta to the right of the spine, and IVC anterior and left of the aorta, which is mirror image of normal situs solitus. VIDEO 40.10 shows a 4-chamber view with mirror image dextrocardia, where the morphologic right ventricle is on the left and the morphologic left ventricle is on the right (marker is kept to patient's left so left side of patient remains on right side of screen). The atrioventricular valves, atria, and ventricles appear normal. Assuming no conotruncal abnormalities, these findings are consistent with situs inversus totalis with mirror image dextrocardia. Situs inversus totalis refers to when left-sided structures of the body including cardiac atria, lungs, and visceral organs are flipped to the right side and right-sided structures switched to the left.

A variety of terminologies are used to describe cardiac location and orientation depending on physician and medical center. Adding a general description to clarify the nomenclature is recommended. One approach is to utilize the base word "position" to describe heart location within the thorax with levoposition, mesoposition and dextroposition referring to left, middle, and right locations. The root word "cardia" can be used to describe orientation of the cardiac apex with levocardia, mesocardia, and dextrocardia referring to apex left, center, or right, respectively. Mirror image dextrocardia is a phrase used when the heart is mirror image from its normal location and orientation. Risk of congenital heart disease or other significant cardiac pathology is not increased in these cases. However, situs inversus totalis is linked with Kartagener syndrome, where disorders of cilia lead to recurrent respiratory infections among other problems. In contrast, dextroversion is a term used to describe dextrocardia without mirror imaging; the left atria and ventricle comprise the left side and the right atria and ventricle comprise the right side of the heart. Dextroversion is typically associated with congenital heart disease.

B, intestinal malrotation can be seen in heterotaxy syndrome but not situs inversus totalis.

C is incorrect as described above.

Right Atrial Isomerism   **Left Atrial Isomerism**

Mid-line liver   Mid-line liver

Gemma Price ©2007

FIGURE **40.5**

D is incorrect. Patients with heterotaxy and splenic dysfunction are at increased risk for infections from encapsulated organisms.

E is incorrect; patients with situs inversus totalis are not at increased risk for dysrhythmias.

Suggested Reading

Eidem et al. *Echocardiography in Pediatric and Adult Congenital Heart Disease.* 2nd ed. Chapter 2. Philadelphia, PA: Wolters Kluwer, 2015.

Answer 6: B. VIDEO 40.11 shows significant flow acceleration by color Doppler at the surgical anastomosis site between a posterior confluence that receives anomalous pulmonary veins in TAPVR (originally draining to the innominate vein via vertical vein) and the posterior wall of the left atrium consistent with significant stenosis (FIG. 40.6). This complication increases pulmonary venous pressures and hydrostatic pressure in the pulmonary capillary beds causing the pulmonary edema seen on CXR and the respiratory symptoms. This patient was taken to the operating room for surgical revision with good outcome. One could not differentiate supracardiac type from others from this image alone. Other anatomical variations of TAPVR include cardiac, infracardiac, and mixed (FIG. 40.7).

A is incorrect. Typically, one or more right-sided pulmonary veins will drain to the SVC in cases of superior sinus venosus ASD. One surgical approach is the Warden procedure where the SVC is resected cephalad to the entrance of the anomalous pulmonary veins and reattached to the right atrial appendage. The remaining anomalous veins entering the proximal portion of the SVC are baffled through an atrial communication to the left atrium. Obstruction to this baffle would be seen in the area of the native SVC or pathway through the atrial septum to LA.

C is incorrect as current surgical approach for D-TGA is the arterial switch operation that does not involve the atria.

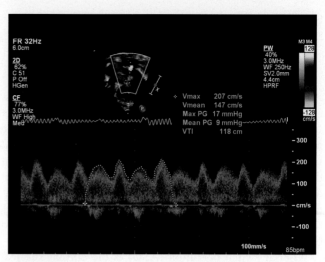

FIGURE 40.6

If an older patient underwent an atrial switch, either Mustard or Senning, systemic venous or pulmonary venous baffles can develop obstruction but would not appear at the border of the left atrial wall and an extracardiac, posterior structure. Instead, the inferior or superior systemic limbs of baffle to the left-sided mitral valve or pulmonary venous baffle to right-sided tricuspid valve would show areas of flow acceleration by color Doppler with increased mean gradient.

D is incorrect as recurrence of supramitral ring or residual obstruction would be seen below the left atrial appendage in closer proximity to the mitral valve annulus.

E is incorrect as the surgical approach to TAPVR to coronary sinus is to unroof the coronary sinus and allow drainage of the anomalous pulmonary veins into the left atrium. Postsurgical obstruction would be located in the vicinity of the dilated coronary sinus as opposed to superior, posterior aspect of the left atrium.

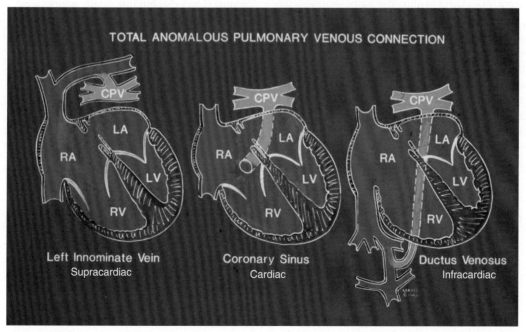

FIGURE 40.7

Suggested Reading

Eidem et al. *Echocardiography in Pediatric and Adult Congenital Heart Disease.* 2nd ed. Chapter 5. Philadelphia, PA: Wolters Kluwer, 2015.

Answer 7: C. TGA is a form of cyanotic congenital heart disease comprised of an aorta arising from a morphologic right ventricle and a pulmonary artery arising from a morphologic left ventricle. In D-TGA, the ventricles are in their normal D-looped position with morphologic left ventricle to the left of the right ventricle and morphologic right ventricle to the right of the left ventricle. Concordance of atrial to ventricular connections with discordance of the ventricular–arterial connections results in two circuits of blood flowing in parallel instead of in series.

Arterial switch operation (ASO) is the current surgical approach involving moving the main pulmonary artery to the aortic valve and the aortic arch to the pulmonary valve to create normal blood flow in series. The coronary arteries must also be moved to the neo-aortic root via "button" technique.

Historically, one of two atrial switch operations was performed to enable blood to flow in parallel. Mustard procedure uses either pericardium or Dacron patch material to create baffles connecting pulmonary blood flow to the tricuspid valve and systemic blood flow to the mitral valve. The Senning procedure accomplishes same redirection of venous flow, however using atrial tissue instead of patch material. These operations leave a systemic morphologic right ventricle, which fails over time as it is not designed to pump against a high resistance systemic circuit. Atrial surgeries also increased risk of significant atrial arrhythmias.

This patient underwent Mustard procedure and developed obstruction of the superior limb of the systemic venous baffle leading to SVC-like syndrome (Video 40.19). Cardiac catheterization confirmed the diagnosis giving limited echo imaging, and stent placement within the baffle relieved the obstruction and her symptoms.

A is incorrect as branch pulmonary arteries are not part of atrial switch procedures. One component of the ASO however is the LeCompte maneuver where the branch pulmonary arteries are pulled anteriorly and can result in stretching and branch pulmonary artery stenosis.

B is incorrect as coronary arteries are not involved in atrial switch operations and symptoms in clinical vignette are not consistent with coronary issue. Evaluation of coronary system however is important after ASO as coronaries are translocated from the native aortic root to the neo-aortic root and can be stretched or kinked. "Button" technique avoids surgery on coronary ostia, and ostial stenosis is not typically encountered.

D is incorrect as obstruction to inferior venous return would not result in swelling of neck and upper extremity.

E is incorrect as obstruction to a pulmonary venous baffle would lead to increased pulmonary venous pressure and hydrostatic pressure within the pulmonary vasculature resulting in pulmonary edema and respiratory symptoms.

Suggested Reading

Eidem et al. *Echocardiography in Pediatric and Adult Congenital Heart Disease.* 2nd ed. Chapter 39. Philadelphia, PA: Wolters Kluwer, 2015.

Answer 8: C. Fontan fenestration is a circular punch that connects the Fontan circuit with the right atrium. This enables maintenance of cardiac output in settings of high pulmonary vascular resistance at the expense of oxygen saturation via right-to-left shunt. Fenestration closure will remove this right-to-left shunt and raise the overall saturation levels. Catheterization cines confirmed absence of significant venovenous collaterals and Fontan baffle leaks. TEE images demonstrate Fontan fenestration (Video 40.14) and subsequent device closure (Video 40.15). Transthoracic imaging can evaluate the IVC and inferior portion of Fontan baffle as well as the Glenn with SVC anastomosis to right pulmonary artery.

A is incorrect as the shunting demonstrated is from Fontan circuit to RA and not across the atrial septum.

B is incorrect as echo imaging does not demonstrate Fontan stenosis or a catheter-based balloon.

D is incorrect as venovenous collaterals are not typically identified by echo but instead by angiograms.

E is incorrect as coronary artery fistula to right atrium would consist of diastolic signal into right atrium and would not cause systemic desaturation.

Suggested Reading

Stout KK, et al. Echocardiographic evaluation of univentricular physiology and cavopulmonary shunts. *Echocardiography* 2015;32(suppl 2):S166–S176. doi:10.1111/echo.12133.

Chapter 41

Heart Diseases in Congenital Syndromes

Majd Makhoul

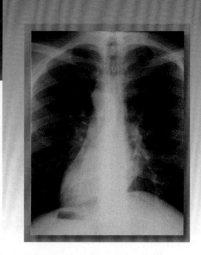

1. A 19-year-old male is evaluated by echocardiography due to a family history of two paternal uncles who died suddenly in their 30s. His height is >95th percentile for age, and he has a pectus excavatum deformity of the sternum and a high-arched palate. Images from his echocardiogram are shown in Figure 41.1 and Video 41.1. Which of the following additional findings would most likely be found?

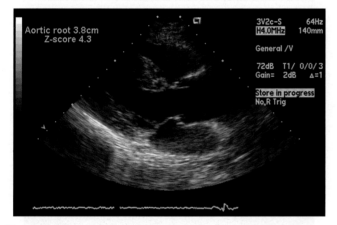

FIGURE 41.1

   A. Fetal genetic screening would have shown 47XY + 21.
   B. An abnormal fibrillin protein.
   C. Six fingers on his right hand.
   D. Supravalvular stenosis in the pulmonary tree with additional focused echo images.
   E. A bifid uvula.

2. An 18-year-old male with Down syndrome (trisomy 21) has recently immigrated to the United States with his family. He showed up in a cardiologist office with no records, but family reports he had open heart surgery at 1 year of age. His 4-chamber echocardiogram clip is shown in Video 41.2. What is the most likely congenital heart defect that he had?

   A. Secundum ASD patch repair
   B. Complete AV canal repair
   C. Partial AV canal repair
   D. TOF repair
   E. Arterial switch for D-TGA

3. Which of the following findings on transthoracic echocardiogram are most consistent with a diagnosis of Noonan syndrome?

   A. Hypertrophic left ventricle and a dysplastic, stenotic pulmonary valve
   B. Nonhypertrophied left ventricle and a secundum ASD
   C. Tetralogy of Fallot with a patent ductus arteriosus
   D. Hypertrophic left ventricle and a dysplastic, stenotic aortic valve
   E. Bicuspid, stenotic aortic valve with coarctation of the aorta

4. A 10-year-old girl with mild dysmorphic features and hypertension is sent for echocardiography (see Fig. 41.2A and B and Videos 41.3A and B). Based on the echo findings seen, the most likely diagnosis from a genetic standpoint is:

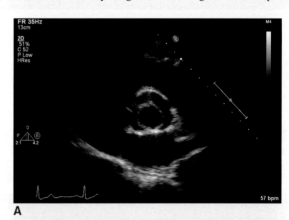

A

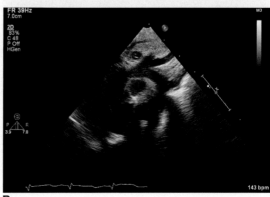

B

FIGURE 41.2

A. Trisomy 21.

B. Williams syndrome.

C. Trisomy 13.

D. Turner syndrome.

E. These echo findings are not associated with a congenital syndrome.

5. An 18-year-old, very outgoing, but dysmorphic young man has a history of severe pulmonary branch stenosis as an infant with subsequent resolution. He had no cardiac follow-up for several years and at most recent PCP evaluation found to have a new murmur. An echocardiogram is performed with the findings shown in Figure 41.3 and Video 41.4.

Based on these images, the most likely genetic diagnosis is:

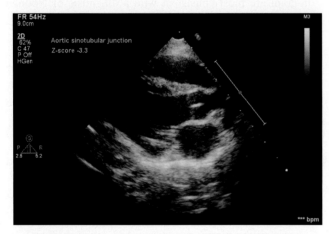

Figure 41.3

A. Trisomy 18

B. DiGeorge syndrome

C. Williams syndrome

D. Noonan syndrome

6. The echocardiographic image in Figure 41.4 and Video 41.5 was obtained in a patient with an absent right thumb. The most likely genetic diagnosis in this patient is:

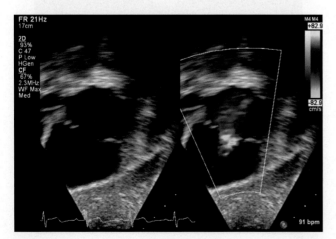

Figure 41.4

A. DiGeorge syndrome

B. Holt-Oram syndrome

C. Ellis-van Creveld syndrome

D. Trisomy 21

7. A 15-year-old patient with dysmorphic features is sent for echocardiography (Fig. 41.5 and Videos 41.6A and B). Based on the findings, the most likely genetic diagnosis is:

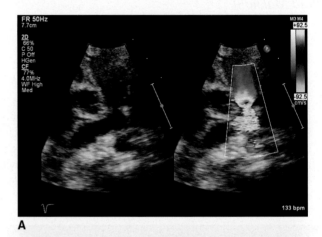

A

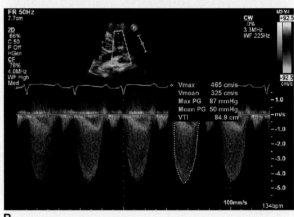

B

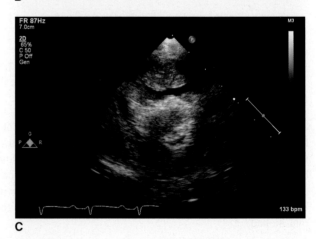

C

Figure 41.5

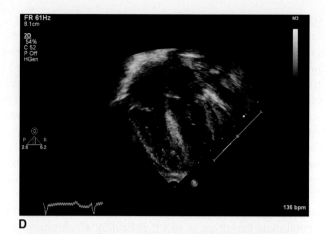

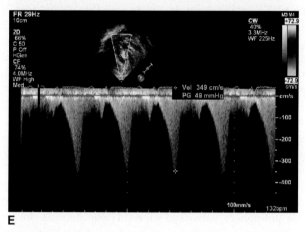

D

E

FIGURE 41.5 *(Continued)*

A. Turner syndrome
B. Williams syndrome
C. Trisomy 13
D. Noonan syndrome

8. You are seeing a 20-year-old male with a history of tracheoesophageal fistula repair in infancy in addition to vertebral anomaly and single kidney. He has history of "hole in the heart" as per his family. They were told that his hole

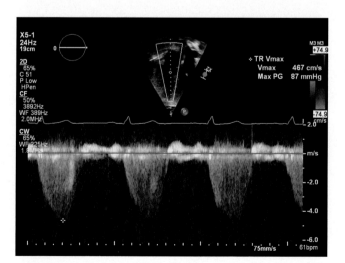

FIGURE 41.6

has naturally closed by extra tissue from one of the valves and would not need surgery. Last cardiac evaluation was at 10 years of age. He has recently developed some exertional SOB, and his PCP heard a new systolic ejection murmur on him so sent him for an echocardiogram. Based on Videos 41.7 and 41.8 and Figures 41.6 and 41.7, what is the likely cause of his murmur?

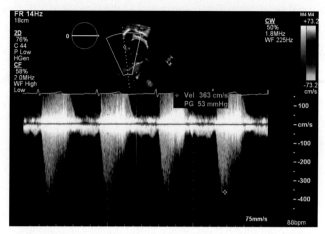

FIGURE 41.7

A. Tricuspid regurgitation from severe pulmonary hypertension
B. Ventricular septal defect with left-to-right shunting
C. Double-chambered right ventricle
D. Pulmonary valve stenosis

9. Which one of the following statements is true regarding 22q11 deletion syndrome?

A. Interrupted aortic arch is the most common CHD associated with it.
B. Conotruncal anomalies are uncommon.
C. Approximately 30% of patients with 22q11 deletion have congenital heart disease.
D. Majority of patients have complete DiGeorge syndrome and impaired immune system.
E. D-transposition of the great arteries is common in this syndrome.

10. Which of the following echocardiographic images should be most carefully investigated in a patient with Williams syndrome?

A. Speckle tracking to assess LV strain
B. Parasternal short-axis imaging of the coronary artery origins
C. Subcostal long-axis imaging of the atrial septum
D. High parasternal angled views to image the branch pulmonary arteries
E. Suprasternal notch imaging of the proximal descending aorta

Questions 11 and 12

An 18-year-old male presents for consultation due to a family history of sudden cardiac death in his brother at age 30. Autopsy showed aortic dissection and tortuous head and neck vessels. He is asymptomatic and physical exam reveals mild hypertension (140/85 mm Hg) and bifid uvula. His femoral pulses are excellent. His echocardiogram shows structurally normal heart with dilated aortic root at the sinuses of Valsalva level with maximal dimension of 38 mm.

11. What is the likely genetic syndrome?

    A. Williams syndrome
    B. Turner syndrome
    C. Noonan syndrome
    D. Loeys-Dietz syndrome

12. What is the best next step in managing this patient?

    A. Renal US with Doppler to evaluate for renal artery stenosis
    B. Karyotype and endocrinology consultation
    C. Cardiac MRI to evaluate branch pulmonary arteries better
    D. Start on ARB and repeat aortic imaging in 6 months

13. An 18-year-old male with a history of recurrent sinusitis, and chronic cough was referred to your clinic due to the abnormality seen on his chest x-ray (see Fig. 41.8).

His echocardiogram shows no structural cardiac defects with one abnormal finding seen in subcostal coronal view (Video 41.9). What is the likely genetic syndrome?

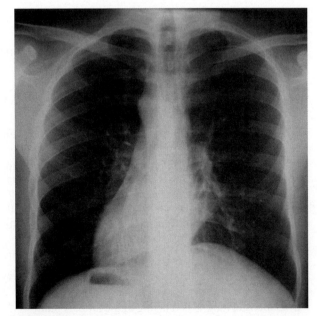

FIGURE 41.8

    A. DiGeorge syndrome
    B. Turner syndrome
    C. Klinefelter syndrome
    D. Noonan syndrome
    E. Kartagener syndrome

Answer 1: B. The image demonstrates a dilated aortic root at the sinuses of Valsalva level (*Z*-score 4.3). In addition, there is evidence of mitral valve prolapse. These findings are most consistent with Marfan syndrome. Marfan syndrome, due to an abnormal fibrillin protein (Option B is single best answer), results in aortic root dilation. This abnormality may progress to an aortic aneurysm. Close observation is essential since progressive dilation leads to risk of aortic dissection. Beta-blocker or ARB therapy may slow progression. Mitral valve prolapse is also common, and with time, significant mitral regurgitation may result in need for mitral valve intervention (Fig. 41.9 and Video 41.10).

Down syndrome is most commonly due to trisomy 21. Normal male karyotype is 46XY, indicating 46 chromosomes with an XY arrangement. In a male with Down syndrome, the extra chromosome (usually located near the 21q22.1-q22.3 region) is written as 47XY + 21. This syndrome is associated with congenital heart disease, most commonly ventricular septal defects and atrioventricular canal defects. Therefore, Option A is incorrect.

Ellis-van Creveld syndrome (also referred to as chondro-ectodermal dysplasia) is an unusual syndrome associated with polydactyly and other skeletal abnormalities such as a sixth digit. The most common cardiovascular abnormality is a large ASD resulting in a common atrium. Therefore, Option C is incorrect.

Patients with Noonan syndrome most commonly demonstrate pulmonary valve and supravalvular stenosis. In addition, Noonan syndrome patients can have abnormalities of the aortic valve and/or hypertrophic cardiomyopathy. Therefore, Option D is incorrect.

Loeys-Dietz syndrome is another connective tissue disorder first described in 2005, with the unusual classic finding of a bifid uvula. Loeys-Dietz syndrome is associated with aortic dilation but also more diffuse arterial pathology. These patients should undergo MRI or CT imaging to identify such pathology and can have dissection at smaller diameters. Therefore, Option E is not the single best answer.

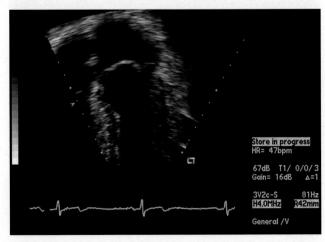

FIGURE 41.9

Suggested Readings

Bruno L, Tredici S, Mangiavacchi M, et al. Cardiac, skeletal and ocular abnormalities in patients with Marfan syndrome and their relatives. Comparison with the cardiac abnormalities in patients with kyphoscoliosis. *Br Heart J* 1984;51:220–230.

Judge DP, Dietz HC. Therapy of Marfan syndrome. *Annu Rev Med* 2008;59:43–59.

Judge DP, Rouf R, Habashi J, et al. Mitral valve disease in Marfan syndrome and related disorders. *J Cardiovasc Transl Res* 2011;4(6):741–747.

Answer 2: B. The video shows inlet VSD patch and primum ASD patch. This patient had complete AV canal repair with ASD closure, VSD closure, and division of common AV valve in addition to cleft left AV valve repair.

A is false. Secundum ASD can be seen in trisomy 21, but the echo images are not consistent with that diagnosis alone.

C is false. Partial atrioventricular canal defect can be seen in trisomy 21, but there is no VSD component with that and the echoes show clearly VSD patch in the inlet portion.

D is false. Tetralogy of Fallot (TOF) is not commonly seen in patients with trisomy 21, although may be present in conjunction with atrioventricular canal (endocardial cushion) defects. Also, the VSD is of different location (anterior malalignment type in TOF).

E is false. D-TGA is not a common lesion in trisomy 21 patients. Also, none of the echo images were suggestive of arterial switch procedure.

Trisomy 21, or Down syndrome, is a genetic syndrome due to complete or partial trisomy of chromosome 21 associated with characteristic facial features, mental retardation, and a simian palmar crease. Approximately 40% to 50% of children born with Down syndrome will have associated congenital heart disease (CHD), with ventricular septal defects being the most common.

Atrioventricular canal (endocardial cushion) defects are also one of the more common types of CHD associated with trisomy 21 and classically are much more common in this population than non–Down syndrome patients and however are not pathognomonic of this genetic syndrome. Atrioventricular canal defects consist of lack of development of the atrioventricular septum resulting in primum-type atrial septal defect and inlet ventricular septal defect in the complete form in addition to common AV valve that consists typically of 5 leaflets.

Partial atrioventricular canal defects (also called primum ASD) have no VSD due to closure by attachments of the AV valves to the ventricular septum. These patients still have a left AV valve cleft. Other relatively common types of CHD seen in trisomy 21 patients include secundum atrial septal defect (ASD) and patent ductus arteriosus (PDA).

Suggested Readings

Dennis J, Archer N, Ellis J, et al. Recognising heart disease in children with Down syndrome. *Arch Dis Child Educ Pract Ed* 2010;95:98–104.

Irving CA, Chaudhari MP. Cardiovascular abnormalities in Down's syndrome: spectrum, management and survival over 22 years. *Arch Dis Child* 2012;97:326–330.

Jones KL. Down syndrome. In: *Smith's Recognizable Patterns of Human Malformation.* 6th ed. Philadelphia, PA: Elsevier Saunders, 2006:7.

Zellers TM, Zehr R, Weinstein E, et al. Two-dimensional and Doppler echocardiography alone can adequately define preoperative anatomy and hemodynamic status before repair of complete atrioventricular septal defect in infants <1 year old. *J Am Coll Cardiol* 1994;24:1563–1570.

Answer 3: A.

A. True. See discussion below.

B. False. These findings may be seen in Noonan syndrome but are not typical for this syndrome and are most common in nonsyndromic patients.

C. False. The pulmonary outflow tract obstruction seen in Noonan syndrome is typically valvular or supravalvular, not subvalvular, due to infundibular obstruction as is commonly seen in tetralogy of Fallot. TOF is not that common in patients with Noonan syndrome too.

D. False. The first part of the question is true: hypertrophic cardiomyopathy is associated with Noonan syndrome. However, the valvular disease in Noonan's typically involves the pulmonary rather than the aortic valve.

E. False. These findings are more consistent with Turner syndrome.

Noonan syndrome is a relatively common genetic syndrome due to a variety of gene mutations in the RAS-MAP pathway. Up to 80% of Noonan syndrome patients have some form of CHD with valvular pulmonary stenosis most common; a supravalvular component may also occur. Hypertrophic cardiomyopathy (HCM) occurs in 15% to 20% of patients. Other less common syndromes in the pathway include LEOPARD syndrome, neurofibromatosis, cardiofaciocutaneous syndrome, and Costello syndrome. All have a high incidence of CHD with defects similar to those seen in Noonan syndrome.

Suggested Readings

Marino B, Digilio MC, Toscano A, et al. Congenital heart diseases in children with Noonan syndrome: an expanded cardiac spectrum with high prevalence of atrioventricular canal. *J Pediatr* 1999;135(6):703–706.

Noonan JA. Hypertelorism with Turner phenotype. A new syndrome with associated congenital heart disease. *Am J Dis Child* 1968;116(4):373–380.

Nugent AW, Daubeney PE, Chondros P, et al. Clinical features and outcomes of childhood hypertrophic cardiomyopathy: results from a national population-based study. National Australian Childhood Cardiomyopathy Study. *Circulation* 2005;112(9):1332–1338.

Tartaglia M, Zampino G, Gelb BD. Noonan syndrome: clinical aspects and molecular pathogenesis. *Mol Syndromol* 2010;1:2–26.

Zenker M. Clinical manifestations of mutations in RAS and related intracellular signal transduction factors. *Curr Opin Pediatr* 2011;23:443–451.

Answer 4: D.

A. False. Trisomy 21 is associated with congenital heart disease (most commonly VSDs and atrioventricular canal defects), but isolated aortic arch issues are unusual (except in cases of unbalanced, RV-dominant AV canal defect in association with LV outflow tract obstruction).

B. False. Williams syndrome is associated with supravalvular aortic stenosis and pulmonary branch stenosis.

C. False. Trisomy 13 is often associated with a variety of congenital heart lesions, most commonly septal defects. Survival into late childhood is very unlikely.

D. True. The echocardiographic images show a bicuspid aortic valve and coarctation of aorta. Of the syndromes listed, Turner syndrome is most likely in this scenario. See discussion below.

E. False. Although BAV and coarctation may be nonsyndromic, the patient had dysmorphic features and her cardiac defects are consistent with Turner syndrome.

Turner syndrome is a sex chromosome abnormality with absence of all or part of the X chromosome and is one of the most common chromosomal anomalies. Cardiac defects are very common including bicuspid aortic valve, coarctation of the aorta, and hypoplastic left heart syndrome. Patients are at risk for aortic dissection in adulthood.

Suggested Readings

Gotzsche CO, Krag-Olsen B, Nielsen J, et al. Prevalence of cardiovascular malformations and association with karyotypes in Turner's syndrome. *Arch Dis Child* 1994;71:433–436.

Sachdev V, Matura LA, Sidenko S, et al. Aortic valve disease in Turner syndrome. *J Am Coll Cardiol* 2008;51:1904–1909.

Sybert VP. Cardiovascular malformations and complications in Turner syndrome. *Pediatrics* 1995;101(1):e11.

Sybert VP, McCauley E. Turner's syndrome. *N Engl J Med* 2004;351:1227–1238.

Answer 5: *C.* The figure and video show narrowed aortic sinotubular junction creating supravalvular aortic stenosis, a finding commonly seen in Williams syndrome.

Williams syndrome is a genetic disorder due to mutation of the elastin gene, resulting in a high incidence of supravalvular aortic stenosis. Arterial stenosis of the renal, coronary, and branch pulmonary arteries, coarctation of the aorta, and mitral valve anomalies also can occur. Interestingly, the pulmonary branch stenosis tends to improve with time, but the supravalvular aortic stenosis is often progressive. Classic phenotypic features of Williams syndrome also include so-called "elfin" facies and a "cocktail" personality. A familial form of supravalvular aortic stenosis also occurs in which the abnormal elastin gene is transmitted from one affected parent to half of the offspring.

Option A is false. Congenital heart disease is common in trisomy 18 (over 50%) with most common lesions being ventricular septal defects and valvular abnormalities (may be polyvalvular). This syndrome has a very high mortality in infancy, and long-term survival is unusual.

Options B and D are false. DiGeorge syndrome and Noonan syndrome are neither typically associated with the echo findings seen on this image. Both are discussed in details elsewhere.

Suggested Readings

Burch TM, McGowan FX Jr, Kussman BD, et al. Congenital supravalvular aortic stenosis and sudden death associated with anesthesia: what's the mystery? *Anesth Analg* 2008;107(6):1848–1854.

Eronen M, Peippo M, Hiippala A, et al. Cardiovascular manifestations in 75 patients with Williams syndrome. *J Med Genet* 2002;39:554–558.

Pober B. Williams-Beuren syndrome. *N Engl J Med* 2010;362:239–252.

Answer 6: *B.* The figure and video demonstrate a secundum ASD with concomitant right atrial dilation.

The association of absent radii (absent thumb) and secundum atrial septal defects is classic for Holt-Oram syndrome.

DiGeorge or 22q11 deletion syndrome is a genetic syndrome associated with conotruncal defects and aortic arch abnormalities, including VSDs, truncus arteriosus, and interrupted aortic arch. These patients also have abnormalities of calcium metabolism and immunologic deficiencies. Partial forms exist. Therefore, Option A is incorrect.

Ellis-van Creveld syndrome is associated with a common atrium, not a simple secundum atrial septal defect. These patients also have extra digits and no absent thumb or radii. Therefore, Option C is incorrect.

Down syndrome is associated with CHD in 40% to 50% of patients, with ventricular septal and atrioventricular canal defects being most common. It is not associated with absent radii. Therefore, Option D is incorrect.

Suggested Readings

Basson CT, Cowley GS, Soloman SD, et al. The clinical and genetic spectrum of the Holt-Oram syndrome (heart-hand syndrome). *N Engl J Med* 1994;330(13):885–891.

Hills CB, Kochilas L, Schimmenti LA, et al. Ellis-van Creveld syndrome and congenital heart defects: presentation of an additional 32 cases. *Pediatr Cardiol* 2011;32:977–982.

Huang T. Current advances in Holt-Oram syndrome. *Curr Opin Pediatr* 2002;14:691–695.

Momma K. Cardiovascular anomalies associated with chromosome 22q11.2 deletion syndrome. *Am J Cardiol* 2010;105:1617–1624.

Answer 7: *D.* The figures demonstrate evidence of a stenotic, hypoplastic pulmonary valve with moderate to severe stenosis by Doppler and evidence of hypertrophic cardiomyopathy. These findings taken together are most consistent with the diagnosis of Noonan syndrome. Over 80% of patients with Noonan syndrome have evidence of congenital heart disease, most commonly pulmonary valve stenosis, which may also include a supravalvular component. Hypertrophic cardiomyopathy occurs in 15% to 20% of Noonan syndrome patients. Less commonly, aortic valve abnormalities or other CHD are seen.

Option A is incorrect, since Turner syndrome is associated with aortic anomalies including bicuspid aortic valve and coarctation of the aorta.

Option B is incorrect since Williams syndrome is associated with supravalvular aortic stenosis and pulmonary branch stenosis.

Option C is incorrect since trisomy 13 is most commonly associated with ventricular septal defects and carries very poor prognosis with most patients passing away in early childhood.

Suggested Readings

Marino B, Digilio MC, Toscano A, et al. Congenital heart diseases in children with Noonan syndrome: an expanded cardiac spectrum with high prevalence of atrioventricular canal. *J Pediatr* 1999;135(6):703–706.

Nugent AW, Daubeney PE, Chondros P, et al. Clinical features and outcomes of childhood hypertrophic cardiomyopathy: results from a national population-based study. National Australian Childhood Cardiomyopathy Study. *Circulation* 2005;112(9):1332–1338.

Tartaglia M, Zampino G, Gelb BD. Noonan syndrome: clinical aspects and molecular pathogenesis. *Mol Syndromol* 2010;1:2–26.

Zenker M. Clinical manifestations of mutations in RAS and related intracellular signal transduction factors. *Curr Opin Pediatr* 2011;23:443–451.

Answer 8: *C.* This young man has likely some form of VACTERL association. This includes combination of vertebral, anal, cardiac, tracheoesophageal, renal, and limb abnormalities. This is a rare association (1:40,000 births) and usually diagnosed in early infancy. TE fistula usually requires surgical repair early in life, and most vertebral abnormalities are not that serious (fused vertebrae). Renal abnormalities like single kidney or horseshoe kidney can be seen in about 50% of patients.

Cardiac defects occur in about 50% of patients too, and the majority has septal defects like ASDs and/or VSDs. This patient likely had a perimembranous VSD that was partially closed by tricuspid valve accessory tissue, which is not uncommon. This can grow and completely block the hole and eliminate the shunt. Due to the VSD shunt that was directed at the RV free anterior wall, some patients develop overgrowth of muscle bundles that lead to narrowing in the middle of the RV cavity and practically divide the RV into an inlet proximal chamber with high pressure (connected to the TV) and outlet distal chamber with low pressure (connected to the pulmonary valve), hence the name double-chambered RV (DCRV).

VIDEO 41.7 is from a parasternal short-axis view that shows color flow acceleration below the RV outflow tract. VIDEO 41.8 is another useful view to evaluate this condition and is obtained from subcostal window with marker pointing at 6 o'clock (subcostal sagittal). FIGURE 41.6 shows increased TR velocity reflecting elevated RV pressure of 87 mm Hg plus RA pressure. Only inlet RV chamber is under that high pressure in this patient though. FIGURE 41.7 shows increased velocity underneath the RVOT with peak gradient of 53 mm Hg, which means that the distal RV chamber and pulmonary artery systolic pressure is much lower than the inlet chamber one. This scenario can be misinterpreted as severe pulmonary hypertension if the reader is not familiar with DCRV physiology and if the RV cavity and RVOT are not thoroughly evaluated.

Answer A is incorrect. This patient has some TR but as explained above does not have severe pulmonary hypertension. Also, TR murmur is expected to be holosystolic and not systolic ejection.

Answer B is incorrect. There is no shunt across the VSD since the patient was 10 years old. Also, VSD murmur is usually holosystolic and not systolic ejection in nature.

Answer D is incorrect. This is the hardest option to eliminate as valvular PS will cause similar murmur to DCRV. VIDEO 41.7 though shows the pulmonary valve moving well with no abnormalities and the color flow acceleration starting in the RV cavity, well below the valve and RVOT.

Suggested Readings

Michelfelder EC, Border WL. Abnormalities of right ventricular outflow. In: Eidem M, Cetta F, O'Leary PW, eds. *Echocardiography in Pediatric and Adult Congenital Heart Disease*. 2nd ed. Philadelphia, PA: Wolters Kluwer; 2014:256–259.

Solomon BD. VACTERL/VATER Association. *Orphanet J Rare Dis* 2011;6:56.

Answer 9: *A.*

A. True. See discussion below.
B. False. Conotruncal anomalies, including interrupted aortic arch, are the most common category of congenital heart lesions in 22q11 deletion syndrome.
C. False. Approximately 70% to 75% of patients with 22q11 deletion syndrome have congenital heart disease.
D. False. Approximately 10% of patients with 22q11 deletion syndrome have complete form of DiGeorge syndrome with significant immunodeficiency.
E. False. D-transposition of the great arteries is rare in 22q11 deletion syndrome.

22q11 deletion syndrome, used to be called velocardiofacial syndrome (VCFS), is a genetic condition due to a microdeletion of chromosome 22q11.2 that is characterized by abnormal pharyngeal arch development. It is associated with developmental abnormalities of the parathyroid glands, thymus, and conotruncal region of the heart. It has an incidence of associated cardiac lesions of 70% to 75%, including most commonly interrupted aortic arch type B (~50%), truncus arteriosus (~35%), and tetralogy of Fallot (~16%).

Other cardiac defects also occur, including pulmonary atresia with ventricular septal defect, ventricular septal defects in association with aortic arch anomalies, aortic stenosis, and pulmonary artery anomalies. D-transposition of the great arteries is uncommon.

Approximately 10% of patients with 22q11 deletion syndrome will have complete DiGeorge syndrome, defined as having at least two of the following: (a) conotruncal cardiac anomaly, (b) immunodeficiency due to thymic aplasia, and (c) hypoparathyroidism with variable hypocalcemia.

Suggested Readings

Jones KL. Deletion 22q11.2 syndrome (Velo-cardio-facial syndrome, DiGeorge syndrome, Shprintzen syndrome). In: *Smith's Recognizable Patterns of Human Malformation*. 6th ed. Philadelphia, PA: Elsevier Saunders, 2006:298.

Momma K. Cardiovascular anomalies associated with chromosome 22q11.2 deletion syndrome. *Am J Cardiol* 2010;105:1617–1624.

Shihui Y, Graf WD, Shprintzen RJ. Genomic disorders on chromosome 22. *Curr Opin Pediatr* 2012;24:665–671.

Answer 10: *D.* Williams syndrome is a rare contiguous gene deletion syndrome on chromosome 7 that affects the elastin (ELN) gene. Supravalvular aortic stenosis is noted in nearly half of patients with Williams syndrome, and peripheral pulmonary artery stenosis is noted in over 1/3 (20% of these patients have both lesions). Therefore, the pulmonary artery branches need to be investigated systematically with 2D, color, and spectral Doppler (therefore, Answer D is the single best answer).

Mild supravalvular aortic stenosis should not result in LVH with impaired strain (Answer A is not the single best answer).

While coronary anomalies can occur in Williams patients, they are rare (Answer B is not the single best answer).

Echo investigation for an atrial septal defects (Answer C) and coarctation of the aorta (Answer E) are important aspects of a complete congenital TTE, but these congenital heart defects are not as common as branch pulmonary artery stenosis in individuals with Williams syndrome.

Other common cardiac lesions in Williams syndrome patients include mitral valve prolapse and regurgitation (15%), ventricular septal defect (13%), and supravalvular pulmonary stenosis (12%).

Suggested Reading
Collins RT II, Kaplan P, Somes GW, et al. Long-term outcomes of patients with cardiovascular abnormalities and Williams syndrome. *Am J Cardiol* 2010;105(6):874–878.

Answer 11: D. This patient likely has some form of Loeys-Dietz syndrome (LDS). It is characterized by vascular findings (cerebral, thoracic, and abdominal arterial aneurysms and/or dissections) and skeletal manifestations (pectus excavatum or pectus carinatum, scoliosis, joint laxity, arachnodactyly). Bifid uvula and cleft palate are also common findings. The natural history of LDS is characterized by aggressive arterial aneurysms (mean age at death 26.1 years). Diagnosis is suspected clinically and confirmed by molecular genetic testing to look for mutation in TGFBR1 and TGFBR2 in addition to other less common ones.

Answer A is incorrect. Williams syndrome is associated with supravalvular aortic stenosis in addition to branch pulmonary artery stenosis. Those patients have some mental retardation and cocktail party–like personality.

Answer B is incorrect. Turner syndrome is associated with BAV, coarctation of the aorta, and early aortic dissection. It is seen in females only though and due to 45XO karyotype. These females are usually short with webbed neck and no menstrual cycles (ovarian failure).

Answer C is incorrect. Noonan syndrome is associated with valvular pulmonary stenosis and hypertrophic cardiomyopathy. Aortic root dilation is not common in these patients. These patients have some dysmorphic features including a deep groove in the area between the nose and mouth (long philtrum), widely spaced eyes, low-set ears that are rotated backward, and high arched palate.

Suggested Readings
Hemelrijk, et al. The Loeys–Dietz syndrome: an update for the clinician. *Curr Opin Cardiol* 2010;25(6):546–551.
Milewicz DM. Genetic aspects of congenital heart disease. In: Willerson JT, Wellens HJJ, Cohn JN, et al., eds. *Cardiovascular Medicine*. London: Springer, 2007.

Answer 12: D. In LDS, aortic dissection occurs at smaller aortic diameters than observed in Marfan syndrome, and vascular disease is not limited to the aortic root. This is why imaging with MRI/MRA is important to get baseline of arterial tree from head to pelvis. Due to the aggressive nature of this disease, close follow-up with repeat echo in 6 months is recommended to determine rate of aortic root growth; and if it exceeds 5 mm per year, surgical intervention might be indicated.

Also, beta-adrenergic blockers or other medications like ARBs are used to reduce hemodynamic stress especially if patients are hypertensive. Aneurysms are amenable to early and aggressive surgical intervention, which is the only effective treatment on the long term.

Answer A is incorrect. There is no indication that this patient has renovascular hypertension. This is a common etiology of secondary hypertension in children and teens. It usually is associated with severe hypertension and might require stenting of stenotic vessels.

Answer B is incorrect. As discussed in previous question answers, Turner syndrome is not the diagnosis here as it is only seen in females. If Turner syndrome was the suspected diagnosis, karyotype and endocrine consultation will be indicated.

Answer C is incorrect. Chest MRA will be needed at some point here as part of evaluating the whole arterial tree as discussed in previous question. The main goal though is not to evaluate the branch pulmonary arteries as they usually are not involved in LDS. If the diagnosis was Noonan syndrome, this would be the correct answer.

Suggested Readings
Hemelrijk, et al. The Loeys–Dietz syndrome: an update for the clinician. *Curr Opin Cardiol* 2010;25(6):546–551.
Genetic aspects of congenital heart defects. *Chapter 3 from Moss and Adams Heart diseases in Infants, Children and Adolescents.* 9th ed.

Answer 13: E. Kartagener syndrome is an autosomal recessive disorder that includes situs inversus totalis and immobility of cilia in the respiratory tract. Those patients have frequent upper and lower respiratory infections leading to bronchiectasis. Chest x-ray shows cardiac apex pointing to the right and stomach bubble on the right side too. The echocardiogram is from subcostal long-axis view showing the cardiac apex pointing to the right also. Patient with situs inversus totalis usually have dextrocardia with mirror image distribution of structures and no significant heart defects.

Answer A is incorrect. DiGeorge syndrome can be associated with increased risk of infection due to T-cell dysfunction. These patients usually have abnormal faces and more complex congenital heart defects including tetralogy of Fallot, truncus arteriosus, and interrupted aortic arch.

Answer B is incorrect. Turner syndrome is due to 45XO karyotype and is not known to be associated with increased risk of infection. These patients are usually females with short stature and ovarian failure (no menstrual cycles).

Answer C is incorrect. Klinefelter syndrome is due to 47 XXY karyotype. There is no increased risk of infection, but these males are usually tall with learning difficulties and sexual developmental issues.

Answer D is incorrect. Noonan syndrome has been discussed in other questions in this chapter.

Suggested Readings
Ozkaya S, et al. Bronchiolitis as a feature of kartagener syndrome. A case report. *J Bronchol Intervent Pulmonol* 2011;18(1):88–90.
Shakya K. Kartagener syndrome: a rare genetic disorder. *J Nepal Med Assoc* 2009;48(173):62–65.

Chapter 42

Fetal Echocardiography for the Boards

Kristopher M. Cumbermack

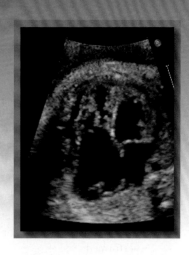

1. You are a high-risk maternal–fetal medicine provider performing an initial evaluation of a 22-year-old G2P1 female who is presently 23 weeks' pregnant. You are recording her current and past medical and family history. Which of the following is not an indication for a fetal echocardiogram to be performed?

   A. She has been on lithium for 5 years for manic depression.
   B. There is a family history of gestational diabetes in her sister.
   C. The fetus' father had repair of a ventricular septal defect at 2 years of age.
   D. She has been taking aspirin for headaches daily for the past 3 weeks.
   E. Amniocentesis performed earlier demonstrates trisomy 21 in the fetus.

2. The fetal echocardiographic image in FIGURE 42.1 and VIDEO 42.1 was obtained during a routine obstetric screening in a 42-year-old G3P2 pregnant female. Which of the following genetic diagnoses is most likely associated with the finding shown?

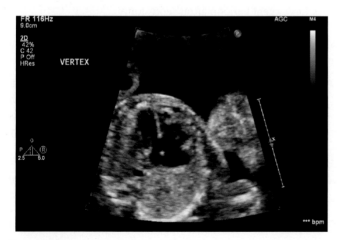

FIGURE 42.1

   A. Turner syndrome
   B. Trisomy 18
   C. Williams-Beuren (or Williams) syndrome
   D. Trisomy 21 (Down syndrome)
   E. Noonan syndrome

3. A G1P0 23-year-old pregnant female with a history of Wolff-Parkinson-White (WPW) syndrome is sent for evaluation secondary to concern for an abnormal fetal heart rhythm noted on routine OB screening. The fetal M-mode tracing in FIGURE 42.2 (VIDEO 42.2) was obtained from the fetus. This tracing demonstrates:

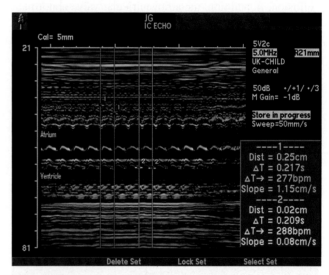

FIGURE 42.2

   A. Fetal ventricular tachycardia
   B. Benign premature atrial contractions
   C. Supraventricular tachycardia
   D. Normal fetal heart rate
   E. Sinus tachycardia

4. A normal fetal echocardiographic four-chamber view excludes which of the following congenital heart lesions in the fetus?

   A. D-transposition of the great arteries
   B. Coarctation of the aorta
   C. Partial anomalous pulmonary venous return
   D. Pulmonary valve stenosis
   E. Hypoplastic left heart syndrome

5. On routine fetal echocardiographic evaluation of a 24-week gestation fetus, a small, circumferential pericardial effusion is noted. The fetal heart is structurally normal with normal Doppler evaluation, including the umbilical vessels. There is normal cardiac rhythm, heart rate, and ventricular function. No other extravascular fluid collections are identified in the fetus. The pregnancy is otherwise uncomplicated.

Which of the following is correct regarding this effusion?

A. This fetus has "hydrops fetalis."
B. Follow-up evaluation for cardiac fibroma should be performed.
C. Although follow-up is indicated, this effusion will most likely resolve.
D. Although small, this effusion indicates a greatly increased risk of fetal demise.
E. Immediate delivery is indicated to prevent intrauterine demise.

6. The fetal four-chamber image in FIGURE 42.3 (VIDEO 42.3) was obtained from a patient on chronic lithium therapy. There is evidence of LV noncompaction and a small pericardial effusion. In addition, the atrioventricular valve abnormality demonstrated is:

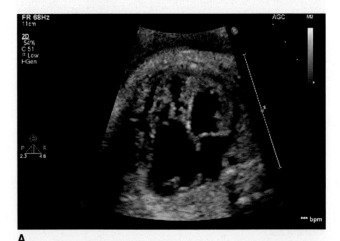

A

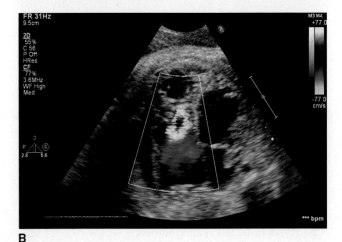

B

FIGURE 42.3

A. Tricuspid atresia
B. Mitral valve prolapse
C. Common atrioventricular valve
D. Ebstein anomaly of the tricuspid valve

7. A 29-year-old G2P1 female with no significant past medical history presents for fetal cardiac consultation due to an abnormal obstetrical screening ultrasound. Her medications include prenatal vitamins. She smokes ½ pack of cigarettes per day but denies other teratogen exposure. When developing your differential diagnosis, which of the following diagnoses would NOT be expected to cause the abnormality seen in VIDEO 42.4?

A. Severe tricuspid valve regurgitation
B. Severe pulmonary regurgitation
C. Severe pulmonary stenosis
D. Coarctation of the aorta
E. Arteriovenous malformation

8. A 26-year-old G3P2 female with a history of BAV presents at 24 WGA for fetal cardiology consultation due to an inability to see the left ventricle and left ventricular outflow tract. She has no prior surgical history. Delivery is planned at their local hospital in their small community. Fetal echocardiography as shown in VIDEOS 42.5 TO 42.8 is obtained. How is delivery planning impacted by these findings?

A. No changes to delivery planning needed.
B. Delivery should always occur no later than 37 weeks' gestational age.
C. Delivery should always be via C-section due to the suspected congenital heart disease.
D. Delivery can be arranged at any center with a neonatal intensive care unit.
E. Relocation to an area near a congenital heart surgical center should occur at 35 to 37 WGA with plans for emergent balloon atrial septostomy.

Answer 1: B. There is a family history of gestational diabetes in her sister.

A. Lithium exposure in the first trimester is associated with Ebstein anomaly of the tricuspid valve in the fetus, which can be identified on fetal echocardiography. Severe forms with significant tricuspid regurgitation may require early postnatal treatment.
B. Maternal diabetes mellitus, not a *family history* in a maternal sibling, is associated with congenital heart disease (CHD) and diabetic cardiomyopathy in the fetus. Most common forms of CHD associated with maternal diabetes are ventricular septal defects (VSDs) and conotruncal anomalies (tetralogy of Fallot, D-transposition of the great arteries).
C. Congenital heart disease in first-degree relatives increases the fetus' risk of CHD by as much as a factor of approximately two to five times, depending on the specific lesion. Most lesions can be identified by fetal echocardiography.

D. Exposure to aspirin can result in constriction or premature closure of the fetal ductus arteriosus with significant deleterious prenatal consequences including right heart failure and pulmonary hypertension. 2D and Doppler assessment by fetal echocardiography is indicated.

E. Forty to fifty percent of fetuses with trisomy 21 (Down syndrome) have CHD. Most common lesions are atrioventricular canal (endocardial cushion) defects and VSDs.

Indications for fetal echocardiography include fetal, maternal, and familial factors.

Primary fetal indications:

- Abnormal obstetric ultrasound suggesting fetal cardiac anomaly (structural or functional)
- Fetal arrhythmia
- Fetal extracardiac anomalies associated with cardiac disease (i.e., omphalocele, diaphragmatic hernia)
- Abnormal fetal karyotype (i.e., trisomies, Turner syndrome)
- Increased nuchal translucency on obstetric screen (increased risk of aneuploidy and CHD)

Most common maternal indications:

- Maternal diabetes (gestational, type 1 or 2)
- Maternal congenital heart disease
- Maternal autoimmune disease (risk of congenital complete heart block in fetuses of mothers with lupus with associated anti-Ro or anti-La antibodies)
- Teratogen exposure (i.e., fetal alcohol syndrome associated with septal defects, lithium associated with Ebstein anomaly, retinoids associated with conotruncal anomalies)

Familial indications include:

- Paternal or sibling congenital heart disease (in general, less than risk with maternal CHD)
- Family history of genetic syndromes associated with CHD

The overall indication with the highest yield is an abnormal obstetric ultrasound, highlighting the importance of high-quality screening for prenatal detection of significant cardiac disease.

Suggested Readings

Hornberger LK. Who should have a fetal heart scan. In: Bader RS, Hornberger LK, Huhta JC, eds. *The Perinatal Cardiology Handbook*. Philadelphia, PA: Mosby, 2008:15–21.

Hornberger LK, Jaeggi E, Trines J. The fetal heart. In: Rumack CM, Wilson S, Charboneau JW, et al., eds. *Diagnostic Ultrasound*. 3rd ed. Philadelphia, PA: Mosby, 2005:1323–1364.

Rychik J, Ayres N, Cuneo B, et al. American Society of Echocardiography guidelines and standards for performance of the fetal echocardiogram. *J Am Soc Echocardiogr* 2004;17:803–810.

Answer 2: D. The fetal echocardiogram is a four-chamber view demonstrating a complete atrioventricular canal defect, which is the most common form of complex congenital heart disease associated with trisomy 21 and is readily identifiable on fetal echocardiography. Down syndrome (DS) is a genetic syndrome due to complete or partial trisomy of chromosome 21 associated with characteristic facial features, mental retardation, and a simian palmar crease. Approximately 40% to 50% of children born with DS will have associated congenital heart disease (CHD), with complete atrioventricular canal defects (also known as endocardial cushion defects) being the most common (~37% to 40% of patients). Multiple lesions are seen in nearly a quarter of patients with DS. It would be appropriate to offer amniocentesis with fetal karyotyping when the diagnosis of fetal atrioventricular canal defect is made.

Option A is incorrect. Turner syndrome (gonadal dysgenesis) is associated with aortic stenosis and coarctation of the aorta, not atrioventricular canal defects.

Option B is incorrect. Although atrioventricular canal defects can be seen in patients with normal chromosomes, they are much more commonly seen in trisomy 21; hence, option D is the single best answer of these choices.

Option C is incorrect. Williams-Beuren or simply Williams syndrome involves an elastin gene defect and is associated with supravalvular aortic stenosis and branch pulmonary artery stenosis.

Option E is incorrect. Noonan syndrome is associated with valvar pulmonary stenosis and hypertrophic cardiomyopathy.

Suggested Readings

Allan LD, Sharland GK, Milburn A, et al. Prospective diagnosis of 1,006 consecutive cases of congenital heart disease in the fetus. *J Am Coll Cardiol* 1994;23(6):1452–1458.

Fesslova V, Villa L, Nava S, et al. Spectrum and outcome of atrioventricular canal defect in fetal life. *Cardiol Young* 2002;12(1):18–26.

Huggon IC, Cook AC, Smeeton NC, et al. Atrioventricular septal defects diagnosed in fetal life: associated cardiac and extra-cardiac abnormalities and outcome. *J Am Coll Cardiol* 2000;36(2):593–601.

Answer 3: C. This fetal M-mode tracing demonstrates supraventricular tachycardia (SVT) with an atrial rate of approximately 277 bpm and a similar ventricular rate with a short V–A interval. SVT is the most common pathologic tachycardia diagnosed in fetal life. Incessant tachycardia may result in fetal cardiac compromise (cardiomegaly, decreased function, and atrioventricular valve regurgitation) with resultant fetal hydrops, necessitating maternal medical therapy. Medical therapy is successful in approximately 80% of patients but may require multiple medications. Of note, WPW can recur in a familial pattern, including at least one form with autosomal dominant inheritance.

Option A is incorrect. Fetal ventricular tachycardia is relatively uncommon and is unlikely here as there is no evidence of atrioventricular dissociation, the atrial rate and ventricular rates are essentially the same, and it appears that atrial activation likely occurs prior to ventricular activation.

Option B is incorrect. The M-mode tracing demonstrates a tachycardia, which is regular. Premature atrial contractions typically are intermittent and irregular. They are extremely common in utero. In the vast majority of cases, they are entirely benign and resolve during pregnancy or in the neonatal period.

Option D is incorrect. Normal fetal heart rates range from approximately 120 bpm to as much as 180 to 200 bpm.

Option E is incorrect. Sinus tachycardia is a normal, appropriate sinus node response, but should not exceed 220 to 230 bpm in the fetus. The fetal tachycardia demonstrated here is much faster than normal, physiologic fetal heart rates.

Suggested Readings

Bader RS. Supraventricular tachycardia. In: Bader RS, Hornberger LK, Huhta JC, eds. *The Perinatal Cardiology Handbook.* Philadelphia, PA: Mosby, 2008:299–324.

Rasiah SV, Ewer AK, Miller P, et al. Prenatal diagnosis, management and outcome of fetal dysrhythmia: a tertiary fetal medicine centre experience over an 8-year period. *Fetal Diagn Ther* 2011;30(2):122–127.

Van Engelen AD, Weijtens O, Brenner JI, et al. Management outcome and follow-up of fetal tachycardia. *J Am Coll Cardiol* 1994;24(5):1371–1375.

Vidaillet HJ, Pressley JC, Henke E, et al. Familial occurrence of accessory atrioventricular pathways (preexcitation syndrome). *N Engl J Med* 1987;317:65–69.

Answer 4: E.

A. False. A fetal four-chamber view does not provide adequate imaging of the left and right ventricular outflow tracts, and hence, the relationships of the great arteries cannot be ascertained from this view.

B. False. The aortic arch is not visualized from a standard four-chamber view on a fetal echocardiogram.

C. False. The pulmonary venous return is not completely evaluated from a standard four-chamber view, although return of some of the pulmonary veins may be demonstrated by either 2D imaging or color Doppler from this view.

D. False. The pulmonary valve is not well visualized from the four-chamber view on a fetal echocardiogram (see A).

E. True. The fetal four-chamber view shows the left ventricular chamber well, and hypoplastic left heart syndrome would be easily identifiable from this view.

The four-chamber view from a fetal echocardiographic perspective clearly demonstrates both atria and ventricles as well as the mitral and tricuspid valves. The ventricular outflow tracts are not well seen in this view as they are more anteriorly and superiorly located. Although at least one pulmonary vein from each side may be seen, partial pulmonary venous anomalies cannot be excluded from the standard four-chamber view. The great arteries and the superior and inferior vena cava are also not well seen from this view. Portions of the atrial and ventricular septae are visualized from the four-chamber view; defects of each septae may be outside of this plane and can be missed. Other defects that may not be apparent include mild Ebstein anomaly of the tricuspid valve, double outlet right ventricle, pulmonary atresia, tetralogy of Fallot, and truncus arteriosus.

Although approximately 90% of congenital heart disease can be detected and the postnatal condition predicted by fetal echocardiography performed by an experienced operator, this question highlights the fact that routine screening using only limited 2D views can miss many significant lesions.

Suggested Readings

Hornberger LK, Jaeggi E, Trines J. The fetal heart. In: Rumack CM, Wilson S, Charboneau JW, et al., eds. *Diagnostic Ultrasound.* 3rd ed. Philadelphia, PA: Mosby, 2005:1323–1364.

Rychik J, Ayres N, Cuneo B, et al. American Society of Echocardiography guidelines and standards for performance of the fetal echocardiogram. *J Am Soc Echocardiogr* 2004;17:803–810.

Wigton TR, Sabbagha RE, Tamura RK, et al. Sonographic diagnosis of congenital heart disease: comparison between the four-chamber view and multiple cardiac views. *Obstet Gynecol* 1993;82:219–224.

Answer 5: C.

A. False. Hydrops fetalis is defined as extravascular fluid collections in at least two fetal compartments (such as ascites, pericardial or pleural effusion, skin edema). Pericardial effusion counts as one site, but alone is not indicative of hydrops.

B. False. Fetal pericardial teratomas are frequently associated with significant pericardial effusions, but cardiac fibromas are not. Cardiac rhabdomyomas are rarely associated with hydrops. Cardiac tumors are readily identifiable on fetal echocardiography.

C. True. See discussion below.

D. False. Small effusions are most commonly benign and self-limited. See discussion below.

E. False. Hydrops fetalis, not isolated small pericardial effusions, would be a potential indication for immediate delivery of fetus.

Small pericardial effusions are not uncommon on fetal echocardiographic evaluation. Congenital heart disease and abnormalities of cardiac rhythm and/or function must be excluded as potential causes, as should other noncardiac causes such as chromosomal anomalies, maternal infections, fetal anemia, and nonimmune hydrops. Isolated, small effusions without other cardiac pathologic findings most commonly are benign and resolve (prenatally or postnatally) without treatment or long-term sequelae. However, pericardial effusions can be a sign of fetal distress and should be followed. Large pericardial effusions are more likely to be seen with structural heart disease, chromosomal anomalies, and cardiac dysfunction. A significantly higher risk of fetal mortality is seen in cases of large effusions associated with extracardiac anomalies or hydrops.

Suggested Readings

Bader RS, Huhta JC. Pericardial effusion. In: Bader RS, Hornberger LK, Huhta JC, eds. *The Perinatal Cardiology Handbook.* Philadelphia, PA: Mosby, 2008:349–364.

Slesnick TC, Ayres NA, Altman CA, et al. Characteristics and outcomes of fetuses with pericardial effusions. *Am J Cardiol* 2005;96(4):599–601.

Yinon Y, Chitayat D, Blaser S, et al. Fetal cardiac tumors: a single-center experience of 40 cases. *Prenat Diagn* 2010;30(10):941–949.

Answer 6: D.

A. False. The image demonstrates apical displacement of the tricuspid valve due to lack of delamination of the septal leaflet. Color Doppler demonstrates significant regurgitation, confirming patency of the valve; there is no evidence of tricuspid atresia. See D.

B. False. The mitral valve appears to be coapting normally without prolapse in this still frame.

C. False. Two separate atrioventricular valves are seen.

D. True. Displacement of the septal leaflet of the tricuspid valve is the classic finding in Ebstein anomaly. There also is significant tricuspid regurgitation, which is common in this lesion. See discussion below.

Ebstein anomaly of the tricuspid valve is a rare form of CHD that occurs in the first trimester of pregnancy due to varying degrees of abnormal delamination of the septal and posterior leaflets of the tricuspid valve. This lesion is associated with lithium teratogenicity though can occur without known cause. Classically, there is significant tricuspid regurgitation, which can result in quite severe enlargement of the right atrium in these patients. The cardiomegaly and valve regurgitation are usually easily identifiable on fetal echocardiography; hence, Ebstein anomaly makes up a greater proportion of prenatally diagnosed CHD than expected based on its prevalence. Pulmonary stenosis or atresia, atrial and ventricular septal defects, left ventricular noncompaction, and arrhythmia are the most common associated findings in patients with Ebstein anomaly. The differential diagnosis includes tricuspid valve dysplasia and functional tricuspid regurgitation.

Suggested Readings

Allan LD, Desai G, Tynan MJ. Prenatal echocardiographic screening for Ebstein's anomaly for mothers on lithium therapy. *Lancet* 1982;2:875–876.

Celermajer DS, Bull C, Till JA, et al. Ebstein's anomaly: presentation and outcome from fetus to adult. *J Am Coll Cardiol* 1994;23(1):170–176.

Hornberger LK, Jaeggi E, Trines J. The fetal heart. In: Rumack CM, Wilson S, Charbonneau JW, et al., eds. *Diagnostic Ultrasound*. 3rd ed. Philadelphia, PA: Mosby, 2005:1323–1364.

Answer 7: C. The fetal echo image in Video 42.4 shows a right ventricle (RV) to left ventricle (LV) size discrepancy with RV appearing significantly larger than the LV. Identification of size discrepancies is a critical part of obstetrical screening leading to fetal cardiology consultation. Volume overload on the right ventricle is one cause of RV enlargement. Tricuspid regurgitation, pulmonary regurgitation, and both cerebral and hepatic arteriovenous malformations increase the volume load on the RV. Coarctation of the aorta can also cause RV enlargement and, in some cases, RV dysfunction. At times, a dilated RV has to be distinguished from a small left ventricle in HLHS; gestational age–based Z scores for ventricular dimensions are helpful in such situations. In addition, constriction of the ductus arteriosus, which can be caused by NSAID use, can lead to an RV–LV discrepancy. Severe pulmonary stenosis or atresia can lead to a small RV but not a dilated RV and is the only one of the listed possibilities that would not cause the RV–LV discrepancy seen in the fetal image provided.

Suggested Reading

Rychik J, et al. Left ventricle to right ventricle size discrepancy in the fetus: the presence of critical congenital heart disease can be reliably predicted. *J Am Soc Echocardiogr* 2009;22(11):1296–1301. doi: 10.1016/j.echo.2009.08.008

Answer 8: E. The fetal echo images are consistent with a fetal diagnosis of hypoplastic left heart syndrome (HLHS). Video 42.5 demonstrates a hypoplastic left ventricle and mitral valve. Video 42.6 shows flow reversal (red) back into a hypoplastic transverse arch supplied by ductal arch (blue) consistent with inadequate systemic blood flow from the left ventricle. Video 42.7 demonstrates abnormal left to right atrial shunting with significant flow acceleration by color Doppler consistent with restrictive atrial septum. As a result, the pulmonary veins shown in Video 42.8 returning to a small left atrium are dilated and demonstrate abnormal flow reversal by color Doppler. This is an extremely high-risk form of HLHS with very high morbidity and mortality potentially requiring emergent atrial septostomy immediately at birth.

Neonates with HLHS can be asymptomatic without murmur at birth. With trend toward earlier discharges, these neonates are at increased risk for being sent home without diagnosis leading to critical illness or sudden cardiac death. However, recent guidelines recommending screening for CHD with pre and postductal O_2 saturation in neonates prior to discharge should significantly decrease this risk. Fetal diagnosis of HLHS allows close monitoring to identify signs of fetal distress and potential high-risk features, such as a restrictive atrial septum with flow reversal within pulmonary veins, that requires special intervention. Fetal diagnosis enables creation of an optimal delivery plan to allow for best possible surgical outcomes should the family choose that option. Delivery at a center other than one that specializes in congenital heart surgery is not recommended as HLHS is a ductal dependent lesion requiring prostaglandin E (PGE) infusion to keep ductus patent and requires pediatric echocardiography expertise, complex neonatal management, and need for surgical intervention typically within first week of life. As early delivery can add morbidity of premature organ systems, it is rarely recommended in fetal congenital heart disease as most forms are well tolerated during fetal circulation. Cases of fetal hydrops or other signs of decompensation associated with CHD would be an exception. Delivery method is rarely determined by fetal CHD alone and is determined by obstetrical or MFM specialists who take into consideration both maternal and fetal factors. Delivery at NICU without expertise in caring for complex CHD or availability of pediatric cardiothoracic surgery is not recommended for ductal dependent or other forms of complex CHD. However, if occurs, PGE can be initiated and patient transferred to appropriate center.

Suggested Readings

Martin GR, et al. Hypoplastic left heart syndrome: current considerations and expectations. *J Am Coll Cardiol* 2012;59(1 suppl):S1–S42. doi: 10.1016/j.jacc.2011.09.022

Holland BJ, et al. Prenatal diagnosis of critical congenital heart disease reduces risk of death from cardiovascular compromise prior to planned neonatal cardiac surgery: a meta-analysis. *Ultrasound Obstet Gynecol* 2015;45(6):631–638. doi: 10.1002/uog.14882

Chapter 43

Pathologic Masses in the Atria

Mikel D. Smith

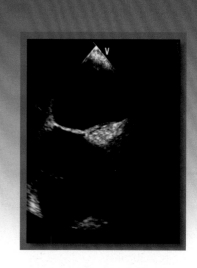

Questions 1 and 2

A 43-year-old female presents to the emergency room with slurred speech. MRI of the brain confirms a stroke. Workup for the stroke includes a transesophageal echocardiogram, and a representative image is shown in FIGURE 43.1 (VIDEO 43.1).

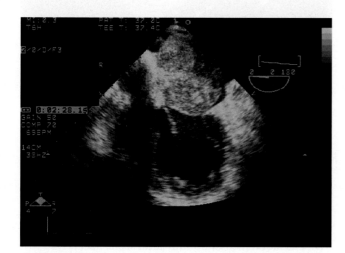

FIGURE 43.1

1. What percentage of these masses is found in the cardiac chamber shown in the image?

   A. 50%

   B. 75%

   C. 95%

   D. 80%

2. Where is the second most common cardiac location for this finding?

   A. Right atrium

   B. Left ventricle

   C. Right ventricle

   D. Mitral valve

Questions 3 to 5

A 56-year-old male presents to his physician's office with complaints of palpitations. His ECG shows new atrial fibrillation. He is started on anticoagulation and then sent for a transesophageal echo (TEE) in anticipation of a cardioversion. He converts to sinus rhythm as the TEE probe is passed. The 2D image reveals a prominent mass in the left atrial appendage that is suspicious for thrombus. Pulsed-wave Doppler assessment of the left atrial appendage is performed and shown in FIGURE 43.2.

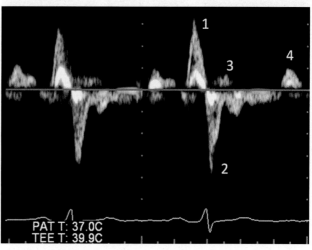

FIGURE 43.2

3. Which wave form is most useful in determining the risk of thrombus?

A. Waveform 1
B. Waveform 2
C. Waveform 3
D. Waveform 4

4. What is the normal velocity of this waveform?

A. 50 cm/s
B. 30 cm/s
C. 20 cm/s
D. 10 cm/s

5. Below what velocity is this waveform associated with an increased risk of thrombus formation?

A. 50 cm/s
B. 40 cm/s
C. 30 cm/s
D. 20 cm/s

6. What phrase best describes the Chiari network?

A. It is the same as the eustachian valve.
B. It serves as the valve of the coronary sinus.
C. It is usually stationary.
D. It can embolize to the lungs.

Questions 7 and 8

A 51-year-old male presents with complaints of profound fatigue. He also notes the inability to increase his heart rate during exercise. ECG reveals AV dissociation suggestive of complete heart block. Echocardiogram revealed a mass in the right atrium and right ventricle (Fig. 43.3, *arrow*, and Video 43.2).

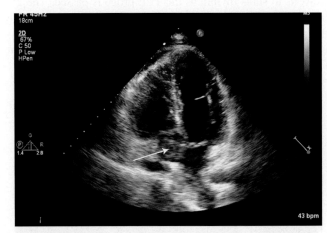

Figure 43.3

7. What is the incidence of biopsy-confirmed primary cardiac lymphoma?

A. 1% to 2%
B. 5% to 10%
C. 10% to 20%
D. 40% to 50%
E. 0.01%

8. Which of the following primary cardiac tumors can be nonmalignant?

A. Fibrosarcoma
B. Angiosarcoma
C. Lymphoma
D. Rhabdomyoma
E. Melanoma

9. A 71-year-old male underwent a transesophageal echo prior to electrical cardioversion (Fig. 43.4, arrow, and Video 43.3). Which of the following underlying conditions may be associated with the finding demonstrated by the arrow? Answer each with (A) yes or (B) not likely.

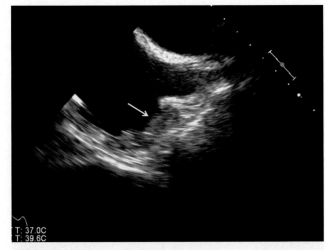

Figure 43.4

A. Atrial fibrillation
B. Pacemaker
C. Migration from the extremities or pelvis
D. Patent foramen ovale with atrial septal aneurysm
E. Chronic indwelling venous catheter

Answers 1: B and *2: A.* Myxomas are the most common benign tumor of the heart. They account for approximately 30% of primary cardiac tumors. They are most commonly found in the left atrium (75% of cases) and most commonly attach to the fossa ovalis. The typical attachment is by a "stalk," and they are commonly encapsulated—features that may be helpful in identifying the mass as a myxoma. The right atrium is the second most common site (15% of cases). Myxomas can also involve the left or right ventricles (5% each). Myxomas are usually single but, less commonly, can also be multiple. After surgical removal, myxomas may recur, so surveillance after surgery is needed. This case demonstrates the importance of TEE in young stroke patients without traditional atherosclerotic risk factors for stroke.

Myxomas can also be associated with the Carney complex and its subsets LAMB syndrome and NAME syndrome. These are autosomal dominant conditions that result in myxomas of the heart and skin, hyperpigmentation of the skin (lentiginosis), and endocrine overactivity (particularly Cushing syndrome). Approximately 7% of myxomas are associated with the Carney complex.

Suggested Readings
Armstrong WF, Ryan T. Chapter 23: masses, tumours, and source of embolus. In: *Feigenbaum's Echocardiography*. 7th ed. Philadelphia, PA: Lippincott Williams & Wilkins, 2010.
Carney J, Gordon H, Carpenter P, et al. The complex of myxomas, spotty pigmentation and endocrine overactivity. *Medicine* 1985;64(4):270–283.
Pinede L, Duhaut P, Loire R. Clinical presentation of left atrial myxoma. A series of 112 consecutive cases. *Medicine* 2001;80(3):159–172.

Answers 3: *A;* ***4:*** *A;* and ***5:*** *D.* Pulsed-wave Doppler of the left atrial appendage (LAA) on TEE is useful for defining the risk of thrombus formation within the appendage. FIGURE 40.2 demonstrates the normal spectral profile of the left atrial appendage flow in a patient in normal sinus rhythm. Waveform 1 represents LAA contraction (emptying velocity). This waveform is the most useful for determining the risk of thrombus formation; waveform 2 demonstrates LAA filling; waveform 3 demonstrates a systolic reflection wave; and waveform 4 demonstrates early diastolic LAA outflow. Normal individuals have an LAA emptying velocity of >50 cm/s. An emptying velocity <20 cm/s is associated with an increased risk of thrombus formation and increased risk of embolic events. The presence of spontaneous echo contrast is also associated with thrombus formation in the LAA.

The "mass" seen during TEE-2D imaging was due a prominent muscle ridge separating a bilobed appendage. Biplane imaging or 3DE can be helpful in distinguishing masses from pectinate muscles and other anatomical variants. An example of biplane TEE imaging of a bilobed appendage is shown here (FIG. 43.5).

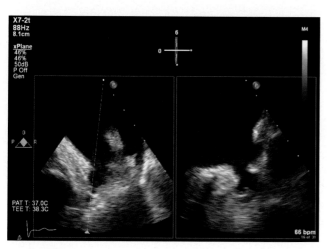

FIGURE 43.5

Suggested Readings
Agmon Y, Khandheria BK, Gentile F, et al. Echocardiographic assessment of the left atrial appendage. *J Am Coll Cardiol* 1999;34:1867–1877.
Armstrong WF, Ryan T. Chapter 23: masses, tumours, and source of embolus. In: *Feigenbaum's Echocardiography*. 7th ed. Philadelphia, PA: Lippincott Williams & Wilkins, 2010.

Answer 6: *B.* The Chiari network is a filamentous structure arising near the orifice of the inferior vena cava. It serves as the valve of the coronary sinus. It is highly mobile. Although sometimes confused with the eustachian valve, a Chiari network is more delicate and more mobile. The eustachian valve is a rigid and protuberant structure that arises along the posterior margin of the inferior vena cava to the border of the fossa ovalis. It served to divert right atrial flow across the fossa ovalis during fetal life. The eustachian valve and Chiari network are not pathologic. Neither of these structures embolize to the lungs.

Suggested Readings
Armstrong WF, Ryan T. Chapter 23: masses, tumours, and source of embolus. In: *Feigenbaum's Echocardiography*. 7th ed. Philadelphia, PA: Lippincott Williams & Wilkins, 2010.
Werner JA, Cheitlin MD, Gross BW, et al. Echocardiographic appearance of the Chiari network: differentiation from right heart pathology. *Circulation* 1981;63(5):1104–1109.

Answers 7: *A* and ***8:*** *D.* Malignant primary tumors of the heart are quite rare and include angiosarcoma, rhabdomyosarcoma, and fibrosarcoma. This patient presented with a primary cardiac lymphoma. Primary cardiac lymphoma is rare, accounting for only 1% to 2% of all primary cardiac tumors. Primary cardiac lymphoma arises most commonly in the right heart (right atrium is the most common). Associated pericardial effusions and conduction abnormalities are common. Tumors can also metastasize to the heart via either direct extension or hematogenous or lymphatic spread. Tumors commonly seen to metastasize to the heart include lung, breast, lymphoma, melanoma, GI tumors, renal cell (via extension of tumor via the IVC), and carcinoid. Rhabdomyomas are the most common cardiac tumor. They may regress and may be diagnosed in utero by fetal ultrasound. Rhabdomyomas are either primary cardiac or noncardiac, are common in patients with tuberous sclerosis, but are benign muscle tumors and do not metastasize to the heart. The remainder of the answers are all primary cardiac malignancies. Therefore, option D is the correct statement.

Suggested Readings
Armstrong WF, Ryan T. Chapter 23: masses, tumours, and source of embolus. In: *Feigenbaum's Echocardiography*. 7th ed. Philadelphia, PA: Lippincott Williams & Wilkins, 2010.
Beghetti M, Gow RM, Haney I, et al. Pediatric benign cardiac tumors: a 15 year review. *Am Heart J* 1997;134:1107–1114.
Nascimento AF, Winters GL, Pinkus GS. Primary cardiac lymphoma: clinical, histologic, immunophenotypic, and genotypic features of 5 cases of a rare disorder. *Am J Surg Pathol* 2007;31(9):1344–1350.
Salcedo EE, Cohen GI, White RD, et al. Cardiac tumors: diagnosis and management. *Curr Probl Cardiol* 1992;17:73–137.

Answers 9A: A (yes); *9B: A* (yes); *9C: B* (not likely); *9D: B* (not likely); and *9E: A* (yes). The figure demonstrates a thrombus in the right atrium, and this can be seen as a result of atrial fibrillation, pacemaker, and indwelling lines. In situ thrombus, as in this case, is most often seen in patients with indwelling lines or pacemaker leads, with the clots seen at the tip of the catheter or in the IVC, due to abraded intima. This particular patient had a pacemaker (leads not shown in image provided) and was in chronic atrial fibrillation.

Migration of thrombi may appear in the RA, but usually appear tangled in the TV or chordal apparatus, or may be seen extending from the IVC (especially in patients with renal cell or other abdominal carcinomas). The mass seen here appears to be broad-based and isolated to the RA appendage.

A patent foramen ovale (especially when associated with an atrial septal aneurysm) may increase the risk of systemic embolization of right-sided thrombi but are not associated with RA appendage clots. Therefore, option D is not likely to occur.

Suggested Readings

Armstrong WF, Ryan T. Chapter 23: masses, tumours, and source of embolus. In: *Feigenbaum's Echocardiography*. 7th ed. Philadelphia, PA: Lippincott Williams & Wilkins, 2010.

de Divitiis M, Omran H, Rabahieh R, et al. Right atrial appendage thrombosis in atrial fibrillation: its frequency and its clinical predictors. *Am J Cardiol* 1999;84:1023–1028.

Ghani MK, Boccalandro F, Denkatas AE, et al. Right atrial thrombus formation associated with central venous catheter utilization in hemodialysis patients. *Intensive Care Med* 2003;29:1829–1832.

Chapter 44

Masses and Tumors of the Ventricles

Vincent L. Sorrell

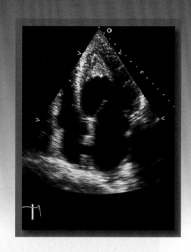

1. Which of the following statements most accurately describes the structure demonstrated with the arrow in the following figure (FIG. 44.1)?

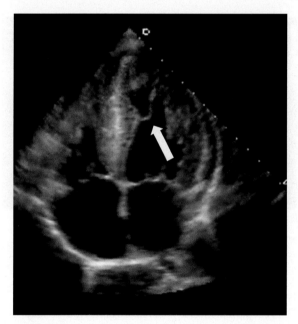

FIGURE 44.1

A. Common course of the right bundle branch
B. A congenital abnormality rarely seen in adults
C. A component of the mitral valve apparatus
D. Commonly associated with idiopathic VT
E. A common nonpathologic finding

2. A 45-year-old patient with ischemic cardiomyopathy is referred for echocardiography for repeat estimation of systolic function prior to internal defibrillator placement. The left ventricular ejection fraction (LVEF) was estimated as 40% by the biplane modified Simpson method. FIGURE 44.2 is the frame of the apical four-chamber view used to calculate end-diastolic volume. Which of the following statements is correct?

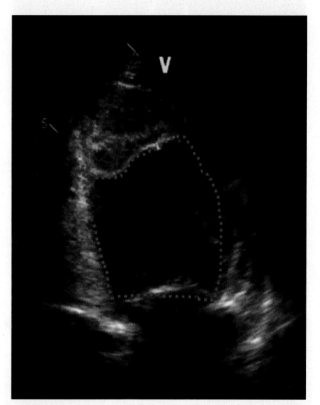

FIGURE 44.2

A. The LVEF is inaccurate as the apical endocardium is excluded.
B. The LVEF is inaccurate as the papillary muscles are excluded.
C. The biplane method cannot be applied in the setting of a large apical thrombus.
D. End of the T wave on ECG identifies end systole.
E. In the setting of an apical thrombus, transesophageal echocardiography is more accurate for LV function measurement.

3. A 45-year-old male with hypertension and significant family history of CAD presented with chest pain for several days. He underwent PCI to the LAD but had no reflow. An ACE inhibitor, beta-blocker, aspirin, and spironolactone were started. After obtaining the echocardiogram as shown in Figure 44.3 and Video 44.1, you decide:

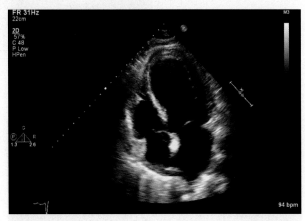

FIGURE 44.3

A. Start heparin as a bridge to Coumadin, keeping an INR of 2 to 3.
B. Increase dose of aspirin to 325 mg.
C. Discharge the patient and have him return in 6 weeks.
D. Aspirin and Plavix should be sufficient.
E. None of the options.

4. Match the transthoracic echocardiogram in Figure 44.4 and Video 44.2 with the single most likely pathologic entity:

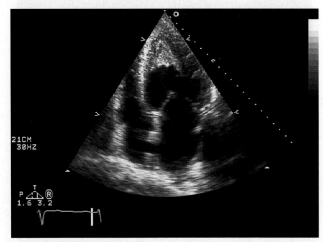

FIGURE 44.4

A. Fabry disease
B. Endomyocardial fibrosis
C. Radiation cardiotoxicity
D. Idiopathic restrictive cardiomyopathy
E. Cardiac sarcoidosis

5. Based on the echo images (Fig. 44.5 and Video 44.3) and the parasternal long-axis and apical four-chamber view, which of the following statements is true?

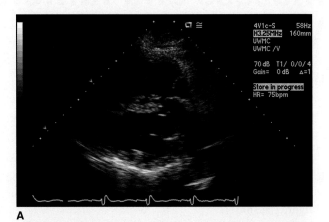

A

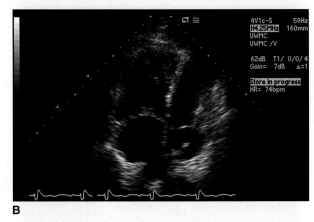

B

FIGURE 44.5

A. The patient has a secundum atrial septal defect.
B. The patient has L-transposition of the great arteries.
C. The patient has a pacemaker/defibrillator lead in the pulmonic ventricle.
D. The pulmonic valve is anterior and to the left of the aortic valve.

6. The echo–bright, linear structure demonstrated in the ventricular apex (Fig. 44.6 and Video 44.4) is most likely which of the following abnormalities?

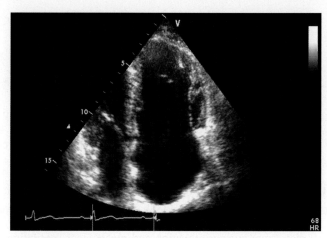

Figure 44.6

A. Aberrant chordae tendineae
B. Apical thrombus
C. Moderator band
D. Redundancy of the tricuspid valve
E. Pacemaker wire

7. A 75-year-old man is referred for an echocardiogram after a bout of paroxysmal atrial fibrillation. The apical four-chamber view is shown in Figure 44.7 and Video 44.5.

Which of the following is most correct?

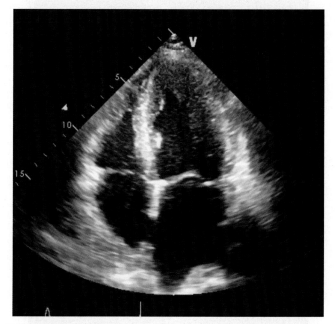

Figure 44.7

A. Parasternal long-axis image is likely normal.
B. Valsalva maneuver should be performed during LVOT Doppler.
C. Correlation with cardiac MRI approaches 100%.
D. Misdiagnosis as an apical aneurysm is possible.
E. Color flow Doppler is rarely helpful in making the diagnosis.

8. The right and left ventricular apexes are well shown in Figure 44.8 and Video 44.6. Based upon these images, which of the following pathologies is most likely responsible for the 2D echo pattern shown?

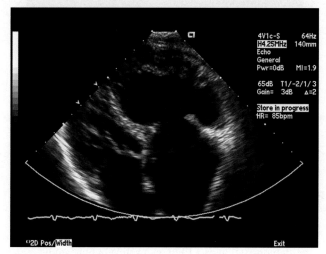

Figure 44.8

A. Endocardial fibroelastosis
B. Hypereosinophilic syndrome
C. Isolated noncompaction
D. Right ventricular volume overload
E. Hypertrophic cardiomyopathy

9. A 60-year-old obese man presents to the medical center with a TIA. His past history is significant for hypertension, hyperlipidemia, and a remote myocardial infarction. His vital signs are stable, and ECG confirms anteroseptal Q waves. Because of poor quality apical images (Fig. 44.9A), he was given an intravenous ultrasound enhancing agent (UEA) for left ventricular opacification (Fig. 44.9B).

Which of the following statements is most correct?

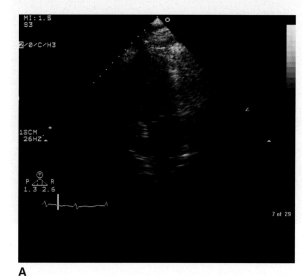

A
Figure 44.9

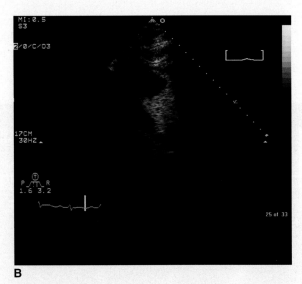

B

FIGURE 44.9 (*Continued*)

A. The UEA should be administered despite the demonstration of a PFO on a saline bubble study.

B. A possible apical thrombus is shown in both figures.

C. Without independent mobility, this apical mass has a low embolic potential.

D. This echo should be reported as possible thrombus, trabeculation, or tumor.

E. The apical myocardial shape is of little consequence in etiology determination.

10. A 40-year-old female presents with mild class II heart failure symptoms and recent left arm "weakness" and "numbness" that lasted for 5 hours. She has no significant past medical history. An echocardiogram was requested and the apical four-chamber images are shown (Fig. 44.10 and Video 44.7).

Which of the following is true?

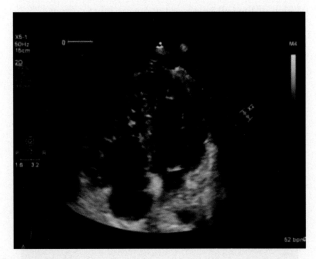

FIGURE 44.10

A. This is a congenital cardiomyopathy with progressive ventricular dysfunction.

B. Conventional heart failure therapy will prevent further LV dysfunction.

C. Cardiovascular MRI is necessary to confirm the diagnosis.

D. This may be acquired, reversible, or found in healthy subjects.

E. A systolic trabecular/compacted myocardial ratio >2.0 is always pathologic.

11. A 49-year-old male presents to the emergency room with 1 week of persistent chest pain and sudden profound dyspnea in the last 3 hours. On exam, he is in severe respiratory distress requiring intubation and mechanical ventilation. His oxygen saturation is 88% on 4 LPM supplementary O_2. SBP = 78 mm Hg, HR = 75 bpm. ECG with diffuse ST depression, R > S in V1 and V2, but no ST elevation. He has rales throughout bilaterally on exam and a soft holosystolic murmur. CXR confirms severe pulmonary edema. Blood work is pending and you perform the following bedside echocardiogram (Fig. 44.11 and Video 44.8).

Which of the following is the next best step in the management of this patient?

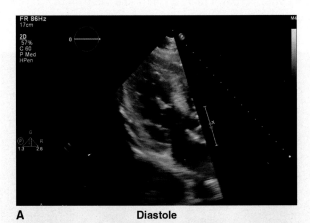

A   **Diastole**

B   **Systole**

FIGURE 44.11

A. Administer fibrinolytic therapy
B. Initiate IV antibiotic therapy
C. Immediate percutaneous coronary intervention
D. Cardiothoracic surgery consultation
E. Perform a CT scan

12. You were asked to review an echo on a 68F patient with a stroke sent to you from a former colleague (Video 44.9).

Based solely upon the parasternal 2D image shown, which of the following conclusions is most accurate?

A. Given the normal biventricular systolic function, this likely represents an aggressive form of Loeffler hypereosinophilic syndrome.
B. With extension beyond the anatomic tissue borders, this would suggest a cardiac malignancy.
C. Thin, echo-bright myocardium next to this mass makes this most likely a large thrombus.
D. The irregular protruding "fingers" suggests myxoma making the search for atrial masses more important.
E. This has the typical appearance of an atypical hypertrophic cardiomyopathy.

Answer 1: E. This is an apical four-chamber view. The left ventricle is identified by recognizing the papillary muscles, increased wall thickness, and more basal mitral valve. A left ventricular band, known by several names including false tendon, are fibromuscular structures in the left ventricle that cross the cavity joining nearby trabeculations or papillary muscles. Chordae tendineae connect the papillary muscles to the mitral valve. The moderator band is located in the right ventricle.

Suggested Readings

Gerlis LM, Dickinson DF. Left ventricular bands: a normal anatomical feature. *Br Heart J* 1984;52(6):641–647.
Gualano SK, Bolling SF, Gordon D, et al. High prevalence of false chordae tendinae in patients without left ventricular tachycardia. *Pacing Clin Electrophysiol* 2007;30(suppl 1):S156–S159.
Kenchaiah S, et al. Epidemiology of left ventricular false tendons: clinical correlates in the Framingham heart study. *J Am Soc Echocardiogr* 2009;22(6):739–745.
Sugiyama M. Echocardiographic features of false tendons in the left ventricle. *Am J Cardiol* 1981;48(1):177–183.

Answer 2: A. The image shows the left ventricle in the apical four-chamber view with a large laminated apical thrombus. When LVEF is measured using the modified Simpson method, the end-systolic and end-diastolic volumes in the four- and two-chamber views are obtained by tracing the endocardium. The endocardial border is traced contiguously excluding papillary muscles, trabeculations, and ventricular thrombi (Fig. 44.12). In the given image, the endocardium has been inaccurately traced excluding the border with overlying thrombus. As LV thrombi form over myocardial segments with wall motion abnormalities (usually aneurysmal, dyskinetic, or akinetic), excluding such segments in LVEF measurement would lead to an inaccurate assessment of LVEF. Hence, option A is correct.

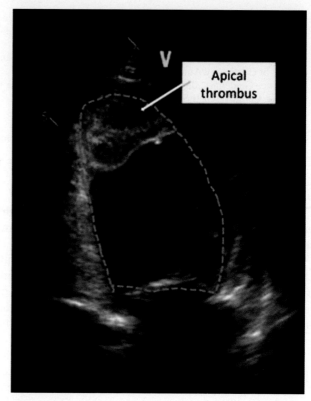

Figure 44.12

Suggested Readings

Lang RM, Bierig M, Devereux RB, et al. Recommendations for chamber quantification. *Eur J Echocardiogr* 2006;7:79–108.
Otterstad JE, Froeland G, St John Sutton M, et al. Accuracy and reproducibility of biplane two-dimensional echocardiographic measurements of left ventricular dimensions and function. *Eur Heart J* 1997;18(3):507–513.

Answer 3: A. Option A is correct. This patient has a laminated thrombus in the left ventricular apex. There is an extensive anteroapical myocardial infarction resulting in apical akinesis.

Option B is incorrect. Aspirin is insufficient to treat left ventricular thrombus.

Option C is incorrect. Even though the left ventricular thrombus is laminated, the apical akinesis leaves the patient at risk for development of further thrombus until there is improved left ventricular function.

Option D is incorrect. Though the patient will be on aspirin and Plavix postmyocardial infarction for secondary prevention and also for the prevention of stent thrombosis, it is insufficient to treat intracavitary thrombus.

Option E is incorrect.

Based on the guidelines for myocardial infarction, those after STEMI who have a large or anterior MI, atrial fibrillation, previous embolus or known LV thrombus, or cardiogenic shock should receive IV unfractionated heparin or low molecular weight heparin. In addition to the treatment of left ventricular thrombus, the purpose of anticoagulation is to prevent stroke (0.75% to 1.2% of MIs).

Suggested Reading

Antman EM, Hand M, Armstrong PW, et al. 2007 focused update of the ACC/AHA 2004 Guidelines for the Management of Patients with ST-Elevation Myocardial Infarction: a report of the American College of Cardiology/American Heart Association Task Force on Practice Guidelines: developed in collaboration with the Canadian Cardiovascular Society endorsed by the American Academy of Family Physicians: 2007 writing group to review new evidence and update the ACC/AHA 2004 Guidelines for the Management of Patients with ST-Elevation Myocardial Infarction, writing on behalf of the 2004 Writing Committee. *Circulation* 2008;117:296–329.

Answer 4: B.

Endomyocardial fibrosis = left ventricular and/or right ventricular apical fibrosis often with superimposed thrombus formation.

Although the other options are difficult to distinguish with echo imaging alone as they mimic other diseases (Fabry with HCM; radiation CM with infiltrative CM and constriction) or are a diagnosis of exclusion (idiopathic CM), this is one of the rare instances where echo can make the diagnosis due to the very distinct 2D appearance.

Endomyocardial fibrosis is a restrictive cardiomyopathy featuring fibrosis of the endocardium especially at the apices of the left and/or right ventricles. This results in impairment in ventricular filling and subsequent congestive heart failure. It was first diagnosed in Uganda and is endemic to tropical areas worldwide, including other central African countries such as Nigeria as well as portions of India and Brazil. It is felt to be the most prevalent restrictive cardiomyopathy in the world. Etiology is not certain although it resembles Loeffler endocarditis (eosinophilic myocarditis) that is linked with eosinophilia. Infectious and environmental etiologies have also been considered. Onset is usually from childhood to young adulthood. In addition to the usual physical findings of congestive heart failure, an exudative ascites without peripheral edema is characteristic, and an exudative pericardial effusion is common. Echocardiographic findings are typical of a restrictive cardiomyopathy but also have characteristic findings of apical obliteration of the left and/or right ventricles due to fibrosis and underlying thrombus. In contradistinction to apical thrombus formation due to hypokinesis or akinesis, the underlying apical myocardium in endomyocardial fibrosis has preserved contractility. Endomyocardial fibrosis also results in papillary muscle dysfunction and commonly some degree of mitral and tricuspid regurgitation. Prognosis is generally poor due to the presentation usually occurring in the end stages of the disease. Symptomatic medical treatment as is common in most restrictive cardiomyopathies is indicated. Surgical treatment with myocardial resection and valvular replacement, if indicated, has been performed and may improve survival in selected cases.

Suggested Readings

Acquatella H, Schiller NB, Puigbo JJ, et al. Value of two-dimensional echocardiography in endomyocardial disease with and without eosinophilia. *Circulation* 1983;67(6):1219–1226.

Berensztein CS, Pineiro D, Marcotegui M, et al. Usefulness of echocardiography and Doppler echocardiography in endomyocardial fibrosis. *J Am Soc Echocardiogr* 2000;13:385–392.

Schneider U, Jenni R, Turina J, et al. Long term follow up of patients with endomyocardial fibrosis: effects of surgery. *Heart* 1998;79:362–367.

Sliwa K, Damasceno A, Mayosi BM. Epidemiology and etiology of cardiomyopathy in Africa. *Circulation* 2005;112:3577–3583.

Answer 5: C. The patient has D-transposition, and the point is to show that the aortic and pulmonic valves are in the same plane in the parasternal long axis. There is no evidence for (option A) atrial septal defect. The patient has D- rather than L-transposition. Option D is wrong because the pulmonic valve is actually anterior and to the right, not left of the aortic valve. The morphologic left ventricle is the pulmonic ventricle since it is pumping blood to the pulmonary system. The morphologic RV is the systemic ventricle (FIG. 44.13).

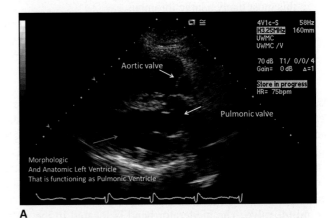

A

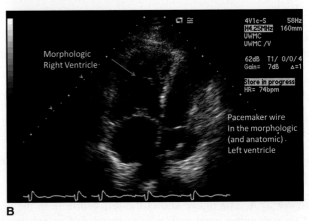

B

FIGURE 44.13 A: Parasternal long-axis view of a patient with D-transposition of the great vessels. The purpose of this image is to show that the aortic and pulmonic valves are in the same plane. **B:** Apical view of a patient with D-transposition of the great arteries. The morphologic right ventricle is enlarged and is functioning as the systemic ventricle, pumping blood through the aortic valve to the systemic circulation.

Suggested Readings

Burchill LJ, Huang J, Tretter JT, et al. Noninvasive imaging in adult congenital heart disease. *Circ Res* 2017;120:995–1014. https://doi.org/10.1161/CIRCRESAHA.116.308983

Houston A, Hillis S, Lilley S, et al. Echocardiography in adult congenital heart disease. *Heart* 1998;80:S12–S26.

Answer 6: D. In order to correctly answer this question, the test-taker must recognize that this is an anatomically correct apical four-chamber view (Mayo display with the right ventricle on the right hand side of the image display). Once this is recognized, then option A is no longer an adequate choice. Options B and C are not good options since they do not adhere to the common appearance of these larger, more mass-like structures. Option E is a possibility, but the video clearly demonstrates that this is not a typical appearance for a pacer wire. Option D is the correct answer, and whether this represents tricuspid valve chordae or actual redundant leaflet is not clear in this one view; however, it is a typical echo finding in Ebstein anomaly.

Suggested Reading
Booker OJ, Nanda NC. Echocardiographic assessment of Ebstein's anomaly. *Echocardiography* 2015;32(suppl 2):S177–S188. doi: 10.1111/echo.12486

Answer 7: D. The images confirm the increasing LV wall thickness from base to apex consistent with an apical variant hypertrophic cardiomyopathy. Although initially discovered in the Japanese population, this is now seen in all ethnicities. It is known to occur at an incidence greater than what is detected with transthoracic echocardiography and cardiovascular MRI is repeatedly providing us with examples of missed cases with echo alone (option C is incorrect). The natural history of this pathology is progressive diastolic dysfunction, dilation of the LA cavity, and commonly, atrial fibrillation as in this patient.

In the parasternal long axis, the apex will be seen at end systole raising the possibility that this diagnosis is present and should be sought in the apical view (option A is incorrect). In cases with a poor quality apical acoustic window, this is even more important. Ultrasound contrast agents can be used in this setting to confirm the "spade-like" systolic pattern. Color flow Doppler can also be used in this manner as a "contrast agent" to improve endocardial visualization (option E is incorrect).

Because the cavity obliteration is apical (or midcavity), there is no systolic anterior motion of the mitral valve and no added value of performing Valsalva (option B is incorrect).

Because of the lack of acoustic mismatch in the myocardial filled LV cavity, no image is created and the reader may misinterpret the epicardial motion as endocardial. Since this moves "outward" during systole, it may be misinterpreted as an apical aneurysm (option D is correct).

Suggested Reading
Stainback RF. Apical hypertrophic cardiomyopathy. *Tex Heart Inst J* 2012;39(5):747–749. PMCID: PMC3461654.

Answer 8: D. There is prominent trabeculation of the RV apex (note: the orientation is displayed with the RV on the right) and the LV, although this is less well seen. Trabeculation meeting the criteria for noncompaction (option C) is common in many patients with alternative pathologic and physiologic explanations (e.g., postinfarction, pregnancy, etc.). In this case, there is clear carcinoid involvement of the tricuspid valve with a fixed TV leaflet in the open (diastolic) position. This results in severe

RV volume overload, which will frequently be associated with this degree of marked trabeculation. The other choices do not have this 2D echo appearance but have patterns that the test-taker should recognize.

Suggested Reading
Almeida AG, Pinto FJ. Non-compaction cardiomyopathy. *Heart* 2013;99:1535–1542. http://dx.doi.org/10.1136/heartjnl-2012-302048

Answer 9: A.

These images show an apical four-chamber view of poor quality (note the increase depth from transducer to LV myocardium consistent with the clinical history of obesity). These patients benefit from the administration of an UEA, especially in the clinical setting of a TIA/stroke. The updated focused ASE guidelines for contrast use denounce the purported increased risk of UEA in patients known to have small right-to-left shunts through a PFO. Based upon this, option A is correct.

Option B is incorrect. The report should reserve "possible" thrombus for echo studies that are not diagnostic. These images clearly demonstrate a large, protruding, filling defect with contrast "creeping" around the edges in an LV apex that is "rounded" (typical LAD remodeling appearance) and would more correctly be interpreted as a "definitive" thrombus. Option E is incorrect since a thrombus will be more commonly seen in an LV apex that is abnormal. Trabeculation can be excluded by off-axis imaging and the appearance of the filling defect. An apical tumor, although rare, can be confirmed with continued contrast imaging demonstrating perfusion (due to arterial flow).

Option C is incorrect since the filling defect/thrombus size alone (>1 cm) is an independent predictor of embolic events. Other embolic features include the protrusion into the lumen, a demonstrated stalk, hypermobility, or other complex features such as multiple "heads" or a pedunculated surface.

Suggested Reading
Porter TR, Mulvagh SL, Abdelmoneim SS, et al. Clinical Applications of Ultrasounic Enhancing Agents in Echocardiography: 2018 American Society of Echocardiography Guidelines Update. *J Am Soc Echocardiogr* 2018;31(3):241–274. doi: 10.1016/j.echo.2017.11.013

Answer 10: D. Although this image has prominent LV trabeculation (in both the LV and the RV), this feature alone is not adequate to make a diagnosis. The clinical history of heart failure and TIA is worrisome for LV noncompaction (isolated, if no other congenital heart defect is found); other etiologies such as ischemia, pregnancy, athletics, etc., should be sought. We continue to learn about this new "cardiomyopathy," and recently, the diagnosis of LVNC is considered best not to coincide with that of a "cardiomyopathy" because it can be observed in healthy subjects with normal LV size and function and it can be acquired and is reversible (option D is correct).

Left ventricular noncompaction (LVNC) describes a ventricular wall anatomy characterized by prominent left ventricular

(LV) trabeculae, a thin compacted layer, and deep intertrabecular recesses. Individual variability is extreme, and trabeculae represent a sort of individual "cardioprinting." Occasionally, LVNC may also be part of a cardiomyopathy, such as in infantile tafazzinopathies.

When the increased trabecular ratio is associated with LV dilation and dysfunction, hypertrophy, or congenital heart disease, the genetic cause may overlap. The prevalence of echo findings consistent with the morphologic features of LVNC in healthy subjects, its reported reversibility in many other conditions, and its incidental finding in the general population suggests that caution should be employed when reporting LVNC cardiomyopathy. Although echo features may fulfill the morphologic criteria, additional echo findings are required to conclude a functional cardiomyopathy.

There are no data to confirm that option B is correct. Option C is also incorrect when the echo images are of adequate quality. Option E is obviously incorrect since the ratio alone cannot make the diagnosis of a cardiomyopathy.

In patients with clinical symptoms of heart failure, stroke, or palpitations/syncope, a search for apical thrombi (use UEA as indicated), careful measurement of LV volumes and function, and ambulatory event recordings are warranted.

Suggested Reading
Arbustini E, et al. Left ventricular noncompaction. A distinct genetic cardiomyopathy? *J Am Coll Cardiol* 2016;68(9):949–966. doi: 10.1016/j.jacc.2016.05.096

Answer 11: D. This patient has presented with a rather typical presentation for a recent, complicated, posterior wall myocardial infarction, likely a few days or weeks old. Papillary muscle complete or partial rupture with acute mitral regurgitation is a catastrophic complication resulting in rapid pulmonary edema and shock. Without urgent recognition and immediate surgery, mortality is high. In my experience, partial rupture, as in this patient, is seen more commonly than complete rupture, likely based upon Darwinian expectations. Echo will frequently demonstrate a hypermobile mass on the chordae that may or may not prolapse into the LA. This papillary muscle head may be partially attached to remaining chords or may get "caught" in the subvalvular apparatus, and therefore, the absence of mass protrusion into the LA should not dissuade the diagnosis. A TEE can confirm the diagnosis whenever uncertain and should be performed immediately upon suspicion.

Suggested Reading
Fradley MG, Picard MH. Rupture of the posteromedial papillary muscle leading to partial flail of the anterior mitral leaflet. *Circulation* 2011;123:1044–1045. https://doi.org/10.1161/CIRCULATIONAHA.110.984724

Answer 12: C. The LV (and RV) systolic function is reduced making option A incorrect. Option B is also incorrect as there is no "extension" beyond the demonstrated anatomic cardiac borders and the mass is entirely within the LV cavity (nearly most of the LV cavity). Option C is the single best answer and is consistent with the motto: "uncommon presentations of common pathologies are more common than common presentations of uncommon pathologies." (**Editor's note:** I apologize for the poetic license of that quote.) Option D is incorrect since ventricular myxomas are not only rare, but usually very apical, often biventricular, and would not (necessarily) be found in the clinical setting of LV dysfunction postinfarction. Finally, option E is incorrect, and this echo should not be misinterpreted as a hypertrophic CM.

Suggested Reading
Srichai MB, Junor C, Rodriguez LL, et al. Clinical, imaging, and pathological characteristics of left ventricular thrombus: a comparison of contrast-enhanced magnetic resonance imaging, transthoracic echocardiography, and transesophageal echocardiography with surgical or pathological validation. *Am Heart J* 2006;152:75–84.

Chapter 45

Pathologic Masses on the Valves

Mikel D. Smith

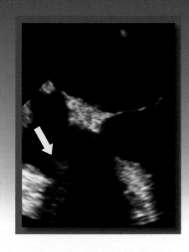

1. You are reading a transthoracic echocardiogram on a 28-year-old intravenous drug user with *Staphylococcus aureus* bacteremia. Which of the following ultrasound features best describes a typical bacterial vegetation?

   A. Irregular-shaped, highly mobile oscillating mass on upstream side of the valve, with independent motion

   B. Smooth, highly mobile spherical mass on the tips of the valve leaflets

   C. Thin, filamentous strands, attached to the upstream side of the valve

   D. Mobile, sessile mass, with broader base, noncontrast enhancing, attached to the upstream side of the valve

2. You are asked to evaluate a 34-year-old young male with a recent history of IVDU who presented with fever and *Streptococcus viridans* bacteremia. His transthoracic echocardiography is shown in Video 45.1. He was started on ceftriaxone pending the results of culture susceptibilities.

   Which of the following is the next best step in management?

   A. Recommend transesophageal echocardiography to confirm the diagnosis.

   B. Continue treatment with antibiotics while pending susceptibility and switch to culture-sensitive antibiotics with a total duration of therapy with 6 weeks.

   C. Continue treatment with current antibiotics for 6 weeks and perform TEE as recommended.

   D. Repeat TTE in few days to document resolution.

   E. Surgical consultation.

3. A 68-year-old male with coronary artery bypass surgery, diabetes, and HTN presented with recurrent TIA-like symptoms. His symptoms resolved by the time he arrived to the ER. His physical exam was unremarkable including neurologic exam. His prior workup (CT scan, carotid duplex, TTE) revealed mild atherosclerosis of the left common carotid artery and grade II atheroma in the aorta, and his ASA dose was increased to 325 mg daily. Due to recurrence of TIA, he underwent TEE, and images are shown in Video 45.2.

   What is the next best course of action?

   A. Add warfarin to his ASA therapy.

   B. Surgical consultation.

   C. Draw blood cultures and initiate broad-spectrum antibiotics.

   D. Reassurance and no further workup needed.

4. A patient presents with *Streptococcus bovis* bacteremia and small vegetation (6 mm) on the anterior mitral leaflet. On further investigation, it is discovered that he was recently diagnosed with colon cancer, underwent partial colectomy, and is now on chemotherapy. He is started on intravenous nafcillin and gentamicin. You are asked to perform a transesophageal echocardiogram. What is the diagnostic accuracy (sensitivity) of transthoracic and transesophageal echocardiography, respectively, in detecting valvular vegetations? (Select the best response.)

   A. <40% and 100%

   B. 40% to 60% and >90%

   C. 60% to 80% and 80% to 90%

   D. <40% and <90%

5. In keeping with the current recommendations of prophylaxis for endocarditis, answer A (yes), B (no), or C (need more information) for each case scenario. Review echocardiography images for each clinical presentation as listed.

   Scenario 5A: A 28-year-old female with congenital repair of VSD, undergoing restorative dental procedure (images shown in Video 45.3 and Fig. 45.1)

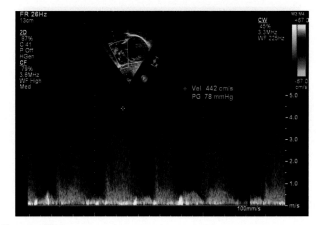

Figure 45.1

Should this patient receive prophylaxis for infective endocarditis?

A. Yes
B. No
C. Need more information

Scenario 5B: A 38-year-old male with corrective surgery for tetralogy of Fallot with RVOT conduit with bioprosthetic PV, undergoing bronchoscopy with biopsy (VIDEO 45.4). Answer A, B, or C.

Scenario 5C: A 45-year-old male with bicuspid aortic valve who is undergoing mechanical aortic valve replacement (VIDEO 45.5). Answer A, B, or C.

Scenario 5D: A 65-year-old female with mitral valve prolapse who is undergoing coronary artery bypass graft surgery for three-vessel coronary artery disease (VIDEO 45.6 and FIG. 45.2). Answer A, B, or C.

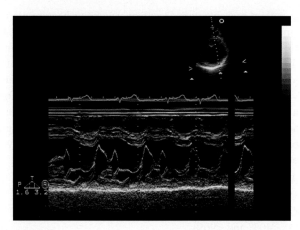

FIGURE 45.2

Scenario 5E: A 57-year-old male who underwent cardiac transplant 2 years ago and on chronic immunosuppressive therapy, who is undergoing root canal surgery (VIDEO 45.7). Answer A, B, or C.

6. Which of the following M-mode finding correlates with acute severe aortic regurgitation?

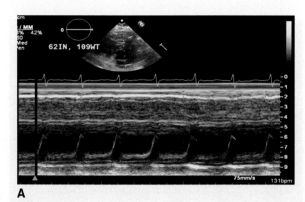

A

FIGURE 45.3

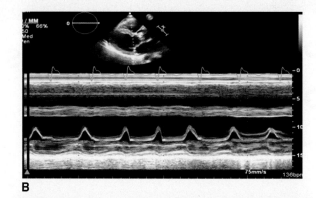

B

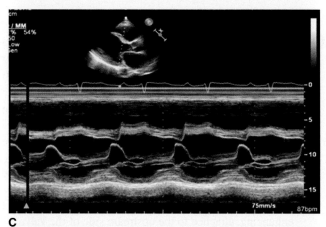

C

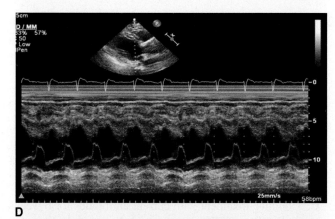

D

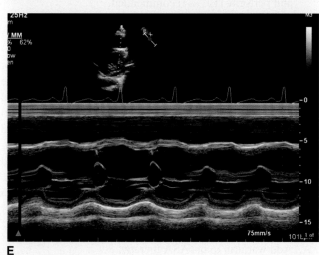

E

FIGURE 45.3 (Continued)

A. FIGURE 45.3A
B. FIGURE 45.3B
C. FIGURE 45.3C
D. FIGURE 45.3D
E. FIGURE 45.3E

7. All of the following echo and Doppler tracings were recorded from patients who had aortic valve endocarditis and regurgitation. Which finding is not predictive of the severity of aortic regurgitation?

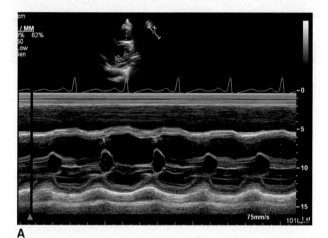

A

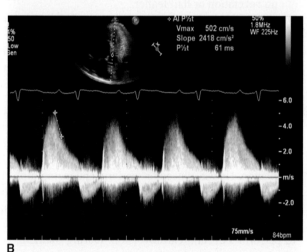

B

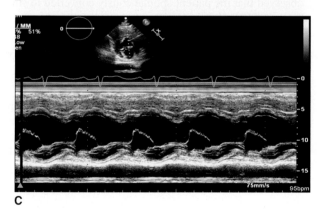

C

FIGURE 45.4

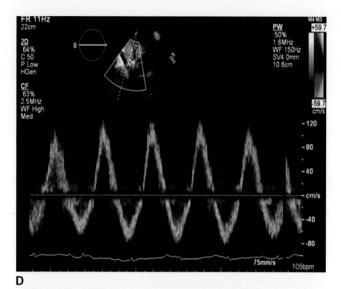

D

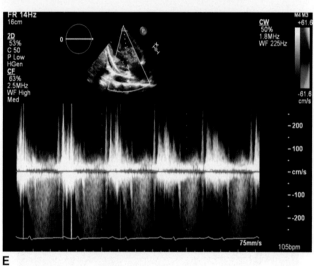

E

FIGURE 45.4 (*Continued*)

A. FIGURE 45.4A
B. FIGURE 45.4B
C. FIGURE 45.4C
D. FIGURE 45.4D
E. FIGURE 45.4E

8. A 42-year-old male who presents with fever to your emergency department is found to have an oscillating intracardiac mass on 2D echocardiography. Which of the following would be sufficient to diagnose infective endocarditis?

A. *Streptococcus viridans* bacteremia in a patient with pharyngitis
B. *Staphylococcus aureus* bacteremia in an intravenous drug user
C. *Acinetobacter* bacteremia in a patient with a post-op sternal infection
D. *Proteus* bacteremia in a patient with urosepsis and indwelling catheter
E. *Enterococcus* bacteremia in a patient with infection at the site of tunneled dialysis catheter

9. Which of the following is not included in the minor criteria in the modified Duke criteria for the diagnosis of infective endocarditis?

A. Predisposing heart condition (uncorrected congenital heart disease)
B. Injectable drug abuse
C. Infected pseudoaneurysm (mycotic aneurysm)
D. Coagulase-negative *Staphylococcus* bacteremia
E. New valvular regurgitation

10. Which of the following findings for left-sided native valve endocarditis is an indication for cardiac surgery?

A. Multivalvular vegetations
B. Congestive heart failure due to regurgitation
C. Preexisting LAHB and RBBB
D. *Staphylococcal aortic valve* endocarditis
E. A mobile mitral vegetation

11. A 34-year-old male with a history of intravenous drug use presented with an aortic valve vegetation. His transthoracic echocardiography images are shown in Video 45.8 and Figure 45.5. Based on your review of the images, which of the following would be a correct statement in your echo report?

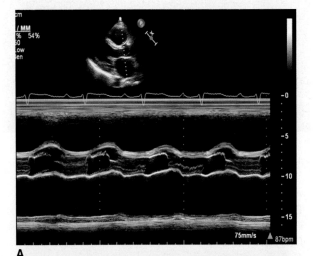

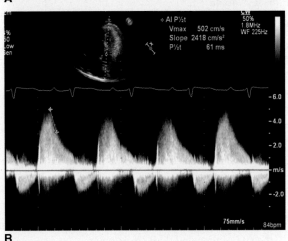

Figure 45.5

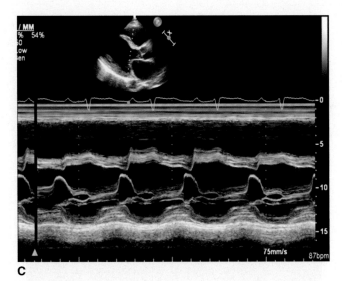

Figure 45.5 (*Continued*)

A. 2D images show a vegetation involving the aortic valve with a flail leaflet, with clear evidence of paravalvular extension of infection suggesting abscess.
B. Color Doppler is not diagnostic of severe aortic regurgitation due to inability to see the origin of the jet.
C. M-mode of the aortic valve shows normal opening and complete closure of the aortic valve suggesting there is no vegetation or flail leaflet.
D. The CW Doppler is not a recording of aortic regurgitation but may represent mitral stenosis.
E. M-mode of the mitral valve shows an A wave in late diastole and is evidence against acute, severe aortic regurgitation.

12. A 78-year-old male with coronary artery bypass surgery, peripheral arterial disease s/p left CEA (carotid endarterectomy), diabetes, and HTN presented with intermittent palpitations and presyncope. He was found to have atrial fibrillation. He was placed on warfarin and metoprolol. His EF was mildly reduced on transthoracic echocardiography. During follow-up after 2 weeks, he continued to be symptomatic, which limited his lifestyle. A decision was made to perform TEE and cardioversion. During imaging, you observed that the patient spontaneously converted to sinus rhythm. TEE did not show LAA thrombus, but you find a small mobile structure on the aortic valve (Video 45.9).

Your recommendation to the referring physician would be:

A. Continue warfarin.
B. Surgical consultation.
C. Draw blood cultures and initiate broad-spectrum antibiotics.
D. Repeat the TEE after 4 weeks of anticoagulation.
E. Stop warfarin; no further anticoagulation is required.

13. Which of the following patients has a definitive diagnosis of infective endocarditis?

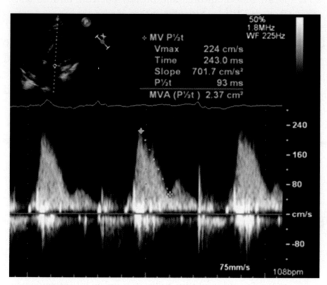

FIGURE 45.6

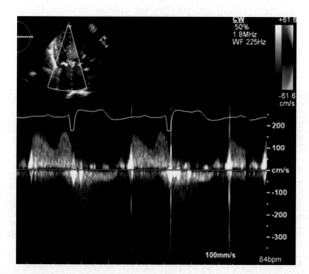

FIGURE 45.7

A. An 82-year-old female for routine follow-up for her history of moderate mitral regurgitation (VIDEO 45.10)

B. A 34-year-old female with substance abuse presented with congestive heart failure (VIDEO 45.11)

C. A 54-year-old female presented with NSTEMI and heart failure (VIDEO 45.12)

D. A 65-year-old female with ESRD and HTN, routine follow-up for heart murmur (VIDEO 44.13 and FIG. 45.6)

E. A 78-year-old female with myxomatous mitral valve disease and torn chord, routine follow-up (VIDEO 45.14 and FIG. 45.7)

14. A 28-year-old male with IVDU presented with acute right hemiparesis. CT scan shows large right MCA territory stroke with midline shift. He undergoes craniotomy as treatment. Echocardiography was performed on admission (VIDEO 45.15 and FIG. 45.8) and repeat exam 7 days later (VIDEO 45.16).

Which of the following is true regarding his endocarditis?

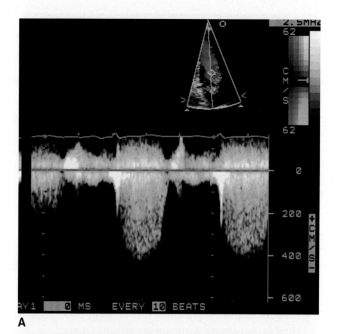

A

B

FIGURE 45.8

A. Embolic risk is not related to vegetation size at presentation.

B. Since most vegetations are mobile structures, high mobility of the vegetation is not predictive of embolic risk.

C. Embolic risk becomes insignificant after the initiation of antibiotic therapy.

D. Embolic risk of a vegetation is the same for mitral and aortic valves.

E. The persistence of a large vegetation after an embolic event makes it more likely to have a recurrence.

15. You are performing a TEE on a patient who is an IVDU who underwent bioprosthetic aortic valve placement 2 years ago. He has now presented again with fevers, chills, and *Staphylococcus aureus* bacteremia. The TEE is shown in Video 45.17 and Figure 45.9.

Which of the following would be the least correct statements in regard to this study?

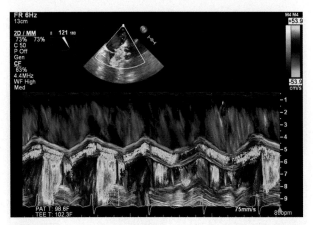

FIGURE 45.9

A. Large mobile mitral valve vegetation with leaflet perforation is present.
B. Color M-mode is diagnostic of fistulous flow.
C. There are no vegetations on the bioprosthetic aortic valve, yet severe aortic regurgitation is noted.
D. There is evidence of severe mitral regurgitation seen on color flow into the left atrium.

16. A 64-year-old male with diabetes, CAD with four-vessel CABG, and recently diagnosed colon cancer (adenocarcinoma) presents with right hemiparesis. He denies any fevers or chills. His initial blood cultures are negative. CT of the brain shows acute left hemispheric infarct. Echocardiography was ordered to rule out a cardiac source of embolism. You are asked to see the patient as he was found to have a murmur of mitral stenosis, and echocardiography is shown in Video 45.18A–C, Figure 45.10, and Video 45.18D–F. Based on your assessment, you recommend which of the following?

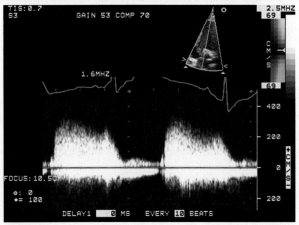

FIGURE 45.10

A. Replace the mitral valve.
B. Observe for clinical symptoms from mitral stenosis.
C. Warfarin therapy.
D. Draw blood cultures and broad-spectrum antibiotics.
E. Repeat TEE in 4 weeks.

17. You are asked to evaluate a 28-year-old young female (IV drug user) who presented with fevers, chills, and *Staphylococcus aureus* bacteremia, and her transthoracic echocardiography is shown in Video 45.19. She was started on broad-spectrum antibiotics pending susceptibility.

Based on your assessment, the diagnosis is:

A. Definite infective endocarditis
B. Possible infective endocarditis
C. Probable infective endocarditis
D. Rejected diagnosis of endocarditis

18. A 58-year-old male who underwent mechanical aortic valve replacement 6 years ago for bicuspid aortic valve presented with pneumonia that was complicated by methicillin-sensitive *Staphylococcus aureus* sepsis. He was started on nafcillin and rifampin with some clinical improvement. His transthoracic echocardiography was limited and difficult to assess mechanical prosthesis; however, it showed mildly elevated gradient across the aortic prosthesis. TEE was performed, and images are shown in Video 45.20 and Figure 45.11. Based on this information and your review of the echo findings, which of the following is the most correct statement?

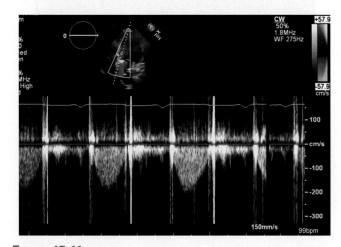

FIGURE 45.11 AV VTI.

V$_{max}$	175 cm/s
V$_{mean}$	122 cm/s
Max PG	12 mm Hg
Mean PG	7 mm Hg
VTI	22.9 cm

A. Prosthetic valve endocarditis is a rare condition (<1% of endocarditis cases) but is associated with 30% to 40% mortality.

B. Due to his multivalvular involvement, he needs urgent replacement of the aortic and mitral valves with bioprostheses.

C. The Duke criteria are equally effective in the diagnosis of native valve and prosthetic valve endocarditis, but its sensitivity falls significantly for mechanical prosthesis.

D. Endocarditis affects mechanical valves at twice the incidence of bioprosthetic valves.

19. A 38-year-old male with a history of HIV and hepatitis presented with bioprosthetic aortic valve endocarditis. His TEE is shown in VIDEO 45.21.

Based on your assessment, which of the following is correct?

A. It is a serious complication but can be treated successfully with conservative medical therapy.

B. Involvement of the mitral valve (rather than the aortic) most often presents with varying degrees of heart block.

C. A mycotic aneurysm in a systemic artery would be much more common than in the aortic root.

D. It involves the aortic valve more commonly than the mitral valve and can lead to fistulous connection to the right atrium, right ventricle, or left atrium.

20. A 28-year-old male with intravenous drug abuse presents with respiratory failure from pulmonary edema. His transthoracic echocardiography is shown in VIDEOS 45.22 AND 45.23 and FIGURE 45.12. His blood cultures show MRSA. He was started on broad-spectrum antibiotics and on heart failure therapy. After being on 3 days of antibiotics, his bacteremia resolved. Mechanical ventilation was no longer required.

At this point, what is the best course of action?

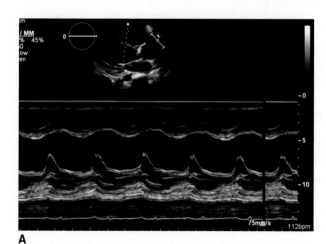

A

FIGURE 45.12

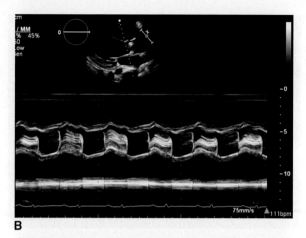

B

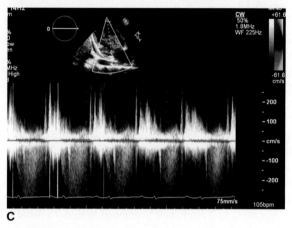

C

FIGURE 45.12 *(Continued)*

A. Continue vancomycin for total of 6 weeks (clinical heart failure and bacteremia resolved).

B. Repeat TTE in 2 weeks to establish resolution of vegetation, valve function, and LV function.

C. Elective surgery in 2 to 4 weeks as early surgical mortality is high during active infection.

D. Surgery as soon as feasible.

21. Clinical presentation and echocardiographic examination are shown in the following images. In each case, assess the indications for valve surgery based on the information and findings as A (yes) or B (no).

A. A 28-year-old male with intravenous drug abuse presented with fever and chills (VIDEO 45.24)

B. A 65-year-old female with bioprosthetic aortic valve and mitral valve replacement for rheumatic heart disease presented with heart failure (VIDEO 45.25)

C. A 38-year-old female with intravenous drug abuse and known tricuspid valve endocarditis who was treated medically for 8 weeks of therapy and successful eradication of bacteremia (VIDEO 45.26 and FIG. 45.13)

D. A 45-year-old with bioprosthetic aortic and mitral valves now presented with *Staphylococcus* bacteremia (VIDEO 45.27)

E. A 48-year-old male with HIV and hepatitis C presented with chronic malaise and weight loss (VIDEO 45.28)

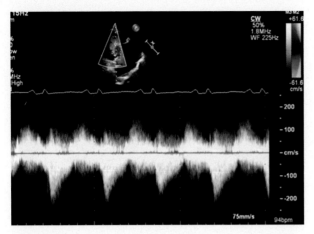

FIGURE 45.13

Answer 1: *A.*

Option A: Typical features of vegetation

Option B: Best describes papillary fibroelastoma

Option C: Best describes Lambl excrescence

Option D: Best describes blood cyst

Echocardiographic features of a typical vegetation include an irregularly shaped, highly mobile mass, oscillating or fluttering, attached to the upstream side of the valve leaflet. They usually have motion that is independent of the valve itself (TABLE 45.1).

Papillary fibroelastoma (PFE) is characterized by a smooth, highly mobile spherical mass usually <1 cm in diameter (but may become 2 to 3 cm in size), attached to mid- to distal valve leaflets or to chordae tendineae. Among the tumors that affect the valves, PFEs are by far the most common, accounting for 85% of valve-associated tumors. These tumors are usually attached to the downstream side of the valve by a small pedicle and are irregularly shaped with delicate frond-like surfaces. They carry a risk of embolization.

Lambl excrescences (fibrous strands) are best described as fine threadlike strands arising on the line of closure (contact surface) of heart valves, which more commonly occur on the mitral, followed by the aortic valve.

Blood cysts are blood-containing cystic structures that usually develop within mitral leaflets. They have a broader base, are sessile, and are less mobile than a fibroelastoma. On contrast echocardiography, they often appear as a filling defect on the valve leaflet.

Table 45.1	Echocardiographic Criteria for Defining a Vegetation	
POSITIVE FEATURE	**NEGATIVE FEATURE**
Low reflectance	High echogenicity
Attached to valve, upstream side	Nonvalvular location
Irregular shape, amorphous	Smooth surface or fibrillar
Mobile, oscillating	Nonmobile
Associated tissue changes, valvular regurgitation	Absence of regurgitation

From Armstrong W, Ryan T. Infective endocarditis. In: *Chapter 14: Feigenbaum's Echocardiography.* 7th ed. Philadelphia, PA: Lippincott Williams & Wilkins, 2009:362, with permission.

Suggested Readings

Abraham KP, Reddy V, Gattuso P, et al. Neoplasms metastatic to the heart: review of 3314 consecutive autopsies. *Am J Cardiovasc Pathol* 1990;3:195–198.

Alam M. Pitfalls in the echocardiographic diagnosis of intracardiac and extracardiac masses. *Echocardiography* 1993;10:181–191.

Gowda RM, Khan IA, Nair CK, et al. Cardiac papillary fibroelastoma: a comprehensive analysis of 725 cases. *Am Heart J* 2003;146:404–410.

Klarich KW, Enriquez-Sarano M, Gura GM, et al. Papillary fibroelastoma: echocardiographic characteristics for diagnosis and pathologic correlation. *J Am Coll Cardiol* 1997;30:784–790.

Narang J, Neustein S, Israel D. The role of transesophageal echocardiography in the diagnosis and excision of a tumor of the aortic valve. *J Cardiothorac Vasc Anesth* 1992;6:68–69.

Sachdev M, Peterson GE, Jollis JG, et al. Imaging techniques for diagnosis of infective endocarditis. *Infect Dis Clin North Am* 2002;16:319–337.

Yamamoto H, Nakatani S, Niwaya K, et al. Giant blood cyst of the mitral valve: echocardiographic and intraoperative images. *Circulation* 2005;112:e341.

Answer 2: *B.* The echocardiogram shown demonstrates a mobile mass (VIDEO 45.1A–C) likely involving the noncoronary leaflet of the aortic valve. Given his IVDU and *Streptococcus* bacteremia, this finding likely represents an endocarditis. There is no mitral or aortic regurgitation (VIDEO 45.1D) and no clear evidence of vegetation involving the tricuspid (VIDEO 45.1E) or pulmonary valve leaflets (VIDEO 45.1F). These transthoracic echocardiographic images are adequate to make the diagnosis of uncomplicated bacterial endocarditis.

Option A: Performing transesophageal echocardiography to confirm the diagnosis is inappropriate, when TTE is definitive for the diagnosis of infective endocarditis. The parasternal images show a vegetation involving the aortic valve (VIDEO 45.1A–C) without significant valvular dysfunction. Therefore, there is no need to confirm the diagnosis. Hence, answer A is incorrect.

Option B: Continuing treatment with ceftriaxone while pending susceptibility and switching to culture-sensitive antibiotic therapy with a total duration of therapy with 6 weeks is the correct answer.

Option C: Continuing treatment with ceftriaxone for 6 weeks is not appropriate, as antibiotic therapy needs to be tailored to susceptibility, and there is no requirement for a TEE at the end of treatment as the transthoracic study demonstrated a vegetation. Hence, answer C is incorrect.

Option D: Repeating TTE in few days to document resolution is not necessary in the absence of high-risk features (such as large vegetations, with size >1 cm, severe valvular insufficiency, abscess cavities or pseudoaneurysms, valvular perforation or dehiscence, and evidence of decompensated heart failure). Repeat echocardiography should be performed if suspicion exists without a diagnosis of IE or with a worrisome clinical course during early treatment of IE. However, it is reasonable to consider routine TTE after the completion of the therapy to establish a new baseline for valve function.

Option E: Surgical consultation is not necessary in the absence of a surgical indication for IE such as a large vegetation or complications such as abscess or heart block.

Echocardiography is central to the diagnosis and management of patients with IE, as it can also help detect complications, such as annular abscess, prosthetic valve partial dehiscence, valve perforation, and valvular regurgitation.

Echocardiography should be performed in all cases of suspected IE (class I, LOE: A). Whether TTE or TEE should be performed first depends on the clinical scenario (see Fig. 45.14). If the clinical suspicion is relatively low or imaging is likely to be of good quality, then it is reasonable to perform TTE. When imaging is difficult or poor (COPD, morbid obesity, etc.), TEE should be considered (1).

If TTE shows a vegetation but the likelihood of complications is low, then a subsequent TEE is unlikely to alter initial medical management. On the other hand, if the clinical suspicion of IE or its complications are high (prosthetic valve, staphylococcal bacteremia, or new atrioventricular block), a negative TTE will not definitely rule out IE or its potential complications, and a TEE should be performed first (as it is more sensitive for the detection of abscesses).

Even though TEE should be the first examination in certain patients with suspected IE, there might be a situation when it is not feasible (uncooperative patient, TEE service not available 24 hours or not immediately available, impending respiratory failure). When TEE is not clinically possible or must be delayed, early TTE should be performed without delay.

Both TEE and TTE may produce false-negative results if vegetations are small or have already embolized. Even TEE may miss initial perivalvular abscesses, particularly when the study is performed early in the patient's illness. Similarly, perivalvular fistulae and pseudoaneurysms develop over time, and negative early TEE images do not exclude the potential for their development.

False-positive results from TEE or TTE studies may occur with previous endocarditis with residual scarring, severe myxomatous change, and even normal degenerative structures such as Lambl excrescences or nodules. As echocardiographic technology improves (higher transducer frequencies and harmonic images), more subtle findings can be recognized and may add to the category of indeterminate findings. One approach to minimizing confusion from these structures is to exploit the high frame rates that are available with current equipment to improve the temporal resolution and better visualize rapidly moving structures such as microcavitations from prosthetic valves or fibrillar components, which can be confounders (Fig. 45.14 and Table 45.2).

Besides some of the complications listed earlier, other features that might point toward disease progression are increase in vegetation size, worsening regurgitation, chamber enlargement, ventricular dysfunction, and evidence of elevated filling pressure. These changes may occur during therapy in the absence of clinical deterioration and often affect management plans. The final decision involves the need for repeat echocardiographic analysis in a patient with an established diagnosis. There are no firm data to support the use of serial echocardiograms in this setting. In most cases, the decision to perform subsequent echocardiograms depends on the clinical course.

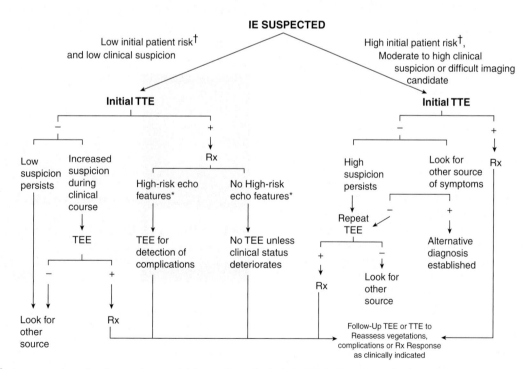

FIGURE 45.14 An approach to the diagnostic use of echocardiography (echo). *High-risk echocardiographic features include large and/or mobile vegetations, valvular insufficiency, suggestion of perivalvular extension, or secondary ventricular dysfunction (see text). †For example, a patient with fever and a previously known heart murmur and no other stigmata of IE. Also, high initial patient risks include prosthetic heart valves, many congenital heart diseases, previous endocarditis, new murmur, heart failure, or other stigmata of endocarditis. Rx indicates antibiotic treatment for endocarditis. (Reproduced from Bayer AS, Bolger AF, Taubert KA, et al. Diagnosis and management of infective endocarditis and its complications. *Circulation* 1998;98(25):2936–2948, with permission.)

Table 45.2 Use of Echocardiography During Diagnosis and Treatment of Endocarditis

Early

Echocardiography as soon as possible (<12 h after initial evaluation)

TEE preferred; obtain TTE views of any abnormal findings for later comparison

TTE if TEE is not immediately available

TTE may be sufficient in small children

Repeat echocardiography

TEE after positive TTE as soon as possible in patients at high risk for complications

TEE 7–10 d after initial TEE if suspicion exists without diagnosis of IE or with worrisome clinical course during early treatment of IE

Intraoperative

Prepump

Identification of vegetations, mechanism of regurgitation, abscesses, fistulas, and pseudoaneurysms

Postpump

Confirmation of successful repair of abnormal findings

Assessment of residual valve dysfunction

Elevated afterload if necessary to avoid underestimating valve insufficiency or presence of residual abnormal flow

Completion of therapy

Establish new baseline for valve function and morphology and ventricular size and function

TTE usually adequate; TEE or review of intraoperative TEE may be needed for complex anatomy to establish new baseline

TEE, transesophageal echocardiography; TTE, transthoracic echocardiography.

From Baddour LM, Wilson WR, Bayer AS, et al. Diagnosis, antimicrobial therapy, and management of complications: a statement for healthcare professionals from the Committee on Rheumatic Fever, Endocarditis, and Kawasaki disease, Council on Cardiovascular Disease in the Young, and the Councils on Clinical Cardiology, Stroke, and Cardiovascular Surgery and Anesthesia, American Heart Association: endorsed by the Infectious Diseases Society of America. Executive summary. *Circulation* 2005;111(23):3167–3184, with permission.

In patients who demonstrate clinical deterioration, repeat testing can be valuable in establishing a cause and in guiding subsequent decision-making. Alternatively, patients who demonstrate a good response to antibiotic therapy based on subsequent blood culture results as well as history and physical examination are unlikely to benefit from any form of additional testing. Some high-risk subsets of patients, such as those with staphylococcal endocarditis involving the aortic valve, may benefit from a second echocardiogram 7 to 10 days after initiation of therapy to exclude complications such as abscess formation.

Reference

1. Baddour LM, Wilson WR, Bayer AS, et al. Diagnosis, antimicrobial therapy, and management of complications: a statement for healthcare professionals from the Committee on Rheumatic Fever, Endocarditis, and Kawasaki disease, Council on Cardiovascular Disease in the Young, and the Councils on Clinical Cardiology, Stroke, and Cardiovascular Surgery and Anesthesia, American Heart Association: endorsed by the Infectious Diseases Society of America. Executive summary. *Circulation* 2005;111:3167–3184.

Suggested Readings

Daniel WG, Mugge A, Grote J, et al. Comparison of transthoracic and transesophageal echocardiography for detection of abnormalities of prosthetic and bioprosthetic valves in the mitral and aortic positions. *Am J Cardiol* 1993;71:210–215.

Heidenreich PA, Masoudi FA, Maini B, et al. Echocardiography in patients with suspected endocarditis: a cost-effectiveness analysis. *Am J Med* 1999;107:198–208.

Lindner JR, Case RA, Dent JM, et al. Diagnostic value of echocardiography in suspected endocarditis: an evaluation based on the pretest probability of disease. *Circulation* 1996;93:730–736.

San Roman JA, Vilacosta I, Zamorano JL, et al. Transesophageal echocardiography in right-sided endocarditis. *J Am Coll Cardiol* 1993;21:1226–1230.

Answer 3: B. Images from TEE show typical features of papillary fibroelastoma (PFE) on the aortic valve. The patient underwent successful surgical removal with valve sparing.

Echocardiographic characteristics of papillary fibroelastomas (also called papilloma, papillary endocardial tumors, cardiac papilloma, or papillary fibroma) are described as a smooth, highly mobile, spherical mass, smaller in size (usually <1 to 1.5 cm), attached to the mid- or distal valve endocardium by a pedicle or stalk, and usually attached to the downstream side of the valve. The lesions may exhibit a refractive appearance with shimmering edges or frond-like surfaces (see FIG. 45.15) and areas of echolucency within the tumor.

PFEs are rare, accounting for 7% to 8% of nonmalignant cardiac tumors. These tumors can form a nidus for platelet and fibrin aggregation and lead to systemic or neurologic emboli. They are more commonly identified on the left-sided valves than the right-sided valves. They have also been found on the chordae and papillary apparatus or other cardiac structures. Rarely, they can occur as multiple tumors.

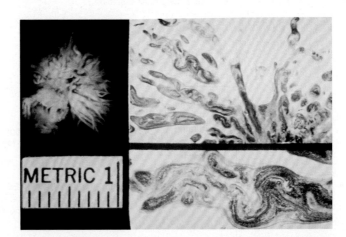

FIGURE **45.15** Pathologic features of PFE of the mitral valve. Gross specimen (**left**) shows multiple frond-like structures (photographed underwater), giving the appearance of a pom-pom or sea anemone. Low-power (**top right**) and higher-power views (**bottom right**) show microscopic features. At the core of each frond is dense elastin (*black*) coated by collagen (*red-pink*) and lined by flat endocardial cells. Elastic van Gieson. **Top right** 318, **bottom right** 354, both reduced by 30%. (Courtesy of Dr. William D. Edwards, Division of Anatomic Pathology, Mayo Clinic. Reprinted from Klarich KW, Enriquez-Sarano M, Gura GM, et al. Papillary fibroelastoma: echocardiographic characteristics for diagnosis and pathologic correlation. *J Am Coll Cardiol* 1997;30(3):784–790, with permission from Elsevier.)

PFEs are associated with embolic events in a high percentage of patients but do not cause significant valvular dysfunction despite the tendency for being located on the valvular endocardium.

A review of echocardiograms at the Mayo Clinic from 1980 to 1995 found 54 patients with echocardiographic diagnosis of PFE; 17 of these patients were confirmed by pathologic diagnosis. They represented 0.019% of all the patients who underwent echocardiographic evaluation during this period of time. TEE was more helpful in identifying the PFE. Most of the tumors (81.5%) were found on the endocardium of left-sided valves. Embolic events were the most common presentation in this series. Surgical resection in this study was curative, with no new embolic events occurring at follow-up.

In general, surgical resection is preferred in symptomatic patients, especially if valvular integrity can be preserved. Anticoagulation therapy has been recommended for patients with asymptomatic PFEs or for nonsurgical candidates. These recommendations are based on anecdotal observations but not clinical trials.

Suggested Readings

Gowda RM, Khan IA, Nair CK, et al. Cardiac papillary fibroelastoma: a comprehensive analysis of 725 cases. *Am Heart J* 2003;146:404–410.

Klarich KW, Enriquez-Sarano M, Gura GM, et al. Papillary fibroelastoma: echocardiographic characteristics for diagnosis and pathologic correlation. *J Am Coll Cardiol* 1997;30:784–790.

Narang J, Neustein S, Israel D. The role of transesophageal echocardiography in the diagnosis and excision of a tumor of the aortic valve. *J Cardiothorac Vasc Anesth* 1992;6:68–69.

Otto C. Echocardiographic evaluation of the patient with a systemic embolic event. In: *The Practice of Clinical Echocardiography*. 5th ed. Philadelphia, PA: Elsevier Saunders, 2013:982–983, Chapter 15.

Yee HC, Nwosu JE, Lii AD, et al. Echocardiographic features of papillary fibroelastoma and their consequences and management. *Am J Cardiol* 1997;80:811–814.

Answer 4: B. Several clinical studies (see TABLE 45.3) have looked at the diagnostic accuracy of transthoracic (TTE) and transesophageal (TEE) echocardiography to detect cardiac involvement with infective endocarditis and its complications.

To use echocardiography in an effective manner, it is important to include an appropriate pretest probability of disease, an understanding of limitations, and a clinical situation in which the diagnostic test results will likely change the management of the patient. The use of harmonic imaging has improved study quality, but not the sensitivity in the visualization of vegetations.

It has also been well recognized that echocardiography is increasingly overused in clinical scenarios with a low (<2% to 3%) pretest probability of disease; its diagnostic utility diminishes in these cases and therefore specificity falls, which can only be improved when used in combination with clinical findings and blood cultures that have been elucidated by the Duke criteria (where echocardiography plays a crucial role, even when blood cultures are negative).

On the other hand, the specificity of echocardiography is related to several factors: the clinical indication and type of population studied, type of the valve (native or prosthetic), and differentiation from noninfectious vegetations such as marantic endocarditis and other confounders (such as valvular thickening or calcifications, torn chordae tendineae, or degenerative nodules).

Vegetation size also affects TTE sensitivity. Lesions <5 mm are difficult to identify by TTE, while sensitivity improves when vegetation size is between 6 and 10 mm. The underlying valve disease may influence the diagnostic accuracy of TTE, such as when myxomatous, sclerotic, or calcified valves are present.

Furthermore, vegetations on prosthetic valves are more difficult to diagnose by TTE, and therefore, TEE should always be used when prosthetic valve endocarditis is suspected. However, there are several factors that can affect the accuracy of TEE, such as sewing ring and support structures of prosthesis (strongly echogenic), shadowing, or suture material. Both thrombus and pannus can have a similar appearance and could be difficult to distinguish from a vegetation.

Diagnostic accuracy also differs when assessing right-sided versus left-sided valves. TTE allows an easy and correct diagnosis of tricuspid vegetations, and both techniques are equally sensitive and specific in detecting TV endocarditis, probably because the majority of patients with tricuspid endocarditis are young intravenous drug abusers with large vegetations. Also, closer imaging proximity of the tricuspid valve to transthoracic imaging window increases sensitivity and specificity.

In native valve endocarditis, TTE sensitivity ranges between 40% and 63% and that of TEE between 90% and 100%, whereas in prosthetic valve endocarditis, TEE has shown an 86% to 94% sensitivity and 88% to 100% specificity for vegetation diagnosis, while TTE sensitivity is only 36% and 69% (1).

Table 45.3	**Studies Comparing the Sensitivity and Specificity of Transthoracic Echocardiography (TTE) and Transesophageal Echocardiography (TOE) in the Diagnosis of Vegetations**				
		SENSITIVITY (%)		SPECIFICITY (%)	
	NO.	TTE	TOE	TTE	TOE
Shapiro et al. (1994)	64	60	87	91	91
Erbel et al. (1988)	96	63	100	98	98
Shively et al. (1991)	66	44	94	98	100

Reproduced from Evangelista A, Gonzalez-Alujas M. Echocardiography in infective endocarditis. *Heart* 2004;90(6):614–617, with permission from BMJ Publishing Group Ltd.

Reference

1. Evangelista A, Gonzalez-Alujas M, et al. Echocardiography in infective endocarditis. *Heart* 2004;90:614–617.

Suggested Readings

Erbel R, Rohmann S, Drexler M, et al. Improved diagnostic value of echocardiography in patients with infective endocarditis by transoesophageal approach. A prospective study. *Eur Heart J* 1988;9:43–53.

Greaves K, Patel A, Celermajer D. Clinical criteria and the appropriate use of transthoracic echocardiography for the exclusion of infective endocarditis. *Heart* 2003;89:273–275.

Hutchison SJ, Rosin BL, Curry S, et al. Transesophageal echocardiographic assessment of lesions of the right ventricular outflow tract and pulmonic valve. *Echocardiography* 1996;13(1):21.

Li JS, Suton DJ, Mick N, et al. Proposed modifications to the Duke criteria for the diagnosis of infective endocarditis. *Clin Infect Dis* 2000;30:633–638.

San Roman JA, Vilacosta I, Zamorano JL, et al. Transesophageal echocardiography in right-sided endocarditis. *J Am Coll Cardiol* 1993;21:1226–1230.

Shapiro SM, Young E, De Guzman S, et al. Transesophageal echocardiography in diagnosis of infective endocarditis. *Chest* 1994;105:377–382.

Shively BK, Gurule FT, Roldan CA, et al. Diagnostic value of transesophageal compared with transthoracic echocardiography in infective endocarditis. *J Am Coll Cardiol* 1991;18:391–397.

Vieira ML, Grinberg M, Pomerantzeff PM, et al. Repeated echocardiographic examinations of patients with suspected infective endocarditis. *Heart* 2004;90:1020–1024.

Answer 5:

Scenario 5A: *Answer: A (yes).*

Transthoracic echocardiography demonstrates an echo bright structure (VIDEO 45.3) in the membranous area of interventricular septum adjacent to the aortic valve consistent with patch repair of her VSD, especially given the history. Color Doppler images also demonstrate evidence of residual VSD leak, and the CW Doppler demonstrates a high-velocity jet in the area of leak (FIG. 45.1). Due to her residual VSD leak, antibiotic prophylaxis is indicated before undergoing restorative dental procedure.

Scenario 5B: *Answer:* **A (yes).**

Images demonstrate an echo bright structure in the membranous area of IVS (VIDEO 45.4A) consistent with his prior surgical repair of VSD and no color Doppler (VIDEO 45.4B) evidence of residual leak, again demonstrated on parasternal short-axis views (VIDEO 45.4C AND D). Successful repair of congenital VSD in and of itself does not warrant an antibiotic prophylaxis; however, given his RVOT conduit with bioprosthetic pulmonary valve, he requires an antibiotic prophylaxis.

Scenario 5C: *Answer:* **A (yes).**

Images are obtained from a patient with bicuspid aortic valve (VIDEO 45.5A AND B), showing diastolic doming of the aortic valve with color Doppler evidence of eccentric aortic regurgitation, again demonstrated on parasternal short-axis views (VIDEO 45.5C AND D). Perioperative prophylactic antibiotics are recommended for the placement of prosthetic valves.

Scenario 5D: *Answer:* **A (yes).**

Echocardiography demonstrates mitral valve prolapse involving the posterior leaflet (VIDEO 45.6A and FIG. 45.2) with color Doppler (VIDEO 45.6B) evidence of mitral valve regurgitation and requires an antibiotic prophylaxis before undergoing cardiac surgery (bypass graft surgery in this case).

Scenario 5E: *Answer:* **B (no).**

The echocardiogram is obtained from a patient with orthotopic heart transplant. Antibiotic prophylaxis is only recommended when there is a valvulopathy in a posttransplant patient. Parasternal long-axis images (VIDEO 45.7A AND B) demonstrate no evidence of significant valvular dysfunction. Interventricular septal motion is consistent with the poststernotomy state. Apical 4Ch view demonstrates large atria suggesting biatrial anastomosis. Qualitatively, RV function is moderately reduced (VIDEO 45.7D AND E). The RA/RV view demonstrates no significant tricuspid regurgitation. There is no evidence of pulmonary valve regurgitation (VIDEO 45.7F AND G). Also note that the main pulmonary artery anastomosis site is clearly visible just superior to the pulmonary valve as a part of cardiac transplant procedure. In all the images shown above, there is no evidence of transplant valvulopathy. Therefore, antibiotic prophylaxis is **not** warranted.

The American Heart Association (AHA) guidelines for prevention of infective endocarditis have been evolving over last several decades, with the most recent key updates providing recommendations for antibiotic prophylaxis published in 2007 (with focused update in 2008), which greatly reduce the patient population for which prophylactic antibiotics are recommended.

The 2007 AHA guidelines committee concluded that only an extremely small number of cases of infective endocarditis might be prevented by antibiotic prophylaxis for dental procedures even if such prophylaxis was 100% effective. Accordingly, the revised guidelines recommend infective endocarditis prophylaxis for dental procedures only for patients with underlying cardiac conditions associated with the highest risk of adverse outcomes from infective endocarditis.

Cardiac conditions associated with the highest risk for which infective endocarditis (IE) prophylaxis with dental procedures is recommended are prosthetic valves, prior endocarditis, congenital heart disease (CHD), unrepaired cyanotic CHD including palliative shunts and conduits, completely repaired CHD with any prosthetic material during the first 6 months after the procedure, repaired CHD with residual defects (which inhibit endothelialization), and cardiac transplantation recipients who develop cardiac valvulopathy.

Dental procedures for which IE prophylaxis is recommended for high-risk patients (as described earlier) are all dental procedures and events that involve manipulation of gingival tissue or the periapical region of teeth or perforation of the oral mucosa except the following: routine anesthetic injections through noninfected tissue, taking dental radiographs, placement of removable prosthodontic or orthodontic appliances, adjustment of orthodontic appliances, and placement of orthodontic brackets, shedding of deciduous teeth, and bleeding from trauma to the lips or oral mucosa.

In select circumstances, the committee also understands that some clinicians and some patients may still feel more comfortable continuing with prophylaxis for infective endocarditis, particularly for those with bicuspid aortic valve or coarctation of the aorta, severe mitral valve prolapse, or hypertrophic obstructive cardiomyopathy. In those settings, the clinician should determine that the risks associated with antibiotics are low before continuing a prophylaxis regimen. Over time, and with continuing education, the committee anticipates increasing acceptance of the new guidelines among both provider and patient communities.

The guidelines recommend a single dose of amoxicillin or ampicillin as the preferred prophylactic agent for individuals who do not have a history of type I hypersensitive reactions to a penicillin. For individuals who are allergic to penicillin or amoxicillin, alternative recommendations include first-generation oral cephalosporins, clindamycin, azithromycin, or clarithromycin.

Antibiotic administration is not recommended for patients undergoing genitourinary or gastrointestinal tract procedures solely for the purpose of preventing endocarditis. Antibiotic prophylaxis for bronchoscopy is not recommended unless the procedure involves incision of the respiratory tract mucosa.

For patients who are undergoing cardiac surgery, a careful preoperative dental evaluation is recommended whenever possible. Patients who undergo surgery for placement of prosthesis (valves or intracardiac materials) are at risk for the development of infection. Because the morbidity and mortality of infection in these patients are high, perioperative prophylactic antibiotics are recommended (class I, LOE B). Prophylaxis at the time of cardiac surgery should be directed primarily against staphylococci (coagulase negative) and should be of short duration. Prophylaxis should be initiated immediately before, during, and up to 48 hours after the surgery.

Suggested Readings

Bonow RO, Carabello B, Chatterjee K, et al. 2008 focused update incorporated into the ACC/AHA 2006 guidelines for the management of patients with valvular heart disease. *Circulation* 2008;118:e1.

Dajani AS, Taubert KA, Wilson W, et al. Prevention of bacterial endocarditis: recommendations by the American Heart Association. *Circulation* 1997;96:363.

Nishimura R, Carabello BA, Faxon DP, et al. ACC/AHA 2008 guideline update on valvular heart disease: focused update on infective endocarditis. *Circulation* 2008;118:887–896.

Wilson W, Taubert KA, Gewitz M, et al. Prevention of infective endocarditis: recommendations by the American Heart Association. *Circulation* 2007;116:1736.

Answer 6: E.

Option A: Shows an M-mode of the mitral valve with fused E and A wave from sinus tachycardia; the mitral valve closes appropriately after QRS.

Option B: M-mode of the mitral valve where A wave is absent due to atrial fibrillation and also notice the beat-to-beat variability.

Option C: M-mode of the mitral valve in a patient with significant chronic aortic regurgitation and a blunted A wave. When correlating with QRS (displayed), the MV completely closes after appropriate delay from electrical activity.

Option D: M-mode of the mitral valve in a patient with significant first-degree AV block, the recording speed of M-mode is also shortened (25 mm/s) that gives an impression of faster heart rate.

Option E: M-mode of the mitral valve showing premature closure of the anterior mitral valve leaflet, before the QRS, consistent with acute severe aortic regurgitation.

Suggested Readings

Armstrong W, Ryan T. Hemodynamics. In: *Chapter 9: Feigenbaum's Echocardiography*. 7th ed. Philadelphia, PA: Lippincott Williams & Wilkins, 2010:217.

Feigenbaum H. Role of M-mode technique in today's echocardiography. *J Am Soc Echocardiogr* 2010;23:240–257.

Panidis I, Ross J, Munley B. Diastolic mitral regurgitation in patients with atrioventricular conduction abnormalities: a common finding by Doppler echocardiography. *J Am Coll Cardiol* 1986;7:768–774.

Answer 7: C.

Option A: M-mode of the mitral valve showing premature closure due to severe acute aortic regurgitation. Note that the closure of the anterior and posterior leaflets precedes the onset of the QRS on ECG.

Option B: CW Doppler through the aortic valve in a patient with severe aortic regurgitation with steep deceleration (pressure half-time of <150 ms) with dense signal. This is due to dissipation of the gradient between diastolic aortic and LV diastolic pressures that occurs with severe acute aortic regurgitation.

Option C: M-mode of the mitral valve showing fluttering of the anterior mitral valve leaflet due to aortic regurgitation (turbulent flow during diastole). These can be seen in even mild to moderate forms of aortic regurgitation and is not necessarily an indicator of severe regurgitation. Therefore, answer C is correct.

Option D: Holodiastolic flow reversal in the descending aorta, which is also associated with severe aortic regurgitation.

Option E: CW Doppler through the mitral valve showing diastolic mitral regurgitation, which is seen in the acute severe aortic regurgitation, from aortic regurgitant flow backward into the left atrium in diastole.

Answers 8: E; 9: E. Not all microorganisms have the same propensity to cause endocarditis; streptococci and *Staphylococcus aureus* are more likely to cause endocarditis than gram-negative rods (*Escherichia coli*, *Proteus*).

Nosocomial enterococcus infection is not included as a major criterion for endocarditis especially when there is a primary focus of infection (infected tunneled dialysis catheter). These types of infections are eradicated once the primary source is removed.

Other microbiologic criteria that are included in modified Duke criteria are as below:

- Typical microorganisms consistent with IE from two separate blood cultures: Viridans streptococci, *Streptococcus bovis*, HACEK group, *Staphylococcus aureus*; or community-acquired enterococci, in the absence of a primary focus; or microorganisms consistent with IE from persistently positive blood cultures, defined as follows: at least two positive blood cultures drawn >12 hours apart or all three or a majority of ≥4 separate blood cultures (with first and last sample drawn at least 1 hour apart)

- Single positive blood culture for *Coxiella burnetii* or antiphase I IgG antibody titer >1:800

Minor criteria

1. Predisposition, predisposing heart condition, or injection drug use
2. Fever (temperature >38°C)
3. Vascular phenomena, major arterial emboli, septic pulmonary infarcts, mycotic aneurysm, intracranial hemorrhage, conjunctival hemorrhages, and Janeway lesions
4. Immunologic phenomena: glomerulonephritis, Osler nodes, Roth spots, and rheumatoid factor
5. Microbiologic evidence: positive blood culture but does not meet a major criterion as noted above or serologic evidence of active infection with organism consistent with IE
6. Echocardiographic minor criteria eliminated

Suggested Reading

Li JS, Sexton DJ, Mick N, et al. Proposed modifications to the Duke criteria for the diagnosis of infective endocarditis. *Clin Infect Dis* 2000;30:633–638.

Answer 10: A. Uncomplicated multivalvular involvement is not considered a class I indication for surgery in left-sided native endocarditis. However, if multivalvular involvement were associated with larger size vegetations (>10 mm), resistant or fungal organisms, abscesses, or embolic complications surgery would be indicated. All of the other options given are class I indication for surgery.

According to the AHA/ACC 2006 guidelines, class I indications for surgery in native valve endocarditis are (a) acute infective endocarditis in patients who present with valve stenosis or regurgitation resulting in heart failure, (b) acute infective endocarditis in patients who present with AR or MR with hemodynamic evidence of elevated LV end-diastolic or left atrial pressures (e.g., premature closure of MV with AR, rapid decelerating MR signal by continuous-wave Doppler [v-wave cutoff sign], or moderate or severe pulmonary hypertension), (c) patients with infective endocarditis caused by fungal or other highly resistant organisms, (d) surgery of the native valve is indicated in patients with infective endocarditis complicated by heart block, annular or aortic abscess, or destructive penetrating lesions (e.g., sinus of Valsalva to the right atrium, right ventricle, or left atrium fistula; mitral leaflet perforation with aortic valve endocarditis; or infection involving the annulus fibrosa).

Transesophageal echocardiography is the preferred imaging technique for the diagnosis and management of IE in adults with either high risk for IE or moderate to high clinical suspicion of IE or in patients in whom imaging by transthoracic

Table 45.4	**Echocardiographic Features That Suggest Potential Need for Surgical Intervention**

Vegetation

Persistent vegetation after systemic embolization

Anterior mitral leaflet vegetation, particularly with size >10 mm[a]

≥1 embolic events during first 2 wk of antimicrobial therapy[a]

Increase in vegetation size despite appropriate antimicrobial therapy[a,b]

Valvular dysfunction

Acute aortic or mitral insufficiency with signs of ventricular failure[b]

Heart failure unresponsive to medical therapy[b]

Valve perforation or rupture[b]

Perivalvular extension

Valvular dehiscence, rupture, or fistula[b]

New heart block[b,c]

Large abscess or extension of abscess despite appropriate antimicrobial therapy[b]

See text for more complete discussion of indications for surgery based on vegetation characterizations.

[a]Surgery may be required because of risk of embolization.

[b]Surgery may be required because of heart failure or failure of medical therapy.

[c]Echocardiography should not be the primary modality used to detect or monitor heart block.

Reprinted from Bonow RO, Carabello BA, Chatterjee K, et al. ACC/AHA 2006 guidelines for the management of patients with valvular heart disease: a report of the American College of Cardiology/American Heart Association Task Force on Practice Guidelines. *J Am Coll Cardiol* 2006;48:e1–e148, with permission from Elsevier.

echocardiography is technically suboptimal or inadequate. Transesophageal echocardiography is more sensitive than transthoracic echocardiography for detecting vegetations and cardiac abscess. The echocardiographic features that suggest the potential need for surgical intervention are listed in Table 45.4.

Answer 11: E.

Option A: The 2D video shows a vegetation involving the aortic valve with a flail leaflet, but there is no clear evidence of perivalvular extension of infection. There is no echolucent area near the annulus or asymmetric thickening that could suggest an abscess. This is an incorrect statement. Transthoracic (TTE) has low sensitivity in detecting abscess (only 28%). Transesophageal echocardiography (TEE) has a much greater likelihood of detecting a myocardial abscess with sensitivity, specificity, and positive and negative predictive values of TEE imaging at around 87%, 95%, 91%, and 92%, respectively.

Option B: The color Doppler jet of aortic regurgitation occupies the entire LV outflow tract area throughout diastole, which is consistent with severe AI (jet/height ratio >0.65). Imaging the jet origin in a perforation or flail leaflet can be difficult by transthoracic imaging and not relevant to the criteria for assessing severity in this case.

Option C: M-mode of the aortic valve showing normal opening and closure does not exclude the possibility of flail leaflet or vegetations. This is an incorrect statement. Note that the systolic fluttering may be due to high flow from severe aortic regurgitation.

Option D: The CW Doppler through the aortic valve does show very steep deceleration along with a high initial velocity, consistent with severe aortic regurgitation due to rapid equalization of LV and aortic diastolic pressures. The systolic envelope represents forward flow through the aortic valve and not mitral regurgitation.

Option E: M-mode of the mitral valve shows an A wave, which indicates a brief reopening of the mitral valve, and is evidence against acute severe aortic regurgitation is a correct statement. Premature closure of the mitral valve in severe aortic regurgitation is usually characterized by the absence of an A wave, since atrial contraction is unable to reopen the valve due to high LV diastolic pressure.

Suggested Readings

Armstrong W, Ryan T. Hemodynamics. In: *Chapter 9: Feigenbaum's Echocardiography*. 7th ed. Philadelphia, PA: Lippincott Williams & Wilkins, 2009:217.

Feigenbaum H. Role of M-mode technique in today's echocardiography. *J Am Soc Echocardiogr* 2010;23:240–257.

Zoghbi W, Enriquez-Sarano M, Foster E, et al. Recommendations for evaluation of the severity of native valvular regurgitation with two-dimensional and Doppler echocardiography. *J Am Soc Echocardiogr* 2003;16:777–802.

Answer 12: **A.** The images are consistent with Lambl excrescences.

Lambl excrescences (fibrin strands, valvular strands, papillary endocardial tumors) are best described as fine thread-like strands arising on the line of closure (contact surface) of any heart valve, but most commonly the mitral followed by the aortic valve. They are acellular strands that contain a fibroelastic core covered by a single layer of endothelium.

They are usually 1 mm or less in thickness and up to >10 mm long. It is important to emphasize that the term "Lambl excrescence" is primarily a histologic and not an echocardiographic description. In recent years, filiform structures on native and prosthetic cardiac valves detected by TEE have also been called "valvular strands" (1).

Lambl excrescences are more common findings with advanced age, especially people over age 60. They are commonly seen in patients with thickened valves. There have been isolated case reports of describing angina pectoris from coronary ostium obstruction from large Lambl excrescences, and surgery in those instances was curative (2,3).

Roldan et al. (4) analyzed the prevalence of excrescences in relation to cardioembolic events. They found no significant difference in prevalence among healthy individuals, individuals with some cardiovascular abnormality other than cardioembolism, and patients with cardioembolic events (38%, 47%, and 41%, respectively). Only 1.4% in the healthy group and 2% of patients with cardiovascular disease other than thromboembolism developed cerebral ischemic events during

an extensive follow-up. Although 41% of patients with a cardioembolic stroke had excrescences, 85% of these patients had another embolic source demonstrated by echocardiography. Based on these results, Roldan et al. concluded that valvular excrescences did not represent a source of cerebral embolism.

References
1. Voros S, Nanda NC, Thakur AC, et al. Lambl's excrescences (valvular strands). *Echocardiography* 1999;16(4):399–414.
2. Freedberg RS, Goodkin GM, Perez JL, et al. Valve strands are strongly associated with systemic embolization: a transesophageal echocardiographic study. *J Am Coll Cardiol* 1995;26:1709–1712.
3. Orsinelli DA, Pearson AC. Detection of prosthetic valve strands by transesophageal echocardiography: clinical significance in patients with suspected cardiac source of embolism. *J Am Coll Cardiol* 1995;26:1713–1718.
4. Roldan CA, Shively BK, Crawford MH. Valve excrescences: prevalence, evolution and risk for cardioembolism. *J Am Coll Cardiol* 1997;30:1308–1314.

Suggested Reading
Otto C. Echocardiographic evaluation of the patient with a systemic embolic event. In: *The Practice of Clinical Echocardiography*. 3rd ed. Philadelphia, PA: Elsevier Saunders, 2007:982–983.

Answer 13: **B.**

Option A: An 82-year-old female for routine follow-up for her history of moderate mitral regurgitation. Her echocardiography shows mitral valve prolapse with a flail segment and at least moderate mitral regurgitation. Clinical features do not suggest infective endocarditis.

Option B: A 34-year-old female with substance abuse presented with congestive heart failure is the correct answer. Her echocardiogram shows a large mitral valve vegetation (involving both leaflets) with perforation of the valve leaflet consistent with complicated infective endocarditis. This image also suggests an intravalvular abscess, which is diagnostic of endocarditis. *Staphylococcus aureus* causes more than 50% of IE occurring in IV drug abusers overall. In patients with IVDU, endocarditis involves the tricuspid valve in 46% to 78%, mitral valve in 24% to 32%, and aortic valve in 8% to 19%; as many as 16% of patients have multivalvular involvement. In the majority of the cases (75% to 93%), the valves were normal before the infection (1).

Option C: A 54-year-old female presented with NSTEMI and heart failure. TEE images show large inferior wall myocardial infarction with ruptured chord and severe mitral regurgitation with anteriorly directed jet. There is no clear mobile mass on the valve leaflets to suggest vegetation.

Option D: A 65-year-old female with ESRD and HTN, routine follow-up for heart murmur. There is significant mitral and aortic annular calcification and shadowing without obvious features to suggest endocarditis. Based on the data available, there is no definite evidence for infective endocarditis (Duke criteria).

Option E: A 78-year-old female with myxomatous mitral valve disease and chordal rupture, for routine follow-up. Her TTE shows a torn chord that overtime can calcify and mimic an old healed calcified vegetation; however, in this patient, the clinical presentation does not suggest endocarditis. There is no significant valve regurgitation. Based on the information available, there is no definite diagnosis of infective endocarditis.

This question addresses the importance of clinical suspicion along with the use of echocardiographic features to make the diagnosis of infective endocarditis. Without clinical information, any of the examples presented (options A, C, D, and E) can mimic infective endocarditis. To use echocardiography in an effective manner, it is important to include an appropriate pretest probability of disease, population studied, understanding the limitations, and clinical variables (as discussed earlier, Duke criteria).

The most commonly encountered abnormal valvular structures include thrombi, vegetations (both infectious and noninfectious), myxomas, fibroelastomas, myxomatous degenerative changes, primary cardiac neoplasms, and metastases. Further differential diagnostic categories are redundant heart valves and valve apparatus and the calcifications associated with the mitral annulus.

Following are some echocardiographic clues to differentiate vegetations from other entities (2,3).

Thrombi on cardiac valves appear as well demarcated, round masses (varying in size, small to large), usually not connected to the valves through a stalk, mostly homogeneous (areas of calcifications in chronic form). It is generally difficult to distinguish thrombi from cardiac tumors. The presence or absence of certain associated findings, however, can help decide between the two. A mass is more likely to be a cardiac thrombus if indicators of a low-flow state are present, such as spontaneous echo contrast or wall motion abnormalities. However, thrombi have been reported on valves in the absence of low cardiac output or hypercoagulable state.

Vegetations. Irregularly shaped, highly mobile mass, an oscillating or fluttering attached to the upstream side of the valve leaflet. They usually have motion that is independent of the valve itself. However, the diagnosis of endocarditis must be made in context of the clinical picture (Duke criteria).

Myxomatous degeneration of cardiac valves. Myxomatous degeneration affects the structure of the valve itself, thickening, and redundancy of the leaflets, which also involves the subvalvular apparatus. The degenerative process is a risk factor for torn chordae, which move independently from the valve leaflet excursions.

Calcification. A relatively nonmobile, heavily calcified annulus and the proximal parts of the posterior mitral valve leaflet. There may be mobile calcified structures attached to the annulus or the valve, which move with annular motion.

Prosthetic sutures. Fibrinized or endothelialized sutures of prosthetic valves can be difficult to differentiate from some of the abovementioned structures. However, they are usually thick, and they are placed in a uniform manner around the prosthetic valves. When these sutures are cut long by the surgeon, they might resemble valvular strands. Also, ruptured sutures may resemble excrescences.

References

1. Murdoch DR, Corey GR, Hoen B, et al. Clinical presentation, etiology, and outcome of infective endocarditis in the 21st century. *Arch Intern Med* 2009;169:463.
2. Sachdev M, Peterson GE, Jollis JG, et al. Imaging techniques for diagnosis of infective endocarditis. *Infect Dis Clin North Am* 2002;16:319–337.
3. Sahasakul Y, Edwards WD, Naessens JM, et al. Age-related changes in aortic and mitral valve thickness: implications for two-dimensional echocardiography based on an autopsy study of 200 normal human hearts. *Am J Cardiol* 1988;62(7):424–430.

Suggested Readings

Mohler ER III. Mechanisms of aortic valve calcification. *Am J Cardiol* 2004;94(11):1396–1402.
Orsinelli D, Pearson A. Detection of prosthetic valve strands by transesophageal echocardiography: clinical significance in patients with suspected cardiac source of embolism. *J Am Coll Cardiol* 1995;26:1713–1718.

Answer 14: *E.* Transthoracic echocardiography demonstrates a large vegetation involving the mitral valve leaflets. On the parasternal long-axis view (VIDEO 45.15A), it is difficult to differentiate it from a large atrial myxoma. However, from apical views (VIDEO 45.15B; apical 4Ch view, VIDEO 45.15C; apical 3Ch view), it is a highly mobile, oscillating mass, attached to the atrial side of the valve leaflet, not attached to interatrial septum with a stalk (characteristic of myxoma), with color Doppler (VIDEO 45.15D) evidence of severe mitral regurgitation. FIGURE 45.8A (CW Doppler across the mitral valve; shows highly dense midpeaking triangular envelope) and FIGURE 45.8B (PW Doppler in the pulmonary vein; shows systolic flow reversal) support the findings of severe mitral regurgitation. Repeat transthoracic echocardiographic images from the same patient 7 days later shows a persistent, large vegetation (VIDEO 45.16) that has been described as a high-risk feature for a future embolic event and likely to be responsible for a recurrent embolic event in patients who already have an event. Therefore, answer E is correct.

Complications can develop in 40% to 50% of patients being treated for active endocarditis and are a major determinant of outcome. Since complications are invariably associated with a worsening prognosis, identifying patients at risk for their development is an important goal. Several investigations have attempted to stratify patients into low- and high-risk subsets and to identify those at risk of complications on the basis of clinical and echocardiographic findings. Most of the parameters that determine high- and low-risk status are clinical, including age, type of organism, and development of heart failure. In addition, stroke occurrence consistently has been a strong negative determinant of outcome in patients with endocarditis (1).

The only echocardiographic parameter that has been consistently associated with an increased risk of complications is vegetation size. In one study (2), there was a strong and nearly linear relationship between vegetation size and the risk of complications. For example, vegetations <7 mm in size accounted for <10% of all complications, whereas those that were >11 mm in size accounted for more than half of the complications, particularly embolic events (three times higher). This association was strong in patients with mitral valve endocarditis (patients with mitral valve endocarditis are more likely to have embolic events than patients with aortic valve endocarditis). Similarly, patients with *Staphylococcus endocarditis* are more likely to have embolic events than patients with *Streptococcus endocarditis* (1,2).

High mobility also predicts embolic risk (62% versus 20% for low mobility), and embolic events were particularly frequent when both severely mobile and very large vegetations were present (83%) (3).

The rate of stroke does fall significantly after the initiation of the antimicrobial therapy, from 4.82 of 1,000 patient-days during 1st week of therapy to 1.71 (65% fall) of 1,000 patient-days ($P < 0.001$). However, echocardiographic predictors of emboli still apply after the initiation of antibiotics. In the large study cited above, only 24% of observed emboli occurred after the start of antibiotic therapy, but greater vegetation length and mobility were still prognostic factors for these later embolic events.

In a TEE study of 83 IE patients, vegetations that enlarged or remained static rather than regressed during 4 to 8 weeks of therapy were associated with an increased incidence of embolic events (45% versus 17%), abscess formation (13% versus 2%), valve replacement (45% versus 2%), and mortality (10% versus 0%) (Figs. 45.16 and 45.17).

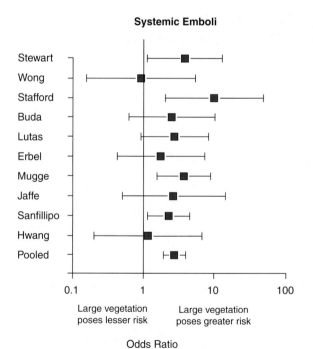

Systemic Emboli

Stewart
Wong
Stafford
Buda
Lutas
Erbel
Mugge
Jaffe
Sanfillipo
Hwang
Pooled

0.1   1   10   100

Large vegetation poses lesser risk   Large vegetation poses greater risk

Odds Ratio

FIGURE 45.16 A meta-analysis of studies that examine whether vegetation size could predict the risk of systemic emboli. The pooled odds ratio for increased risk associated with large vegetation was 2.80 (95% confidence interval 1.95 to 4.02, $P < 0.01$). (Reprinted from Tischler MD, Vaitkus PT. The ability of vegetation size on echocardiography to predict clinical complications: a meta-analysis. *J Am Soc Echocardiogr* 1997; 10(5):562–568. Copyright © 1997 American Society of Echocardiography. With permission.

References

1. Armstrong W, Ryan T. Infective endocarditis. In: *Chapter 14: Feigenbaum's Echocardiography*. 7th ed. Philadelphia, PA: Lippincott Williams & Wilkins, 2009:374–375.
2. Sanfilippo AJ, Picard MH, Newell JB, et al. Echocardiographic assessment of patients with infectious endocarditis: prediction of risk for complications. *J Am Coll Cardiol* 1991;18:1191–1199.
3. Tischler M, Vaitkus P, et al. The ability of vegetation size on echocardiography to predict clinical complications: a meta-analysis. *J Am Soc Echocardiogr* 1997;10(5):562–568.

Suggested Readings

Dickerman SA, Abrutyn E, Barsic B, et al. The relationship between the initiation of antimicrobial therapy and the incidence of stroke in infective endocarditis: an analysis from the ICE Prospective Cohort Study (ICE-PCS). *Am Heart J* 2007;154(6):1086.

Di Salvo G, Habib G, Pergola V, et al. Echocardiography predicts embolic events in infective endocarditis. *J Am Coll Cardiol* 2001;37(4):1069.

Mügge A, Daniel WG, Frank G, et al. Echocardiography in infective endocarditis: reassessment of prognostic implications of vegetation size determined by the transthoracic and the transesophageal approach. *J Am Coll Cardiol* 1989;14(3):631.

Saric M, et al. Guidelines for the use of echocardiography in the evaluation of a cardiac source of embolism. *J Am Soc Echocardiogr* 2016;29:1–42.

Vilacosta I, Graupner C, San Román JA, et al. Risk of embolization after institution of antibiotic therapy for infective endocarditis. *J Am Coll Cardiol* 2002;39(9):1489.

Answer 15: B.

Option A: Large mobile mitral valve vegetation with leaflet perforation is present is incorrect. TEE images show an extension of infection from endocarditis involving a bioprosthetic aortic valve along with a fistulous connection between the abscess cavity and left atrium. There is no definite perforation of mitral valve leaflets seen on the images shown.

Option B: Color M-mode is diagnostic of fistulous flow. This answer is correct. It shows to and fro flow during systole and diastole (M-mode cursors pass through left atrium, fistula tract between LA and aortic sinus [abscess cavity], LV outflow tract area, and anterior septum). If there was a closed abscess cavity, you would expect the flow only during diastole.

Option C: There are vegetations on the bioprosthetic aortic valve and severe aortic regurgitation is noted. There is clear evidence of vegetation involving the bioprosthetic aortic valve (involving all the leaflets) with color Doppler evidence of severe aortic regurgitation. Therefore, this answer is incorrect.

Option D: Aortic paravalvular abscess with dehiscence is present. There is an abscess cavity involving aortic annulus, more obvious anteriorly with expansion during diastole (Video 45.17D, short-axis view of the AV) with rocking motion of the prosthetic valve. However, the large color flow jet into the LA is due to fistulous flow from the aorta, and not mitral regurgitation. This answer is incorrect.

Several echocardiographic features identify patients at high risk for a complicated course or with a need for surgery. These features include large vegetations, severe valvular insufficiency, abscess cavities or pseudoaneurysms, valvular perforation or dehiscence, and evidence of decompensated heart failure. See Tables 45.5 and 45.6.

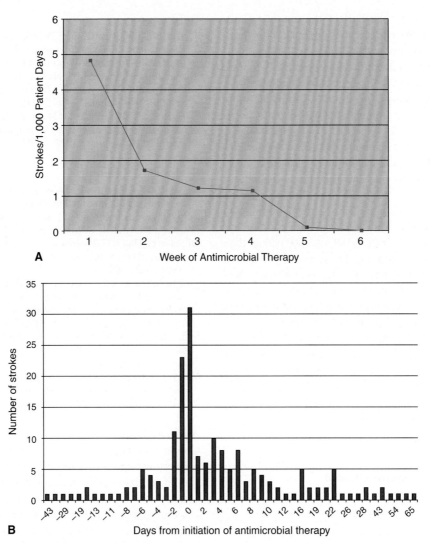

FIGURE 45.17 (Reprinted from Dickerman SA, Abrutyn E, Barsic B, et al. The relationship between the initiation of antimicrobial therapy and the incidence of stroke in infective endocarditis: an analysis from the ICE Prospective Cohort Study (ICE-PCS). *Am Heart J* 2007;154(6):1086–1094. Copyright © 2007 Elsevier. With permission.

Transesophageal echocardiography is the preferred imaging technique for the diagnosis and management of IE in adults with either high risk for IE or moderate to high clinical suspicion of IE or in patients in whom transthoracic echocardiography yields suboptimal images. Transesophageal

Table 45.5 **Complications of Endocarditis**

STRUCTURAL	HEMODYNAMIC
Leaflet rupture	Acute valvular regurgitation
Flail leaflet	Valve obstruction
Leaflet perforation	Heart failure
Abscess	Intracardiac shunt
Aneurysm	Tamponade
Prosthetic valve dehiscence	Perivalvular regurgitation
Embolization	
Pericardial effusion	
Fistula	

From Armstrong W, Ryan T. Infective endocarditis. In: *Chapter 14: Feigenbaum's Echocardiography*. 7th ed. Philadelphia, PA: Lippincott Williams & Wilkins, 2009:369, with permission.

Table 45.6 **Specific Characteristics of Infective Lesions**

LESION	CHARACTERISTICS
Vegetation	Irregularly shaped, discrete echogenic oscillating masses, adherent to and distinct from cardiac surfaces including valves, myocardium, and intracardiac devices
Abscess	Thickened area or mass within the myocardium or annular region with a nonhomogeneous echogenic or echolucent appearance. Aneurysm echolucent space bounded by thin tissue
Fistulae	Systolic shunting of blood identified by flow Doppler technique
Leaflet perforation	Defect in leaflet with flow
Valvular dehiscence	Rocking motion of prosthetic valve with excursion >15 degrees in at least one direction

Reprinted from Sachdev M, Peterson GE, Jollis JG, et al. Imaging techniques for diagnosis of infective endocarditis. *Infect Dis Clin North Am* 2002;16(2):319–337. Copyright © 2002 Elsevier Science (USA). With permission.

echocardiography is more sensitive than transthoracic echocardiography for detecting vegetations and cardiac abscess.

Echocardiographic features that suggest potential need for surgical intervention are categorized as follows:

- **Vegetation:** Persistent vegetation after systemic embolization, anterior mitral leaflet vegetation (particularly with size >10 mm), one embolic event during first 2 weeks of antimicrobial therapy, and increase in vegetation size despite appropriate antimicrobial therapy
- **Valvular dysfunction**: Acute aortic or mitral insufficiency with signs of ventricular failure, heart failure unresponsive to medical therapy, and valve perforation or rupture
- **Perivalvular extension:** Valvular dehiscence, rupture, or fistula, large abscess, or extension of abscess despite appropriate antimicrobial therapy

Suggested Readings

Armstrong W, Ryan T. Infective endocarditis. In: *Chapter 14: Feigenbaum's Echocardiography*. 7th ed. Philadelphia, PA: Lippincott Williams & Wilkins, 2009:374–375.

Bayer AS, Bolger AF, Taubert KA, et al. Diagnosis and management of infective endocarditis and its complications. *Circulation* 1998;98:2936–2948.

Mugge A, Daniel WG, Frank G, et al. Echocardiography in infective endocarditis: reassessment of prognostic implications of vegetation size determined by the transthoracic and the transesophageal approach. *J Am Coll Cardiol* 1989;14:631–638.

Sachdev M, Peterson GE, Jollis JG, et al. Imaging techniques for diagnosis of infective endocarditis. *Infect Dis Clin North Am* 2002;16:319–337.

Steckelberg JM, Murphy JG, Ballard D, et al. Emboli in infective endocarditis: the prognostic value of echocardiography. *Ann Intern Med* 1991;114:635–640.

Answer 16: *C.* Marantic endocarditis, also known as nonbacterial thrombotic endocarditis (NBTE), Libman-Sacks endocarditis, and verrucous endocarditis, usually involves the edge of the valves and results from endothelial damage leading to platelet aggregates interwoven with strands of fibrin on valve leaflets (most often mitral or aortic) in the presence of a hypercoagulable state.

The verrucae consist of accumulations of immune complexes, mononuclear cells, hematoxylin bodies, and fibrin and platelet thrombi. Healing usually leads to fibrosis, scarring, and, in some cases, calcification. If the verrucal lesions are extensive, the healing process can produce deformity of the valve, leading to mitral or aortic regurgitation.

Underlying risk factors for hypercoagulable state in majority of cases are advanced malignancy (common with adenocarcinomas of the pancreas, lung, colon, or prostate), and other causes are antiphospholipid antibodies syndromes (lupus anticoagulant and anticardiolipin). The vegetations vary in size from small (microscopic) to large masses on the valves and typically involve edge of the leaflets ("kissing lesions"). When suspected, workup should include ruling out underlying malignancy, markers of hypercoagulable state including serum levels of lupus anticoagulant and IgG anticardiolipin antibodies.

The major clinical manifestations are from systemic emboli (CNS, spleen, kidney, and extremities) rather than valvular dysfunction. Diagnosis can be challenging as half of the patients do not have murmur on auscultation, and small lesions (<2 mm) may not be identified by echocardiography.

Therapy: 2008 ACCP Guidelines. In patients without evidence for embolic event, antiplatelet or anticoagulation therapy should be considered for those patients with vegetations or significant valvular thickening and certainly for all patients with thromboembolic events. Treatment of the underlying malignancy, often metastatic at the time of diagnosis of NBTE, should be attempted in appropriate patients. Valve surgery is considered in selected cases once the underlying condition is treated with reasonable predicted survival if there is persistence of severe valve dysfunction.

Suggested Readings

Dutta T, Karas MG, Segal AZ, et al. Yield of transesophageal echocardiography for nonbacterial thrombotic endocarditis and other cardiac sources of embolism in cancer patients with cerebral ischemia. *Am J Cardiol* 2006;97(6):894.

Moyssakis I, Tektonidou MG, Vasilliou VA. Libman-Sacks endocarditis in systemic lupus erythematosus: prevalence, associations, and evolution. *Am J Med* 2007;120(7):636.

Rogers LR, Cho ES, Kempin S, et al. Cerebral infarction from non-bacterial thrombotic endocarditis. Clinical and pathological study including the effects of anticoagulation. *Am J Med* 1987;83(4):746.

Salem DN, O'Gara PT, Madias C, et al. Valvular and structural heart disease: American College of Chest Physicians evidence-based clinical practice guidelines (8th Edition). *Chest* 2008;133(suppl 6):593S.

Answer 17: *B.* Diagnosis is possible infective endocarditis, as she has one major (*Staphylococcus* bacteremia) and two minor (IV drug use and fever) criteria. Transthoracic echocardiography (Video 45.19A and B) shows no definite evidence of vegetation involving the aortic or mitral valve, and color Doppler demonstrates no regurgitation. Video 45.19C–E demonstrate normal structure and function of the tricuspid and pulmonary valves (mild TR by color flow). These transthoracic images are adequate and do not demonstrate any echocardiographic evidence of definite endocarditis.

The clinical diagnosis of infective endocarditis has always been challenging without the use of echocardiography. In 1994, the Duke Endocarditis Service published new criteria for the diagnosis of endocarditis that relied heavily on echocardiographic findings. In this original study, 405 cases were retrospectively reviewed and classified as definite, possible, or rejected on the basis of the presence or absence of major and minor criteria. When compared with previously used criteria, the proposed Duke criteria classified significantly more cases as definite endocarditis. Among pathologically proven cases, the Duke criteria were significantly more sensitive (80%) compared with the von Reyn criteria (51%) (Table 45.7).

Although the original criteria were generally accepted as an important advance in the diagnosis of endocarditis, there were limitations that were addressed in a subsequent publication (Li et al., 2000). As described earlier, using major and minor criteria,

Table 45.7 **Comparison of von Reyn and Duke Criteria for Diagnosing Endocarditis**

DUKE DEFINITIONS	VON REYN DEFINITIONS			
	PROBABLE	POSSIBLE	REJECTED	TOTAL (%)
Definite	65	59	11	40
Possible	6	56	87	44
Rejected	0	0	52	15
Total	21%	34%	45%	100

Reprinted from Durack DT, Lukes AS, Bright DK. New criteria for diagnosis of infective endocarditis: utilization of specific echocardiographic findings. *Am J Med* 1994;96(3):200–209. Copyright © 1994. With permission.

patients can be classified as having definite evidence of endocarditis, possible endocarditis, or the diagnosis can be rejected.

The diagnosis of infective endocarditis is definite (two major criteria, or one major + three minor criteria, or five minor criteria), possible (one major + one minor or three minor criteria), and rejected (firm alternate diagnosis explaining evidence of infective endocarditis; or resolution of infective endocarditis syndrome with antibiotic therapy for ≤4 days; or no pathologic evidence of infective endocarditis at surgery or autopsy, with antibiotic therapy for ≤4 days; or does not meet criteria for possible infective endocarditis, as earlier).

This approach has subsequently been endorsed by the American College of Cardiology/American Heart Association practice guidelines for the management of patients with valvular heart disease (Nishimura et al., 2014).

Suggested Readings

Armstrong W, Ryan T. Infective endocarditis. In: *Chapter 14: Feigenbaum's Echocardiography.* 7th ed. Philadelphia, PA: Lippincott Williams & Wilkins, 2009:361–362.

Li JS, Sexton DJ, Mick N, et al. Proposed modifications to the Duke criteria for the diagnosis of infective endocarditis. *Clin Infect Dis* 2000;30:633–638.

Nishimura RA, et al. 2014 AHA/ACC guideline for the management of patients with valvular heart disease. *J Am Coll Cardiol* 2014;63(suppl 22):e57–e105.

Otto C. Echocardiographic evaluation of the patient with a systemic embolic event. In: *The Practice of Clinical Echocardiography.* 3rd ed. Philadelphia, PA: Elsevier Saunders, 2007:506–507.

Answer 18: C. Echocardiography shows a vegetation on the aortic prosthesis (Video 45.20A) and no evidence of paravalvular abscess, regurgitation, or dehiscence (Video 45.20A–C). There is a small vegetation on the anterior mitral valve leaflet without direct extension or complication (such as perforation) and mild mitral regurgitation. The CW Doppler (see Fig. 45.11) demonstrates no significant obstruction across aortic valve prosthesis (peak gradient 12 mm Hg and mean gradient of 7 mm Hg); early peak, normal acceleration time (<100 ms) for aortic prosthesis; and typical opening and closing clicks of a mechanical prosthesis.

It is often difficult to evaluate for prosthetic valve endocarditis especially mechanical prosthesis due to the following: shadowing, signal dropouts from prosthetic material, reverberations (2D and color Doppler), and suture material. The type

and location of prosthesis also impact the diagnostic accuracy. For an example, mitral prostheses are relatively easier to evaluate than aortic prostheses both by TTE and by TEE. Right-sided prosthesis is better assessed by TTE. Thus, the Duke criteria are not as effective as in native valves since vegetations are more difficult to identify.

There is some indirect evidence of prosthetic malfunction that, when present, should make you consider prosthetic valve endocarditis.

When assessing with TTE, the following should be performed for every mechanical prosthesis:

1. Always compare with a previous echocardiogram (when available).
2. CW and PW Doppler assessment (assess the contours, density, acceleration time for aortic and pulmonary prosthesis, pressure half times for mitral and tricuspid prosthesis, opening and closing clicks).
3. Flow across the different valves and stroke volumes should correlate in the absence of significant regurgitation.
4. Know the normal patterns of backflow (color Doppler) in prosthetic valves (e.g., in case of St. Jude prosthesis, color Doppler would show brief, nonturbulent backflow with one central and two peripheral jets, with backflow volume of <5 mL per systole).
5. M-mode evaluation through prosthesis (to assess opening and closing clicks and slope during cardiac cycle).
6. Take advantage of contrast (saline for right-sided prosthesis and echo-contrast LVO [LV opacification] for left-sided prosthesis).
7. Prosthetic valve endocarditis (PVE) is the most severe form of IE; is often difficult to diagnose; occurs in 1% to 6% of patients with a valve prostheses, with an annual incidence of 0.3% to 1.2%; and is associated with poor prognosis (20% to 40% mortality) (1).
8. It accounts for 10% to 30% of all cases of IE and affects mechanical and bioprosthetic valves equally. Early PVE (within 1 year of surgery, common pathogen is coagulase-negative staphylococci, 37%, and *Staphylococcus aureus*, 24%) and late PVE (>1 year, same pathogens as native valve endocarditis) have different microbiologic profiles (1,2). Consequences of PVE include leaflet perforation, regurgitation, obstruction or stenosis of perivalvular abscess, dehiscence, pseudoaneurysms, and fistulae; therefore, TEE plays an essential role in the diagnosis.
9. The Duke criteria have been shown to be helpful for the diagnosis of native valve endocarditis, with a sensitivity of 70% to 80%, but are less useful in PVE, because of their lower sensitivity in this setting. In prosthetic valve endocarditis, TEE has shown an 86% to 94% sensitivity and 88% to 100% specificity for vegetation diagnosis, while TTE sensitivity is only 36% to 69% (3).
10. When evaluating with echocardiography, it is important to recognize the sewing ring and support structures of the prosthesis (strongly echogenic), valvular strands (commonly seen), and pannus formation (all of which can be difficult to differentiate from vegetative growth). Therefore, when available, it is important to review any

prior postsurgical echocardiograms for comparison. Several factors associated with poor prognosis in PVE are advanced age, staphylococcal infection, early PVE, heart failure, stroke, and intracardiac abscess.

11. Surgical strategy (radical debridement including removal of prosthesis, all foreign material, any calcium remaining from prior surgery) is recommended for PVE in high-risk subgroups (heart failure, severe prosthetic dysfunction, abscess, or persistent bacteremia) (4,5). However, this patient has no high-risk features, other than the organism (*Staphylococcus*), so that the initial treatment should be medical. Thus, urgent valve replacement is incorrect. (Early surgery may be needed in *Staphylococcus* or fungi or other highly resistant organisms.) Conversely, patients with uncomplicated nonstaphylococcal and nonfungal late PVE can be managed conservatively. However, patients who are initially treated medically require close follow-up, because of the risk of late events (1).

12. The decision to proceed with surgery is a complex one that must rely on clinical criteria as well as echocardiographic findings (see 2006 AHA/ACC Guidelines for surgery in a patient with prosthetic valve endocarditis; see TABLE 45.8) (6).

Table 45.8	**Surgery for Prosthetic Valve Endocarditis**

Class I

1. Consultation with a cardiac surgeon is indicated for patients with infective endocarditis of a prosthetic valve. *(Level of Evidence C)*
2. Surgery is indicated for patients with infective endocarditis of a prosthetic valve who present with heart failure. *(Level of Evidence B)*
3. Surgery is indicated for patients with infective endocarditis of a prosthetic valve who present with dehiscence evidenced by cine fluoroscopy or echocardiography. *(Level of Evidence B)*
4. Surgery is indicated for patients with infective endocarditis of a prosthetic valve who present with evidence of increasing obstruction or worsening regurgitation. *(Level of Evidence C)*
5. Surgery is indicated for patients with infective endocarditis of a prosthetic valve who present with complications (e.g., abscess formation). *(Level of Evidence C)*

Class IIa

1. Surgery is reasonable for patients with infective endocarditis of a prosthetic valve who present with evidence of persistent bacteremia or recurrent emboli despite appropriate antibiotic treatment. *(Level of Evidence C)*
2. Surgery is reasonable for patients with infective endocarditis of a prosthetic valve who present with relapsing infection. *(Level of Evidence C)*

Class III

Routine surgery is not indicated for patients with uncomplicated infective endocarditis of a prosthetic valve caused by first infection with a sensitive organism. *(Level of Evidence C)*

Reprinted from Bonow RO, Carabello BA, Chatterjee K, et al. ACC/AHA 2006 guidelines for the management of patients with valvular heart disease: a report of the American College of Cardiology/American Heart Association Task Force on Practice Guidelines. *J Am Coll Cardiol* 2006;48:e1–e148, with permission from Elsevier.

References

1. Habib G, Hoen B, Tornos P, et al. Guidelines on the prevention, diagnosis, and treatment of infective endocarditis. The Task Force on the Prevention, Diagnosis, and Treatment of Infective Endocarditis of the European Society of Cardiology (ESC). *Eur Heart J* 2009;30(19):2369–2413.
2. Lopez J, Revilla A, Vilacosta I, et al. Definition, clinical profile, microbiological spectrum, and prognostic factors of early-onset prosthetic valve endocarditis. *Eur Heart J* 2007;28:760–765.
3. Evangelista A, Gonzalez-Alujas M, et al. Echocardiography in infective endocarditis. *Heart* 2004;90:614–617.
4. Tornos P, Almirante B, Olona M, et al. Clinical outcome and long-term prognosis of late prosthetic valve endocarditis: a 20-year experience. *Clin Infect Dis* 1997;24:381–386.
5. Hill EE, Herregods MC, Vanderschueren S, et al. Management of prosthetic valve infective endocarditis. *Am J Cardiol* 2008;101:1174–1178.
6. Nishimura RA et al. 2014 AHA/ACC guideline for the management of patients with valvular heart disease. *J Am Coll Cardiol* 2014;63(suppl 22):e57–e105.

Suggested Readings

Habib G, Derumeaux G, Avierinos JF, et al. Value and limitations of the Duke criteria for the diagnosis of infective endocarditis. *J Am Coll Cardiol* 1999;33:2023–2029.
Habib G, Thuny F, Avierinos JF. Prosthetic valve endocarditis: current approach and therapeutic options. *Prog Cardiovasc Dis* 2008;50:274–281.

Answer 19: D. Images show abscess as evidenced by posterior aortic wall thickening and areas of echolucency in a patient with aortic valve vegetation. Color Doppler demonstrates flow communication with an abscess cavity.

VIDEO 45.21A AND B shows aortic paravalvular extension of infection and annular abscess as evidenced by aortic wall thickening and areas of echolucency within and leaflet disruption from infection. Abscess cavity has ruptured into the RA as evidenced by color Doppler (VIDEO 45.21C).

Periannular extension of infection, or abscess formation, is a localized pocket of infection and is one of the most serious complications of IE. Among patients with IE, the reported incidence of perivalvular abscess at surgery or autopsy has ranged from about 30% to 40%. The aortic valve and its adjacent annulus are more susceptible to abscess formation and the complications of perivalvular extension of infection (41%) than are the mitral valve and ring (6%). Risk factors for perivalvular abscess are *Staphylococcus* or *Enterococcus* bacteremia and injection drug use.

Perivalvular abscess should be suspected when fever persists despite appropriate antimicrobial therapy and/or when conduction abnormalities appear on the ECG. Transesophageal echocardiography (TEE) has a much greater likelihood of detecting a myocardial abscess than transthoracic echocardiography (TTE). The sensitivity, specificity, and positive and negative predictive values of TEE imaging were 87%, 95%, 91%, and 92%, respectively (1,2). The sensitivity of TTE was much lower (28% versus 87%), although the specificity was 99% (2). However, some perivalvular abscesses may be missed by TEE. Patients with perivalvular abscesses appear to have higher rates of systemic embolization and fatal outcomes.

In one study comparing outcomes of patients with and without perivalvular abscesses, the rate of embolization was approximately twice as high (64% versus 30%). These patients also have a higher mortality rate (23% versus 14% in those without abscesses).

Perivalvular abscess can extend into adjacent cardiac conduction tissues (leading to various forms of heart block), or it can affect the valve function leading to regurgitation. Involvement of the conducting system is most common with infection of the aortic valve, especially when there is involvement of the valve ring between the right and noncoronary cusp (this anatomic site overlies the intraventricular septum that contains the proximal ventricular conduction system). Rarely, perivalvular infection can result in extrinsic coronary compression and can cause acute coronary syndrome. An abscess may rupture to allow communication with one of the cardiac chambers. Echocardiographically, this can be detected as a fistulous connection between two chambers of the heart (such as the right and left ventricles) or between the aortic root and a chamber (i.e., between a sinus of Valsalva and the left or right atrium), and color Doppler may demonstrate flow within the abscess cavity, within the fistula, and its connection to another chamber. Depending on which aortic sinus of Valsalva is involved, the location of the fistula varies widely and may communicate with any of the cardiac chambers.

Mycotic aneurysms (MAs), defined as an echolucent outpouching of the vessel wall, are uncommon complications of infective endocarditis that result from septic embolization of vegetations to the arterial vasa vasorum or direct contact from the aortic valve into the nearby coronary cusp, with subsequent spread of infection through the intima and outward through the vessel wall. Arterial branching points favor the impaction of emboli and are the most common sites of development of MAs. MAs caused by IE occur most frequently in the intracranial arteries, followed by the visceral arteries; rarely, it involves the aortic root or aortic sinuses and is similar in many ways to abscesses. It is usually connected through a single channel with the vessel from which it arises. As such, it can be either filled with infectious material or contain free-flowing blood. Such aneurysms may rupture to produce an intracardiac shunt or may undermine the function of the aortic valve.

References

1. Daniel WG, Mügge A, Martin RP, et al. Improvement in the diagnosis of abscesses associated with endocarditis by transesophageal echocardiography. *N Engl J Med* 1991;324(12):795.
2. Evangelista A, Gonzalez-Alujas M, et al. Echocardiography in infective endocarditis. *Heart* 2004;90:614–617.

Suggested Readings

Armstrong W, Ryan T. Infective endocarditis. In: *Chapter 14: Feigenbaum's Echocardiography*. 7th ed. Philadelphia, PA: Lippincott Williams & Wilkins, 2009:369–373.
Cosmi JE, Tunick PA, Kronzon I, et al. Mortality in patients with paravalvular abscess diagnosed by transesophageal echocardiography. *J Am Soc Echocardiogr* 2004;17(7):766.
Omari B, Shapiro S, Ginzton L, et al. Predictive risk factors for periannular extension of native valve endocarditis. Clinical and echocardiographic analyses. *Chest* 1989;96(6):1273.
Otto C. Echocardiographic evaluation of the patient with a systemic embolic event. In: *The Practice of Clinical Echocardiography*. 3rd ed. Philadelphia, PA: Elsevier Saunders, 2007:502–515.
Wilson WR, Lie JT, Houser OW, et al. The management of patients with mycotic aneurysm. *Curr Clin Top Infect Dis* 1981;2:151–183.

Answer 20: D. Surgery as soon as feasible. He has multiple high-risk clinical predictors of mortality such as *Staphylococcus aureus* bacteremia, heart failure, perivalvular abscess, large vegetation, and severe valvular regurgitation.

VIDEO 45.22 shows a large vegetation involving aortic valve leaflets and anterior mitral valve leaflet with color Doppler evidence of severe aortic valve regurgitation. There appears to be also perforation of the aortic valve leaflet as evidenced by multiple peripheral jets (away from closure line). He also has premature closure of the mitral valve (see FIG. 45.12A) and diastolic mitral regurgitation (see FIG. 45.12C) from severe aortic regurgitation and backward flow into the left atrium during late diastole. These findings are also present on VIDEO 45.22 but difficult to appreciate as the temporal resolution of 2D (40 to 60 frame/s) and color Doppler is poor (15 to 30 frames/s). However, M-mode with its higher temporal resolution (1,000 to 2,000 frames/s) clearly demonstrates the premature closure of the mitral valve. TEE images as shown (VIDEO 45.23) confirm the findings shown by TTE; in addition, it also demonstrates paravalvular extension of the infection and aortic valve leaflet perforation with color Doppler showing origins of the multiple jets of aortic regurgitation.

Medical therapy or waiting with repeat TEE exam or elective surgery is not a good option as his prognosis is poor without early surgical intervention. Surgery in this situation (complicated infective endocarditis with heart failure and abscess) is a class I indication (2006 AHA/ACC Guidelines for surgery in a patient with infective endocarditis).

Predictors of death—Several studies have demonstrated predictors of death in patients with infective endocarditis (IE), infection with *Staphylococcus aureus*, heart failure, embolic events, perivalvular abscess, larger vegetation size (>10 mm), contraindication to surgery or poor surgical candidacy, and persistent bacteremia (1,2).

Mortality rates for large series of patients with native valve endocarditis treated since 1980 ranged from 13% to 20%. Death from IE has been associated with increased age (>65 to 70 years), underlying diseases, infection involving the aortic valve, development of CHF, nosocomial origin, *S. aureus* infection, renal failure, and central nervous system complications (2). Early surgical treatment in patients with CHF due to valve dysfunction has decreased the mortality associated with CHF. As a result, neurologic events, uncontrolled infection, and myocardial abscess have accounted for a larger proportion of deaths in recent series.

Outcomes for patients with prosthetic valve endocarditis (PVE), as contrasted with native valve endocarditis (NVE), have been less favorable. Mortality is significantly higher for

PVE with onset <2 months after surgery, 70% versus 45% for later onset (>2 months). With the recognition that PVE outcome would benefit from surgical intervention, mortality rates have decreased to 14% to 36% (3). Long-term survival was adversely affected by the presence of moderate or severe CHF at discharge.

Among patients with NVE (nonaddicts) discharged after medical or medical surgical therapy, survival was 71% to 88% at 5 years and 61% to 81% at 10 years. Among patients treated surgically for NVE, survival at 5 years ranged from 70% to 80% (4).

In those patients who need urgent surgery, persistent infection and renal failure are predictors of mortality. Predictably, patients with an indication for surgery who cannot proceed due to prohibitive surgical risk have the worst prognosis (5).

References

1. Wang A, Athan E, Pappas PA. Contemporary clinical profile and outcome of prosthetic valve endocarditis. *JAMA* 2007;297(12):1354.
2. Wallace SM, Walton BI, Kharbanda RK, et al. Mortality from infective endocarditis: clinical predictors of outcome. *Heart* 2002;88(1):53.
3. Bonow R, Mann D, Zipes D, et al. Infective endocarditis. In: Karchmer AW, ed. *Braunwald's Heart Disease: A Textbook of Cardiovascular Medicine.* 9th ed. Philadelphia, PA: Saunders Elsevier, 2011:1540–1560.
4. Hill EE, Herijgers P, Claus P, et al. Infective endocarditis: changing epidemiology and predictors of 6-month mortality: a prospective cohort study. *Eur Heart J* 2007;28(2):196.
5. Habib G, Hoen B, Tornos P, et al. Guidelines on the prevention, diagnosis, and treatment of infective endocarditis. The Task Force on the Prevention, Diagnosis, and Treatment of Infective Endocarditis of the European Society of Cardiology (ESC). *Eur Heart J* 2009;30(19):2369–2413.

Suggested Readings

Chu VH, Cabell CH, Benjamin DK Jr, et al. Early predictors of in-hospital death in infective endocarditis. *Circulation* 2004;109(14):1745.
Murdoch DR, Corey GR, Hoen B, et al. Clinical presentation, etiology, and outcome of infective endocarditis in the 21st century. *Arch Intern Med* 2009;169:463.

Answer 21:

Scenario 21A: *Answer:* **A (yes).**

Scenario A is an example of a 28-year-old male with intravenous drug use who presented with fever and chills with echocardiography (Video 45.24) showing mitral valve aneurysm and perforation from infective endocarditis. This is a class I indication for surgery (complicated infective endocarditis) (1).

Scenario 21B: *Answer:* **B (no).**

Scenario B is an example of a 65-year-old female with bioprosthetic aortic valve and mitral valve replacement for rheumatic heart disease who presented with heart failure. Her echocardiography (Video 45.25) shows suture material of the prosthetic valve that can be difficult to differentiate from vegetation. As discussed earlier, however, they are fibrinized or endothelialized, thick structures and are placed in a uniform manner around the prosthetic valves. When these sutures are cut "long" by the surgeon, they might resemble valvular strands

(2,3). Clinical presentation may help differentiate it from true infectious process. Sometimes, it is useful to have old postsurgical echocardiography for side-by-side comparison.

Scenario 21C: *Answer:* **A (yes).**

Scenario C is an example of a 38-year-old female with intravenous drug use and known tricuspid valve endocarditis who was treated medically for 8 weeks of therapy and successful eradication of bacteremia, and her echocardiography shows chronic vegetation (calcification) of tricuspid valve and severe wide-open tricuspid regurgitation with malcoaptation of leaflets. Given her severe tricuspid valve dysfunction with poor RV function, she would need tricuspid valve surgery. Echocardiographic images from the same patient during acute phase of tricuspid valve endocarditis are shown in Video 45.29.

Endocarditis involving the tricuspid valve is most commonly seen in the setting of intravenous drug abuse or in association with an indwelling catheter in the right ventricle (a pacer lead). In one series (4), involving 121 intravenous drug abusers, a tricuspid valve vegetation was seen in all cases, whereas the pulmonary valve was involved in only four.

Vegetation size tends to be greater in right-sided endocarditis, and tricuspid regurgitation of varying severity is generally present. Even after successful antibiotic therapy, when infection is no longer clinically active, masses on the tricuspid valve often remain (3).

Pulmonary valve vegetations are less common and can be difficult to visualize. The superiority of transesophageal echocardiography is less well established in right-sided endocarditis. Because the tricuspid valve is well seen from the transthoracic windows and because right-sided vegetations are typically large, transthoracic echocardiography is often adequate for diagnosis and both techniques have demonstrated high sensitivity (3,4). Below is an example of a 32-year-old female with a modified ROSS procedure in childhood and recent use of intravenous drugs presenting bioprosthetic pulmonary valve vegetation and pulmonary stenosis (see Video 45.30 and Fig. 45.18).

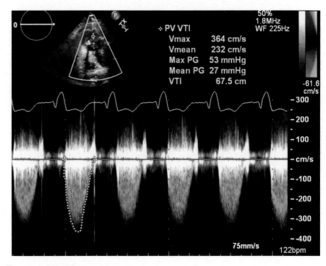

Figure 45.18

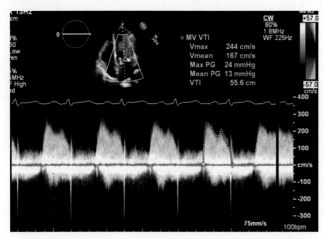

FIGURE **45.19**

Scenario 21D: *Answer:* **A (yes).**

Scenario D is an example of a 45-year-old with bioprosthetic aortic and mitral valve who presented with *Staphylococcus* bacteremia. His echocardiography shows prosthetic valve dehiscence (rocking motion of prosthetic valve with excursion >15 degrees), a large vegetation involving bioprosthesis and valve stenosis. CW Doppler image is shown in FIGURE 45.19 from the same patient. Surgery is indicated for patients with infective endocarditis of a prosthetic valve who present with dehiscence evidenced by cine fluoroscopy or echocardiography (class I, Level of Evidence B) (1).

Scenario 21E: *Answer:* **A (yes).**

Scenario E is an example of a 48-year-old male with HIV and hepatitis C who presented with chronic malaise and weight loss. His echocardiography demonstrates a large vegetation involving the aortic valve, with flail aortic valve leaflets, abscess involving aortic annulus, aortomitral intervalvular fibrosa, and fistulous connection with right atrium. All of these findings are associated with increased mortality. Surgery is indicated in patients with infective endocarditis complicated by heart block, annular or aortic abscess, or destructive penetrating lesions (e.g., sinus of Valsalva to right atrium, right ventricle, or left atrium fistula; mitral leaflet perforation with aortic valve endocarditis; or infection in annulus fibrosa) (class I, Level of Evidence B) (1).

References

1. Bonow RO, Carabello BA, Chatterjee K, et al. ACC/AHA 2006 guidelines for the management of patients with valvular heart disease: A report of the American College of cardiology/American Heart Association Task Force on Practice Guidelines. *J Am Coll Cardiol* 2006;48:e1–e148.
2. Otto C. Echocardiographic evaluation of the patient with a systemic embolic event. In: *The Practice of Clinical Echocardiography.* 3rd ed. Philadelphia, PA: Elsevier Saunders, 2007:502–515.
3. Armstrong W, Ryan T. Infective endocarditis. In: *Chapter 14: Feigenbaum's Echocardiography.* 7th ed. Philadelphia, PA: Lippincott Williams & Wilkins, 2009:361–385.
4. Hecht SR, Berger M. Right-sided endocarditis in intravenous drug users. Prognostic features in 102 episodes. *Ann Intern Med* 1992;117:560–566.

Suggested Reading

Habib G, Hoen B, Tornos P, et al. Guidelines on the prevention, diagnosis, and treatment of infective endocarditis. The Task Force on the Prevention, Diagnosis, and Treatment of Infective Endocarditis of the European Society of Cardiology (ESC). *Eur Heart J* 2009;30(19):2369–2413.

Chapter 46

Normal and Abnormal Pericardial Findings

Steve Leung

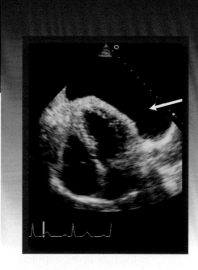

1. Which of the following is true regarding pericardial effusion?

A. Pericardial effusion remains unchanged despite change in patient position.

B. Without trauma, stranding in the pericardial space is seen only in patients who have malignant pericardial effusions.

C. Pericardial effusion can accumulate around the great vessels.

D. All pericardial effusions that can be visualized by echocardiogram can be safely drained with echocardiographic guidance.

E. Pericardial effusion that can be visualized by echocardiography is pathologic and requires further evaluation.

2. In the evaluation of pericardial thickness:

A. Transthoracic echocardiography can identify a normal and thickened pericardium accurately.

B. Transesophageal echocardiography has better accuracy in identifying a thickened pericardium compared to transthoracic echocardiography.

C. Normal pericardial thickness rules out constrictive pericarditis.

D. A thickness of >2 mm is considered diagnostic for constrictive pericarditis.

E. During measurement of pericardial thickness by echocardiography, only the visceral pericardium is being measured.

3. What is the M-mode finding of a physiologic amount of pericardial effusion in the parasternal long-axis view?

A. An echo-free space between the posterior epicardium and pericardium that is seen throughout the cardiac cycle.

B. An echo-free space between the posterior epicardium and pericardium that is only seen during systole.

C. An echo-free space between the posterior epicardium and pericardium that is only seen during diastole.

D. An echo-free space between the anterior epicardium and pericardium that is seen during inspiration.

E. It is not normal to see pericardial fluid with an M-mode technique.

4. A 73-year-old male presents to the echo lab for assessment of left ventricular function assessment after a recent STEMI and received a coronary stent in the left circumflex artery, 2 days ago. He is currently asymptomatic and hemodynamically stable. His ECG demonstrates normal sinus rhythm and normal axis without any ST-segment changes. On his echocardiogram, he had normal left ventricular systolic function and chamber size. There was no pericardial effusion. He also had 20% respiratory variation in the tricuspid inflow, but no respiratory variation in the mitral inflow pattern. In the parasternal long-axis view, you noticed that the posterior pericardium appears bright (Fig. 46.1). What is the likely explanation of this finding?

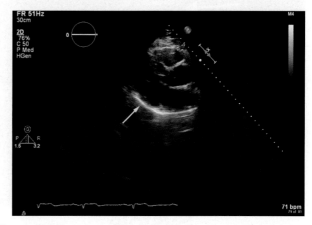

Figure 46.1

A. Dressler syndrome
B. Calcified pericardium due to constrictive pericarditis
C. Inflammation of the myocardium from his NSTEMI
D. Acute pericarditis
E. Normal finding of a pericardium, as the pericardium is a highly reflective structure

5. Which of the following clinical scenarios is a *rarely appropriate* indication for echocardiographic evaluation of the pericardium?

A. A 76-year-old female with a history of prosthetic aortic valve replacement a year ago with a small pericardial effusion presents for her yearly echocardiogram for surveillance.
B. A 48-year-old female with a history of breast cancer and underwent lumpectomy, radiation therapy, and chemotherapy presents for evaluation due to medically refractory lower extremity edema.
C. A 56-year-old male with an anterior STEMI 6 weeks ago presents with atypical chest pain.
D. A 62-year-old male driver involved in a motor vehicle accident. He is hypotensive despite fluid resuscitation.
E. A 68-year-old female with a moderate-sized pericardial effusion of unknown etiology undergoing pericardiocentesis for diagnosis.

6. A 50-year-old patient presents following a motor vehicle accident. An echocardiogram is ordered to evaluate for shortness of breath. What is indicated by the arrow in FIGURE 46.2 (and VIDEOS 46.1 AND 46.2)?

A. Hemorrhagic pericardial effusion
B. Chest wall
C. Intramyocardial hemorrhage
D. Epicardial fat
E. Right ventricular wall

7. A 55-year-old male with atypical chest pain and dyspnea on exertion presents for an echocardiogram. He has no past medical or surgical history and is not on any medications. Physical exam revealed normal blood pressure, a 2/6 systolic murmur heard at the left lower sternal border, and an extremely laterally displaced PMI. His ECG demonstrates normal sinus rhythm, normal axis, incomplete right bundle branch block, and poor R-wave progression. Echocardiography demonstrated a normal-sized left ventricle with hyperdynamic function. There is abnormal motion of the septum. The right ventricle is moderately dilated with normal function. The tricuspid valve appeared normal with mild tricuspid regurgitation. The peak velocity across the valve during systole was 2.2 m/s. The aortic, mitral, and pulmonic valves appear normal. The inferior vena cava is <2 cm and collapses during inspiration. What is the most likely diagnosis for this patient?

A. Silent myocardial infarction
B. Ebstein anomaly
C. D-transposition of the great arteries
D. Congenital absence of the pericardium
E. Presence of a right-to-left shunt

8. A 38-year-old male presents for evaluation of a murmur. During his echocardiographic exam, he was found to have a round echo-free area approximately 4 cm in diameter lateral to his right atrium near the atrioventricular groove. Color Doppler did not demonstrate significant flow. What should be the immediate next step?

A. Manufactured microbubble contrast/agitated saline bubble injection
B. Recommend PET
C. Recommend cardiac CT
D. Recommend cardiac MRI
E. Recommend cardiac catheterization

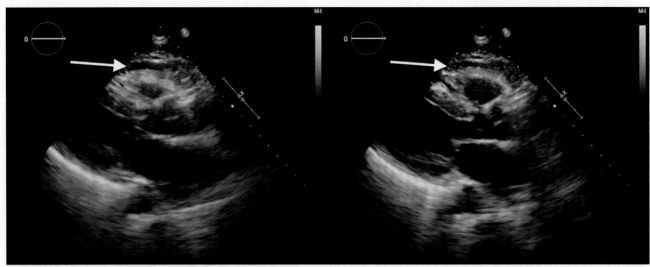

Systole **Diastole**

FIGURE 46.2

9. A 45-year-old male with no significant past medical history presents for evaluation of dyspnea on exertion. An echocardiogram was performed. The patient was placed in the left lateral decubitus position. The technologist noted a normal-appearing sternal and thoracic musculoskeletal appearance and tried to obtain a parasternal long-axis view. However, despite several attempts, no good echocardiographic window was obtained until she moved her probe laterally near the left midaxillary line. There was no atrioventricular discordance or ventriculoarterial discordance. What is the most likely diagnosis?

A. Marfan syndrome
B. Chronic obstructive pulmonary disease
C. Congenital absence of the pericardium
D. Dextrocardia
E. Ebstein anomaly

10. A 52-year-old asymptomatic female was referred for echocardiogram prior to start of chemotherapy for breast cancer. She was noted to have this echo finding (Fig. 46.3, Video 46.3). Color Doppler did not reveal any flow. Agitated saline and echocardiographic contrast did not opacify this structure. What is the likely diagnosis of this structure?

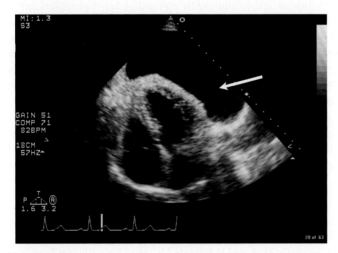

FIGURE 46.3 2D echocardiogram still frame, parasternal long axis, demonstrating the pericardial fat, pericardium, and epicardial fat. The visceral and parietal pericardia are very thin in normal patients. Without pericardial effusion, the two layers cannot be discerned. Movie—2D echocardiogram, parasternal long axis, demonstrating the pericardial fat, pericardium, and epicardial fat.

A. Persistent left superior vena cava
B. Metastatic breast cancer mass
C. Left ventricular pseudoaneurysm
D. Emphysematous change (bleb)
E. Pericardial cyst

Answer 1: C. Pericardial effusion can be positional but can also be loculated and remains unchanged despite changing patient's position. Stranding in the pericardial space can be seen in patients with infected pericardial effusion, uremic pericarditis, as well as chronic inflammatory effusions. Pericardial effusion can accumulate around the proximal portion of the great vessels due to the reflection of the pericardium. This is also the reason why patients with acute ascending aortic dissection can present with hemopericardium. Occasionally, pericardial effusion may be located only near the inferolateral wall or behind the atria and cannot be reached safely with apical or subxiphoid approaches. If indicated, these would require surgical drainage. Everyone has pericardial effusion within the pericardium. A normal amount can be visualized with echocardiography during diastole, but not during systole (1).

Reference

1. Horowitz MS, Schultz CS, Stinson EB, et al. Sensitivity and specificity of echocardiographic diagnosis of pericardial effusion. *Circulation* 1974;50:239–247.

Answer 2: B. The sensitivity of transthoracic echocardiogram in the evaluation of pericardial thickness is low (ranging from 46% to 63%) (1, 2). In a study performed by Ling LH et al., transesophageal echocardiography was 95% sensitive and 86% specific in identifying a thickened pericardium (≥3 mm), with electron beam computed tomography as the reference standard (3). In a study evaluating pericardial thickness in constrictive pericarditis, approximately 82% had increased pericardial thickness, and 18% of patients had normal pericardial thickness (4). Therefore, Options C and D are incorrect. Pericardial thickness of >4 mm assists in the diagnosis of constrictive pericarditis. In the absence of a pericardial effusion, echocardiography cannot discern the visceral and parietal pericardium. Therefore, Option E is incorrect.

References

1. Engel PJ. Echocardiographic findings in pericardial disease. In: Fowler NO, ed. *The Pericardium in Health and Disease*. Armonk, NY: Futura, 1985:99–151.
2. Hinds SW, Reisner SA, Amico AF, et al. Diagnosis of pericardial abnormalities by 2D echo: a pathology-echocardiography correlation in 85 patients. *Am Heart J* 1992;123:143–150.
3. Ling LH, Oh JK, Tei C, et al. Pericardial thickness measured with transesophageal echocardiography: feasibility and potential clinical usefulness. *J Am Coll Cardiol* 1997;29(6):1317–1323.
4. Talreja DR, Edwards WD, Danielson GK, et al. Constrictive pericarditis in 26 patients with histologically normal pericardial thickness. *Circulation* 2003;108:1852–1857.

Answer 3: B. A physiologic pericardial effusion can be seen during systole in the M-mode posterior to the left ventricle and not during diastole (Fig. 46.4). Based on the Horowitz classification, in patients with an echo-free space between the posterior epicardium and pericardium seen only during systole, the volume of pericardial effusion was <16 mL (1).

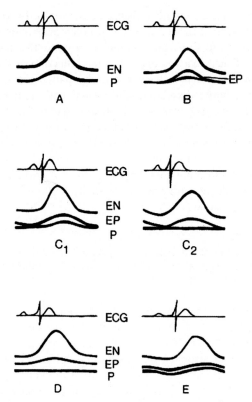

FIGURE 46.4 Patterns of posterior epicardial and pericardial movement in the presence and absence of pericardial effusions. Patterns A, B, and C1 were found in patients with <16 mL of pericardial fluid. C2 represents a small effusion by this criterion, especially in the presence of a large heart. D is the classic pattern for pericardial effusion. E represents a thickened pericardium (Horowitz MS, Schultz CS, Stinson EB, et al. Sensitivity and specificity of echocardiographic diagnosis of pericardial effusion. *Circulation* 1974;50:239–247).

Reference

1. Horowitz MS, Schultz CS, Stinson EB, et al. Sensitivity and specificity of echocardiographic diagnosis of pericardial effusion. *Circulation* 1974;50:239–247.

Answer 4: E. The normal parietal pericardium is a highly reflective structure (1). This finding is seen in most patients with good echo windows. Dressler syndrome (Option A) usually occurs weeks after myocardial infarction or postpericardiotomy for bypass operation and not days. Patients with Dressler syndrome would have typical symptoms of acute pericarditis such as chest pain and can have pericardial effusion on echocardiography. A calcified pericardium (Option B) is difficult to diagnose on echocardiography and generally is not well visualized. Also, there is no mitral inflow respiratory variation, which is expected in constrictive pericarditis (>25%) (2). Echocardiography cannot routinely diagnose inflammation of the myocardium or pericardium based on echogenicity (Options C and D). The most common abnormal finding for acute pericarditis is pericardial effusion; however, without any clinical symptoms or signs for acute pericarditis, this is unlikely.

References

1. Armstrong W, Ryan T. Chapter 10: Pericardial diseases. *Feigenbaum's Echocardiography.* 7th ed. Philadelphia, PA: Lippincott Williams & Wilkins, 2009:247.

2. Oh JK, Hatle LK, Seward JB, et al. Diagnostic role of Doppler echocardiography in constrictive pericarditis. *J Am Coll Cardiol* 1994;23:154–162.

Answer 5: A. Repeat echocardiography in patients with small pericardial effusions or a recently replaced prosthetic valve (<3 years) with no change in clinical status is a rarely appropriate indication (1). Option B is a patient with a history of radiation exposure and clinical symptoms suspicious for constrictive pericarditis, which is an appropriate indication for echocardiography. Option C is a patient who presents with possible Dressler syndrome and may have a pericardial effusion causing dyspnea on exertion. Option D is a patient who may have suffered cardiac contusion and possibly hemorrhage into the pericardial space. Option E is a patient who would benefit from an echocardiogram to assist and guide the diagnostic pericardiocentesis.

Reference

1. ACCF/ASE/AHA/ASNC/HFSA/HRS/SCAI/SCCM/SCCT/SCMR 2011. Appropriate use criteria for echocardiography. *J Am Soc Echocardiogr* 2011;24:229–267.

Answer 6: D. The arrow indicates a space anterior to the right ventricle, which is of mixed echogenicity. This is a typical finding in individuals with epicardial fat. Epicardial fat is generally seen in between the right ventricular wall and chest wall. It is an area that is almost echo-free and moves with the right ventricle (Video 46.2) (1). CT scan of the same patient clearly delineates this structure as epicardial fat due to its low Hounsfield units (dark appearance). A pericardial effusion is usually echo-free, although a pericardial hematoma can have mixed echogenicity (Option A). The chest wall (Option B) is anterior to the structure indicated by the arrow. Pericardial tumors (Option C) are generally associated with a pericardial effusion. Right ventricular wall (Option E) is posterior to the structure. The presence of epicardial fat has been associated with increased incidence of coronary artery disease (2).

References

1. Iacobellis G, Assael F, Ribaudo MC, et al. Epicardial fat from echocardiography: a new method for visceral adipose tissue prediction. *Obes Res* 2003;11:304–310.
2. Iacobellis G, Bianco AC. Epicardial adipose tissue: emerging physiological, pathophysiological and clinical features. *Trends Endocrinol Metab* 2011;22(11):450–457.

Answer 7: D. This patient most likely has congenital absence of a pericardium. The laterally displaced apex, normal-sized left ventricle, paradoxical motion of the septum, and dilated right ventricle are signs of absence of a pericardium (1). Echo windows are generally laterally displaced due to the displacement of the heart. Silent myocardial infarction (Option A) would not cause a laterally deviated apex. There should be evidence of tricuspid valve abnormalities such as apical displacement of the septal leaflet in Ebstein anomaly (Option B). In D-transposition of the great arteries (Option C), the right ventricle has to support systemic pressures, which would cause the peak velocity across the tricuspid valve to be much higher than just 2.2 m/s. Presence of right-to-left shunt (Option E) is unlikely to cause a dilated right ventricle with a normal RVSP.

Reference

1. Connolly HM, Click RL, Schattenberg TT, et al. Congenital absence of the pericardium: echocardiogram as a diagnostic tool. *J Am Soc Echocardiogr* 1995;8:87–92.

Answer 8: A. The patient likely has a pericardial cyst or coronary aneurysm. At this juncture, transthoracic echo can differentiate this area as vascular or not by injection of a manufactured microbubble contrast agent (either Definity or Optison) or by agitated saline bubble injection. Agitated saline microbubble injection is useful for the evaluation of right-to-left shunts. The microbubbles are generally trapped in the pulmonary capillaries and do not appear into the left cardiac chambers unless there is a right-to-left intracardiac or intrapulmonary shunt. If the patient does have a right-to-left shunt, but not enough bubbles traveled to the left side of the heart for evaluation of the cystic structure, then one should consider using manufactured microbubble contrast agent. The ultrasound contrast agents are structurally smaller than agitated saline microbubbles and able to travel through the pulmonary circulation and into the systemic arterial system (1). If the patient has a coronary aneurysm, then the center of the structure should be filled with the contrast agent. However, if this structure is avascular, then it should remain echo-free. These contrast studies should be performed prior to ordering additional imaging modalities such as cardiac CT, cardiac MRI, or cardiac catheterization (Options C, D, and E). PET scan does not have a significant role in the evaluation of pericardial cyst (Option B).

Reference

1. Sieswerda GT, Kamp O, Visser CA. Myocardial contrast echocardiography: clinical benefit and practical issues. *Echocardiography* 2000;17(6 Pt 2):S25–S36.

Answer 9: C. In congenital absence of the pericardium, the ventricular axis is shifted to the left (Fig. 46.5). With the ventricles rotated to the left, the technologist needs to understand that the cardiac axis may be shifted significantly and may require to image from the midaxillary line or beyond (1). Patients with Marfan syndrome (Option A) and chronic obstructive pulmonary disease (Option B) have increased the thoracic cavity length and are likely to create a more vertical axis of the heart without significantly affecting the parasternal view too much. Patients with marked pectus deformities, which may be seen in Marfan syndrome, may shift the heart and cardiac axis, but this patient had a normal sternum. Dextrocardia (Option D) would be difficult to image from the left parasternal window, as this patient, but should not be able

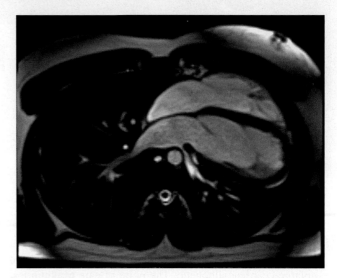

FIGURE 46.5 Cardiac MRI axial image of a patient with congenital absence of a pericardium demonstrating the extreme leftward axis that these patients may have. Echocardiographic imaging of these patients requires technologists to search for the best unconventional windows.

to obtain any echocardiographic window from the left midaxillary line. Ebstein anomaly (Option E) should only appear to have an atrialization of the right ventricle and not a complete shift of the cardiac axis.

Reference

1. Connolly HM, Click RL, Schattenberg TT, et al. Congenital absence of the pericardium: echocardiography as a diagnostic tool. *J Am Soc Echocardiogr* 1995;8:87–92.

Answer 10: E. This patient has a pericardial cyst. The most common location of a pericardial cyst is near the right atrioventricular groove (1). This pericardial cyst is located next to the lateral wall/apex of the left ventricle (Fig. 46.3). The structure is echo-lucent, and thus, it is unlikely to be a metastatic breast cancer mass. Persistent left superior vena cava is generally located in the left atrioventricular groove and has low velocity Doppler signal. If a peripheral IV is placed in the right upper extremity, it may not be opacified by agitated saline; however, it should opacify with echocardiographic contrast. Similarly, left ventricular pseudoaneurysm should opacify with echocardiographic contrast. The mass is able to transduce ultrasound to the posterior area; thus, it is unlikely to be filled with air (bleb), but rather fluid.

Reference

1. Khandaker MH, Espinosa RE, Nishimura RA, et al. Pericardial disease: diagnosis and management. *Mayo Clin Proc* 2010;85(6):572–593.

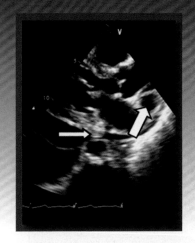

Chapter 47

Pericardial Effusions

Steve Leung

1. A 44-year-old patient presents to the emergency department with chest pain and hypotension. A chest x-ray reveals an enlarged cardiac silhouette. The point of care troponin test is 3.4 ng/dL. The emergency department physician orders a stat echocardiogram suspecting tamponade to be the likely reason of hypotension.

The most appropriate response would be:

A. An echocardiogram is not indicated now as the patient needs to be taken for emergent pericardiocentesis, and echocardiography could be performed at that time but should not delay this procedure.

B. The cardiac silhouette is not usually enlarged on a chest x-ray unless the pericardial effusion is at least 200 mL in volume. However, urgent echocardiography is indicated to confirm the presence of pericardial fluid and hemodynamic significance.

C. Initially, an attempt of IV fluid should be given. If the BP increases, the echocardiogram is no longer necessary.

D. The abnormally elevated cardiac biomarker makes the diagnosis of pericardial tamponade highly unlikely.

E. An immediate bedside pericardiocentesis should be attempted prior to echocardiography.

2. Five different patients were referred to your echocardiography laboratory with a complaint of dyspnea on exertion, and each was found to have a small- to moderate-sized pericardial effusion. Which patient profile is least likely to be associated with a pericardial effusion on echocardiography?

A. A 32-year-old female who is 34 weeks' pregnant

B. A 55-year-old female with class III pulmonary hypertension

C. A 72-year-old male with hemodynamically severe aortic stenosis

D. A 21-year-old male on conventional epilepsy therapy

E. A 45-year-old female with sarcoidosis

3. Which of the following is the reason for the development of this patient's pericardial effusion (Fig. 47.1, Video 47.1)?

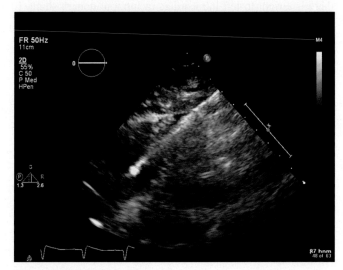

FIGURE 47.1 Subcostal view.

A. Bacterial pericarditis

B. Metastatic melanoma

C. Pacemaker lead perforation

D. Uremic pericarditis

E. Volume overload

4. A 50-year-old patient with metastatic melanoma presents with hypotension and tachycardia. He has jugular venous distention and clear lungs. This spectral Doppler pattern was recorded (Fig. 47.2). Which of the following comorbid condition can be seen in cardiac tamponade patients with this Doppler pattern?

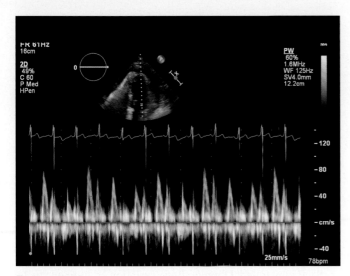

FIGURE 47.2

A. Atrial septal defect
B. Severe aortic regurgitation
C. Chronic severe left ventricular systolic dysfunction
D. Renal failure
E. Positive pressure ventilation

5. A 72-year-old patient with breast cancer presents to the emergency department with generalized fatigue. A CT scan of the chest reveals a large pericardial effusion, and a stat echocardiogram is performed (Fig. 47.3). The cardiologist concludes that the patient has a large pericardial effusion with 2D echocardiographic features of tamponade. Which of the following 2D echo findings is most consistent with the cardiologist's interpretation?

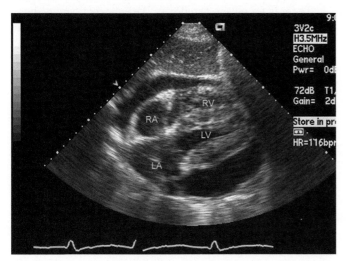

FIGURE 47.3 From Feigenbaum H, Armstrong WF, Ryan T. *Chapter 10: Feigenbaum's Echocardiography.* 6th ed. Philadelphia, PA: Lippincott Williams & Wilkins, 2004.

A. A 1.5-cm pericardial effusion in diastole with late ventricular systolic RVOT collapse
B. A 1.8-cm pericardial effusion in diastole with early ventricular systolic RA collapse
C. A 2.2-cm pericardial effusion in diastole with ventricular diastolic LA collapse
D. A 2.5-cm pericardial effusion in systole with ventricular systolic LA collapse
E. A 1.8-cm pericardial effusion in systole with late atrial diastolic RA collapse

6. Which of these is the least likely a reason for the pericardial effusion seen in Figure 47.4?

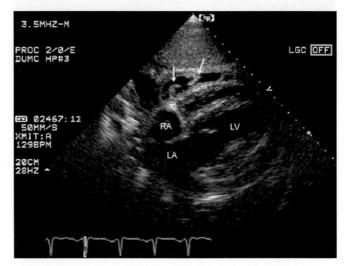

FIGURE 47.4

A. Uremia from poorly compliant peritoneal dialysis
B. Bacterial pericarditis
C. Chronic effusion from any etiology
D. Metastatic melanoma
E. Pregnancy associated with preeclampsia

Questions 7 and 8

See Figure 47.5 and Video 47.2.

7. The posterior echo-free space indicated by the arrow in Figure 47.5 was diagnosed as a pleural effusion. Which of the following statements supports this diagnosis?

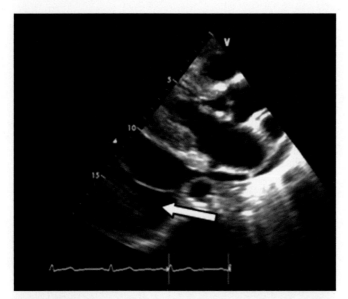

FIGURE 47.5

A. Fluid noted *only* behind the left atrium is more likely a pericardial, rather than a pleural, effusion.

B. Fluid that extends posterior to the thoracic aorta is a pleural effusion.

C. The visceral pericardium separates pleural effusion from pericardial effusion and, in this patient, can be demonstrated to be normal thickness.

D. The presence of fibrinous strands indicates a probable pericardial effusion.

E. An echo-free space parallel to the cardiac contour is most likely a pleural effusion.

8. FIGURE 47.5 and VIDEO 47.2 have two additional relatively common echocardiographic findings that warrant recognition. Which of the following options most accurately identifies both the echo-dense (narrow arrow) and the echo-free (wide arrow) structures marked in FIGURE 47.6, respectively?

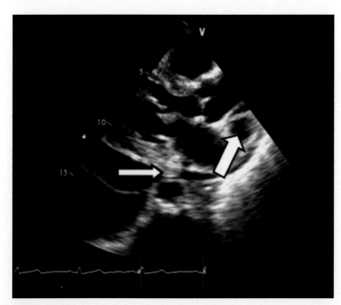

FIGURE 47.6 (Answer 11): Transthoracic echocardiogram, subcostal view, demonstrating the echogenic hemorrhagic pericardial effusion (*white arrow*).

A. Fibrinous mass and loculated pericardial effusion

B. Malignant pericardial metastasis and a normal right PA branch

C. Benign pericardial fat mass and a dilated right PA branch

D. Benign pericardial fat mass and a coronary artery aneurysm

E. Malignant pericardial fat mass and a dilated pulmonary vein

9. Which of the following statements is accurate regarding respiratory variation of spectral Doppler flow patterns in pericardial tamponade?

A. Mitral and tricuspid inflow variation with respiration is an exaggeration of the normal physiologic response to changes in intrathoracic pressure seen only in constrictive pericarditis.

B. Exaggerated Doppler flow variation is unlikely to be present in patients suffering from status asthmaticus.

C. The spectral Doppler flow variation observed across the mitral inflow is less obvious than the variation that is seen across the tricuspid inflow.

D. Respiratory variation of Doppler flows is a specific but not a sensitive sign for cardiac tamponade.

E. End-inspiratory mitral inflow is higher than expiratory mitral inflow in tamponade.

10. A 65-year-old female with lung cancer presents with shortness of breath and dizziness. She was seen by her primary care physician a week prior and was started on diuretic therapy to treat suspected heart failure since she was noted on physical examination to have elevated jugular venous pressure (JVP) and ankle swelling. On presentation today, her heart rate is 92 bpm, BP 87/55 mm Hg, and JVP 6 cm. There is no pulsus paradoxus. An echocardiogram shows normal LV systolic function. A moderate pericardial effusion is present. The IVC is 1.4 cm and completely collapses with inspiration. Which of the following statements is most correct regarding this patient?

A. The small IVC with inspiratory collapse essentially rules out tamponade.

B. The pericardial effusion is likely a side effect of the diuretics.

C. A fluid challenge may elicit typical clinical signs of tamponade.

D. The 2D findings of the right heart seen in tamponade are unlikely to be present.

E. Doppler findings in tamponade are unlikely to be present.

11. A 22-year-old intravenous drug user presented with MSSA infective endocarditis identified on transthoracic echo to be involving the mitral and tricuspid valves. He underwent tricuspid and mitral valve replacement operation. Postoperative day 1, the patient became progressively hypotensive and hypoxic. FIGURE 47.7 (VIDEO 47.3) shows bedside echo images from subcostal view. Which of the following is the cause of the patient's change in status?

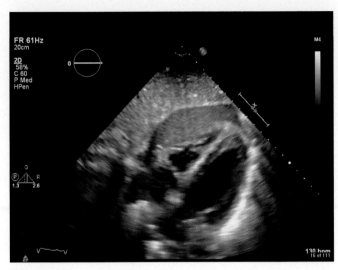

FIGURE 47.7

A. The patient developed hemopericardium and caused compression of the right ventricle.

B. The patient had an undiagnosed metastatic malignancy that was incidentally identified on this bedside echo.

C. This is a benign finding of epicardial fat on the right ventricular free wall and is not the cause of the patient's change in clinical status.

D. The echo findings appear to be retained surgical material within the pericardium, causing patient to have septic shock.

E. Patient developed postpericardiotomy pericarditis.

12. A 65-year-old female presents with cardiac tamponade. Her echo demonstrates this finding (Fɪɢ. 47.8, Vɪᴅᴇᴏ 47.4). Which of the following is a comorbid condition that she can potentially have?

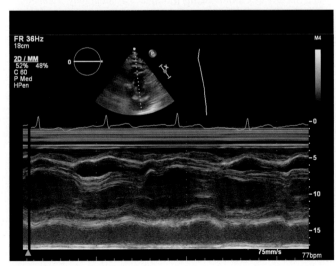

FIGURE 47.8

A. Loculated postoperative hemorrhagic effusion behind the left atrium

B. Severe pulmonary hypertension

C. Chronic venous thromboembolic disease

D. Eisenmenger syndrome

E. Acute viral pericarditis

13. A 45-year-old diabetic male presents with 6 days of fever, cough, and substernal chest pain that is worse on lying supine. He is noted to have a large pericardial effusion with collapse of the RV and RA. The patient is taken emergently to the catheterization lab, where an echocardiographically guided drainage of the pericardial effusion is undertaken. After the procedure, the patient has a repeat echocardiogram that shows resolution of the effusion with abnormal ventricular septal motion and dilation of the inferior vena cava. The medial mitral annulus e′ velocity = 20 cm/s. What should your next step be?

A. Repeat the pericardiocentesis that is likely loculated and missed on echo.

B. Perform an immediate percutaneous pericardiotomy.

C. Refer for a surgical pericardiotomy.

D. Initiate a course of NSAID Rx.

E. Diagnose this patient with a diabetic cardiomyopathy.

14. Collapse of the right atrium seen in tamponade is most likely to be seen in which segment of the cardiac cycle?

A. End atrial systole

B. End atrial diastole

C. Early atrial systole

D. Early atrial diastole

15. Which of the following is an absolute contraindication for echocardiographically guided pericardiocentesis in the setting of fulminant cardiac tamponade?

A. Uncorrected coagulopathy.

B. Severe thrombocytopenia <50,000/μL.

C. Acute type I aortic dissection.

D. Loculated pericardial effusion.

E. There are no absolute contraindications to pericardiocentesis.

16. In which of the following clinical scenarios would transesophageal echocardiography be most helpful when evaluating for tamponade?

A. A 50-year-old patient with chronic relapsing pericarditis

B. A 65-year-old male 4-hour status post coronary artery bypass surgery

C. A 75-year-old female with chronic hypothyroidism

D. An 18-year-old male with angiosarcoma

E. A 60-year-old female with esophageal cancer

Answer 1: B. Chest pain and hypotension of indeterminate etiology are an appropriate indication for echocardiography as this combination could occur in many conditions including pericardial tamponade, myocardial infarction, congestive heart failure, pulmonary embolism, and acute dissection. Each of these is a life-threatening condition requiring different types of lifesaving interventions. Chest x-ray is not a diagnostic test for tamponade. Hence, delaying bedside echocardiography and planning an intervention in the absence of a definite diagnosis would be incorrect. Therefore, Answers A and E are incorrect.

The cardiac silhouette would not be enlarged on chest x-ray due to a pericardial effusion unless the volume of pericardial fluid is approximately >200 mL. Tamponade more often occurs due to rapid accumulation of a small volume of pericardial fluid, thereby rapidly increasing intrapericardial pressure. In large effusions, the slow accumulation allows for pericardial stretch and compensation delaying hemodynamic collapse. However, urgent echocardiography is indicated to evaluate for tamponade. Answer B is the single most correct option.

In a situation with low blood pressure of unknown etiology, a trial of crystalloid bolus is reasonable. However, unexplained hypotension, regardless of response to IV fluid administration, remains an appropriate indication for echocardiography and can exclude potentially life-threatening pathologies or assist in volume status determination. Answer C is therefore incorrect.

An abnormal cardiac biomarker or troponin value does not exclude tamponade as myopericarditis may be present, resulting in a pericardial effusion leading to tamponade and myocyte damage. Hence, Answer D is wrong.

Suggested Readings

Maisch B, Seferović PM, Ristić AD, et al. Guidelines on the diagnosis and management of pericardial diseases executive summary; Task Force on the Diagnosis and Management of Pericardial Diseases of the European Society of Cardiology. *Eur Heart J* 2004;25(7):587–610.

Spodick DH. Acute cardiac tamponade. *N Engl J Med* 2003;349(7):684–690.

Answer 2: C. Pregnancy can cause the development of echocardiographically visible pericardial effusions. A pericardial effusion in pulmonary hypertension, though uncommon, is a known poor prognostic sign. Along with hydralazine, isoniazid, and minoxidil, phenytoin is a known iatrogenic cause of pericardial effusions. Sarcoidosis has been described as a cause of pericardial and pleural effusions. Aortic stenosis, even if hemodynamically severe, is not a known cause of a pericardial effusion, and another etiology should be considered in these patients.

Suggested Readings

Currie GP, Kerr K, Buchan K, et al. A rare cause of recurrent massive pericardial and pleural effusions. *Q J Med* 2008;101(12):989–990.

Haiat R, Halphen C. Silent pericardial effusion in late pregnancy: a new entity. *Cardiovasc Intervent Radiol* 1984;7(6):267–269.

Answer 3: C. This patient had recent pacemaker implantation, and the subcostal view demonstrates the right ventricular pacemaker lead perforating through the right ventricular wall defined by the long linear echo-dense object. The white arrow delineates where the lead perforated through the right ventricle. The red arrow is where the lead pierced through the epicardial fat and into the pericardial space. In patients who have unexplained chest pain after cardiac intervention, it is reasonable to evaluate further with echocardiogram for pericardial effusion. In cases with intracardiac lead placement, it is important to note the location of the lead (FIG. 47.9).

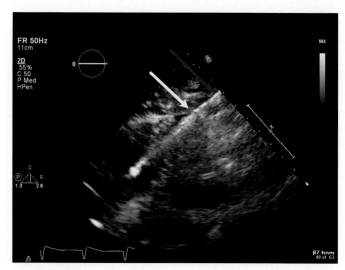

FIGURE 47.9

Answer 4: C. The spectral Doppler pattern is mitral inflow with respiratory variation in a patient with cardiac tamponade. The E-wave peak velocity decreases with inspiration and increases with expiration. Patients with atrial septal defect, elevated left ventricular diastolic pressure (severe aortic insufficiency, severe left ventricular systolic dysfunction), or positive pressure ventilation may not have respiratory variation despite being in cardiac tamponade. Patients with other comorbid conditions can generally have respiratory variation when in tamponade. Significant respiratory variation, when present, does not necessary indicate cardiac tamponade. Patients who are dyspneic and change their intrathoracic pressure greatly (e.g., status asthmaticus, morbid obesity, pulmonary embolism) or have constrictive pericarditis can also have respiratory variation.

Suggested Reading

Klein AL, Abbara S, Agler DA, et al. American Society of Echocardiography clinical recommendations for multimodality cardiovascular imaging of patients with pericardial disease: endorsed by the Society for Cardiovascular Magnetic Resonance and Society of Cardiovascular Computed Tomography. *J Am Soc Echocardiogr.* 2013;26(9):965–1012.

Answer 5: B. Pericardial effusion size is measured in diastole. The width of the echo-free space (at maximum diameter) on M-mode has been used to quantify pericardial effusion. It must be recognized that these are not universally accepted, and CT and MRI may be more useful for accurate quantification. By convention, a large circumferential pericardial effusion by 2D echocardiography measures more than 2 cm in diastole.

Many criteria by 2D and Doppler are described as findings of tamponade. The following is a list of these echo findings: 2D:

1. Early diastolic RV collapse
2. RA collapse in atrial diastole (or ventricular systole)
3. LA collapse in atrial diastole
4. Dilated IVC with loss of respiratory collapse
5. Ventricular interdependence
6. Swinging heart
7. LV "pseudohypertrophy" (LV wall thickening that resolves following pericardiocentesis and is hypothesized to be due

to myocardial venous congestion in the setting of increased pericardial pressure)

Respiratory variation in Doppler flow:

1. Inspiratory decrease in mitral inflow E-wave velocity >25%.
2. Expiratory decrease in tricuspid inflow E-wave velocity >40%.
3. Hepatic veins: expiratory increase in diastolic flow reversal.
4. Superior vena cava forward flow is predominantly systolic, with decrease or loss of the diastolic component and increased flow reversals on expiration.
5. Left-sided isovolumetric relaxation time is increased in inspiration.
6. Pulmonary veins: inspiratory decrease in velocity.

Therefore, of the echo findings listed above, the only answers that describe a large pericardial effusion are Options B, C, and D. Options A and E are incorrect since the pericardial effusion is not classically considered large. Option A is also incorrect since the RVOT collapse is not diastolic. Option E is concerning for tamponade and would be correct, except it is not the single best answer since, in addition to being <2.0 cm, the collapse is occurring late and the hemodynamic significance would be less than if the collapse occurred early in the cardiac cycle. Although the finding in Option D indicates a very large pericardial effusion, with no other echo information, this does not necessarily confirm that the patient has tamponade. Option C is incorrect since the LA collapse is noted in ventricular diastole that occurs during atrial systole (normal atrial systolic contraction), and careful evaluation of timing should be considered so as not to be misinterpreted as "hemodynamic compression."

Diastolic RA collapse is a 2D finding in tamponade. Therefore, Option B is the correct answer.

Suggested Readings

Horowitz MS, Schulz CS, Stinson EB, et al. Sensitivity and specificity of echocardiographic diagnosis of pericardial effusion. *Circulation* 1974;50:239–247.

Maisch B, Seferović PM, Ristić AD, et al.; Task Force on the Diagnosis and Management of Pericardial Diseases of the European Society of Cardiology. Guidelines on the diagnosis and management of pericardial diseases executive summary; The Task force on the diagnosis and management of pericardial diseases of the European society of cardiology. *Eur Heart J* 2004;25(7):587–610.

Segni ED, Beker B, Arbel Y, et al. Left ventricular pseudohypertrophy in pericardial effusion as a sign of cardiac tamponade. *Am J Cardiol* 1990;66(4):508–511.

Answer 6: E. The figure shows a large pericardial effusion with fibrinous strands. This echocardiographic morphology is characteristic of an inflammatory or malignant effusion and usually signifies that the effusion is chronic. A small pericardial effusion can occur during pregnancy, but this is usually transudative and not associated with stranding seen on 2D echocardiography. Complications from pericardial effusion in pregnancy are rare.

Suggested Readings

Enein M, Aziz A, Zima A, et al. Echocardiography of the pericardium in pregnancy. *Obstet Gynecol* 1987;69:851–855.

Haiat R, Halphen C. Silent pericardial effusion in late pregnancy: a new entity. *Cardiovasc Intervent Radiol* 1984;7(6):267–269.

Answer 7: B. The potential pericardial space behind the left atrium is restricted due to pericardial reflections surrounding the pulmonary veins. Hence, the fluid noted *only* behind the left atrium is likely a pleural effusion and less likely to be a pericardial effusion. Hence, Answer A is incorrect.

In the parasternal long-axis view, the descending thoracic aorta, which is an extra pericardial structure, is visualized anterior to a pleural effusion and posterior to a pericardial effusion. Hence, Answer B is correct (Fig. 47.10).

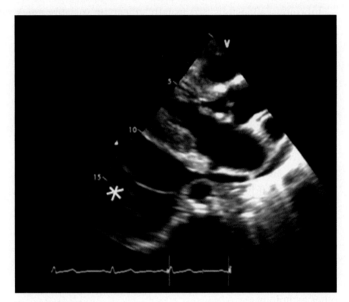

FIGURE 47.10

A pericardial effusion accumulates between the visceral and parietal layers of the pericardium. While the *visceral pericardium is adherent to the epicardium*, the parietal pericardium is the external layer. When concomitant pleural and pericardial effusions are present, the *parietal pericardium* serves as the demarcating layer. The thickness of the parietal pericardium could be more readily measured when it is bordered by pleural and pericardial effusions. In this patient, it is normal thickness. Hence, Answer C is wrong.

Fibrinous strands (or "stranding") may be seen in a purulent pericardial or pleural effusion and are characteristic of an inflammatory or malignant effusion and are usually chronic. In the image shown, the echo-dense structure (see asterisk in figure below) within the pleural effusion is lung tissue (likely atelectasis) and does not represent "stranding." Hence, Answer D is incorrect.

While the echo-free space depicting a pericardial effusion is usually parallel to the cardiac contour due to its constraints within the pericardial layers, a pleural effusion does not necessarily follow the cardiac contour. Hence, Answer E is incorrect.

Suggested Reading

Armstrong WF, Ryan T. Aortic valve disease. In: Feigenbaum H, Armstrong WF, Ryan T, eds. *Chapter 10: Feigenbaum's Echocardiography*. 6th ed. Philadelphia, PA: Lippincott Williams & Wilkins, 2005:271–305.

Answer 8: C. The echo-dense "mass" attached at the posterior AV groove is a common location for fat. When a pericardial effusion is present, this fat is readily visualized and needs to be recognized as a normal variant. The tissue characterization has the appearance of the fat and does not appear to cross tissue planes or have other malignant features.

The echo-free circular structure posterior to the aorta is the common location for the right pulmonary artery branch as it courses under the aortic arch. When this is normal sized, it is not usually seen on a parasternal long-axis view, but when dilated, it can be readily visualized. Therefore, Option C is most correct.

Fibrinous adhesions are usually linear or variably thick filamentous echo-dense structures within the effusion. They do not appear as single structures as seen on this figure. Furthermore, although a loculated pericardial effusion could be located in this region, it would not appear circular (vascular) and would be unlikely present given the extent of the posterior circumferential effusion also seen. Therefore, Option A is incorrect.

Metastatic tumors can occur in this location and are commonly associated with pericardial effusions. However, these effusions are exudative, frequently only "partially" echo-free, and often have fibrinous adhesions. Furthermore, these masses are commonly multiple, cross tissue borders, and are misshapen (not smooth bordered as in this case example). Therefore, Options B and E are incorrect.

Option D is incorrect since the dilated right pulmonary artery branch needs to be recognized and not misinterpreted as a coronary artery aneurysm, the sinus of Valsalva aneurysm, or other pathology.

Suggested Reading

Pressman G, Verma N. Pericardial fat masquerading as tumor. *Echocardiography* 2010;27:E18–E20.

Answer 9: C.

Respiratory variation in flow across cardiac valves noted on Doppler echocardiography is an exaggeration of the normal physiologic response to lowering intrathoracic pressure necessary to inhale. This can be seen in patients with cardiac tamponade and constrictive pericarditis. Normal individuals may have some degree of respiratory variation in the absence of any pathologic conditions. Hence, Answer A is incorrect.

In status asthmaticus, clinical pulsus paradoxus and echo Doppler inflow variation may be seen due to the exaggerated respiratory effort and resultant exaggerated changes in intrathoracic pressure with respiration. Hence, Answer B is incorrect.

The variation across the tricuspid inflow is usually more than mitral inflow in normal individuals. This is further exaggerated in tamponade physiology. Although different authors have used different degrees of variation as significant, an acceptable change is 40% respiratory variation across the tricuspid inflow and 25% across the mitral inflow. Therefore, the respiratory variation across the tricuspid inflow is more obvious than the mitral inflow, making Answer C the correct option.

Doppler variation is more sensitive and less specific than 2D findings in tamponade. Doppler changes are found in many other conditions, including asthma, COPD, obesity, pulmonary emboli, cardiogenic shock, and tension pneumothorax. Hence, Answer D is incorrect. In cardiac tamponade, the peak mitral inflow is higher during expiration than inspiration in patients. During expiration, the increased intrathoracic pressure forces blood out of the pulmonary circulation and increases flow through the mitral valve. Thus, Answer E is incorrect.

Suggested Reading

Oh JK, Seward JB, Tajik AJ, eds. *The Echo Manual*. 3rd ed. Philadelphia, PA: Lippincott Williams & Wilkins, 2006.

Answer 10: C. The patient in the above clinical scenario likely has low-pressure tamponade. This is a hemodynamic condition seen in patients who are volume depleted due to overdiuresis, hemorrhage, or hemodialysis, with a pericardial effusion causing tamponade. The classic clinical signs seen in tamponade including tachycardia, elevated JVP, and pulses paradoxus are not seen in low-pressure tamponade. However, a fluid challenge may unmask these signs. Hence, Answer C is most correct given the choices.

Although classical clinical signs are absent in low-pressure tamponade, the 2D echocardiogram will usually demonstrate right atrial and/or right ventricular collapse as well as typical respiratory Doppler variation seen in tamponade. IVC plethora is not seen in this patient but may be present. Therefore, Answers D and E are incorrect. Answer A is incorrect since the exception to the rule that IVC plethora must be present for tamponade to exist is this relatively uncommon situation of low-pressure tamponade. Answer B is incorrect as diuretics are not known to cause a pericardial effusion.

Patients with low-pressure tamponade show significant improvement in symptoms with pericardiocentesis.

Suggested Readings

Antman EM, Cargill V, Grossman W. Low-pressure cardiac tamponade. *Ann Intern Med* 1979;91:403–406.
Sagristà-Sauleda J, Angel J, Sambola A, et al. Low-pressure cardiac tamponade: clinical and hemodynamic profile. *Circulation* 2006;114:945.

Answer 11: A. The subcostal view of this transthoracic echo demonstrates an echogenic pericardial effusion (arrow) (Fig. 47.11). This is seen in acute hemopericardium and likely a complication from the recent operation. The patient had tamponade physiology and was taken to the OR for evacuation and providing hemostasis. Answer B is unlikely as this would have been identified preoperatively during the diagnosis of his infective endocarditis. Answer C is not true, as epicardial fat is generally more echo-lucent with linear echoes within the fat that moves with ventricular motion. Answer D is unlikely as the appearance of the echodensity is fairly uniform to be foreign material. Answer E usually occurs weeks after the pericardiotomy and not acutely like this. Also, it would not cause such an echogenic density in the pericardial space.

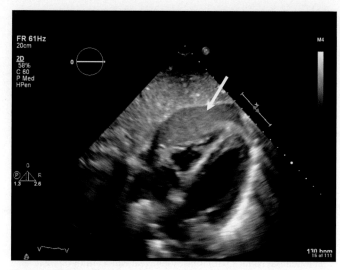

FIGURE 47.11

Answer 12: E. The patient has RV diastolic collapse seen in patients with cardiac tamponade. Any condition that decreases the compressibility of the RV could theoretically lead to the absence of the echocardiographic feature of RV diastolic collapse despite high intrapericardial pressures. Chronic venous thromboembolism often causes chronic pulmonary hypertension and secondary RV hypertrophy, and this may prevent the expected collapse of the RV (since the intraventricular pressure is equally as high as the elevated intrapericardial pressure). In this situation, the more compliant LV might collapse first leading ultimately to decreased cardiac output and hemodynamic collapse. Similarly, patients with Eisenmenger syndrome have elevated right ventricular pressure that could prevent diastolic collapse of the RV. Loculated pericardial effusion behind the left atrium can also cause hemodynamic compromise in post-cardiotomy patients, without causing RV diastolic collapse. Acute infective pericarditis, malignant effusions, uremia, and myxedema are known to cause pericardial effusions, but RV diastolic collapse would still be expected to be seen with increased pericardial pressure since these diseases are not commonly associated with pulmonary hypertension.

Suggested Readings

Gollapudi RR, Yeager M, Johnson AD. Left ventricular cardiac tamponade in the setting of cor pulmonale and circumferential pericardial effusion. Case report and review of the literature. *Cardiol Rev* 2005;13(4):214–217.
Plotnick GD, Rubin DC, Feliciano Z, et al. Pulmonary hypertension decreases the predictive accuracy of echocardiographic clues for cardiac tamponade. *Chest* 1995;107(4):919–924.

Answer 13: D. The pericardial effusion appears resolved, and it would not be common to have an associated loculated effusion and a circumferential effusion in the same patient. Therefore, Answer A is not the most correct option.

In some patients, after drainage of the underlying effusion, a constrictive physiology appears. This is called effusive–constrictive pericarditis. Given that there is noted abnormal septal motion, a "septal bounce" should be considered. The TDE e' velocity of the septal mitral annulus is rapid, and this may be

seen in patients with constriction since it acts to longitudinally compensate for the lateral wall "tethering" from the adjacent pericardial inflammation.

In a subset of these patients, the constrictive physiology is temporary (transient constrictive pericarditis). Inflammation of the pericardium is responsible for the phenomenon, and NSAIDs (followed by corticosteroids if necessary) might reverse the pathophysiology and clinical consequence. Therefore, Answer D is most correct.

It would be prudent to wait 2 to 3 months before considering definitive therapy for constriction, which is surgical pericardiectomy. Answer C is incorrect.

Case reports point that in patients with effusive constriction, the CRP levels and erythrocyte sedimentation levels may not be elevated. In addition to echocardiography, cardiac MRI would be of value as it could show moderate diffuse pericardial delayed hyperenhancement with gadolinium.

If the TDE e' velocity was low, this would raise the likelihood for a cardiomyopathy and is one method to distinguish constriction from restriction. Answer E is incorrect.

Suggested Readings

Haley JH, Tajik AJ, Danielson GK, et al. Transient constrictive pericarditis: causes and natural history. *J Am Coll Cardiol* 2004;43(2):271–275.
Zurick AO III, Klein AL. Effusive-constrictive pericarditis. *J Am Coll Cardiol* 2010;56(1):86.

Answer 14: B. Buckling and collapse of the right atrium occur when the right atrial volume (and consequently the right atrial pressure) is minimal and the pericardial pressure is maximal, causing a significant pressure gradient. This typically occurs in end atrial diastole.

Suggested Reading

Gillam LD, Guyer DE, Gibson TC, et al. Hydrodynamic compression of the right atrium: a new echocardiographic sign of cardiac tamponade. *Circulation* 1983;68(2):294–301.

Answer 15: E. There are no absolute contraindications to pericardiocentesis in the emergency setting for cardiac tamponade. There is an increased risk of converting a typical pericardial effusion into a hemorrhagic one in many patients, including coagulopathies or thrombocytopenia. In patients with type A aortic dissection and associated tamponade, there is a theory that because the decrease in cardiac output secondary to pericardial tamponade might prevent propagation of the aortic dissection, it might also decrease bleeding into the pericardium from the aorta because of a decrease in the pressure gradient between the aorta and pericardial space. However, in a dying patient, pericardiocentesis can be a temporizing procedure as the patient gets prepared for definitive therapy. The risks versus benefits should always be weighed prior to performing the procedure.

Suggested Readings

Cruz I, Stuart B, Caldeira D, et al. Controlled pericardiocentesis in patients with cardiac tamponade complicating aortic dissection: experience of a centre without cardiothoracic surgery. *Eur Heart J Acute Cardiovasc Care* 2015;4(2):124–128.

Isselbacher EM, Cigarroa JE, Eagle KA. Cardiac tamponade complicating proximal aortic dissection: is pericardiocentesis harmful? *Circulation* 1994;90:2375–2379.

Silvestry FE, Kerber RE, Brook MM, et al. Echocardiography-guided interventions. *J Am Soc Echocardiogr* 2009;22(3):213–231.

Answer 16: B. Transesophageal echocardiography is often not necessary to diagnose tamponade. However, when the imaging quality is poor or focal tamponade is suspected, transesophageal echocardiography may be of value.

A patient who undergoes CABG surgery 4 hours prior would usually have poor transthoracic windows due to air in the thoracic cavity, sternal incisions, and dressings as well as pain due to which positioning and imaging could be limited. Further, these patients are prone to regional tamponade with isolated chamber compression due to a loculated hematoma that may not be visualized with TTE. Hence, if a TEE is not performed, the diagnosis of tamponade may be missed.

In addition to standard Doppler evaluations, respiratory variation of the pulmonary veins could be studied when TEE is performed in this patient. Therefore, TEE is most helpful in this scenario, and Answer B is correct. Regional tamponade may also be present after blunt chest trauma or loculated pericardial effusions.

While Answers A, C, and D list known causes of pericardial effusions, there is no definite benefit in TEE, unless the image quality is poor due to other reasons.

Esophageal cancer is an absolute contraindication for TEE due to the high risk of esophageal perforation. Answer E is incorrect.

Suggested Reading

Troianos CA, Porembka DT. Assessment of left ventricular function and hemodynamics with transesophageal echocardiography. *Crit Care Clin* 1996;12(2):253–272.

Chapter 48

Pericardial Constraint

Vincent L. Sorrell

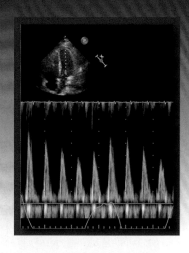

1. A 64-year-old male with a history of coronary artery disease s/p PCI, lymphoma s/p chemotherapy, and radiation therapy presents to your clinic with progressive dyspnea on exertion and lower extremity edema. ECG was unremarkable. Echo tech attempted some parasternal views but had difficulty obtaining an optimal window. Four-chamber view is shown in VIDEO 48.1. What is the likely diagnosis?

   A. Malnourished/cachexia
   B. Constrictive pericarditis
   C. Chronic obstructive pulmonary disease
   D. Morbid obesity
   E. Acute pericarditis with tamponade physiology

2. A 47-year-old male presents to the hospital with progressive shortness of breath and fatigue. He underwent coronary artery bypass grafting, MAZE procedure, and left atrial appendage isolation 2 weeks ago. He was discharged in good condition. An echocardiogram was performed (FIG. 48.1/VIDEO 48.2). The patient did not have right atrial inversion or right ventricular diastolic collapse. What is the cause of this patient's shortness of breath/fatigue?

   A. Recurrent atrial fibrillation
   B. Cardiac tamponade
   C. Aortic dissection
   D. Atrial dissection
   E. Acute coronary bypass graft failure

3. Which of the following mitral inflow Doppler patterns/tissue Doppler patterns is likely to be present in the patient described in Question 1?

   A. E/A ratio < 0.8
   B. Septal E/e' > 20
   C. Septal e' < 6 cm/s
   D. Fixed isovolumetric relaxation time
   E. Fixed response to volume loading

4. Which of the following pulsed-wave (PW) Doppler spectral patterns would be *least likely seen* in a patient with chronic constrictive physiology?

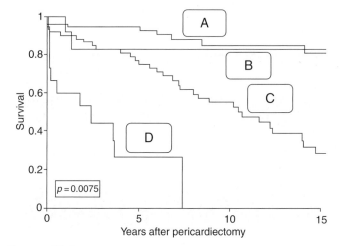

FIGURE 48.1 Modified from Bertog SC, Thambidorai SK, Parakh K, et al. Constrictive pericarditis: etiology and cause-specific survival after pericardiectomy. *J Am Coll Cardiol* 2004;43(8):1445–1452. Copyright © 2004 American College of Cardiology Foundation. With permission.

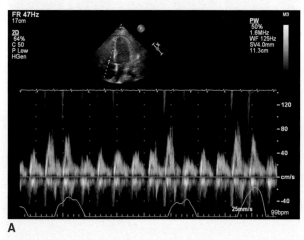

FIGURE 48.2 From Armstrong WF, Ryan T. *Feigenbaum's Echocardiography.* 7th ed. Philadelphia, PA: Lippincott Williams & Wilkins, 2010, with permission.

405

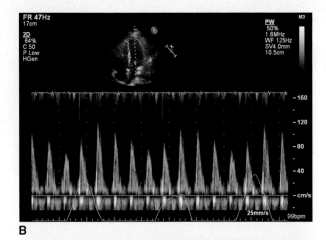

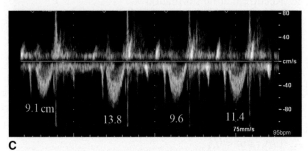

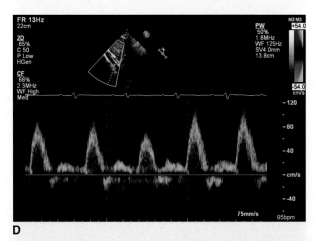

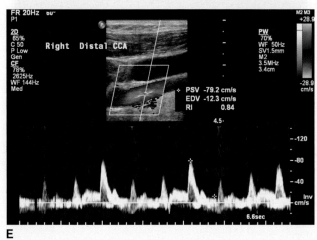

FIGURE 48.2 (*Continued*)

A. Tricuspid valve inflow (FIG. 48.2A)
B. Mitral valve inflow (FIG. 48.2B)
C. LV outflow tract (FIG. 48.2C)
D. Descending abdominal aorta (FIG. 48.2D)
E. Distal right common carotid artery (FIG. 48.2E)

5. Which one of the following M-mode displays would be least likely seen in a patient with chronic constrictive physiology?

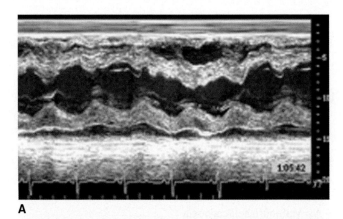

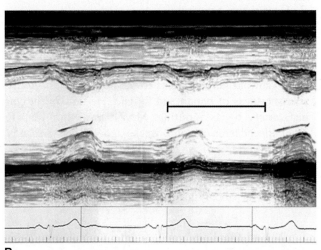

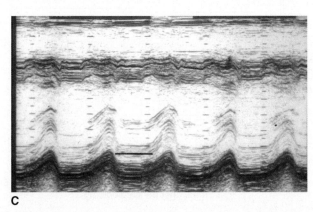

FIGURE 48.3 **A:** From Armstrong WF, Ryan T. *Feigenbaum's Echocardiography.* 7th ed. Philadelphia, PA: Lippincott Williams & Wilkins, 2010, with permission. **B:** From Armstrong WF, Ryan T. *Feigenbaum's Echocardiography.* 7th ed. Philadelphia, PA: Lippincott Williams & Wilkins, 2010, with permission.

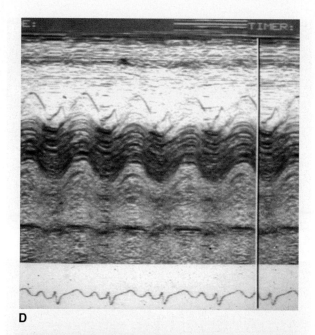

D

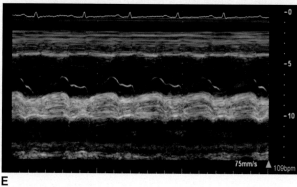

E

FIGURE 48.3 (*Continued*)

A. FIGURE 48.3A
B. FIGURE 48.3B
C. FIGURE 48.3C
D. FIGURE 48.3D
E. FIGURE 48.3E

6. Which of the following color M-mode displays *best describes* the pattern most likely to be seen in a patient with chronic constrictive pericarditis?

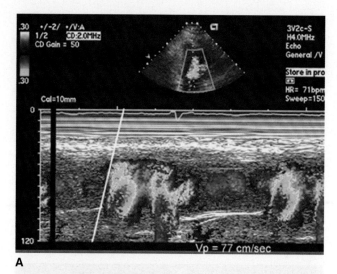

A

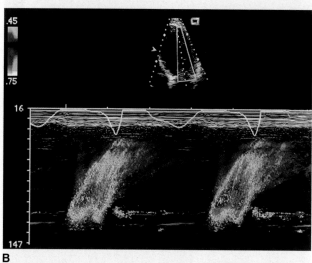

B

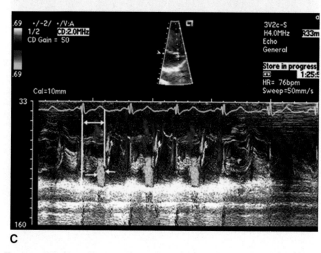

C

FIGURE 48.4 **A:** From Armstrong WF, Ryan T. *Feigenbaum's Echocardiography.* 7th ed. Philadelphia, PA: Lippincott Williams & Wilkins, 2010, with permission. **C:** From Armstrong WF, Ryan T. *Feigenbaum's Echocardiography.* 7th ed. Philadelphia, PA: Lippincott Williams & Wilkins, 2010, with permission.

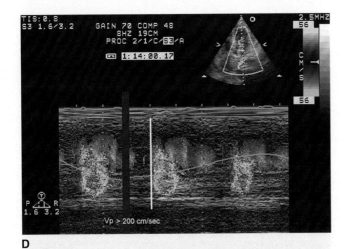

D

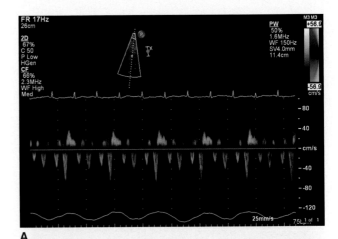

A

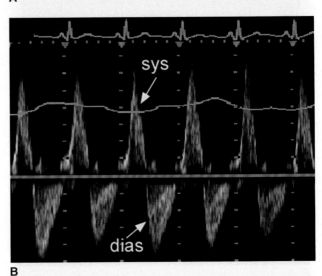

B

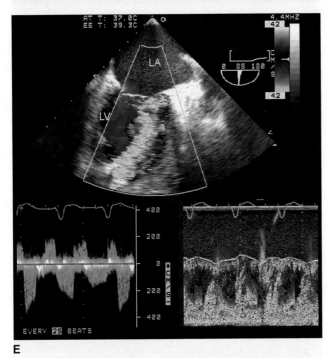

E

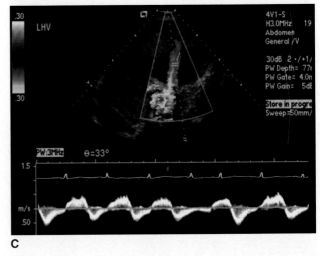

C

FIGURE **48.4** (*Continued*) **D:** From Armstrong WF, Ryan T. *Feigenbaum's Echocardiography*. 7th ed. Philadelphia, PA: Lippincott Williams & Wilkins, 2010, with permission. **E:** From Armstrong WF, Ryan T. *Feigenbaum's Echocardiography*. 7th ed. Philadelphia, PA: Lippincott Williams & Wilkins, 2010, with permission.

A. Vp = 77 cm/s (FIG. 48.4A)
B. Vp = 35 cm/s (FIG. 48.4B)
C. Vp = 89 cm/s (FIG. 48.4C)
D. Vp = 200 cm/s (FIG. 48.4D)
E. Vp = 95 cm/s (FIG. 48.4E)

7. Which one of the following pulsed-wave Doppler flow patterns from the hepatic vein is *most likely* from a patient with chronic constrictive physiology?

FIGURE **48.5** **B:** From Armstrong WF, Ryan T. *Feigenbaum's Echocardiography*. 7th ed. Philadelphia, PA: Lippincott Williams & Wilkins, 2010, with permission. **C:** Reproduced from Scheinfeld MH, Bilali A, Koenigsberg M. Understanding the spectral Doppler waveform of the hepatic veins in health and disease. *Radiographics* 2009;29:2081–2098.

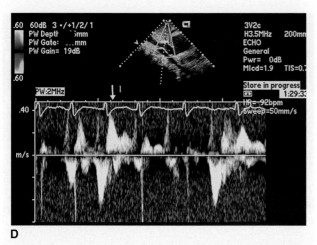

D

FIGURE 48.5 (*Continued*) **D:** From Armstrong WF, Ryan T. *Feigenbaum's Echocardiography.* 7th ed. Philadelphia, PA: Lippincott Williams & Wilkins, 2010, with permission.

A. FIGURE 48.5A
B. FIGURE 48.5B
C. FIGURE 48.5C
D. FIGURE 48.5D

Questions 8 and 9

A 33-year-old female presents with palpitations, chest pain, fatigue, and generalized malaise of several weeks' duration. Her physical examination reveals dilated neck veins with failure to collapse during inspiration, but no significant pulsus paradoxus. She has bibasilar crackles. Her transthoracic echocardiogram is shown in VIDEO 48.3A–C and FIGURE 48.6A. A pericardiocentesis was performed, which revealed an exudative pericardial effusion with unremarkable cytology, Gram stain, and culture. She had significant improvement in her clinical symptoms of chest pain, dyspnea, and fatigue.

A repeat echocardiogram (48 hours later) is shown in VIDEO 48.2D–H and FIGURE 48.6B–E.

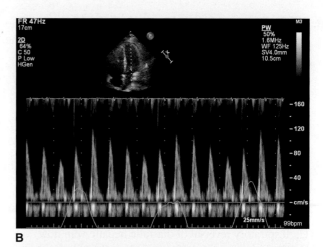

B

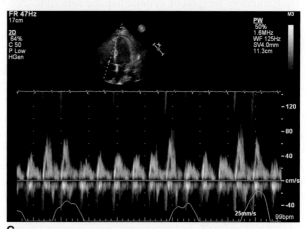

C

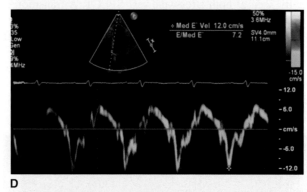

D

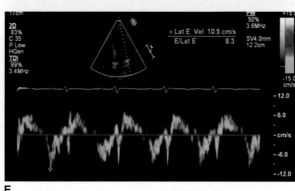

E

FIGURE 48.6 (*Continued*) **B:** PW Doppler through the mitral valve. **C:** PW Doppler through the mitral and tricuspid valves. **D:** Tissue Doppler velocity from the medial annulus. **E:** Tissue Doppler velocity from the lateral annulus.

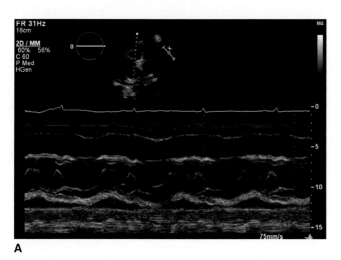

A

FIGURE 48.6 **A:** M-mode through short-axis view at the mitral valve level.

8. Based upon her clinical presentation and serial echocardiograms, which of the following is most consistent with her
likely diagnosis?

 A. Chronic constrictive pericarditis
 B. Exudative–restrictive pericarditis
 C. Exudative effusive–constrictive pericarditis
 D. Restrictive cardiomyopathy
 E. Mixed constrictive–restrictive cardiomyopathy

9. Which of these is the correct respiratory pattern of hepatic
vein flow in constrictive pericarditis?

 A. Inspiratory reversal of systolic hepatic vein flow
 B. Expiratory reversal of diastolic hepatic vein flow
 C. Inspiratory reversal of diastolic hepatic vein flow
 D. Expiratory reversal of systolic hepatic vein flow

Questions 10 and 11

A 64-year-old female with a history of hypertension, diabetes
mellitus, and systemic scleroderma presents to you for a second opinion with dyspnea on exertion and chest pain for the
past few months. Her current medications include lisinopril,
metoprolol, and metformin. She also takes dipyridamole to
reduce symptoms from her Raynaud phenomenon. On physical examination, she has bilateral lower extremity edema. Her
primary care physician requested a nuclear stress test that did
not reveal any evidence of significant ischemia. However, this
test reported a mildly reduced LV systolic function with a calculated LVEF of 0.47 and prominent right ventricular radio-
activity seen at both stress and rest SPECT. A transthoracic
echocardiogram was obtained and confirmed a mildly reduced
LV systolic function with Doppler findings concerning for
pericardial constriction.

Her cardiovascular evaluation and diagnostic testing were
performed in a community hospital in her hometown. Based on
these results, she was referred to you for a second opinion prior

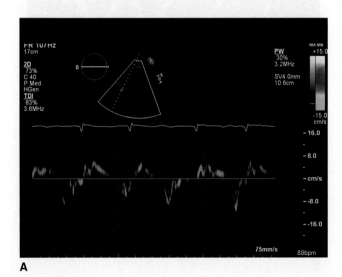

A

Figure 48.7

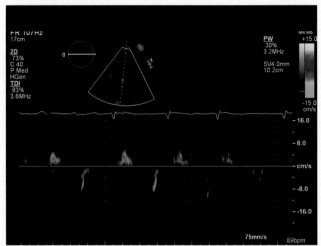

B

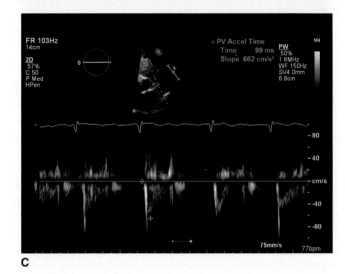

C

Figure 48.7 (Continued)

to consideration for surgical pericardial stripping. Her transthoracic echocardiographic images are shown in Video 48.4 and
Figure 48.7.

10. Based upon your review of these images, you should recommend which of the following next steps?

 A. Perform an ECG-gated cardiac CT angiogram to
 evaluate the coronary arteries as well as the pulmonary
 parenchyma.
 B. Perform an invasive coronary angiogram before
 proceeding with the presumed necessary pericardial
 stripping procedure.
 C. She does not have pericardial constriction, and no
 further workup is immediately necessary.
 D. Perform a right heart catheterization and vasodilator
 challenge.

11. Which of the following statements is *most accurate* regarding the differences most commonly noted between *constriction and restriction*?

    A. The lateral wall E′ velocity is usually exaggerated in *restriction*.

    B. The mitral valve E-wave deceleration time is usually short (<160 ms) in *both* constriction and restriction.

    C. The RV-to-RA transvalvular gradient is usually increased in *constriction*.

    D. The hepatic vein flow demonstrates systolic blunting in *constriction*.

    E. The color M-mode Vp is usually >55 cm/s in *restriction*.

Answer 1: B. This patient has a calcified pericardium consistent with constrictive pericarditis, which is the likely etiology of his symptoms (FIG. 48.8). The echo images demonstrate a shield of calcium that prevented the ultrasound from reaching the lateral wall of the myocardium. Cachexia can cause decreased soft tissue between rib spaces, and thus, it would be a probe contact issue. Chronic obstructive pulmonary disease is likely to cause expansion of lung space. Morbid obesity causing technical difficulties would be due to the distance from the probe to the myocardium. Acute pericarditis should not present with calcified pericardium. Tamponade physiology was not demonstrated in this echo image; however, this patient likely has other signs that may be similar to tamponade (e.g., respiratory variation, chamber size change with respiration, IVC plethora).

Answer 2: B. This patient has cardiac tamponade. He did not have right atrial inversion or right ventricular diastolic collapse due to the loculated nature of his pericardial effusion. This mainly affected his left cardiac chambers, and thus left atrial inversion is seen (FIG. 48.9).

Answer 3: E. This patient has pericardial constriction. Because of pericardial constraint, there is impaired diastolic cardiac filling, akin to the "rigid box" analogy often described in the literature, with rapid early diastolic filling followed by an abrupt cessation of diastolic filling as diastolic pressures rise (i.e.,

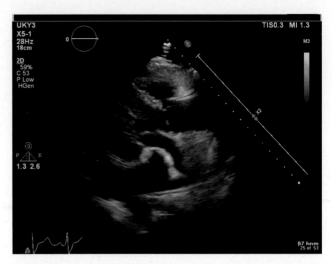

FIGURE 48.9 (Answer 2): Transthoracic echocardiogram, parasternal long axis view, demonstrating the left atrium free wall is inverted into the chamber. There is also a large pericardial effusion as well.

when the "box" is full). Because of the relative pressure difference across the mitral valve imposed by the less compliant pericardium limiting diastolic filling, there is an initial rapid early diastolic filling period (exaggerated E-wave velocity) due to the high left atrial to left ventricular gradient, with a resultant exaggerated E/A ratio of mitral inflow (unlikely to have a ratio of <0.8). Because of the relatively high LV pressures, however, this early diastolic LV filling is truncated prematurely (short deceleration time). Although these findings are nonspecific and may be seen in any pathologic condition with significant constrictive or restrictive physiology including primary pulmonary disease or severe diastolic dysfunction, the presence of an exaggerated variation in E-wave velocity with respiration is highly specific for constriction, especially if this variation is ≥25%. This ventricular interdependence manifests as enhanced right-sided filling and decreased left-sided filling with inspiration and is directly related to the external rigidity of the pericardium. As a result, evaluation of mitral inflow patterns may also reveal respiratory variation in the isovolumetric relaxation time of the left ventricle, with prolongation during inspiration

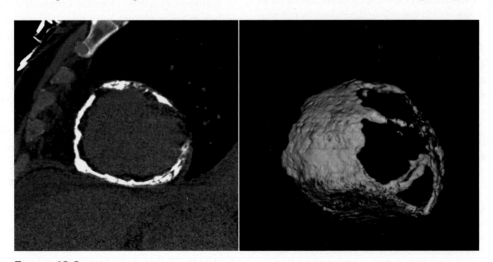

FIGURE 48.8 (Answer 1): CT chest without contrast demonstrating the calcified pericardium surrounding the myocardium in this patient. 3D rendering of the CT image showing how the calcified pericardium surrounds most of the myocardium.

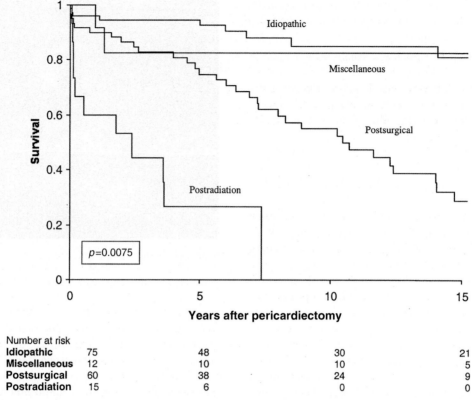

FIGURE 48.10 Reprinted from Bertog SC, Thambidorai SK, Parakh K, et al. Constrictive pericarditis: etiology and cause-specific survival after pericardiectomy. *J Am Coll Cardiol* 2004;43(8):1445–1452. Copyright © 2004 American College of Cardiology Foundation. With permission.

and shortening with expiration. It is thought that the more classic findings of pericardial constriction are most prominent when the patient is euvolemic and if the clinical suspicion is high despite lack of echocardiographic evidence and provocative maneuvers including volume loading or head-up tilt positioning to unmask the aforementioned classic findings in patients with hypovolemia (FIG. 48.10). Regarding tissue Doppler findings, patients with constrictive pericarditis have preserved tissue velocities. As opposed to restrictive cardiomyopathy, patients with constriction have e' > 6 cm/s. Although the left atrial pressure in constrictive pericarditis is elevated (around 20s), due to the preserved e', the E/e' (<15) usually underestimates the true LA pressure. This phenomenon is called annulus paradoxus. Due to the constrictive nature of the pericardium, this prevents the rapid relaxation of the lateral mitral annulus relative to the unconstrained septal mitral annulus. Normally, the lateral mitral annulus moves more than the septal; however, it is reversed in constrictive pericarditis (annulus reversus).

Suggested Readings

Abdalla IA, Murray RD, Lee JC, et al. Does rapid volume loading during transesophageal echocardiography differentiate constrictive from restrictive cardiomyopathy? *Echocardiography* 2002;19(2):125–134.

Armstrong W, Ryan T. Pericardial diseases. In: *Chapter 10: Feigenbaum's Echocardiography*. 7th ed. Philadelphia, PA: Lippincott Williams & Wilkins, 2009:217.

Catherine M, Otto MD. Pericardial diseases. In: Goldberger E, ed. *Chapter 10: Textbook of Clinical Cardiology*. 4th ed. Philadelphia, PA: Saunders Elsevier, 2009.

Maisch B, Seferovic P, Ristic A, et al. Guidelines on the diagnosis and management of pericardial diseases. *Eur Heart J* 2004;25:587–610.

Ha JW, Oh JK, Lieng H, et al. Annulus paradoxus. *Circulation* 2001;104:976–978.

Answer 4: *C.* Images A, B, D, and E are obtained from the same patient with chronic constrictive pericarditis as a result of radiation therapy for lymphoma. Cardiac hemodynamics and their relationship to Doppler patterns in constrictive physiology are depicted in FIGURE 48.11.

Image A is a PW Doppler obtained from tricuspid valve inflow from a patient with constrictive pericarditis demonstrating >50% variation in tricuspid valve inflow E-wave with normal respiration. During inspiration, there is increase in the right-sided flow as evidenced by increase in velocity of the tricuspid inflow E-wave. Due to rigid pericardium, which restricts the filling of inflow to the right ventricle, the ventricular septum moves toward the left. The opposite septal response occurs during expiration as depicted in FIGURE 48.11.

Image B is a PW Doppler recorded from the same patient. The mitral valve inflow E-wave velocity increases during expiration, and the opposite occurs during inspiration.

Image C is obtained from a patient with severe left ventricular systolic dysfunction and reduced cardiac output. There is beat-to-beat variability in both the peak velocity and TVI (stroke volume), which is the Doppler correlate of pulsus alternans. In a patient with constrictive physiology, there is phasic variation in the stroke volume (SV), but this is not beat

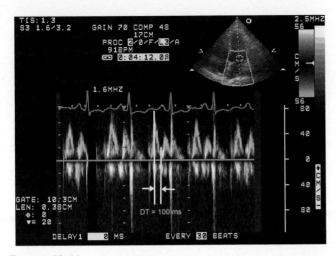

FIGURE 48.11 Pulsed Doppler recording of mitral valve inflow in a 65-year-old patient with constrictive pericarditis. Note the inappropriately elevated E/A ratio and the short deceleration time (DT), which averaged 100 ms in this example. (From Armstrong WF, Ryan T. *Feigenbaum's Echocardiography*. 7th ed. Philadelphia, PA: Lippincott Williams & Wilkins, 2010, with permission.)

to beat but rather varies based on respiratory rate. Furthermore, the SV is usually normal or even increased (during expiration). This reciprocal and phasic variation with respiration is manifested clinically as pulsus paradoxus on physical exam.

Image D is a PW Doppler interrogation from the descending abdominal aorta obtained from the same patient in *images A and B* and demonstrates a normal high-resistance triphasic Doppler waveform with respiratory variation (increases during expiration). These phasic variations are transmitted to the periphery as shown in *image E* recorded from the right distal common carotid artery in the same patient. As opposed to the *high*-resistance flow noted in *image D*, this figure demonstrates *low*-resistance flow (persistence of forward flow during diastole) with respiratory variation (increase in the flow during expiration).

Doppler echocardiography has provided a window into the pathophysiology of the intracardiac blood flow in constriction and offers substantial diagnostic insight. The classic Doppler findings of pericardial constriction are an exaggerated E/A ratio of mitral valve inflow with a short deceleration time and exaggerated respiratory variation in E-wave velocity (>25% for mitral E-wave velocity and >35% to 40% for tricuspid E-wave velocity, which normally varies <10%). In current practice, it is not uncommon to see less typical patterns due to variable volume status or other associated conditions such as coexistent restrictive cardiomyopathy or pulmonary hypertension.

The following caveats are valuable to learn and remember:

1. Abovementioned phasic variations in inflow patterns are typically seen in normal, nonlabored respiration in patients with constrictive pericarditis.
2. The elevated E/A ratio with a short deceleration time can be seen in any disease state with restrictive or constrictive physiology.
3. Exaggerated phasic variation can also be seen in primary respiratory distress from other nonconstrictive etiologies (especially the tricuspid inflow). Evaluation of mitral inflow

patterns may also reveal exaggerated respiratory variation in the isovolumic relaxation time of the left ventricle.
4. Classically described Doppler findings of constrictive physiology are prominent when the patient is euvolemic. If hypovolemia is suspected, one can repeat the Doppler evaluation after volume loading (or leg lifting).
5. Some of the above-described Doppler findings can be absent in patients with localized forms of constriction or in patients with significant concurrent valve disease.

Suggested Readings

Armstrong W, Ryan T. Pericardial diseases. In: *Chapter 10: Feigenbaum's Echocardiography*. 7th ed. Philadelphia, PA: Lippincott Williams & Wilkins, 2009:217.

Ha JW, Ommen SR, Tajik AJ, et al. Differentiation of constrictive pericarditis from restrictive cardiomyopathy using mitral annular velocity by tissue Doppler echocardiography. *Am J Cardiol* 2004;94:316.

LeWinter MM, Tischler MD. Pericardial diseases. In: Bonow RO, Mann DL, Zipes DP, et al., eds. *Chapter 75: Braunwald's Heart Disease: A Textbook of Cardiovascular Medicine*. 9th ed. Philadelphia, PA: Saunders Elsevier, 2011.

Little WC, Freeman GL. Pericardial disease. *Circulation* 2006;113:1622.

Answer 5: E. The M-mode echocardiogram in *image A* demonstrates respiratory variation in the RV and LV cavities (expiration is depicted by a longer white arrow and inspiration by a shorter white arrow, FIG. 48.12). Note that the interventricular septum (IVS) bulges toward the LV during inspiration and the opposite occurs during expiration. These findings confirm *ventricular interdependence*, common in patients with pericardial constriction. This M-mode display also demonstrates an early systolic downward motion of the IVS (precedes the peak posterior wall motion), which can be seen in patients with LBBB pattern on ECG (FIG. 48.13). The lack of phasic variability of the IVS on this figure helps to differentiate constrictive physiology from LBBB.

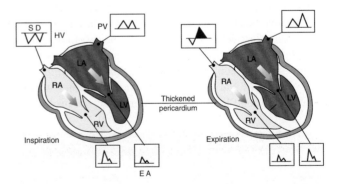

FIGURE 48.12 Schematic representation of transvalvular and central venous flow velocities in constrictive pericarditis. During inspiration, the decrease in left ventricular filling results in a leftward septal shift, allowing augmented flow into the right ventricle. The opposite occurs during expiration. (D, diastole; EA, mitral inflow; HV, hepatic vein; LA, left atrium; LV, left ventricle; PV, pulmonary venous flow; RA, right atrium; RV, right ventricle; S, systole.) (Reprinted from LeWinter MM, Tischler MD. Pericardial diseases. In: Bonow RO, Mann DL, Zipes DP, et al., eds. *Braunwald's Heart Disease: A Textbook of Cardiovascular Medicine*. 9th ed. Philadelphia, PA: Saunders Elsevier, 2011. Copyright © 2011 Elsevier. With permission.)

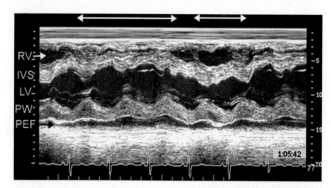

The M-mode echocardiogram displayed in *image B* was recorded in a patient with constrictive pericarditis and a thickened posterior pericardial echo (dark line, Fig. 48.14). To the right of this display, marked by the black bracket, damping has been increased to suppress the fainter myocardial echoes. Note that the pericardial echo has not been suppressed. Also note the flat motion of the posterior wall after the initial rapid posterior motion (black arrow, Fig. 48.14) of the endocardium and *loss of the so-called a-dip* that follows atrial contraction (after P wave).

The M-mode echocardiogram from *image C* was recorded in a patient with constrictive pericarditis and a thickened pericardium. Similar echo features as described previously in image B are again noted (thickened posterior pericardium, flat posterior wall motion, loss of a-dip). An additional M-mode feature that can be seen in patients with constrictive pericarditis is *inadequate LV filling during diastole*, which is demonstrated by the height of the posterior motion of the posterior wall over diastole (only 2.7-mm diastolic descent).

This M-mode echocardiogram is from the same patient after surgical pericardiectomy and demonstrates normalization of LV filling and a visible a-dip that follows atrial contraction during late diastole (Fig. 48.15). Note the 4.0-mm diastolic descent.

The M-mode echocardiograms in *images D and E* are of the pulmonic valve (PV) from the parasternal window. Usually, only one leaflet can be intersected by the M-mode

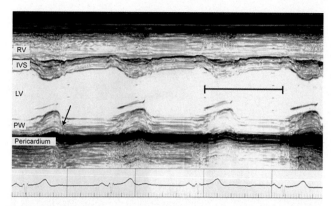

interrogation beam. In patients with constrictive pericarditis, the heart is encased in a rigid pericardium, which does not allow proper filling of the RV during diastole. During inspiration, the *PV opens early* (prior to RV systole) to accommodate this increased right-sided flow as the septum deviates toward the left. This is depicted by a vertical line on image D and Fig. 48.16. In image E, however, the PV opens as normal after electrical ventricular systole. Therefore, Option E is incorrect.

Characterization of PV motion provided one of the earliest echo clues to the presence of pulmonary hypertension and indirect evidence of other right heart diseases. Normal PV motion (Fig. 48.17) is characterized by presystolic A-wave motion (relatively low-amplitude excursion, <6 mm) with atrial systole (absent in atrial fibrillation). It requires a relatively low PA diastolic pressure so that the atrial contraction is able to overcome the driving force for partial opening of the pulmonary valve. The A-wave is followed by a box-like opening of the PV leaflet during ventricular systole. It is not uncommon to have incomplete visualization of PV on M-mode.

Answer 6: *D.* Images shown represent color M-mode echocardiographic imaging techniques. This technique uses pulsed Doppler interrogation along a single line of interrogation.

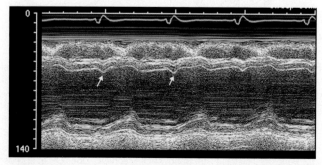

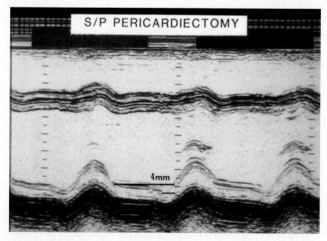

FIGURE 48.16

PREMATURE PV OPENING

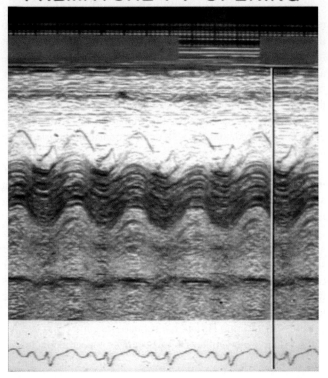

FIGURE 48.17

Unlike M-mode echocardiography, the Doppler velocity shift is recorded and then color encoded and superimposed on the M-mode image. This process results in high temporal resolution data on the direction and timing of flow events. Since this is a pulsed-wave Doppler technique, as with color-flow Doppler imaging, velocity resolution is limited.

Acquisition is performed in any transthoracic window. A narrow color sector should be used, and gain should be adjusted to avoid noise. The high temporal resolution of this technique has been used to assist in determining the velocity of propagation of left ventricular inflow (Vp), a marker of diastolic function of the left ventricle. Other clinical instance in which color Doppler M-mode imaging plays a role is in the assessment of an abnormal flow signal over time such as the timing and width of an aortic insufficiency jet, the duration of mitral regurgitation, fistulous flow, and the cannula flow of mechanical support devices (FIG. 48.18).

This color Doppler M-mode echocardiogram demonstrates aortic regurgitation from a transesophageal echocardiogram (see inserted schematic for orientation).

The color Doppler M-mode display in *image D* is from a patient with constrictive pericarditis. With this technique, the velocity with which the mitral inflow races toward the apex in diastole is considered normal (>55 cm/s). As is often seen in constriction, the Vp is exaggerated and steep (>200 cm/s). By comparison, the Vp is abnormally reduced in restriction (<50 cm/s).

The color M-mode from *image E* is a TEE color M-mode recorded in a patient with a pulsatile LVAD used as bridge to transplant. For this device, flow is unidirectional and moves from an apical cannula into a pulsatile device and is then pumped to the ascending aorta. Failure of the inlet biologic valve results in LVAD regurgitation of the *pulsatile* pump and is readily detected using color M-mode as *continuous* (not phasic) flow. Note the continuous antegrade and retrograde flow at the apical cannula (arrows, FIG. 48.19). Both the color Doppler M-mode and CW Doppler confirm bidirectional continuous rather than phasic flow consistent with acute failure of the inlet cannula valve.

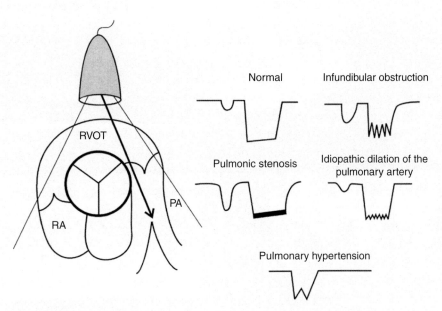

FIGURE 48.18 Pulmonary valve M-mode. (From Armstrong WF, Ryan T. *Feigenbaum's Echocardiography.* 7th ed. Philadelphia, PA: Lippincott Williams & Wilkins, 2010, with permission.)

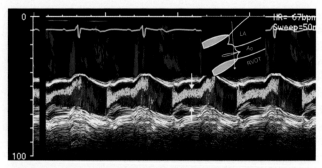

Figure 48.19 Aortic regurgitation color M-mode. (From Armstrong WF, Ryan T. *Feigenbaum's Echocardiography*. 7th ed. Philadelphia, PA: Lippincott Williams & Wilkins, 2010, with permission.)

Color Doppler M-mode images recorded in patients with mitral regurgitation are useful for obtaining the exact timing of regurgitation. Both tracings in Figure 48.20 were recorded from the LV apex. The image (A) was recorded in a patient with *mitral valve prolapse, and regurgitation* was confined to the latter 40% of systole (*image C*). The two vertical white lines indicate the duration of mechanical systole (double-headed arrow). The image (B) was recorded in a patient with holosystolic mitral regurgitation.

Acquisition technique of Vp:

M-mode interrogation scan line is positioned through the center of the LV inflow blood column from the mitral valve to the LV apex. Color-flow baseline is shifted to lower the Nyquist limit so that the central highest velocity slope can be best visualized. Flow propagation velocity (Vp) is measured as the slope of the first aliasing velocity during early filling, measured from the mitral valve plane to 4 cm distally into the LV cavity.

Alternatively, the slope of the transition from no color to color is measured, and Vp > 50 cm/s is considered *normal* (see *image A*).

Similar to transmitral Doppler filling patterns, normal LV intracavitary filling is dominated by an early wave and an atrial-induced filling wave, and it changes markedly during delayed relaxation with myocardial ischemia and LV failure.

The slope of early flow propagation velocity (Vp) provides a semiquantitative marker of diastolic function where a reduced slope and lower velocity are consistent with *decreased chamber compliance* (see *image B*). Vp also predicts LV filling pressures when used in conjunction with transmitral Doppler E-wave. The ratio of peak E′ velocity to Vp (≥2.5) is directly proportional to LA pressure (15 mm Hg) with reasonable accuracy and is especially valuable when other Doppler indices appear inconclusive.

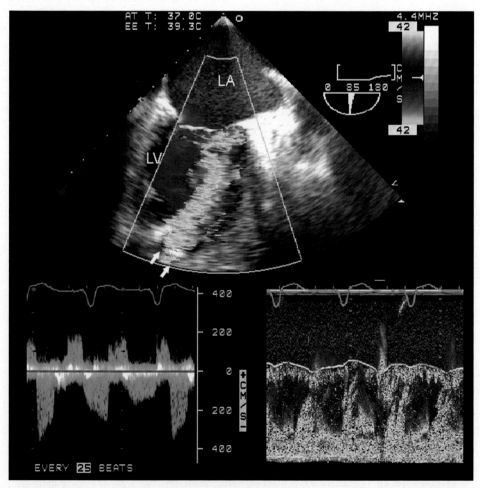

Figure 48.20 From Armstrong WF, Ryan T. *Feigenbaum's Echocardiography*. 7th ed. Philadelphia, PA: Lippincott Williams & Wilkins, 2010, with permission.

Suggested Readings

Armstrong W, Ryan T. Specialized echocardiographic techniques and methods. In: *Chapter 3: Feigenbaum's Echocardiography.* 7th ed. Philadelphia, PA: Lippincott Williams & Wilkins, 2009:217.

Brun P, Tribouilloy C, Duval AM, et al. Left ventricular flow propagation during early filling is related to wall relaxation: a color M-mode Doppler analysis. *J Am Coll Cardiol* 1992;20:420–432.

Garcia MJ, Ares MA, Asher C, et al. An index of early left ventricular filling that combined with pulsed Doppler peak E velocity may estimate capillary wedge pressure. *J Am Coll Cardiol* 1997; 29:448–454.

Nagueh SF, Appleton CP, Gillebert TC, et al. Recommendations for the evaluation of left ventricular diastolic function by echocardiography. *J Am Soc Echocardiography* 2009;22:107–133.

Takatsuji H, Mikami T, Urasawa K, et al. A new approach for evaluation of left ventricular diastolic function: spatial and temporal analysis of left ventricular filling flow propagation by color M-mode Doppler echocardiography. *J Am Coll Cardiol* 1996;27:365–371.

***Answer 7:** A.* Doppler assessment of hepatic vein (HV) flow has clinical relevance beyond the estimation of right atrial (RA) filling pressure. As a general rule, these abnormal flow patterns are complementary to other echo findings and should not be used alone as diagnostic findings. The normal HV waveform has two antegrade waves—a larger systolic "*S wave*" and a smaller diastolic "*D wave*"—and a small retrograde flow reversal from atrial contraction "*A-wave*" (Figs. 48.21 and 48.22). HV flow is respiratory cycle dependent (*normally increased*

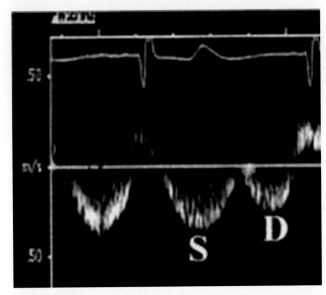

FIGURE 48.22 Normal hepatic vein flow PW Doppler spectrum, zoomed example. (Reprinted from Zoghbi W, Enriquez-Sarano M, Foster E, et al. Recommendations for evaluation of the severity of native valvular regurgitation with two-dimensional and Doppler echocardiography. *J Am Soc Echocardiogr* 2003;16(7):777–802. Copyright © 2003 American Society of Echocardiography. With permission.)

during inspiration, decreased during expiration with some retrograde flow). Several disease states result in characteristic abnormalities of HV flow, such as abnormalities in RA and RV relaxation and compliance (RV failure, constrictive or restrictive cardiomyopathies), tricuspid regurgitation, and atrial fibrillation. In patients with *severe tricuspid regurgitation*, flow reversal during ventricular systole is transmitted into the RA and then into the hepatic veins, and the normal antegrade systolic flow is replaced by a *prominent retrograde S wave*. This prominent retrograde wave is tall (>50 cm/s), and early peaking (Figs. 48.23 and 48.24) when RV systolic function is preserved, and in case of severe RV systolic dysfunction, retrograde flow has a delayed and diminutive peak (<50 cm/s) (Fig. 48.25). The sensitivity of flow reversal for severe TR is 80%, while specificity is not well established.

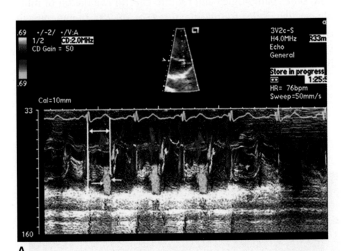

A

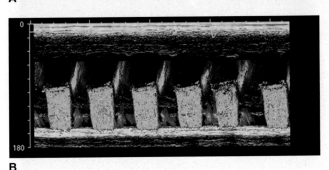

B

FIGURE 48.21 Mitral regurgitation color M-mode. (From Armstrong WF, Ryan T. *Feigenbaum's Echocardiography.* 7th ed. Philadelphia, PA: Lippincott Williams & Wilkins, 2010, with permission.)

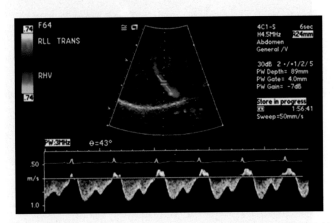

FIGURE 48.23 Normal hepatic vein flow. (Reproduced from Scheinfeld MH, Bilali A, Koenigsberg M. Understanding the spectral Doppler waveform of the hepatic veins in health and disease. *Radiographics* 2009;29:2081–2098, with permission.)

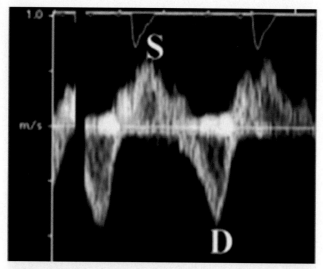

FIGURE 48.24 Hepatic vein flow severe TR with normal RV function, zoomed example. (Reprinted from Zoghbi W, Enriquez-Sarano M, Foster E, et al. Recommendations for evaluation of the severity of native valvular regurgitation with two-dimensional and Doppler echocardiography. *J Am Soc Echocardiogr* 2003;16(7):777–802. Copyright © 2003 American Society of Echocardiography. With permission.)

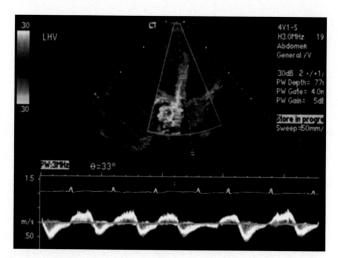

FIGURE 48.26 Hepatic vein flow severe TR with reduced RV function. (Reproduced from Scheinfeld MH, Bilali A, Koenigsberg M. Understanding the spectral Doppler waveform of the hepatic veins in health and disease. *Radiographics* 2009;29:2081–2098, with permission.)

For comparison with *constrictive physiology*, the hepatic vein pulsed-wave spectral Doppler flow recorded from a patient with documented, *restrictive cardiomyopathy* is provided below to demonstrate the variability in HV inflow patterns (FIG. 48.27). Note the *loss of smooth multiphasic flow* out of the hepatic vein and the *distinct inspiratory reversal* of flow (downward-pointing arrow), which is difficult to appreciate in these patients prone to atrial fibrillation (see FIG. 48.5D). In patients with restrictive cardiomyopathy and normal sinus

rhythm, there is *systolic blunting to systolic reversal* with *each cardiac cycle* depending on the severity of diastolic dysfunction (FIG. 48.26), and there is *prominent inspiratory or complete loss of phasic variations* seen. Be aware that the presence of atrial fibrillation alone can cause variability (erratic) spectral Doppler flow signals in the hepatic veins that may be confused with other pathologies and require careful evaluation of multiple cardiac cycles for clarification (FIG. 48.28). In patients with *constrictive physiology*, there is reversal of forward flow *during expiration* as the RV becomes less compliant and LV filling is increased (septum moves rightward) (see FIG. 48.5A).

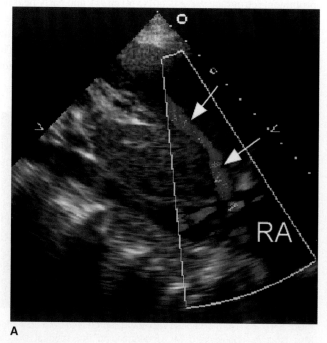

A

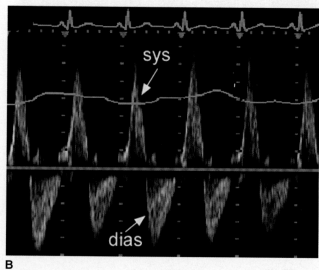

B

FIGURE 48.25 Hepatic vein flow severe TR with normal RV function. (From Armstrong WF, Ryan T. *Feigenbaum's Echocardiography.* 7th ed. Philadelphia, PA: Lippincott Williams & Wilkins, 2010, with permission.)

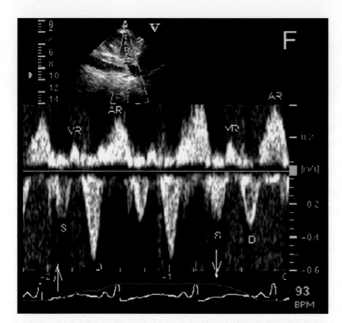

FIGURE 48.27 Hepatic vein flow restrictive cardiomyopathy and normal sinus rhythm. (Reproduced from Cotroneo J, Sleik K, Rodriguez E, et al. Hydroxychloroquine-induced restrictive cardiomyopathy. *Eur J Echocardiogr* 2007;8(4):247–251. Reproduced by permission of The European Society of Cardiology.)

Suggested Readings

Armstrong W, Ryan T. Pericardial diseases. In: *Chapter 10: Feigenbaum's Echocardiography*. 7th ed. Philadelphia, PA: Lippincott Williams & Wilkins, 2009:217.

Cotroneo J, Sleik K, Rodriguez E, et al. Hydroxychloroquine-induced restrictive Cardiomyopathy. *Eur J Echocardiography* 2007;8:247–251.

Scheinfeld MH, Bilali A, Koenigsberg M. Understanding the spectral Doppler waveform of the hepatic veins in health and disease. *Radiographics* 2009;29:2081–2098.

Zoghbi W, Enriquez-Sarano M, Foster E, et al. Recommendations for evaluation of the severity of native valvular regurgitation with two-dimensional and Doppler echocardiography. *J Am Soc Echocardiogr* 2003;16:777–802.

Answers 8: **C.** The two-dimensional echo images demonstrate a *large pericardial effusion without tamponade* (VIDEO 48.2A–C). This is also demonstrated on M-mode echo through the RV and LV short axis at the level of the mitral valve (note the echo-free space anterior to RV free wall and posterior pericardial space). On 2D and M-mode images, there is no RV free wall *diastolic collapse* suggestive of hemodynamic significance (tamponade). Repeat echocardiography after pericardiocentesis shows *marked interventricular septal bounce* during inspiration and *ventricular interdependence* (VIDEO 48.2D–G). On these 2D images, note the partially echo-free space (fixed throughout the cardiac cycle—distinguishes this from pericardial fluid), which is consistent with a *severely thickened pericardium.* VIDEO 48.2H demonstrates a dilated IVC with no evidence of collapse during inspiration (plethora).

Pulsed-wave Doppler of the mitral and tricuspid valve inflow demonstrates phasic variation in the Doppler velocity (>25% variability across mitral inflow and >50% variability across tricuspid valve inflow) as shown in FIGURE 48.6B AND C. These patients have an increase in the tricuspid valve velocity during inspiration and increase in mitral valve velocity during expiration. FIGURE 48.6D AND E from the same patient demonstrates higher tissue Doppler E-wave velocity of the medial annulus relative to the normally higher E-wave velocity of the lateral annulus ("*annulus reversus*") commonly seen in patients with constrictive physiology. This is thought to be due to the physical constraint on the lateral annulus applied by the adjacent pericardium and the compensatory free longitudinal septal motion. Since this patient's hemodynamics after pericardiocentesis failed to resolve and the pericardial fluid was consistent with an exudative effusion, the correct answer is *Option C* (exudative effusive–constrictive pericarditis).

This patient's presentation demonstrates typical findings of effusive constrictive pericarditis, which is a relatively uncommon pericardial syndrome. It is characterized by impaired diastolic filling from elements of both the hemodynamically significant pericardial effusion and constriction by an inflamed pericardium.

Although hemodynamic embarrassment and tamponade may be present, the thickening of the visceral pericardium may prevent right ventricular (RV) or right atrial (RA) free wall collapse. This results in a decreased accuracy of individual 2D echocardiographic or Doppler flow patterns for the conventional diagnosis of hemodynamic compromise. The diagnosis is often made when jugular venous distension persists and hemodynamics (invasive or Doppler) fail to normalize after pericardiocentesis. Once a pericardiocentesis is performed, the effusive component resolves and the remaining hemodynamic findings appear more similar to constrictive physiology. The most common causes of effusive constrictive pericarditis are idiopathic, malignancy, and radiation therapy.

The prevalence of this condition, based on a series reported by Sagrista-Sauleda (1), is 8% in consecutive patients undergoing pericardiocentesis. In their series, they defined effusive–constrictive pericarditis as a failure of the RA pressure to decline by at least 50% to a level below 10 mm Hg when the pericardial pressure is reduced to near 0 mm Hg by pericardiocentesis. In this era, the diagnosis of effusive–constrictive pericarditis can be easily made by noninvasive imaging modalities (echocardiography or cardiac magnetic resonance imaging [CMR]).

Echocardiography performed after pericardiocentesis not only will confirm effective removal of pericardial fluid but will also enable screening for the presence of residual constrictive physiology. However, the presence of abnormal pericardial thickening and ventricular interdependence is best demonstrated by CMR (VIDEO 48.5A). Furthermore, contrast-enhanced CMR is able to confirm an inflammatory component. Clinically, this is important since invasive pericardial stripping should not proceed during active inflammation.

Similar to transient constrictive pericarditis (common after cardiac surgery), patients with idiopathic effusive–constrictive pericarditis may have marked improvement with anti-inflammatory agents. Therefore, all patients with transient constrictive pericarditis or effusive–constrictive pericarditis should be treated with an initial trial of anti-inflammatory drugs. Failure to respond to NSAID treatment may require steroid therapy with a very slow taper

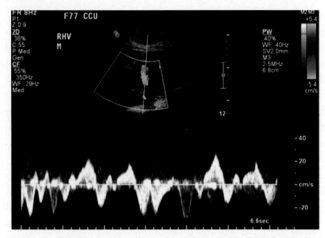

FIGURE 48.28 Hepatic vein flow in atrial fibrillation. (Reproduced from Scheinfeld MH, Bilali A, Koenigsberg M. Understanding the spectral Doppler waveform of the hepatic veins in health and disease. *Radiographics* 2009;29:2081–2098, with permission.)

over months. Serial echocardiography plays an important role by documenting resolution of the echocardiographic features of constrictive physiology, and in addition, CMR is helpful in confirming the resolution of the inflammatory process (FIG. 48.29).

A follow-up serial echocardiogram was obtained after 3 months of NSAID and steroid treatment and is shown in VIDEO 48.4B–D. The previously noted pericardial thickening and constrictive physiology have now resolved.

Reference

1. Sagrista-Sauleda J, Angel J, Sanchez A, et al. Effusive-constrictive pericarditis. *N Engl J Med* 2004;350:469–475.

Suggested Readings

Armstrong W, Ryan T. Pericardial diseases. In: *Chapter 10: Feigenbaum's Echocardiography.* 7th ed. Philadelphia, PA: Lippincott Williams & Wilkins, 2009:217.
LeWinter MM, Tischler MD. Pericardial diseases. In: Bonow RO, Mann DL, Zipes DP, et al., eds. *Chapter 75: Braunwald's*

Heart Disease: A Textbook of Cardiovascular Medicine. 9th ed. Philadelphia, PA: Saunders Elsevier, 2011.
Wang ZJ, Reddy GP, Gotway MB, et al. CT and MR imaging of pericardial disease. *Radiographics* 2003;23:S167–S180.

Answer 9: *B.* In pericardial constriction, right heart filling during expiration is impaired, resulting in increased expiratory reversal of diastolic hepatic vein flow. A similar Doppler pattern may also be seen in pericardial tamponade, chronic lung disease, pulmonary embolism, and right ventricular infarction. In restrictive cardiomyopathy, there is inspiratory decrease and/or flow reversal during systole.

Suggested Reading

Oh JK, Hatle LK, Seward JB, et al. Diagnostic role of Doppler echocardiography in constrictive pericarditis. *J Am Coll Cardiol* 1994;23:154–162.

Answers 10: *D; 11: B.* She has *systemic scleroderma* with *Raynaud phenomenon.* It is known that up to 40% of patients with *diffuse scleroderma* can develop pulmonary hypertension, either isolated or in association with interstitial lung disease. Pulmonary hypertension in a patient with systemic sclerosis is an important cause of morbidity and mortality with a *2-year survival of only 40%* (versus 80% *without* pulmonary hypertension). Early recognition and treatment of this associated disease in scleroderma are therefore critically important.

Echocardiography plays a major role in identification of right and left ventricular function and can demonstrate evidence of pulmonary hypertension. Transthoracic echo images shown in this case example demonstrate moderately reduced LV systolic function, moderately reduced RV systolic function with moderately dilated RV cavity (VIDEO 48.3), and a reduced pulmonary acceleration time of <100 ms consistent with pulmonary hypertension (see FIG. 48.7C).

FIGURE 48.7A AND B are tissue Doppler velocity spectral profiles recorded from the lateral and medial annulus and demonstrate reduced systolic velocities (S′) and early

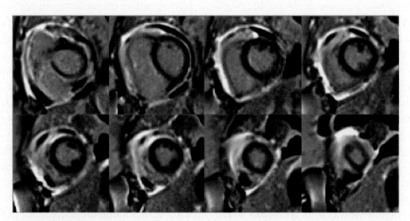

FIGURE 48.29 CMR; late gadolinium contrast enhancement images from the same patient demonstrate residual trace pericardial effusion and contrast enhancement of the pericardium consistent with active inflammation.

Table 48.1	Differences between Constrictive and Restrictive Physiology	
	CONSTRICTION	**RESTRICTION**
Atrial size	Normal	Dilated
Pericardial appearance	Thick/bright	Normal
Septal motion	Abnormal	Normal
Mitral E/A	Increased ≥2.0	Increased ≥2.0
Deceleration time	Short (<150 ms)	Short (<160)
Annular E′	Normal/ exaggerated	Reduced (<8 cm/s)
Pulmonary HTN	Rare	Frequent
Mitral/tricuspid regurgitation	Infrequent	Frequent (TR>MR)
IVRT	Varies with respiration	Stable with respiration
Respiratory variation of mitral E velocity	Exaggerated (≥25%)	Normal
Color M-mode mitral Vp	Increased (>55 cm/s)	Reduced
Hepatic vein flow	Exp. diastolic reversal	Systolic blunting
Strain	Normal	Reduced
BNP	Normal or low	Increased
Ventricular filling	Discordance	Concordance

Modified from Armstrong WF, Ryan T. *Feigenbaum's Echocardiography*. 7th ed. Philadelphia, PA: Lippincott Williams & Wilkins, 2010, with permission.

diastolic velocities (E′). *Option D* is the correct answer (right heart catheterization and vasodilator challenge) since this enables the managing physician to (a) confirm the diagnosis of and (b) explore treatment options for *pulmonary hypertension*. *Option A* is a reasonable option to noninvasively evaluate for coronary artery disease, but this option does not provide specific information about pulmonary hemodynamics. *Options B and C* are incorrect, as this patient does not demonstrate any evidence of pericardial constriction. Patients with pulmonary HTN can also demonstrate a *septal bounce* with each cardiac cycle, and this finding can be more prominent during inspiration. Therefore, it is important to maintain an open differential diagnosis and to recognize this finding from constrictive physiology. Table 48.1 illustrates some important differences between constrictive and restrictive physiology.

Suggested Readings

Armstrong W, Ryan T. Pericardial diseases. In: *Chapter 10: Feigenbaum's Echocardiography*. 7th ed. Philadelphia, PA: Lippincott Williams & Wilkins, 2009:217.

MacGregor A, Canavan R, Knight C, et al. Pulmonary hypertension in systemic sclerosis: risk factors for progression and consequences for survival. *Rheumatology (Oxford)* 2001;40(4): 453–459.

Stupi A, Steen V, Owens G, et al. Pulmonary hypertension in the CREST syndrome variant of systemic sclerosis. *Arthritis Rheum* 1986;29(4):515–524.

Chapter 49

Echo of the Normal and Diseased Aorta

Aiden Abidov

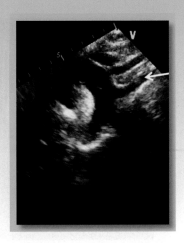

1. Regarding aortic atheromas, which of the following statements is true?

A. Mild aortic plaque demonstrates intimal thickness of ≤2 mm.

B. Severe aortic plaque is defined by intimal thickness of ≥5 mm.

C. Plaques with evidence of clot, ulceration, or intimal thickness of ≥4 mm are defined as complex plaques.

D. Increased risk of embolic events is determined by the presence of clot or ulceration and not the intimal thickness.

2. Which of the following is true regarding the condition causing the Doppler signal shown in FIGURE 49.1?

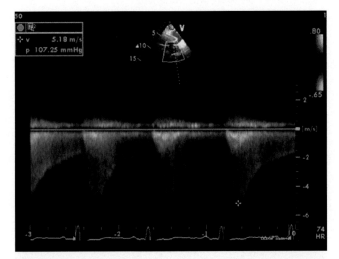

FIGURE **49.1** Reproduced with permission from the Edinburgh Cardiovascular Imaging Web site, http://cvsimaging.mvm.ed.ac.uk

A. Aortic luminal narrowing is a result of inflammation and secondary intimal hyperplasia.

B. Greater than 50% of patients may have aortic valve abnormalities.

C. A peak systolic gradient must be ≥40 mm Hg to be considered hemodynamically significant.

D. Presence of diastolic gradient indicates severe disease.

3. You are performing a TEE in a 75-year-old male patient with diagnosis of TIA. On one of the midesophageal views, you see a 3-mm-thick small partially calcified atheroma with a single small mobile component. Please grade the severity of your finding using the modified FAP study criteria.

A. Grade 3

B. Grade 4

C. Grade 5

D. Cannot grade the atheroma based on the provided information

4. Which one of the following TEE views allows best visualization of the entire aortic root and the proximal ascending aorta?

A. Mid- to upper esophageal 45 to 60 degrees

B. Midesophageal 0 degree

C. Mid- to upper esophageal 110 to 150 degrees

D. Upper esophageal 0 degree

5. What is the structure identified by a solid white arrow in FIGURE 49.2?

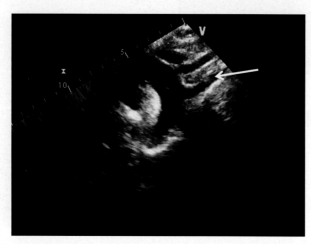

FIGURE 49.2

A. Left common carotid artery
B. Right common carotid artery
C. Left subclavian artery
D. Innominate artery

6. A 32-year-old female with Turner syndrome undergoes an exercise test to evaluate dyspnea. She exhibits significant shortness of breath at low levels of exertion and a hypertensive response. The images in FIGURE 49.3 were noted on an echocardiogram performed on the same day.

Which of the following is true?

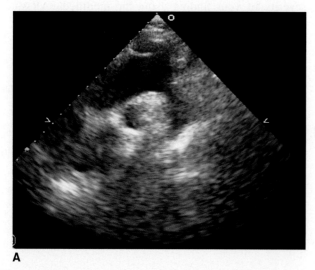

A

FIGURE 49.3 Reproduced from Chavhan GB, Parra DA, Mann A, et al. Normal Doppler spectral waveforms of major pediatric vessels: specific patterns. *Radiographics* 2008;28(3):691–706, with permission.

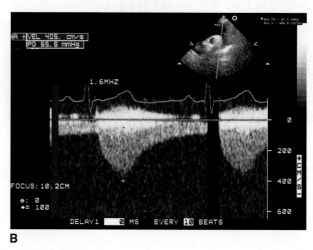

B

FIGURE 49.3 (*Continued*)

A. While typically noted at birth, most of these lesions are observed rather than treated.
B. Right heart failure and left-to-right shunting are frequently associated with this lesion.
C. Turner syndrome is associated with a defect in the production of type III collagen.
D. Mitral valve prolapse is likely to be associated with this defect.
E. Turner syndrome is associated with a lower risk of aortic dissection than Loeys-Dietz syndrome.

7. A 22-year-old female presents to the emergency department with fatigue and night sweats, transient vision loss, and left arm pain and weakness. Physical examination reveals that the radial pulse is absent and the brachial pulse is diminished on the left side. There is a high-pitched systolic murmur on cardiac exam. The neurologic exam is now normal. Embolic disease is suspected, and TEE is planned. The transthoracic image in FIGURE 49.4 was obtained.

Which of the following is true?

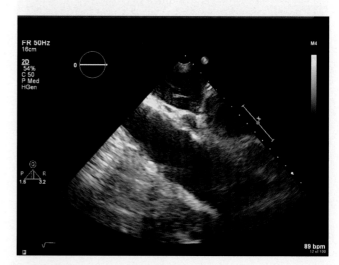

FIGURE 49.4 Reproduced with permission from Addetia K, Therrien J. Spot diagnosis using pulse wave Doppler interrogation of the abdominal aorta. *J Cardiovasc Ultrasound* 2012;20(2):112–113. Copyright © 2012 Korean Society of Echocardiography.

A. Acute bacterial endocarditis is the most likely diagnosis.

B. Temporal arteritis should be considered and a temporal artery biopsy planned.

C. Polymyalgia rheumatica is the likely diagnosis, and corticosteroids should be administered.

D. A large vessel granulomatous disease should be suspected.

E. Mitral valve prolapse is likely.

8. What is true in description of the sinus of Valsalva aneurysms?

A. A sinus of Valsalva aneurysm may occur in any of the coronary sinuses; however, the most frequent location is a noncoronary sinus.

B. Most frequently, rupture of the aneurysm is seen in patients younger than age 35.

C. The best views to visualize both ruptured and unruptured aneurysms on TTE are the parasternal long- and midparasternal short-axis views.

D. Use of agitated saline contrast does not improve diagnostic accuracy of the TTE in the sinus of Valsalva aneurysm rupture, since the rupture leads to a predominantly left-to-right shunting.

9. A 24-year-old male presents to your clinic for evaluation of dyspnea on exertion. An echo was performed, and the parasternal long-axis view is shown in Video 49.1. Suprasternal views revealed normal-sized arch and proximal descending aorta. Which of the following is the most likely diagnosis?

A. Marfan syndrome

B. Bicuspid aortic valve

C. Sinus of Valsalva aneurysm

D. Coarctation of the aorta

E. Infective endocarditis

10. Which of the following findings may be seen with pulse-waved Doppler flow in the abdominal aorta on subcostal views?

A. A low-resistance flow in fasting patients.

B. Very early diastolic flow reversal and late-diastolic flow usually represent abnormal findings.

C. The steep rise and narrow width of the aortic pulsation are suggestive of high cardiac output state.

D. Blunted and delayed systolic upstroke and diastolic flow reversal with persistent forward flow throughout diastole are suggestive of a hemodynamically significant coarctation of the aorta.

11. An extra chamber is seen next to the left atrium in the apical three-chamber view (Video 49.2). The structure measures 3.5 × 3.0 cm. An intravenous catheter could not be established in this patient. Color Doppler was applied, which demonstrates <1 m/s pulsatile flow during systole. What is this structure most likely to be?

A. Dilated coronary sinus due to persistent left superior vena cava

B. Dilated coronary sinus due to anomalous pulmonary vein

C. Dilated descending aorta

D. Pericardial cyst

E. Malignant mass

Answer 1: C.

Option A: False. Aortic plaques are defined as mild when the intimal thickness is ≤3 mm.

Option B: False. Severe plaques demonstrate a thickness of ≥4 mm.

Option C: True. See discussion below.

Option D: False.

Plaques with evidence of clot, ulceration, or intimal thickness of ≥4 mm are defined as complex plaques. The risk of embolization is directly related not only to high-risk features (ulcerations, thrombus) but also to a plaque thickness ≥4 mm. The adjusted odds ratio for ischemic stroke of an aortic plaque with thickness ≥4 mm was found to be 9.1 compared to odds ratio of 4.4 in plaques with thickness of 1 to 3.9 mm. Location of plaque in the ascending aorta and the aortic arch and the presence of large complex plaques (those with ulcerations or mobile components) are associated with a higher risk.

Suggested Readings

Amarenco P, Cohen A, Tzourio C, et al. Atherosclerotic disease of the aortic arch and the risk of ischemic stroke. *N Engl J Med* 1994;331:1474–1479.

Cohen A, Tzourio C, Bertrand B, et al. Aortic plaque morphology and vascular events. A follow-up study in patients with ischemic stroke. *Circulation* 1997;96:3838–3841.

Di Tullio MR, Russo C, Jin Z, et al. Aortic arch plaques and risk of recurrent stroke and death. *Circulation* 2009;119:2376–2382.

Answer 2: D.

Option A: False.

Option B: False.

Option C: False.

Option D: True. See discussion below.

Coarctation of the aorta is a congenital stenosis of the descending aorta involving most frequently the lumen distally to the origin of the left subclavian artery. Etiology of this disease is likely related to a primary aortopathy with structural derangement of collagen and elastin in the media and secondary intimal hypoplasia. There is a close association with the presence of the bicuspid aortic valve (25% to 46% of patients with coarctation will have bicuspid aortic valve). Peak systolic gradient of >20 mm Hg across the coarctation site is considered significant. Presence of delayed systolic upstroke and persistent diastolic flow across the coarctation indicates a severe degree of luminal narrowing at the level of coarctation.

Suggested Readings

Isner JM, Donaldson RF, Fulton D, et al. Cystic medial fibrosis in coarctation of the aorta: a potential factor contributing to adverse consequences observed after percutaneous balloon angioplasty of coarctation sites. *Circulation* 1987;75:689–695.

Lang RM, et al. Coarctation of the aorta. In: Lang R, Goldstein S, Kronzon I, et al., eds. *Dynamic Echocardiography.* St. Louis, MO: Saunders, 2011:460–461, Chapter 110.

Answer 3: *C.*

Option A: False.
Option B: False.
Option C: True. See discussion below.
Option D: False.

The original FAP (French Study of Aortic Plaques) used the following classification of the aortic plaques (1):

Group 1	No plaques, wall thickness <1 mm
Group 2	Plaques 1–3.9 mm
Group 3	Plaques ≥4 mm

Modified FAP study classification (2) took into consideration the presence of plaque mobility and defined thoracic aortic atheromas as follows:

Group 0	No atheroma or atheroma <1 mm
Group 1	Plaques 1–3.9 mm
Group 2	Plaques ≥4 mm
Group 3	Any plaque with obvious component

Most recent classification (3) (based on older 1996 publication of Hartman et al. (4)) suggests the following perioperative TEE-based classification to grade aortic atheromas.

Grade 1	Normal aorta
Grade 2	Extensive aortic thickening
Grade 3	Protruding plaques <5 mm
Grade 4	Protruding plaques ≥5 mm
Grade 5	Mobile atheroma

References

1. The French Study of Aortic Plaques in Stroke Group. Atherosclerotic disease of the aortic arch as a risk factor for recurrent ischemic stroke. *N Engl J Med* 1996;334:1216–1221.
2. Ferrari E, Vidal R, Chevallier T, et al. Atherosclerosis of the thoracic aorta and aortic debris as a marker of poor prognosis: benefit of oral anticoagulants. *J Am Coll Cardiol* 1999;33:1317–1322.
3. Savage RM, Aronson S, Sherman SK. *Comprehensive Textbook of Perioperative Transesophageal Echocardiography.* Philadelphia, PA: Lippincott Williams & Wilkins, 2011:594.
4. Hartman GS, Yao FS, Bruebach M III, et al. Severity of aortic atheromatous disease diagnosed by transesophageal echocardiography predicts stroke and other outcomes associated with cardiac surgery: a prospective study. *Anesth Analg* 1996;83(4):701–708.

Answer 4: *C.*

Option A: False
Option B: False
Option C: True
Option D: False

The so-called midesophageal AV long-axis view is used to measure the AV annulus, LVOT, aortic root, and proximal ascending aorta. Visualization of the proximal and midascending aorta will require withdrawing the TEE probe into a higher position and rotating in a more vertical plane (toward 90 degrees) in order to obtain a better vessel view. Remaining views mentioned in this question would demonstrate the following structures (in an average normal patient):

Mid- to upper esophageal 45- to 60-degree view—short axis of the aortic root/sinuses of Valsalva and the RV outflow with the pulmonary valve
Midesophageal 0-degree view—four-chamber view
Upper esophageal 0-degree view—aortic arch (long-axis view) and right pulmonary artery (short-axis view)

Suggested Readings

Armstrong WF, Ryan T. *Feigenbaum's Echocardiography.* 7th ed. Philadelphia, PA: Lippincott Williams & Wilkins, 2010.
Savage RM, Aronson S, Sherman SK. *Comprehensive Textbook of Perioperative Transesophageal Echocardiography.* Philadelphia, PA: Lippincott Williams & Wilkins, 2011:218–222.
Shanewise JS, et al. ASE/SCA guidelines for performing a comprehensive intraoperative multiplane transesophageal echocardiography examination: recommendations of the American Society of Echocardiography, Council for Intraoperative Echocardiography and the Society of Cardiovascular Anesthesiologists Task Force for Certification in Perioperative Transesophageal Echocardiography. *J Am Soc Echocardiogr* 1999;12:884–900.

Answer 5: *C.*

Option A: False.
Option B: False.
Option C: True. See discussion below.
Option D: False.

This figure demonstrates a suprasternal view, allowing evaluation of the aortic arch and the arch branching pattern. Most common in humans is a three-vessel arch with innominate, left common carotid and left subclavian arteries (right to left) originating from separate ostia. The so-called bovine arch describes a normal anatomic variant with a two-vessel aortic arch, a common origin of the innominate and left common carotid arteries.

Suggested Readings

Armstrong WF, Ryan T. *Feigenbaum's Echocardiography.* 7th ed. Philadelphia, PA: Lippincott Williams & Wilkins, 2010.
Layton KF, Kallmes DF, Cloft HJ, et al. Bovine aortic arch variant in humans: clarification of a common misnomer. *Am J Neuroradiol* 2006;27:1541–1542.

Answer 6: *E.*

In FIGURE 43.5, a transthoracic view of the aortic root suggests dilation of the aortic arch and a stenotic area beyond the take off of the left subclavian artery. In FIGURE 49.3B, continuous-wave Doppler analysis indicates a peak velocity of 404 m/s and a peak gradient of 65 mm Hg in this area. This is consistent with flow acceleration in this region of the aorta. Taken together, these findings are consistent with coarctation of the aorta in the setting of Turner syndrome. Turner syndrome arises from the complete, or partial, absence of one sex chromosome. Short stature and ovarian failure are the most commonly observed characteristics, though early death from aortic and cardiovascular disease is noted. Coarctation of the aorta is found in approximately 8% of patients, and between 10% and 20% have a bicuspid aortic valve. The risk of aortic dissection in the setting of Turner syndrome is lower than among patients with Marfan syndrome or Loeys-Dietz syndrome and is associated with other risk factors for dissection such as systemic hypertension. The risk of dissection among patients with Turners syndrome increases when accompanied by a bicuspid aortic valve or coarctation of the aorta.

Coarctation of the aorta is also relatively common in the general population. Most lesions are noted at birth and are treated soon thereafter. Later in life, these patients are more likely to present with heart failure, exercise-induced hypertension, and intracranial hemorrhage. The prognosis for patients in which a coarctation of the aorta goes untreated is poor due to aortic dissection, heart failure, and intracranial hemorrhage. Surgical repair is the traditional treatment approach, but endovascular balloon dilation and stent placement have also been utilized.

Suggested Readings

Hiratzka LF, Bakris GL, Beckman JA, et al. ACCF/AHA/AATS/ ACR/ASA/SCA/SCAI/SIR/STS/SVM Guidelines for the diagnosis and management of patients with thoracic aortic disease. A report of the American College of Cardiology Foundation/ American Heart Association Task Force on Practice Guidelines, American Association for Thoracic Surgery, American College of Radiology, American Stroke Association, Society of Cardiovascular Anesthesiologists, Society for Cardiovascular Angiography and Interventions, Society of Interventional Radiology, Society of Thoracic Surgeons, and Society for Vascular Medicine. *J Am Coll Cardiol* 2010;55:e27–e129.

Pinsker JE. Clinical review. Turner syndrome: updating the paradigm of clinical care. *J Clin Endocrinol Metab* 2012;97:E994–E1003.

Answer 7: D. A transthoracic echocardiogram from the subcostal window indicates an enlarged aorta with evidence of calcific or atherosclerotic change. In this clinical setting, a vasculitis, likely Takayasu arteritis, is suspected. Takayasu arteritis is associated with vasculitis of the elastic arteries. Diagnostic criteria include age of onset <40 years, intermittent claudication, diminished brachial pulse, subclavian or aortic bruit, systolic blood pressure variation of >10 mm Hg between the arms, and angiographic evidence of aortic or branch vessel stenosis. When three criteria are met, the diagnosis is quite likely (sensitivity 90.5%, specificity 97.8%). Aneurysms are common in the aortic arch or root, abdomen, and other thoracic segments, and stenosis of the aorta is more common than dilation and aneurysm formation (Fig. 49.5).

Temporal arteritis, also known as giant cell arteritis, occurs among older patients, typically older than 50 years. As with Takayasu arteritis, the disease affects women more commonly than men. Diagnostic criteria include age older than 50 years, recent onset of localized headache, temporal artery pulse attenuation or tenderness, an erythrocyte sedimentation rate of >50 mm/h, and a biopsy demonstrating necrotizing vasculitis. When three or more criteria are met, the diagnostic sensitivity and specificity are >90%. There is extracranial vascular involvement in 25% of patients, and aortic aneurysm

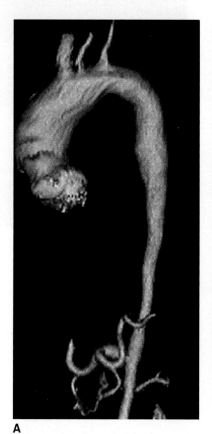
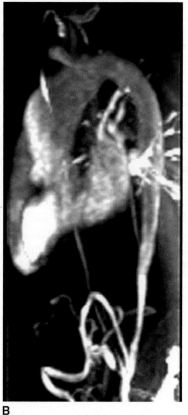

A   **B**

FIGURE 49.5 Magnetic resonance angiography (MRA) showing the dilated ascending aorta with diffuse narrowing of the left sided great arteries and the descending aorta.

and dissection are possible. In the case described above, temporal arteritis or polymyalgia rheumatic is unlikely due to the patient's age. Mitral valve prolapse, while found in association with Marfan syndrome, is not a part of the constellation of findings associated with Takayasu arteritis.

Suggested Reading
Raman SV, Aneja A, Jarjour WN. CMR in inflammatory vasculitis. *J Cardiovasc Magn Reson* 2012;14:82.

Answer 8: B.
Option A: False.
Option B: True. See discussion below.
Option C: False.
Option D: False.

The sinus of Valsalva aneurysms indeed may occur in any of the coronary sinuses. However, the most frequent location is the right coronary sinus. Rupture of the aneurysm is seen more often in young patients. The rupture most frequently causes communication to the right ventricle or right atrium. The best views to visualize both ruptured and unruptured aneurysms on TTE are parasternal long- and **basal** short-axis views. Agitated saline may significantly improve diagnostic accuracy of the test while screening for ruptured sinus of Valsalva aneurysms by creating a "negative contrast" phenomenon in the right heart structures.

Suggested Reading
Armstrong WF, Ryan T. *Feigenbaum's Echocardiography.* 7th ed. Philadelphia, PA: Lippincott Williams & Wilkins, 2010.

Answer 9: A.
Option A: True
Option B: False
Option C: False
Option D: False
Option E: False

The parasternal long-axis view shows a dilated aortic root with effacement of the sinotubular junction. The focal involvement of the aortic root alone or in combination with the sinotubular junction and ascending aorta and sparing the rest of the aorta are typical findings in Marfan syndrome. In patients with bicuspid aortic valves, the aneurysmal portion is generally in the midascending aorta and likely to present later in life. The dilation appears to involve more than just the sinus of Valsalva; thus, it is not sinus of Valsalva aneurysm. Coarctation is not visualized in this patient, and it is more commonly associated with bicuspid aortic valve. There are no vegetations or systemic signs to suggest infective endocarditis.

Answer 10: D.
Option A: False.
Option B: False.
Option C: False.
Option D: True. See discussion below.

A high-resistance flow with very early diastolic flow reversal as well as late-diastolic flow with normal-appearing

systolic upstroke can represent a normal Doppler pattern in the aorta with rapid elastic recoil (Fig. 49.3 (1), a normal pediatric patient), especially in fasting patients. Doppler waveform may demonstrate variable flow pattern in nonfasting patients (Fig. 49.4A, a normal adult patient). Holodiastolic flow reversal is seen in patients with severe aortic regurgitation (Fig. 49.4B). The steep rise and narrow width of the aortic pulsation are usually suggestive of low cardiac output state (Fig. 49.4D—a patient with tricuspid atresia and failed Fontan operation demonstrating a low cardiac output and increased peripheral vasoconstriction). Finally, blunted and delayed systolic upstroke and diastolic flow reversal with continuous diastolic flow are suggestive of a hemodynamically significant coarctation of the aorta.

Answer 11: C.
The patient has a dilated descending aorta, which runs next to the left atrioventricular groove. Pulsed wave Doppler in the the subcostal view of this aorta is shown (Fig. 49.6). Dilated coronary sinus has more continuous type flow, as it receives venous flow. It is lower in pressure and less likely to be round in shape. Unlike dilated coronary sinus, the descending aorta does not move with the left atrioventricular groove during the cardiac cycle. Since there is flow in this echolucent structure, it is unlikely to be pericardial cyst (no flow) or malignant mass (echogenic).

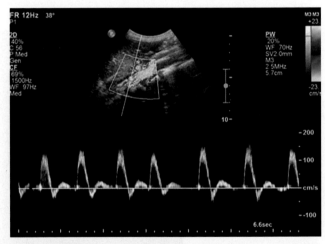

FIGURE 49.6 Pulsed wave Doppler of the descending aorta seen in the subcostal view.

Reference
1. Chavhan GB, Parra DA, Mann A, et al. Normal Doppler spectral waveforms of major pediatric vessels: specific patterns. *Radiographics* 2008;28(3):691–706.

Suggested Readings
Addetia K, Therrien J. Spot diagnosis using pulse wave Doppler interrogation of the abdominal aorta. *J Cardiovasc Ultrasound* 2012;20(2):112–113.
Armstrong WF, Ryan T. *Feigenbaum's Echocardiography.* 7th ed. Philadelphia, PA: Lippincott Williams & Wilkins, 2010.

Chapter 50

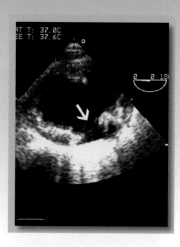

Acute Aortic Syndromes

Steve Leung

1. A 75-year-old male with hypertension and coronary artery disease suddenly develops back and chest discomfort and shortness of breath. Emergency medical services are summoned. On arrival, the patient is found unresponsive with a systolic blood pressure of 75 mm Hg. Upon arrival at the emergency department, an electrocardiogram is performed that indicates an acute inferior myocardial infarction. Soon thereafter, the patient develops a cardiac arrest and expires. Echocardiography is performed during the resuscitation attempt. The images in FIGURE 50.1 are obtained.

Which of the following answers best explains this scenario?

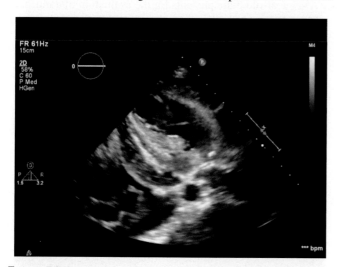

FIGURE 50.1 Bedside transthoracic images of a 75-year-old male with chest pain and shock.

A. An acute inferior myocardial infarction with rupture of the coronary artery into the pericardial space
B. An acute inferior myocardial infarction followed by rupture of the ventricular free wall into the pericardial space
C. Myocardial tamponade due to a malignant pericardial effusion with associated myocardial ischemia from hypotension
D. Acute aortic dissection with extension to the aortic root and hemorrhage into the pericardium
E. Purulent pericarditis with the development of myocardial ischemia due to hypotension

2. A 48-year-old male presents to the emergency department with abdominal pain. He has a history of hypertension and coronary artery disease and an aortic valve replacement. Recently, he has noticed difficulty walking long distances due to thigh pain. In the emergency department, the patient is noted to be in moderate distress. His heart rate is 103 bpm, and blood pressure is found to be 190/70 mm Hg, and he has normal oxygen saturations. He has moderate abdominal tenderness on examination with a normal cardiac exam. An electrocardiogram is performed showing sinus tachycardia. A chest x-ray shows a slightly widened mediastinum and a small left pleural effusion. His initial laboratory values show a serum creatinine level of 1.1 mg/dL. While waiting for a computed tomographic study to be performed, a transthoracic echocardiogram is performed. The images in FIGURE 50.2 are obtained.

Which of the following statements describes the scenario and a reasonable "next step" in the management of the patient?

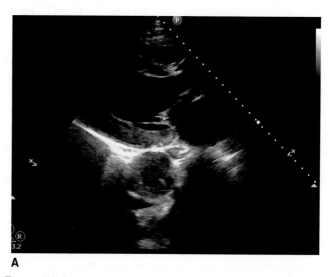

A

FIGURE 50.2 Transthoracic echocardiogram of a patient with abdominal pain.

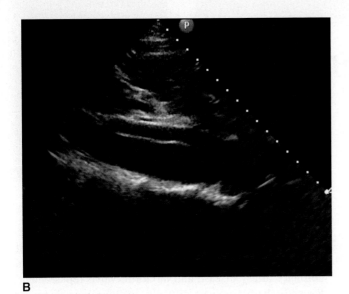

B

FIGURE 50.2 (Continued)

A. A type B dissection is suspected. Medical therapy with a beta-blocker is indicated, and a surgical intervention is unlikely to be of benefit.

B. A type A dissection is noted. Immediate consultation with a thoracic surgeon is recommended, and transfer to the operating room for surgical repair is indicated.

C. An aortic dissection is noted, and the extent is unknown. A surgical intervention is eminent. Transfer to the operating room following the initiation of medical therapy is recommended with intraoperative transesophageal echocardiography employed to determine the extent of the dissection.

D. An aortic dissection is noted. Initiation of medical therapy with sodium nitroprusside is reasonable, followed by emergent transesophageal echocardiography to determine the extent of the dissection.

E. An aortic dissection in the descending aorta is noted. The initiation of medical therapy with a beta-blocker and sodium nitroprusside is reasonable followed by the use of computed tomography or magnetic resonance imaging to determine the extent of the dissection is warranted.

3. A 72-year-old male with a long history of tobacco use and chronic renal insufficiency presents with chest and back pain. The patient's electrocardiogram shows sinus tachycardia, and a left bundle-branch block is also noted on previous studies. The serum creatinine is 4.7 mg/dL. A transesophageal echocardiogram was performed, and the image in FIGURE 50.3 was obtained.

Which of the following best explains the findings above?

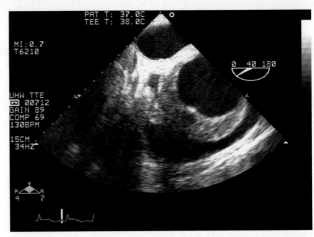

FIGURE 50.3 From Meredith EL, Masani ND. Echocardiography in the emergency assessment of acute aortic syndromes. *Eur J Echocardiogr* 2009;10(1):i31–i39. Reproduced by permission of Oxford University Press.

A. An acute dissection of the ascending aorta with an intimal tear

B. An intramural hematoma

C. An aortic abscess

D. An aortic pseudoaneurysm

E. Traumatic aortic dissection

4. A 45-year-old male presents for the evaluation of a murmur. In addition to findings consistent with a thoracic aortic aneurysm, the image in FIGURE 50.4 was obtained.

Which of the following statements is accurate?

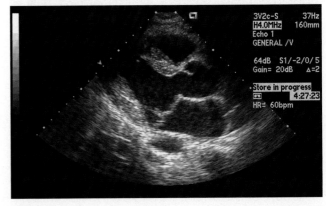

FIGURE 50.4 From Armstrong WF, Ryan T. *Feigenbaum's Echocardiography.* 7th ed. Philadelphia, PA: Lippincott Williams & Wilkins, 2010, with permission.

A. This disorder represents a sporadic mutation in 25% of patients, in particular the FBN1 gene.

B. A bicuspid aortic valve is also commonly noted in this condition.

C. Treatment with beta-blockade precludes the need for surveillance imaging of the aortic root.

D. Repair of the dilated aortic root is typically performed at a diameter of 6.0 cm.

E. A typical genotype for patients with this disorder is 45 X.

5. Loeys-Dietz syndrome is associated with which of the following abnormalities?

A. Coarctation of the aorta
B. Ovarian failure
C. Tissue fragility
D. Gastrointestinal bleeding
E. Early rupture of aortic aneurysms

6. A 12-year-old female is noted to have a loud diastolic heart murmur. Echocardiography reveals a bicuspid aortic valve. Which of the following is true?

A. The aortic root and ascending aorta are typically spared in this condition.
B. Surgical repair of a bicuspid aortic valve is unreasonable in the setting of aortic regurgitation.
C. Aortic stenosis is more common among young patients with a bicuspid valve than aortic regurgitation.
D. The likelihood of finding a BAV during aortic dissection repair is greater than the likelihood of identifying Marfan syndrome.
E. The most common site of leaflet fusion is the noncoronary and right coronary commissures.

7. An 80-year-old female with severe aortic stenosis undergoes transcatheter aortic valve replacement (TAVR). Prior to balloon valvuloplasty, intraoperative transesophageal echocardiogram demonstrated this finding (FIG. 50.5, VIDEO 50.1).

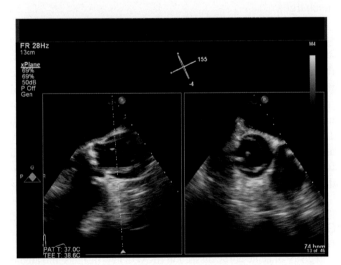

FIGURE 50.5

A. Hemorrhagic pericardial effusion in the transverse sinus
B. Type A dissection caused by transaortic access
C. Balloon valvuloplasty being performed
D. Wire crossing a bioprosthetic valve
E. A pigtail catheter curled up and around in the aortic root

8. A 32-year-old female presents after a syncopal episode. ECG demonstrated transient complete heart block. Which of the following is the cause of this patient's syncope (FIG. 50.6, VIDEO 50.2)?

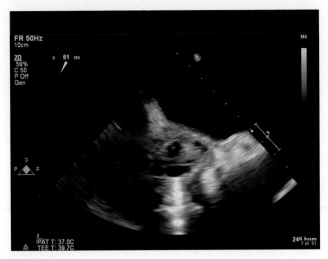

FIGURE 50.6

A. Aortic root abscess/infective endocarditis
B. Intracardiac malignancy
C. Sarcoidosis
D. Severe aortic stenosis due to unicuspid valve
E. Lyme disease

9. A 45-year-old male is brought to the emergency department following an automobile accident during which he received a penetrating injury to his chest. He is unconscious and hypotensive, with diminished pulses throughout. A transthoracic echocardiogram is performed (FIG. 50.7).

Which of the following statements is true?

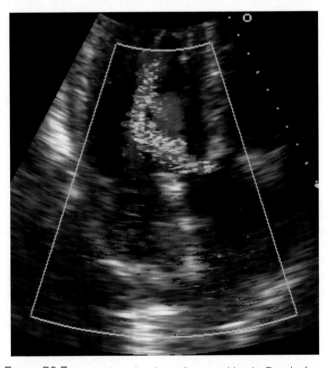

FIGURE 50.7 A transthoracic echocardiogram with color Doppler from the apical three-chamber view.

A. The image indicates a traumatic injury at the aortic isthmus.

B. TEE should be undertaken immediately to characterize the degree of aortic insufficiency.

C. Blunt chest trauma often results in injury to the aortic valve.

D. Survival to discharge among patients who are hospitalized with traumatic aortic injuries is >50%.

E. Aortic insufficiency is more common in the setting of penetrating trauma than blunt traumatic injuries.

10. A 64-year-old male with a history of coronary artery disease and hypertension is known to have an ascending thoracic aortic aneurysm. Which of the following statements is true?

A. Asymptomatic patients with a dilated ascending aorta of >5.0 cm should be considered for surgical intervention.

B. Patients with Marfan syndrome should be treated with long-acting calcium channel blockers to reduce progression of aortic disease.

C. Among patients with an ascending aortic aneurysm, referral for surgery should be made if the growth rate of the aorta exceeds 1.5 cm in 1 year.

D. Patients undergoing aortic valve replacement with an aortic root dimension of >4.5 cm should be considered for concomitant repair of the aorta.

E. Patients with a thoracic aortic aneurysm should be treated with statins to achieve an LDL cholesterol level of 100 mg/dL.

11. A 55-year-old female presents with sudden onset of chest pain. Initial ECG demonstrates sinus tachycardia. First troponin was negative, and serial troponins are pending. As part of the evaluation, the patient underwent an echocardiogram (Videos 50.3 and 50.4). Which of the following is the cause of the patient's chest pain?

A. Anomalous left coronary artery off the pulmonary artery (ALCAPA)

B. Pulmonary embolism

C. Descending aortic dissection

D. Pericarditis causing tamponade

E. Patent ductus arteriosus

Answer 1: D. The elderly hypertensive male in the scenario above has likely suffered an acute aortic syndrome (AAS) dissection of the ascending aorta (AAD). In Figure 50.1A, a parasternal long-axis view is depicted, showing an anterior clear space consistent with a pericardial effusion. In Figure 50.1B, an apical four-chamber view is depicted, demonstrating an echo-free space around the right ventricle and the apex consistent with a pericardial effusion. In the setting of acute aortic dissection and pericardial tamponade, even a small pericardial effusion can cause hemodynamic embarrassment.

An acute myocardial infarction with rupture in the pericardial space, as is described in answer B, is more likely following percutaneous intervention than at presentation. Ventricular free wall rupture with tamponade is also a possibility, though typically this is a late presentation of acute myocardial infarction. The sudden onset of symptoms in the patient described above makes this ventricular free wall rupture an unlikely cause of the patient's pericardial effusion. Malignant pericardial effusions typically arise slowly and present with progressive, rather than acute, symptoms. The lack of infectious symptoms makes purulent pericarditis unlikely. The best answer is answer D.

Aortic dissections are classified using the Stanford criteria (type A or type B) or the DeBakey criteria (type I, II, or III). Type A dissections involve the ascending aorta, and type B dissections affect the aorta distal to the left subclavian artery. The less often utilized DeBakey criteria include type I dissections in which the tear begins in the ascending aorta and extends to the arch and descending aorta. DeBakey type II dissections involve only the ascending aorta and type III dissections the descending aorta (Fig. 50.8). The majority of patients presenting with an AAS have a type A dissection (62%). The overall mortality of patients treated with type A dissections is 27.4%. Surgical intervention appears to be associated with improved survival (26.6% versus 58%). Type B dissections are less common and are typically treated with antihypertensive therapy. Uncomplicated type B dissections treated medically have a 90% likelihood of survival to discharge.

A history of hypertension is found in most patients who suffer AAS. The mortality associated with untreated AAD is approximately 75% at 2 weeks. In the emergency department, the mortality is 1% to 2% per hour. The electrocardiographic findings represent the evidence that the dissection has extended into the right coronary ostium, causing the acute inferior myocardial infarction. Abnormal ECG findings are present in up to 19% of AAD. The echocardiographic findings during attempts at resuscitation indicate the presence of a pericardial effusion found in 20% to 30% of AAD and 6% of descending aortic dissections.

Suggested Readings

Hagan PG, Nienaber CA, Isselbacher EM, et al. The international registry of acute aortic dissection (IRAD): new insights into an old disease. *JAMA* 2000;283:897–903.

Meredith EL, Masani ND. Echocardiography in the emergency assessment of acute aortic syndromes. *Eur J Echocardiogr* 2009;10:i31–i39.

Suzuki T, Mehta RH, Ince H, et al. Clinical profiles and outcomes of acute type b aortic dissection in the current era: lessons from the international registry of aortic dissection (IRAD). *Circulation* 2003;108(suppl 1):II312–II317.

Upadhye S, Schiff K. Acute aortic dissection in the emergency department: diagnostic challenges and evidence-based management. *Emerg Med Clin North Am* 2012;30:307–327, viii.

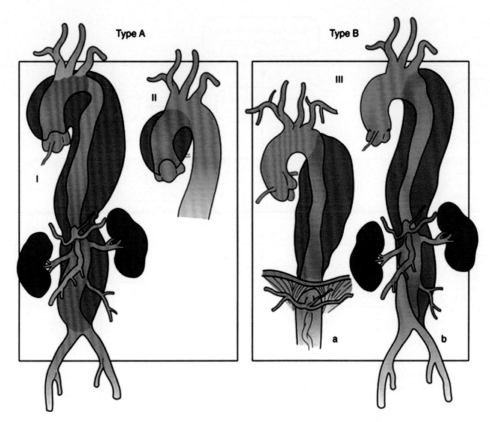

FIGURE 50.8 Classification scheme for aortic dissections using the Stanford criteria (types A and B) and the DeBakey criteria (type I, II, or III). (Reprinted from Upadhye S, Schiff K. Acute aortic dissection in the emergency department: diagnostic challenges and evidence-based management. *Emerg Med Clin North Am* 2012;30(2):307–327. Copyright © 2012 Elsevier. With permission.)

Answer 2: E. In FIGURE 50.2A, a parasternal long-axis image indicates left ventricular hypertrophy and left atrial enlargement, likely due to long-standing hypertension. There is also evidence of a dissection in the descending aorta with associated thrombus. In FIGURE 50.2B, subcostal images from a transthoracic echocardiogram show a dissection flap within the descending aorta. The appropriate treatment strategy involves medical therapy for the acute aortic syndrome (AAS) and a diagnostic evaluation to determine the extent of the dissection. The images do not fully characterize the dissection. Extension of the dissection into the ascending aorta would affect the management strategy. It is premature to assume the dissection is confined to the descending aorta; thus, answer A is incorrect. The presence of the dissection flap in the descending aorta makes answer B incorrect. Answers C, D, and E outline different methods of managing a large dissection. Transfer of the patient to the operating room followed by transesophageal echocardiography may be necessary when the patient presents in extremis, but this approach robs the surgical team of valuable information that could be obtained from CT or MRA, so answer C is not optimal. With respect to the best approach for imaging in AAS, transesophageal echocardiography (TEE) is rapidly available and does not expose the patient to contrast dye. TEE has a reported sensitivity of 94% to 100% and a specificity of 77% to 100% for identifying an intimal flap in an ascending aortic dissection. Additionally, TEE will demonstrate aortic insufficiency and pericardial effusions. Limitations include poor visualization of the branches of the aorta and the descending aorta. Other strategies include MRI and CT. These modalities show similar diagnostic abilities and have some advantages with respect to the complete characterization of the aorta and its branches. The American College of Cardiology and the American Heart Association have developed a diagnostic algorithm for the emergent evaluation of suspected aortic dissection (FIG. 50.9). In the case outlined above, the patient is hemodynamically stable and would benefit from careful imaging to determine the best course of therapy. CT or MRA offers the best assessment of the extent of the dissection; thus, answer E is correct.

Suggested Readings

Hiratzka LF, Bakris GL, Beckman JA, et al. 2010 ACCF/AHA/AATS/ACR/ASA/SCA/SCAI/SIR/STS/SVM guidelines for the diagnosis and management of patients with thoracic aortic disease. A report of the American College of Cardiology Foundation/American Heart Association Task Force on Practice Guidelines, American Association for Thoracic Surgery, American College of Radiology, American Stroke Association, Society of Cardiovascular Anesthesiologists, Society for Cardiovascular Angiography and Interventions, Society of Interventional Radiology, Society of Thoracic Surgeons, and Society for Vascular Medicine. *J Am Coll Cardiol* 2010;55:e27–e129.

Meredith EL, Masani ND. Echocardiography in the emergency assessment of acute aortic syndromes. *Eur J Echocardiogr* 2009;10:i31–i39.

Upadhye S, Schiff K. Acute aortic dissection in the emergency department: diagnostic challenges and evidence-based management. *Emerg Med Clin North Am* 2012;30:307–327, viii.

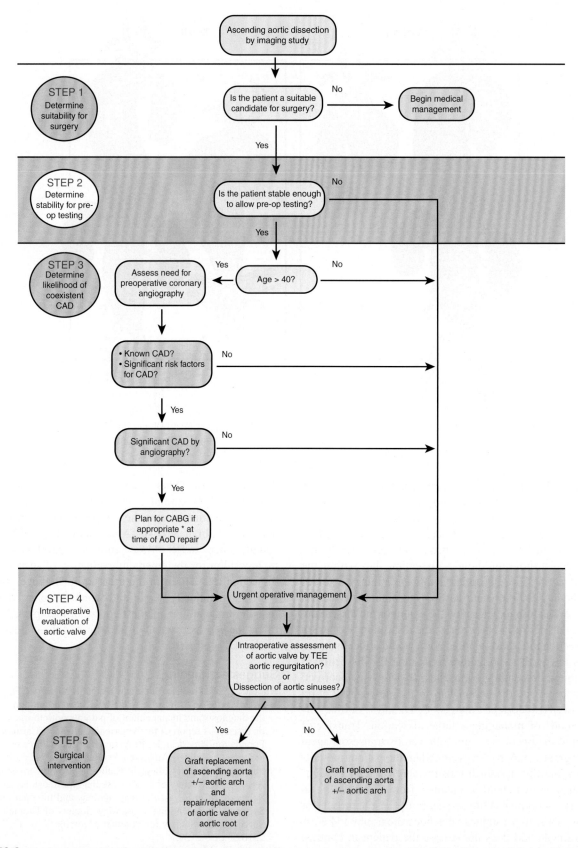

Figure 50.9 Diagnostic algorithm for the management of suspected acute aortic syndrome. (Reprinted from Hiratzka LF, Bakris GL, Beckman JA, et al. 2010 ACCF/AHA/AATS/ACR/ASA/SCA/SCAI/SIR/STS/SVM guidelines for the diagnosis and management of patients with thoracic aortic disease: a report of the American College of Cardiology Foundation/American Heart Association Task Force on Practice Guidelines, American Association for Thoracic Surgery, American College of Radiology, American Stroke Association, Society of Cardiovascular Anesthesiologists, Society for Cardiovascular Angiography and Interventions, Society of Interventional Radiology, Society of Thoracic Surgeons, and Society for Vascular Medicine. *J Am Coll Cardiol* 2010;55(14):e27–e129. Copyright © 2010 American College of Cardiology Foundation and the American Heart Association, Inc. With permission.)

Answer 3: B. In FIGURE 50.3, the aorta is visualized in a transesophageal echocardiogram. A discrete crescentic area of thrombus that partially surrounds the aorta is noted, consistent with an intramural hematoma. There are several types of intimal tears responsible for AAS (FIG. 50.10A). Classically, 10% to 20% of patients with an AAS are thought to present with an intramural hematoma (IMH, FIG. 50.10B). IMH is defined as hemorrhage into the intimal media without a tear in the intimal lining. This is in contrast to a penetrating aortic ulcer in which an atherosclerotic plaque erodes into the media, causing hemorrhage (FIG. 50.10C). More recently, an analysis from the International Registry of Acute Aortic Dissection found IMH to be present among 6.3% of patients presenting with AAS. Propagation of the IMH may lead to

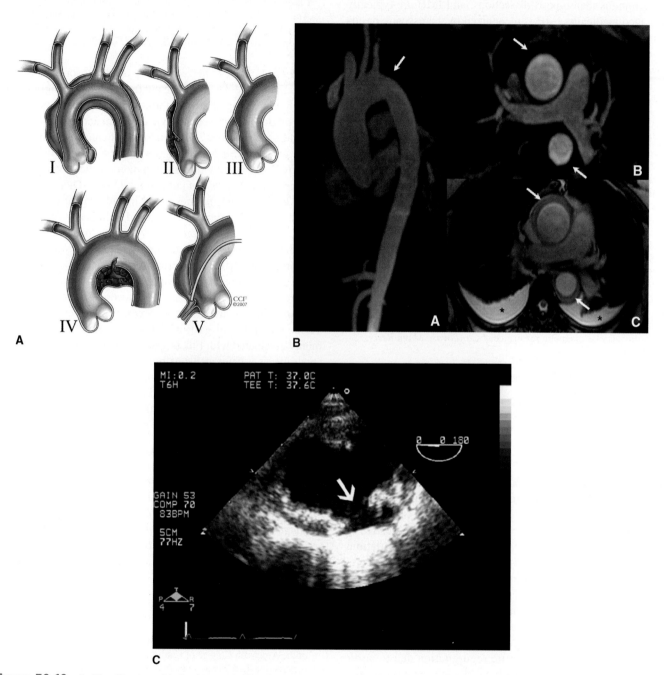

FIGURE 50.10 **A:** Classification of intimal tears. I: Classic aortic dissection. II: Intramural hematoma. III: Intimal tear without a hematoma. IV: Penetrating atherosclerotic ulcer. V: Iatrogenic (catheter-induced or traumatic) dissection. (From Hiratzka LF, Bakris GL, Beckman JA, et al. 2010 ACCF/AHA/AATS/ACR/ASA/SCA/SCAI/SIR/STS/SVM guidelines for the diagnosis and management of patients with thoracic aortic disease. A report of the American College of Cardiology Foundation/American Heart Association Task Force on Practice Guidelines, American Association for Thoracic Surgery, American College of Radiology, American Stroke Association, Society of Cardiovascular Anesthesiologists, Society for Cardiovascular Angiography and Interventions, Society of Interventional Radiology, Society of Thoracic Surgeons, and Society for Vascular Medicine. *J Am Coll Cardiol* 2010;55(14):e27–e129. Reprinted with permission from the Cleveland Clinic Foundation.) **B:** Magnetic resonance imaging of an intramural hematoma (*arrows*) and a pleural effusion (*asterisk*). (From Ma X, Zhang Z, Fan Z, et al. Natural history of spontaneous aortic intramural hematoma progression: six years follow-up with cardiovascular magnetic resonance. *J Cardiovasc Magn Reson* 2010;12:27, with permission.) **C:** Transesophageal images depicting a penetrating aortic ulcer.

symptoms indistinguishable from an aortic dissection. Most occur in the descending aorta and are more common among older patients. Among patients with IMH in the ascending aorta, patients in the IRAD analysis were most often managed surgically in a manner similar to AAD. Among the small number managed medically, the inpatient mortality was 40%. Among type B IMH, the prognosis appears to be somewhat less ominous than type B dissections, and IMH are typically managed medically. IMH is recognized by a crescentic or circumferential thickening of the aortic wall without evidence of an entry point or dissection flap. The ACC/AHA guidelines specify a maximal thickness of 7 mm on TEE without evidence of an intimal flap or tear or the presence of longitudinal flow within the false lumen.

Suggested Readings

Hiratzka LF, Bakris GL, Beckman JA, et al. 2010 ACCF/AHA/AATS/ACR/ASA/SCA/SCAI/SIR/STS/SVM guidelines for the diagnosis and management of patients with thoracic aortic disease. A report of the American College of Cardiology Foundation/American Heart Association Task Force on Practice Guidelines, American Association for Thoracic Surgery, American College of Radiology, American Stroke Association, Society of Cardiovascular Anesthesiologists, Society for Cardiovascular Angiography and Interventions, Society of Interventional Radiology, Society of Thoracic Surgeons, and Society for Vascular Medicine. *J Am Coll Cardiol* 2010;55:e27–e129.

Ma X, Zhang Z, Fan Z, et al. Natural history of spontaneous aortic intramural hematoma progression: six years follow-up with cardiovascular magnetic resonance. *J Cardiovasc Magn Reson* 2010;12:27.

Meredith EL, Masani ND. Echocardiography in the emergency assessment of acute aortic syndromes. *Eur J Echocardiogr* 2009;10:i31–i39.

Upadhye S, Schiff K. Acute aortic dissection in the emergency department: diagnostic challenges and evidence-based management. *Emerg Med Clin North Am* 2012;30:307–327, viii.

Answer 4: A. A parasternal long-axis image is presented. The image shows what is likely mild left ventricular hypertrophy, an enlarged aortic root at the sinotubular junction, and mitral valve prolapse. The combination of a dilated ascending aorta and mitral valve prolapse is suggestive of Marfan syndrome. Marfan syndrome results from mutations in the FBN1 gene. Approximately 25% of patients represent new cases due to sporadic mutations. The FBN gene encodes fibrillin-1, an extracellular matrix protein. The cardinal features of the syndrome involve cardiovascular, ocular, and skeletal abnormalities. Aortic disease is ubiquitous. Concomitant mitral valve prolapse is most common, but patients may present with aortic regurgitation due to aortic root dilation. Treatment with beta-blockers may slow progression of the aortic root dilation but is not curative, so patients may continue to experience enlargement of the aorta or rupture. There is a lower threshold for surgical repair of a dilated aortic root or ascending aorta. Typically, repair is performed at a threshold diameter of 5.0 cm, or when there is evidence of rapid growth (0.5 cm/y), a family history of a dissection at a diameter of <5.0 cm, or significant aortic regurgitation.

Suggested Reading

Hiratzka LF, Bakris GL, Beckman JA, et al. 2010 ACCF/AHA/AATS/ACR/ASA/SCA/SCAI/SIR/STS/SVM guidelines for the diagnosis and management of patients with thoracic aortic disease. A report of the American College of Cardiology Foundation/American Heart Association Task Force on Practice Guidelines, American Association for Thoracic Surgery, American College of Radiology, American Stroke Association, Society of Cardiovascular Anesthesiologists, Society for Cardiovascular Angiography and Interventions, Society of Interventional Radiology, Society of Thoracic Surgeons, and Society for Vascular Medicine. *J Am Coll Cardiol* 2010;55:e27–e129.

Answer 5: E. Loeys-Dietz syndrome is an autosomal dominant connective tissue disorder. The condition is increasingly recognized as consisting of arterial tortuosity and aneurysms, craniofacial malformations such as hypertelorism and bifid uvula, and skeletal abnormalities. The syndrome is caused by mutations in the gene for transforming growth factor–beta. Dilation and dissection of the aortic root are common. Aortic root aneurysms have been noted in 98% of patients with Loeys-Dietz syndrome. Other cardiac abnormalities noted include patent ductus arteriosus, bicuspid aortic valve, bicuspid pulmonary valve, mitral valve prolapsed, and coronary artery aneurysms. The high likelihood of aortic dissection among these patients when the aortic diameter is <5.0 cm has prompted the recommendation that repair occurs earlier. Turner syndrome arises from the complete, or partial, absence of one sex chromosome. Short stature and ovarian failure are the most commonly observed characteristics. Tissue fragility and gastrointestinal bleeding are more commonly associated with Ehlers-Danlos syndrome. Ehlers-Danlos syndrome is a heterogeneous group of inherited disorders that affect the connective tissue leading to hyperextensibility, tissue fragility, and scarring. Also noted is the tendency for rupture of the gastrointestinal tract and for the rupture of the thoracic and abdominal arteries, including the abdominal aorta.

> **Editor's Note:** We are continuing to learn about this relatively recently identified aortic syndrome—LDS. Early surgical repair is becoming the recommendation with aortic dimensions smaller than other aortic syndromes due to the higher dissection risk. A significant number of previously diagnosed patients with Marfan syndrome are being newly recognized as LDS (often with typical bifid uvula and other features), and this should always be considered a possibility.

Suggested Readings

Hiratzka LF, Bakris GL, Beckman JA, et al. 2010 ACCF/AHA/AATS/ACR/ASA/SCA/SCAI/SIR/STS/SVM guidelines for the diagnosis and management of patients with thoracic aortic disease. A report of the American College of Cardiology Foundation/American Heart Association Task Force on Practice Guidelines, American Association for Thoracic Surgery, American College of Radiology, American Stroke Association, Society of Cardiovascular Anesthesiologists, Society for Cardiovascular Angiography and Interventions, Society of Interventional Radiology, Society of Thoracic Surgeons, and Society for Vascular Medicine. *J Am Coll Cardiol* 2010;55:e27–e129.

Kalra VB, Gilbert JW, Malhotra A. Loeys-Dietz syndrome: cardiovascular, neuroradiological and musculoskeletal imaging findings. *Pediatr Radiol* 2011;41:1495–1504; quiz 1616.

Parapia LA, Jackson C. Ehlers-Danlos syndrome—a historical review. *Br J Haematol* 2008;141:32–35.

Answer 6: *D.* A bicuspid aortic valve is found in 1% to 2% of the general population. Bicuspid valves may be inherited in an autosomal dominant manner and may be associated with aortic root dilation and thoracic aortic aneurysm formation. Among 2,000 patients undergoing surgery for a bicuspid aortic valve, 20% had a concurrent ascending aortic aneurysm repair. The most common site of leaflet fusion is the left and right coronary commissures. Aortic regurgitation is common among young patients with a bicuspid valve, and aortic stenosis more common among older patients. Repair of a bicuspid valve in the setting of aortic regurgitation has excellent long-term results. Aortic dissection is more common among patients with a bicuspid aortic valve than in patients with Marfan syndrome.

Suggested Reading

Svensson LG, Kim KH, Blackstone EH, et al. Bicuspid aortic valve surgery with proactive ascending aorta repair. *J Thorac Cardiovasc Surg* 2011;142:622–629, e621–e623.

Answer 7: *B.* In FIGURE 50.5/VIDEO 50.1, a transesophageal echocardiogram in biplane demonstrates an ascending aortic dissection. This is most likely caused by transaortic access. The false lumen surrounds the true lumen in the cross-sectional view with a guidewire in the center and pigtail catheter resting against the true lumen wall anteriorly. This patient did not have a pericardial effusion, and the left coronary artery flow did not appear obstructed on color Doppler. Balloon valvuloplasty is generally performed with contrast injected into the balloon, causing echogenic brightness within the balloon itself. Also, the balloon should cross the aortic valve when it is inflated; thus, leaflets should not be touching.

Suggested Reading

Généreux P, Webb JG, Svensson LG, et al. Vascular complications after transcatheter aortic valve replacement: insights from the PARTNER (Placement of AoRTic TraNscathetER Valve) trial. *JACC* 2012;60(12):1043–1052. doi: 10.1016/j.jacc.2012.07.003

Answer 8: *A.* This patient had an aortic root abscess due to infective endocarditis, which is also the cause of her complete heart block as the infection invaded to the AV node. The image demonstrates a thickening around the aortic root, which extends into the LVOT. This is not seen in cardiac sarcoidosis (may present with focal aneurysms), malignancy, unicuspid aortic valve, or Lyme disease.

Suggested Reading

Choussat R, Thomas D, Isnard R, et al. Perivalvular abscesses associated with endocarditis: clinical features and prognostic factors of overall survival in a series of 233 cases. Perivalvular Abscesses French Multicenter Study. *Eur Heart J* 1999;20(3):232–241.

Answer 9: *E.* A transapical, three-chamber view is provided, with color flow Doppler consistent with aortic insufficiency. While it is difficult to judge the severity of aortic insufficiency from this image, in the setting of a motor vehicle accident with penetrating trauma to the chest, severe acute aortic regurgitation should be considered. Among patients with blunt trauma,

the aortic isthmus is a common site of injury with the ascending aorta and aortic valve more commonly involved in the setting of penetrating trauma. Overall, acute valvular disease is not common among patients with traumatic aortic injury, occurring in only 12% of patients in one European series. The most effective method of characterizing a traumatic aortic dissection is undetermined, but CTA is the best-studied modality. Still, some recommend surgical exploration. TEE has potential advantages in that it can identify valvular, myocardial, and pericardial injuries but at the expense of incomplete characterization of the aorta and no information about extravascular injuries. The prognosis of patients presenting with traumatic rupture of the aorta is quite poor with just 9% to 14% of patients surviving to reach the hospital and only 2% surviving hospitalization.

Suggested Readings

Mosquera VX, Marini M, Muniz J, et al. Blunt traumatic aortic injuries of the ascending aorta and aortic arch: a clinical multicentre study. *Injury* 2013;44(9):1191–1197.

Patterson BO, Holt PJ, Cleanthis M, et al. Imaging vascular trauma. *Br J Surg* 2012;99:494–505.

Richens D, Kotidis K, Neale M, et al. Rupture of the aorta following road traffic accidents in the United Kingdom 1992–1999. The results of the co-operative crash injury study. *Eur J Cardiothorac Surg* 2003;23:143–148.

Answer 10: *D.* Among asymptomatic patients with a thoracic aortic aneurysm, medical therapy should include antihypertensive medications to achieve a systolic blood pressure of <140 mm Hg for most patients. Patients with Marfan syndrome may benefit from treatment with beta-blockers or from treatment with angiotensin receptor blockers. Aggressive management of lipids with a statin is recommended. The target LDL cholesterol level is <70 mg/dL. Asymptomatic patients with a thoracic aneurysm should be referred for surgery when the ascending aorta or aortic sinus diameter is 5.5 cm or greater. Patients with Marfan syndrome are referred when the diameter of the aorta or sinus exceeds 5.0 cm. Additionally, if the aneurysm has a growth rate of >0.5 cm/y, it is also reasonable to consider surgery.

Suggested Readings

Braverman AC. Medical management of thoracic aortic aneurysm disease. *J Thorac Cardiovasc Surg* 2013;145:S2–S6.

Hiratzka LF, Bakris GL, Beckman JA, et al. 2010 ACCF/AHA/AATS/ACR/ASA/SCA/SCAI/SIR/STS/SVM guidelines for the diagnosis and management of patients with thoracic aortic disease. A report of the American College of Cardiology Foundation/American Heart Association Task Force on Practice Guidelines, American Association for Thoracic Surgery, American College of Radiology, American Stroke Association, Society of Cardiovascular Anesthesiologists, Society for Cardiovascular Angiography and Interventions, Society of Interventional Radiology, Society of Thoracic Surgeons, and Society for Vascular Medicine. *J Am Coll Cardiol* 2010;55:e27–e129.

Answer 11: *C.* The transthoracic echo images are from suprasternal view. The 2D imaging demonstrates a dissection flap. The color Doppler shows to and from flow in the descending aorta, which is through the true lumen during early systole (FIG. 50.11A, blue color and down the aorta) and false lumen

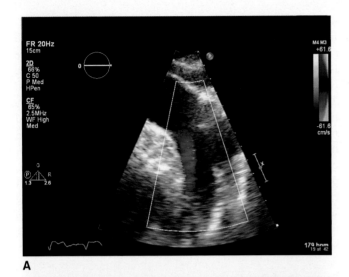

A

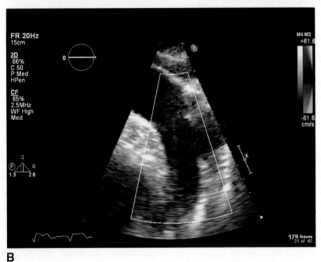

B

FIGURE 50.11

during late systole/early diastole (FIG. 50.11B, red color and up the aorta). At times, the dissection flap cannot be clearly identified due to either artifact or not perpendicular to the ultrasound beam. Color Doppler can be helpful in evaluation of flow in

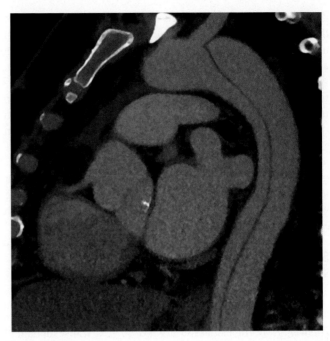

FIGURE 50.12

these scenarios. ALCAPA is generally identified much earlier in age and presents with heart failure. Doppler should demonstrate abnormal flow from the pulmonary artery. Patent ductus arteriosus should have continuous high-velocity flow into the pulmonary artery from the aorta. In cases of severe pulmonary hypertension, there can be reversal of flow from the pulmonary artery and back into the aorta; however, this would not cause the flow to go retrograde in the aorta. There are no findings from these suprasternal views to suggest pulmonary embolism or pericarditis/tamponade. FIGURE 50.12 is a CT image showing the type B dissection that this patient had.

Suggested Reading

Evangelista A, Flachskampf FA, Erbel R, et al. Echocardiography in aortic diseases: EAE recommendations for clinical practice. *Eur J Echocardiogr* 2010;11(8):645–658. https://doi.org/10.1093/ejechocard/jeq056

Chapter 51

59 Case Examples Using Recent Echo-Relevant Guidelines and Consensus Documents

Vincent L. Sorrell

The following questions were developed from the recently published guidelines, consensus documents, special reports, and recommendations created or endorsed by the ASE and many times cowritten with other major (imaging) societies. Where noted, the references **highlight** whether the document was a **guideline** or **other document**. Although some of these questions read more as a general cardiology topic, the material is either based upon or derived from an echocardiographic parameter or criterion.

1. Which of the following are the primary reasons that 3D echocardiography has become an increasingly utilized and important tool in evaluating children with congenital heart diseases as compared with older adults?

   A. Noninvasive nature of technique and improved acoustic windows
   B. Cross-plane (or X-plane) capabilities and higher-frequency probes
   C. Real-time nature of technique and improved LV volumes and LVEF
   D. Ability to obtain 2D and 3D datasets with the same probe and noninvasive nature of technique
   E. Improved acoustic windows and value in presurgical planning

2. When performing 3D echocardiography, the operator has the unique option of displaying the echo images in any orientation. Which of the following correctly describes the "surgical view" of an **atrial septal defect** as opposed to the more commonly displayed "anatomic view"?

   A. Is projected as if the patient is standing upright.
   B. Should be akin to the lead surgeon's view operating from the left side of the patient.
   C. Results in an "en face" view of the right side of the atrial septum rotated 90 degrees clockwise.
   D. Results in an "en face" view of the left side of the atrial septum rotated 90 degrees clockwise.
   E. Instead of the coronary sinus being seen at a 6 o'clock position, it will be seen at a 3 o'clock position.

3. Compared with 2D echocardiography, which of the following statements is most true regarding 3D echocardiography in congenital heart diseases?

   A. Multiple randomized trials have proven its procedural success.
   B. Morbidity and mortality have been proven to be reduced.
   C. Valvular lesions and septal defects have been primarily responsible for its growth.
   D. There is a greater consistency across institutions regarding its application.
   E. 3D is likely to replace 2D as the primary echo tool in the near future.

4. A 30-year-old male is seen in the adult echo lab for follow-up of his congenital heart disease. He states that he had a Mustard operation as a child. No other records are available. Which of the following is most likely correct?

A. This patient likely had the most common cyanotic heart defect in newborns.

B. His mother had an increased likelihood for diabetes.

C. He will most commonly have a known genetic mutation or syndrome.

D. Coronary ischemia is an important complication and should be evaluated.

E. It is unusual that this patient has an XY chromosomal pattern.

5. You were asked to review selected still frame images of an echocardiogram that a colleague brought to you. You are told that these were obtained in their newborn grandson. In addition to showing these to your congenital heart imaging team, which of the following findings would be expected if this was from a baby with D-TGA?

A. A subaortic conus was seen.

B. A subpulmonic conus was seen.

C. Bilateral conus was seen.

D. Mitral-to-aortic fibrous continuity was confirmed.

E. Tricuspid to pulmonary fibrous discontinuity was confirmed.

6. A 25-year-old male presents to clinic with palpitations and frequent PVCs noted on ECG. He has a history of D-TGA and an arterial switch operation as a child. He describes mild, but new, dyspnea on exertion; he denies chest pain or syncope. A transthoracic echocardiogram demonstrates images consistent with the reported clinical history. Reported cardiac dimensions are within normal limits except for the neoaorta, which was mildly dilated at 3.9 cm. The global LV and RV function is normal with mild anteroseptal LV hypokinesis. There is mild TR with a maximal RV to RA velocity of 2.8 m/s.

Which of the following would be most important next step in the management of this patient?

A. TEE examination

B. Right heart catheterization

C. Stress echocardiogram

D. Ambulatory event monitor

E. Cardiothoracic surgery consultation

7. A 72-year-old female with long-standing, poorly controlled hypertension is evaluated with transthoracic echocardiography. The LV diastolic dimension is normal, LV mass is 105 g/m^2, and LVEF > 60% without wall motion abnormality. LAVI = 44 cm/m^2. RV size and function are normal. Mild TR with a maximal velocity of 3.2 m/s is recorded. The mitral inflow pattern reveals an E wave of 110 cm/s and an A wave of 50 cm/s. The septal e′ = 5.8 cm/s and the lateral e′ = 6.5 cm/s. The sonographer asks the patient to perform a Valsalva maneuver.

Which of the following is the most likely change in mitral inflow pattern that would be seen?

A. No change in Doppler findings.

B. E/A ratio will increase.

C. E/e′ ratio will increase.

D. E/A ratio will decrease.

E. E/e′ ratio will decrease.

8. Which of the following is considered the most correct method of properly performing a Valsalva maneuver during Doppler echocardiography of the mitral inflow?

A. The patient should be asked to "bear down" as long as possible.

B. The maneuver should be held for 3 to 5 seconds and echo imaging obtained at release.

C. The maneuver should be held for 10 seconds and Doppler recorded after 5 seconds.

D. The maneuver should be held for 10 seconds and continuous mitral inflow Doppler recorded.

E. If the LAP is high, dramatic changes are seen immediately regardless of the method.

9. A 68-year-old female with a dilated cardiomyopathy is seen in the heart failure clinic. She has known CAD with previous myocardial infarction and a reported LVEF 35%. She complains of mild dyspnea, which has not significantly changed despite titration of her heart failure medications to their maximal doses more than 3 months earlier. Physical examination reveals BP 108/62 mm Hg, HR 72 bpm; PMI wide and displaced laterally; 2/6 holosystolic murmur; no diastolic murmur. No gallops or rubs.

You were asked by your heart failure colleague to estimate her LA pressure based upon the following echo Doppler findings obtained today:

E = 48 cm/s; A = 64 cm/s

Which of the following is the best estimate of this patient's mean LAP?

A. LAP cannot be estimated without tissue Doppler findings.

B. LAP cannot be estimated without knowing the LAVI.

C. LAP is either normal or low.

D. LAP is moderately increased.

E. LAP is severely increased.

10. A 43-year-old-male patient presents with worsening symptoms of dyspnea to your clinic. An echocardiogram is obtained (see Video 51.1).

Which of the following summarizes best the assessment of LV diastolic function in this patient?

A. Echo Doppler cannot be used to estimate diastolic function in this patient.

B. Conventional Doppler measures do not correlate with LV filling pressures.

C. E/e′ ratio does not predict adverse outcomes in this population.

D. LAVI does not predict adverse outcomes in this population.

E. A restrictive filling pattern, when present, is associated with poor clinical outcomes.

11. Recognizing the known limitations to conventional echo Doppler parameters in this clinical population, which of the following additional measures should be included and has been shown to have the best correlation with LV filling pressures?

A. Pulmonary vein S/D ratio <1.0

B. Pulmonary vein Ar velocity >30 cm/s

C. Pulmonary vein Ar minus mitral A-wave duration >30 ms

D. DT of mitral E velocity <150 ms

E. Color M-mode velocity flow propagation (Vp) >40 cm/s

12. Which of the following statements is true regarding the assessment of diastolic function in patients with Valvular heart diseases?

A. Mitral stenosis renders assessment of LV diastolic function impossible.

B. IVRT/TE-e′ ratio can be used to estimate LAP in patients with MR and normal LVEF.

C. E/e′ ratio remains accurate in patients with MR and normal LVEF.

D. Severe mitral annular calcification does not preclude the predictive value of the E/e′ ratio.

E. Severe AS precludes the conventional assessment of LV diastolic function.

13. A 45-year-old male with recently diagnosed hypertension presents to clinic with dyspnea on exertion. He states that he has been physically active until the past 3 months where he has reduced his walking from 3 miles/day most days of the week to <1 mile duration 1 or 2 days/week. He denies chest pain, palpitations, or syncope. He does not smoke cigarettes and denies history of substance abuse, including ETOH. He denies diabetes or a family history of CAD. His lipid profile was recently normal.

His medications include lisinopril 40 mg daily and Advil occasionally.

On exam, height 72 inches; weight 190 pound; BP 140/88 mm Hg; HR 72 bpm. JVP is normal. No carotid bruits. Cardiac exam is normal, except for a soft S4.

ECG is within normal limits.

Echocardiography findings: excellent image quality. Normal LV and RV dimensions; borderline increased LV myocardial mass index. LAVI = 32 cm/m². Normal LVEF; normal RVEF. No wall motion abnormalities. No valve regurgitation or stenosis.

E = 68 cm/s

A = 80 cm/s

Medial e′ = 6 cm/s

Lateral e′ = 9 cm/s

Which of the following is most appropriate next step?

A. Exercise nuclear myocardial perfusion imaging SPECT stress test.

B. Dobutamine echocardiography with Doppler.

C. Transesophageal echocardiography.

D. Diastolic exercise testing.

E. Right and left heart catheterization.

F. Consider noncardiovascular etiologies.

14. A 72-year-old female presents to your emergency department with a stroke. Workup did not find an etiology. An echocardiogram is performed. Which of the following findings on 2D echo is considered a low (not high) embolic potential risk?

A. Left atrial myxoma

B. Small aortic valve papillary fibroelastoma

C. Atrial flutter rhythm

D. Giant Lambl excrescences

E. Nonvalvular endocarditis

15. During hospitalization, this patient developed paroxysmal atrial fibrillation. If this patient undergoes a TEE examination, which of the following best describes the correct order (from **highest to lowest**) of TEE findings to predict subsequent stroke?

A. LV systolic dysfunction > dilated LAVI > LAA thrombus

B. LAA thrombus > low LAA peak velocity (<27 cm/s) > mobile aortic plaques

C. Mobile aortic plaque > LAA thrombus > low LAA peak velocity (<27 cm/s)

D. LAA thrombus > mobile aortic plaques > low LAA peak velocity (<27 cm/s)

E. Spontaneous echo contrast > low LAA velocity (<27 cm/s) > LAA thrombus

16. A 32-year-old male patient has a long history of intravenous drug abuse and presents to the ER with high fever and new murmur. He last injected 72 hours ago and has been too ill to "use" since then. His fever has been present for a week. He has no previous history of endocarditis. On examination, he appears ill. He is diaphoretic and responds weakly to questions. HR is 110 bpm, BP 90/68 mm Hg. JVP is prominent and elevated, best noted in systole. He has a 3/6 holosystolic murmur. No gallop. No rub. Blood cultures have been drawn and are pending.

Which of the following findings would support performing a transthoracic echocardiogram over a first-line transesophageal echocardiogram?

A. Severe TR is suspected.

B. Positive blood cultures for *Staphylococcus aureus*.

C. Suspicion for leaflet perforation on POCUS.

D. Prosthetic valve endocarditis suspected.

E. Transient AV block is noted on telemetry.

17. A 66-year-old male with chronic, poorly controlled hypertension, previous percutaneous coronary intervention for ACS 2 years ago, and tobacco abuse presents to the urgent care facility with TIA symptoms. The patient states that he was in the shower when he noted slight visual changes and then mild left arm numbness and weakness that resolved after 2 hours. Examination reveals laterally displaced PMI. BP 200/104 mm Hg; HR 90 bpm and regular; normal JVP without bruits; normal S1, S2, and loud S4. No murmurs, rubs, or S3 gallop. ECG with sinus rhythm, LAE, and LVH with associated repolarization changes.

A POCUS is performed and demonstrates normal LV and RV dimensions and function. A basal parasternal short-axis image is seen in VIDEO 51.2.

Which of the following statements regarding this patient is true?

A. Mitral annular calcification (MAC) is mild and unlikely to be a cause of the TIA.

B. The MAC is severe and an associated infective endocarditis lesion is present.

C. Without a mobile component, MAC is not considered a cardioembolic source.

D. The severe MAC is ulcerated and a superimposed thrombus was the likely stroke cause.

E. Paroxysmal AF may be a more likely TIA source if the MAC is severe.

18. A 43-year-old female with a history of breast cancer and recently completed chemotherapy presents to your clinic with increasing dyspnea. She denies CP, syncope, or palpitations. She has no history of stroke, CAD, diabetes or hypertension. Her chemotherapy (>200 mg/m² doxorubicin) was completed 1 week ago. Examination reveals BP 128/78 mm Hg, HR 86 bpm. JVP = 10 cm H₂O. No neck bruits. No murmurs, rubs, or gallops on cardiac auscultation. Evidence of left mastectomy is noted. Normal peripheral pulses. 1+ bilateral lower extremity edema.

ECG = sinus rhythm with nonspecific ST changes. Baseline MUGA = LVEF 59%.

Echocardiogram performed today:

Good-quality images. LVEF 50% (biplane Simpson); mild global hypokinesis; no regional wall motion abnormalities; no valve regurgitation or stenosis; no pericardial effusion.

Which of the following is true regarding the diagnosis of CTRCD (cancer therapeutic–related cardiac dysfunction) in this patient?

A. There is no difference between the reported MUGA and echo LVEF.

B. This fulfills the criteria for CTRCD.

C. A repeat echocardiogram should be performed in the next 2 to 3 weeks.

D. A repeat MUGA should be immediately performed.

E. Perform a dobutamine stress echocardiogram.

19. A repeat, limited 2D echocardiogram was performed 2 weeks after the reported LVEF of 50%. The sonographer obtained 2D images with and without manufactured contrast and also acquired 3D full-volume datasets. The following results were obtained:

LVEF (visual) = 55%	LVEF (Teicholz) = 68%
LVEF (biplane Simpson) = 56%	LVEF (3DE full volume) = 58%
LVEF (biplane Simpson with contrast) = 42%	LVEF (3DE with contrast) = 44%

Which of the following options best explains the reported variation in LVEF values?

A. The LVEF has markedly worsened and now fulfills the criteria for CTRCD.

B. The LVEF is unchanged from the previous study.

C. The LVEF has returned normal.

D. Given the extreme variations in LVEF, this data is not reliable.

E. The most accurate LVEF to report is 44%.

20. You performed myocardial strain assessment on the previous echo and compared results to this newly obtained, repeat study. The following selected results were reported on myocardial mechanics assessment:

BASELINE ECHO	
Global longitudinal strain = −14%	Global radial strain = +38%
REPEAT ECHO	
Global longitudinal strain = −19%	Global radial strain = +40%

Which of the following is the best interpretation of this data?

A. Baseline LV global function was abnormal, but repeat echo is now normal.

B. Baseline and follow-up LV global function is abnormal.

C. Cannot interpret the findings due to the marked variability of reported results.

D. Unable to report without knowing the ultrasound machine and software platform.

E. These values are all normal and within the reported variability of strain.

21. A 72-year-old female patient presents to the ER with dyspnea, fever, and hypotension. She is found to have pneumonia and bacterial sepsis requiring mechanical ventilation and admission to the ICU. Examination reveals BP 88/50 mm Hg and HR 118 bpm. Her past medical history is significant for HFpEF and renal insufficiency. You were asked to perform a POCUS to estimate her volume status as they initiate therapy.

Which of the following findings would best suggest hypovolemia as a cause of hypotension?

A. LV internal diameter at end diastole <4.4 cm

B. LV internal diameter at end systole <2.0 cm

C. IVC = 1.8 cm at expiration and 0.5 cm at inspiration

D. Hyperdynamic LVEF with midcavity gradient >25 mm Hg

E. LVOT velocity time integral <18 cm

22. A 58-year-old male admitted overnight to the observation unit was found to have serially increasing cardiac biomarkers and persistent chest pain despite therapy for ACS. ECG reveals nonspecific T-wave changes in the precordial leads. You recommend an urgent revascularization strategy and perform an echocardiogram while awaiting transfer of the patient to the cardiac catheterization laboratory.

At coronary angiography, 3V CAD is found and the patient undergoes a CABG operation. On postop day 7, the patient has progressed extremely well and is awaiting discharge when a repeat echocardiogram is performed. The results of the two serial echo studies are compared.

Which of the following changes is considered a clinically important change?

A. LV internal diameter at diastole changed from 56 to 53 mm.
B. RV TAPSE changed from 19 to 14 mm.
C. E/A ratio changed from 2.1 to 0.8.
D. E/e′ ratio changed from 13 to 9.
E. RVSP changed from 55 to 40 mm Hg.

23. A 24-year-old female presents to your clinic with a history of murmur noted on exam. She denies chest pain, syncope, palpitations, or dyspnea, but comments that she seemed to never be able to keep up with her childhood friends' sports activities. On exam, BP 118/72 mm Hg; HR 78 bpm with respiratory variation. JVP not elevated. Normal S1; wide, fixed split S2; P2 normal. No S3. No S4. Soft 2/6 systolic ejection murmur is best heard at the base.

Echocardiography demonstrates a normal LV and RV size and function and confirms a secundum ASD. You are asked if heart surgery is required and whether a percutaneous ASD closure device should be placed. Which of the following is true?

A. There is no indication for ASD closure.
B. Percutaneous ASD closure device should be placed if defect diameter is >38 mm.
C. Percutaneous ASD closure device should be placed if >1 of 4 septal rims exceeds 5 mm.
D. Surgical ASD closure should be performed if an anomalous pulmonary vein is seen.
E. Surgical ASD closure should be performed if there is >1 defect.

24. The patient above returned to your ER 48 hours after successful percutaneous closure device placement with abrupt chest pain and syncope. BP = 80/56 mm Hg; HR = 122 bpm. A pericardial friction rub is noted on exam. An urgent TTE is performed and demonstrates a moderate pericardial effusion that is partially echo-free. Which of the following is the most appropriate next step in management?

A. Colchicine and NSAID Rx
B. Urgent TEE
C. Urgent cardiac catheterization
D. Emergency pericardiocentesis
E. Cardiac surgery

25. An 86-year-old male is seen in clinic for routine follow-up of hypertension, which has been mostly controlled (carvedilol 25 mg bid; losartan 40 mg). He has no other significant past medical history. He denies any complaints. He states that he had an echocardiogram performed during his last visit and wants to know how the results of this recent TTE compared to his first echo more than 20 years earlier. On exam, BP 144/82 mm Hg. HR 72 bpm regular. JVP normal. S1 normal and S2 paradoxically split. No murmur or gallop. ECG = sinus, normal axis, and LBBB pattern.

	ECHO (THIS YEAR)	ECHO (20 YEARS EARLIER)
IVS	10.8 mm	12.0 mm
PW	10.1 mm	12.0 mm
LVIDd	5.4 cm	4.6 cm
LVEF	60%	65%
LV mass	212 g	188 g
LVd volume	108 mL	96 mL

Assuming that each of these measurements is accurately obtained, which of the serial changes between these two echo studies would suggest a pathologic worsening?

A. None of these serial changes represent pathologic worsening.
B. LV wall thickness.
C. LVEF.
D. LV mass.
E. LV diastolic volume.

26. A 36-year-old male with hypertension is seen in clinic. He takes enalapril 20 mg bid and states this has controlled his BP for the past 2 years. He is a competitive athlete and recently completed a 26.2 mile race in under 3 hours. His personal best was under 2 hours and 30 minutes when he was 24 years old. He denies any symptoms, but was noted to have a health screening abnormal ECG (reported as high QRS voltage and nonspecific ST changes).

Results of his echocardiogram are listed below:

IVS = 12 mm

PWD = 12 mm

LVDd = 62

Relative wall thickness = 0.39

LV volume index = 78 mL/m^2

LV mass index = 112 mg/m^2

Which of the following left ventricular geometric patterns does this best represent?

A. Normal geometry
B. Concentric hypertrophy
C. Eccentric hypertrophy
D. Physiologic hypertrophy
E. Mixed hypertrophy

27. A 60-year-old man with hypertension was seen for follow-up in your clinic. He has had hypertension for over 10 years and has been treated to goal BP for the past 3 years. He currently takes losartan 40 mg, amlodipine 10 mg, and HCTZ 25 mg once daily. During his initial evaluation, an ECG and 2D echocardiogram were performed and demonstrated moderate concentric LVH. He asks to have a repeat echocardiogram to see if his LVH has "gone away."

Which of the following is the best response to this patient?

A. Perform repeat 2D echo to confirm LV regression.
B. Perform a 3D echo to confirm LV regression.
C. Perform repeat 2D echo since progressive LVH warrants increased antihypertensive treatment.
D. Do not perform repeat 2D echo since the test–retest variability limits any use of the results.
E. Do not perform repeat 2D echo since LVH regression does not correlate with prognosis.

28. You are called by a junior sonographer in your echocardiography lab since the technical director was unavailable. She wants to know if she is placing herself at personal risk if she performs the requested TTE on a patient who just received a radioisotope injection as part of a 2-day nuclear myocardial perfusion imaging SPECT test. The indication for the TTE was to evaluate global and regional LV function in a patient with chest pain. The study was considered urgent, but not emergent.

Which of the following would be the most appropriate response?

A. There is zero risk to the sonographer.
B. The TTE should be delayed 48 hours.
C. If pregnant, she should ask a nonpregnant colleague to complete the exam.
D. The sonographer should wear a lead apron during the examination.
E. The TTE exam should be performed right-handed.

29. A TTE was ordered on a 60-year-old male with severe obesity and respiratory failure on mechanical ventilation in the medical intensive care unit. The study is planned as a portable exam. Which of the following is most accurate regarding the image quality in this patient?

A. Image quality may be good.
B. The sonographer should travel with LV-manufactured contrast for LV opacification.
C. Contrast can be added on a subsequent study if it is demonstrated to be necessary.
D. Ultrasound contrast would be considered a contraindication in this patient.
E. If a previous echo demonstrates that contrast was not used, it will not be needed on this exam.

30. You are consulted on a 42-year-old male with a stroke. His history is significant for a previous cryptogenic stroke 8 months earlier. MRI confirms three different vascular territory small ischemic events with different ages. He had a normal ECG and 60-day transient event monitor at the time of his previous stoke. He also had a reportedly normal TTE and peripheral vascular ultrasound although these were not available for review by you. He was treated with aspirin upon discharge and was progressing well with his rehabilitation until this event. The neurology team is strongly suspicious of an embolic event and requests a repeat echocardiogram.

Which of the following combinations of options listed below results in the **highest likelihood** to detect a patent foramen ovale?

ULTRASOUND METHOD	PHYSIOLOGIC MANEUVER	CONTRAST/ BUBBLE OPTION	INJECTION ROUTE
1. 2D TTE TH	7. Resting	10. Normal saline	13. Right arm
2. 2D TTE FI	8. Valsalva maneuver	11. Bacteriostatic saline	14. Left arm
3. 2D TEE	9. Valsalva release	12. Bacteriostatic/ blood mixture	15. Leg vein
4. TTE CFD			
5. TEE CFD			
6. TCD			

TH, tissue harmonics; FI, fundamental imaging; CFD, color-flow Doppler; TCD, transcranial Doppler.

A. 1 + 8 + 10 + 13
B. 2 + 7 + 11 + 14
C. 5 + 9 + 10 + 13
D. 3 + 9 + 12 + 15
E. 6 + 8 + 12 + 15
F. 4 + 7 + 11 + 14

TTE-agitated saline macrobubble study performed via a **lower extremity** injection **during the release of the Valsalva maneuver.**

31. A 55-year-old male is seen in the emergency department because of chest pain. ECG reveals nonspecific inferolateral ST and T-wave changes. His pain decreased from 9/10 severity to 3/10 after the first sublingual nitro and completely resolved after the second. You were consulted and at the bedside immediately after his CP resolved. Exam reveals BP 144/86 mm Hg; HR 86 bpm; normal S1 and S2. A soft S4 is noted. No murmurs or rubs.

You perform a bedside 2D echo for wall motion assessment (see Videos 51.3 to 51.6).

Which of the following is the most correct interpretation of this echo?

A. Unable to measure the WMSI
B. WMSI = 1.0 to 1.1
C. WMSI = 1.2 to 1.4
D. WMSI = 1.5 to 1.7
E. WMSI = 1.8 to 2.0

32. Which of the following statements is most correct?

   A. A wall motion score index of 1.0 in a high-quality study predicts a very low (<1%) risk of an acute myocardial infarction.

   B. A regional wall motion abnormality is ≥10× more likely than normal motion to be found in a patient with an acute myocardial infarction.

   C. A wall motion score index >1.5 predicts a very poor clinical outcome.

   D. It is most important to use a 17-segment model to measure the wall motion score index.

   E. Since his chest pain was not resolved, there is no added value in performing echo.

33. A 58-year-old female with poorly controlled hypertension undergoes an echocardiogram for progressive dyspnea. Based upon FIGURE 51.1, which of the following statements is most accurate?

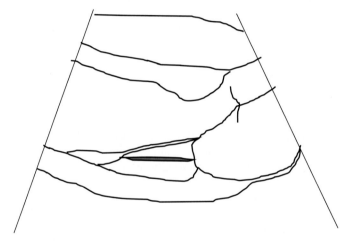

FIGURE 51.1

   A. An M-mode–derived LV mass of 90 g/m² would be abnormal.

   B. 2D would be more accurate than M-mode.

   C. Short axis would likely be more accurate than long axis.

   D. The 2D measure should be performed in the mid LV.

   E. A 3D-derived LV mass value would be necessary.

34. As the echo lab director, you were asked to resolve a discrepancy on the reported LA size in a 60-year-old male patient that presented with new, paroxysmal atrial fibrillation. Your EP colleague is considering various approaches to optimal management, but these options are based upon the LA size.

PSLAX LA 2D diameter (diastole)	4.6 cm
PSSAX LA M-mode diameter (systole)	5.0 cm
LA indexed volume (ellipsoid)	35 mL/m²
LA indexed volume (disk summation)	49 mL/m²
TEE SAX LAD	4.2 cm
TEE indexed volume	30 mL/m²

Which of the following is the most accurate statement to tell your EP colleague?

   A. The LA diameter is within normal limits.

   B. The LA diameter is mildly increased.

   C. The LA volume index is normal.

   D. The LA volume index is mild to moderately increased.

   E. The LA volume index is severely dilated.

35. An asymptomatic 62-year-old male with stage B mitral stenosis (valve area = 1.6 cm²) and normal LV systolic function on a transthoracic echocardiogram last year is seen in clinic.

Which of the following is most correct regarding follow-up?

   A. A repeat TTE should be performed during this visit.

   B. He should be scheduled for a repeat echo next year.

   C. He won't need another echo for 2 more years unless symptoms develop.

   D. He won't need another clinic visit for 2 more years.

   E. A TEE should be performed within the next year.

36. An 82-year-old female with recent light-headedness and near syncope is seen in clinic. She recalls a lengthy history of a heart murmur. She denies frank syncope, heart failure, or chest pain. She has not undergone cardiac testing in the past. On examination, BP 150/78 mm Hg; HR 78 bpm; normal JVP; normal carotid upstroke without bruits. Normal S1 and normally split S2; no gallops. 3/6 harsh systolic murmur at the base. No diastolic murmur.

Echocardiography reveals normal LV size and function. V1 = 1.2 m/s; V2 = 3.6 m/s.

Which of the following is the next best step in the management of this patient?

   A. Arrange serial follow-up.

   B. Perform TEE.

   C. Perform cardiac cath.

   D. Perform exercise stress test.

   E. Recommend TAVR/SAVR evaluation.

37. An 83-year-old female with stage D AS is evaluated by the heart valve multidisciplinary team for possible TAVR after being refused SAVR at her local hospital. She was in good health until breast cancer requiring mastectomy and chemo/hormonal therapy 2 years earlier. She has since recovered and said to be cancer free. Her oncologist states her life expectancy is >12 months. She has no other major comorbidities but would greatly prefer a nonthoracotomy intervention.

Which of the following is the most appropriate recommendation?

   A. Close follow-up.

   B. Perform Surgical AVR.

   C. Perform TAVR.

   D. Perform percutaneous balloon valvuloplasty.

   E. Recommend palliative medicine.

38. A 52-year-old asymptomatic male with aortic regurgitation is seen in clinic for annual follow-up. He denies dyspnea or chest pain and states he walks for 30 minutes at a time, 4 days each week without symptoms. On exam, BP 135/82 mm Hg; HR 82 bpm; 2/6 SEM at the base with an ejection click; 3/4 holodiastolic murmur at the LSB. An echo performed 1 month ago revealed a bicuspid AV, no stenosis, and moderate to severe AR; effective regurgitant volume = 0.35 cm^2; regurgitant fraction = 55%; LVEF = 45% to 50% and the LV cavity was mildly dilated.

Which of the following is the most appropriate next step in management?

A. Schedule annual follow-up
B. Exercise stress test
C. Dobutamine stress echo with Doppler
D. Nifedipine 30 mg daily
E. Aortic valve replacement

39. A 29-year-old female recently emigrated from Bangladesh is seen for the first time in your clinic with a complaint of severe dyspnea on exertion. She admits to having a known cardiac murmur since a prolonged illness as a preadolescent. She denies syncope, but describes chest tightness with her dyspnea on <1 block exertion or <1 flight of stairs. Exam is consistent with severe mitral stenosis and mild mitral regurgitation. BP 118/70 mm Hg; HR 70 bpm. ECG = atrial fibrillation with controlled rate. Medications include digoxin 0.25 mg daily. You perform echocardiography, which confirms normal LV size and function, normal RV size and function, normal RVSP, rheumatic MV changes (Wilkins score = 6), and mild MR; a small, mobile thrombus is seen in the posterior left atrium.

Mitral inflow demonstrates PHT = 178 ms; MVA = 1.2 cm^2 (averaged over 10 beats).

Which of the following is the most appropriate next step in management?

A. IV heparin, oral warfarin, and elective cardioversion in 4 weeks
B. Cardiac catheterization
C. Transesophageal echocardiography
D. Percutaneous MV balloon commissurotomy
E. Mitral valve replacement

40. A 58-year-old male patient with stage D mitral regurgitation is seen in clinic with complaints of progressive dyspnea. Cardiac catheterization reveals normal coronary arteries. Echocardiography confirms normal LVEF = 65%; mildly dilated LV cavity; the Carpentier MV classification is type II, P2; ERO = 0.5 cm^2; regurgitant volume = 75 mL; LAVI = 50 mL/m^2. The cardiac surgeon is planning on a mitral valve replacement operation using a pericardial bioprosthesis.

Which of the following is the best approach to this patient's management?

A. Suggest that he proceed with the currently planned surgery.
B. Recommend that the surgeon instead uses a bileaflet mechanical MVR.
C. Recommend that the surgery be performed by another cardiac surgeon.
D. Perform a transesophageal echocardiogram prior to surgery.
E. Postpone surgery and arrange close follow-up after initiation of lisinopril.

41. A 66-year-female with palpitations is seen in urgent care and found to have new-onset atrial fibrillation on ECG. Regarding the appropriateness of echocardiography in this patient, which of the following statements is most accurate?

A. TTE is always appropriate in atrial fibrillation regardless of symptoms.
B. TTE would only be appropriate if the patient had chest pain.
C. TTE would only be appropriate if ECG demonstrated abnormal findings.
D. TEE would be considered appropriate regardless of symptoms.
E. TEE would be appropriate if the patient had stroke symptoms.

42. This patient was in good health and asymptomatic, except for her recent 2-day complaint of palpitations, and she denies hypertension, coronary artery disease, hyperlipidemia, or diabetes. Cardiac examination reveals BP 150/90 mm Hg; HR 120 bpm irregular; normal JVP; no murmurs, rubs, or S3 gallop. Her echocardiogram was reported as normal LV size and function, no LV wall thickening, and the LAVI = 30 mL/m^2. Mitral valve has moderate mitral annular calcification, but there is no LA to LV gradient.

Which of the following is most accurate?

A. This patient has lone atrial fibrillation.
B. Most likely, her cause for AF will be revealed by measuring her TSH lab value.
C. Most likely, etiology for AF is undiagnosed hypertension.
D. Elective immediate cardioversion is indicated and considered safe.
E. Lifelong anticoagulation is warranted due to the dilated LA and abnormal MV.

43. Subsequent evaluation of this patient resulted in the detection of 3V CAD and scheduled CABG surgery with maze operation. She also underwent LAA ligation (stapling exclusion) at the time of the surgery and is now being seen in your clinic. ECG reveals atrial fibrillation. She has tolerated warfarin and has no bleeding risks. Which of the following statements is most accurate?

A. Anticoagulation is no longer necessary.

B. A routine TEE should be performed to determine the need to continue anticoagulation.

C. Anticoagulation should be continued despite the LAA ligation.

D. A wave >50 cm/s on TTE Doppler mitral inflow would be adequate to avoid warfarin.

44. A 44-year-old male is seen for routine follow-up in your ambulatory clinic. His past history is significant for coarctation repair as a child and hypertension treated with lisinopril 40 mg and atenolol 100 mg daily. He states he is well and denies any symptoms. Family history is normal. Examination reveals BP 128/80 mm Hg (right arm = left arm); HR 62 bpm; JVP normal without bruit. PMI is normal; 2/6 SEM; soft ejection click; no gallop. Normal peripheral pulses. Trace pedal edema.

Echocardiography reveals normal LV and RV function; mild LV wall thickening; bicuspid aortic valve with no stenosis; mild AR; aortic root (leading edge-leading edge method) = 56 mm; ascending aorta = 48 mm; arch = 25 mm. These measures were consistent with a CTA scan performed 6 months earlier.

Which of the following is next most appropriate step in management?

A. Aortic valve replacement.

B. Aortic root replacement.

C. Add HCTZ 25 mg daily.

D. Repeat CTA.

E. Close follow-up in 6 months.

45. A 66-year-old man with chest pain is seen in clinic. He is known to have CAD and underwent circumflex PCI 2 years ago. His symptoms are consistent with typical angina. He denies rest symptoms and states that his chest pain has not been progressive, but occurs consistently with activities. Medications (unchanged in past year) include baby aspirin, Lipitor 20 mg, Norvasc 10 mg, and Imdur 30 mg daily. Exam reveals BP 128/78 mm Hg; HR 62 bpm; normal focused CV exam. ECG normal. He had an adequate quality stress echocardiogram 3 months ago that was reportedly normal after 8 minutes of exercise on a Bruce protocol.

Which of the following would be the most appropriate next step in management of this patient?

A. Continue current medical therapy.

B. Increase Imdur or add beta-blocker.

C. Schedule coronary angiography.

D. Perform exercise stress ECG.

E. Repeat exercise stress echocardiography.

46. An active 68-year-old woman is seen in your clinic seeking clearance prior to starting an exercise and diet weight loss program. She has a history of hypertension and takes losartan 40 mg daily. She walks 3 to 4 miles/daily and swims for 1 hour/day on weekends. She describes chest pressure at her peak heart rate, but denies frank chest pain. Occasional dyspnea is also noted with the pressure, but this always resolves "quickly when I rest." ECG and echocardiogram have been obtained.

Which of the following options would be the best approach to risk stratify this patient?

A. No further diagnostic investigation is warranted.

B. Exercise stress echocardiography.

C. Exercise nuclear SPECT MPI.

D. Pharmacologic stress echocardiography.

E. Invasive coronary angiography.

47. The use of exercise testing instead of pharmacologic stress in this patient would result in which of the following?

A. Increased likelihood of a false-negative nuclear SPECT result.

B. Increased likelihood of a false-negative stress echocardiography result.

C. Higher rate of anteroseptal and apical wall motion abnormalities.

D. Reduced diagnostic sensitivity and specificity.

E. A normal test result would confer an excellent clinical outcome.

48. You are asked to consult on a 72-year-old female in the hospital for risk assessment prior to urgent, nonemergent, hip surgery. Due to limited mobility and a heart murmur, the surgeon obtained an echocardiogram.

Which of the following findings would predict the highest short-term cardiovascular event rate?

A. Heart failure symptoms and a global LVEF > 50%

B. Asymptomatic with a reduced global LVEF < 50%

C. Asymptomatic LV diastolic dysfunction

D. Mild-to-moderate AS

E. Mild-to-moderate MR

49. A 51-year-old female is seen in the emergency department with moderate heart failure symptoms. She has no past medical history and denies alcohol or other substance abuse. An echocardiogram confirms a dilated cardiomyopathy with global LV systolic dysfunction and LVEF = 28%. No regional wall motion abnormalities or more than mild valve regurgitation. She states that her younger sister also has a cardiomyopathy and the sister was told it was "idiopathic."

ECG = IVCD; nonspecific ST changes.

Nuclear SPECT MPI = normal perfusion; LV dilatation; reduced global LVEF = 30%.

In addition to GDMT, which of the following would be considered most appropriate in this patient?

A. Coronary angiography
B. Cardiac CTA
C. Screening echo on all asymptomatic siblings
D. Dobutamine echocardiography
E. ICD placement
F. Cardiac resynchronization therapy

50. A 54-year-old male with increasing episodic chest pain was seen in clinic. His past history is significant for CABG 10 years earlier. His chest pain is described as substernal, exertional, and lasts 15 to 20 minutes despite recent efforts to maximize his GDMT. Chest pain resolves with rest or 1 to 2 s/l ntg pills. He underwent a dobutamine stress echocardiogram and the results are as follows:

BASELINE FINDINGS

BP = 128/80 mm Hg

HR = 72 bpm

WMSI = 2.25

LOW-DOSE FINDINGS (10 mcg/kg/min)

BP = 130/78 mm Hg

HR = 76 bpm

WMSI = 1.52

PEAK STRESS FINDINGS (40 mcg/kg/min; 1.0 mg atropine)

BP = 118/70 mm Hg

HR = 154 bpm

WMSI = 2.48

In addition to GDMT, which of the following would be the most appropriate?

A. Refer to exercise rehab program.
B. Coronary angiography.
C. Cardiac CTA.
D. Resting thallium SPECT MPI.
E. PET scan.

51. Three-vessel CAD is found on coronary angiography for the patient in Question 40, and the heart team determines that there are adequate targets for revascularization.

Which of the following would be the most appropriate next step in management?

A. Refer to exercise rehab program alone.
B. Perform cardiac MRI scan.
C. Perform PET scan.
D. Redo CABG surgery.
E. Single-vessel PCI to the most severe lesion.
F. Transplant and/or device evaluation.

52. The patient is considering his options for revascularization or GDMT alone. He would like additional information regarding his risks/benefits of surgery to help him decide.

Which of the following statements is most accurate based upon his clinical presentation and DSE results?

A. Coronary angiography will likely demonstrate a coronary plaque rupture.
B. The peak dose WMSI is only possible with multivessel ischemia.
C. The improved low-dose WMSI implies high likelihood of LVEF recovery after surgery.
D. The rest to low to peak dose WMSI pattern implies a favorable clinical outcome.
E. The severely reduced LVEF makes CABG surgery very high risk.

53. A 29-year-old male undergoes TTE for abnormal ECG and murmur. A representative parasternal long-axis image is displayed in Video 51.1. Continuous-wave Doppler maximal LV outflow velocity = 240 cm/s.

Which of the following is the most accurate diagnosis?

A. Equivocal for hypertrophic cardiomyopathy.
B. Athlete's heart.
C. Hypertrophic nonobstructive cardiomyopathy.
D. Hypertrophic obstructive cardiomyopathy.
E. Additional Doppler info is required.

54. A repeat Doppler cursor was placed in the LVOT during a Valsalva maneuver and the continuous-wave Doppler maximal LV outflow velocity = 410 cm/s.

Which of the following is most correct?

A. A mean gradient >30 mm Hg at rest or provocation warrants interventional treatments.
B. A peak gradient >30 suggests HOCM.
C. Absence of a peak gradient >50 mm Hg at rest requires no further treatment.
D. Gradients may vary based upon the time of the day and food intake.
E. Low-dose dobutamine is an excellent method for gradient provocation.
F. Exercise is considered a contraindication.

55. You are supervising a 40-year-old male with hypertrophic CM and a resting LVOT gradient of 25 mm Hg. He is scheduled to undergo a stress Doppler echo using a Bruce protocol. He completes stage 2 and stops due to dyspnea at 7 minutes of total exercise.

Which of the following is most accurate regarding his blood pressure to exercise?

A. A drop in SBP > 20 mm Hg at peak exercise is a common finding.
B. An increased pulse pressure is associated with sudden cardiac death.
C. Increased SBP > 20 mm Hg in stage I is a low-risk finding regardless of subsequent BP.
D. A flat SPB response (<20 mm Hg total increase) is a high-risk finding.
E. A modified Bruce protocol is preferred over a Bruce protocol.

56. Stress echocardiography is traditionally used to assess known or suspected ischemic heart disease. Separate from the detection of myocardial ischemia, which of the following stress echo parameters and clinical condition combinations adds proven clinical value?

A. Mean transmitral gradient increase >5 mm Hg in MV prosthesis
B. Mean transmitral gradient increase >4 mm Hg after MV repair
C. Change in global longitudinal strain <5% in primary MR
D. Reduction in TAPSE < 19 mm in primary MR
E. Increase LVEF < 10% in primary MR

57. Exercise is the preferred method of stress for the provocation of ischemia during stress echocardiography. Which of the following statements is most correct regarding the hemodynamic impact of exercise in a normal volunteer?

A. Heart rate increases ≥4×.
B. Systolic blood pressure increases ≥2×.
C. Systemic vascular resistance increases ≥50%.
D. Pulmonary artery systolic pressure falls.
E. Coronary blood flow increases ≥3×.

58. A 45-year-old male with hypertrophic cardiomyopathy undergoes a stress Doppler echocardiogram. Past history is significant for symptomatic LVOT obstruction with a resting gradient >50 mm Hg. With metoprolol 100 mg twice daily, the resting gradient decreased to <20 mm Hg and symptoms improved until recently. The referring physician is now wanting to assess changes with exercise.

Which of the following echo findings during exercise echocardiography are associated with poor clinical outcomes and not just markers of poor exercise tolerance.

A. Increase in postexercise LVOT gradient >50 mm Hg despite holding metoprolol.
B. Increased exercise LVOT gradient >40 mm Hg on metoprolol.
C. A paradoxical decrease in the LVOT gradient from 40 to 25 mm Hg.
D. Increase in MR from mild to moderately severe.
E. Systolic BP increases from 120 to 125 mm Hg at peak exercise.
F. E/e' ratio changes from 10 to 20.

59. A 39-year-old female with heart failure (LVEF 30%) from a suspected nonischemic etiology undergoes a pharmacologic stress echocardiogram.

Which of the following findings are more consistent with a nonischemic than an ischemic response to stress echo?

A. WMSI at baseline = 2.3; peak dobutamine = 1.8
B. Seven akinetic wall segments noted at peak dobutamine
C. Biphasic response to dobutamine
D. Coronary flow reserve increase >2.0 with vasodilator

Answer 1: E. This question specifically asks why 3D is more commonly used in children compared with adults and did not ask why 3D is preferred over 2D.

Choice A is incorrect since it is a noninvasive tool in both adults and children.

Choice B is incorrect for the same reason as A—"crossplane" capabilities available in both populations.

Choice C is incorrect as well since "real-time nature of technique and improved LV volumes and LVEF" apply to both populations.

Choice D similarly applies to the specific question being asked—"ability to obtain 2D and 3D datasets with the same probe and noninvasive nature of technique" apply across populations.

Choice E is correct: children have improved acoustic windows compared to most larger adults, and therefore, the 3D dataset is better quality. Also, with enhanced spatial relationships and greater anatomic understanding, 3DE is critically important in "presurgical planning." Older adults have often been palliated and "presurgical planning" is less commonly the critical issue.

Suggested Reading
Simpson J, et al. Three-dimensional echocardiography in congenital heart disease: an expert consensus document from the European Association of Cardiovascular Imaging and the American Society of Echocardiography. *J Am Soc Echocardiogr* 2017;30(1):1–27. http://dx.doi.org/10.1016/j.echo.2016.08.022

Answer 2: E. The term "surgical" view is used to describe 3D projections reflecting the surgeon's view during an operation. The surgical view is projected as if the patient is lying supine with the lead surgeon operating from the right side of the patient. The "anatomic" view is projected as if the person is standing upright. The effect of this is that an anatomic en face view of the right side of the atrial or ventricular septum would be *rotated counter clockwise 90 degrees* when projecting a "surgical" view.

Option A is incorrect since it is projected as if the patient is lying **supine**.

Option B is incorrect since it is akin to the lead surgeon's view operating from the **right** side of the patient.

Option C is incorrect as it results in an "en face" view of the **right** side of the atrial septum rotated 90 degrees **counterclockwise**.

Option D is therefore also incorrect.

Option E is the only correct option, and moving from the 6 o'clock position to a 3 o'clock position is the same as rotating counterclockwise 90 degrees.

Answer 3: C. 3D echo should be regarded as a technique that complements rather than replaces 2D echo for assessment of congenital heart diseases. 3DE use has increased as technology has improved, but there is wide institutional variability. There are *no randomized trials* relating to procedural success, morbidity, or mortality related to the application of 3D echo; it has been adopted into practice on the basis of a clinical need to provide additional diagnostic information. 3D echo is reported to be most valuable in valvular lesions and atrial/ventricular septal defects (e.g., decision-making in patients with DORV where surgical planning is determined based upon the size and location of the VSD relative to the position of the great arteries. With 3D, the added *depth of field* from a full-volume acquisition improves visualization of the position and size of the VSD relative to the great arteries).

Option A is incorrect as there are **no randomized clinical trials** comparing 2D to 3D.

Option B is incorrect, since given A, morbidity and mortality cannot have been studied.

Option C is correct. Valvular lesions and septal defects have been primarily responsible for its clinical utilization and growth of application. Also, complex anatomic relationships may be improved with 3D compared with 2D.

Option D is clearly incorrect as there is a much greater **inconsistency** across institutions regarding its application.

Option E is incorrect as 3D should be considered complementary to 2D similar to the use of Doppler with 2D. It is not intended to replace 2D, and even if the entire study is obtained using a 3D probe, the reader will need to take advantage of single-cut planes (2D) displays for optimal interpretation.

Suggested Readings

Charakida M, Qureshi S, Simpson JM. 3D echocardiography for planning and guidance of interventional closure of VSD. *JACC Cardiovasc Imaging* 2013;6:120–123.

Pushparajah K, Miller OI, Simpson JM. 3D echocardiography of the atrial septum: anatomical features and landmarks for the echocardiographer. *JACC Cardiovasc Imaging* 2010;3:981–984.

Saric M, Perk G, Purgess JR, et al. Imaging atrial septal defects by real-time three-dimensional transesophageal echocardiography: step-by-step approach. *J Am Soc Echocardiogr* 2010;23:1128–1135.

Sivakumar K, Singhi A, Pavithran S. Enface reconstruction of VSD on RV septal surface using real-time 3D echocardiography. *JACC Cardiovasc Imaging* 2012;5:1176–1180.

Answer 4: *B.* Option B is correct since TGA is associated with maternal diabetes.

Option A is incorrect. This patient had transposition of the great arteries (TGA), which is often palliated with an atrial switch operation (either Mustard or Senning). This is the SECOND most common cyanotic heart defect in newborns (TOF is the most common).

Option C is incorrect since there is no known genetic mutation or common genetic syndrome associated, although it is highly likely that a genetic etiology exists.

Option D is incorrect since coronary ischemia is NOT a common complication. Certainly, coronary anomalies may coexist, but ischemia is not common. Conversely, the arterial switch operation (ASO, or Jatene repair) is at more of a risk for coronary ischemia from the necessity to reimplant the coronaries and the associated risk of coronary kinking from maneuvering the pulmonary artery branches anteriorly to the aorta and tucking the aorta behind the PA (LeCompte maneuver).

Option E is incorrect since males are effected with TGA more than females in a >2:1 ratio.

Suggested Readings

Cohen MS, et al. Multimodality imaging guidelines of patients with transposition of the great arteries: a report from the American Society of Echocardiography Developed in Collaboration with the Society for Cardiovascular Magnetic Resonance and the Society of Cardiovascular Computed Tomography. *J Am Soc Echocardiogr* 2016;29:571–621.

Lisowski LA, Verheijen PM, Copel JA, et al. Congenital heart disease in pregnancies complicated by maternal diabetes mellitus. An international clinical collaboration, literature review, and meta-analysis. *Herz* 2010;35:19–26.

Answer 5: *A.* This basic anatomic, congenital question requires the reader to understand what a "conus" is and how this differs in TGA versus a normally developed heart (e.g., the most common adult echo). A subaortic conus (muscle remnant) should not be seen in the normal heart, but this conal anatomy (aka mitral-to-aortic discontinuity) is seen in the great majority of patients with TGA.

Transposition of the great arteries represents a conotruncal malformation or anomaly. During development of the normal heart, the conotruncus (representing the primitive outflow tracts and semilunar valves) rotates such that the pulmonary artery is aligned with the right ventricle and the aorta is aligned with the left ventricle (ventricular–arterial discordance).

Conus is defined as the ring of muscle that sits entirely under a great vessel. Conus can be present under one, both, or neither great artery. In the normal heart, *subpulmonary conus* is present (muscular separation between the tricuspid and pulmonary valves; aka *tricuspid to pulmonic fibrous discontinuity*), and there is no *subaortic conus* (aka *mitral-to-aortic fibrous continuity*). The most common conal morphology in patients with TGA is persistence of the subaortic conus with regression of the subpulmonary conus (seen in 88% to 96% of patients with TGA). Bilateral conus is rare and seen in approximately 5% of TGA.

Option B is incorrect as a subpulmonic conus is seen in normal development (aka tricuspid to pulmonic discontinuity).

Option C is incorrect since a bilateral conus is a rare finding.

Option D is incorrect since mitral-to-aortic fibrous continuity is expected in normal hearts.

Option E is incorrect since tricuspid to pulmonary fibrous discontinuity is seen in normals.

Answer 6: *C.* This question requires the reader to **understand the "late" complications after ASO** procedures, which include pulmonary hypertension, LV dysfunction, pulmonary stenosis, supravalvular aortic stenosis, neoaortic (or pulmonic) valve regurgitation, aortopulmonary collateral vessels, and, importantly, coronary artery kinking and stenosis. Since this patient has new dyspnea on exertion, PVCs on ECG, and anteroseptal hypokinesis on echo, *ischemia should be strongly considered.*

Transection of the great arteries with translocation and reanastomosis, along with translocation of the CAs (Jatene; ASO), has potential consequences that require long-term transthoracic echocardiographic evaluation. These include RV outflow tract obstruction and branch pulmonary artery stenosis, complications of the neoaortic root and valve, subaortic obstruction, and late complications of the CAs.

Patients with coronary stenosis or occlusion may be asymptomatic, and the findings on TTE are often subtle. Regional wall motion abnormalities or progressive ventricular dilation and dysfunction may be clues to coronary stenosis or occlusion. Stress echocardiography can be used as a screening tool to evaluate for regional wall motion abnormalities. Ventricular ectopy late after ASO is unusual and should prompt investigation for CA ischemia.

Option A is not the best answer since TEE is not the initial study to evaluate for ischemia, even though a high-quality TEE examination may be able to demonstrate coronary kinking or obstruction (with pulsed Doppler velocity >60 cm/s). This procedure may be used if the primary concern was aortic or pulmonic valve disease in a poor-quality TTE.

Option B is incorrect since right heart catheterization cannot exclude coronary ischemia. This procedure may be used to assess for supravalvular stenosis, either pulmonic or aortic.

Option C is the best option as stress echocardiography is the only listed option primarily used to assess for myocardial ischemia. Cardiac CTA might be considered an appropriate alternative first-line diagnostic testing option at many institutions.

Option D is not the best first-line option, although ambulatory event monitoring may be important once ischemia is excluded. Had the patient experienced syncope with palpitations, then this option may have been considered an earlier diagnostic choice.

Option E is incorrect since until more diagnostic information is known, cardiothoracic surgery is not currently indicated.

Suggested Reading

Tsuda T, Bhat AM, Robinson BW, et al. Coronary artery problems late after arterial switch operation for transposition of the great arteries. *Circ J* 2015;79:2372–2379.

Answer 7: *D.* This question emphasizes the echo findings in patients with a **pseudonormal** mitral inflow pattern. Despite the limited details of this patient's echo Doppler findings, there is sufficient evidence of an elevated LAP (E/A ratio 2.2; E/e′ > 14; LAVI > 34 cm/m^2; TR max V > 2.8 m/s).

Option A is incorrect and would only occur if the patient is unable to perform an adequate Valsalva.

Options B and C are incorrect as the E wave velocity is expected to be reduced.

Option D is the most correct answer.

Option E is not incorrect (as the E velocity falls, the E/e′ ratio may also slightly decrease), but this ratio will not drop below the diagnostic threshold, and this ratio "change" is not used for diagnostic purposes.

Not every patient can perform this maneuver adequately. The patient must generate and sustain a sufficient increase in intrathoracic pressure, and the examiner needs to maintain the correct sample volume location between the mitral leaflet tips during the maneuver.

The E/e′ ratio is very rarely >14 in normal individuals and does not significantly alter with age. However, changes in mitral inflow velocities do change with aging, but can be exposed as pathologic with a Valsalva maneuver. The Valsalva maneuver can help distinguish normal LV filling from pseudonormal filling and can clarify whether a restrictive LV filling pattern is fixed or reversible. A decrease in E/A ratio of >50% is highly specific for increased LV filling pressures and supports the presence of diastolic dysfunction.

The procedure should be standardized by continuously recording mitral inflow using pulsed-wave Doppler for 10 seconds during the straining phase of the maneuver.

When Valsalva is used with a bubble study to provoke right-to-left shunting across a PFO, it has been demonstrated that the "release" phase exacerbates the greatest atrial septal shift and this should be timed to maximal RA bubble opacification.

Suggested Reading

Nagueh SF, et al. Recommendations for the evaluation of left ventricular diastolic function by echocardiography: an update from the American Society of Echocardiography and the European Association of Cardiovascular Imaging. *J Am Soc Echocardiogr* 2016;29:277–314.

Answer 8: *D.* See discussion accompanying the answer to Question 7.

Options A, B, and C are incorrect as a standardized protocol should be attempted to become most expert at the hemodynamic alteration(s) that ensues.

Option D is the recommended method to standardize this technique: the maneuver should be held for 10 seconds while continuous mitral inflow Doppler is recorded. This provides the best opportunity to see if the LAP is indeed elevated. This should be considered in any patient with an E/A ratio >1.2 (e.g., pseudonormal, restrictive, and normal patterns).

Option E is incorrect since changes in mitral inflow may be subtle or delayed depending upon the individual's ability to perform and hold a Valsalva maneuver. Therefore, the standard protocol is recommended so that misinterpretation may be reduced.

Suggested Reading

Nagueh SF, et al. Recommendations for the evaluation of left ventricular diastolic function by echocardiography: an update from the American Society of Echocardiography and the European Association of Cardiovascular Imaging. *J Am Soc Echocardiogr* 2016;29:277–314.

Answer 9: *C.* This patient has a reduced LVEF, known myocardial disease, and E/A ratio <0.8 with a maximal E velocity <50 cm/s.

In patients with a *depressed LVEF* or with *normal LVEF but evidence of myocardial disease*, an E/A ratio <0.8 with a peak E velocity of <50 cm/s, the mean LAP is either normal or low. This patient also has grade I diastolic dysfunction. In these patients, an E/A ratio >2.0 implies the LA mean pressure is elevated and also has grade III diastolic dysfunction.

In these patients, an E/A ratio <0.8 (but peak E velocity >50 cm/s) or an E/A ratio between 0.8 and 2.0 is insufficient to estimate the LAP, and additional parameters are required (maximal TR velocity, E/e′ ratio, and the LAVI).

If more than half of these *measurable* variables are abnormal (two-thirds or three-fourths), then the LAP is considered to be elevated and grade II diastolic dysfunction is present. If more than half of these *measurable* variables are normal (2/3 or 3/4), then the LAP is considered to be normal.

In cases of limited *measurable* parameters or equivocal 50% discordant findings, the LAP cannot be estimated and the echo results are considered inconclusive. In these cases, the pulmonary vein S/D ratio should be obtained and used as an additional parameter. A ratio <1.0 is abnormal.

Option A is incorrect since the LAP can still be estimated based upon the mitral inflow alone when certain patterns are seen (and the LV myocardium is diseased; LVEF is low).

Option B is incorrect (see option A discussion).

Option C is correct and the LAP is either normal or low in this specific pattern.

Options D and E are incorrect since the LAP is NOT likely to be increased in this pattern.

Answer 10: E. This patient has a hypertrophic cardiomyopathy based upon Video 51.1.

A comprehensive approach is recommended for assessment of LV diastolic function and filling pressures in patients with hypertrophic cardiomyopathy. This includes E/e′ ratio, LA volume index, pulmonary vein atrial reversal velocity, and peak velocity of TR jet by CW Doppler. In general, individual variables have modest correlations with LV filling pressures in patients with HCM, likely related to variability in phenotype, muscle mass, amount of myocardial fiber disarray, and obstructive versus nonobstructive physiology. This leads to different combinations of altered relaxation and compliance and resultant variations of mitral inflow patterns. Aside from assessment of LV filling pressure, 2D and Doppler indices of LV diastolic function provide incremental prognostic information in this population. An enlarged left atrium, abnormal E/e′ ratio, and restrictive LV filling pattern have each been shown to have a worse clinical outcome in adults with HCM.

Option A is incorrect since echo Doppler parameters, although imperfect, can still be used to estimate diastolic function and highlight poor prognostic findings.

Option B is not the best options since conventional measures used to estimate LV filling pressures are modestly accurate.

Options C and D are incorrect since the E/e′ ratio, LAVI, and restrictive filling patterns predict adverse outcomes in patients with HCM.

Option E is correct since a restrictive filling pattern is not universally present and, when noted, predicts adverse outcomes.

Answer 11: C. Doppler parameters recommended for the evaluation of diastolic function in patients with HCM are averaged E/e′ ratio (>14), LA volume index (>34 mL/m²), pulmonary vein atrial reversal velocity (Ar-A duration >30 ms), and peak velocity of TR jet by CW Doppler (>2.8 m/s). These parameters can be applied irrespective of the presence or absence of dynamic obstruction and MR, except for patients with more

than moderate MR, in whom *only Ar-A duration and peak velocity of TR* jet remain valid.

There are different methods for measuring mitral-to-apical flow propagation (Vp). In patients with normal LV volumes and LVEF but elevated LV filling pressures, Vp can be misleadingly normal. Furthermore, Vp has a lower feasibility and reproducibility since angulation between M-mode cursor and flow results in erroneous measurements.

In patients with depressed LVEFs and a dilated LV, Vp is a valuable measure that correlates with LV filling pressures. Combined with mitral inflow E wave, an E/Vp > 2.5 predicts PCWP > 15 mm Hg with reasonable accuracy (in low LVEF patients).

Options A and B are incorrect since the pulmonary vein S/D ratio and Ar maximal velocity are not very specific in HCM.

Option C is the best answer since the pulmonary vein Ar minus mitral A-wave duration (>30 ms) has been studied in HCM.

Option D is not accurate since a shortened DT of mitral E velocity <150 ms is not very accurate as an LAP estimate in patients with normal LV function.

Option E is also incorrect since color M-mode velocity flow propagation (Vp) has been shown to be inaccurate in HCM (and other normal LVEF populations).

Suggested Readings

Biagini E, et al. Prognostic implications of the Doppler restrictive filling pattern in hypertrophic cardiomyopathy. *Am J Cardiol* 2009;104:1727–1731.

Nagueh SF, et al. Doppler estimation of left ventricular filling pressures in patients with hypertrophic cardiomyopathy. *Circulation* 1999;99:254–261.

Answer 12: B. Understand how to measure LAP in patients with mitral and aortic valve disease.

Mitral stenosis renders assessment of LV diastolic function more challenging, but IVRT, TE-e′, and mitral inflow peak velocity at early and late diastole can be of value in the semi-quantitative prediction of mean LAP. The time interval Ar-A and IVRT/TE-e′ ratio may be applied for estimation for prediction of LV filling pressures in patients with MR and normal LVEF, whereas E/e′ ratio may be considered only in patients with MR and depressed EF. The guidelines in patients without valvular heart disease can be applied to patients with aortic stenosis, irrespective of severity of valvular stenosis. This excludes patients with heavy MAC. In patients with severe AR, be it acute or chronic, premature closure of mitral valve, diastolic MR, LA enlargement, average E/e′ ratio >14, and TR peak velocity >2.8 m/s are consistent with elevated LV filling pressures.

Moderate and severe MR leads to an elevation of peak E velocity and a decrease in pulmonary venous systolic velocity and thus the S/D ratio in pulmonary venous flow. In severe MR, pulmonary venous flow reversal can be seen in late systole. Thus, MR per se can induce changes in transmitral and pulmonary venous flow patterns resembling advanced LV diastolic dysfunction, with the possible exception of the difference in duration between Ar and mitral A velocity.

MR velocity recording by CW Doppler can provide a highly specific, though not sensitive, sign of increased LAP with early peaking ("triangle-shaped") and usually a reduced LV–LA gradient. The utility of E/e′ in predicting LV filling pressures in the setting of moderate or severe MR is more complex. In patients with depressed EFs, an increased E/e′ ratio has a direct significant relation with LAP and predicts hospitalizations and mortality. *E/e′ does not appear to be useful in patients with primary MR and normal EFs.* IVRT and the ratio of IVRT to TE-e′ correlate reasonably well with mean PCWP, regardless of EF. An IVRT/TE-e′ ratio <3 readily predicts PCWP > 15 mm Hg in this patient subgroup.

In patients with moderate to severe MAC, mitral orifice area is decreased, leading to increased diastolic transmitral velocities, while lateral or posterior e′ may be decreased due to restriction of the posterior mitral leaflet excursion. Thus, an increase in E/e′ ratio occurs due to the mechanical effect of mitral calcification.

Option A is incorrect since the assessment of LV diastolic function, although difficult, remains possible in patients with mitral stenosis.

Option B is the best option since the IVRT/TE-e′ ratio can be used to estimate LAP in patients with MR and normal LVEF.

Option C is incorrect since the E/e′ ratio is not accurate in patients with MR and a normal LVEF.

Option D is incorrect since severe mitral annular calcification grossly lowers the tissue Doppler e′ and lowers the predictive value of the E/e′ ratio as an estimate of the LV filling pressure.

Option E is incorrect since even severe AS adheres to the conventional assessment of LV diastolic function and has been demonstrated to remain an accurate estimate.

Suggested Reading

Soeki T, et al. Mitral inflow and mitral annular motion velocities in patients with mitral annular calcification: evaluation by pulsed Doppler echocardiography and pulsed Doppler tissue imaging. *Eur J Echocardiogr* 2002;3:128–134.

Answer 13: D. This patient has grade I diastolic function and a normally estimated LAP *at rest*. Importantly, though, his e′ velocities are <7 (septal) and <10 (lateral).

The most appropriate patient population for diastolic exercise testing is the group of symptomatic patients with a resting grade 1 diastolic dysfunction indicating delayed myocardial relaxation with normal resting LV filling pressures.

Diastolic stress testing is indicated when resting echocardiography does not explain the symptoms of heart failure or dyspnea, especially with exertion. In general, patients with completely normal hearts and diastolic function at rest with preserved e′ velocity (>7 cm/s for septal e′, >10 cm/s for lateral e′) need not undergo stress testing as it is highly unlikely that they will develop diastolic dysfunction and elevated filling pressures with exercise. Likewise, patients with abnormal findings at baseline consistent with elevated LV filling pressures should not be referred for diastolic stress testing as the cardiac etiology for dyspnea has already been established and

their filling pressures will almost certainly increase further with exercise.

The test is considered abnormal when all of the following three conditions are met during exercise: average E/e′ > 14 or septal E/e′ ratio > 15, peak TR velocity > 2.8 m/s, and septal e′ velocity <7 cm/s.

Option A is incorrect. An exercise nuclear myocardial perfusion imaging SPECT stress test would only assess for CAD, and this patient has a relatively low pretest probability. Furthermore, his ECG is normal (stress ECG is considered a class I indication in this population), and his echo images were "excellent quality" (allowing for a nonirradiating option had imaging been required).

Option B is incorrect as this patient has proven he can exercise and a pharmacologic stress test, such as dobutamine echocardiography (with or without Doppler), is not warranted.

Option C is wrong and there is no good indication for a transesophageal echocardiography.

Option D is the best option. Diastolic exercise testing is *reserved for patients with grade I diastolic filling parameters at rest, but worsening symptoms of dyspnea* suggesting an exertional increase in LV filling pressures.

Option E is not the best option at this time, but a right (and left) heart catheterization may become necessary if additional diagnostic information is suggestive of PAH or severe ischemia.

Option F is not the best option at this point since this patient has newly diagnosed hypertension and may very likely be experiencing increased LA pressures during exercise providing an opportunity to medication adjustment to improve symptoms.

Answer 14: D. The following are considered *high embolic potential*:

- Atrial fib/flutter
- Recent apical infarct
- Chronic LV aneurysm with clot
- Dilated cardiomyopathy
- Left heart prosthetic valves
- Native, prosthetic, and nonvalve endocarditis
- Intracardiac tumors
- Aortic atheroma (especially highly protruding and mobile)

The following considered *low embolic potential*:

- LA/LAA spontaneous echo contrast (smoke)
- LV aneurysm without clot
- MV prolapse
- Mitral annular calcification
- Calcific AS
- Fibrin strands and Lambl excrescences (even if giant)
- Septal defects/anomalies including PFO, ASD, and ASA

Options A, B, C, and E are each considered HIGH RISK for embolization.

Option D, Lambl excrescences, regardless of size (e.g., "giant") is not considered a high embolic risk.

Answer 15: *D.* Understand TEE findings and their relative risk of embolic potential.

The basis of imaging in atrial fibrillation centers on identifying one of the many underlying cardiac causes of atrial fibrillation, such as valvular heart disease, ventricular dysfunction, and hypertension.

Once an associated etiology of atrial fibrillation has been identified or ruled out, attention turns to details of LA anatomy, specifically whether the left atrium is enlarged and, if so, how severely. LA enlargement has significance relative to thromboembolic risk, maintenance of sinus rhythm, and prognosis. Although thrombus can be identified by TTE and the specificity is high, the sensitivity of TTE is unacceptably low, in part because most atrial thrombi are located in the LAA rather than the main LA cavity. LAVI is superior to LA diameters, and atrial volumes have significant prognostic value relative to stroke risk, mortality, atrial fibrillation recurrence after electrical cardioversion, ablation, and cardiac surgery.

The SPAF trial (Stroke Prevention in Atrial Fibrillation trial) randomized patients to warfarin versus aspirin for primary stroke prophylaxis. A substudy looked at the LAA data obtained by TEE and found independent predictors of thromboembolism: presence of LAA clot (RR, 3.5), aortic plaque (RR, 2.1), and low LAA peak flow velocity <27 cm/s (RR, 1.7).

Options A, C, and E are incorrect since it is presumed that the highest risk for stroke is an actual thrombus seen in the LAA.

Options B and D place the highest risk (LAA clot) first and, therefore, either could be the correct option.

Option B incorrectly lists atrial velocity (relative risk 1.7) ahead of aortic plaque (with a slightly higher RR of 2.1).

Answer 16: *A.* Recognize the important indications for performing a TEE as first-line procedure over a TTE in patients with endocarditis.

Sensitivity and specificity for native leaflet or cusp perforation diagnosis have been estimated at 45% and 98%, respectively, for TTE and 95% and 98%, respectively, for TEE. Therefore, TEE is considered a first-line modality when suspecting endocarditis complications (perforation, abscess), prosthetic valve endocarditis, *Staphylococcus aureus* bacteremia, and intracardiac devices (i.e., pacemakers) and when transthoracic echocardiographic images are suboptimal.

TTE is the first-line modality for all other situations and may be sufficient to suggest searching for another source of infection if the clinical suspicion for endocarditis is low and the test results are negative (note: the specificity of TTE and TEE is similarly excellent).

In the setting of intermediate or high clinical suspicion for endocarditis, negative results on TTE should always be followed by TEE. Furthermore, repeat TEE at an interval of approximately 7 days is reasonable if the clinical suspicion of IE remains high even after negative results on initial TEE.

Option A is the best choice through the process of elimination (all other options are considered appropriate options for TEE as a first-line procedure over TTE).

Options B to E are incorrect since each option is considered an appropriate situation for TEE as a first-line test of choice.

Answer 17: *E.* Understand the significance of mitral annular calcification and its risk of stroke.

Severe MAC involves more than two-thirds of the C-shaped annulus and is best seen on parasternal long-axis and short-axis views by TTE. The parasternal short-axis view reveals a thick, lumpy, and highly echogenic rim that surrounds the external perimeter of the posterior mitral leaflet. Acoustic shadowing from the dense, calcium-laden material is also seen, particularly in the apical views by TTE (midesophageal long-axis view by TEE). The presence, extent, and severity of MAC are best evaluated by TTE, and MAC may conceal a posterior annular abscess in endocarditis on TEE.

When evaluating MAC, attention must be paid to low echogenic mobile components (vegetation, thrombus), as well as to highly echogenic (calcific) mobile components. MAC may serve as nidus for IE and is related to significant carotid artery obstruction, is an independent predictor of the presence of severe aortic atheroma, and has been associated with stroke in multiple population studies.

Possible mechanisms of stroke related to MAC:

- IE-related vegetation embolization
- Atherosclerotic risk marker for ischemic–thrombotic stroke
- Ulcerated MAC with superimposed thrombus
- MAC-associated calcific mobile components that embolize
- Increased transmitral gradient with LA dilation and (paroxysmal) atrial fibrillation

Option A is incorrect as the mitral annular calcification shown in the video is moderate to severe, and not mild.

Option B confirms the MAC is severe, but no associated endocarditis is present on the images.

Option C is incorrect since there are multiple proposed mechanisms for the known increase risk of stroke demonstrated in multiple population studies.

Option D is correct in that the MAC is severe, but it does not demonstrate ulceration or superimposed thrombus. This is important to search for a warrant an echo "sweep" to exclude.

Option E is the best choice. Paroxysmal (or chronic) AF is more likely to occur in patients with a dilated LA and/or elevated LA pressures. Severe MAC (but not lesser degrees of MAC) may be associated with an increased mitral valve gradient (degenerative mitral stenosis), and this would be a more likely TIA source than the MAC itself.

Suggested Readings

Benjamin EJ, et al. Mitral annular calcification and the risk of stroke in an elderly cohort. *N Engl J Med* 1992;327:374–379.

Kizer JR, et al. Mitral annular calcification, aortic valve sclerosis, and incident stroke in adults free of clinical cardiovascular disease: the Strong Heart Study. *Stroke* 2005;36:2533–2537.

Saric M, et al. Guidelines for the use of echocardiography in the evaluation of a cardiac source of embolism. *J Am Soc Echocardiogr* 2016;29:1–42.

Shohat-Zabarski R, et al. Mitral annulus calcification with a mobile component as a possible source of embolism. *Am J Geriatr Cardiol* 2001;10:196–198.

Answer 18: C. Be able to diagnose cancer therapeutic–related cardiac dysfunction (CTRCD).

Option A is incorrect. Although there are differences in the technique and the variability between MUGA and TTE, a reduction of 9% points in a symptomatic patient after a type I agent (doxorubicin), combined with the comment that there is mild global hypokinesis, is very suspicious for CTRCD (although does not meet strict criteria). Another perspective is that the MUGA value was above the lower limit of normal (for MUGA 55%), and the echo was below this threshold (54% for females).

Option B is incorrect since this DOES NOT strictly fulfill the criteria for CTRCD (10% point fall confirmed on repeat imaging 2 to 3 weeks later).

Option C is the most accurate option since by definition of CTRCD (and good clinical practice), a repeat echocardiogram should be performed in the next 2 to 3 weeks. The subsequent LVEF may have returned to normal or may have worsened.

Option D is not correct as a repeat MUGA immediately performed should only be considered if the image quality was poor. Repeating the LVEF too soon will not alter management.

Option E is incorrect as there is no suspicion for ischemia at this time and a viability assessment is not warranted.

Answer 19: C. This series of data emphasizes the importance of understanding how the LVEF is obtained and the limitations of various methods to measure this value.

Options A and B are incorrect since the most reliable reported LVEF techniques (expert "visual" assessment, 2D biplane, and 3D without contrast) each reported a normal LVEF value.

Option C is the correct option given the normal LVEF with each of the three techniques of visual assessment, biplane MOD, and 3DE full volume (in this "high-quality" echocardiogram).

Option D is not correct since the extreme variations in LVEF can be explained (Teicholz, single-plane method is not accurate; contrast was not necessary for the 2D images [reported good quality]; and contrast was shown to be inferior for LVEF assessment with 3D methods).

Option E is incorrect since the LVEF 44% was from 3DE with contrast.

Answer 20: A. This question requires the reader to know that the GLS (global longitudinal strain) is the consensus method giving the best likelihood for meaningful data. Global regional strain ("thickening" value and therefore a "+"-reported value) is less reproducible.

Although not a **guideline** document, the **consensus committee** defined CTRCD as a decrease in the LVEF of >10 percentage points, to a value <53% (as this is the "averaged" lower limit of normal reference value for males [52%] and females [54%]). This decrease should be *confirmed by repeated cardiac imaging performed 2 to 3 weeks* after the baseline diagnostic study showing the initial decrease in LVEF.

LVEF decrease may be further categorized as *symptomatic* or *asymptomatic*, or with regard to reversibility:

- **Reversible**: to within 5 percentage points of baseline
- **Partially reversible**: improved by >10 percentage points from the nadir but remaining >5 percentage points below baseline
- **Irreversible**: improved by <10 percentage points from the nadir and remaining >5 percentage points below baseline
- **Indeterminate**: patient not available for re-evaluation

Option A is correct. The baseline LV global function was abnormal (−14% would be considered abnormal regardless of the gender, age, or vendor), and the markedly improved value (more negative at −19%; total change of 26%) is now normal.

Option B is incorrect as the follow-up LV global function is normal.

Option C is incorrect as the reported results are consistent and interpretable within the framework of the question and the other reported LVEF findings.

Option D is incorrect, although it is important to know the ultrasound machine and software platform (use the same system for serial studies) as well as the age, gender, and image quality.

Option E is incorrect as a value of −14% should not be considered a normal result.

Suggested Reading

Plana JC, et al. Expert consensus for multimodality imaging evaluation of adult patients during and after cancer therapy: a report from the American Society of Echocardiography and the European Association of Cardiovascular Imaging. *J Am Soc Echocardiogr* 2014;27:911–939.

Answer 21: C. Ability to estimate volume status in an ICU patient.

Cardiac chambers can be measured serially during a focused examination of volume status. A small LV internal diameter at end diastole (LVIDD) can be indicative of hypovolemia; care should be taken to not mistake a low LV internal diameter at end systole (LVIDs) with hypovolemia. Hypovolemia is best monitored using end-diastolic measurements, because a low LVIDs could also depict decreased systemic vascular resistance (SVR), increased inotropic state, or decreased ventricular filling. In hypovolemia, both LVIDd and LVIDs are decreased, while in the setting of decreased SVR, LVIDd is normal and LVIDs is decreased. Both RV and LV internal diameters can be measured serially to monitor response to fluids. Reference ranges for LVIDd are 3.9 to 5.3 cm in women and 4.2 to 5.9 cm in men.

Option A is incorrect. Although it is correct that the LV internal diameter is the most important parameter used to assess volume status, an end-diastolic diameter of 4.4 cm is normal for females (<3.9 cm would suggest hypovolemia).

Option B is incorrect since the LV internal diameter at end systole is a better marker of systemic vascular resistance (afterload). A value of 2.0 cm is small and consistent with sepsis.

Option C is the best option in this patient. A small, collapsing IVC in a mechanically ventilated patient strongly suggests hypovolemia. However, the "reverse" is not true: a dilated IVC in an intubated patient is not predictive of volume status.

Option D is incorrect since there are other causes of a hyperdynamic LVEF with midcavity gradient >25 mm Hg beyond hypovolemia (e.g., inotropic therapy, hypertrophic cardiomyopathy).

Option E is incorrect as the LVOT velocity time integral is a marker of the LV stroke volume. This may be low (<18 cm) for other reasons beyond hypovolemia.

Answer 22: C. Understand the concept of coefficient of variance as it relates to echo measures.

This question requires the reader to understand the concept of interobserver variability and coefficients of variation (CoV). Many echo parameters are hindered by poor variability, and therefore, the echo reader must be alert to changes that represent "real" changes compared to differences that are merely reported variations within the known CoV.

As you likely realized quickly, this question was rather typical for some Boards-like material. All that was required to "answer" the question correctly was reading the short prompt prior to the options, but the entire "question" was not required (it was only used to set up the prompt and place it in context).

Because echocardiographic monitoring is currently used in a wide range of clinical settings, it is imperative that the person using quantitative echocardiography to guide therapeutic decision-making (whether an anesthesiologist, a cardiologist, or an emergency room physician) understand the interobserver variability of each of the quantitative measurements and have the technical expertise required to ensure the serial measurements are obtained accurately.

Some common **interobserver variability (IOV)** and/or **meaningful changes** are listed below:

IVC collapsibility index		Meaningful change = <50% to >50%; >50% to <50%
E/A ratio	IOV = 6%	Meaningful change = <1.0 to 1–2 to >2.0
E/e' ratio:	IOV = 8%	Meaningful change = <8 to 9–14 to >15
LVOT VTI	IOV = 6%	
RVSP	IOV = 3%	Meaningful change = <40 to 40–60 to >60 mm Hg
LVIDd	IOV = 8%	

Options A, D, and E are within the expected variability for the reported parameter and should therefore, on their own, not be considered as meaningful changes. The LV internal diameter changed from 56 to 53 mm (<8% change), and the E/e' and RVSP both remained within the "intermediate" ranges for these values.

Option B is incorrect since the RV TAPSE parameter is known to be falsely reduced after CABG surgery. Otherwise, a change from 19 (normal) to 14 mm (moderately reduced) would be considered meaningful.

Option C is the correct choice as an E/A ratio change from 2.1 (restrictive) to 0.8 (impaired) would likely represent a meaningful difference between these two values.

Suggested Reading
Porter TR, et al. Guidelines for the use of echocardiography as a monitor for therapeutic intervention in adults: a report from the American Society of Echocardiography. *J Am Soc Echocardiogr* 2015;28:40–56.

Answer 23: D. It is now believed that most ASDs should be closed soon after diagnosis if no contraindications exist, regardless of size and shunt ratio; however, the closure of PFOs and very small ASDs (Qp/Qs < 1.5:1) or those with no signs of RV volume overload can be debated.

Limitations to percutaneous closure include:

- A single defect too large for closure (>38 mm)
- Multiple ASDs unsuitable for percutaneous closure
- Defect too close to the SVC, IVC, pulmonary veins, AV valves, or coronary sinus
- Defect with **any** insufficient anterior, posterior, superior, or inferior rims <5 mm
- Patients with associated abnormal pulmonary venous drainage
- Associated congenital abnormality requiring cardiac surgery
- Severe PAH and bidirectional or right-to-left shunting (Eisenmenger syndrome)
- Intracardiac thrombi diagnosed by TEE

Option A is incorrect because there is no indication for ASD closure.

Option B is incorrect because percutaneous ASD closure device should be placed if defect diameter is >38 mm.

Option C is incorrect because percutaneous ASD closure device should be placed if more than one of four septal rims exceeds 5 mm.

Option D is the correct answer, because surgical ASD closure should be performed if an anomalous pulmonary vein is seen.

Option E is incorrect because surgical ASD closure should be performed if there is more than one defect.

Answer 24: E. This patient has a complication after device placement. The most serious concern is device erosion presenting as cardiac hemopericardium and tamponade.

Complications of percutaneous septal closure devices are rare but serious and include device embolization, cardiac perforation, tamponade, and device erosion. Device embolization occurs in approximately 0.1% to 0.4% of cases and is most common with ASD closure devices. Device embolization (readily diagnosed with routine TTE) is a potential life-threatening complication requiring immediate removal by percutaneous or surgical intervention. Risk factors for **device embolization** include an undersized ASD device, deficient rims of surrounding tissue, and device malpositioning.

Device erosion is a rare but potentially fatal event; estimated rate of erosion is 0.1% to 0.3%. This may occur at the RA, LA, or aorta and result in hemopericardium, tamponade, aortic fistula, and/or death. Device erosion can begin as a subclinical event, with the device impinging on the surrounding structures, tenting the atrial or aortic tissue, or resulting in a subclinical pericardial effusion. Erosion can also manifest clinically with chest pain, syncope, shortness of breath, the development of a hemopericardium, cardiac tamponade, hemodynamic compromise, and death.

Most cases occur within 72 hours of device implantation, but **late erosion** has been reported >6 years after deployment. Due to the infrequency of this dire complication, the etiology remains poorly understood, but *device oversizing* (present in up to 40% cases), the *complete absence of the aortic rim*, a *high/superior septal location* of the defect, and a *deficient anterior rim with associated insufficiency of the posterior rim* are each considered likely causes. Malalignment of the defect with the aorta, a dynamic ASD (one that changes size more than 50% throughout the cardiac cycle), a deficient or an absent aortic rim (present in up to 90% of cases), and a device that straddles or splays around the aorta are also considered potential risk factors for erosion.

Option A is incorrect since treatment for acute pericarditis would not be sufficient to treat this patient's emergency complication.

Option B is incorrect, although incremental information may be gained if the TTE was suboptimal. Certainly, at the time of cardiac surgery, an intraoperative TEE would be performed.

Option C is incorrect and would delay cardiac surgery with potential devastating consequences. Urgent cardiac catheterization and device retrieval may be considered in patients with device embolization.

Option D is incorrect since an emergency pericardiocentesis would not eliminate the underlying cause of the hemopericardium and may only serve to delay the primary treatment.

Option E is the correct option.

Suggested Readings
Amin Z, et al. Erosion of Amplatzer septal occluder device after closure of secundum atrial septal defects: review of registry of complications and recommendations to minimize future risk. *Catheter Cardiovasc Interv* 2004;63:496–502.
Silvestry FE, et al. Guidelines for the echocardiographic assessment of atrial septal defect and patent foramen ovale: from the American Society of Echocardiography and Society for Cardiac Angiography and Interventions. *J Am Soc Echocardiogr* 2015;28:910–958.

Answer 25: A. This question requires the reader to understand the normal changes that occur with the aging heart. This patient has concentric remodeling of the LV with a relative wall thickness now >42%, but an LV mass that is normal.

LV volumes (V) are inversely associated with age. LV mass (M) decreases with age as well, albeit to a more limited extent than volume. As a consequence, relative wall thickness (RWT) and M/V ratios increase. There is an age-related development of a concentric remodeling with systolic and diastolic dysfunction.

Concentric LV remodeling is a late-stage response of the LV and can be caused by chronic pressure, volume overload, or MI. It is most commonly associated with coronary artery disease, but is also associated with long-standing hypertension, especially untreated hypertension. Echocardiographic features show normal or small LV cavity size, usually increased LV wall thickness and normal LVM. Concentric remodeling is also associated with changes in the shape of the LV—for example, LV sphericity changes—and becomes more rounded, rather than bullet shape.

Option A is the best choice since these serial changes are expected in the normal aging heart.

Option B is incorrect since the LV wall thickness normally increases with aging.

Option C is incorrect and suggests no significant interval change (LVEF difference of 5% is within the observer variability).

Options D and E are incorrect since both the LV mass and the LV diastolic volume normally decrease with age.

Suggested Reading
Rosen BD, et al. Left ventricular remodeling is associated with decreased global and regional systolic function. *Circulation* 2005;112:984–991.

Answer 26: D. This patient has a mildly dilated left ventricle, mild LVH, and normal RWT.

CHARACTERIZATION OF LV GEOMETRY BASED ON LVM, LV VOLUME, AND RWT

LV GEOMETRIC PATTERN	LV VOLUME INDEX (ML/M²)	LVM INDEX (G/M²)	RWT
Normal ventricle	≤75	≤115 (men) or <95 (women)	0.32–0.42
Physiologic hypertrophy	>75	>115 (men) or >95 (women)	0.32–0.42
Concentric remodeling	≤75	≤115 (men) or #95 (women)	>0.42
Eccentric remodeling	>75	≤115 (men) or #95 (women)	<0.32
Concentric hypertrophy	≤75	>115 (men) or >95 (women)	>0.42
Mixed hypertrophy	>75	>115 (men) or >95 (women)	>0.42
Dilated hypertrophy	>75	>115 (men) or >95 (women)	0.32–0.42
Eccentric hypertrophy	>75	>115 (men) or >95 (women)	<0.32

The limitation of the classical categories is the suboptimal categorization of dilated ventricles. Recently, a new subdivision of LV geometry was suggested based upon LV mass, LV volume, and RWT. Using this approach, the **nondilated ventricle** is characterized as having normal morphology, concentric remodeling, or concentric hypertrophy, based on LVH and RWT (>0.42). **Dilated ventricles without LVH** are described as having eccentric remodeling if the RWT is <0.32. **Dilated ventricles with LVH** are described as having eccentric hypertrophy (RWT < 0.32), mixed hypertrophy (RWT > 0.42), or physiologic hypertrophy (RWT 0.32 to 0.42). See FIGURE 51.2.

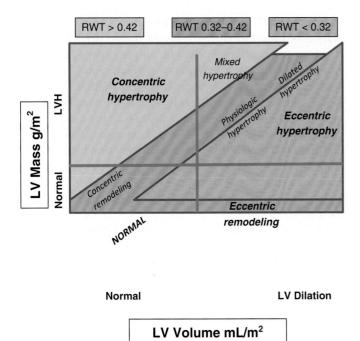

FIGURE 51.2

Options A, B, C, and E are incorrect and represent other variations of LV size, LV mass, and relative wall thickness.

Option D, physiologic hypertrophy, is the most correct option and is consistent with the clinical history of an athlete's heart (and chronic, but controlled, hypertension).

Suggested Readings
Gaasch WH, Zile MR. Left ventricular structural remodeling in health and disease: with special emphasis on volume, mass, and geometry. *J Am Coll Cardiol* 2011;58:1733–1740.
Marwick TH, et al. Recommendations on the use of echocardiography in adult hypertension: a report from the European Association of Cardiovascular Imaging (EACVI) and the American Society of Echocardiography (ASE). *J Am Soc Echocardiogr* 2015;28:727–754.

***Answer 27:** D.* This question warrants an understanding of LVH progression and regression and its impact on patient management.

Decisions regarding the initiation, intensification, or monitoring of response to antihypertensive therapies are made entirely on clinical (not echo) parameters. Given the progressive nature of hypertensive cardiomyopathy, periodic evaluation of cardiac function and morphology by echocardiography may be warranted, especially if symptoms change.

LVH represents an important end organ consequence of hypertension. Population-based studies using echocardiography (and ECG) have demonstrated that LVH is closely linked with stroke, renal impairment, LV dysfunction, atrial and ventricular arrhythmias, and sudden cardiac death.

The use of repeat echo to document changes in LVM has been difficult to incorporate into clinical practice due to the inherent variability of LV mass measurements and the fact that hypertension is not the only cause of LVH (present in one-third of hypertensive subjects). LVH is also influenced by obesity, diabetes, renal impairment, and other unknown genetic factors.

Although a reduction in LVH is associated with improved clinical outcomes, large populations are required to overcome the variability of measurement. Because of this test–retest limitation of 2D echo, CMR is considered more accurate to demonstrate this effect. 3D echo partly overcomes this problem, but requires high-quality images.

Option A is not correct, and despite the population-based knowledge that LVH is associated with worse outcomes and regression demonstrates improved prognosis, repeat 2D echo to confirm LV regression has not been incorporated to the individual patient.

Option B is incorrect since the initial echo was performed with 2D, and although 3D is more accurate to measure LV mass (compared with cardiac MRI), comparison with an earlier 2D echo method would not necessarily be accurate to confirm LV regression.

Option C is incorrect since a repeat 2D echo that demonstrates progressive LVH would not in itself warrant an increase in antihypertensive treatment. This patient is at goal BP and the echo would not be used to further guide therapy.

Option D is a true statement and the best choice. There is significant variation in LVH measurement and the test–retest variability limits any use of the results in the individual patient.

Option E is an incorrect statement and LVH regression does correlate with prognosis in all population studies.

Suggested Reading
Nadour W, Biederman RW. Is left ventricular hypertrophy regression important? Does the tool used to detect it matter? *J Clin Hypertens* 2009;11:441–447.

***Answer 28:** C.* This question raises the importance of understanding the risk of radiation exposure and the steps taken to minimize this risk.

Sonographers sit very close to their "hot" patients and frequently drape their arms and bodies over patients who have recently received radioactive agents for diagnostic nuclear studies, thereby rendering the patients transiently radioactive. Proximity to this radioactive source and the relatively long duration of the exposure are two important determinants of potential radiation dose absorption by sonographers.

Sonographers may also perform TTE or assist with TEE during structural heart procedures (e.g., transcatheter aortic valve replacement, percutaneous mitral valve repair, left atrial occluder device implantation, and atrial septal device closures) and spend significant time in the cardiac catheterization and electrophysiology laboratories. This places the sonographer in close proximity to x-ray sources, which are actively emitting radiation. This source of radiation is much greater than the risk from exposure to a "hot patient" and requires much greater understanding of the risks and steps for risk reduction (including wearing lead aprons and proper positioning to maximize distance from the source).

Option A is incorrect since the patient is considered "hot," and there is a small, but not "zero," risk of radiation exposure to the sonographer.

Option B is incorrect since the TTE should not be delayed 48 hours in a patient with an "urgent" indication for echocardiography. Furthermore, the most commonly used radioisotope for SPECT testing is technetium-based, and with a half-life of 6 hours, no more than 24 hours would be necessary to consider the patient as no longer "hot."

Option C is the best choice since the greatest risk would be to the unprotected fetus who should be kept away from all radiation sources.

Option D is not the best choice and simply not necessary due to the very low risk. Delaying the time from injection of the radiation source and then keeping your distance from the source would be simpler and more important steps.

Option E is not the best choice since a right-handed examination requires greater patient contact and proximity to the radiation source (the heart) than a left-handed–performed exam.

Suggested Reading

McIlwain EF, et al. Special report: radiation safety for the cardiac sonographer: recommendations of the Radiation Safety Writing Group for the Council on Cardiovascular Sonography of the American Society of Echocardiography. *J Am Soc Echocardiogr* 2014;27:811–816.

Answer 29: B. This question requires understanding of the indications and workflow for using UCA in the echo lab.

Option A is not the best option as it is highly unlikely that all echo windows will be of a good quality and much more likely that at least one acoustic window will benefit from UCA.

Option B is the best choice. In preparation of this echo, the sonographer should travel with LV-manufactured contrast for LV opacification.

Option C is incorrect since requiring that a subsequent study be performed would not be the best workflow. Also, having the sonographer interrupt image acquisition to go get UCA or having to return for additional images is an inefficient workflow.

Option D is not correct since contrast is not a contraindication in this patient.

Option E is not the best answer, although previous echo studies should always be reviewed prior to serial examinations. If a previous echo demonstrates that contrast was not used, it does not exclude that it either should have been used on the earlier exam and does not exclude that the image quality is now worsened due to respiratory failure.

Answer 30: D. This question emphasizes the importance of technique to perform a saline bubble study.

Option D is the most correct option as it emphasizes *TEE over TTE, harmonics over fundamental, 2D with contrast over CFD, Valsalva release over resting, a bacteriostatic saline–air–blood admixture over normal saline–air alone,* and *lower extremity over upper extremity.*

Although transcranial Doppler (TCD) is sensitive at detecting even small amounts of right-to-left shunting, it does not locate the origin of the shunt. Right arm is superior over left arm as most patients are in a left lateral decubitus position, and this increases the chance for an obstructed venous route from either line kinking or venous pressure from body weight. Lower extremity is superior to upper extremity owing to the

anatomic direction of the PFO shunt (along the IVC/eustachian valve toward the SVC).

ULTRASOUND METHOD	PHYSIOLOGIC MANEUVER	CONTRAST/BUBBLE OPTION	INJECTION ROUTE
1. 2D TTE **TH**	7. Resting	10. Normal saline	13. **Right** arm
2. 2D TTE FI	8. Valsalva maneuver	11. Bacteriostatic saline	14. Left arm
3. 2D **TEE**	9. **Valsalva release**	12. **Bacteriostatic/ blood mixture**	15. **Leg vein**
4. TTE CFD			
5. TEE CFD			
6. TCD			

TH, tissue harmonics; FI, fundamental imaging; CFD, color-flow Doppler; TCD, transcranial Doppler.

A saline contrast injection is indicated to rule out an intrapulmonary or intracardiac right-to-left shunt. A PFO has been associated with stroke, paradoxical emboli, decompression sickness, platypnea, and orthodeoxia. Although the clinical significance of detecting a PFO by echocardiography is controversial, studies to evaluate these disease states routinely include saline contrast injections. The literature has clearly shown the advantage of transesophageal echocardiography (TEE) over transthoracic echocardiography (TTE) in detecting these shunts, but screening procedures have still used TTE.

Saline contrast is primarily used to assess for right-to-left shunting and to detect residual shunts after defect closure. Bolus injection of sterile saline contrast macroscopic bubbles that do not normally cross the pulmonary circuit is the method of choice to screen for a PFO. It is recommended that the saline contrast be composed of >8 mL of *bacteriostatic* normal saline agitated with 0.5 mL of room air, agitated back and forth between two sterile syringes using a three-way stopcock just before IV bolus injection through a forearm (or, less desirable, hand) vein.

Specific physiologic maneuvers and admixtures of saline with the patient's blood have been proposed to optimize the contrast produced. It is important that release of a Valsalva maneuver or coughing (to transiently increase right atrial pressure) occurs when the saline contrast bolus arrives in the right atrium. It is optimal to have >20-gauge cannula access in an antecubital vein (preferably on the patient's right side). Optimal visualization of the interatrial septum and use of tissue harmonic imaging improve the sensitivity.

Both right- and left-arm saline contrast injections should be used whenever a persistent left-sided superior vena cava or unroofed coronary sinus is suspected. Although femoral venous injections improve flow directed to the septum, these are too invasive for routine sonographer use in detecting a PFO.

Although typically an intracardiac shunt will demonstrate left heart bubbles within three beats, it is important to note that bubbles may appear sooner with pulmonary arteriovenous shunts in high-output states and may occur later than three beats if there is delayed coughing or Valsalva maneuvers.

Also, false-negative saline contrast studies can occur if the interatrial septum is persistently bowed toward the right atrium during agitated saline injection, as a PFO can be held closed with the septum in this position. If there is still suspicion that a PFO exists after negative results, a repeat saline contrast injection should be performed using a blood–saline–air mixture or a more appropriately timed Valsalva or cough maneuver to ensure that the results are truly negative. With TEE, direct visualization of the septum secundum and septum primum is recommended during saline contrast injection, to document the location and size of any right-to-left shunt. Image acquisition should be timed to begin just before the appearance of saline contrast in the right atrium and continue for at least 10 cardiac cycles after contrast appearance.

Suggested Readings

Attaran RR, et al. Protocol for optimal detection and exclusion of a patent foramen ovale using transthoracic echocardiography with agitated saline microbubbles. *Echocardiography* 2006;23(7): 616–622. doi:10.1111/j.1540-8175.2006.00272.x

Gin KG, et al. Femoral vein delivery of contrast medium enhances transthoracic echocardiographic detection of patent foramen ovale. *J Am Coll Cardiol* 1993;22:1994–2000.

Porter TR, et al. Guidelines for the cardiac sonographer in the performance of contrast echocardiography: a focused update from the American Society of Echocardiography. *J Am Soc Echocardiogr* 2014;27:797–810.

Soliman O II, et al. The use of contrast echocardiography for the detection of cardiac shunts. *Eur J Echocardiogr* 2007;8:S2–S12.

Answer 31: **C (1.2 to 1.4).** This question requires the reader to calculate the WMSI (score 1 = normal; score 2 = hypokinesis; score 3 = akinesis; score 4 = dyskinesis; index = total score/# wall segments measured). Example: all segments seen and normal = total score 16/16 segments = 1.0.

From the review of the 4 videos, all 16 myocardial segments can be seen. In the parasternal long axis, the mid inferolateral segment is not well seen, but it is normal in the parasternal short axis view. All regional wall segments can be seen to thicken normally (wall score = 1.0) except for two segments: the basal inferior (akinetic) and inferoseptal (akinetic) segments. This is typical for an inferior wall myocardial infarction. These two segments should be scored as 3.0 providing a total wall score of 20. The WMSI in this case is therefore 20/16 = 1.25.

Answer 32: **B.** This question requires understanding of the prognostic value of the WMSI.

For the assessment of regional LV function, the ventricle is divided into segments. Segmentation schemes should reflect coronary perfusion territories, result in segments with comparable myocardial mass, and allow standardized communication within echocardiography and with other imaging modalities. Accordingly, a 17-segment model is commonly used.

Beginning at the anterior junction of the interventricular septum and the RV free wall and continuing counterclockwise, basal and midventricular segments should be labeled as anteroseptal, inferoseptal, inferior, inferolateral, anterolateral, and anterior. In this 17-segment model, the apex is divided into five segments, including septal, inferior, lateral, and anterior segments, as well as the "apical cap," (the myocardium beyond the end of the LV cavity).

The 17-segment model is used for myocardial perfusion studies or when comparing between different imaging modalities, specifically single photon emission computed tomography, positron emission tomography, and CMR. When using this 17-segment model to assess wall motion, the 17th segment (the apical cap) should not be included.

In echocardiography, regional myocardial function is assessed on the basis of the observed wall thickening and endocardial motion of the myocardial segment. Because myocardial motion may be caused by adjacent segment tethering or overall LV displacement, regional deformation (thickening, shortening) should be the focus of the analysis. However, it must be recognized that deformation can also be passive and therefore may not always accurately reflect myocardial contraction.

It is recommended that each segment be analyzed individually in multiple views. A semiquantitative wall motion score can be assigned to each segment to calculate the LV wall motion score index as the average of the scores of all segments visualized. The following scoring system is recommended: (1) normal or hyperkinetic, (2) hypokinetic (reduced thickening), (3) akinetic (absent or negligible thickening, e.g., scar), and (4) dyskinetic (systolic thinning or stretching, e.g., aneurysm).

Option A is not correct as a wall motion score index (1.0), even in a high-quality study, will predict a low (<3%) risk of an acute myocardial infarction, but not very low (<1%) risk. Therefore, it is not entirely suitable for a simple triage and ER discharge technique alone.

Option B is correct. A regional wall motion abnormality is ≥10× more likely than normal motion to be found in a patient with an acute myocardial infarction.

Option C is not the best answer. Although a wall motion score index >1.5 predicts a worse clinical outcome than a WMSI 1.0, it does not predict a very poor prognosis (usually reserved for WMSI > 2.5 or 2.2).

Option D is incorrect since it is most accurate to use a 16-segment model to measure the wall motion score index (17-segment models used for perfusion).

Option E is not the best option since severe ischemia will result in prolongation of the regional wall motion abnormality (myocardial "stunning"). This is the principle used in exercise stress echo that images after termination of stress.

Suggested Readings

Lang RM, et al. Recommendations for cardiac chamber quantification by echocardiography in adults: an update from the American Society of Echocardiography and the European Association of Cardiovascular Imaging. *J Am Soc Echocardiogr* 2015;28:233–270.

Editor's Note: This "update" was created to improve normal values for all cardiac chambers using new technology (e.g., 3D echo) and using larger published normal subject databases.

Sabia P, et al. Value of regional wall motion abnormality in the emergency room diagnosis of acute myocardial infarction. A prospective study using two-dimensional echocardiography. *Circulation* 1991;84:I85.

Shiina A, et al. Prognostic significance of regional wall motion abnormality in patients with prior myocardial infarction: a prospective correlative study of two-dimensional echocardiography and angiography. *Mayo Clin Proc* 1986;61(4):254–262.

Answer 33: **E.** This question requires the reader to recognize the **basal septal hypertrophy** and understand how this impacts the cardiac dimensions and LV mass calculation.

In patients with basal septal hypertrophy, the linear dimension methods, which use basal ventricular measurements, result in overestimation of the true mass, because the thickest region of the interventricular septum is incorporated in the measurement. In contrast, the area–length method, which uses midventricular measurements, underestimates LV mass, because the thickest part of the interventricular septum is not included in the measurement. The 3D method has the advantage of accommodating regional differences in wall thickness and therefore can provide the most accurate measurements of LV mass in this setting.

In the normally shaped left ventricle, both M-mode and 2D echocardiographic formulas to calculate LV mass can be used. Reference upper limits of normal LV mass by linear measurements are 95 g/m^2 in women and 115 g/m^2 in men. Reference upper limits of normal LV mass by 2D measurements are 88 g/m^2 in women and 102 g/m^2 in men with 2D methods. Upper normal limits of 3D echocardiographic LV mass data are insufficient to substantiate recommendations for reference values.

Option A is incorrect. An M-mode–derived LV mass >95 g/m^2 would be abnormal (>88 by 2D). Also, an M-mode value in this patient should be considered with caution due to the basal focal septal wall thickening (not a reflection of the entire LV wall thickening).

Option B is not entirely accurate as a 2D measure would still be inaccurate due to the proximal septal thickening.

Option C is not correct, and a short-axis orientation has the same limitations of a single-dimensional, non-2D–guided M-mode and may not precisely align the basal IVS and PW with the true alignment of the LV.

Option D is incorrect. Moving the 2D measure from the recommended basal LV segments to the mid LV to get beyond the basal focal LV wall thickening raises additional limitations regarding the LV diameter (which is cubed for LV mass measures). This is a common error used by sonographers.

Option E is the best choice since a 3D-derived LV mass value would be more precise in abnormally shaped LV cavities and patients with regional LV wall thickening.

Answer 34: *E.* This question requires the reader to understand the different methods to measure the LA size and understand their strengths and limitations.

With TEE, the entire left atrium frequently cannot be fit in the image sector. Accordingly, TEE should not be used to assess LA size. LA size should be measured at the end of LV systole, when the LA chamber is at its greatest dimension. While acquiring images to measure LA size and volumes, care should be taken to avoid foreshortening of the left atrium. Because the longitudinal axes of the left ventricle and left atrium frequently lie in different planes, dedicated acquisitions of the left atrium from the apical approach should be obtained for optimal LA volume measurements. As a routine quality check, using the biplane disk summation method, the length measured in the two- and four-chamber views should be similar.

When tracing the borders of the left atrium, the confluences of the pulmonary veins and the LA appendage should be excluded. The atrioventricular interface should be represented by the mitral annulus plane, not by the tip of the mitral leaflets.

AP linear dimension from the PSLAX should not be used as the sole measure of LA size. Compared with AP diameter, LA volume has a stronger association with outcomes in cardiac patients and can readily be measured using the biplane Simpson method (disk summation algorithm, similar to LV volume). Two-dimensional echocardiographic LA volumes are typically smaller than those reported from computed tomography or CMR.

Options A and B are incorrect as the LA diameter, whether normal or not, is less accurate and less correlative with prognosis than LA volumes (indexed to BSA). It is important to realize that all techniques are limited by foreshortened images and TEE is not recommended for LA assessment.

Options C and D are incorrect since the most accurate method to measure the LA volume index is the biplane summation of disks (Simpson method).

Option E is the best choice since this technique is most reliable, and using this method, the LA volume index is severely dilated (>48 mL/m^2).

Suggested Reading
Pritchett AM, et al. Left atrial volume as an index of left atrial size: a population-based study. *J Am Coll Cardiol* 2003;41:1036–1043.

Answer 35: *C.* Understand the indications for serial echocardiography in mitral stenosis.

STAGE
A At risk to develop VHD
B Progressive VHD (mild-to-moderate severity and asymptomatic)[a]
C Asymptomatic severe[b]
C1: Ventricle compensated
C2: Ventricle decompensated
D Symptomatic severe

[a]Follow-up echocardiography: Mild asymptomatic disease every 3 years; moderate asymptomatic disease annually.

[b]Follow-up echocardiography: May be required more frequent than annual, especially if the ventricle is starting to decompensate.

After initial evaluation of an asymptomatic patient with valvular heart disease (VHD), the clinician may decide to continue close follow-up. The purpose of close follow-up is to prevent the irreversible consequences of severe VHD that primarily affect the status of the ventricles and pulmonary circulation (but may occur in the absence of symptoms). At a minimum, the follow-up should consist of a yearly history and physical examination. Periodic TTE monitoring provides important prognostic information. The frequency of an echocardiography is based on the type and severity of the valve pathology, the known rate of progression, and the effect on the affected ventricle.

Option A is incorrect as a repeat TTE is not indicated during this visit.

Option B is not correct and a repeat annual echo is not warranted in a patient with stage B MS.

Option C is the most correct statement as he won't need another echo for 2 more years unless symptoms develop.

Option D is not correct. Although the echo is not required annually, patients with stage B valve disease warrant clinical follow-up at least annually.

Option E is not correct and a TEE is not indicated at this time.

Suggested Reading

Nishimura RA, et al. 2014 AHA/ACC guideline for the management of patients with valvular heart disease. *J Am Coll Cardiol* 2014;63(22):e57–e185. http://dx.doi.org/10.1016/j.jacc.2014.02.536

Answer 36: *A.* Recognize the physical exam and echo findings of "non–severe" aortic stenosis.

Most patients with AS are first diagnosed when cardiac auscultation reveals a systolic murmur or after a review of TTE requested for other indications. Physical examination findings are specific but not sensitive for evaluation of stenosis severity. The classic findings of a loud (grade 3/6), late-peaking systolic murmur that radiates to the carotid arteries, a single or paradoxically split second heart sound, and a delayed and diminished carotid upstroke confirm the presence of severe AS. However, carotid upstroke may be normal in elderly patients because of the effects of aging on the vasculature, and the murmur may be soft or may radiate to the apex. **The only physical examination finding that is reliable in excluding the possibility of severe AS is a normally split second heart sound.**

Option A is the best option. This patient has stage B AS (progressive, moderate, asymptomatic). Given the examination with a normally split S2, this physical finding essentially excludes severe AS and is consistent with her echo findings (peak gradient = 52 mm Hg; dimensionless ratio = 0.33 [1.2/3.6]).

Options B, C, and D are incorrect and should be reserved for suboptimal echo or discrepant findings with clinical exam (or when additional information is required). If there are questions regarding the clinical symptoms, then exercise testing is valuable in experienced hands using careful monitoring (may unmask symptoms in one-third of asymptomatic severe AS stage C patients).

Option E should be reserved for stage D AS (and occasionally stage C2).

Answer 37: *C.* Recognize the indications/contraindications for TAVR, many of which are echo-/Doppler-based parameters.

TAVR is a class I indication in patients who meet an indication for AVR for AS who have a prohibitive surgical risk and a predicted post-TAVR survival >12 months.

Decision-making is complex in the patient at high surgical risk with *severe symptomatic AS*. The decision to perform surgical AVR and TAVR or to forgo intervention requires input from a heart valve team. The primary cardiologist is aware of coexisting conditions that affect risk and long-term survival,

the patient's disease course, and the patient's preferences and values. **Cardiac imaging specialists** who are knowledgeable about AS and TAVR provide evaluation of aortic valve anatomy and hemodynamic severity, vascular anatomy, aortic annulus size, and coronary anatomy, including the annular–ostial distance. Interventional cardiologists help determine the likelihood of a successful transcatheter procedure. The cardiac surgeon can provide a realistic estimate of risk with a conventional surgical approach, at times in conjunction with a cardiac anesthesiologist. An expert in VHD, typically a cardiologist or cardiac surgeon with expertise in imaging and/or intervention, provides the continuity and integration needed for the collaborative decision-making process. Nurses and other members of the team coordinate care and help with patient education.

Option A is incorrect as a patient with stage D AS warrants intervention for risk reduction.

Option B is incorrect since the patient is requesting a non-surgical approach and there is adequate clinical trial evidence that this approach is reasonable.

Option C is the best choice for a patient with stage D AS and a life expectancy >12 months.

Option D is incorrect and should be reserved for a limited clinical population as this technique is not associated with more than short-term clinical improvement and may have catastrophic procedural risks (acute AR from a flail valve leaflet or stroke). As a bridge to a more permanent operation (TAVR or SAVR), this is considered class IIb.

Option E is incorrect, although this choice is an important consideration in patients with stage D AS and no TAVR or SAVR option.

Suggested Reading

Kodali SK, Williams MR, Smith CR, et al. Two-year outcomes after transcatheter or surgical aortic-valve replacement. *N Engl J Med* 2012;366:1686–1695.

Answer 38: *E.* This question requires an understanding of the indications for AVR in chronic AR, including stage C2 disease (severe AR with EF < 50%).

The most common causes of chronic AR in developed countries are now bicuspid aortic valve and calcific valve disease (replacing annuloectatic aortic dilatation as the previously reported most common etiology of AR). Another cause of AR is rheumatic heart disease (the leading cause in many developing countries). In the majority of patients with AR, the disease course is chronic and slowly progressive with increasing LV volume overload and LV adaptation via chamber dilation and hypertrophy. Management of patients with AR depends on accurate diagnosis of the cause and stage of the disease process.

The stages of AR range from patients at risk of AR (stage A) or with progressive mild-to-moderate AR (stage B) to severe asymptomatic (stage C) and symptomatic AR (stage D). Each of these stages is defined by valve anatomy, valve hemodynamics, severity of LV dilatation, and LV systolic function, as well as by patient symptoms. Numerous studies (*N* > 1,150) have consistently shown that measures of LV systolic function (LVEF or fractional shortening) and LV end-systolic dimension (LVESD) or volume are associated with development of HF symptoms or death in initially asymptomatic patients (stages B and C1). Moreover, in symptomatic patients undergoing AVR (stage D), preoperative LV systolic function and end-systolic dimension or volume are significant determinants of survival and functional results after surgery. Symptomatic patients (stage D) with normal LVEF have significantly better long-term postoperative survival than those with depressed systolic function.

Option A is incorrect as this patient has class I indication for AVR.

Option B is incorrect, but an exercise stress test is reasonable to confirm symptoms if the LVEF was normal.

Option C is incorrect, and dobutamine stress echo with Doppler is not a proven technique to evaluate patients with chronic AR.

Option D is not the best choice and also nifedipine vasodilator Rx is reasonable in chronic AR; this patient already meets class I surgical indications.

Option E is the best option and an aortic valve replacement should be performed since the LVEF is low (<50%).

Suggested Reading

Nishimura RA, et al. 2014 AHA/ACC guideline for the management of patients with valvular heart disease. *J Am Coll Cardiol* 2014;63(22):e57–e185. http://dx.doi.org/10.1016/j.jacc.2014.02.536

Answer 39: E. This question requires the reader to understand the indications/contraindications to PMVBC in severe symptomatic mitral stenosis (stage D).

Option A is incorrect since this option does not deal with the class I indication for MVR.

Options B and C are not the best answers, but would be indicated if there was discrepancy of the data and clinical findings or if planning for PMVBC.

Option D is incorrect. Although the Wilkins score confirms a favorable MV morphology for PMVBC and the patient certainly has stage D MS warranting intervention, the presence of an LA thrombus should be considered a contraindication (as would moderate or greater MR; or a Wilkins score >12).

Option E is the best option in this patient.

Suggested Reading

Nishimura RA, et al. 2014 AHA/ACC guideline for the management of patients with valvular heart disease. *J Am Coll Cardiol* 2014;63(22):e57–e185. http://dx.doi.org/10.1016/j.jacc.2014.02.536

Answer 40: C. This question emphasizes the importance of understanding the MV anatomy that predicts successful MV repair.

MV replacement surgery **should not be performed** for treatment of isolated severe primary MR *limited to less than one-half of the posterior leaflet* unless MV repair has been attempted and was unsuccessful. Surgical repair of MR has been remarkably successful, particularly in the treatment of chronic primary MR. Repair of isolated degenerative mitral disease, when leaflet dysfunction is sufficiently limited that

only annuloplasty and repair of the posterior leaflet are necessary, has led to outcomes distinctly superior to biologic or mechanical MVR: operative mortality of <1%, long-term survival equivalent to that of age-matched general population, approximately 95% freedom from reoperation, and >80% freedom from recurrent moderate or severe MR at 15 to 20 years after operation. As much as one-half of the posterior leaflet may be excised, plicated, or resuspended. Posterior leaflet repair has become sufficiently standardized in this situation that repair rather than MVR is the standard of care. Execution of this procedure with a success rate >90% should be the expectation of every cardiac surgeon who performs mitral valve procedures.

Options A and B are class III recommendations unless an attempted MV repair has failed. Option C is the best option and may be necessary to provide a MV repair procedure. Any other replacement surgery is considered class III.

Option D is incorrect as it is not necessary if the TTE is of high quality. Based upon the details of the report, enough information is available, but a TEE would also be performed intraoperatively to confirm morphology (and assist with postop repair assessment).

Option E is incorrect in a patient with stage D MR disease.

Suggested Reading

Nishimura RA, et al. 2014 AHA/ACC guideline for the management of patients with valvular heart disease. *J Am Coll Cardiol* 2014;63(22):e57–e185. http://dx.doi.org/10.1016/j.jacc.2014.02.536

Answer 41: A. Understand the AUC for echocardiography in atrial fibrillation.

Option A is the best option since at least one TTE study is always considered appropriate in new-onset atrial fibrillation regardless of symptoms. Echo is useful to assess the LA size, the LV function, and the mitral valve morphology. However, repeated serial echo for repeated visits of palpitations would be unnecessary or rarely necessary (depending on change in symptoms or exam).

Options B and C are incorrect due to the discussion above under option A.

Option D is incorrect as TEE is reserved for the evaluation of patients with atrial fibrillation and abnormal findings on TTE or in preparation for DCCV to shorten the total duration of anticoagulation.

Option E is not entirely correct. Although a TEE may be appropriate in some patients with stroke symptoms, it may not be indicated in others. Certainly a TEE is not warranted to search for an embolic source once the diagnosis of AF has been made.

Answer 42: C. This question raises the importance of understanding the etiology of AF and echo is sometimes helpful in this regard.

The four most common comorbidities in patients with atrial fibrillation is the same for those >65 as it is for those <65 years old: hypertension (>80%), CAD (64%), hyperlipidemia (>60%), and heart failure (>50%). Lone AF is reserved for patients without clinical or echo evidence of cardiopulmonary disease, hypertension, or diabetes. This term should no longer be used to guide Rx. LA dilatation, reduced LV fractional shortening, and increased LV wall thickness are echo risk factors for atrial fibrillation.

In patients with AF clearly of <48 hours' duration, it is common practice to perform cardioversion without TEE or antecedent anticoagulation. No RCTs comparing anticoagulation strategies in patients with AF duration of <48 hours exist. If high-risk features are present, such as mitral stenosis or prior history of thromboembolism, long-term anticoagulation should be considered. Decisions about whether to initiate long-term systemic anticoagulation at the time of cardioversion in a patient with AF of <48 hours' duration should be based on the patient's long-term risk of stroke using the CHA2DS2-VASc risk score.

Option A is incorrect. This patient has lone atrial fibrillation.

Option B would be unlikely since thyrotoxicosis would be less common without other symptoms.

Option C is the most correct option since it is well known that the most likely etiology for AF is undiagnosed hypertension.

Option D is not accurate as elective immediate cardioversion is not indicated and without initial anticoagulation, regardless of the suspected (unproven) short duration of AF symptoms, would not be considered safe and would subject the patient to undue risks of a stroke.

Option E is not correct as there are no indications that lifelong anticoagulation is warranted (a mildly dilated LA and moderate MAC is not in itself an indication for lifelong anticoagulation).

Suggested Reading
Klein AL, et al. Use of transesophageal echocardiography to guide cardioversion in patients with atrial fibrillation. *N Engl J Med* 2001;344:1411–1420.

Answer 43: *C.* Understand the success rate of surgical closure of the LAA and need for continued anticoagulation.

The results of surgical occlusion of the LAA remain suboptimal, with echocardiographic follow-up suggesting incomplete occlusion in >50% of subjects. In first-generation devices and surgical closure, this is certainly the case. However, with new-generation percutaneous devices and TEE guidance, the results are better.

In 137 patients (1993–2004) that underwent a surgical attempt at LAA occlusion (52 excision; 85 suture or stapling exclusion), TEE-defined unsuccessful closures were characterized by either persistent flow into the LAA or a remnant stump of >1.0 cm of the LAA in 82/137 (60%). Success rate for stapling was 0%. Particularly noteworthy is that thrombus was identified in >25% of patients with unsuccessful LAA occlusion. This latter finding constitutes important data guiding the continued need for anticoagulation in patients who have undergone surgical LAA ligation.

Option A is incorrect and anticoagulation should be considered after LAA ligature.

Option B is not correct. Although a routine TEE might demonstrate a high-risk finding (e.g., remaining flow, thrombus,

exposed stump/LAA lobe), even a normal postsurgical TEE warrants anticoagulation in low-risk patients.

Option C is the most correct, and anticoagulation should be continued despite the LAA ligation due to the persistence of clot/embolic risks.

Option D is not correct, and an A wave >50 cm/s on TTE Doppler mitral inflow is not adequate to avoid other indications for warfarin.

Suggested Readings
January CT, et al. 2014 AHA/ACC/HRS guideline for the management of patients with atrial fibrillation. *J Am Coll Cardiol* 2014;64:e1–e76.
Kannel WB, et al. Prevalence, incidence, prognosis, and predisposing conditions for atrial fibrillation: population-based estimates. *Am J Cardiol* 1998;82:2N–9N.

Answer 44: *B.* This question requires the reader to understand the aortic dilatation threshold for surgical repair in *asymptomatic patients with BAV*.

Two guidelines differ with regard to the recommended threshold of aortic dilatation that would justify surgical intervention in patients with bicuspid aortic valves. The ACC and AHA therefore convened a subcommittee representing members of the two guideline writing committees to review the evidence, reach consensus, and draft a statement of clarification for both guidelines. This statement of clarification provides recommendations that replace those contained in the *thoracic aortic disease* guideline and the *valvular heart disease* guideline.

Operative intervention to repair or replace the aortic root (sinuses) or replace the ascending aorta is indicated in **asymptomatic patients with BAV** if the diameter of the aortic root or ascending aorta is *5.5 cm or greater*. There is uncertainty about whether patients with BAV should undergo aortic repair at diameters smaller than those recommended for patients with ascending aortic aneurysms in the setting of a tricuspid aortic valve. Both the histology and mechanical properties of the ascending aorta differ between those with BAV and those with tricuspid aortic valves, raising the possibility that the aortic wall may be more vulnerable to dissection in those with BAV.

Suggested Reading
Hiratzka LF, et al. Surgery for aortic dilatation in patients with bicuspid aortic valves: a statement of clarification from the American College of Cardiology/American Heart Association Task Force on Clinical Practice Guidelines. *J Am Coll Cardiol* 2016;67:264–231.

Answer 45: *B.* This question requires the reader to understand the approach to the low-risk patient with suspected ischemic heart disease and the timing of stress testing.

If the low-risk patient with suspected ischemic heart disease has known CAD and previous revascularization, then it is important to review previous stress tests. If recent (<1 year) and not "high risk," then continued GDMT is the most important strategy in care. If high risk, then revascularization should be considered in addition to GDMT. If stress test was remote (>1 year), then stress testing may again be considered. If able to exercise and ECG is normal, then stress ECG is consider class I regardless of known/unknown CAD and/or previous PCI procedure.

Option A is not the best choice since this patient is having typical angina, which would benefit from additional treatment.

Option B is the best option, and increasing either his Imdur or adding a beta-blocker (in place of amlodipine if BP warrants) for additional antianginal effect may resolve his stable symptoms.

Option C is not correct at this time, although, if typical angina persists, coronary angiography would be warranted as another option (invasive approach) to treat his symptoms.

Option D is not correct. The fact that he underwent a recent, adequate quality, stress echo, and the results suggested a low-risk finding, repeat stress ECG is not considered appropriate.

Option E is not correct as a repeat exercise stress echocardiography within 1 year of the previous normal test findings would not likely reveal a different result. However, the previous stress echo should be reviewed by you with specific attention to the posterior (inferolateral) region given his previous circumflex PCI.

Suggested Reading

Fihn SD, et al. 2012 ACCF/AHA/ACP/AATS/PCNA/SCAI/STS guideline for the diagnosis and management of patients with stable ischemic heart disease. *J Am Coll Cardiol* 2012;60:e44–e164.

Answer 46: D. This question requires the reader to know the best approach to SIHD in patients with a LBBB pattern on ECG.

Option A is not the best choice. A 68F with hypertension and angina symptoms should consider risk stratification prior to initiation into an exercise program.

Options B and C are incorrect since this lady has a LBBB.

Option D is the best option available. Pharmacologic stress imaging is considered class I approach to risk stratify patients with LBBB. Some institutions believe that vasodilator MPI is superior to inotropic echocardiography, but this head-to-head trial has not been performed and both tests have proven accurate in skilled hands.

Option E is incorrect since an invasive coronary angiography should be reserved for moderate- to high-risk results (ISCHEMIA trial pending) or persistent angina symptoms after Rx. A noninvasive coronary angiogram (cardiac CTA) may be considered a reasonable alternative, however.

Answer 47: E. Understand the value added with pharmacologic protocols compared with exercise protocols in patients with LBBB.

In patients with LBBB on baseline ECG, dobutamine stress echocardiography is *less sensitive* but *more specific* than nuclear MPI in detecting coronary stenosis and provides prognostic information that is incremental to clinical findings. One meta-analysis demonstrated that abnormal stress nuclear MPI and stress echocardiography **each confer an up to 7-fold** increased risk of adverse cardiovascular events.

The patient's pretest likelihood of CAD also influences cost-effectiveness such that exercise echocardiography is more cost-effective in lower-risk patients (with annual risk of death or MI < 2%) than in higher-risk patients, in whom nuclear MPI is more cost-effective.

Isolated "false-positive" reversible perfusion defects of the septum on nuclear MPI due to abnormal septal motion causing a reduction in diastolic filling time have been reported in patients with LBBB without significant coronary stenosis. Compared to patients without LBBB, use of exercise stress in patients with LBBB or ventricular pacing substantially reduced diagnostic specificity. Although a normal nuclear perfusion scan in this clinical setting is highly accurate in indicating the absence of a significant coronary stenosis and a low risk of subsequent cardiac events, an abnormal study can be nondiagnostic.

Pharmacologic stress with either nuclear MPI or echocardiography is recommended for risk assessment in patients with SIHD who have LBBB on ECG, regardless of ability to exercise to an adequate workload is considered a **class I indication**.

Options A and B are not correct since exercise results in an increased likelihood of a false-positive, not false-negative, nuclear SPECT and stress echo result.

Option C is not correct. There is a higher rate of septal perfusion defects and wall motion abnormalities. However, this should NOT extend into the anterior wall, the anteroseptal or inferoseptal walls, or the apical region. This is where clinical expertise is valuable—recognize the "expected" from the "unexpected" patterns. Furthermore, abnormal "motion" without abnormal "wall thickening" is the typical pattern in LBBB. Abnormal "wall thickening" raises the likelihood for ischemia.

Option D is not the best option. Although there is reduced diagnostic specificity, sensitivity is either increased or unchanged.

Option E is the best option since a normal exercise stress imaging test result would still confer an excellent clinical outcome despite the LBBB pattern on ECG.

Suggested Readings

Cortigiani L, et al. Prognostic value of pharmacologic stress echocardiography in patients with left bundle branch block. *Am J Med* 2001;110:361–369.

Fihn SD, et al. 2012 ACCF/AHA/ACP/AATS/PCNA/SCAI/STS guideline for the diagnosis and management of patients with stable ischemic heart disease. *J Am Coll Cardiol* 2012;60:e44–e164.

Answer 48: A. This question emphasizes the importance of clinical symptoms over markers of LV function in isolation.

The relationship between measures of resting LV systolic dysfunction and perioperative events in noncardiac surgery has been evaluated, and an LVEF < 35% is considered risky for perioperative heart failure exacerbation. LVEF has only modest incremental predictive power over clinical risk factors, and patients with a history of HF demonstrated that preoperative LVEF < 30% was needed to demonstrate an increased risk of perioperative complications.

In 1,005 consecutive patients undergoing elective vascular surgery at a single center, LV dysfunction (LVEF < 50%) was present in 50% of patients, of whom 80% were asymptomatic. The 30-day cardiovascular event rate was highest in patients with symptomatic HF (49%), followed by those with asymptomatic systolic LV dysfunction (23%), asymptomatic diastolic LV dysfunction (18%), and normal LV function (10%).

Option A is the best answer since this includes heart failure symptoms.

Options B and C are incorrect since these patients are asymptomatic.

Options D and E are incorrect since less than severe AS or MR are not considered high risk.

Suggested Readings

Fleisher LA, et al. 2014 ACC/AHA guideline on perioperative cardiovascular evaluation and management of patients undergoing noncardiac surgery. *J Am Coll Cardiol* 2014;64:e77–137.

Flu W-J, et al. Prognostic implications of asymptomatic left ventricular dysfunction in patients undergoing vascular surgery. *Anesthesiology* 2010;112:1316–1324.

Answer 49: *C.* This question requires the reader to understand the indications for screening family members of patients with *familial cardiomyopathies.*

It is increasingly being recognized that as many as one-third patients with an idiopathic DCM have a *familial cardiomyopathy* (defined as two closely related family members who meet the criteria for idiopathic DCM). Consideration of familial cardiomyopathies includes the increasingly important discovery of noncompaction cardiomyopathies. Genetic screening and counseling should also be considered.

First-degree relatives of patients with a familial DCM should undergo **serial echocardiographic screening** with assessment of LV function and size. *Frequency of screening* is uncertain, but every 3 to 5 years is reasonable.

Patients with idiopathic DCM should inform first-degree relatives of their diagnosis. Relatives should update their clinicians and discuss whether they should undergo screening by echocardiography.

Options A and B are not the best options as this patient has no CAD symptoms or CAD risk factors, and the normal perfusion on SPECT lowers CAD likelihood. If symptoms exist, or patient had diabetes, or there was suspicion for "balanced ischemia" on SPECT, then either invasive or noninvasive coronary imaging would be considered a class I indication.

Option C is the correct choice, and screening echo on all asymptomatic siblings is considered appropriate for familiar cardiomyopathies.

Option D is not correct, and dobutamine echocardiography would be important for either viability or ischemia assessment, which would not be required at this time.

Options E and F are incorrect at this time, although either may be considered important after stabilization of medical therapy, repeat LV function assessment, and monitoring of symptom response to Rx.

Suggested Readings

Hershberger RE, Siegfried JD. Update 2011: clinical and genetic issues in familial dilated cardiomyopathy. *J Am Coll Cardiol* 2011;57:1641–1649.

Yancy CW, et al. 2013 ACCF/AHA guideline for the management of heart failure: a report of the American College of Cardiology Foundation/American Heart Association Task Force on Practice Guidelines. *J Am Coll Cardiol* 2013;62:e147–e239.

Answer 50: *B.* This question highlights the importance of DSE interpretation. This DSE is consistent with a biphasic response (improved WMSI at low dose and worsening at peak stress). Significant myocardial viability and significant myocardial ischemia are thus demonstrated.

Option A is usually a correct option, but, in this instance, would be premature and referral to an exercise rehab program would be associated with undue risks given the high-risk findings on stress echo.

Option B is the most correct option, and coronary angiography would be necessary prior to considering revascularization options.

Option C is incorrect as a cardiac CTA is rarely (if ever) indicated for a patient 10 years after CABG surgery.

Options D and E are not the best options since these are both viability tests, which this patient has already completed. If the dobutamine echo was not "biphasic" or there was an inadequate or suboptimal result, then resting thallium or PET scan may be considered alternative options.

Answer 51: *D.* This question highlights the continued clinical importance of myocardial viability assessment in the post-STICH trial era.

Option A is incorrect (see discussion to Question 40).

Options B and C are incorrect since viability testing has already been performed.

Option D is the most correct option and the only choice that offers the potential for complete revascularization.

Option E is not the best option since single-vessel PCI to the most severe lesion would result in incomplete revascularization. If staged with PCI intervention to the other ischemic coronary arteries, then this option may be correct (but as written, it is incorrect).

Option F is incorrect since transplant and/or device evaluation should be reserved for persistent heart failure symptoms on OMT.

Answer 52: *D.* The "biphasic pattern" has been one of the most important noninvasive markers to predict LV functional recovery after revascularization.

Option A is the best option since the clinical presentation does not suggest an unstable or ACS presentation. At times, a plaque rupture may be found despite stable angina clinical presentation, but this is less common.

Option B is not entirely correct. The peak dose WMSI is reported as 2.48. In a normal resting echo, multivessel ischemia would be required to achieve a WMSI > 2.0 (severe ischemia in a wraparound LAD with large diagonal branch approaches WMSI ~ 2.0). However, there are multiple ways to obtain a WMSI 2.48 without MV ischemia by including LV scar or aneurysms.

Option C is not correct as the improved low-dose WMSI implies high likelihood of myocardial viability (relative to scar), but this does not prove ischemia, and therefore, LVEF may not recovery after surgery aimed at relief of ischemia.

Option D is most correct. The rest to low to peak dose WMSI pattern (biphasic pattern) implies a favorable clinical outcome (and high likelihood for LV functional recovery).

Option E is not the best option. Although the severely reduced LVEF is an important factor in determining surgical outcome, the good coronary targets, biphasic LV response (and relatively large region of myocardium in jeopardy—based upon WMSI difference), relatively low age, and generalized good health of the patient balance the surgical risks.

The assessment of myocardial viability in patients with CAD and HF remains a class IIa recommendation. Myocardial viability indicates the likelihood of improved outcomes with either surgical or medical therapy but does not identify patients with greater survival benefit from revascularization. Decisions about revascularization in patients with moderate to severely reduced LV function should be made jointly by the heart team. The most important considerations in the decision to proceed with a surgical or interventional approach include coronary anatomy that is amenable to revascularization and appropriate concomitant GDMT.

Candidates for coronary revascularization who present with a high suspicion for obstructive CAD should undergo coronary angiography. Stress nuclear imaging or echocardiography may be an acceptable option for assessing ischemia in patients presenting with HF who have known CAD and no angina unless they are ineligible for revascularization.

Although the results of the STICH (Surgical Treatment for Ischemic Heart Failure) trial have cast doubt on the role of myocardial viability assessment to determine the mode of therapy, the data are nevertheless predictive of a positive outcome. When these data are taken into consideration with multiple previous studies demonstrating the usefulness of this approach, it becomes reasonable to recommend viability assessment when treating patients with HFrEF who have known CAD.

Suggested Reading
Bonow RO, et al. Myocardial viability and survival in ischemic left ventricular dysfunction. *N Engl J Med* 2011;364:1617–1625.

Answer 53: *E.* Understand the importance of provocation maneuvers when assessing HCM and the resting Doppler max gradient is <30 mm Hg.

Although the resting max gradient <30 mm Hg (echo tip: 250 cm/s = 25 mm Hg), provocation is warranted, and resting Doppler data alone are not adequate to diagnose or exclude "obstructive" HCM.

Option A is not correct as the severity of the LV wall thickness would be nearly pathognomonic for hypertrophic cardiomyopathy (>25 mm).

Option B is not correct. An athlete's heart may at times be confused with HCM, but LV wall thickness would rarely ever exceed 13 to 15 mm.

Options C and D are not the best options since the hypertrophic cardiomyopathy cannot be categorized as obstructive or nonobstructive until provocation maneuvers have been performed.

Option E is the best option since additional Doppler info (during provocation) is required.

Answer 54: *D.* This question requires an understanding of the diagnosis and gradient values warranting consideration for interventional therapies.

For HCM, it is the *peak instantaneous LV outflow gradient* rather than the mean gradient that influences treatment decisions.

Obstruction to LV outflow is dynamic, varying with loading conditions and contractility of the ventricle. Increased myocardial contractility, decreased ventricular volume, or decreased afterload increases the degree of obstruction. Patients with little or no gradient at rest can generate large LVOT gradients under conditions such as exercise, the strain phase of the Valsalva maneuver, or during pharmacologic provocation.

There is often large spontaneous variation in the severity of the gradient throughout the day or with diet (exacerbation of symptoms during the postprandial period is common). It has been well established that LVOT obstruction contributes to the symptoms and outcomes.

One-third of patients with HCM will have obstruction at rest (gradients >30 mm Hg). Another one-third will have provoked gradients (<30 mm Hg at rest and ≥30 mm Hg with physiologic provocation). Other patients will have the nonobstructive form of HCM (gradients <30 mm Hg at rest and with provocation; "tricks": this may be referred to as "NOCM" to differentiate from "HOCM"). Gradients >50 mm Hg, either at rest or with provocation, represent the conventional threshold for intervention (surgical or percutaneous) if symptoms cannot be controlled with medications.

Provocation with dobutamine infusion during Doppler echocardiography is no longer recommended; however, for equivocal cases, cardiac catheterization with isoproterenol may be used to elicit a provocable gradient. The peak-to-peak gradient obtained with catheterization most closely approximates the peak instantaneous gradient by continuous-wave Doppler echocardiography.

Option A is incorrect. A mean gradient >30 mm Hg at rest signifies an obstructive HCM, but is not a value used to consider intervention. Also, important to know that in HCM, it is the "maximal" gradient (not the "mean") that is used for risk stratification.

Option B is not the best answer, although a peak gradient >30 mm Hg at rest would suggest an obstructive HCM.

Option C is not correct. Absence of a peak gradient > 50 mm Hg at rest warrants careful Doppler assessment with provocation.

Option D is the best answer as gradients do often vary based upon the time of the day and food intake.

Option E is incorrect since dobutamine (any dose) is contraindicated as a method of gradient provocation since it is known to potentially cause gradients even in patients without HCM.

Option F is incorrect. Exercise (noncompetitive) is now considered important in patients with HCM. Exercise Doppler is also a diagnostic option for provocation.

Suggested Reading

Gersh BJ, et al. 2011 ACCF/AHA guideline for the diagnosis and treatment of hypertrophic cardiomyopathy. *J Am Coll Cardiol* 2011;58:e212–e260.

Answer 55: D. This question emphasizes the importance of understanding the normal and pathologic Doppler response to exercise.

Exercise testing is helpful in the risk assessment of patients with hypertrophic cardiomyopathy. An abnormal blood pressure response to exercise (defined as either a **failure to increase by at least 20 mm Hg** or a **drop of at least 20 mm Hg during effort**) has been demonstrated to be one factor associated with risk of sudden arrhythmic death. Most published studies examining exercise blood pressure response use symptom-limited treadmill exercise testing with a Bruce protocol.

Option A is incorrect and a drop in SBP > 20 mm Hg at peak exercise should be considered a high-risk finding.

Option B is incorrect as an increased pulse pressure is expected in a normal BP response to exercise (the SBP increases more than the DBP; therefore, the pulse pressure widens).

Option C is not the best answer. Although an increased SBP > 20 mm Hg in stage I may be normal, patients with HOCM may develop marked LVOT gradients, and associated SBP drops relatively suddenly at later exercise stages (peak exercise).

Option D is the best option since a flat SPB response (<20 mm Hg total increase) is a high-risk finding and one of the potential markers of sudden cardiac death.

Option E is incorrect. Most investigators and reports have performed symptom-limited exercise stress with a Bruce protocol.

Suggested Readings

Gersh BJ, et al. 2011 ACCF/AHA guideline for the diagnosis and treatment of hypertrophic cardiomyopathy. *J Am Coll Cardiol* 2011;58:e212–e260.
Olivotto I, et al. Prognostic value of systemic blood pressure response during exercise in a community-based patient population with hypertrophic cardiomyopathy. *J Am Coll Cardiol* 1999;33:2044–2051.

Answer 56: D. This question asks the reader to know the "other" echo/Doppler parameters that can be monitored during stress echocardiography for nonischemic clinical investigations.

Option A is incorrect since a mean transmitral gradient increase >5 mm Hg in MV prosthesis is considered normal and should be >10 mm Hg to be considered pathologic increase.

Option B is incorrect since a mean transmitral gradient increase >4 mm Hg after MV repair may be normal, but >7 mm Hg is considered the pathologic cutoff value.

Option C is also incorrect since the value of change is not correctly listed. A change in global longitudinal strain of 3% to 5% in primary MR would be considered normal and must be <2% (essentially, negligible) to be considered a pathologic response.

Option D is the correct answer. Any reduction in TAPSE to a value below the normal range (<19 mm) in primary MR would be considered an abnormal response and likely represents an impact from the regurgitant volume and transient pulmonary hypertension.

Option E is incorrect as an increase in the LVEF of 5% to 10% in primary MR would be considered a normal response and must be <4% to 5% to be considered pathologic.

Suggested Reading

Lancellotti P, et al. The clinical use of stress echocardiography in non-ischaemic heart disease: recommendations from the European Association of Cardiovascular Imaging and the American Society of Echocardiography. *J Am Soc Echocardiogr* 2017;30(2):101–138. http://dx.doi.org/10.1016/j.echo.2016.10.016

Answer 57: E. This question requires the reader to understand the normal hemodynamic impact of exercise during stress echocardiography.

Options A and B are incorrect since the heart rate and BP values increase by less degrees.

Options C and D are not correct since the systemic vascular resistance decreases and the PA systolic pressure increases during exercise.

Option E is the best answer as the coronary blood flow increases ≥3 to 5× in normal individuals without cardiovascular disease.

During exercise stress echo (treadmill or bike), the heart rate will increase 2 to 3×, LV contractility 3 to 4×, and systolic blood pressure by half. However, the systemic vascular resistance will fall. Initially, due to increased peripheral venous return, the LV end-diastolic volume increases, but at higher HR will decrease.

In the supine bike position compared with upright treadmill, the HR and exercise tolerance are lower and the LV end-diastolic volume and mean arterial blood pressure are higher. These differences contribute to a higher wall stress, an increase in myocardial oxygen demand, and higher filling pressures.

Coronary blood flow increases 3 to 5× in normal subjects and <2× in many patients with nonischemic dilated or HCM. In these patients with a reduced CFR, the regional myocardial oxygen–supply mismatch (subendocardial ischemia) may result in regional LV systolic dysfunction despite angiographically normal coronary arteries (as seen in dilated and HCM).

Suggested Reading

Lancellotti P, et al. The clinical use of stress echocardiography in non-ischaemic heart disease: recommendations from the European Association of Cardiovascular Imaging and the American Society of Echocardiography. *J Am Soc Echocardiogr* 2017;30(2):101–138. http://dx.doi.org/10.1016/j.echo.2016.10.016

Answer 58: E. This question asks the reader to understand the normal and abnormal echo changes during exercise in a patient with HCM. Also, this question asks the test taker to recognize the differences in clinical outcome prediction versus poor exercise tolerance prediction.

Option A is incorrect. An increase in postexercise LVOT gradient >50 mm Hg is considered a pathologic response only when the metoprolol is not held.

Option B is not correct since an increased exercise LVOT gradient to 40 mm Hg does not reach the pathologic threshold for intervention of >50 mm Hg.

Exercise SE is an important method to monitor the response to therapy in patients with HCM. Dynamic LVOT obstruction (>50 mm Hg) can be easily assessed. Abnormal BP response to exercise, blunted contractile (systolic) and diastolic reserve, and worsened MR are associated with poor exercise capacity and outcome. SE is not indicated when a gradient >50 mm Hg is present at rest or with Valsalva maneuver.

A limited exercise capacity, an abnormal blood pressure response (hypotensive or blunted response), significant ST depression, inducible wall motion abnormalities, blunted coronary flow reserve (dipyridamole test), exercise LVOTO (>50 mm Hg), and blunted systolic function reserve are all parameters of *worse prognosis*.

Dynamic increase in MR, often in relation to systolic anterior motion of the mitral valve, blunted changes in e′ (no diastolic reserve), increase in E/e′, and PH at exercise are all markers of *poor exercise tolerance*; some patients can display a paradoxical decrease in LVOTO during exercise, which is associated with a *more favorable outcome* and suggests alternative reasons for dyspnea.

Option C is not true. A paradoxical decrease in the LVOT gradient has been associated with good clinical outcomes.

Options D and F are predictors of poor exercise tolerance (increased LA pressure), but do not predict outcome.

Option E is the most correct choice. A systolic BP increase from 120 to 125 mm Hg at peak exercise would be considered a pathologic, blunted increase and has been demonstrated to predict poor clinical outcomes.

Suggested Reading

Lancellotti P, et al. The Clinical use of stress echocardiography in non-ischaemic heart disease: recommendations from the European Association of Cardiovascular Imaging and the American Society of Echocardiography. *J Am Soc Echocardiogr* 2017;30(2):101–138. http://dx.doi.org/10.1016/j.echo.2016.10.016

Answer 59: A. This question requires the reader to consider the various pharmacologic stress echo responses in ischemic versus nonischemic cardiomyopathy.

Differentiating nonischemic from ischemic cardiomyopathy is challenging, especially with severely dilated hearts with a very low LVEF. Patients with a nonischemic cardiomyopathy often have regional wall motion abnormalities, experience angina, and have ECG evidence of myocardial infarction. It has been shown that patients with an ischemic cardiomyopathy, compared to dilated, nonischemic CM, are more likely to display >6 akinetic segments at peak dobutamine test, demonstrated less improvement in regional wall motion at low-dose dobutamine, and are more likely to have a biphasic response.

Answer A is the best available option. A WMSI at baseline of 2.3 that improves to a peak dobutamine WMSI of 1.8 is a significant increase in LVEF and LV inotropic reserve more common in dilated, nonischemic etiologies. However, this could also be found in a pt with CAD (previously treated and nonischemic).

Option B is not correct as >6 akinetic wall segments noted at peak dobutamine have been shown to be more common in ischemic CM than nonischemic CM.

Option C is incorrect, and a biphasic response to dobutamine is one of the best predictors of underlying CAD, inotropic reserve, and improvement after revascularization.

Option D is not the best answer. A coronary flow reserve increase >2.0 during vasodilator stress demonstrates adequate coronary flow, but this could be found in either etiology and not discriminatory.

Suggested Reading

Lancellotti P, et al. The Clinical use of stress echocardiography in non-ischaemic heart disease: recommendations from the European Association of Cardiovascular Imaging and the American Society of Echocardiography. *J Am Soc Echocardiogr* 2017;30(2):101–138. http://dx.doi.org/10.1016/j.echo.2016.10.016

Chapter 52

3-Dimensional Echocardiography

Paul Anaya

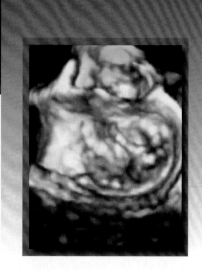

1. FIGURE 52.1 demonstrates a full-volume acquisition for 3D estimation of the LV ejection fraction. Current 3D echocardiography systems allow for optimized real-time imaging, full-volume acquisition, and 3-dimensional zoom imaging, each with its own pyramidal 3D data set.

For estimation of LV systolic function, which of the following pyramidal 3D data set sizes would be appropriate?

A. 90 degrees × 90 degrees
B. 30 degrees × 30 degrees
C. 60 degrees × 60 degrees
D. 60 degrees × 30 degrees

2. Which of the following features of real-time 3D echocardiography compared to standard 2D echocardiography is **least advantageous**?

A. Immediate display of volumetric images
B. Enhanced understanding of anatomical relationships
C. Reduced spatial resolution
D. Enhanced accuracy of LVEF quantitation
E. Improved temporal resolution

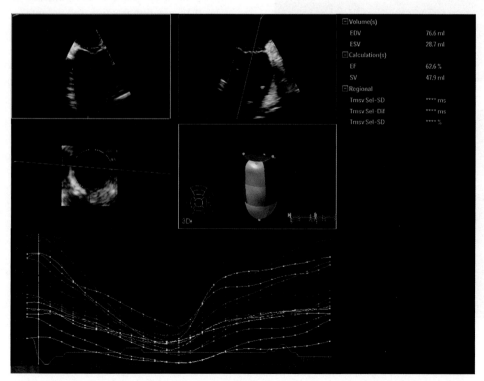

FIGURE 52.1 Full-volume acquisition for 3D estimation of the LV ejection fraction.

3. 3D echocardiography has been validated and should be clinically incorporated in each of the following clinical settings, **except**

A. Evaluation of cardiac LV volumes and systolic function
B. Assessment of RV volume and function
C. Evaluation of left atrial size
D. Volumetric evaluation of regurgitant lesions and shunts
E. Presentation of realistic views of heart valves

4. A 54-year-old male with a history of ischemic cardiomyopathy presents with atrial fibrillation and rapid ventricular response. He requires a TEE for evaluation prior to cardioversion. Which of the 3DE acquisition modes will result in images with a high likelihood of artifacts?

A. Real-time 3DE imaging
B. Live 3D zoom mode
C. Live 3D wide angle/full volume
D. ECG-triggered multiple-beat 3DE imaging

5. Which of the following steps to reduce the demonstrated artifact encountered during acquisition of this wide-volume 3DE image is **least likely** to be corrective (Fig. 52.2 and Video 52.1)?

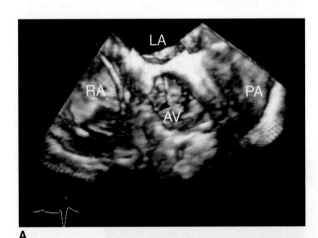

A

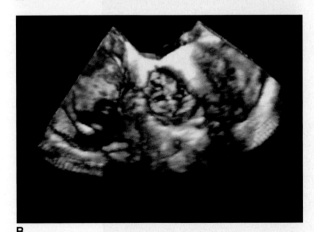

B

Figure 52.2

A. It is impossible to eliminate gating artifacts due to ectopy.
B. Suspend respiration and reacquire image.
C. Increase the line density to increase the temporal resolution.
D. Increase the gain since the major artifact is image "dropout."
E. Display in a different reference plane that is parallel to the sweep plane as this is a display artifact and not an acquisition artifact.

6. Which of the following structures has been most studied with real-time 3D echocardiography?

A. Right ventricle
B. Left ventricle
C. Right atrium
D. Left atrium
E. Aorta

7. A 73-year-old male who presents with chest pain was found to have ST elevations in the inferior leads, with subsequent right ventricular heart failure. Which of the imaging modalities has the greatest interstudy reproducibility regarding the assessment of right ventricular systolic function?

A. 3D echocardiography.
B. 2D echocardiography.
C. Cardiac MRI.
D. Cardiac CT.
E. 2D with contrast, 3DE, and cardiac MRI are equally reproducible.

8. What are the two most critical anatomic landmarks used in 3D echocardiography to determine an accurate left ventricular (LV) ejection fraction and volume?

A. Left ventricle trabeculae and papillary muscles
B. Mitral annulus and aortic annulus
C. Interventricular septum and left ventricular apex
D. Mitral annulus and left ventricular apex
E. RV insertion points

9. Which of the following statements is true regarding 3D transesophageal echocardiography (TEE) in comparison to 2D TEE in the assessment of mitral stenosis?

A. The optimal timing of the cardiac cycle to measure planimetry for mitral stenosis in 3D TEE is midsystole.
B. 2D TEE tends to overestimate mitral valve area (MVA) in comparison to 3D TEE.
C. Mitral valve commissural fusion is overestimated with 2D TEE.
D. 3D TEE provides limited information on the degree of commissural calcification.
E. Reproducibility of 2DE measurements of mitral valve area is higher than with 3DE.

10. Which of the following is **least demonstrated** in this 3D TEE (Fig. 52.3 and Video 37.2) of the mitral valve?

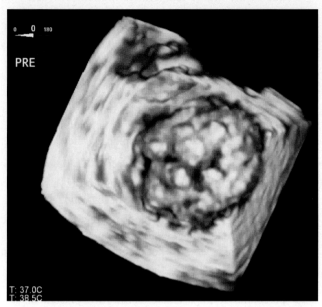

Figure 52.3 Adapted from Silvestry FE, Kerber RE, Brook MM, et al. Echocardiography-guided interventions. *J Am Soc Echocardiogr* 2009; 22(3):213–231; quiz 316–317. Copyright © 2009 American Society of Echocardiography. With permission.

A. Multiscallop billowing and prolapse
B. Annular enlargement
C. Left atrial enlargement
D. Severe mitral regurgitation
E. Elevated zone of coaptation

11. The patient with shortness of breath and a loud precordial holosystolic murmur shown in Figure 52.4 and Video 52.3 has which of the following?

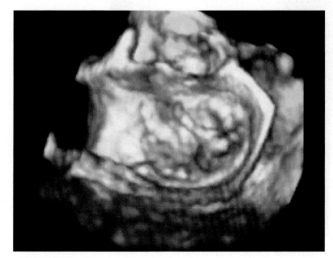

Figure 52.4

A. Anterior mitral valve leaflet prolapse
B. Flail P1 scallop of the posterior mitral leaflet viewed from the LV
C. Flail P2 scallop of the posterior mitral leaflet viewed from the LV
D. Flail P3 scallop of the posterior mitral leaflet viewed from the LA
E. Flail A2 scallop of the anterior mitral leaflet viewed from the LA

12. Figure 52.5 and Video 52.4 in this patient with normal cardiac loop formation are most consistent with

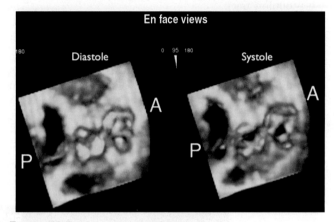

Figure 52.5 A, anterior; P, posterior.

A. Mitral valve stenosis
B. Aortic valve stenosis
C. Pulmonic valve stenosis
D. Tricuspid valve stenosis
E. Superior vena cava stenosis

13. When evaluating aortic stenosis by echocardiography, 3DE has potentially an incremental value over 2DE due to all of the following **except**

A. Substituting LVOT diameter–derived LVOT area with planimetered LVOT area measured from 3DE
B. Improved image spatial anatomy and spatial resolution
C. Substituting 3DE-derived LV stroke volume with LVOT-derived stroke volume (velocity–time integral method)
D. Direct planimetry of the aortic valve area on 3DE datasets
E. Determination of the effect of valve shape on pressure gradients and effective orifice areas

14. Which of the following below **is false** in regard to the LVOT, aortic valve, and aortic root?

A. 3DE allows effective measurement of the distance between the annulus and leaflet tips to the coronary ostia, which is crucial for optimal placement of prosthetic valves by the percutaneous route.

B. 2DE parasternal long-axis view of the aortic valve and root often underestimates LV outflow tract area, as it presumes a circular shape.

C. 3DE enables multiplane imaging of the aortic valve (e.g., simultaneous display of the valve in both the long and short axes), demonstrating the true shape of the LV outflow tract.

D. Aortic annular diameter was initially reported from computed tomographic studies to be more round than oval.

E. 3D echocardiography measures of aortic annulus dimensions can be accurately obtained compared to CT.

15. A 60-year-old female patient presented with signs of right heart failure. Which of the following statements is most accurate regarding the assessment of the tricuspid valve function in these 3DE images (Fig. 52.6 and Video 52.5)?

A. The geometric changes of the tricuspid annulus can be less accurately assessed with 3D compared to 2D due to the higher temporal resolution provided with multibeat full-volume acquisition.

B. Although 3D-derived vena contracta can be measured, it is unlikely to be different than the 2D vena contracta measurement.

C. 3D images are considered standard images and are always required for accurate surgical planning.

D. 3D echo provides incremental diagnostic value over 2DE with regard to location of leaflet pathology.

E. By adding color flow Doppler to the 3D image, temporal resolution is improved over 2DE.

16. Which of the following statements is true with regard to the recommended clinical practice of 3D echo?

A. Both tricuspid and pulmonic valve regurgitations have been the least studied by 3D echo.

B. LV ejection fraction is not recommended to be used in clinical practice.

C. There is no role of 3D echo in the assessment of percutaneous transcatheter aortic valve placement.

D. Infective endocarditis has been well validated in 3D echo.

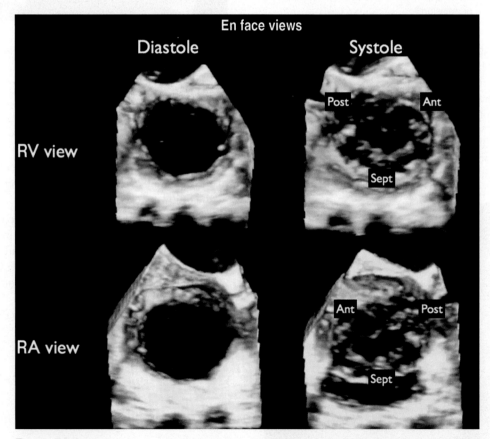

Figure 52.6 Ant, anterior tricuspid valve leaflet; post, posterior tricuspid valve leaflet; sept, septal tricuspid valve leaflet.

17. Compared with cardiac MRI, 3D echocardiographic measures of left ventricular volumes, ejection fraction, and mass tend to be:

	LV VOLUME	LVEF	LV MASS
A	Underestimated	Accurate	Accurate
B	Overestimated	Overestimated	Overestimated
C	Accurate	Accurate	Underestimated
D	Accurate	Accurate	Accurate
E	Overestimated	Accurate	Accurate

18. 3D echocardiography is a validated technique, providing useful clinical information not available with 2D echocardiography in all of the following clinical settings except?

A. Evaluation of cardiac LV volumes and systolic function
B. Assessment of RV volume and function
C. Evaluation of left atrial size
D. Quantitative evaluation of regurgitant lesions and shunts
E. Presentation of realistic views of the heart valves

19. A 24-year-old female presents with generalized malaise, fevers, and nausea and vomiting of 1-week duration. PMH is significant for mitral valve endocarditis for which she underwent a mitral valve replacement approximately 9 months ago. Vital signs on presentation include the following: BP 95/70 mm Hg, HR 120 bpm, temp 38.2°C, resp rate 28/min, and SpO$_2$ 92% on 3 L O$_2$ via nasal cannula. Physical examination shows an acutely ill-appearing young female in mild respiratory distress. There are audible bilateral and diffuse expiratory wheezes on lung exam; cardiac exam is significant for the mechanical sound of her mitral valve prosthesis and a 2/6 systolic murmur at the lower left sternal edge; abdominal exam is normal and there is no evidence of peripheral edema. ECG demonstrates sinus tachycardia and a CXR shows cardiomegaly but no lung pathology. Laboratory values include a leukocytosis. Urinalysis shows leukocytes and positive nitrite. Blood cultures demonstrate G(-) rods. She is admitted to the hospital and a TEE is performed. 3D images from the TEE are shown in FIGURES 52.7 TO 52.9. The images in FIGURES 52.7 TO 52.9 and VIDEO 52.1 demonstrate which of the following:

A. A normal functioning MV bioprosthesis
B. A normal functioning mechanical MV prosthesis
C. Prosthetic MV dehiscence
D. Prosthetic MV abscess

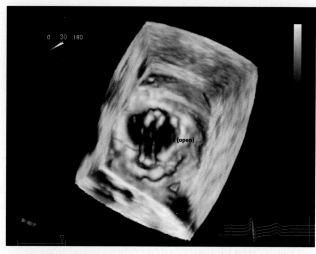

FIGURE 52.7

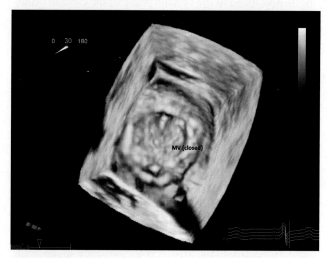

FIGURE 52.8

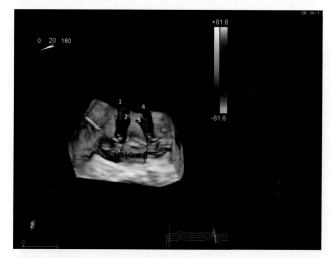

FIGURE 52.9

20. A 67-year-old female is being evaluated for shortness of breath and new-onset atrial fibrillation. Her past medical history is significant for CKD-4 and hypertension. Her symptoms have progressed over the last 6 months and more recently are associated with palpitations lasting several minutes. Physical examination reveals a woman appearing older than her stated age in mild respiratory distress at rest on room air. There is marked jugular venous distention, bibasilar crackles over the lung fields bilaterally, a 2/6 SM at the apex, and a harsh diastolic murmur heard over the left 4th intercostal space at the midclavicular line. CXR shows mild pulmonary edema and evidence of biatrial enlargement. Calcification over the mitral valve area is visible. The ECG shows atrial fibrillation, incomplete RBBB, left atrial abnormality, and right atrial enlargement. In comparison to 2D TEE, 3D TEE performed to evaluate mitral stenosis

A. Is less reproducible due to limitations from stitch artifact
B. Is best timed to the systolic phase of the cardiac cycle
C. Underestimates mitral valve area
D. Is not suited to assess the severity of commissural calcification

21. A 72-year-old female with a history of atrial fibrillation and mild–moderate aortic valvular stenosis undergoes an emergent surgical procedure. She was previously anticoagulated with apixaban, which was discontinued at the time of her surgery. Her recovery from surgery has been complicated by GI bleeding, and a thorough invasive investigation revealed the presence of a bleeding ulcer within the duodenum treated endoscopically. As a result, all anticoagulation therapy has been stopped. On postoperative day 9, the patient is noted to have a right-sided weakness and expressive aphasia. Head CT reveals no evidence of hemorrhage. A brain MRI reveals evidence of an acute stroke involving the left middle cerebral artery vascular territory. A TEE is performed, which shows the following (Figs. 52.10 to 52.13 and Video 52.7).

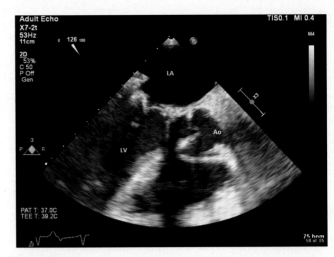

FIGURE 52.11

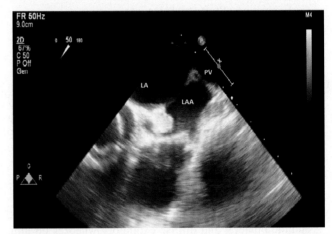

FIGURE 52.12

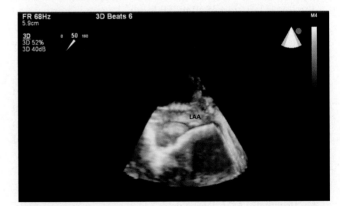

FIGURE 52.13

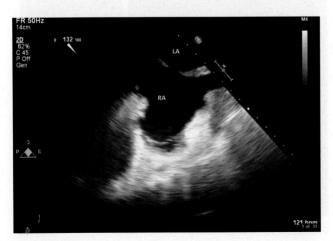

FIGURE 52.10

The most likely etiology for the patient's stroke is

A. A left atrial myxoma
B. A left atrial appendage thrombus
C. Ischemic cerebrovascular disease
D. Hypoperfusion due to recent blood loss

22. Referring to the previous question, the patient eventually recovers enough to be discharged to a rehabilitation facility. She completes 2 months of physical rehabilitation and returns for a follow-up clinic visit. She was placed on warfarin anticoagulation therapy with a target INR of 2.0 to 2.5. She has had no recurrent bleeding complications. Despite this, the patient informs you that she fears having another bleeding event and prefers not to have to take any anticoagulants. She learned about a new procedure being offered at your hospital from a fellow resident at the rehabilitation center that would essentially prevent clots from escaping into the bloodstream and is interested in pursuing this further. You review the criteria for the Watchman device and agree that the patient would be an excellent candidate. A TEE is performed and after volume loading to a LA pressure of 12 mm Hg, the following measurements are made: 1.73 cm × 1.53 cm × 1.83 cm at 30 degrees, 60 degrees, and 90 degrees.

Based on these measurements, you advise the patient to:

A. Watchman device implantation.
B. Surgical LAA ligation and MAZE.
C. Surgical AVR, LAA ligation, and MAZE.
D. Perform CTA to more accurately size the LAA.
E. Perform CTA after volume loading and remeasure the LAA.

23. In the preparation for implantation of the Watchman device, largest to smallest measurements for the LAA orifice size by available imaging modalities are as follows:

A. CTA → 3DTEE → 2DTEE → fluoroscopy
B. 3DTEE → CTA → fluoroscopy → 2DTEE
C. Fluoroscopy → CTA → 3DTEE → 2DTEE
D. Fluoroscopy → 2DTEE → 3DTEE → CTA

Answer 1: A. Current 3D matrix–array transducers contain approximately 3,000 individual transducer elements capable of acquiring differently sized pyramidal 3D volume sets within a single heartbeat (Figs. 52.14 to 52.16). Full-volume acquisition mode requires the largest acquisition sector possible, which is a matrix size of 90 degrees × 90 degrees. In contradistinction with other acquisition modes, full-volume acquisition must be ECG gated. The resulting image represents a compilation of four separate sectors acquired over 4 heartbeats, which are then merged to form the larger sector. Answer B is incorrect as the sector size would be too small to accommodate the larger structure of the left ventricle. However, this sector width is ideal for viewing smaller structures such as the cardiac valves as it permits a more focused and better resolved view. Answers C and D are incorrect for the similar reason that the pyramidal sizes would be too small for the left ventricle. Nevertheless, a

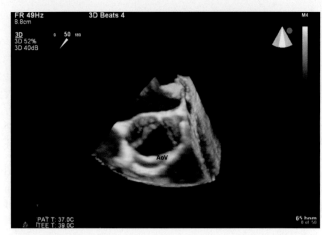

Figure 52.14

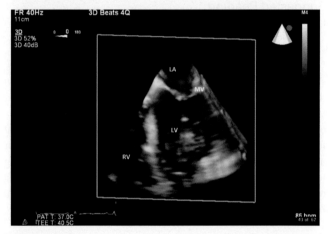

Figure 52.15

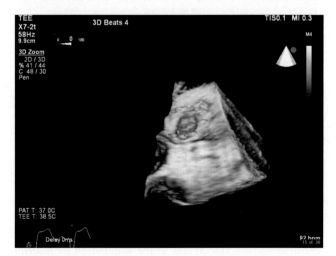

Figure 52.16

sector volume of no more than 50 to 60 degrees × 30 degrees seems best suited for real-time, 3D imaging. Any 3D volume can be adjusted by size, line density, and number of beats acquired to maximize temporal and spatial resolution, keeping in mind the inverse relation between sector size and spatial resolution and direct relationship between line density and spatial resolution.

Suggested Reading

Lang RM, BAdano LP, Tsang W, et al. EAE/ASE recommendations for image acquisition and display using three-dimensional echocardiography. *J Am Soc Echocardiogr* 2012;25:3–46.

Answer 2: E. RT-3DE has inferior temporal resolution over standard 2DE. Temporal resolution is the inherent image acquisition speed per unit time. This can also be thought of in terms of frame rate (or volume rate, in the case of 3D). Real-time 3DE allows for immediate display of 3DE datasets, allows for enhanced understanding of anatomical relationships, and allows for a greater degree of LV volume and systolic function quantitation. Spatial resolution is dependent on the number of scan lines per volume (density) but is generally inferior to standard 2DE.

Suggested Reading

Lang RM, BAdano LP, Tsang W, et al. EAE/ASE recommendations for image acquisition and display using three-dimensional echocardiography. *J Am Soc Echocardiogr* 2012;25:3–46.

Answer 3: B. The usefulness of 3D echocardiography has been demonstrated in (a) the evaluation of LV chamber volumes and function, (b) left atrial size, (c) presentation of realistic views of heart valves, and (d) volumetric evaluation of regurgitant lesions and shunts with 3DE color Doppler imaging. 3DE for assessment of RV size and systolic function is a promising technique, and despite a number of encouraging studies in this regard, it is currently not adequately validated to be sufficient for routine clinical use.

Suggested Readings

Hung J, Lang R, Flachskampf F, et al. 3D echocardiography: a review of the current status and future directions. *J Am Soc Echocardiogr* 2007;20:213–233.

Iwakura K, Ito H, Kawano S, et al. Comparison of orifice area by transthoracic three-dimensional Doppler echocardiography versus proximal isovelocity surface area (PISA) method for assessment of mitral regurgitation. *Am J Cardiol* 2006;97:1630–1637.

Jenkins C, Bricknell K, Marwick TH. Use of real-time three-dimensional echocardiography to measure left atrial volume: comparison with other echocardiographic techniques. *J Am Soc Echocardiogr* 2005;18:991–997.

Ota T, Fleishman CE, Strub M, et al. Real-time, three dimensional echocardiography: feasibility of dynamic right ventricular volume measurement with saline contrast. *Am Heart J* 1999;137:958–966.

Answer 4: D. Currently, there are two different methods for 3DE data acquisition: real-time/live 3DE imaging and electrocardiographically triggered multiple-beat 3DE imaging. Real-time or live 3DE refers to the acquisition of multiple pyramidal datasets per second in a single heartbeat. Most ultrasound systems have real-time 3DE volume imaging available in the following modes: live 3D narrow volume, live 3D zoomed, live 3D wide-angled (full volume), and live 3D color Doppler. Although this methodology overcomes the limitations imposed by rhythm disturbances or respiratory motion, it is limited by lower temporal (lower frame/volume rates) and spatial (lower image quality) resolution. In contrast, multiple-

beat 3D echocardiography provides images of higher temporal resolution. This is achieved through multiple acquisitions of narrow volumes of data over several heartbeats (ranging from two to six cardiac cycles) that are subsequently stitched together to create a single volumetric dataset. However, gated imaging of the heart is inherently prone to imaging artifacts known as "stitching artifacts" created by the patient or respiratory motion or irregular cardiac rhythms such as atrial fibrillation.

Suggested Reading

Lang RM, BAdano LP, Tsang W, et al. EAE/ASE recommendations for image acquisition and display using three-dimensional echocardiography. *J Am Soc Echocardiogr* 2012;25:3–46.

Answer 5: D. The acquisition artifact (Fig. 52.17 and Video 52.7, shown in red arrows in Fig. 52.17B) is termed a gating artifact or "stitch artifact" and is due to an irregular cardiac rhythm with variations in RR interval length. Potential solutions include waiting for a semiconstant rhythm (in the case of isolated extrasystoles) and asking the patient to breath-hold as this artifact may also occur due to chest wall movement. Gating artifacts are most prominent when the volumetric dataset is viewed from

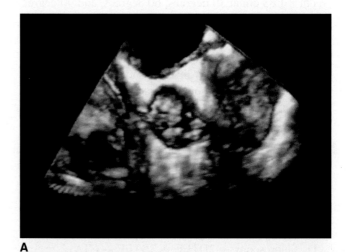

A

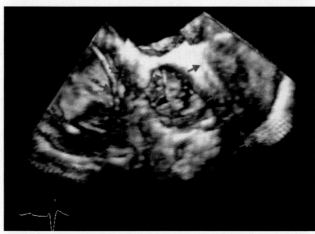

B

Figure 52.17

a cut plane perpendicular to the sweep plane. Therefore, using a reference plane parallel to the sweep plane is an additional method of minimizing this artifact. Increasing line density will reduce the volume rate and reduce temporal resolution but have no effect on gating artifacts. The method least likely to produce an artifact-free image is changing the overall gain. Image "dropout" is as a result of an undergained image, which does not appear to be the case in this example. The reacquired image without stitch artifacts is seen in FIGURE 52.17A.

Answer 6: B. LV chamber and mass quantification have been studied extensively using 3D echocardiography. Initial 3DE methods with manual rotational techniques to measure LV volumes used reconstruction techniques that, although more accurate and reproducible than 2DE methods, required long acquisition and postprocessing times. Moreover, the accuracy of the volume calculations was highly dependent on image quality. The introduction of RT-3DE systems that use matrix phased-array transducers with increased processing elements has significantly improved image quality and reduced acquisition time. LV quantification software is now widely available and is increasingly robust and accurate compared to cardiac MRI. With exception to recent work related to transcatheter aortic valve replacement (TAVR), limited data exist on the use of 3DE for quantifying aortic size. The degree of correlation between 3D echocardiography to cardiac MRI for the assessment of RV volumes and ejection fraction has been shown in recent studies but requires specialized, noncommercially available software. In a limited number of studies, left atrial volume has been accurately quantified by 3D echocardiography. These methods have been shown to correlate well with MRI and have accuracy comparable to 2D left atrial volume methods. 3D echocardiography–based measures of right atrial volume have yet to be validated against an independent reference technique such as CMR.

Suggested Readings

Bauer F, Shiota T, White RD, et al. Determinant of left atrial dilation in patients with hypertrophic cardiomyopathy: a real-time 3-dimensional echocardiographic study. *J Am Soc Echocardiogr* 2004;17:968–975.

Hung J, Lang R, Flachskampf F, et al. 3D echocardiography: a review of the current status and future directions. *J Am Soc Echocardiogr* 2007;20:213–233.

Jenkins C, Bricknell K, Marwick TH. Use of real-time three-dimensional echocardiography to measure left atrial volume: comparison with other echocardiographic techniques. *J Am Soc Echocardiogr* 2005;18:991–997.

Mor-Avi V, Jenkins C, Kuhl HP, et al. Real-time 3D echocardiographic quantification of left ventricular volumes: multicenter study for validation with magnetic resonance imaging and investigation of sources of error. *J Am Coll Cardiol Imaging* 2008;1:413–423.

Otani K, Takeuchi M, Kaku K, et al. Assessment of the aortic root using real-time 3D transesophageal echocardiography. *Circ J* 2010;74(12):2649–2657.

Answer 7: C. Assessment of RV function is of great interest in cardiovascular medicine, especially congenital heart disease and pulmonary hypertension. Due to its widespread availability, 2D echocardiography is used as the first-line imaging modality for the assessment of RV size and RV function. The tricuspid annular plane systolic excursion (TAPSE) has typically been used as a surrogate for RV performance with 2DE. The quantitative assessment of RV size and function has been hampered by the complex RV anatomy. Initial studies comparing 3DE to CMR revealed little convincing concordance in the assessment of RV volumes and RVEF. However, with the development of more specialized software specifically for this purpose, more recent studies have shown a higher degree of correlation. In addition, 3DE measurements have been shown to be more accurate than those from standard 2DE. 2D echocardiography with contrast has not been shown to be equally reproducible to 3D echocardiography nor cardiac MRI.

Suggested Readings

Bleeker GB, Steendijk P, Holman ER, et al. Assessing right ventricular function: the role of echocardiography and complementary technologies. *Heart* 2006;92(suppl 1):i19–i26.

Jenkins C, Chan J, Bricknell K, et al. Reproducibility of right ventricular volumes and ejection fraction using real-time three-dimensional echocardiography: comparison with cardiac MRI. *Chest* 2007;131:1844–1851.

Kjaergaard J, Petersen CL, Kjaer A, et al. Evaluation of right ventricular volume and function by 2D and 3D echocardiography compared to MRI. *Eur J Echocardiogr* 2005;7:430–438.

Niemann PS, Pinho L, Balbach T, et al. Anatomically oriented right ventricular volume measurements with dynamic three-dimensional echocardiography validated by 3-Tesla magnetic resonance imaging. *J Am Coll Cardiol* 2007;50:1668–1676.

Prakasa KR, Dalal D, Wang J, et al. Feasibility and variability of three dimensional echocardiography in arrhythmogenic right ventricular dysplasia/cardiomyopathy. *Am J Cardiol* 2006;97:703–709.

Answer 8: D. 3D echocardiography imaging of the left ventricle can provide volume and ejection fraction measurements independent of geometric assumptions regarding LV shape. The anatomic landmarks used for this process are the mitral annulus and LV apex, which are used to initiate edge detection by semiautomated quantification software. The mitral annulus avoids underestimating the basal plane of the LV, and the LV apical endocardium allows for definition of the true length of the LV cavity by avoiding foreshortening errors.

Other anatomic features of importance are the LV trabeculae and papillary muscles, which ideally should be included within the LV cavity for the calculation of LV volumes. The other options mentioned are not typically used for LV analysis.

Answer 9: D. A recent study showed the feasibility of mitral valve morphology and valve area assessment using real-time 3D transesophageal imaging. According to that study, 3D TEE measurements of the mitral valve orifice area (MVA) in patients with rheumatic mitral stenosis can be obtained in 95% of patients. The MVA by 3DE demonstrated the best agreement with MVA by the continuity equation followed by MVA by 2D planimetry and lastly MVA by pressure half-time method. 2D TEE was found to underestimate commissural fusion in 19% of cases. Although 3D TEE has the ability to show en face views of the mitral valve from left atrial (Fig. 52.18 and Video 52.8) and left ventricular viewpoints, thus providing the degree of commissural fusion, it is unable to provide reliable information on the degree of commissural calcification. The optimal timing of the cardiac cycle to measure planimetry is middiastole for both 2DE and 3DE.

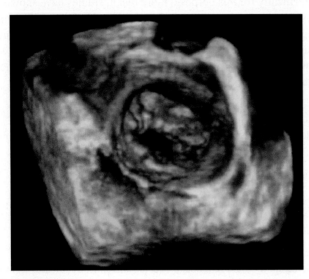

FIGURE 52.18

Suggested Readings

Anwar AM, Attia WM, Nosir YF, et al. Validation of a new score for the assessment of mitral stenosis using real-time three-dimensional echocardiography. *J Am Soc Echocardiogr* 2010;23:13–22.

Schlosshan D, Aggarwal G, Mathur G, et al. Real-time 3D transesophageal echocardiography for the evaluation of rheumatic mitral stenosis. *J Am Coll Cardiol Imaging* 2011;4:580–588.

Weyman AE. Assessment of mitral stenosis: role of real-time 3D TEE. *J Am Coll Cardiol Imaging* 2011;4(6):589–591.

Answer 10: *D.* This is a 3D TEE en face image of the mitral valve in a patient with degenerative mitral valve disease, also known as Barlow disease. There is evidence of multiple areas of leaflet prolapse with an elevated coaptation zone between the anterior and posterior leaflets. There is also a circular, enlarged mitral annulus and suggestion of left atrial enlargement. Without the addition of color Doppler, mitral regurgitation per se cannot be quantified on this image alone.

> ***Editor's Note:*** *Had a flail leaflet been demonstrated, then the question would be more difficult to answer since a flail leaflet implies severe MR (regardless of color flow Doppler). However, a multisegment MVP (Barlow disease) may have any degree of MR and in my experience is often overestimated due to the drastic 2D or 3D leaflet pathologic appearance.*

Suggested Readings

Barlow JB, Bosman CK. Aneurysmal protrusion of the posterior leaflet of the mitral valve. An auscultatory-electrocardiographic syndrome. *Am Heart J* 1966;71(2):166–178.

Lang RM, Tsang W, Weinert L, et al. Valvular heart disease: the value of dimensional echocardiography. *J Am Coll Cardiol* 2011;58:1933–1944.

Answer 11: *D.* The 3D TEE dataset demonstrates a flail P3 scallop (red arrow, Fig. 52.19) due to a ruptured chordae tendineae (yellow arrow). This will typically result in malcoaptation at the posteromedial commissure and result in severe anteriorly directed mitral regurgitation. Hence, murmurs from flail posterior segments tend to be loudest anteriorly. Conversely, flail anterior leaflets will result in posteriorly directed mitral regurgitant jets with murmurs that radiate into the back posteriorly. Compared to 2D TEE, 3D TEE has equal reliability in identifying functional mitral regurgitation. However, 3D TEE has the advantage of better localizing the diseased or flail scallop.

> ***Editor's Note:*** *As with any still image, there may be misinterpretation until visualized in motion. This still image looks like a flail P2 segment with attached torn chord. Either way, the answer can only be D since it is a 'posterior leaflet pathology' and is 'viewed from the LA'.*

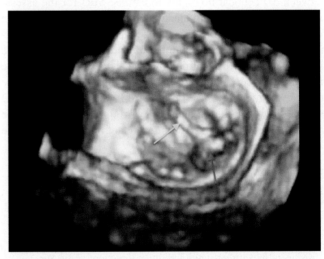

FIGURE 52.19

Suggested Reading

Ben Zekry S, et al. Comparative accuracy of two- and three-dimensional transthoracic and transesophageal echocardiography in identifying mitral valve pathology in patients undergoing mitral valve repair: initial observations. *J Am Soc Echocardiogr* 2011;24(10):1079–1085.

Answer 12: *C.* The image shown is an en face view of the aortic and pulmonic valves from the orientation of the great vessels (pulmonary artery and aorta, respectively). There is severe thickening, doming, and stenosis of the pulmonic valve commissures and leaflets (red arrows, Fig. 52.20) consistent with congenital pulmonic valve stenosis. As can be seen, this patient underwent a balloon valvuloplasty with reduction in peak gradients from 45 mm Hg to 16 mm Hg and improvement in systolic leaflet excursion (green arrow). The 3D TEE image was obtained using a cropped real-time wide-volume mode. With 3DE, the number of cusps, thickness, and mobility of the pulmonic valve leaflets could be measured, and closure lines were visualized in 70% of patients. However, due to the early-stage data, the ASE/EAE guidelines do not currently support the routine use of 3D transthoracic echocardiography or transesophageal echocardiography for the evaluation of pulmonic valve disease.

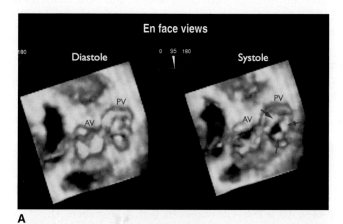

A

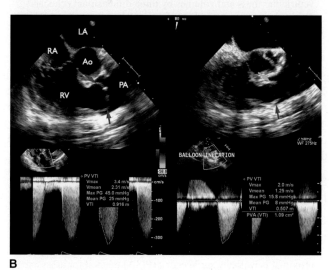

B

FIGURE 52.20

Suggested Readings

Anwar AM, Soliman O, van den Bosch AE, et al. Assessment of pulmonary valve and right ventricular outflow tract with real-time three-dimensional echocardiography. *Int J Cardiovasc Imaging* 2007;23:167–175.

Lang RM, BAdano LP, Tsang W, et al. EAE/ASE recommendations for image acquisition and display using three-dimensional echocardiography. *J Am Soc Echocardiogr* 2012;25:3–46.

Answer 13: *B.* Spatial resolution with 3DE is based on several system factors and is not ubiquitously improved over standard 2DE. However, there is evidence to suggest that the LVOT area is not usually circular, and therefore using LVOT diameter–derived areas may potentially underestimate aortic valve area. Furthermore, substituting LVOT-derived area from direct planimetry of 3DE images provides a more accurate assessment of stenosis severity. Likewise, substituting 3DE-derived left ventricular stroke volume for the endocardial detection method (at end systole and end diastole) for LVOT-derived VTI measures (continuity equation method) of stroke volume also improves the accuracy of aortic stenosis severity. Direct planimetry of AVA is feasible and relatively accurate when compared to invasive techniques and likely is superior to 2DE. Finally, valve shape is an important determinant of pressure loss in patients with aortic stenosis (with smaller effective areas and higher pressure gradients for flatter valves).

Suggested Readings

Gilon D, Cape EG, Handschumacher MD, et al. Effect of three-dimensional valve shape on the hemodynamics of aortic stenosis: three-dimensional echocardiographic stereolithography and patient studies. *J Am Coll Cardiol* 2002;40:1479–1486.

Goland S, Trento A, Iida K, et al. Assessment of aortic stenosis by three-dimensional echocardiography: an accurate and novel approach. *Heart* 2007;93:801–807.

Gutierrez-Chico JL, Zamorano JL, Prieto-Moriche E, et al. Real-time three-dimensional echocardiography in aortic stenosis: a novel, simple, and reliable method to improve accuracy in area calculation. *Eur Heart J* 2008;29:1296–1306.

Khaw AV, von Bardeleben RS, Strasser C, et al. Direct measurement of left ventricular outflow tract by transthoracic real-time 3D-echocardiography increases accuracy in assessment of aortic valve stenosis. *Int J Cardiol* 2009;136:64–71.

Answer 14: *D.* The 2DE parasternal long-axis view of the aortic valve and root often underestimates LV outflow tract area, as it presumes a circular shape. Three-dimensional echocardiography enables multiplane imaging of the aortic valve (e.g., simultaneous display of the valve in both the long and short axes), demonstrating the true shape of the LV outflow tract. As well, 3D echocardiography often confirms normal and abnormal findings when structures visualized in one plane can be examined in real time by checking a second orthogonal plane. 3DE can measure the distance between the annulus and leaflet tips to the coronary ostia, which is crucial for optimal placement of prosthetic valves by the percutaneous route. Aortic annular diameter was initially reported from computed tomographic studies to be more oval than round. 3D echocardiography measures of aortic annulus dimensions have been highly correlated with both CMR and CT, while 2D echocardiography has been shown to underestimate aortic annular diameters.

Suggested Readings

Hung J, Lang R, Flachskampf F, et al. 3D echocardiography: a review of the current status and future directions. *J Am Soc Echocardiogr* 2007;20:213–233.

Silvestry FE, et al. Echocardiography-guided interventions. *J Am Soc Echocardiogr* 2009;22(3):213–231.

Zamorano JL, et al. EAE/ASE recommendations for the use of echo-cardiography in new transcatheter interventions for valvular heart disease. *J Am Soc Echocardiogr* 2011;24:937–965.

Answer 15: *D.* The image shown above demonstrates a dilated tricuspid valve annulus and central malcoaptation of the tricuspid leaflets resulting in a large anatomic regurgitant orifice in ventricular systole. 3DE enhances visualization of TV leaflet morphology and the associated geometrical changes of the TV annulus. In addition, surgical planning can be enhanced by a detail description regarding the level of leaflet attachment and coaptation, subchordal anatomy, and accurate quantification of regurgitant jets. 3D echocardiography images of the tricuspid valve are not always required, especially in case where 2D imaging is satisfactory. In a small study of 29 patients with a variety of TV pathologies, 3DE provided incremental diagnostic value over 2DE with regard to the etiology and location of the abnormal leaflet segments. Functional TR is associated with enlargement of the TV annulus and with an increase in the planarity and circularity. Like mitral regurgitation, 3DE can also be used to find planes perpendicular to the TV leaflets for quantification of TR by vena contracta. Similar to vena contracta studies in MR, this has led to the recognition that the vena contracta in TR is elliptical and not circular. With the addition of color Doppler to 3DE on current systems, volume rates and temporal resolution are likely to be reduced to levels inferior to 2DE.

Suggested Readings

Pothineni KR, Duncan K, Yelamanchili P, et al. Live/real time three-dimensional transthoracic echocardiographic assessment of tricuspid valve pathology: incremental value over the two-dimensional technique. *Echocardiography* 2007;24:541–552.

Song JM, Jang MK, Choi YS, et al. The vena contracta in functional tricuspid regurgitation: a real-time three-dimensional color Doppler echocardiography study. *J Am Soc Echocardiogr* 2011;24:663–670.

Sugeng L, Weinert L, Lang RM. Real-time 3-dimensional color Doppler flow of mitral and tricuspid regurgitation: feasibility and initial quantitative comparison with 2-dimensional methods. *J Am Soc Echocardiogr* 2007;20:1050–1057.

Ton-Nu TT, Levine RA, Handschumacher MD, et al. Geometric determinants of functional tricuspid regurgitation: insights from 3-dimensional echocardiography. *Circulation* 2006;114:143–149.

Answer 16: *A.* LVEF is a routine clinical measure that has been used to estimate the severity of LV systolic performance. It appears from prior studies that LVEF by 3DE correlates well with cardiac MRI. 3DE has an important role to play in the assessment and intraprocedural evaluation of patients undergoing transcatheter aortic valve replacement. The detection of vegetations by 3DE has received little attention, and preliminary data suggest that it may be helpful in aiding diagnosis but has not been well validated to date. TABLE 52.1 lists the current indications of 3D echo according to the American Society of Echocardiography.

Suggested Readings

de Isla LP, et al. Usefulness of real-time 3-dimensional echocardiography in the assessment of infective endocarditis. *J Ultrasound Med* 2005;24:231–233.

Lang RM, Badano LP, Tsang W, et al. EAE/ASE recommendations for image acquisition and display using three-dimensional echocardiography. *J Am Soc Echocardiogr* 2012;25:3–46.

Answer 17: *A.* 3D echocardiography compares favorably with cardiac MRI for estimation of LVEF and LV mass despite the fact that it tends to underestimate the LV volumes. Underestimation of LV volume is believed to reflect differences in techniques used for endocardial border recognition between the two imaging modalities. 3D echocardiography shows greater correlation with cardiac MRI measures of LV volumes, mass, and ejection fraction as compared to 2D echocardiography.

Suggested Readings

Gutierrez-Chico JL, Zamorano JL, Perez de Isla L, et al. Comparison of left ventricular volumes and ejection fractions measured by three-dimensional echocardiography versus by two-dimensional echocardiography and cardiac magnetic resonance in patients with various cardiomyopathies. *Am J Cardiol* 2005;95:809–813.

Kuhl HP, Schreckenberg M, Rulands D, et al. High-resolution transthoracic real-time three-dimensional echocardiography: quantitation of cardiac volumes and function using semi-automatic border detection and comparison with cardiac magnetic resonance imaging. *J Am Coll Cardiol* 2004;43:2083–2090.

Pouleur AC, le Polain de Waroux JB, et al. Assessment of left ventricular mass and volumes by three-dimensional echocardiography in patients with or without wall motion abnormalities: comparison against cine magnetic resonance imaging. *Heart* 2008;94:1050–1057.

Answer 18: *B.* The usefulness of 3D echocardiography has been demonstrated in the evaluation of LV chamber volumes and function, left atrial size, quantitative volumetric evaluation of regurgitant lesions and shunts, and the presentation of realistic views of the heart valves. However, it is currently not adequately validated for the assessment of right ventricular size and function.

Suggested Readings

Hung J, Lang R, Flachskampf F, et al. 3D echocardiography: a review of the current status and future directions. *J Am Soc Echocardiogr* 2007;20:213–233.

Iwakura K, Ito H, Kawano S, et al. Comparison of orifice area by transthoracic three-dimensional Doppler echocardiography versus proximal isovelocity surface area (PISA) method for assessment of mitral regurgitation. *Am J Cardiol* 2006;97:1630–1637.

Jenkins D, Bricknell K, Marwick TH. Use of real-time three-dimensional echocardiography to measure left atrial volume: comparison with other echocardiographic techniques. *J Am Soc Echocardiogr* 2005;18:991–997.

Ota T, Fleishman CE, Strub M, et al. Real-time, three dimensional echocardiography: feasibility of dynamic right ventricular volume measurement with saline contrast. *Am Heart J* 1999;137:958–966.

Table 52.1	Summary of Indications for 3D Echocardiography			
	RECOMMENDED FOR CLINICAL PRACTICE	**PROMISING CLINICAL STUDIES**	**AREAS OF ACTIVE RESEARCH**	**UNSTUDIED**
Left ventricle functional assessment				
Volume	✓			
Shape			✓	
Ejection fraction	✓			
Dyssynchrony			✓	
Mass		✓		
Right ventricle functional assessment				
Volume		✓		
Shape				✓
Ejection fraction		✓		
Left atrial assessment				
Volume			✓	
Right atrial assessment				
Volume				✓
Mitral valve assessment				
Anatomy	✓			
Stenosis	✓			
Regurgitation			✓	
Tricuspid valve assessment				
Anatomy				✓
Stenosis				✓
Regurgitation				✓
Pulmonic valve assessment				
Anatomy				✓
Stenosis				✓
Regurgitation				✓
Aortic valve assessment				
Anatomy		✓		
Stenosis		✓		
Regurgitation				✓
Infective endocarditis				✓
Prosthetic valves			✓	
Guidance of transcatheter procedures[a]	✓			

[a]Mitral clips, mitral valvuloplasty, transcatheter aortic valve implantation, paravalvular leak closure, atrial septal defect closure, ventricular septal defect closure, and left atrial appendage closure.

Reprinted from Lang RM, Badano LP, Tsang W, et al. EAE/ASE recommendations for image acquisition and display using three-dimensional echocardiography. *J Am Soc Echocardiogr* 2012;25:3–46. Copyright © 2012 Elsevier. With permission.

Answer 19: B. The images shown in Figures 52.7 to 52.9 are of a normal functioning St. Jude mechanical MV prosthesis. The video file demonstrates no valvular vegetation, masses/thrombus, or pannus formation. The bileaflet mechanical valve opens well. A trace amount of regurgitation is normally seen with these valves and is known as backflow jets, which are typically narrow and of short duration. Answer A is incorrect since the prosthetic valve shown is not bioprosthetic but mechanical. Answer C is incorrect since there are no signs indicating that the prosthetic MV is unstable. On the contrary, the mechanical MV appears well seated. Answer D is incorrect since there is no evidence suggestive of a mobile mass/abscess or vegetation on the mechanical MV prosthesis.

Suggested Readings

Pibarot P, Demsnil JG. Prosthetic heart valves: selection of the optimal prosthesis and long term management. *Circulation* 2009;119:1034–1048.

Zoghbi WA, Chambers JB, Dumesnil JG, et al. Recommendations for evaluation of prosthetic valves with ecocardiography and Doppler ultrasound. *J Am Soc Echocardiogr* 2009;22:975–1014.

Answer 20: D. 3D transesophageal echocardiography measurements of the mitral valve orifice area in patients with rheumatic mitral stenosis can be obtained in 95% of patients. The mitral valve area by 3D echocardiography demonstrated the best agreement with mitral valve area by the continuity equation, followed by 2D planimetry. 3D echocardiography did not correlate as well with valve area obtained by the pressure half-time method. 2D transesophageal echocardiography was found to underestimate commissural fusion in 19% of cases. Although 3D TEE has the ability to show en face views of the mitral valve from the left atrial and left ventricular viewpoints, thus providing the degree of commissural fusion, it is not able to provide reliable information regarding the severity of commissural calcification. The optimal timing of the cardiac cycle to measure planimetry is middiastole for both 2D echocardiography and 3D echocardiography.

Suggested Readings

Anwar AM, Attia WM, Nosir YF, et al. Validation of a new score for the assessment of mitral stenosis using real-time three-dimensional echocardiography. *J Am Soc Echocardiogr* 2010;23:13–22.

Schlosshan D, Aggarwal G, Mathur G, et al. Real-time 3D transesophageal echocardiography for the evaluation of rheumatic mitral stenosis. *J Am Coll Cardiol Imaging* 2011;4:580–588.

Weyman AE. Assessment of mitral stenosis: role of real-time 3D TEE. *J Am Coll Cardiol Imaging* 2011;4:589–591.

Answer 21: **B.** This question is meant to illustrate the utility of 3D echocardiography in the evaluation of the left atrial appendage. The patient has a history of atrial fibrillation and based on the available information has a strong indication for long-term anticoagulation therapy. Given her unfortunate circumstance, cessation of her anticoagulation was necessary, and over the ensuing time, she developed the complication depicted in the 2D and 3D echocardiography images representing a large thrombus. Answers A, C, and E can also be causes of stroke through mechanisms of embolic occlusion from an intracardiac mass such as an atrial myxoma or fibroelastoma or from occlusive atherosclerosis of the intracerebral arteries. However, the images presented make it clear that the most likely etiology for this patient's stroke is the LAA thrombus (FIGS. 52.21 AND 52.22). Acute hypoperfusion of the brain due to massive blood loss can result in symptoms resembling a stroke, although more global cerebral dysfunction would also be expected. Provided rapid resuscitation and replacement of blood loss are achieved, these effects would furthermore be expected to be transient.

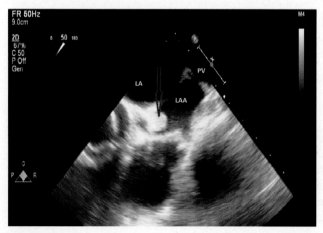

FIGURE 52.21

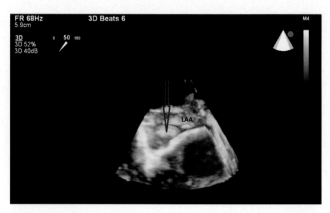

FIGURE 52.22

Suggested Readings

Karakus G, Kodali V, Inamdar V, et al. Comparative assessment of left atrial appendage by transesophageal and combined two- and three-dimensional transthoracic echocardiography. *Echocardiography* 2008;25:918–924.

Khan GN, Dairywala IT, Liu Z, et al. Three dimensional echocardiography of left atrial appendage thrombus. *Echocardiography* 2001;18:163–166.

Nakajima H, Seo Y, Ishizu T, et al. Analysis of the left atrial appendage by three-dimensional transesophageal echocardiography. *Am J Cardiol* 2010;106:885–892.

Answer 22: **A.** Percutaneous closure of the left atrial appendage has become an accepted treatment modality for patients with atrial fibrillation and a contraindication to the long-term use of oral anticoagulants. This is largely based on the results of the PROTECT-AF trial, which demonstrated that percutaneous implantation of a left atrial appendage occlude was feasible, safe, and associated with favorable outcomes and low risk of subsequent stroke as compared to warfarin anticoagulation therapy. Sizing of the LAA using cardiac imaging is an important part of the planning for such procedures. Traditionally, 2D TEE has been used to image the LAA from four standard views—20 to 30 degrees, 45 to 60 degrees, 90 degrees, and 120 to 135 degrees. Measurements are performed in the setting of normal LA pressure and at end diastole when the LAA is at its largest size. Real-time 3D TEE imaging of the LAA has been shown to be more accurate than 2D TEE for the assessment of LAA orifice size. The obtained measurements demonstrate that the patient's LAA is able to accommodate a Watchman device and the patient fits the criteria for LAA occlusion on clinical grounds. Currently, no studies comparing the efficacy of the Watchman device compared to surgical ligation of the AA have been completed. The LAAOS study is evaluating the efficacy of routine LAA ligation in patients undergoing elective CABG surgery. Given the promising 5-year results of the PROTECT-AF trial and the unclear benefit of surgical LAA ligation, answer B is incorrect. Answer C is similarly incorrect. Additionally, the patient does not have severe aortic valvular stenosis and therefore would not warrant AVR. Although CTA can provide more accurate sizing of the LAA, it is clear from the 2D measurements that the LAA can accommodate a Watchman device and assessment of leakage can be performed in real time prior to deployment to ensure proper sizing. There is no need in this case to pursue CTA to confirm the size of the LAA. Therefore, both D and E are incorrect. Sizing of the LAA should be done with the patient adequately hydrated.

Suggested Readings

Onlan O, Crystal E. Left atrial appendage exclusion for stroke prevention in patients with nonrheumatic atrial fibrillation. *Stroke* 2007;38:624–630.

Rajwani A, Nelson AJ, Shirazi MG, et al. CT sizing for left atrial appendage closure is associated with favourable outcomes for procedural safety. *Eur Heart J Cardiovasc Imaging* 2017;18:1361–1368.

Wiebe J, Franke J, Lehn K, et al. Percutaneous left atrial appendage closure with the Watchman device. Long-term results up to 5 years. *J Am Coll Cardiol Interv* 2015;8:1915–1921.

Answer 23: A. According to a study by Saw et al., CT angiography is feasible for sizing the LAA in preparation for percutaneous LAA occlusion. The measurements obtained by CT angiography may offer advantages over other imaging modalities (TEE, fluoroscopy) due to the ability to generate 3-dimensional reconstructions, which can be manipulated to find the largest dimensions. LAA measures obtained by CTA are typically larger than those obtained by echocardiography, although 3-dimensional echocardiography correlates best with measurements obtained by CT angiography. For Watchman device measurements, CTA correlated best with TEE for the ostium width as compared to fluoroscopy ($R = 0.74$ versus 0.65, respectively) and more modestly for appendage depth ($R = 0.56$ versus 0.28, respectively). Mean differences between CTA and TEE measures were 0.7 mm for the ostium width and 3 mm for LAA depth. While fluoroscopy can be used to measure the left atrial appendage at the time of left atrial appendage occlusion, measurements typically are smaller when compared to either echocardiography or CT angiography.

Suggested Readings

Nucifora G, Faletra FF, Regoli F, et al. Evaluation of the left atrial appendage with real-time 3-dimensional transesophageal echocardiography. Implications for catheter-based left atrial appendage closure. *Circ Cardiovasc Imaging* 2011;4:514–523.

Saw J, Fahmy P, Spencer R, et al. Comparing measurements of CT angiography, TEE, and fluoroscopy of the left atrial appendage for percutaneous closure. *Cardiovasc Electrophysiol* 2016;27:414–422.

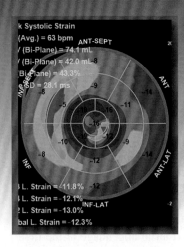

Chapter 53

Echo Strain for the Boards

Paul Anaya

1. Each of the following statements regarding strain imaging are true **except**

  A. Strain refers to the lengthening, shortening, or thickening of a region of the myocardium.

  B. Strain rate describes the distance over which deformation occurs.

  C. With tissue Doppler imaging (TDI), the direction of the myocardial velocity denotes contraction or elongation.

  D. Tissue Doppler imaging (TDI) parameters of velocity are used to calculate strain rate.

  E. Strain is calculated by integrating strain rate values over time.

2. Which of the following is true of strain imaging?

  A. Strain imaging provides a method to objectively quantify regional myocardial function independently of translational motion.

  B. Strain imaging can only be performed using tissue Doppler imaging (TDI).

  C. Strain is measured in units of cm/s.

  D. TDI-based longitudinal, radial, circumferential, and rotational strains are best measured from the apical windows.

  E. Longitudinal strain should be the same at all points along the septum in a normal heart.

3. A patient with a history of a remote myocardial infarction is being evaluated for angina and potential revascularization. You are trying to determine if the myocardium is ischemic and/or viable. Which of the following is true regarding strain analysis for myocardial ischemia and viability?

  A. Strain imaging can improve the sensitivity and specificity of detecting ischemia in response to dobutamine when compared to conventional stress echo.

  B. Speckle tracking echocardiography can reliably predict the transmural extent of myocardial infarction.

  C. TDI strain rate analysis can provide incremental value over wall motion scoring alone to determine the viability of the myocardial segments in dobutamine stress echo.

  D. Speckle tracking echocardiography strain analysis can accurately predict viable myocardium from transmural scar tissue.

  E. All of the options are true.

4. Which of the following is false regarding strain imaging?

  A. Strain imaging can help distinguish hypertrophic cardiomyopathy (HCM) from the "athlete's heart."

  B. Strain imaging can help distinguish HCM from left ventricular hypertrophy (LVH) related to hypertension.

  C. Strain imaging can help distinguish the cardiac hypertrophy of Friedreich ataxia (FA) from HCM.

  D. Strain imaging can help determine the cardiac involvement in light-chain amyloidosis before the onset of clinical symptoms.

  E. Strain rate imaging can provide additional data to predict prognosis in light-chain amyloidosis beyond established 2-D echo and TDI modalities.

5. For valvular heart disease, which of the following is true regarding strain imaging?

  A. Strain imaging does not offer additional clinical utility in patients with severe aortic stenosis (AS) and normal ejection fraction (EF) when compared to age-matched patients with LVH.

  B. In patients with asymptomatic moderate to severe AS, strain imaging during exercise testing can identify a group of patients with a "normal" exercise test but with evidence of subclinical systolic dysfunction.

  C. The addition of STE strain imaging to standard echo evaluation did not change the ability to predict the development of symptoms or worsening LV function in patients with moderate to severe aortic regurgitation (AR) managed conservatively.

  D. In patients with chronic, severe mitral regurgitation, the addition of strain imaging does not improve the ability to predict postoperative declines in EF.

  E. Strain analysis did not improve risk prediction for postoperative mortality in patients referred for cardiac surgery when compared to standard surgical risk prediction.

6. A 65-year-old male presents to the cardiology clinic for follow-up. He has a known cardiomyopathy with ejection fraction of 25%. His ECG reveals a normal sinus rhythm as well as a left bundle-branch block (QRS > 120 ms). He is on optimal medical therapy with a beta-blocker, ACE inhibitor, and spironolactone at the highest tolerated doses. He remains symptomatic with significant shortness of breath and a New York Heart Association functional class of III. He has an echo with longitudinal strain analysis performed using STE (Fig. 53.1). Which of the following statements is true?

A. He is likely to benefit from CRT based on the strain analysis.
B. He is likely to benefit from CRT based on clinical variables, and the strain analysis did not add clinically meaningful data.
C. He is unlikely to benefit from CRT based on the strain analysis.
D. He is unlikely to benefit from CRT based on clinical variables, and the strain analysis did not add clinically meaningful data.

7. The strain map seen in Figure 53.2 demonstrates which of the following?

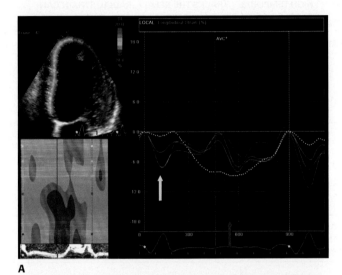

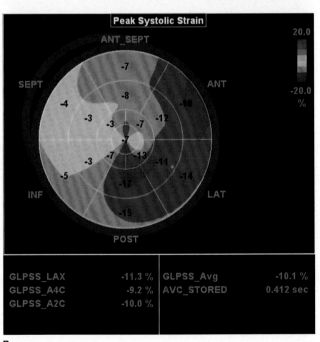

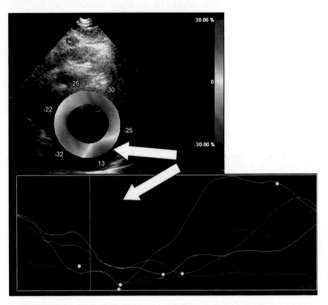

Figure 53.2 Circumferential strain of the left ventricle at the basal short-axis level.

A. Normal left ventricular function
B. Anterior wall hypokinesis
C. Septal wall hypokinesis
D. Lateral wall hypokinesis
E. Inferolateral wall akinesis

8. A 48-year-old male is admitted to the hospital overnight to evaluate complaints of chest pain. The patient reported the onset of chest pain 2 days prior to admission, occurring initially as he walked to retrieve his mail after dinner, but now is present constantly with no apparent exacerbation with exertional activity. The intensity of the pain waxes and wanes and he localizes it to the midchest. Past medical history is otherwise not significant. Physical exam findings are normal. The electrocardiogram and laboratory studies are also normal. With treatment, the patient's symptoms have subsided. He is transported to the echo lab for a dobutamine

Figure 53.1 From Teske AJ, De Boeck BW, Melman PG, et al. Echocardiographic quantification of myocardial function using tissue deformation imaging, a guide to image acquisition and analysis using tissue Doppler and speckle tracking. *Cardiovasc Ultrasound* 2007;5:27. Available at: http://www.cardiovascularultrasound.com/content/5/1/27. © 2007 Teske et al.; licensee BioMed Central Ltd.

stress test. Which of the following components of myocardial contractility can be ascertained by visual evaluation of wall motion using echocardiography?

A. Wall thickening in all myocardial wall segments can be accurately measured using two-dimensional echocardiography.

B. Myocardial twist function can be determined from long-axis views of the LV.

C. Radial deformation can be ascertained from short-axis and long-axis views of the LV.

D. LV shortening can be measured using two-dimensional echocardiography.

9. Two methods used to perform myocardial deformation imaging and obtain strain are tissue Doppler imaging (TDI) and speckle tracking imaging. In comparison to TDI, speckle tracking is characterized by which of the following?

	TRACKS ACOUSTIC MARKERS EQUALLY DISTRIBUTED WITHIN THE MYOCARDIUM	DEPENDENT ON US ANGLE OF INCIDENCE	TRACKS ALL MYOCARDIAL WALL SEGMENTS SIMULTANEOUSLY	REQUIRES NARROW, CENTRAL SECTOR WITH A HIGH FRAME RATE	HIGH TEMPORAL RESOLUTION	TRACKS THE RELATIVE VELOCITY OF MOTION	RADIAL STRAIN CAN ONLY BE APPLIED TO ANTERIOR AND INFERIOR WALL SHORT-AXIS VIEWS
A	Y	N	N	N	Y	Y	N
B	Y	N	Y	N	N	N	N
C	N	Y	N	Y	Y	Y	Y
D	Y	N	Y	Y	N	N	N

10. Which of the following descriptions most accurately characterizes strain imaging?

	EXPRESSED AS UNITS OF LENGTH	PROVIDES INFORMATION ON SUBENDOCARDIAL LV MECHANICS	RELATES TO MID-MYOCARDIAL LV MECHANICS	MEASURES TRANSMURAL LV MECHANICS	IDENTIFIES EXTENT OF MYOCARDIAL DISEASE	PROVIDES NO INFORMATION ON MYOCARDIAL PATHOPHYSIOLOGY
A	N	N	Y	N	N	Y
B	Y	N	N	Y	N	N
C	N	Y	Y	Y	Y	N
D	Y	Y	N	N	Y	Y

11. A 45-year-old male presents to the emergency department after experiencing acute chest pain. He states that the pain was sharp in nature, lasting approximately 10 min, and occurred shortly after returning home from a late night of working. The patient smokes 1 to 2 packs of cigarettes per day and occasionally smokes marijuana. He drinks alcohol about three times per week, usually with lunch or dinner while meeting clients. He has no significant family history to report. Past medical history is otherwise unremarkable. Vital signs show BP 170/95 mm Hg, HR 97 bpm, RR 22, and BMI 34. Physical examination reveals an obese male in no acute distress. There is no visible jugular venous distention and peripheral pulses are normal. Cardiac exam reveals a regular rate, normal S1S2, +S4 gallop, and no audible murmurs. Abdominal and extremity exams are normal.

Laboratory chemistries and CBC are normal except for a urine drug screen positive for cocaine. Cardiac biomarkers are normal. ECG shows normal sinus rhythm, rate 89 bpm, and no evidence of acute ischemia or previous infarction. CXR is normal.

An echocardiogram is performed at rest and reports a peak longitudinal strain rate value of -0.8 s^{-1} and peak early diastolic strain rate of 0.9^{-1} in the anterior wall segments compared with -1.0 and 1.1 s^{-1}, respectively, in the remaining wall segments.

Longitudinal strain values are as follows: inferior -19, lateral -22, anterior -14, and septal -16. Postsystolic negative strain was noted in the anterior wall segments. Regional wall motion and LV systolic function are visually normal. Left ventricular hypertrophy is detected.

Which of the following is the most likely explanation for the patient's chest pain?

A. Microvascular disease

B. Acute pulmonary embolus

C. Acute aortic dissection

D. Epicardial coronary artery disease

12. A 57-year-old female presents to the outpatient echo lab for a previously scheduled dobutamine stress test to evaluate atypical chest pain. Throughout the study, the patient reports no symptoms and no electrocardiographic abnormalities are detected. Target heart rate is reached and two-dimensional echocardiographic scans are obtained at rest, low, peak, and recovery periods using standard views. Speckle tracking–derived longitudinal strain segmental values are also obtained using apical views. No regional wall motion abnormalities are detected and LV function is normal.

The following strain tracing is obtained (Fig. 53.3).

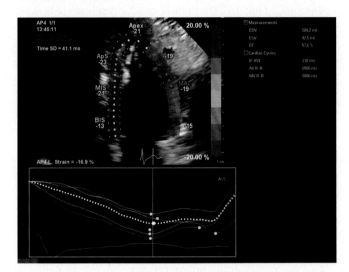

FIGURE 53.3 LV global longitudinal strain obtained from the apical four-chamber view immediately postexercise stress.

Which of the following choices is the best explanation to explain these findings?

A. Normal longitudinal strain values associated with normal LV wall motion and function
B. Cardiac translation artifact from respiration
C. Normal dobutamine stress findings and noise artifact of the strain acquisition
D. Abnormal dobutamine stress test demonstrating lateral wall ischemia

13. Consider the following patient clinical profiles:

Patient A is a 68-year-old male who presents to the emergency department with acute chest pain, which began 60 min ago and is diagnosed with an acute anterior STEMI for which he undergoes emergent PCI. Door-to-balloon time was estimated to be 95 minutes. Peak troponin T level was 8.0 µg/dL. Global longitudinal strain for the LV was −16.

Patient B is a 70-year-old male who presents to the emergency department with acute chest pain, which has been intermittent for the past 3 hours and is diagnosed with an acute anterior STEMI for which he undergoes emergent

PCI. Door-to-balloon time was estimated to be 80 min. Peak troponin T level was 10 µg/dL. Global longitudinal strain for the LV was −10.

What is the likely clinical outcome of patient A compared to patient B?

A. Patient A is more likely to have ischemia-mediated arrhythmias due to the longer door-to-balloon time.
B. Patient B is likely to have the same or better outcome based on similar levels of peak troponin detected, similar GLS values, and shorter door-to-balloon time.
C. Patient A is likely to have less myocardial damage and therefore less adverse cardiac remodeling compared to patient B.
D. Patient B is more likely to require dual antiplatelet therapy for more than 1 year due to a higher rate of recurrent MI following PCI.

14. A 48-year-old female has been undergoing treatment for a rare form of CML over the past year. Treatments have included various combinations of chemotherapy, including anthracycline-based regimens. Since her original diagnosis, she has developed anemia and has reported complaints of shortness of breath with exertion, generalized fatigue, and weakness. The severity of these symptoms has been variable over the course of her treatment. An echocardiogram obtained prior to her treatment with chemotherapy demonstrated normal findings, and normal LV systolic function characterized by a 3DE-based ejection fraction of 65% and speckle tracking–derived global longitudinal strain (GLS) value of −22. A second echocardiogram obtained 3 months later after completing 2 cycles of an earlier chemotherapy cocktail showed a 3DE-based LV ejection fraction of 62% and a speckle tracking–derived GLS value of −20. Since the patient reported no changes in her symptoms, she has not undergone another echocardiogram until now. She is scheduled to undergo yet another cycle of chemotherapy next week, and in preparation for it, she undergoes a complete echocardiogram. Her current echocardiographic findings demonstrate normal LV and RV morphology, normal cardiac valvular function and morphology, grossly normal LV systolic function with a 3DE-based LV ejection fraction of 55%, and speckle tracking–derived GLS value of −17.

Based on these findings, what advice would you provide to the patient's treating physician?

A. Continue treatment with the current chemotherapy regimen.
B. Add metoprolol titrated to the maximal tolerated dose and continue chemotherapy.
C. Halt further treatment with the current chemotherapy regimen, closely monitor the patient, and repeat the echocardiogram in 3 months.
D. Add metoprolol and enalapril titrated to the maximal tolerated dose.
E. Continue treatment, but change to a different chemotherapy regimen.

15. A 62-year-old ex-marathon runner presents to your clinic with complaints of left arm/hand tingling. The patient is of African American heritage and states that until recently he was the "picture of health." On a routine visit with his primary care provider 3 months ago, lab studies were obtained, which revealed an abnormally elevated serum creatinine level. Repeat testing over the ensuing 3 months has consistently demonstrated the same abnormality, prompting his primary care provider to obtain additional tests. The patient states that he gave up marathon running 5 years ago following an injury. Since then, he has had intermittent swelling of lower extremities, which he has attributed to his previous injury. Aside from this, he has generally felt fine and currently takes no medications. Family history is significant for hypertension. He is aware of one uncle on his mother's side who died suddenly from unexplained causes. Vitals include a BP 150/85, HR 50 bpm, RR 18/min, and BMI 24. Physical examination findings are pertinent for distended jugular veins to approximately 8 cm while lying supine at 45 degrees, clear lung fields bilaterally, regular rate, soft S1S2, no S3 gallops, +S4 gallop, and a 2/6 SM at midupper sternum. Valsalva maneuver and squatting/standing maneuvers did not elicit any appreciable changes in the murmur. Peripheral pulses are normal. CXR shows cardiomegaly. A 12-lead ECG demonstrates sinus bradycardia, 55 bpm, and no evidence of myocardial infarction or acute ischemia. Low voltage was noted in the limb leads. A complete echocardiogram was performed demonstrating the following findings (Fig. 53.4).

What is the most likely diagnosis, which explains the patient's presentation and findings?

A. Hypertensive heart disease
B. Hypertrophic cardiomyopathy—nonobstructive type
C. Cardiac amyloidosis
D. Fabry disease of the heart

Answer 1: B.

Option A: True. If this is considered in one dimension for simplicity, strain (ε) may be described as $\varepsilon = (L - L_0)/L_0$, where L = the original length and L_0 = the final length (Fig. 53.5).

Option B: False. Strain rate describes the speed at which deformation occurs. It is measured in units of 1/s.

Option C: True. In TDI, systolic contraction leads to upward (positive) velocities (S) and diastolic elongation to negative velocities (E') (Fig. 53.6B).

Option D: True. TDI produces data regarding myocardial velocity. Strain rate (SR) can be calculated by $SR = (V_2 - V_1)/L$ and is measured in 1/unit time (Figs. 53.6 AND 53.7).

Option E: True. As such, strain is a unitless measurement.

Suggested Readings

D'hooge J, Heimdal A, Jamal F, et al. Regional strain and strain rate measurements by cardiac ultrasound: principles, implementation and limitations. *Eur J Echocardiogr* 2000;1:154–170.

Mirsky I, Parmley WW. Assessment of passive elastic stiffness for isolated heart muscle and the intact heart. *Circ Res* 1973;33:233–243.

Mor-Avi V, Lang RM, et al. Current and evolving echocardiographic techniques for the quantitative evaluation of cardiac mechanics: ASE/EAE consensus statement on methodology and indications. *J Am Soc Echocardiogr* 2011;24:277–313.

Answer 2: A.

Option A: True. Strain is a measure of the deformation of tissue. With strain imaging, deformation in a segment of myocardium is assessed in reference to a nearby segment. This removes the potential errors that can be seen with translational motion.

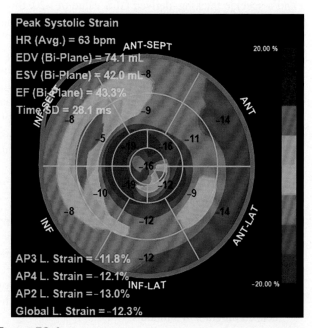

FIGURE 53.4 LV global longitudinal strain map of patient described in Question 15.

$$\varepsilon = \frac{L - L_0}{L_0} = \frac{\Delta L}{L_0}$$

FIGURE 53.5 In simplest terms, strain (ε) is a measure of the elastic properties of cardiac muscle when confronted by a stress or how much a muscle can elongate or shorten. As such, strain represents the percent change from the original, or unstressed, dimension. The time interval over which this change occurs is not a component of strain. In the image above, the unstressed length L_0 elongates to a total length of L. Thus, the change in length (ΔL) divided by the unstressed length (L_0) represents strain. (From Teske AJ, De Boeck BW, Melman PG, et al. Echocardiographic quantification of myocardial function using tissue deformation imaging, a guide to image acquisition and analysis using tissue Doppler and speckle tracking. *Cardiovasc Ultrasound* 2007;5:27. Available at: http://www.cardiovascularultrasound.com/content/5/1/27. © 2007 Teske et al.; licensee BioMed Central Ltd.)

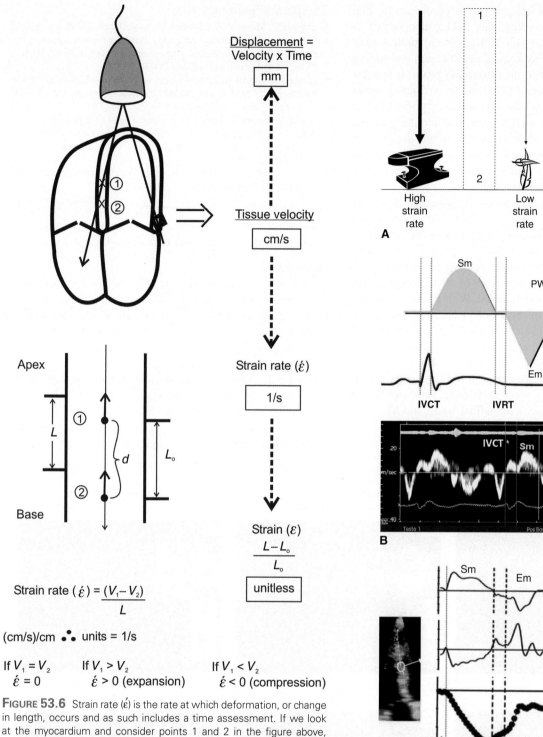

Figure 53.6 Strain rate ($\dot{\varepsilon}$) is the rate at which deformation, or change in length, occurs and as such includes a time assessment. If we look at the myocardium and consider points 1 and 2 in the figure above, we can measure a distance between these two points (mm). We can also measure the tissue velocity at each time point (cm/s). If we go one step further and measure the speed at which this change in distance has occurred, then we have measured strain rate. If we measure only the percent change from the original dimension (without time), we have measured strain. (From Armstrong WF, Ryan T. *Feigenbaum's Echocardiography.* 7th ed. Philadelphia, PA: Lippincott Williams & Wilkins, 2010, with permission.)

Figure 53.7 **A:** Another way to think about the differences in strain versus strain rate would be to consider an anvil and a feather traveling from point 1 to point 2. The distance traveled is the same for both and represents strain. However, the speed at which this change occurs is different and represents strain rate. **B,C:** Tissue Doppler imaging (TDI)-based myocardial velocity and association with strain and strain rate. (From Citro R, Bossone E, Kuersten B, et al. Tissue Doppler and strain imaging: anything left in the echo-lab? *Cardiovasc Ultrasound* 2008;6:54. Available at: http://www.cardiovascularultrasound.com/content/6/1/54. © 2008 Citro et al.; licensee BioMed Central Ltd.)

Option B: False. Strain imaging can be performed by TDI or speckle tracking echocardiography (STE), also known as 2-D strain. Strain analysis with TDI has been studied more extensively but is limited to areas of myocardium that have a low angle of incidence with the ultrasound beam. It focuses mostly on longitudinal strain from the apical four-chamber views and radial strain from the parasternal short-axis views. Speckle tracking is a newer application of strain analysis and is not dependent on the angle of incidence but depends on high-resolution two-dimensional images and optimal frame rates (generally 40 to 80 frames/second with normal heart rates) to accurately track regions of interest.

Option C: False. Strain is a unitless measure. It is described as a percentage of change from the original dimension and is a positive value when lengthening occurs and a negative value when shortening occurs (see FIG. 53.7).

Option D: False. Myocardial regional mechanics have been described primarily by four types of strain: longitudinal, radial, circumferential, and rotational. With TDI imaging, the measurement is subject to the Doppler angle of incidence. Based on this, longitudinal strain is measured from the apical views, while radial, circumferential, and rotational strains are all best measured from the parasternal views (FIG. 53.8).

Option E: False. When measured in healthy adults, longitudinal systolic velocities show decreasing values from the base to the apex. Likewise, longitudinal strain and SR show a segmental increase from the base to the apex (-15.78 ± 3.63 versus −24.00 ± 5.87, *P* = 0.0001 and −0.83 ± 0.21 versus −1.44 ± 0.37, *P* = 0.0001) (FIG. 53.9).

Suggested Readings

Bussadori C, Moreo A, Di Donato M, et al. A new 2D-based method for myocardial velocity strain and strain rate quantification in a normal adult and paediatric population: assessment of reference values. *Cardiovasc Ultrasound* 2009;13(7):8.

D'hooge J, Heimdal A, Jamal F. Regional strain and strain rate measurements by cardiac ultrasound: principles, implementation and limitations. *Eur J Echocardiogr* 2000;1:154–170.

Geyer H, Giuseppe C, Haruhiko A. Assessment of myocardial mechanics using speckle tracking echocardiography: fundamentals and clinical applications. *J Am Soc Echocardiogr* 2010;23:351–369.

Gorcsan J, Hidekazu T. Echocardiographic assessment of myocardial strain. *J Am Coll Cardiol* 2011;58:1401–1413.

Mor-Avi V, Lang RM, Badano LP. Current and evolving echocardiographic techniques for the quantitative evaluation of cardiac mechanics: ASE/EAE consensus statement on methodology and indications. *J Am Soc Echocardiogr* 2011;24:277–313.

Answer 3: E.

Option A: True. Peak systolic strain rate of the myocardium increases in response to dobutamine. In an ischemic myocardium, the increase in peak systolic strain rate and strain is blunted. When added to conventional two-dimensional stress echo imaging, strain rate imaging improved sensitivity/specificity from 81%/82% to 86%/90%.

Option B: True. STE has been shown to correlate significantly with CMR for determining the extent of infarction in a myocardial segment. Radial strain allowed differentiation of transmural infarction from nontransmural infarction with a sensitivity of 70.0% and a specificity of 71.2%.

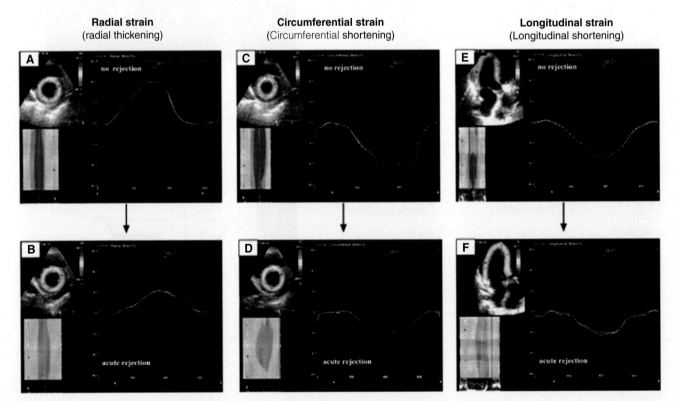

Radial strain (radial thickening)   **Circumferential strain** (Circumferential shortening)   **Longitudinal strain** (Longitudinal shortening)

FIGURE 53.8 Republished with permission of Bentham Science Publishers Ltd. from Dandel M, Lehmkuhl H, Knosalla C, et al. Strain and strain rate imaging by echocardiography—basic concepts and clinical applicability. *Curr Cardiol Rev* 2009;5(2):133–148; permission conveyed through Copyright Clearance Center, Inc. Copyright © 2009 Bentham Science Publishers Ltd.

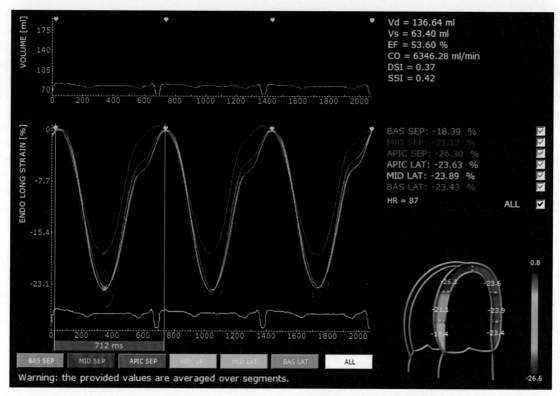

FIGURE 53.9 In the image, both strain and strain rate increase from the base to the apex of the septum. This is displayed by color-coded segments (basal septum, *pink*; midseptum, *purple*; apical septum, *dark blue*). (From Bussadori C, Moreo A, Di Donato M, et al. A new 2D-based method for myocardial velocity strain and strain rate quantification in a normal adult and paediatric population: assessment of reference values. *Cardiovasc Ultrasound* 2009;7:8. Available at http://www.cardiovascularultrasound.com/content/7/1/8. © 2009 Bussadori et al.; licensee BioMed Central Ltd.)

Option C: True. Strain imaging increases the sensitivity of dobutamine stress echo in predicting viability of the myocardium from 73% to 82% when compared to conventional wall motion analysis. Specificities were comparable.

Option D: True. When using contrast-enhanced MRI as the reference standard, STE strain analysis could discriminate between viable myocardium and transmural scar with a sensitivity of 81.2% and specificity of 81.6%.

Option E: All of the answers are true as described.

Suggested Readings

Becker M, Hoffmann R, Kühl HP. Analysis of myocardial deformation based on ultrasonic pixel tracking to determine transmurality in chronic myocardial infarction. *Eur Heart J* 2006;27:2560–2566.

Hanekom L, Jenkins C, Jeffries L, et al. Incremental value of strain rate analysis as an adjunct to wall-motion scoring for assessment of myocardial viability by dobutamine echocardiography: a follow-up study after revascularization. *Circulation* 2005;112:3892–3900.

Roes SD, Mollema SA, Lamb HJ, et al. Validation of echocardiographic two-dimensional speckle tracking longitudinal strain imaging for viability assessment in patients with chronic ischemic left ventricular dysfunction and comparison with contrast-enhanced magnetic resonance imaging. *Am J Cardiol* 2009;104:312–317.

Voigt J, Exner B, Schmiedehausen K. Strain-rate imaging during dobutamine stress echocardiography provides objective evidence of inducible ischemia. *Circulation* 2003;107:2120–2126.

Answer 4: C.

Option A: True. Early diastolic strain rates have been shown to be lower in patients with HCM when compared to those with athlete's heart. When measured in early diastole, a SR < 7/s gave a positive predictive value of 0.96 and a negative predictive value of 0.94 in differentiating patients with hypertrophic cardiomyopathy from athlete's heart. This differentiation was seen in all age groups. This differentiation between athlete's heart and HCM is of utmost importance clinically as HCM can be associated with increased risk of SCD. While the 2-D echo imaging may appear similar in athlete's heart and HCM, other measures such as diastolic function, strain, and strain rate are generally quite different. These evaluations become useful in differentiating these two entities with very different clinical outcomes.

Option B: True. When strain analyses were performed using TDI, mean systolic strain of <10.6% was able to discriminate between HCM and LVH from hypertension with a sensitivity of 85.0%, a specificity of 100.0%, and a predictive accuracy of 91.2%.

Option C: False. Children with asymmetric septal HCM, concentric HCM, and Friedreich ataxia associated with concentric HCM were evaluated by echo. Evaluation of the children with HCM revealed reduced early diastolic and systolic myocardial velocities and peak systolic SR compared with controls. There were no differences in any echocardiographic variable between patients with isolated concentric HCM and Friedreich ataxia–related HCM. Strain imaging was not helpful in distinguishing the children with FA from others with concentric HCM.

Option D: True. Cardiac amyloidosis causes an early impairment in systolic function at a time when fractional shortening remains normal and precedes clinical symptoms of heart failure. Basal peak systolic SR was statistically different in patients with known amyloidosis and no cardiac involvement ($-19\% \pm 4\%$), cardiac involvement but no heart failure (HF) ($-15\% \pm 4.5\%$), and cardiac involvement with HF ($-8.0\% \pm 5\%$).

Option E: True. When studied in patients with known AL amyloidosis, the mean basal strain was a powerful predictor of clinical outcome and was superior to the established methods of standard two-dimensional echocardiographic, Doppler flow measurements, and simple tissue velocity indexes.

Suggested Readings

Ganame J, Pignatelli RH, Eidem BW. Myocardial deformation abnormalities in paediatric hypertrophic cardiomyopathy: are all aetiologies identical? *Eur J Echocardiogr* 2008;9(6):784–790.

Kato TS, Noda A, Izawa H. Discrimination of nonobstructive hypertrophic cardiomyopathy from hypertensive left ventricular hypertrophy on the basis of strain rate imaging by tissue Doppler ultrasonography. *Circulation* 2004;110:3808–3814.

Koyama J, Falk RH. Prognostic significance of strain Doppler imaging in light-chain amyloidosis. *J Am Coll Cardiol Imaging* 2010;3:333–342.

Koyama J, Ray-Sequin PA, Falk RH. Longitudinal myocardial function assessed by tissue velocity, strain, and strain rate tissue Doppler echocardiography in patients with AL (primary) cardiac amyloidosis. *Circulation* 2003;107:2446–2452.

Palka P, Lange A, Fleming AD, et al. Differences in myocardial velocity gradient measured throughout the cardiac cycle in patients with hypertrophic cardiomyopathy, athletes and patients with left ventricular hypertrophy due to hypertension. *J Am Coll Cardiol* 1997;30:760–768.

Answer 5: B.

Option A: False. In patients with moderate to severe AS and preserved EF, decreased longitudinal strain and SR by 2-D-STE were observed versus healthy, age-matched controls and patients with LVH. After aortic valve replacement, these parameters improved while EF remained unchanged. Thus, subclinical systolic dysfunction could be appreciated using strain analysis prior to any change in EF.

Option B: True. Using 2-D-STE, patients with AS have reduced longitudinal myocardial function at rest and at peak exercise compared to controls. Changes in LV global longitudinal strain during exercise were lower in AS patients with a "normal" response to exercise versus controls (-17.4 ± 3.9 versus -25 ± 3.7; $P < 0.05$). Thus, subclinical systolic dysfunction can be identified by strain imaging with exercise in patients with asymptomatic AS.

Option C: False. In patients with moderate to severe AR managed conservatively, STE-based measures of strain and SR predicted the development of symptoms or worsening LV function. Significantly reduced myocardial systolic strain and systolic SR were predictive of disease progression during conservative management, while conventional parameters of LV function and size were not.

Option D: False. Speckle tracking echo–based longitudinal SR measured preoperatively strongly predicted a postoperative decline in EF of >10% when using the midinterventricular septum and a cutoff value of <0.80/second. The predictive capacity of SR was better than preoperative LV volume, EF, or dP/dt. Longitudinal strain rate predicted changes in EF with a 60% sensitivity and a 96.5% specificity.

Option E: False. Strain analysis by STE improved risk stratification in patients referred for coronary artery bypass grafting, aortic valve surgery, or mitral valve surgery when compared to the standard of care, EuroSCORE. In patients with similar EuroSCOREs and a preserved EF, the rate of postoperative death was 2.4-fold higher (11.8% versus 4.9%, $P = 0.04$) when global longitudinal strain was impaired.

Suggested Readings

de Isla LP, de Agustin A, Rodrigo JL, et al. Chronic mitral regurgitation: a pilot study to assess preoperative left ventricular contractile function using speckle-tracking echocardiography. *J Am Soc Echocardiogr* 2009;22:831–838.

Delgado V, Tops LF, van Bommel RJ, et al. Strain analysis in patients with severe aortic stenosis and preserved left ventricular ejection fraction undergoing surgical valve replacement. *Eur Heart J* 2009;30:3037–3047.

Donal E, Thebault C, O'Connor K, et al. Impact of aortic stenosis on longitudinal myocardial deformation during exercise. *Eur J Echocardiogr* 2011;12:235–241.

Olsen NT, Sogaard P, Larsson HB, et al. Speckle-tracking echocardiography for predicting outcome in chronic aortic regurgitation during conservative management and after surgery. *JACC Cardiovasc Imaging* 2011;3:223–230.

Ternacle J, Berry M, Alonso E, et al. Incremental value of global longitudinal strain for predicting early outcome after cardiac surgery. *Eur Heart J Cardiovasc Imaging* 2013;14(1):77–84.

Answer 6: A.

Option A: Strain imaging can help predict response to cardiac resynchronization therapy (CRT). In this example, the strain analysis shows a clearly significant delay in septal peak systolic strain compared to lateral peak systolic strain (425 ms) by STE. A recent paper used a longitudinal strain delay index to predict response to CRT. This strain delay index correlated with reverse remodeling in both the ischemic ($r = -0.68$, $P < 0.0001$) and nonischemic ($r = -0.68$, $P < 0.0001$) population.

Responders would be expected to improve the delay from the septal peak systolic strain to the lateral peak systolic strain as seen in this example of the former patient post-CRT (Fig. 53.10). The delay is now -60 ms, and there is improvement in the ejection fraction.

Option B: In contemporary studies, about one-third of all CRT patients do not respond to therapy. The current criteria for CRT are based on clinical parameters (symptoms, functional status), ventricular function, and QRS duration. Thus, there is a need for improved predictors for successful response to CRT. The strain analysis shows a clearly significant delay in septal peak systolic strain compared to lateral peak systolic strain (425 ms) by STE. This would suggest a clinical response to CRT; however, this is currently not an accepted method of determining candidacy for CRT-based therapy.

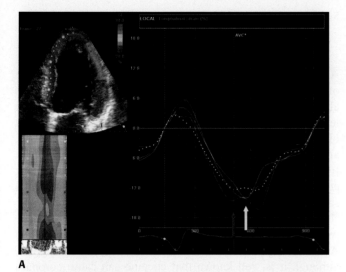

A

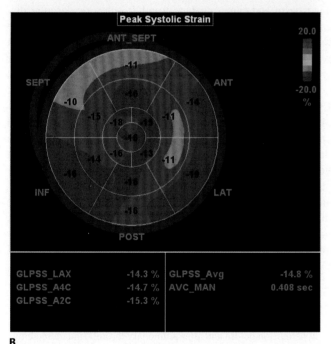

B

FIGURE **53.10** From Teske AJ, De Boeck BW, Melman PG, et al. Echocardiographic quantification of myocardial function using tissue deformation imaging, a guide to image acquisition and analysis using tissue Doppler and speckle tracking. *Cardiovasc Ultrasound* 2007;5:27. Available at: http://www.cardiovascularultrasound.com/content/5/1/27. © 2007 Teske et al.; licensee BioMed Central Ltd.

Option C: Based solely on clinical variables, this patient meets criteria for CRT. He has all of the clinical variables that qualify him for CRT therapy: a QRS > 120 ms, reduced ejection fraction, and clinical symptoms despite adequate medical therapy. However, the strain analysis shows a significant delay, which would suggest a higher likelihood of benefit.

Option D: Again, this patient meets criteria based on clinical, echo, and ECG criteria. The strain analysis suggests he may obtain a benefit from CRT.

Suggested Readings

Gorcsan J III, Abraham T, Agler DA, et al. Echocardiography for cardiac resynchronization therapy: recommendations for performance and reporting—a report from the American Society of Echocardiography Dyssynchrony Writing Group endorsed by the Heart Rhythm Society. *J Am Soc Echocardiogr* 2008;21:191–213.

Lim P, Buakhamsri A, Popovic ZB, et al. Longitudinal strain delay index by speckle tracking imaging: a new marker of response to cardiac resynchronization therapy. *Circulation* 2008;118:1130–1137.

Answer 7: E.

Option A: As the ventricle contracts, muscle fibers shorten in the longitudinal and circumferential directions and thicken or lengthen in the radial direction. The myocardium in this image has been color coded with a scale that corresponds to circumferential strain percent. With negative strain (shortening), the myocardium is red (−30% red), and with positive strain (lengthening), the myocardium is blue (30% blue). There is clearly a difference in color coding of the wall segments; thus, normal left ventricular wall motion cannot be true.

Option B: The best motion is seen in the basal anterior, septal, and lateral walls, which have the darkest red coloring and are plotted on the graph as the lines with a marked negative percent strain during systole. This answer is therefore incorrect.

Option C: The best motion is seen in the basal anterior, septal, and lateral walls, which have the darkest red coloring and are plotted on the graph as the lines with a marked negative percent strain during systole. This answer is therefore incorrect.

Option D: The best motion is seen in the basal anterior, septal, and lateral walls, which have the darkest red coloring and are plotted on the graph as the lines with a marked negative percent strain during systole. This answer is therefore incorrect.

Option E: The inferolateral wall shows akinesis based on the blue coloring and the relatively flat plot of the strain curve. This is indicative of lack of shortening with systole.

Suggested Readings

Dandel M, Lehmkuhl H, Knosalla C, et al. Strain and strain rate imaging by echocardiography—basic concepts and clinical applicability. *Curr Cardiol Rev* 2009;5(2):133–148.

Perk G, Tunick PA, Kronzon I. Non-Doppler two-dimensional strain imaging by echocardiography—from technical considerations to clinical applications. *J Am Soc Echocardiogr* 2007;20:234–243.

Answer 8: C. Although contractility consists of wall thickening, shortening, and twist, only radial deformation can be assessed visually using 2-D echocardiography. Wall thickening can be estimated from all regional wall segments, but is dependent on visualization of the epicardial border, which is challenging along the medial and lateral walls where image resolution is dependent of beam width and line density. Myocardial twist function cannot be determined by visual evaluation of wall motion by 2-D echocardiography. LV shortening can be assessed using 2-D echocardiography but only in the radial direction. LV shortening in the longitudinal direction is not easily assessed using 2-D echocardiography.

Suggested Readings

Geyer H, Caracciolo G, Abe H, et al. Assessment of myocardial mechanics using speckle-tracking echocardiography: fundamentals and clinical applications. *J Am Soc Echocardiogr* 2010;23:351–369.

Heimdal A, Stoylen A, Torp H, et al. Real-time strain rate imaging of the left ventricle by ultrasound. *J Am Soc Echocardiogr* 1998;11:1013–1019.

Perk G, Tunick PA, Kronzon I. Non-Doppler two-dimensional strain imaging by echocardiography—from technical considerations to clinical applications. *J Am Soc Echocardiogr* 2007;20:234–243.

Answer 9: D. Non-Doppler strain imaging known as speckle tracking echocardiography (STE) involves the frame-by-frame tracking of natural acoustic markers, which are equally distributed throughout the myocardium. STE analyzes displacement from a single point of reference within tissue over space and time (Lagrangian strain), whereas tissue Doppler imaging–based (TDI) strain measures the relative velocity of motion at a defined location within tissue over time (Eulerian strain). Both Doppler and non-Doppler strain imaging methods require a narrow angle, central sector, and high frame rate for optimal quality. Unlike STE, TID strain is dependent on the ultrasound angle of incidence and therefore requires that the line of axis is parallel to the ultrasound beam path. Therefore, TDI strain analysis can only be applied to apical views for longitudinal strain and middle anterior and inferior short-axis views for radial strain. The superior temporal resolution of TDI as compared to STE results in more accurate strain rate analysis.

Suggested Readings

Gilman G, Khandheria BK, Hagen ME, et al. Strain rate and strain: a step-by-step approach to image and data acquisition. *J Am Soc Echocardiogr* 2004;17:1011–1020.

Perk G, Tunick PA, Kronzon I. Non-Doppler two-dimensional strain imaging by echocardiography—from technical considerations to clinical applications. *J Am Soc Echocardiogr* 2007;20:234–243.

Answer 10: C. Strain, as applied to myocardial mechanics, is a measure of the shortening and stretch properties of the myocardium known as deformation. It is determined by measuring the change in length ($\Delta L = L - L_0$) of an object and dividing by the original length (L_0). The result is a dimensionless measure of deformation, which is expressed as a fractional or percentage change from baseline. Advantages of using strain include the ability to derive information related to subendocardial, mid-myocardial, and transmural myocardial function by measuring global longitudinal strain, circumferential strain, and LV torsion or twist, respectively. Such information has provided valuable insight into subclinical changes in LV function as a result of myocardial ischemia, infiltrative disease states, and exposure to cardiotoxic agents.

Suggested Readings

Gilman G, Khandheria BK, Hagen ME, et al. Strain rate and strain: a step-by-step approach to image and data acquisition. *J Am Soc Echocardiogr* 2004;17:1011–1020.

Perk G, Tunick PA, Kronzon I. Non-Doppler two-dimensional strain imaging by echocardiography—from technical considerations to clinical applications. *J Am Soc Echocardiogr* 2007;20: 234–243.

Sutherland GR, Di Salvo G, Claus P, et al. Strain and strain rate imaging: a new clinical approach to quantifying regional myocardial function. *J Am Soc Echocardiogr* 2004;17:788–802.

Answer 11: D. Strain rate represents the temporal derivative of strain and is a measure of the rate of deformation. It is also a surrogate measure for the shortening velocity per fiber length. Evidence from several studies indicates that measures of longitudinal strain, postsystolic strain, systolic strain rate, and early diastolic strain rate can predict myocardial ischemia from significant coronary artery disease. In one study, Liang et al. (2006), the combination of abnormal peak longitudinal strain rate below the cutoff of -0.83 s^{-1} and early diastolic strain rate of <0.96 s^{-1} predicted coronary stenosis of $>70\%$ with a sensitivity of 94% and a specificity of 64%. Answers A and B cannot be ascertained with the information given, although it is well known that cocaine can cause coronary vasospasm and can contribute to atherosclerotic vascular disease at both the macro- and microvascular levels. It is possible that the patient has some degree of microvascular disease, but whether this fully explains his clinical presentation is unclear without demonstrating the absence of obstructive epicardial coronary artery disease. Abnormal speckle tracking–derived LV circumferential and radial strain values have been associated with chronic thromboembolic disease and response to endarterectomy, although no role for strain imaging has been defined for the evaluation of acute pulmonary embolus. Right ventricular (RV) strain measures can be useful in the evaluation of RV function in the setting of pulmonary hypertension. Similarly, there is no defined role for LV strain in the diagnosis or management of acute aortic dissection. There is no evidence provided to support either an acute pulmonary embolus or acute aortic dissection. Therefore, answers B and C are incorrect.

Suggested Readings

Olson N, Brown JP, Kahn AM, et al. Left ventricular strain and strain rate by 2D speckle tracking in chronic thromboembolic pulmonary hypertension before and after pulmonary thromboendarterectomy. *Cardiovasc Ultrasound* 2010;8:43–51.

Liang HY, Cauduro S, Pellikka P, et al. Usefulness of two-dimensional speckle strain for evaluation of left ventricular diastolic deformation in patients with coronary artery disease. *Am J Cardiol* 2006;98:1581–1586.

Shan Y, Villarraga HR, Pislaru C, et al. Quantitative assessment of strain and strain rate by velocity vector imaging during dobutamine stress echocardiography to predict outcome in patients with left bundle branch block. *J Am Soc Echocardiogr* 2009;22:1212–1219.

Voigt J-U, Exner B, Schmiedehausen K, et al. Strain-rate imaging during dobutamine stress echocardiography provides objective evidence of inducible ischemia. *Circulation* 2003;107:2120–2126.

Answer 12: D. Postsystolic shortening is a phenomenon of myocardial shortening that occurs after the ejection phase of the cardiac cycle. Therefore, despite the apparent contraction of the affected wall segments, there is no contribution of this to systolic function. Although the precise mechanisms governing PSS are not well understood, evidence suggests that it is largely a passive consequence of the interaction between ischemic myocardial regions and surrounding nonischemic regions. Since PSS is closely associated with the myocardial ischemic cascade, it has shown promise as an early marker of myocardial ischemia measurable by current speckle tracking strain imaging. The application of strain imaging to dobutamine stress testing has been shown to enhance the sensitivity and specificity of dobutamine stress echo to identify myocardial ischemia (blunted peak systolic strain and strain rate, postsystolic shortening), determine the extent of infarction (radial strain versus longitudinal strain), and predict myocardial viability as compared to conventional wall motion analysis.

Suggested Readings

Becker M, Hoffmann R, Kuhl HP. Analysis of myocardial deformation based on ultrasonic pixel tracking to determine transmurality in chronic myocardial infarction. *Eur Heart J* 2006;27:2560–2566.

Hanekom L, Jenkins C, Jeffries L, et al. Incremental value of strain-rate analysis as an adjunct to wall-motion scoring for assessment of myocardial viability by dobutamine echocardiography: a follow-up study after revascularization. *Circulation* 2005;112:3892–3900.

Roes SD, Mollema SA, Lamb HJ, et al. Validation of echocardiographic two-dimensional speckle tracking longitudinal strain imaging for viability assessment in patients with chronic ischemic left ventricular dysfunction and comparison with contrast-enhanced magnetic resonance imaging. *Am J Cardiol* 2009;104:312–317.

Voigt J, Exner B, Schmiedehausen K. Strain-rate imaging during dobutamine stress echocardiography provides objective evidence of inducible ischemia. *Circulation* 2003;107:2120–2126.

Answer 13: *C.* Studies have demonstrated a relationship between peak systolic longitudinal strain values and cardiac troponin T, making abnormal peak systolic longitudinal strain a marker of myocardial damage following an acute MI. Both factors are closely related to time to reperfusion quantified as the time from symptom onset to time of balloon inflation. Abnormal peak longitudinal strain following reperfusion for an acute MI is also associated with a higher risk of adverse LV remodeling and possibly worse clinical outcomes in the form of subsequent heart failure development and death. Therefore, the correct answer is C. Answer A is not correct because the door-to-balloon time is not so protracted as to expect significantly worse outcomes compared to guideline-recommended door-to-balloon times of 90 minutes. Answer B is not correct since the relationship between troponin T level and peak systolic longitudinal strain and symptom-to-balloon time would predict a worse outcome for patient B. Answer D is incorrect since there is no current evidence linking abnormal peak systolic longitudinal strain to the duration of DAPT.

Suggested Readings

Asanuma T, Nakatani S. Myocardial ischaemia and post-systolic shortening. *Heart* 2015;101:509–516.

Becker M, Hoffmann R, Kuhl HP. Analysis of myocardial deformation based on ultrasonic pixel tracking to determine transmurality in chronic myocardial infarction. *Eur Heart J* 2006;27:2560–2566.

Hung C-L, Verma A, Uno H, et al. Longitudinal and circumferential strain rate, left ventricular remodeling, and prognosis after myocardial infarction. *J Am Coll Cardiol* 2010;56:1812–1822.

Park YH, Kang S-J, Song J-K, et al. Prognostic value of longitudinal strain after primary reperfusion therapy in patients with anterior-wall acute myocardial infarction. *J Am Soc Echocardiogr* 2008;21:262–267.

Shehata M. Value of two-dimensional s train imaging in prediction of myocardial functional recovery after percutaneous revascularization of infarct-related artery. *Echocardiography* 2015;32:630–637.

Thambyrajah J, Vijayalakshmi K, Graham RJ, et al. Strain rate imaging pre- and post-percutaneous coronary intervention: a potential role in the objective detection of ischaemia in exercise stress echocardiography. *Eur J Echocardiogr* 2008;9:646–654.

Answer 14: *C.* Cardiotoxicity related to exposure to chemotherapy has been defined by a decrease in LV ejection fraction by ≥5% in the presence of symptoms of heart failure or a decrease of ≥10% in the absence of such symptoms. The balance of continuing treatment for a potentially life-threatening malignancy and the risk of causing a potentially irreversible toxin-induced cardiomyopathy must be carefully determined by treating physicians, and changes in LV systolic function influence such clinical decision-making. Although the definition of chemotherapy-related cardiotoxicity is rooted in LVEF estimation, more sensitive markers of LV systolic function such as global longitudinal strain have shown promise in identifying patients at risk for cardiotoxicity even before an actual decline in LVEF is demonstrated. In one study, a cutoff value for GLS of <−17.5 was associated with an increased risk of cardiotoxicity. The inclusion of clinical cardiology consultants as part of a multidisciplinary medical team, cardiac biomarker assessment following chemotherapy, and treatment with heart failure–directed medical therapy have also been studied and show promise in preventing or treating the cardiotoxic effects of chemotherapy, but are not yet considered standard of care. Answers A and B are incorrect since there has been a more than 10% decrease in the baseline LVEF since treatment was begun. Accordingly, further chemotherapeutic treatment should be halted. There is no evidence to support continuation of chemotherapeutic treatment even after initiating beta-blocker or ACE inhibitor therapy. Therefore, answer D is incorrect. Finally, answer E is incorrect as all chemotherapeutic agents carry the potential of having cardiotoxic effects and switching to a different regimen is unlikely to improve LV systolic function and, more likely, will worsen it.

Suggested Readings

Ali MT, Yucel E, Bouras S, et al. Myocardial strain is associated with adverse clinical cardiac events in patients treated with anthracyclines. *J Am Soc Echocardiogr* 2016;29:522–527.

Charbonnel C, Convers-Domart R, Rigaudeau S, et al. Assessment of global longitudinal strain at low dose anthracycline-based chemotherapy for the prediction of subsequent cardiotoxicity. *Eur Heart J Cardiovasc Imaging* 2017;18:392–401.

Thavendiranathan P, Grant AD, Negishi T, et al. Reproducibility of echocardiographic techniques for sequential assessment of left ventricular ejection fraction and volumes. Application to patients undergoing cancer chemotherapy. *J Am Coll Cardiol* 2013;61:77–84.

Thavendiranathan P, Poulin F, Lim K-D, et al. Use of myocardial strain imaging by echocardiography for the early detection of cardiotoxicity in patients during and after cancer chemotherapy: a systematic review. *J Am Coll Cardiol* 2014;63:2751–2768.

Editor's Note: in 2014, the term CTRCD (cancer therapeutics-related cardiac dysfunction) was included in the expert consensus document published by the American Society of Echocardiography and the European Association of Cardiovascular Imaging. See Plana JC, et al. *J Am Soc Echocardiogr* 2014;27(9):911–939. In this document, the experts established the following definition to standardize our approach to this complex patient population: LVEF decrease >10% points, to a value <53%; confirmed by repeat imaging in 2 to 3 weeks after initially detected drop in LVEF. Furthermore, the role of the cardiologist is as a consultant to the oncologist and final decisions regarding the continuation of chemotherapies is multifactorial.

Answer 15: C. In a study of patients with cardiac amyloidosis conducted by Phelan et al., regional variation in measures of longitudinal strain was discovered and characterized as a gradient of strain values with the lowest values found at the cardiac base and the highest values seen at the apex. This apical sparing pattern is consistent and easily recognizable, allowing this entity to be distinguished from other cardiomyopathies and causes of left ventricular hypertrophy. In contrast, no consistent pattern of longitudinal strain values distinguishes hypertrophic cardiomyopathy (HCM) from other pathologic and physiologic causes of left ventricular hypertrophy. However, patients with HCM are characterized with lower values of global longitudinal strain as compared to hypertensive heart disease. Strain rate imaging may be better suited to distinguish HCM from hypertensive heart disease or physiologic causes of LVH (athlete's heart). Similarly, strain rate imaging has been applied to the evaluation of patients with Fabry disease with those patients with cardiac involvement demonstrating lower strain rate values in the lateral myocardial wall segments despite preserved global longitudinal strain.

Suggested Readings

Kato TS, Noda A, Izawa H. Discrimination of nonobstructive hypertrophic cardiomyopathy from hypertensive left ventricular hypertrophy on the basis of strain rate imaging by tissue Doppler ultrasonography. *Circulation* 2004;110:3808–3814.

Liu D, Niemann M, Hu K, et al. Echocardiographic evaluation of systolic and diastolic function in patients with cardiac amyloidosis. *Am J Cardiol* 2011;108:591–598.

Palka P, Lange A, Fleming AD, et al. Differences in myocardial velocity gradient measured throughout the cardiac cycle in patients with hypertrophic cardiomyopathy, athletes and patients with left ventricular hypertrophy due to hypertension. *J Am Coll Cardiol* 1997;30:760–768.

Phelan D, Collier P, Thavendiranathan P, et al. Relative apical sparing of longitudinal strain using two-dimensional speckle-tracking echocardiography is both sensitive and specific for the diagnosis of cardiac amyloidosis. *Heart* 2012;98:1442–1448.

Shanks M, Thompson RB, Paterson ID, et al. Systolic and diastolic function assessment in Fabry disease patients using speckle-tracking imaging and comparison with conventional echocardiographic measurements. *J Am Soc Echocardiogr* 2013;26:1407–1414.

Sun JP, Stewart WJ, Yang XS, et al. Differentiation of hypertrophic cardiomyopathy and cardiac amyloidosis from other causes of ventricular wall thickening by two-dimensional strain imaging echocardiography. *Am J Cardiol* 2009;103:411–415.

Chapter 54

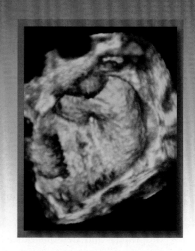

Echocardiography during Interventional Procedures

Paul Anaya

1. FIGURE 54.1 and VIDEO 54.1 demonstrating the right atrial aspect of an atrial septal defect (ASD) were obtained from a 72-year-old female during evaluation for possible percutaneous closure. The dotted yellow line represents the largest ASD diameter (30 mm), while the solid yellow line represents the ASD's aortic rim (7 mm). Other ASD rims were also measured and deemed sufficient for ASD closure.

Additionally, echocardiography demonstrated an enlarged right heart and no significant pulmonary arterial hypertension.

Which of the following is the correct answer?

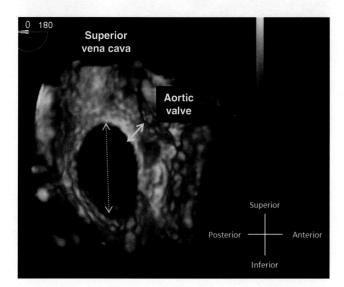

FIGURE 54.1

A. ASD is too large for device closure.
B. ASD anatomy is favorable for device closure.
C. The patient is too old for device closure.
D. The aortic rim of ASD is too small for device closure.
E. The patient does not have a secundum ASD.

2. FIGURE 54.2 and VIDEO 54.2 were obtained from a 23-year-old male with an atrial septal defect (ASD) referred for possible percutaneous closure.

Panel A demonstrates the left atrial aspect of an ASD (asterisk); its diameters were measured at 18 × 12 mm.

Panel B and VIDEO 54.2 demonstrate the left ventricular side of the patient's mitral valve.

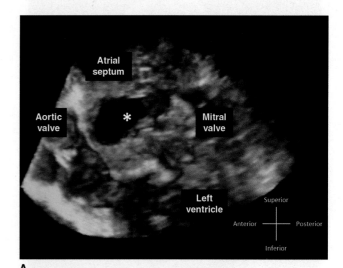

A

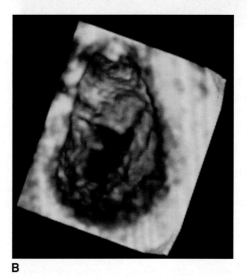

B

FIGURE 54.2

Echocardiography also demonstrated moderate mitral regurgitation, enlarged right heart, no pulmonic stenosis, and a peak systolic gradient of the tricuspid regurgitant jet of 25 mm Hg. Right atrial pressure was estimated at 3 mm Hg.

You recommend cancelation of percutaneous ASD closure in this patient because:

A. ASD is too small.

B. The patient has pulmonary hypertension.

C. The secundum ASD is not amenable to percutaneous closure.

D. The right heart is dilated.

E. There is mitral valve pathology.

3. FIGURE 54.3 was obtained by 3D transesophageal echocardiography and demonstrates the left atrial aspect of the mitral valve in the so-called surgical view.

What structure is marked by the arrow?

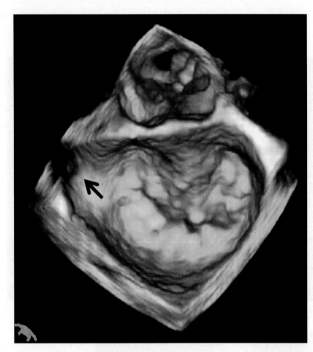

FIGURE 54.3

A. Left atrial appendage

B. Atrial septal defect

C. Right pulmonary artery

D. Aortic root

E. Left upper pulmonary vein

4. FIGURE 54.4 was obtained by transesophageal echocardiography (TEE) in a 67-year-old male with atrial fibrillation and two embolic strokes who underwent percutaneous exclusion of the left atrial appendage (LAA) using an LAA occluder (black arrow in Panel A and yellow arrow in Panel B).

Panel A demonstrates the 3D TEE appearance of the LAA occluder (black arrow) seen from the left atrial side. Panel B is the color Doppler 2D TEE image obtained at 45 degrees; the yellow arrow points to the location of the LAA occluder. The width of the jet shown in Panel B is 6 mm.

Which of the following is the correct statement?

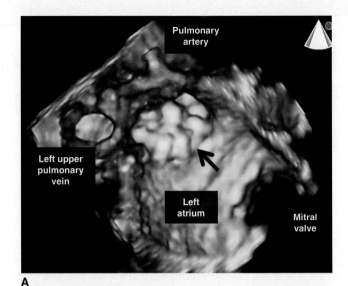

A

B

FIGURE 54.4

A. The occluder is placed too deep into the LAA.

B. The LAA occluder is not inferior to anticoagulation in preventing further embolic strokes.

C. The patient may stop anticoagulation immediately post percutaneous LAA occlusion.

D. LAA thrombus is an indication for LAA occluder implantation.

E. There is a large residual leak around the occluder.

5. FIGURE 54.5 was obtained by 3D transesophageal echocardiography and demonstrates the left atrial aspect of the mitral valve in the so-called surgical view.

What structure is marked by the arrow?

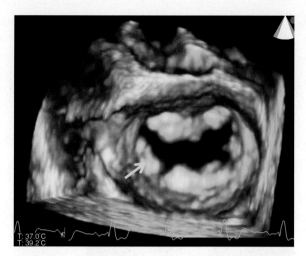

FIGURE 54.5

A. Scallop A1
B. Lateral commissure
C. Scallop P1
D. Scallop A2
E. Accessory scallop

6. The pair of images in FIGURE 54.6 demonstrates the same anatomic structure before (Panel A; peak systole) and after an intervention (Panel B; diastole).

What procedure was performed?

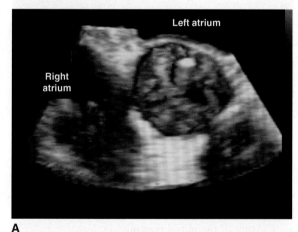

A

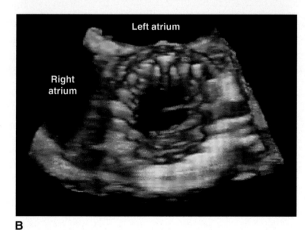

B

FIGURE 54.6

A. Aortic valve balloon valvuloplasty only
B. Surgical aortic valve repair
C. Transcutaneous aortic valve replacement
D. Valve-in-valve implantation to treat bioprosthetic valve regurgitation
E. Type A aortic dissection endovascular graft

7. The pair of images in FIGURE 54.7 demonstrates spectral Doppler tracings from the same anatomic structure before (Panel A) and after a successful intervention (Panel B).

What percutaneous procedure was performed?

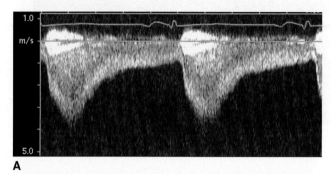

A

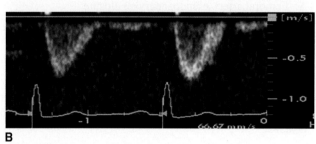

B

FIGURE 54.7

A. Patent ductus arteriosus occlusion
B. Endovascular graft for type B aortic dissection
C. Atrial septal defect occlusion
D. Aortic coarctation repair
E. Aortic transection repair

8. Panel A and Panel B of FIGURE 54.8 demonstrate spectral Doppler tracings from the vascular structure depicted in Panel C. Panel A is obtained before and Panel B after an intervention.

What procedure was performed?

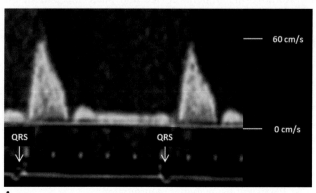

A

FIGURE 54.8

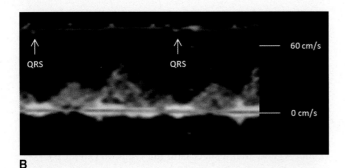

B

C

FIGURE 54.8 (*Continued*)

A. Femoral artery pseudoaneurysm closure
B. Internal carotid artery stenting
C. Ligation of dialysis access atrioventricular shunt
D. Coronary artery bypass grafting
E. Balloon angioplasty of the renal artery

9. After reviewing the echocardiographic images with your critical care team, you decide that the next best action to take is:

A. Advance the Impella device under echocardiographic guidance from an LV long-axis view through the aortic valve to a position approximately 3.5 to 4.5 cm from the aortic valve plane.
B. Advance the Impella device until flow from the LV is detected on the Impella module.
C. Call cardiothoracic surgery for immediate surgical correction of a mechanical complication.
D. Advance the Impella device under echocardiographic guidance from an LV long-axis view through the aortic valve to a position at the midpapillary muscle or approximately 5 to 6 cm from the aortic valve plane.
E. Remove the Impella device and place the patient on ECMO support.

10. Shortly after the completion of a paravalvular leak closure procedure, the patient acutely becomes progressively tachycardic and hypotensive. Upon review of the postprocedure TEE, which of the following echo findings should be routinely carefully demonstrated to exclude this as a potential cause for the clinical presentation?

A. A new interatrial shunt
B. Mitral regurgitation
C. A new pericardial effusion.
D. Persistent paravalvular regurgitation
E. Left atrial appendage thrombus

11. The pair of images in FIGURE 54.9 demonstrates the surgical view of the mitral valve before (Panel A) and after an intervention (Panel B).

What procedure was performed?

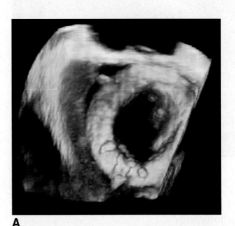

A

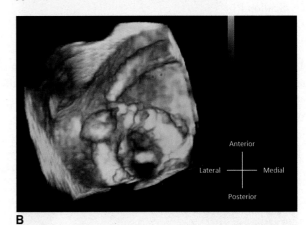

B

FIGURE 54.9

A. Mitral balloon valvuloplasty
B. Mitral valve clipping
C. The bioprosthetic valve replaced with mechanical one
D. Device closure of the left atrial appendage
E. Closure of the mitral paravalvular leak

12. The pair of images in FIGURE 54.10 demonstrates the same anatomic structure before (Panels A1 and A2 on the left) and after an intervention (Panels B1 and B2 on the right). VIDEO 54.3 is obtained prior to the procedure and VIDEO 54.4 after the procedure.

What procedure was performed?

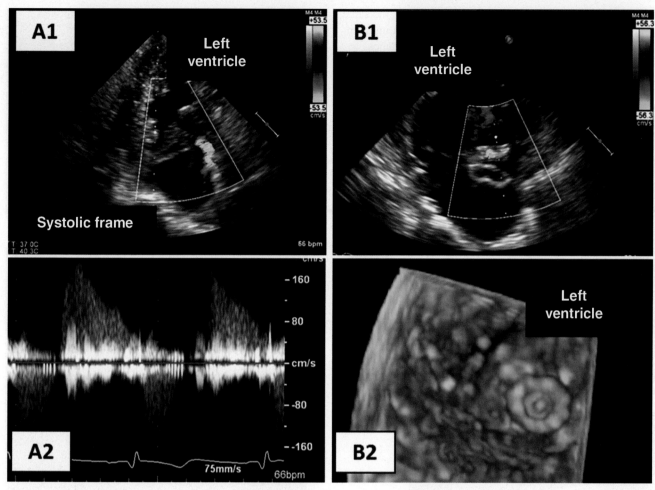

FIGURE 54.10

A. Ventricular septal defect closure
B. Left ventricular pseudoaneurysm closure
C. Insertion of the left ventricular assist device cannula
D. Transapical mitral commissurotomy
E. Ventricular septal ablation

13. The pair of images in FIGURE 54.11 demonstrates the same anatomic structure before (Panel A) and after an intervention (Panel B). VIDEO 54.5 demonstrates the lesion prior to the intervention.

FIGURE 54.11 (*Continued*)

What procedure was performed?

A. Ventricular septal ablation
B. Insertion of the left ventricular assist device cannula
C. Left ventricular pseudoaneurysm closure
D. Ventricular septal defect closure
E. Transcutaneous aortic valve replacement

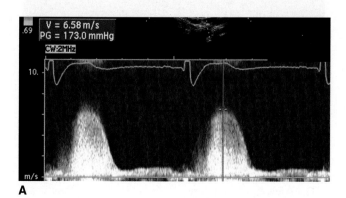

FIGURE 54.11

14. The pair of images in FIGURE 54.12 demonstrates the same anatomic structure before (Panel A) and after an intervention (Panel B). Both panels represent diastolic frames.

What procedure was performed?

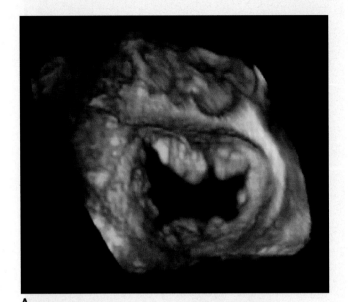

A

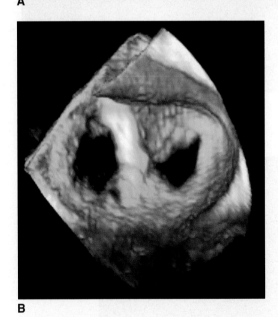

B

FIGURE 54.12

A. Mitral valve clipping
B. Mitral balloon valvuloplasty
C. Atrial septal defect closure
D. Mechanical valve replaced with bioprosthetic one
E. Closure of the mitral paravalvular leak

15. The images in FIGURE 54.13 demonstrate a finding before (Panel A), during (Panel B), and after an intervention (Panel C). VIDEO 54.6 corresponds to Panel A and VIDEO 54.7 corresponds to Panel C.

Which of the following is the most likely explanation for the interval change?

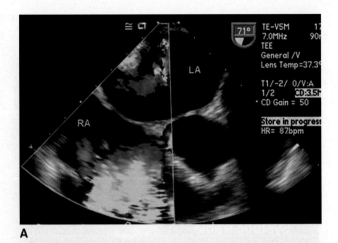

A

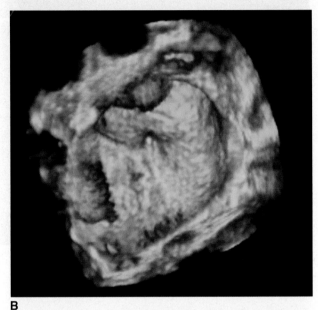

B

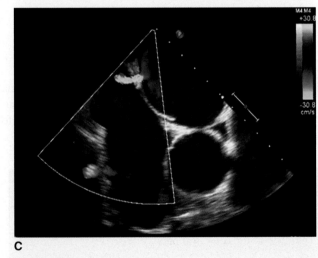

C

FIGURE 54.13

A. New primum atrial septal defect
B. Right atrial free wall perforation
C. Coronary sinus fistula
D. Transseptal puncture
E. Superior vena cava–type sinus venosus atrial septal defect

16. The pair of images in FIGURE 54.14 demonstrates the same anatomic structure before (Panel A) and after an intervention (Panel B). In each panel, the distance between dots on the grid is 5 mm.

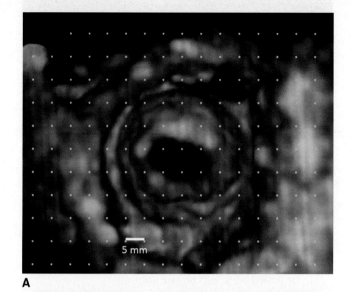

5 mm

A

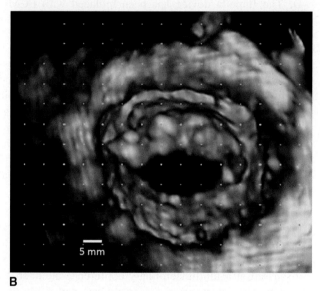

5 mm

B

FIGURE 54.14

Which procedure was performed?

A. Mitral valve clipping
B. Alfieri stitch
C. Mitral balloon valvuloplasty
D. Atrial septostomy
E. Closure of the mitral paravalvular leak

17. The pair of images in FIGURE 54.15 demonstrates the same anatomic structure before (Panel A, VIDEO 54.8) and after an intervention (Panel B).

Which defect was treated during the procedure?

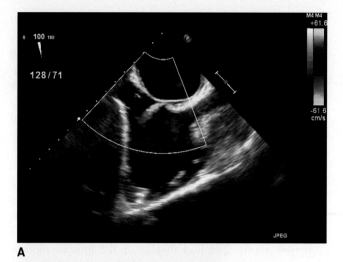

A

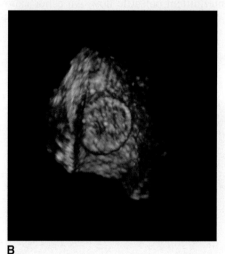

B

FIGURE 54.15

A. Sinus venosus atrial septal defect
B. Patent foramen ovale
C. Primum atrial septal defect
D. Secundum atrial septal defect
E. Unroofed coronary sinus

18. A 50-year-old male presented to an outside hospital with severe shortness of breath, dizziness, and nausea. Evaluation in the emergency department revealed an obese male in moderate respiratory distress, cool and clammy skin, a rapid, irregular heart rate, and distended jugular veins. ECG demonstrated atrial fibrillation, heart rate 135 bpm, ST elevation, and absent R waves in the anterior precordial leads. BP was 82/50 mm Hg, pulse 140 bpm, respiratory rate 33 breaths per minute, and SpO$_2$ 87% on 4 L O$_2$ via nasal cannula. CXR showed evidence of vascular congestion. Laboratory studies included a comprehensive metabolic profile, which was significant for a sCr level of 2.3, BUN 30, K 5.2, AST 120, ALT 135, bilirubin 2.5, and alkaline phosphatase 240. Troponin I level was 0.1 ng/dL. ABG was 7.25/30/65.

The patient is taken to the cardiac catheterization lab where he is intubated and placed on mechanical ventilatory support. A diagnostic cardiac catheterization is performed and PCI completed on a proximal LAD occlusion. An Impella 5.0 is inserted for mechanical support, 4.5 L/min support is confirmed, and hemodynamics improved. Systemic anticoagulation with heparin is started.

The patient is transported to the cardiac intensive care unit and transferred to a hospital bed. However, for the next few hours, the patient's condition worsens and he is hypotensive despite escalation of vasopressor support. He is now anuric. The flow display on the Impella module demonstrates intermittent pulsatile flow. An echocardiogram is obtained and the following image is shown (see Fig. 54.16).

The figure demonstrates which of the following:

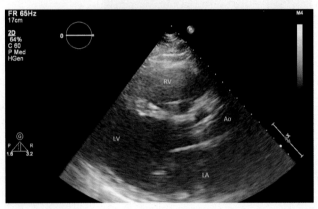

FIGURE 54.16

A. The Impella device is appropriately positioned passed the aortic valve.
B. The Impella device is dislodged and penetrated the aorta, entering the RV outflow tract.
C. The Impella device is inappropriately positioned passed the aortic valve.
D. The Impella device has thrombosed.

19. The patient described in the previous question is taken to the cardiac catheterization lab, and a subsequent echocardiographic view is obtained (Fig. 54.17). You conclude the following:

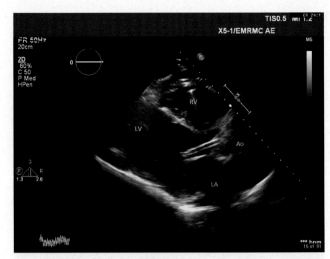

FIGURE 54.17

A. The Impella device must be further advanced.
B. The Impella device is in the proper position and should be sutured securely in place.
C. The Impella device was advanced too far and now must be pulled back into proper position.
D. The Impella device has been replaced with ECMO cannulae.

20. A 55-year-old female with a history of severe mitral stenosis undergoes a mitral valve replacement with a bioprosthetic mitral valve. She has an uneventful recovery and is discharged home. You have followed her in your clinic over the ensuing 3 years. For most of that time, she has been doing well, but in the last year, she developed progressive dyspnea with exertion. Three months ago, she noted occasional swelling in her lower extremities and palpitations. A Holter monitor study showed paroxysmal atrial fibrillation.

A repeat echocardiogram performed at that time revealed the presence of moderate–severe paravalvular mitral regurgitation. The patient states that she does not want to undergo another surgery if it can be avoided. Her case is discussed at a multidisciplinary conference attended by general and interventional cardiologists and cardiothoracic surgeons. A consensus is reached that the patient is a suitable candidate for percutaneous closure of the paravalvular leak.

Figures 54.18 and 54.19 (Videos 54.9 and 54.10) show the bioprosthetic MV and associated paravalvular mitral defect and regurgitation. Figures 54.20 to 54.23 show intraprocedural images as well as the final result (red arrow = catheter; yellow arrow = plug; blue arrow = paravalvular [PV] defect).

Based on the echo images shown at the start of the procedure, the trajectory of the catheter as it crosses the interatrial septum is:

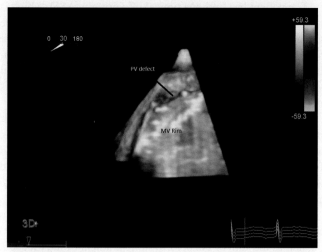

FIGURE 54.18

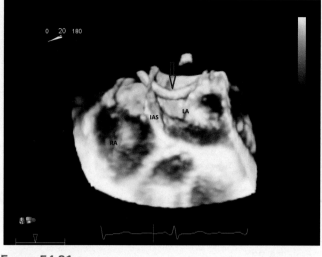

FIGURE 54.21

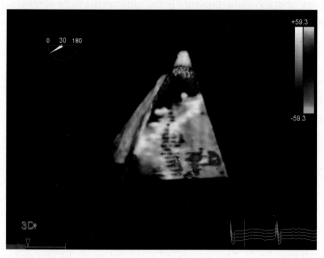

FIGURE 54.19

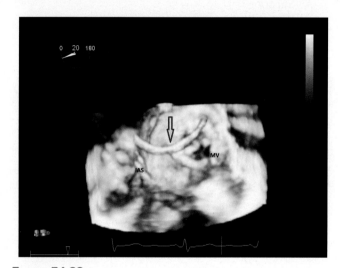

FIGURE 54.22

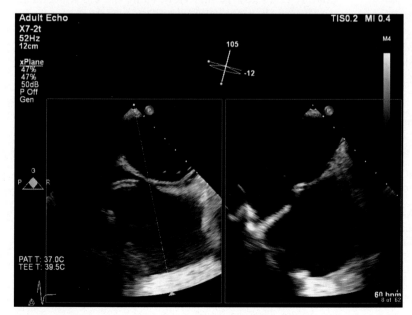

FIGURE 54.20

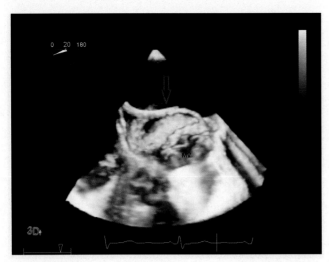

FIGURE 54.23

A. Superior
B. Posterior
C. Inferior
D. Inferior and posterior

Answer 1: *B.* In the United States, ASD occluders are currently approved only for secundum ASDs. The patient has findings typical of a secundum ASD.

Contraindications for device closure of a secundum ASD include ASD diameter of >38 mm and insufficiency of the aortic rim (<3 mm) or other ASD rims (<5 mm). In addition, device closure should not be performed:

- In patients with preexisting intracardiac thrombus (since thrombus can be dislodged by catheters and other hardware used in percutaneous ASD closure)
- In patients who have contraindications to antiplatelet therapy (since antiplatelet therapy is given for several weeks post device implantation)

The patient's age is not a contraindication for device closure of ASD.

Since the patient has a secundum ASD with a diameter of 30 mm and a sufficient aortic rim, her ASD is amenable to percutaneous ASD closure. Thus, the correct answer is B.

Suggested Readings

Dehghani H, Boyle AJ. Percutaneous device closure of secundum atrial septal defect in older adults. *Am J Cardiovasc Dis* 2012;2(2):133–142.

Saric M, Perk G, Purgess J, et al. Imaging atrial septal defects by real-time 3D transesophageal echocardiography: step-by-step approach. *J Am Soc Echocardiogr* 2010;23(11):1128–1135.

Warnes CA, Williams RG, Bashore TM, et al. ACC/AHA 2008 guidelines for the management of adults with Congenital Heart Disease: Executive Summary: a report of the American College of Cardiology/American Heart Association task force on practice guidelines. *Circulation* 2008;118:2395–2451.

Answer 2: *E.* In the United States, percutaneous ASD occluders are currently approved only for secundum ASDs.

The patient has findings typical of a primum ASD, which is located in the portion of the interatrial septum adjacent to the atrioventricular (tricuspid and mitral) valves as shown in Figure 54.2A. Primum ASD is typically part of the endocardial cushion defect spectrum and may be associated with cleft mitral valve and partial or complete atrioventricular canal defect. This patient has a cleft mitral valve as shown in Figure 54.2B.

Because of their location and associated mitral valve pathology, primum ASDs are not amenable to percutaneous closure, and appropriate patients with such defects should be referred for surgical closure of ASD (as well as repair of associated anomalies). Given the primum ASD and cleft mitral valve, the correct answer is E.

Patient has normal pulmonary artery systolic pressure. In this patient, the right ventricular systolic pressure can be calculated as the sum of the peak systolic gradient of the tricuspid regurgitant jet (25 mm Hg) and the right atrial pressure (3 mm Hg). Since the patient does not have pulmonic stenosis, pulmonary artery systolic pressure is the same as the right ventricular systolic pressure, that is, 28 mm Hg.

Right heart dilatation is a hallmark of all ASDs with significant left-to-right shunt; right heart dilatation is an indication rather than a contraindication for ASD closure.

Suggested Readings

Perk G, Ruiz C, Saric M, et al. Real-time three-dimensional transesophageal echocardiography in transcutaneous, catheter-based procedures for repair of structural heart diseases. *Curr Cardiovasc Imaging Rep* 2009;2(5):363–374.

Warnes CA, Williams RG, Bashore TM, et al. ACC/AHA 2008 guidelines for the management of adults with Congenital Heart Disease: Executive Summary: a report of the American College of Cardiology/American Heart Association task force on practice guidelines. *Circulation* 2008;118:2395–2451.

Answer 3: *A.* The so-called surgical view of the mitral valve shows the mitral valve the way surgeons see the valve (FIG. 54.23). In this view, using the clockface analogy, the aortic valve is located at 12 o'clock, the left atrial appendage at 9 o'clock, and the interatrial septum at 3 o'clock.

The 3D image structure marked by arrow in this patient is the left atrial appendage. Thus, the correct answer is A.

Suggested Readings

Garcia Fernandez MA, Perk G, Saric M, et al. Chapter 12. Real-time three-dimensional transesophageal echocardiography for guidance of catheter based interventions. In: Badano LP, Lang RM, Zamorano JL, eds. *Textbook of Real-Time Three-Dimensional Echocardiography*. 1st ed. Springer, 2011:121–134.

Perk G, Ruiz C, Saric M, et al. Real-time three-dimensional transesophageal echocardiography in transcutaneous, catheter-based procedures for repair of structural heart diseases. *Curr Cardiovasc Imaging Rep* 2009;2(5):363–374.

Answer 4: *E.* Figure 54.4A demonstrates a Watchman device placed into the LA appendage at appropriate depth; the device is neither too deep nor too superficial relative to the LA appendage ostium. Thus, answer A is incorrect.

Percutaneous exclusion of the LA appendage (LAA) using the so-called Watchman device has been shown in a randomized clinical trial to be noninferior to chronic warfarin treatment in prevention of systemic thromboembolism in patients with atrial fibrillation (1). Thus, percutaneous LAA exclusion might provide an alternative strategy to chronic warfarin therapy for stroke prophylaxis in patients with nonvalvular atrial fibrillation. Thus, answer B is incorrect.

Adult patients with nonvalvular atrial fibrillation were eligible for inclusion in this multicenter, randomized noninferiority trial if they had at least one of the following: previous stroke or transient ischemic attack; congestive heart failure, or diabetes; hypertension; or were 75 years or older.

After implantation of the Watchman device, all patients are expected to take warfarin therapy for 6 weeks, clopidogrel for 6 months, and aspirin for life. Thus, answer C is incorrect.

LAA thrombus is a contraindication of implantation of an LAA exclusion device as the thrombus may be dislodged during the procedure and cause an acute thromboembolic event. Thus, answer D is incorrect.

Other exclusion criteria for Watchman device placement include contraindications to warfarin, comorbidities other than atrial fibrillation that require chronic warfarin use, LAA thrombus, a patent foramen ovale with atrial septal aneurysm and right-to-left shunt, mobile aortic atheroma, and symptomatic carotid artery disease.

Unfortunately, there is a large (>5 mm) residual peridevice leak seen in Figure 54.4B. Thus, the correct answer is E. This patient would be expected to continue warfarin therapy as there was incomplete exclusion of the LA appendage.

Reference

1. Holmes DR, Reddy VY, Turi ZG; PROTECT AF Investigators, et al. Percutaneous closure of the left atrial appendage versus warfarin therapy for prevention of stroke in patients with atrial fibrillation: a randomised non-inferiority trial. *Lancet* 2009;374(9689):534–542.

Suggested Readings

Garcia Fernandez MA, Perk G, Saric M, et al. Chapter 12. Real-time three-dimensional transesophageal echocardiography for guidance of catheter based interventions. In: Badano LP, Lang RM, Zamorano JL, eds. *Textbook of Real-Time Three-Dimensional Echocardiography*. 1st ed. Springer, 2011:121–134.

Perk G, Biner S, Kronzon I, et al. Catheter-based left atrial appendage occlusion procedure—role of echocardiography. *Eur Heart J Cardiovasc Imaging* 2012;13(2):132–138.

Perk G, Ruiz C, Saric M, et al. Real-time three-dimensional transesophageal echocardiography in transcutaneous, catheter-based procedures for repair of structural heart diseases. *Curr Cardiovasc Imaging Rep* 2009;2(5):363–374.

Answer 5: *C.* The so-called surgical view of the mitral valve (Fig. 54.5) shows the mitral valve the way surgeons see the valve. In this view using the clockface analogy, the aortic valve is located at 12 o'clock, the left atrial appendage at 9 o'clock, and the interatrial septum at 3 o'clock.

The mitral leaflet adjacent to the aortic valve is the anterior mitral leaflet; the other leaflet is the posterior mitral leaflet. The lateral commissure is located at approximately

10 o'clock and the medical commissure at approximately 2 o'clock.

Each leaflet typically consists of three scallops, which are numbered in this view from left to right as 1, 2, and 3. Thus, scallop 1 of the either mitral leaflet is located laterally (adjacent to the left atrial appendage), while scallop 3 is located medially (close to the interatrial septum).

The arrow points to the P1 scallop of the posterior mitral leaflet. Thus, the correct answer is C.

Suggested Readings

Garcia Fernandez MA, Perk G, Saric M, et al. Chapter 12. Real-time three-dimensional transesophageal echocardiography for guidance of catheter based interventions. In: Badano LP, Lang RM, Zamorano JL, eds. *Textbook of Real-Time Three-Dimensional Echocardiography*. 1st ed. Springer, 2011:121–134.

Perk G, Ruiz C, Saric M, et al. Real-time three-dimensional transesophageal echocardiography in transcutaneous, catheter-based procedures for repair of structural heart diseases. *Curr Cardiovasc Imaging Rep* 2009;2(5):363–374.

Answer 6: *C.* Figure 54.6A demonstrates severe senile calcific aortic stenosis of a trileaflet valve. Figure 54.6B shows a 3D TEE appearance of transcutaneous aortic valve replacement with a CoreValve. Both are viewed from the ascending aorta side of the valve.

In the United States, two percutaneous aortic valves are being used: Medtronic CoreValve and Edwards SAPIEN valve. The CoreValve consists of a nitinol wire mesh and bioprosthetic aortic valve leaflets. In Panel B, a crown of CoreValve nitinol wires is seen along the inside perimeter of the ascending aorta; the thin line inside the lumen represents bioprosthetic leaflets. Thus, the correct answer is C.

Prior to transcutaneous aortic valve replacement, aortic balloon valvuloplasty is performed. Immediately thereafter, transcutaneous prosthetic aortic valve is implanted. Thus, answer A is incorrect.

Figure 54.6B does not have an appearance of either a surgically implanted bioprosthetic or a mechanical prosthesis. Thus, answer B is incorrect.

Surgically implanted aortic bioprostheses typically have three struts. No struts are seen in Figure 54.6A, which demonstrates a native aortic valve. Furthermore, valve-in-valve implantation is not a currently approved indication for the use of transcutaneous aortic valves. Thus, answer D is incorrect.

Figure 54.6B may bear some resemblance to an ascending aortic endograft. However, Figure 54.6A demonstrates no aortic dissection; instead, it shows severe native aortic stenosis. Thus, answer E is incorrect.

Suggested Readings

Garcia Fernandez MA, Perk G, Saric M, et al. Chapter 12. Real-time three-dimensional transesophageal echocardiography for guidance of catheter based interventions. In: Badano LP, Lang RM, Zamorano JL, eds. *Textbook of Real-Time Three-Dimensional Echocardiography*. 1st ed. Springer, 2011:121–134.

Perk G, Ruiz C, Saric M, et al. Real-time three-dimensional transesophageal echocardiography in transcutaneous, catheter-based procedures for repair of structural heart diseases. *Curr Cardiovasc Imaging Rep* 2009;2(5):363–374.

Answer 7: D. Figure 54.7A demonstrates typically spectral Doppler tracings of a patient with severe coarctation of the aorta. Note the very high peak systolic velocity (almost 4 m/s) as well as the abnormal persistence of antegrade flow during diastole. After percutaneous balloon dilation of the aortic coarctation, the spectral Doppler flow in the descending thoracic aorta normalizes. Note the normal peak systolic velocity (in this patient <1 m/s) as well as the normal absence of holodiastolic antegrade flow. Thus, the correct answer is D.

Figure 54.7A may bear some resemblance to systolic and diastolic antegrade flow across a patent ductus arteriosus. However, a successful percutaneous closure of PDA would result in a complete cessation of flow across the PDA, which is not the case in Figure 54.7B. Thus, answer A is incorrect.

Prior to intervention, neither type B aortic dissection nor the atrial septal defect is characterized by such high systolic and diastolic flow velocities shown in Figure 54.7A. Thus, neither answer B nor D is correct.

Aortic transection, which typically results from a deceleration injury, is a medical emergency. It requires immediate surgical rather than percutaneous intervention. Thus, answer E is incorrect.

Suggested Readings

Garcia Fernandez MA, Perk G, Saric M, et al. Chapter 12. Real-time three-dimensional transesophageal echocardiography for guidance of catheter based interventions. In: Badano LP, Lang RM, Zamorano JL, eds. *Textbook of Real-Time Three-Dimensional Echocardiography.* 1st ed. Springer, 2011:121–134.

Perk G, Ruiz C, Saric M, et al. Real-time three-dimensional transesophageal echocardiography in transcutaneous, catheter-based procedures for repair of structural heart diseases. *Curr Cardiovasc Imaging Rep* 2009;2(5):363–374.

Saric M, Kronzon I. Chapter 110. Coarctation of the aorta. In: Lang R, Goldstein SA, Kronzon I, et al., eds. *Dynamic Echocardiography: A Case-Based Approach.* 1st ed. St. Louis, MO: Springer, 2010:459–461.

Answer 8: D. Figure 54.8C demonstrates a color Doppler recording from the left internal mammary artery (LIMA). The flow velocity pattern of a native (nongrafted) LIMA is shown in Figure 54.8A. Native (nongrafted) LIMA demonstrates the typical high-resistance flow of an artery that supplies skeletal muscles; note that antegrade flow occurs primarily in systole and that there is very little antegrade runoff during diastole.

Figure 54.8B demonstrates a change of flow velocity pattern after LIMA is grafted to the left descending coronary artery during coronary artery bypass surgery. LIMA now assumes the flow velocity pattern that is typically seen in the left coronary artery: (a) significant antegrade flow occurs in both systole and diastole, and (b) diastolic flow is more prominent than the systolic one. Thus, the correct answer is D.

Femoral pseudoaneurysm has a characteristic to-and-fro flow (antegrade in systole, retrograde in diastole). Since this is not seen in Figure 54.8A, answer A is incorrect.

Post successful stenting, internal carotid artery flow velocity pattern would have normalized, that is, it would have assumed a low-resistance flow velocity pattern characterized by a combination of a predominantly systolic antegrade flow and a significant antegrade runoff during diastole. Since this is not seen in Figure 54.8B, answer B is incorrect.

Dialysis access shunt, being an atrioventricular shunt, would have demonstrated high-velocity antegrade flow during both systole and diastole at baseline. Since this is not seen in Figure 54.8A, answer C is incorrect.

Post successful balloon angioplasty, renal artery flow velocity pattern would have normalized, that is, it would have assumed a low-resistance flow velocity pattern characterized by a combination of predominantly systolic antegrade flow and a significant antegrade runoff during diastole. Since this is not seen in Figure 54.8B, answer E is incorrect.

Suggested Reading

Kasliwal R, Mittal S, Shrivastava S, et al. Echocardiography in minimally invasive direct coronary artery bypass. *Echocardiography* 1999;16(6):603–610.

Answer 9: A. Positioning of percutaneous ventricular assist devices such as the Impella devices can be done with echocardiographic guidance. Ideally, the Impella device should be positioned approximately 3.5 to 4.5 cm from the aortic valve plane in order to function properly. Therefore, answer D is incorrect. Flow from the device is detected and displayed on an external module. Display of flow on the monitor, however, depends on having the inflow portion of the device within the LV and the outflow port within the aorta. In the event that both ports are colocalized within the LV or aorta, no display of flow will appear on the monitor. Once placed in the proper position, the Impella device is sutured securely to prevent inadvertent device migration. In the current case, the Impella device likely migrated out of the LV during the patient transfer from the gurney to the hospital bed, resulting in a return of his symptoms and abnormal hemodynamics.

Figure 54.16 depicts the Impella device as seen from a parasternal long-axis view. The Impella is largely within the aorta with only a small portion protruding from the aortic valve plane. This may have provided a signal of flow on the Impella module, although it may have been suboptimal as the LVAD inflow port migrated intermittently between the LV and the aorta. This position would not have provided adequate support to the LV. For this reason, answer B is incorrect. Proper repositioning would likely have restored the favorable hemodynamics seen at the time of original placement in the cardiac catheterization lab. Therefore, switching to a different mechanical support strategy would is not indicated. There is no evidence to support a mechanical complication requiring surgical intervention. Therefore, answers C and E are incorrect.

Suggested Reading

Catena E, Milazzo F, Merli M, et al. Echocardiographic evaluation of patients receiving a new left ventricular assist device: the Impella recover 100. *Eur J Echocardiogr* 2004;5:430–437.

Answer 10: C. The TEE operator has the responsibility of providing echocardiographic imaging guidance to the interventional cardiologist during a percutaneous intracardiac procedure. Once the procedure is completed, however, the responsibilities of the TEE operator do not cease. Rather, it is imperative that a careful imaging review of the structures involved in the procedure is carried out using two-dimensional, three-dimensional, and Doppler techniques. For any percutaneous interventional procedure involving the cardiac valves, it is important to comprehensively assess the function of those valves, as well as adjacent valvular structures. Any intracardiac shunts created during the procedure such as the interatrial shunt created to gain access to the mitral valve through penetration of the interatrial septum should be re-evaluated in terms of its morphologic features and potential hemodynamic impact. In cases where closure of an intrinsic intracardiac shunt is the objective, assessing the location and stability of the closure device and its effectiveness in eliminating the shunt is necessary.

An overview of LV and RV systolic function and wall motion can be helpful in the identification of periprocedural myocardial ischemia or infarction. Finally, as for any intracardiac procedure, a careful assessment for the development of a pericardial effusion, with particular attention to size, distribution, and impact on cardiac function and hemodynamics, is imperative.

Although each of the listed Options A through E can be found as a consequence of structural heart manipulations (like paravalvular closure repair), the most likely cause for acute hypotension and tachycardia would be development of a new (even small) pericardial effusion.

Suggested Readings

Perk G, Lang RM, Garcia-Fernandez MA, et al. Use of real time three-dimensional transesophageal echocardiography in intracardiac catheter based interventions. *J Am Soc Echocardiogr* 2009;22:865–882.
Smith LA, Monaghan MJ. Monitoring of procedures: peri-interventional echo assessment for transcatheter aortic valve implantation. *Eur Heart J Cardiovasc Imaging* 2013;14:840–850.
Zamorano JL, Badano LP, Bruce C, et al. EAE/ASE recommendations for the use of echocardiography in new transcatheter interventions for valvular heart disease. *J Am Soc Echocardiogr* 2011;24:937–965.

Answer 11: E. Both Figure 54.9A and B demonstrate the left atrial aspect of a bioprosthetic mitral valve in the so-called surgical view. In this view using the clockface analogy, the aortic valve is located at 12 o'clock, the left atrial appendage at 9 o'clock, and the interatrial septum at 3 o'clock.

Figure 54.9A demonstrates a paravalvular dehiscence at approximately 11 o'clock. The dehiscence (seen on color Doppler as a paravalvular mitral regurgitant leak) is closed percutaneously with a vascular plug seen in Figure 54.9B lateral to the mitral bioprosthetic sewing ring at 11 o'clock. In Figure 54.9B, the catheter used to deliver the plug is still seen. The catheter was subsequently removed, and the procedure was completed. Thus, the correct answer is E.

Percutaneous mitral balloon valvuloplasty of a stenosed bioprosthetic valve is done infrequently. Had that been the procedure, Figure 54.9B would have shown a valvuloplasty balloon

inside the sewing ring of the mitral bioprosthesis. Thus, answer A is incorrect.

Mitral valve clipping is a percutaneous procedure used to treat native (not prosthetic) mitral valve regurgitation. It resembles the surgical Alfieri stitch; the clip is typically placed between A2 and P2 scallops of the native mitral valve. Thus, answer B is incorrect.

Both Figure 54.9A and B show the typical sewing ring of mitral bioprosthetic ring. Since there is no change in the appearance of the mitral prosthesis from Figure 54.9A to Figure 54.9B, answer C is incorrect.

Device closure of the left atrial appendage is accomplished by a percutaneous placement of a plug in the ostium of the left atrial appendage. In Figure 54.9A and B, the native left atrial appendage with no plug is seen at approximately 9 o'clock. Thus, answer E is incorrect.

Suggested Readings

Garcia Fernandez MA, Perk G, Saric M, et al. Chapter 12. Real-time three-dimensional transesophageal echocardiography for guidance of catheter based interventions. In: Badano LP, Lang RM, Zamorano JL, eds. *Textbook of Real-Time Three-Dimensional Echocardiography*. 1st ed. Springer, 2011:121–134.
Perk G, Biner S, Kronzon I, et al. Catheter-based left atrial appendage occlusion procedure—role of echocardiography. *Eur Heart J Cardiovasc Imaging* 2012;13(2):132–138.

Answer 12: B. Figure 54.10A1 demonstrates a systolic color flow that leaves the left ventricle during systole. Figure 54.10A2 further characterizes the flow and demonstrates the to-and-fro pattern characteristic of a pseudoaneurysm (the flow exits the left ventricle into the pseudoaneurysm during systole and returns into the left ventricle from the pseudoaneurysm during diastole). VIDEO 54.3 demonstrates the to-and-fro flow on color Doppler imaging.

Based on Figures 54.10A1 and A2, as well as VIDEO 54.3, one can establish the diagnosis of left ventricular pseudoaneurysm in this patient with recent infarction of the anterior wall. Figures 54.10B1 and B2, as well as VIDEO 54.4, demonstrate that the left ventricular pseudoaneurysm was closed percutaneously with a closure device. Thus, the correct answer is B.

Ventricular septal defect (VSD) would have had a different flow velocity pattern in Figure 54.10A2. Typical VSD does not show a to-and-fro flow velocity pattern. Instead, in an uncomplicated VSD, the flow from the left ventricle to the right ventricle occurs almost exclusively during systole albeit a small amount of flow into the right ventricle occurs during diastole as well. Thus, answer A is incorrect.

Figure 54.10B2 demonstrates a closure device. An inflow cannula of a left ventricular assist device is typically placed in the left ventricular apex and would have demonstrated a central lumen in Figure 54.10B2. Thus, answer C is incorrect.

Mitral valve is not seen in any of the attached still images or the videos. Thus, answer D is incorrect.

During ventricular septal ablation, alcohol is injected into a septal coronary artery branch. Figure 54.10A2 is not consistent with a coronary artery flow (flow in the coronary arteries is antegrade in systole and diastole). Thus, answer E is incorrect.

Suggested Readings

Dudiy Y, Jelnin V, Einhorn BN, et al. Percutaneous closure of left ventricular pseudoaneurysm. *Circ Cardiovasc Interv* 2011;4(4):322–326.

Garcia Fernandez MA, Perk G, Saric M, et al. Chapter 12. Real-time three-dimensional transesophageal echocardiography for guidance of catheter based interventions. In: Badano LP, Lang RM, Zamorano JL, eds. *Textbook of Real-Time Three-Dimensional Echocardiography*. 1st ed. Springer, 2011:121–134.

Perk G, Ruiz C, Saric M, et al. Real-time three-dimensional transesophageal echocardiography in transcutaneous, catheter-based procedures for repair of structural heart diseases. *Curr Cardiovasc Imaging Rep* 2009;2(5):363–374.

Answer 13: *D.* Figure 54.11A demonstrates the typical spectral Doppler flow velocity pattern of uncomplicated VSD. Note that the flow from the left ventricle to the right ventricle occurs almost exclusively during systole albeit a small amount of flow into the right ventricle occurs during diastole as well. The VSD was subsequently closed with a percutaneous closure device. The left ventricular side of the VSD closure device is seen in Figure 54.11B. Thus, answer D is correct.

During ventricular septal ablation, alcohol is injected into a septal coronary artery branch. Figure 54.11A is not consistent with a coronary artery flow (flow in the coronary arteries is antegrade in systole and diastole). Thus, answer A is incorrect.

An inflow cannula of a left ventricular assist device is (a) typically placed in the left ventricular apex and (b) would have demonstrated a central lumen in Figure 54.11B. Since neither is the case, answer B is incorrect.

Flow velocity pattern in Figure 54.11A is not consistent with a left ventricular pseudoaneurysm. Pseudoaneurysms have a characteristic to-and-fro flow pattern (flow leaves the left ventricle into the pseudoaneurysm during systole and returns from the pseudoaneurysm into the left ventricle during diastole). Thus, answer C is incorrect.

Aortic stenosis is characterized by an elevated systolic gradient. However, the systolic antegrade flow in aortic stenosis is not holosystolic but rather occurs only during the ejection phase. In contrast, the systolic flow in Figure 54.11A is holosystolic. In other words, the onset of aortic stenosis flow occurs after QRS on the ECG; the flow of VSD starts at QRS on the ECG. Furthermore, Figure 54.11B demonstrates a device adjacent to and not in the aortic valve. Thus, answer E is incorrect.

Suggested Readings

Garcia Fernandez MA, Perk G, Saric M, et al. Chapter 12. Real-time three-dimensional transesophageal echocardiography for guidance of catheter based interventions. In: Badano LP, Lang RM, Zamorano JL, eds. *Textbook of Real-Time Three-Dimensional Echocardiography*. 1st ed. Springer, 2011:121–134.

Perk G, Ruiz C, Saric M, et al. Real-time three-dimensional transesophageal echocardiography in transcutaneous, catheter-based procedures for repair of structural heart diseases. *Curr Cardiovasc Imaging Rep* 2009;2(5):363–374.

Saric M, Kronzon I. Chapter 107. Ventricular septal defect and Eisenmenger syndrome. In: Lang R, Goldstein SA, Kronzon I, et al., eds. *Dynamic Echocardiography: A Case-Based Approach*. 1st ed. St. Louis, MO: Springer, 2010:446–450.

Answer 14: *A.* Both Figures 54.12A and B demonstrate the left atrial aspect of a native mitral valve in the so-called surgical view. In this view using the clockface analogy, the aortic valve is located at 12 o'clock, the left atrial appendage at 9 o'clock, and the interatrial septum at 3 o'clock.

Figure 54.12B demonstrates the characteristic appearance of a mitral valve clip between A2 and P2 scallops. This percutaneous procedure is equivalent to the surgical Alfieri stitch and is used to treat severe degenerative or functional mitral regurgitation. Thus, the correct answer is A.

Percutaneous mitral balloon valvuloplasty is the treatment of choice for rheumatic mitral stenosis. Figure 54.12A does not demonstrate mitral stenosis. Furthermore, the mitral valve would have still had one diastolic orifice postvalvuloplasty. In contrast, Figure 54.12B demonstrates two separate diastolic orifices; this is a typical finding post mitral clipping. Thus, answer B is incorrect.

The atrial septum is well seen at 3 o'clock in Figure 54.12B. No device associated with the atrial septum is seen. Thus, answer C is incorrect.

Both Figures 54.12A and B demonstrate a native (nonprosthetic) mitral valve. Thus, neither answer D nor answer E is correct.

Suggested Readings

Garcia Fernandez MA, Perk G, Saric M, et al. Chapter 12. Real-time three-dimensional transesophageal echocardiography for guidance of catheter based interventions. In: Badano LP, Lang RM, Zamorano JL, eds. *Textbook of Real-Time Three-Dimensional Echocardiography*. 1st ed. Springer, 2011:121–134.

Perk G, Ruiz C, Saric M, et al. Real-time three-dimensional transesophageal echocardiography in transcutaneous, catheter-based procedures for repair of structural heart diseases. *Curr Cardiovasc Imaging Rep* 2009;2(5):363–374.

Answer 15: *D.* Figure 54.13A and Video 54.6 demonstrate an intact interatrial septum on 2D TEE color Doppler. Figure 54.13B shows the left atrial aspect of the interatrial septum on 3D TEE during transseptal puncture. Figure 54.13C and Video 54.7 demonstrate a small iatrogenic atrial septal defect (ASD) in the posterior portion of the atrial septum, a residual of the transseptal puncture.

Transseptal puncture is an obligatory step in many percutaneous procedures involving the left heart (such as percutaneous mitral balloon valvuloplasty, left atrial appendage occlusion, and paravalvular mitral prosthetic leak closure). In this patient, a deflated balloon used in mitral valvuloplasty was delivered first transvenously into the right atrium and then across the previously created transseptal puncture into the left atrium and across the mitral valve. After removal of all transseptal catheters, it is not unusual to see a small residual iatrogenic atrial septal defect. Thus, the correct answer is D.

The location of the ASD in the posterior portion of the atrial septum seen in Figure 54.13B is not consistent with a primum ASD. Primum ASDs are located near the atrioventricular (mitral and tricuspid) valves. Thus, answer A is incorrect.

Figure 54.13B demonstrates puncture of the interatrial septum and not of the right atrial free wall. Thus, answer B is incorrect.

The location of the ASD in the posterior portion of the atrial septum seen in Figure 54.13B is not consistent with the anatomic location of either the coronary sinus or the superior vena cava. Thus, neither answer D nor answer E is correct.

Suggested Readings

Garcia Fernandez MA, Perk G, Saric M, et al. Chapter 12. Real-time three-dimensional transesophageal echocardiography for guidance of catheter based interventions. In: Badano LP, Lang RM, Zamorano JL, eds. *Textbook of Real-Time Three-Dimensional Echocardiography*. 1st ed. Springer, 2011:121–134.

Perk G, Ruiz C, Saric M, et al. Real-time three-dimensional transesophageal echocardiography in transcutaneous, catheter-based procedures for repair of structural heart diseases. *Curr Cardiovasc Imaging Rep* 2009;2(5):363–374.

Saric M, Perk G, Purgess J, et al. Imaging atrial septal defects by real-time 3D transesophageal echocardiography: step-by-step approach. *J Am Soc Echocardiogr* 2010;23(11):1128–1135.

Answer 16: C. Both Figure 54.14A and B show the 3D transesophageal echocardiographic appearance of a rheumatic mitral valve from the left ventricular perspective. Figure 54.14A demonstrates severe rheumatic mitral stenosis with a valve area of approximately 0.6 cm². Post mitral balloon valvuloplasty, the mitral valve area in Figure 54.14B doubled to approximately 1.2 cm². Thus, the correct answer is C.

In mitral valve clipping or after Alfieri stitch, the mitral orifice is divided into two or more holes due to placement of either a clip or a stitch typically between A2 and P2 scallops of the mitral valve. Since in both Figure 54.14A and B there is single mitral orifice, neither answer A nor answer B is correct.

Atrial septostomy is a creation of a de novo large atrial septal defect to treat cyanotic congenital heart disease such as the D-transposition of the great arteries. Historically, atrial septostomy was the very first percutaneous procedure for the treatment of structural heart disease. It was introduced in 1966 by the American physician William Rashkind (1922 to 1986) at the Children's Hospital of Philadelphia. Neither Figure 54.14A nor B has the appearance of an atrial septal defect. Thus, answer D is incorrect.

Both Figure 54.14A and B show native mitral valve. Paravalvular leaks occur with prosthetic mitral valves. Thus, answer E is incorrect.

Suggested Readings

Bonow RO, Carabello BA, Chatterjee K, et al. 2008 focused update incorporated into the ACC/AHA 2006 guidelines for the management of patients with valvular heart disease: a report of the American College of Cardiology/American Heart Association Task Force on Practice Guidelines (Writing Committee to revise the 1998 guidelines for the management of patients with valvular heart disease). Endorsed by the Society of Cardiovascular Anesthesiologists, Society for Cardiovascular Angiography and Interventions, and Society of Thoracic Surgeons. *J Am Coll Cardiol* 2008;52(13):e1–e142.

Garcia Fernandez MA, Perk G, Saric M, et al. Chapter 12. Real-time three-dimensional transesophageal echocardiography for guidance of catheter based interventions. In: Badano LP, Lang RM, Zamorano JL, eds. *Textbook of Real-Time Three-Dimensional Echocardiography*. 1st ed. Springer, 2011:121–134.

Inoue K, Owaki T, Nakamura T, et al. Clinical application of transvenous mitral commissurotomy by a new balloon catheter. *J Thorac Cardiovasc Surg* 1984;87(3):394–402.

Perk G, Ruiz C, Saric M, et al. Real-time three-dimensional transesophageal echocardiography in transcutaneous, catheter-based procedures for repair of structural heart diseases. *Curr Cardiovasc Imaging Rep* 2009;2(5):363–374.

Rashkind WJ, Miller WW. Creation of an atrial septal defect without thoracotomy. A palliative approach to complete transposition of the great arteries. *JAMA* 1966;196(11):991–992.

Wilkins GT, Weyman AE, Abascal VM, et al. Percutaneous balloon dilatation of the mitral valve: an analysis of echocardiographic variables related to outcome and the mechanism of dilation. *Br Heart J* 1988;60:299–308.

Answer 17: B. Figure 54.15A represents a 2D transesophageal echocardiographic image obtained in the bicaval view with the superior vena cava on the right, the inferior vena cava on the left, the left atrium on the top, and the right atrium on the bottom of the image. Color Doppler demonstrates a small shunt across the patent foramen ovale (PFO), which in this patient is in the left-to-right direction. In general, flow across PFO can be predominantly unidirectional (left to right or right to left) or bidirectional depending on pressure differences between the two atria. Figure 54.15B shows the right atrial aspect of a PFO closure device. Thus, the correct answer is B.

All the remaining answers are related to non-PFO types of atrial septal defect. Figure 54.15A demonstrates the typical appearance of PFO, a small defect between the two layers of the atrial septum. Thus, the other answers are incorrect.

Suggested Readings

Garcia Fernandez MA, Perk G, Saric M, et al. Chapter 12. Real-time three-dimensional transesophageal echocardiography for guidance of catheter based interventions. In: Badano LP, Lang RM, Zamorano JL, eds. *Textbook of Real-Time Three-Dimensional Echocardiography*. 1st ed. Springer, 2011:121–134.

Perk G, Ruiz C, Saric M, et al. Real-time three-dimensional transesophageal echocardiography in transcutaneous, catheter-based procedures for repair of structural heart diseases. *Curr Cardiovasc Imaging Rep* 2009;2(5):363–374.

Saric M, Perk G, Purgess J, et al. Imaging atrial septal defects by real-time 3D transesophageal echocardiography: step-by-step approach. *J Am Soc Echocardiogr* 2010;23(11):1128–1135.

Answer 18: C. The image demonstrates a dilated LV and the conspicuous absence of an Impella inflow cannula within the LV cavity. In fact, the Impella device has dislodged proximally and is now located within the aortic root. Answer A is incorrect since the Impella device is not in the correct position. Answer B is incorrect since there is no evidence indicating penetration of the aorta. Answer D is incorrect as there is no evidence of thrombosis. Thrombosis is unlikely given that the patient is receiving systemic anticoagulation therapy. The pulsatile nature of the flow displayed on the Impella module is not consistent with a thrombosed Impella device, which is more likely to show a dampened waveform or no flow. Flow display on the Impella module depends on the inflow and outflow ports on the Impella cannula being localized in separate chambers, namely the LV and aorta. If both ports colocalize within the same chamber, flow display becomes flatlined. Given the intermittent display of flow on the Impella module, it is likely that the Impella device is intermittently sliding between the LVOT and the proximal aorta such that the inflow port periodically is within the LV cavity long enough to register flow.

Suggested Reading

Scalia GM, McCarthy PM, Savage RM, et al. Clinical utility of echocardiography in the management of implantable ventricular assist devices. *J Am Soc Echocardiogr* 2000;13:754–763.

Answer 19: B. Following from the previous question, the next best action would be to reposition the Impella device, especially given that while it was in the proper position in the cardiac catheterization lab, the hemodynamics were observed to improve. It would be important, however, that the Impella device be advanced to the ideal position of approximately 3.5 to 4.5 cm from the aortic valve plane. Echocardiography is well suited to guide repositioning of the Impella device. FIGURE 54.17 shows the end result of this manipulation and now demonstrates an Impella device in the proper position. There is no need for further advancement or retraction. The only reasons to consider a different mechanical circulatory support device are (a) inadequate support provided by the Impella device or (b) a complication related to the use of the Impella device (e.g., hemolytic anemia, acute kidney injury related to hemolysis, device thrombosis).

Suggested Readings

Catena E, Milazzo F, Merli M, et al. Echocardiographic evaluation of patients receiving a new left ventricular assist device: the Impella recover 100. *Eur J Echocardiogr* 2004;5:430–437.

Patel KM, Sherwani SS, Baudo AM, et al. The use of transesophageal echocardiography for confirmation of appropriate Impella 5.0 device placement. *Anesth Analg* 2012;114:82–85.

Rasalingam R, Johnson SN, Bilhorn KR, et al. Transthoracic echocardiographic assessment of continuous-flow left ventricular assist devices. *J Am Soc Echocardiogr* 2011;24:135–148.

Scalia GM, McCarthy PM, Savage RM, et al. Clinical utility of echocardiography in the management of implantable ventricular assist devices. *J Am Soc Echocardiogr* 2000;13:754–763.

Answer 20: D. The image depicted in FIGURE 54.20 is a biplane view of the left and right atria and interatrial septum. They clearly demonstrate the trajectory of the catheter, emanating from an inferior position and directed posteriorly as denoted by its position in relation to the IVC (inferiorly) and the left atrium (posteriorly). The 3D images show the catheter from a perspective looking down onto the mitral valve in sequence as the paravalvular leak is closed with a closure device.

Suggested Reading

Perk G, Lang RM, Garcia-Fernandez MA, et al. Use of real time three-dimensional transesophageal echocardiography in intracardiac catheter based interventions. *J Am Soc Echocardiogr* 2009;22:865–882.

Chapter 55

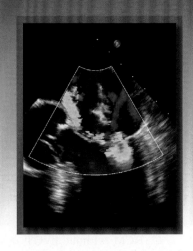

Intraoperative Echocardiography for the Boards

Vincent L. Sorrell

Questions 1 to 4

A 60-year-old female with a history of hypertrophic cardiomyopathy (HCM) is listed for cardiac surgery. Her pre-pump intraoperative transesophageal echo (TEE) images (Figs. 55.1 to 55.4 and Video 55.1) show that the left ventricle (LV) is hyperdynamic without regional wall motion abnormality.

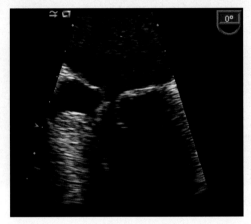

FIGURE 55.1

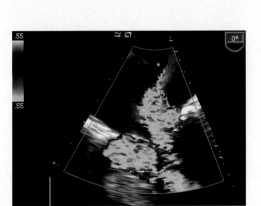

FIGURE 55.2

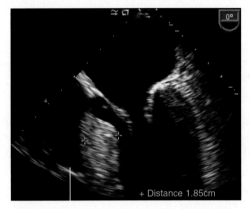

FIGURE 55.3

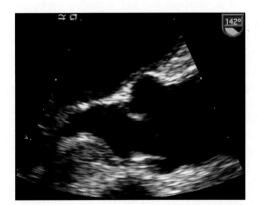

FIGURE 55.4

1. What is the diagnosis, and what are your recommendations to the surgeon?

   A. HCM with LV outflow tract (OT) obstruction and at least moderate mitral regurgitation (MR). Recommend septal myectomy, and the patient will probably require mitral valve repair/replacement.

   B. HCM with LVOT obstruction and at least moderate MR. Recommend septal myectomy, and the patient will probably *not* require mitral valve repair/replacement.

   C. HCM without LVOT obstruction and an abnormal mitral valve. Recommend mitral valve repair/replacement only.

   D. HCM with midcavitary obstruction and MR. Recommend mitral valve repair/replacement with papillary muscle debulking.

   E. Ventricular septal defect (VSD) with severe MR. Recommend mitral valve repair/replacement and VSD repair.

2. When is surgery in HCM recommended?

   A. Mean outflow tract gradient of >40 mm Hg

   B. SAM resulting in MR

   C. Peak outflow tract gradient of >50 mm Hg

   D. Presyncope during moderate exertion on beta-blocker therapy at resting HR of 52 bpm

   E. HCM with malpositioned papillary muscles

3. During postpump intraoperative TEE assessment, what intervention might be useful to provoke inducible SAM and LVOT obstruction?

   A. Isoproterenol

   B. Amyl nitrite

   C. Phenylephrine

   D. Perindopril

   E. Propranolol

4. Which of the statements is true regarding septal myectomy?

   A. It is associated with high (>5%) postoperative mortality even in experienced centers.

   B. Shunts between the resected intramyocardial vessels and the LV cavity are common.

   C. Rates of heart block requiring pacemaker insertion are higher than for septal ablation.

   D. It results in intramyocardial scarring close to the site of resection on delayed gadolinium-enhanced magnetic resonance imaging.

   E. There are randomized control trial (RCT) data demonstrating the beneficial effects of septal myectomy on both symptoms and survival.

Questions 5 to 8

A 55-year-old male presents with shortness of breath for mitral valve surgery. Figures 55.5, 55.6, and 55.7 show his intraoperative TEE images.

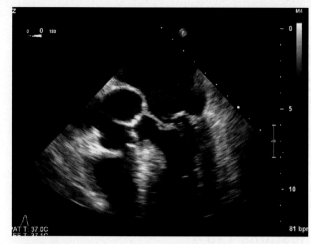

Figure 55.5

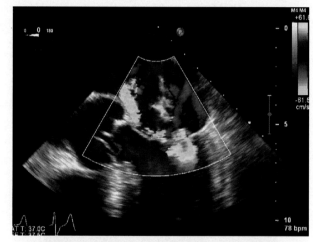

Figure 55.6

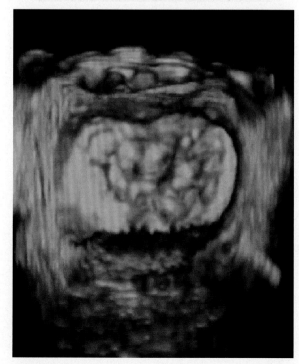

Figure 55.7

5. Based on the still images and the 3D cine reconstruction seen in VIDEO 55.2, what is the mitral valve pathology?

A. Flail of P1/P2
B. Flail of P2/P3
C. Flail of A1/A2
D. Prolapse of P2/P3
E. Restriction of the anterior mitral valve leaflet

6. According to the Carpentier functional classification of mitral valve disease, what class is displayed in this case?

A. Class I
B. Class II
C. Class IIIa
D. Class IIIb
E. Class IV

7. In the operating room, which of the following findings is most supportive of your suspicion that this is severe MR?

A. A proximal flow convergence radius of 0.8 cm at a Nyquist limit of 40 cm/s
B. A calculated regurgitant volume of 55 mL
C. A vena contracta width of 0.6 cm
D. A moderately dilated LA and LV
E. Systolic flow reversal in the pulmonary veins

8. What finding might be an indication to recommend surgery in an asymptomatic patient with severe MR?

A. Pulmonary artery pressures of >40 mm Hg at rest
B. Severely dilated left atrium
C. EF 25% with chordal preservation unlikely
D. LV end-systolic diameter of 45 cm
E. Right ventricular dysfunction

Questions 9 to 11

A 72-year-old male presents for replacement of an aneurysmal ascending aorta. On routine preoperative TEE, a number of unexpected findings were noted (VIDEOS 55.3 TO 55.5 and FIGS. 55.8 AND 55.9).

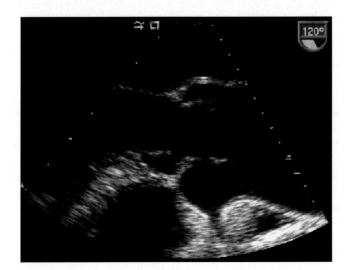

FIGURE 55.8

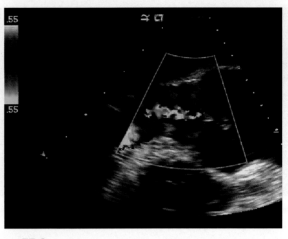

FIGURE 55.9

9. What is the most likely diagnosis?

A. Carney complex
B. Shone syndrome
C. Atrial myxoma and partial subvalvular membrane
D. Atrial thrombus and partial subvalvular membrane
E. Papillary fibroelastomas in the left atrium and LVOT

10. In this case, what is the most likely complication to occur if these previously undiagnosed entities were not removed?

A. Severe aortic incompetence
B. Severe aortic stenosis
C. Infective endocarditis
D. Sudden cardiac death
E. Embolization

11. How might these findings change the surgical approach?

A. Change to a left posterolateral thoracotomy.
B. Use bicaval cannulation instead of the right atrium for cardiopulmonary bypass (CPB).
C. Use retrograde cardioplegia.
D. Avoid the use of protamine postoperatively.

Questions 12 and 13

A 58-year-old female is undergoing redo open heart surgery for coronary artery bypass surgery. VIDEOS 55.6 AND 55.7 and FIGURE 55.10 are the prepump intraoperative TEE images of her descending aorta.

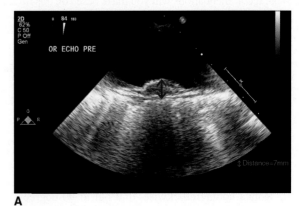

A

FIGURE 55.10

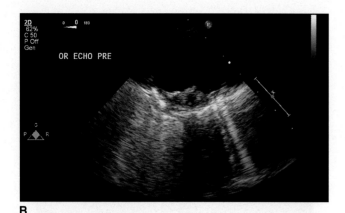

B

Figure 55.10 (Continued)

12. What is the unexpected diagnosis in this prepump intraoperative TEE?

    A. Moderate atheroma of the descending aorta
    B. Severe atheroma of the descending aorta
    C. Aortic hematoma
    D. Malignant neoplasm of the descending aorta
    E. Aortic dissection

13. Regarding this patient, which of the following statements is true?

    A. There is no increase in risk of stroke, mortality, or length of stay in hospital.
    B. Performing an endarterectomy is advisable to reduce the risk of intraoperative stroke.
    C. It is advisable to avoid minimally invasive port-access techniques.
    D. The use of statin therapy has a level of evidence A.
    E. The use of anticoagulation has a level of evidence A.

Questions 14 and 15

A 55-year-old male undergoes a prepump intraoperative TEE for coronary artery bypass grafting and a mitral valve repair. No prior preoperative TEE had been performed. The coronary sinus is noted on the intraoperative TEE to be dilated (1.8-cm diameter). A left-arm bubble study reveals no PFO, but bubbles are noted in the coronary sinus prior to arrival in the right atrium.

14. What recommendations will you make based on this finding?

    A. Use antegrade cardioplegia.
    B. Use retrograde cardioplegia.
    C. Use both antegrade and retrograde cardioplegia.
    D. Use the left subclavian vein to place a Swan-Ganz catheter preoperatively.
    E. The patient is asymptomatic, so this finding should not alter the management.

15. From a midesophageal four-chamber view, how would you best visualize the coronary sinus?

    A. Retract the probe, and anteflex at 0 degrees.
    B. Rotate counterclockwise, dial out to 90 degrees, and retract the probe.

    C. Advance the probe to a deep transgastric position in full anteflexion at 0 degrees.
    D. Rotate counterclockwise and dial out to 45 degrees.
    E. Advance the probe tip to the gastroesophageal junction, and gently anteflex at 0 degrees.

16. An 85-year-old frail male with a history of recurrent falls presents with symptoms of congestive cardiac failure after an episode of infective endocarditis, which affected his mitral valve. After reviewing the images post pump (Videos 55.8 and 55.9), what will you advise the surgeon?

    A. There is mild persistent MR; request a bolus of isoproterenol to fully assess the true severity.
    B. There is at least moderate persistent MR; advise to order follow-up TTE in a few days under normal loading conditions.
    C. There is the expected degree of MR post repair; advise to order follow-up TTE in a few days under normal loading conditions.
    D. Advise to go back on pump, and replace the mitral valve with a bioprosthesis if further repair is not possible.
    E. Advise to go back on pump, and replace the mitral valve with a mechanical valve if further repair is not possible.

Answer 1: **B**

Option A: False. See below.

    Option B: **True.** There is severe septal hypertrophy with severe systolic anterior motion (SAM) of the mitral valve, resulting in LVOT obstruction at rest as indicated by marked flow acceleration in the LVOT. There is a characteristic pattern seen in obstructive HCM with a posteriorly directed jet of MR that results from the SAM, presumably by the anterior tension on the mitral leaflet tips. Notably, there is no sign of mitral myxomatous degeneration (leaflet prolapse, flail, or redundancy), and the patient has normal LV function. The relatively normal mitral valve morphology makes SAM the most likely cause of the MR. Ruling out other causes for MR is a class Ib indication for the use of intraoperative TEE in surgery for HCM. After myectomy, in most cases like this one, the MR resolves, and mitral valve repair/replacement is not necessary.

    Option C: False. The mitral valve leaflets appear normal.

    Option D: False. There is no midcavitary obliteration shown in these images.

    Option E: False. There is no VSD shown in these images.

Answer 2: D. Appropriate selection of patients for surgical myectomy is of vital importance and a predictor of outcomes. While a peak gradient of 50 mm Hg at rest or with provocation is a necessary component indicating utility of myectomy, surgery is usually reserved for patients with obstruction and severe symptoms refractory to medical management. Myectomy should be performed by an experienced surgeon in a high-volume center (class Ic indication). The obstruction in HCM is dynamic; therefore, the peak gradient is used as a discriminator and not the mean gradient; therefore, response A is incorrect. Response B would be correct if the patient was on maximum medical therapy and symptomatic; however, this is not stated. HCM with malposition of the papillary muscles resulting in obstruction, which are amenable to surgical intervention, is a reason to choose surgical intervention over septal ablation. In those cases, the papillary muscle surgery is an important component of the surgery, but the patient must still fulfill the gradient and symptom requirements described above. Therefore, response E is only partially correct, as the answer does not state the gradient and symptom requirements have been fulfilled.

Answer 3: *A*

Option A: **True.** Isoproterenol is a potent nonselective beta-adrenergic agonist that has strong positive inotropic and chronotropic effects on the myocardium, which often exacerbates the degree of resting outflow tract obstruction, SAM, and MR. This assessment of provoked gradient is useful in ruling out significant inducible obstruction, which can cause persistence of symptoms and clinical events after myectomy.

Option B: False. Amyl nitrite is a potent vasodilator that causes a drop in afterload and results in exacerbation of SAM and obstruction. However, it is inhaled and, therefore, not amenable to use in an intubated patient.

Option C: False. Phenylephrine is a vasoconstrictor and therefore will improve outflow tract obstruction.

Option D: False. Perindopril would not be suitable for this purpose as it is slow acting, reduces afterload, and is available only in an oral formula.

Option E: False. Propranolol is a nonselective beta-blocker and, as a peripheral vasoconstrictor, will theoretically reduce SAM and dynamic obstruction.

Answer 4: *B*

Option A: False. While some older series from the 1980s did report operative mortalities as high as 5%, it is now generally accepted that mortality risk is rare (<1%) in high-volume institutions.

Option B: **True.** Small diastolic shunts seen by color Doppler at the site of resection are common and are—as a result of transection of small septal perforators—rarely of any clinical significance because the amount of the shunt is tiny. They may persist for weeks to years postoperatively.

Option C: False. The rate of heart block requiring pacemaker insertion post septal ablation ranges between 10% and 25%. This is substantially higher than after surgical myectomy. A recent meta-analysis described an almost threefold increased risk of requiring a pacemaker post septal ablation compared to surgical myectomy.

Option D: False. Alcohol septal ablation may result in intramyocardial scarring on delayed gadolinium-enhanced imaging on cardiac magnetic resonance. Septal myectomy does not.

Option E: False. While there are good observational studies of this therapy, there has been no randomized clinical trial assessing the effects of septal myectomy on survival.

Suggested Readings

Cavalcante JL, Barboza JS, Lever HM. Diversity of mitral valve abnormalities in obstructive hypertrophic cardiomyopathy. *Prog Cardiovasc Dis* 2012;54(6):517–522.

Fifer MA, Vlahakes GJ. Management of symptoms in hypertrophic cardiomyopathy. *Circulation* 2008;117:429–439.

Gersh BJ, Maron BJ, Bonow RO, et al.; American College of Cardiology Foundation/American Heart Association Task Force on Practice Guidelines. 2011 ACCF/AHA guideline for the diagnosis and treatment of hypertrophic cardiomyopathy: a report of the American College of Cardiology Foundation/American Heart Association Task Force on Practice Guidelines. Developed in collaboration with the American Association for Thoracic Surgery, American Society of Echocardiography, American Society of Nuclear Cardiology, Heart Failure Society of America, Heart Rhythm Society, Society for Cardiovascular Angiography and Interventions, and Society of Thoracic Surgeons. *J Am Coll Cardiol* 2011;58(25):e212–e260.

Nishimura RA, Holmes DR Jr. Clinical practice. Hypertrophic obstructive cardiomyopathy. *N Eng J Med* 2004;350:1320–1327.

Answer 5: *B*

Editor's Note: *Another typical criterion for flail versus prolapse is the direction toward which the leaflet tip is pointing. If this is pointing toward the LV, it is flail. If this leaflet tip is curved back and facing the LA, then this is considered prolapsing (despite the extent of tissue within the LA which may be quite marked).*

- From the 2D still images, a flail segment of the posterior mitral valve leaflet with a severe jet of anteriorly directed MR is seen. Because of the hypermobile portion of the leaflet, this would be termed flail, rather than prolapse. Therefore, answer D is less correct because in prolapse without flail, the mobile portion would not be seen.
- The Carpentier MV leaflet morphologic description is critically important to allow optimal communication between the imaging specialist and the interventional cardiologist or surgeon: A1 is the lateral portion of the anterior leaflet, A2 is the middle portion of the anterior leaflet, P1 is the lateral scallop of the posterior leaflet, P2 is the middle scallop of the posterior leaflet, and P3 is the medial scallop of the posterior leaflet.
- Considering the 2D image is a long-axis view with the aortic valve in view, it is likely that the P2 segment is affected as A2–P2 segments are usually visualized when the aortic valve is seen in the long axis. The scallops involved are clarified on the 3D imaging (Fig. 55.11), which shows that the flail is at the junction of P2 and P3. The 3D image shows the mitral valve in the "surgeon's view" orientation, with the aortic valve on top and the anterolateral commissure on the left of the screen. P3 is the medial scallop (to the right on the figure), while P1 is the lateral scallop (to the left on the figure). Hence, responses A and C are incorrect as the A1, A2, and P1 segments are not involved.

Editor's Note: *Identification of the mitral valve segments requires practice and a careful understanding of the correlation between long-axis and short-axis 2D images with 3D data. Normally, anteflexion of the TEE probe (which moves from a 4-chamber to a 5-chamber view) will add (a portion of) the P1 segment to the already seen P2 segment. However, as seen in this case, all orientations must be considered and no single view should be used for your final conclusion. The 3D SAX orientation clearly demonstrates P2 with P3 (rather than P1).*

- Restriction of the anterior mitral leaflet would also cause anteriorly directed MR; however, these images do not show restriction of the anterior mitral leaflet. Therefore, response E is wrong.

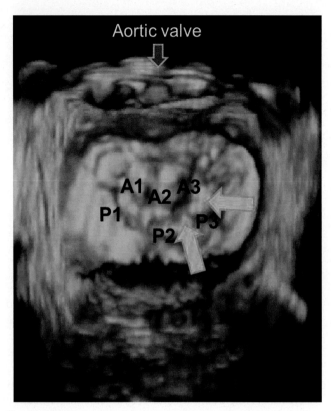

FIGURE 55.11 *Yellow arrows* indicate the flail segment.

Answer 6: B

- The Carpentier **functional classification** of mitral valve disease is used to describe the mechanism of valvular dysfunction and is based on the opening and closing motions of the mitral leaflets.
- Class I—normal leaflet motion. Example: leaflet perforation
- Class II—excess leaflet motion. Example: prolapse or flail, usually due to myxomatous degeneration
- Class III—restricted leaflet motion
  ○ Class IIIa—diastolic- and systolic-restricted leaflet motion. Example: rheumatic heart disease or postradiation
  ○ Class IIIb—relative restriction of normal leaflets. Example: ischemic heart disease with apical tethering of the leaflets due to left ventricular enlargement, also called functional MR
- Class IV—does not exist in the Carpentier system

Answer 7: E. This question assesses familiarity with the American Society of Echocardiography guidelines for the quantification of MR and the parameters that define severe from moderately to severe or less MR.

Option A: False. At a Nyquist limit of 40 cm/s, one can use the abbreviated formula of $r^2/2$, which gives an effective regurgitant orifice area of 0.32 cm^2, which is in the moderately severe range (severe is >0.4 cm^2, presuming the MR is pansystolic). Besides the Nyquist limit of 40 cm/s, other assumptions made when using this simplified calculation include a systolic

V_{max} of 500 cm/s, a hemispheric shape of the aliasing zone, and lack of wall constraint. This abbreviated formula should be only used as a general screening tool.

Option B: False. A regurgitant volume of ≥60 mL is considered severe.

Option C: False. A vena contracta width of ≥0.7 cm with a large central MR jet (area 40% of LA) in a pansystolic jet without wall-impinging morphology is considered severe.

Option D: False. While a moderately dilated LA and LV may be seen in severe MR, it is not the most supportive finding as these are nonspecific and are often seen in cardiomyopathy with less severe or no MR.

Option E: **True.** A number of factors (atrial fibrillation, elevated LA pressures) other than MR may result in systolic blunting of the pulmonary veins. However, systolic flow reversal in one or more veins is quite specific for severe MR. It is worth noting that this finding is not 100% sensitive for severe MR.

Answer 8: D

Option A: False. Mitral valve surgery has a class IIa level of evidence C in asymptomatic patients with pulmonary artery pressures of ≥50 mm Hg at rest or 60 mm Hg with stress.

Option B: False. Severe LA enlargement is not an indication for surgery.

Option C: False. EF ≤30% without likelihood of chordal preservation is an indication for medical management.

Option D: **True.** The LV end-systolic diameter of ≥40 mm and/or of LVEF of ≤60% and ≥30% is a class Ib indication for mitral valve surgery. These findings are associated with improved long-term LV function and longevity after surgery.

Option E: False. RV dysfunction is not an indication for surgery in the guidelines.

Suggested Readings

Bonow RO, Carabello BA, Chatterjee K, et al.; American College of Cardiology/American Heart Association Task Force on Practice Guidelines. 2008 focused update incorporated into the ACC/AHA 2006 guidelines for the management of patients with valvular heart disease: a report of the American College of Cardiology/American Heart Association Task Force on Practice Guidelines (Writing Committee to revise the 1998 guidelines for the management of patients with valvular heart disease). Endorsed by the Society of Cardiovascular Anesthesiologists, Society for Cardiovascular Angiography and Interventions, and Society of Thoracic Surgeons. *J Am Coll Cardiol* 2008;52(13):e1–e142.

Lang RM, Badano LP, Tsang W, et al.; American Society of Echocardiography; European Association of Echocardiography. EAE/ASE recommendations for image acquisition and display using three-dimensional echocardiography. *J Am Soc Echocardiogr* 2012;25(1):3–46.

Sparano DM, Ward RP. Management of asymptomatic, severe mitral regurgitation. *Curr Treat Options Cardiovasc Med* 2012;14(6):575–583.

Stewart WJ. Choosing the "golden moment" for mitral valve repair. *J Am Coll Cardiol* 1994;24(6):1544–1546.

Zoghbi WA, Enriquez-Sarano M, Foster E, et al.; American Society of Echocardiography. Recommendations for evaluation of the severity of native valvular regurgitation with two-dimensional and Doppler echocardiography. *J Am Soc Echocardiogr* 2003;16(7):777–802.

Answer 9: C

Option A: False. Carney complex is an autosomal dominant disorder comprising myxomas of the heart and skin, hyperpigmentation of the skin, and endocrine disorders. In this case, there is only a single myxoma, and no reference is made in the stem to the other extracardiac findings.

Option B: False. Shone syndrome comprises of the supravalvular mitral membrane, parachute mitral valve, subaortic stenosis, and coarctation of the aorta—none of which are seen in this patient.

Option C: **True.** Incidental findings of a left atrial mass and a partial subaortic membrane. Myxomas are a common type of benign cardiac tumor. Most commonly, myxomas are attached by a stalk to the interatrial septum at the fossa ovalis, in the right or left atrium. About 80% of myxomas are located in the left atrium. In addition, this patient was found on the prepump intraoperative TEE to have a partial subaortic membrane that was easily removed during the procedure. The myxoma seen here is atypical as it is somewhat broad based and multilobed; however, given its location and the presence of a stalk, myxoma is still the most likely diagnosis. Of note, there is no known association between the myxomas, subaortic membranes, and aortic aneurysms. The purpose of this case was to highlight the not uncommon scenario of discovering incidental pathologies on a prepump TEE.

Option D: False. This is very unlikely to be a thrombus given the location and the fact that the patient is in sinus rhythm (visible atrial activity on 2D echo).

Option E: False. The left atrial mass actually could be a papillary fibroelastoma or some other histopathology. One does not know the tissue type until histologic evaluation. More likely, the LA mass is a myxoma (a tumor, usually benign) because of its location and solid appearance. Papillary fibroelastomas tend to be very fluid and flowery, like a sea anemone. The LVOT mass could also have been a papillary fibroelastoma, but on histologic evaluation, it was found to be fibrotic tissue and not a fibroelastoma. In addition, it does not display the typical characteristics of a papillary fibroelastoma, which usually involve the valves and have a peripheral "shimmer" on a 2D echocardiography secondary to the small frond-like projections seen on histopathology.

Answer10: E

Option A: False. Aortic incompetence (AI) is a common complication of subvalvular membranes associated with outflow tract turbulence. However, no gradient was present in this case; the membrane was not causing any obstruction, and the AI is mild.

Option B: **False.** The aortic valve leaflets are not thickened or calcified and display relatively normal systolic excursion. Progression to severe AS is not the most likely complication in this case.

Option C: **False.** Infective endocarditis involving a subaortic membrane is a rare complication numbering a few case reports; embolization is the most likely complication in this patient.

Option D: **False.** Myxoma is an unusual cause of sudden death and not the most likely complication in the case.

Option E: **True.** Embolization is the most common complication of atrial myxomas (between 11% and 29%). Therefore, surgical resection is often advised, especially when another indication for cardiac surgery is present, as in this case.

Answer 11: B

Option A: False. Given the complexity of this operation, a median sternotomy would be the incision of choice.

Option B: **True.** To access the left atrium for the resection of the atrial myxoma, the surgeon will likely approach by retracting the right side of the heart anteriorly, so bicaval cannulation would be necessary. For aortic surgery alone, the surgeon would typically use a single venous cannula through the right atrial appendage, but this cannula would impede access to the left atrium now that the myxoma has been found.

Option C: False. These findings will not alter the means of cardioplegia.

Option D: False. Protamine is given to reverse the heparin and restore normal coagulation post CPB in all cardiac surgeries.

Suggested Readings

Burke A, Jeudy J Jr, Virmani R. Cardiac tumours: an update: cardiac tumours. *Heart* 2008;94(1):117–123.

Murphy MC, Sweeney MS, Putnam JB Jr, et al. Surgical treatment of cardiac tumors: a 25-year experience. *Ann Thorac Surg* 1990;49(4):612–617; discussion 617–618.

Pinede L, Duhaut P, Loire R. Clinical presentation of left atrial cardiac myxoma. A series of 112 consecutive cases. *Medicine (Baltimore)* 2001;80(3):159–172.

Stratakis CA, Kirschner LS, Carney JA. Clinical and molecular features of the Carney complex: diagnostic criteria and recommendations for patient evaluation. *J Clin Endocrinol Metab* 2001;86(9):4041–4046.

St. Louis JD, Bannan MM, Lutin WA, et al. Surgical strategies and outcomes in patients with Shone complex: a retrospective review. *Ann Thorac Surg* 2007;84(4):1357–1362; discussion 1362–1363.

Answer 12: B

Option A: False. See below.

Option B: **True.** Early case series used a cutoff of ≥5 mm thickness to classify severe atheroma. The French Aortic Plaque in Stroke (FAPS) identified plaque thickness of ≥4 mm as significantly associated with an increased risk of stroke. In one series, intraoperative TEE could differentiate areas of minimal intimal thickness from more complex atheromas 93% of the time.

Option C: False—findings most consistent with atheroma.

Option D: False—findings most consistent with atheroma.

Option E: False—no dissection flap is seen in these images.

Answer 13: C

Option A: False. The risk of intraoperative stroke in patients with severe aortic atheroma of the ascending aorta and aortic arch is five- to sevenfold higher than in those without aortic atheroma. This is associated with a significantly increased mortality.

Option B: False. Endarterectomy is necessary in some patients with very severe atheroma, but the surgery is associated with an increased risk of intraoperative stroke.

Option C: **True.** The intra-aortic endoclamp may cause additional atheroemboli and therefore cannot be safely advanced in these patients. While the surgeon will not actually be cross-clamping the aorta in the location of the descending aorta shown, atherosclerosis is a generalized disease, increasing the risks of atheroembolization of debris to the brain and peripheries resulting in great morbidity. Off-pump surgery is sometimes a good option. When "on-pump" surgery is done on such patients, intraoperative epicardial echo can help to guide placement of arterial cannulae.

Option D: **False.** However, statins have been demonstrated to reduce the risk of stroke in a meta-analysis of randomized clinical trials in the prevention of myocardial infarction. Although it makes sense that statins would help patients with severe atheroma, the level of evidence is not at a high level. Statins probably cause plaque stabilization/regression and the reduction of thrombin generation by platelets.

Option E: **False.** The role of anticoagulation in aortic atheroma has been found to be helpful in some series, but it remains controversial.

Suggested Readings

American Society of Anesthesiologists and Society of Cardiovascular Anesthesiologists Task Force on Transesophageal Echocardiography. Practice guidelines for perioperative transesophageal echocardiography. An updated report by the American Society of Anesthesiologists and the Society of Cardiovascular Anesthesiologists Task Force on Transesophageal Echocardiography. *Anesthesiology* 2010;112(5):1084–1096.
Katz ES, Tunick PA, Rusinek H, et al. Protruding aortic atheromas predict stroke in elderly patients undergoing cardiopulmonary bypass: experience with intraoperative transesophageal echocardiography. *J Am Coll Cardiol* 1992;20(1):70–77.
Vaduganathan P, Ewton A, Nagueh SF, et al. Pathologic correlates of aortic plaques, thrombi and mobile "aortic debris" imaged in vivo with transesophageal echocardiography. *J Am Coll Cardiol* 1997;30(2):357.

Answer 14: A

Option A: **True.** This patient has a congenital anomaly called a persistent left-sided superior vena cava (SVC), in which the systemic venous drainage from the left internal jugular and left subclavian veins returns to the heart via the coronary sinus. This makes standard retrograde cardioplegia less effective, because the cardioplegia would be distributed to veins of the left arm and left cerebral veins, and an inconsistent amount of cardioplegia would go to the myocardium.

Option B: **False.** See above.

Option C: **False.** See above.

Option D: **False.** Access to the right ventricle can be very difficult in these cases.

Option E: **False.** Most patients with persistent left-sided SVCs are asymptomatic unless associated with more clinically relevant congenital anomalies. Almost 40% of these patients have other associated cardiac anomalies.

Answer 15: E

Option A: **False.** This action may bring the pulmonary arteries/bifurcation into view.

Option B: **False.** This action may bring the left-sided pulmonary veins into view.

Option C: **False.** This action may bring the LVOT and aortic valve into view and is the one method to obtain perpendicular alignment to the AV for accurate assessment of gradients across the LVOT/AV.

Option D: **False.** This action may bring the left atrial appendage into view.

Option E: **True.** This is one method for obtaining a view of the coronary sinus; alternatively, from a bicaval view, rotate to 100 to 140 degrees, and turn counterclockwise.

Suggested Readings

Sarodia B, Stoller J, et al. Persistent left superior vena cava: case report and literature review. *Respir Care* 2000;45(4):411–416.
Savage RM, Aronson S, Thomas JD, et al. *Comprehensive Textbook of Intraoperative Transesophageal Echocardiography.* Philadelphia, PA: Lippincott Williams & Wilkins, 2011.
Shanewise JS, Cheung AT, Aronson S, et al. Guidelines for performing a comprehensive intraoperative multiplane transesophageal echocardiographic examination: recommendations of the American Society of Echocardiography council on intraoperative echocardiography. *Anesth Analg* 1999;89:870–884.
Winter F. Persistent left superior vena cava; survey of world literature and report of thirty additional cases. *Angiology* 1954;5(2):90–132.

Answer 16: D

Option A: **False.** There is at least moderate MR that was in fact severe after complete interrogation.

Option B: **False.** Deciding about advising a second pump run is based on the residual regurgitation post repair:

- 0 to 1+: no further surgery
- 2+: will likely require further surgery (if no contraindication)
  - Reasonable to observe without decannulating
  - Reasonable to perform a phenylephrine challenge
- 3+ to 4: further repair or replacement necessary

Option C: **False.** The patient has severe MR post repair—this is never the expected or desirable outcome.

Option D: **True.** Repair is preferable given the documented improved outcomes with this strategy; however, if it is not possible, replacement with a bioprosthesis is preferable to significant persistent MR, especially given the patient's age and risk of falls (Video 55.10).

Option E: **False.** This option may be reasonable in a younger patient or if the patient is taking anticoagulation for other indications, but given the age profile and risk of falls, if further repair is not possible, replacement with a bioprosthesis would be more advisable than a mechanical valve.

Suggested Readings

Savage RM, Shiota T, Stewart W, et al. *Comprehensive Textbook of Intraoperative Transesophageal Echocardiography.* Philadelphia, PA: Lippincott Williams & Wilkins, 2011:443–512.
Zurick AO, Stewart WJ, Griffin BF. Intraoperative echocardiography in surgical and transcatheter mitral valve repair. In: Otto CM, ed. *The Practice of Clinical Echocardiography.* 4th ed. Philadelphia, PA: Elsevier-Saunders, 2012.

Chapter 56

Invasive Echo for the Boards

Vincent L. Sorrell

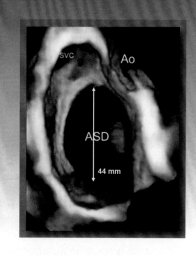

1. Which of the following statements is false of intracardiac echocardiography (ICE) compared to transesophageal echocardiography (TEE) for echocardiographic guidance of interventional cardiac procedures?

   A. ICE requires general anesthesia similar to TEE.

   B. ICE provides similar or superior image quality for near-field structures as TEE.

   C. ICE can provide direct visualization of the endocardium and the ablation catheter, which can be identified by the highly specific fan-shaped echocardiographic artifact of the large tip of the ablation electrode.

   D. Risks of ICE are low (<1% to 2%) but include vascular trauma, hematoma, retroperitoneal bleed, cardiac perforation, and arrhythmia.

2. In FIGURE 56.1 and VIDEO 56.1 of an echocardiography-guided pericardiocentesis procedure, the location of the pericardiocentesis needle is:

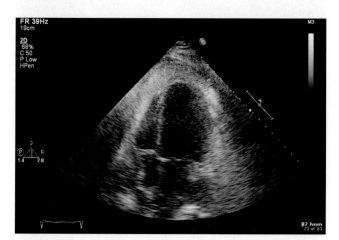

FIGURE 56.1

   A. In the right ventricle
   B. In the right atrium
   C. In the pericardial space
   D. In the pleural space

3. An 89-year-old male with severe aortic stenosis undergoes a transcatheter aortic valve implantation with an Edwards SAPIEN transcatheter heart valve. FIGURE 56.2 and VIDEO 56.2 are obtained by transesophageal echocardiography immediately after deployment of a transcatheter aortic valve. Which of the following statements is true?

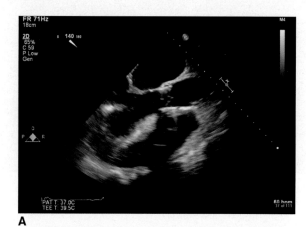

A

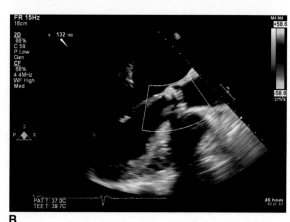

B

FIGURE 56.2

A. The transcatheter aortic valve is deployed and functioning well.
B. Supplementary balloon dilation is necessary for the paravalvular aortic regurgitation.
C. The patient needs an emergent surgical aortic valve replacement.
D. The prosthesis is oversized.

4. A 56-year-old male with hypertrophic obstructive cardiomyopathy is undergoing alcohol septal ablation with TEE guidance. After verification of the correct balloon position and the hemodynamic effect of balloon occlusion, 1 to 2 mL of diluted echocardiographic contrast agent followed by a 1- to 2-mL saline flush is injected through the inflated balloon catheter, and the image obtained is shown in FIGURE 56.3.

The image shows:

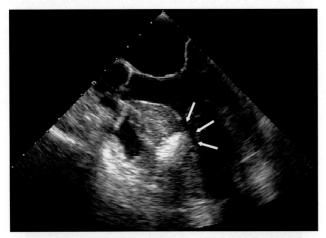

FIGURE 56.3 Adapted from Silvestry FE, Kerber RE, et al. Echocardiography-guided interventions. *J Am Soc Echocardiogr* 2009;22(3):213–231; quiz 316–317.

A. The selected septal perforator is optimal for alcohol septal ablation.
B. The selected septal perforator is too apical for alcohol septal ablation.
C. The selected coronary branch supplies the posteromedial papillary muscle and is therefore not optimal for alcohol septal ablation.
D. There is inadequate myocardial opacification after contrast injection.

5. Which of the following interventional procedures can be guided by transthoracic echocardiography (TTE) alone, without the use of transesophageal echocardiography (TEE) or intracardiac echocardiography (ICE)?

A. Transcatheter aortic valve implantation
B. Percutaneous left ventricular assist device placement
C. Percutaneous mitral valve repair
D. Alcohol septal ablation

6. A 56-year-old female with symptomatic paroxysmal atrial fibrillation refractory to medical management is undergoing a radiofrequency pulmonary vein ablation procedure with intracardiac echocardiography (ICE) guidance. While radiofrequency energy is being delivered, a dense shower of microbubbles is noted on ICE. What does this represent?

A. Perforation of the left atrial tissue being ablated
B. Lack of tissue contact by the ablation catheter
C. Tissue heating to unsafe levels
D. A normal occurrence during radiofrequency ablation procedures

7. An 88-year-old male with severe aortic stenosis undergoes a transcatheter aortic valve implantation with an Edwards SAPIEN transcatheter heart valve. The valve is deployed, and immediate transesophageal echocardiography reveals mild paravalvular aortic regurgitation (FIG. 56.4 and VIDEO 56.3). The patient's blood pressure suddenly starts to decrease and drops from 110/60 mm Hg to 65/34 mm Hg. The heart rate is 98 bpm. Transesophageal echocardiography from the deep gastric window immediately after the decrease in blood pressure reveals the images shown in FIGURE 56.5 and VIDEO 56.4. What should be the next best step in management?

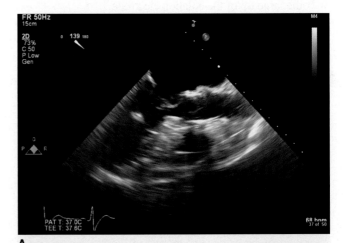

A

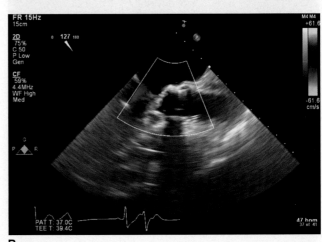

B

FIGURE 56.4

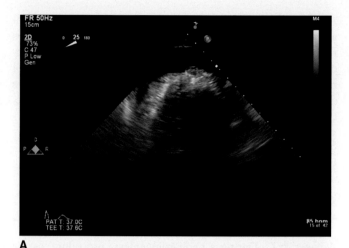

A

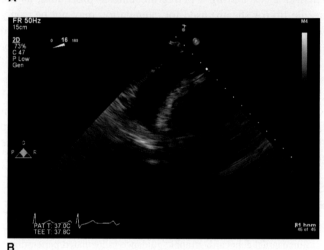

B

FIGURE 56.5

A. Immediate supplementary balloon dilation
B. Emergent pericardiocentesis
C. Emergent sternotomy and surgical aortic valve replacement
D. Administration of IV pressors

8. A 73-year-old male with permanent atrial fibrillation and a history of embolic stroke develops recurrent gastrointestinal bleeding precluding systemic anticoagulation. He is morbidly obese and also has obstructive sleep apnea, achalasia, and cervical spondylosis. He is referred for percutaneous occlusion of the left atrial appendage (LAA). Which of the following would be the best option for echocardiographic guidance of LAA closure?

A. Transesophageal echocardiography (TEE)
B. Intracardiac echocardiography (ICE) with the catheter in the right atrium
C. Intracardiac echocardiography (ICE) with the catheter in the left atrium after a transseptal puncture
D. Transthoracic echocardiography (TTE)

9. Real-time 3D echocardiography may provide incremental value over 2D echocardiography for the planning of many interventional procedures. Which of the following percutaneous interventional procedures has yet to demonstrate a benefit of 3D over 2D?

A. Percutaneous mitral valve repair
B. Closure of atrial septal defect
C. Pulmonary stenosis valvuloplasty
D. Right ventricular biopsy

10. The mitral scallop (by the Carpentier classification) shown by the arrows in the 3D transesophageal echocardiogram view of a mitral valve from a "surgical" view (FIG. 56.6) is:

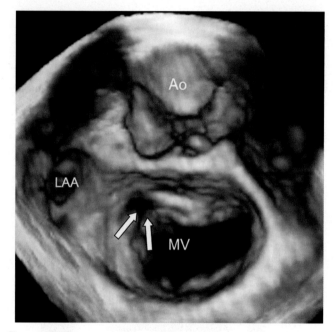

FIGURE 56.6

A. P3 scallop
B. A1 scallop
C. P1 scallop
D. A3 scallop

11. A 91-year-old male presents with 1 week of dyspnea on minimal exertion and lower extremity edema. Heart rate was 112 bpm, and blood pressure was 85/35 mm Hg. Examination revealed inaudible heart sounds. An urgent echocardiogram showed a large pericardial effusion (FIG. 56.7 and VIDEO 56.5). The patient is referred for pericardiocentesis for cardiac tamponade. Which of the following windows should be used for the pericardiocentesis?

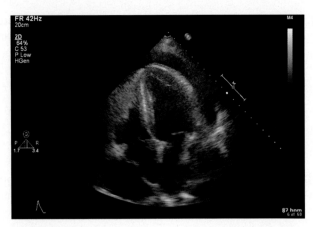

FIGURE 56.7

A. Apical window
B. Subxiphoid window
C. Parasternal window
D. Any of the above

12. A 19-year-old male with an ASD and right heart enlargement is referred for percutaneous closure. 3D imaging preprocedure shows the image in FIGURE 56.8. What is the best choice for ASD closure for this patient?

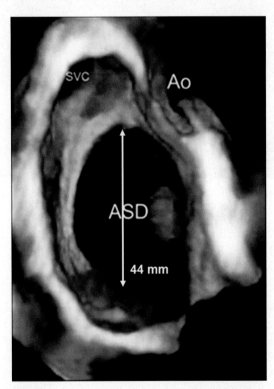

FIGURE 56.8

A. Percutaneous closure with the Amplatzer Septal Occluder
B. Percutaneous closure with the Gore HELEX Septal Occluder
C. Percutaneous closure with the Amplatzer Multi-Fenestrated Septal Occluder
D. Surgical closure with a patch

Answer 1: A. With the use of TEE for guidance, general anesthesia and endotracheal intubation are almost always required, given the length of interventional cardiac procedures. General anesthesia or endotracheal intubation is not required for ICE, which decreases the overall procedure time and increases patient comfort and tolerance of the procedure. Choices B, C, and D are true.

Suggested Readings

Hijazi ZM, Shivkumar K, et al. Intracardiac echocardiography during interventional and electrophysiological cardiac catheterization. *Circulation* 2009;119(4):587–596.

Silvestry FE, Kerber RE, et al. Echocardiography-guided interventions. *J Am Soc Echocardiogr* 2009;22(3):213–231; quiz 316–317.

Answer 2: C. During a pericardiocentesis procedure, as the needle tip (or sheath) used for cannulation may not be easily visualized on echocardiography, after a small amount of fluid (i.e., 10 mL) is withdrawn, confirmation that the needle or sheath is in the pericardial space is achieved by the injection of a small amount of agitated saline as microbubbles that are easily visualized by echocardiography. FIGURE 56.1 and VIDEO 56.1 show that the agitated saline is in the pericardial space, confirming the correct location of the pericardiocentesis needle in the pericardial space. Choices A, B, and D are incorrect since the agitated saline is not visualized in those locations.

Suggested Readings

Betts TR, Radvan JR. Contrast echocardiography during pericardiocentesis. *Heart* 1999;81(3):329.

Pandian NG, Brockway B, et al. Pericardiocentesis under two-dimensional echocardiographic guidance in loculated pericardial effusion. *Ann Thorac Surg* 1988;45(1):99–100.

Silvestry FE, Kerber RE, et al. Echocardiography-guided interventions. *J Am Soc Echocardiogr* 2009;22(3):213–231; quiz 316–317.

Tsang TS, Enriquez-Sarano M, et al. Consecutive 1127 therapeutic echocardiographically guided pericardiocenteses: clinical profile, practice patterns, and outcomes spanning 21 years. *Mayo Clin Proc* 2002;77(5):429–436.

Answer 3: A. The images show a well-deployed transcatheter aortic valve with trace central and trace paravalvular regurgitation. Paravalvular regurgitation, not infrequently with multiple jets, is common following TAVI, though trace to mild, and with a benign stable course in the majority of patients. On the other hand, severe aortic regurgitation may occur as a consequence of incomplete expansion or incorrect positioning of the device, restricted cusp motion, or inappropriate prosthetic size. An undersized prosthesis is expected to be associated with paravalvular aortic regurgitation. In contrast, an oversized prosthesis may result in suboptimal stent expansion, impaired cusp mobility, and central aortic regurgitation. In the case of moderate paravalvular aortic regurgitation, supplementary balloon dilation can be performed. Choices B, C, and D are incorrect because the patient has only trace to mild paravalvular regurgitation.

Suggested Reading

Zamorano JL, Badano LP, et al. EAE/ASE recommendations for the use of echocardiography in new transcatheter interventions for valvular heart disease. *J Am Soc Echocardiogr* 2011;24(9):937–965.

Answer 4: B. Figure 56.3 shows a midesophageal four-chamber view after the injection of contrast (arrows), demonstrating that the site of perfusion of the selected septal perforator is too apical from the site of the septal contact of the mitral valve and therefore not optimal for alcohol septal ablation. Choice A is therefore incorrect. The optimal target territory of the basal septum should include the portion of the septum adjacent to the area of maximal flow acceleration on color Doppler and the area of systolic anterior motion–septal contact. Myocardial contrast echocardiography (transthoracic or transesophageal) is used to confirm that the presumed target septal perforator perfuses the desired region of the basal septum and no other cardiac structures, before alcohol is infused. Choice C is incorrect since the contrast opacification is in the hypertrophied septum. Choice D is incorrect since the area of the myocardium supplied by the selected septal perforator appears to opacify well with contrast injection.

Suggested Readings

Silvestry FE, Kerber RE, et al. Echocardiography-guided interventions. *J Am Soc Echocardiogr* 2009;22(3):213–231; quiz 316–317.
Sorajja P, Ommen SR, Holmes DR Jr, et al. Survival after alcohol septal ablation for obstructive hypertrophic cardiomyopathy. *Circulation* 2012;126(20):2374–2380.

Answer 5: D. Echocardiography during alcohol septal ablation requires visualization of the septum, which can be achieved by transthoracic echocardiography (TTE) as well as with transesophageal echocardiography (TEE) or intracardiac echocardiography (ICE). TTE is the conventional approach used in many institutions. Some institutions prefer TEE because it provides more precise imaging of the subaortic anatomy of the left ventricle than TTE. If TTE is used, apical four-chamber and three-chamber (long-axis) views should be used. These views may be supplemented with parasternal long-axis and short-axis views. If TEE is used, the apical four-chamber view (at 0 degree) and the longitudinal view (usually 120 to 130 degrees) should be used. These views may be supplemented by the transgastric short-axis view to help ensure that no erroneous perfusion of the papillary muscles occurs. Other procedures where TTE can offer similar guidance as TEE include balloon or blade atrial septostomy, endomyocardial biopsy, and pericardiocentesis. Choices A, B, and C are incorrect because guidance by TEE or ICE has distinct advantages over guidance by TTE for these procedures.

Suggested Reading

Silvestry FE, Kerber RE, et al. Echocardiography-guided interventions. *J Am Soc Echocardiogr* 2009;22(3):213–231; quiz 316–317.

Answer 6: C. During radiofrequency ablation of atrial fibrillation, ICE guidance helps with clarification of the branching patterns of the right pulmonary vein, guides the positioning of interventional catheters, verifies catheter tip–tissue contact, assesses underlying pulmonary vein physiology, helps in the positioning of balloon-type catheters for ablative interventions, and monitors for excessive tissue heating as manifested by the occurrence of microbubbles. Dense microbubbles suggest steam formation and occur only at tissue temperatures higher than 60°C. When dense showers of microbubbles are seen, energy delivery is terminated immediately. Occurrence of dense microbubbles may be even more accurate than catheter tip temperature

monitoring for the assessment of heat generation during ablation. Microbubbles seen on ICE directly correlate with cerebral microembolic events detected by transcranial Doppler, tissue disruption, and char formation. Restricting power output to avoid microbubble formation on ICE raises the efficacy of pulmonary vein isolation while minimizing the risk of severe pulmonary vein stenosis and cerebroembolic complications.

Suggested Readings

Silvestry FE, Kerber RE, et al. Echocardiography-guided interventions. *J Am Soc Echocardiogr* 2009;22(3):213–231; quiz 316–317.
Wood MA, Shaffer KM, Ellenbogen AL, et al. Microbubbles during radiofrequency catheter ablation: composition and formation. *Heart Rhythm* 2005;2(4):397–403.

Answer 7: B. The initial images reveal a well-deployed prosthetic aortic valve with mild paravalvular regurgitation. Subsequent images from the deep gastric window show a large pericardial effusion. The patient's sudden hypotension is likely secondary to the acute, large pericardial effusion leading to cardiac tamponade. The next best step in management is emergent pericardiocentesis. During a transcatheter aortic valve implantation, acute severe hypotension could result from cardiac tamponade due to wire perforation of the left or right ventricle, left ventricular dysfunction, or severe aortic regurgitation. Left ventricular dysfunction with acute wall motion abnormalities may be secondary to coronary ostial occlusion by fragment embolization or by an obstructive portion of the valve frame, sealing cuff, or native cusp. Choice A is incorrect since the prosthetic valve appears to be well deployed with only mild paravalvular aortic regurgitation, which is not responsible for the acute, severe hypotension. Choice C is incorrect for the same reason. Choice D is incorrect since the definitive management of acute cardiac tamponade is pericardiocentesis and not pressors. This patient had emergent pericardiocentesis with drainage of 700 mL of oxygenated blood, with immediate improvement in hemodynamics. He stabilized without emergent surgery. The etiology of the acute pericardial effusion was felt to be due to wire perforation of the left ventricle.

Suggested Reading

Zamorano JL, Badano LP, et al. EAE/ASE recommendations for the use of echocardiography in new transcatheter interventions for valvular heart disease. *J Am Soc Echocardiogr* 2011;24(9):937–965.

Answer 8: C. The current modality of choice for echocardiographic guidance of percutaneous occlusion of the left atrial appendage (LAA) is transesophageal echocardiography (TEE). However, in this patient, a TEE is contraindicated due to several reasons—obstructive sleep apnea, achalasia, and cervical spondylosis. Hence, Choice A is incorrect. A transthoracic echocardiogram (TTE) is suboptimal for visualization of the LAA. Hence, Choice D is incorrect. Intracardiac echocardiography (ICE) is used for echocardiographic guidance of percutaneous occlusion of the LAA; however, far-field structures such as the LAA may not be completely visualized with the ICE catheter in the right atrium due to poor image quality from the depth of structures imaged and foreshortening. Therefore, Choice B is incorrect and Choice C is the correct answer. ICE imaging of the LAA has been shown to be optimal from within the LA itself, as the closer proximity of atrial structures to the ICE probe allows the use of a higher ultrasound frequency, which provides higher image resolution without sacrificing the depth of ultrasound tissue penetration. ICE imaging from the proximal pulmonary artery or right ventricular outflow tract can provide better visualization of the distal LAA in cross-section. This approach also avoids a second transseptal puncture.

Suggested Readings

Chue CD, de Giovanni J, et al. The role of echocardiography in percutaneous left atrial appendage occlusion. *Eur J Echocardiogr* 2011;12(10):i3–i10.

Silvestry FE, Kerber RE, et al. Echocardiography-guided interventions. *J Am Soc Echocardiogr* 2009;22(3):213–231; quiz 316–317.

Answer 9: C. Real-time 3D echocardiography offers the potential for incremental value over 2D echocardiography for interventional procedures such as right ventricular biopsy, percutaneous mitral valve repair, and closure of atrial septal defects and patent foramen ovale. Bioptome position can be better confirmed with a 3D view than 2D alone, and visualization of the bioptome in multiple simultaneous planes allows accurate localization of the biopsy site. Mitral valve anatomy may be better studied with 3D imaging than with 2D imaging, and therefore, 3D imaging can play a significant role in the planning of percutaneous mitral valve repair. Similarly, real-time 3D echocardiography allows for accurate anatomic assessment before closure of an atrial septal defect or patent foramen ovale and can localize the closure device during the procedure in relation to other cardiac structures potentially enhancing success and possibly decreasing the complication rate. The ASE position paper on standards and guidelines for 3D echo guidance of transcatheter procedures lists mitral clips, mitral valvuloplasty, TAVI, paravalvular leak closures, ASD closures, VSD closures, and LA appendage closure as "recommended for clinical practice." To date, there is no evidence that 3D is superior to 2D in TV and PV interventions, and the ASE lists these as "unstudied" (Table 56.1.)

Table 56.1 Summary of Indications for 3D Echocardiography

	RECOMMENDED FOR CLINICAL PRACTICE	PROMISING CLINICAL STUDIES	AREAS OF ACTIVE RESEARCH	UNSTUDIED
Left ventricle functional assessment				
Volume	✓			
Shape			✓	
Ejection fraction	✓			
Dyssynchrony			✓	
Mass		✓		
Right ventricle functional assessment				
Volume		✓		
Shape				✓
Ejection fraction		✓		
Left atrial assessment				
Volume			✓	
Right atrial assessment				
Volume				✓
Mitral valve assessment				
Anatomy	✓			
Stenosis	✓			
Regurgitation			✓	
Tricuspid valve assessment				
Anatomy				✓
Stenosis				✓
Regurgitation				✓
Pulmonic valve assessment				
Anatomy				✓
Stenosis				✓
Regurgitation				✓
Aortic valve assessment				
Anatomy		✓		
Stenosis		✓		
Regurgitation				✓
Infective endocarditis				✓
Prosthetic valves			✓	
Guidance of transcatheter procedures[a]	✓			

[a]Mitral clips, mitral valvuloplasty, transcatheter aortic valve implantation, paravalvular leak closure, atrial septal defect closure, ventricular septal defect closure, and left atrial appendage closure.

Reprinted from Lang RM, Badano LP, Tsang W, et al. EAE/ASE recommendations for image acquisition and display using three-dimensional echocardiography. *J Am Soc Echocardiogr* 2012;25(1):3–46, with permission from Elsevier.

Suggested Readings

Lang RM, Badano LP, Tsang W, et al. EAE/ASE recommendations for image acquisition and display using three-dimensional echocardiography. *J Am Soc Echocardiogr* 2012;25(1):3–46.

Magni G, Hijazi ZM, et al. Two- and three-dimensional transesophageal echocardiography in patient selection and assessment of atrial septal defect closure by the new DAS-Angel Wings device: initial clinical experience. *Circulation* 1997;96(6):1722–1728.

McCreery CJ, McCulloch M, et al. Real-time 3-dimensional echocardiography imaging for right ventricular endomyocardial biopsy: a comparison with fluoroscopy. *J Am Soc Echocardiogr* 2001;14(9):927–933.

Silvestry FE, Kerber RE, et al. Echocardiography-guided interventions. *J Am Soc Echocardiogr* 2009;22(3):213–231; quiz 316–317.

Answer 10: *B.* The most appealing and informative view on 3D transesophageal echocardiography of the mitral valve is the atrial perspective (or the so-called "surgical view"). This view is obtained rotating the image so that the aorta is positioned at about 12 o'clock on an imaginary clock face, the left atrial appendage and lateral commissure are on the left, while the medial commissure is on the right of the observer (FIG. 56.9). The free margin of the posterior leaflet has two indentations that divide the leaflet in three segments called scallops: lateral or P1, central or P2, and medial or P3. By convention, the correspondent areas of the anterior leaflet are named A1, A2, and A3 although the free edge has no indentations at all. The indentations are the normal anatomical configuration of the mitral valve and allow a greater opening in diastole. This "Carpentier" classification facilitates valve analysis, and it is the most used. In FIGURE 56.6, the arrows

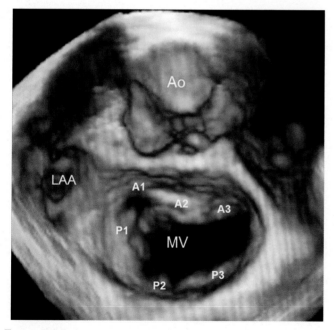

FIGURE 56.9

point to the A1 scallop (FIG. 56.9). Therefore, Choice B is correct and Choices A, C, and D are incorrect.

Suggested Reading

Faletra FF, de Castro S, Pandian NG, et al. *Atlas of Real Time 3D Transesophageal Echocardiography*. London, UK: Springer, 2010.

Answer 11: *D.* In this patient with a large circumferential pericardial effusion, any of the above windows can be used to enter the pericardial space for pericardiocentesis. Choice of the window should be based on the experience of the proceduralist. Echocardiography helps in identification of the ideal entry site and needle trajectory for pericardiocentesis. The ideal site of needle entry is the point on the chest wall at which the largest fluid collection is closest to the skin and from which a straight needle trajectory avoids vital structures. The subxiphoid approach is used most commonly, with a long needle directed toward the left shoulder at a 30-degree angle to the skin. This route is extrapleural and avoids the coronary, pericardial, and internal mammary arteries. Other approaches are apical, left axillary, left parasternal, and right parasternal. This patient had pericardiocentesis performed via the subxiphoid window, and 550 mL of exudative pericardial fluid was drained. The etiology of his pericardial effusion was subsequently determined to be viral pericarditis.

Suggested Readings

Maisch B, Seferovic PM, et al. Guidelines on the diagnosis and management of pericardial diseases executive summary; The Task force on the diagnosis and management of pericardial diseases of the European society of cardiology. *Eur Heart J* 2004;25(7):587–610.

Silvestry FE, Kerber RE, et al. Echocardiography-guided interventions. *J Am Soc Echocardiogr* 2009;22(3):213–231; quiz 316–317.

Tsang TS, Enriquez-Sarano M, et al. Consecutive 1127 therapeutic echocardiographically guided pericardiocenteses: clinical profile, practice patterns, and outcomes spanning 21 years. *Mayo Clin Proc* 2002;77(5):429–436.

Answer 12: *D.* The ASD shown in FIGURE 56.8 measures 44 × 32 mm. Contraindications for percutaneous closure of ASDs include large defects that are >38 mm in diameter, insufficient septal rims, or insufficient LA size to accommodate a device. The device sizes for the Amplatzer devices ranges from 4 to 38 mm, which corresponds to the atrial septal defect diameter. The Gore HELEX Septal Occluder is available in diameters ranging from 15 to 35 mm, in 5-mm increments. For an ASD measuring 44 mm in diameter, surgical closure with a patch is the only option. Hence, Choice D is the correct answer and Choices A, B, and C are incorrect.

Suggested Reading

Tobis J, Shenoda M. Percutaneous treatment of patent foramen ovale and atrial septal defects. *J Am Coll Cardiol* 2012;60(18):1722–1732.

Chapter 57

Echo as It Relates to Multimodal Imaging

Vincent L. Sorrell

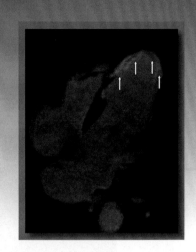

1. A 42-year-old male with a history of borderline hypertension was seen in your clinic due to an abnormal EKG during his last routine physical exam. You ordered a 2D echocardiogram to evaluate LV function and LV mass. This study was limited due to poor acoustic windows. The left ventricular function was noted to be normal with poor endocardial definition and without significant valvular abnormalities. The patient was sent for cardiac MRI for further evaluation (Fig. 57.1). What is the next best step based on these findings?

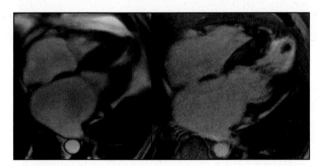

FIGURE 57.1

A. Initiate long-term anticoagulation.
B. Initiate beta-blocker/ACE-I therapy to regress the LVH.
C. Refer this patient for an ICD implant.
D. Schedule the patient for an endomyocardial biopsy.
E. Schedule the patient for an alcohol septal ablation procedure.

2. A 41-year-old male with no significant past medical history presented with new-onset atrial fibrillation. The transthoracic echocardiogram showed unexplained right ventricular dilation without a clear source of intracardiac shunt. The patient was referred for cardiac MRI, and the images are shown in FIGURE 57.2. Which of the following conditions best explains these findings?

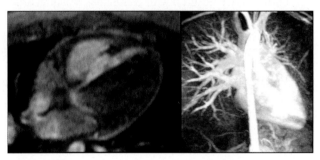

FIGURE 57.2

A. A partial anomalous pulmonary vein without ASD
B. A partial anomalous pulmonary vein with ASD
C. Ebstein anomaly
D. Congenitally corrected transposition of the great arteries

3. A 44-year-old male with a past medical history significant for borderline dyslipidemia was referred by his cardiologist for coronary CT angiography based on complaints of atypical chest pain. His coronary angiography showed minimal disease in the left anterior descending coronary artery; however, the abnormality in FIGURE 57.3 was noted. Based on the presence of this abnormality, which of the following Doppler abnormality on echocardiogram is expected?

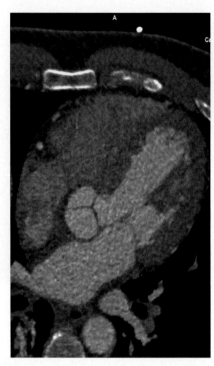

FIGURE 57.3

A. Elevated velocity at the level of left ventricular outflow tract (LVOT), with continuous wave recording demonstrating a peak velocity during late systole
B. The continuous wave (CW) Doppler of the descending aorta demonstrating persistent turbulent jet throughout diastole
C. Elevated velocity at the level of LVOT, with continuous wave recording demonstrating a peak velocity during midsystole
D. Systolic flow reversal noted in the hepatic vein
E. The CW Doppler in the LVOT that includes the IVCT and IVRT periods as well as the systolic ejection period

4. A 64-year-old male with a past medical history significant for hypertension and hyperlipidemia was referred for coronary CT angiography for evaluation of atypical chest pain. His CCTA images are shown in FIGURE 57.4. Should the patient be referred for dobutamine stress echocardiography, one would expect?

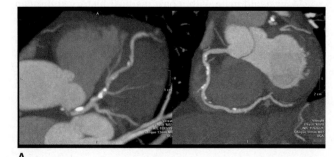

A

FIGURE 57.4

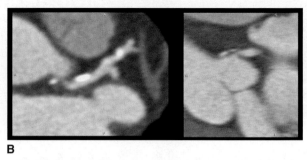

B

FIGURE 57.4 (Continued)

A. Abnormal anterior wall motion
B. Abnormal inferior wall motion
C. Abnormal inferolateral wall motion
D. Abnormal wall motion in multiple coronary artery territories

5. A 29-year-old female was referred for cardiac MRI after being diagnosed with hypertrophic cardiomyopathy on a 2D echocardiography. The cardiac MRI (CMR) images are shown in FIGURE 57.5. In addition to the CMR demonstrated diagnosis, which of the following alternative diagnostic tests would have been the least likely to have arrived at the same pathology?

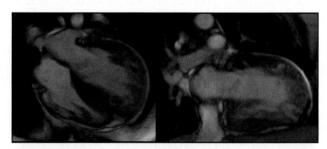

FIGURE 57.5

A. Invasive left ventriculography
B. Computed tomography
C. Three-dimensional echocardiography
D. Manufactured ultrasound contrast echocardiography
E. Agitated saline bubble contrast echocardiography

6. A 32-year-old male with a history of hypertension and systolic ejection click on physical exam was referred for cardiac MRI after his transthoracic echocardiogram demonstrated a possible bicuspid aortic valve with mild aortic regurgitation. The cardiac MRI image is shown in FIGURE 57.6. A pulsed-wave Doppler spectrum from the suprasternal notch with the sample volume position in the descending thoracic aorta 3.0 cm distal to the origin of the left subclavian artery origin.

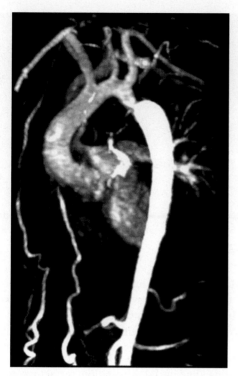

FIGURE 57.6

A. High systolic velocity, which continues throughout the cardiac cycle (diastolic tail)
B. Significant diastolic flow reversal
C. High systolic velocity, with no flow during diastole
D. Reduced systolic flow, with a characteristically low peak velocity, and prolonged acceleration and deceleration times

7. A 51-year-old male with a past medical history significant for hypertension and dyslipidemia was referred for coronary CT angiography for evaluation of chest pain. The abnormality shown in FIGURE 57.7 was incidentally noted. To confirm this diagnosis by echocardiography, the best step would be

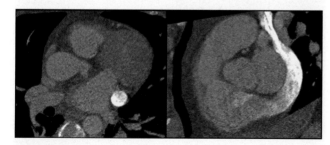

FIGURE 57.7

A. Inject agitated saline via right peripheral IV and evaluate the interatrial septum
B. Obtain mitral valve inflow Doppler velocity to obtain diagnosis
C. Obtain maximal velocity across the tricuspid valve using continuous wave Doppler
D. Inject agitated saline via left peripheral IV while obtaining images in the parasternal long-axis view

8. A 60-year-old male with a history of hypertension was referred for an echocardiogram based on complaints of shortness of breath. He was referred for further evaluation by cardiac MRI based on abnormal findings on his echocardiogram. The images were obtained during diastole (FIG. 57.8, left) and systole (FIG. 57.8, right). Based on these images, one would expect the following abnormality on echocardiogram.

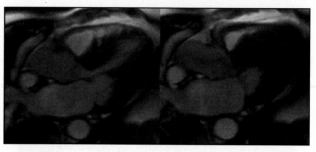

FIGURE 57.8

A. Elevated velocity at the level of left ventricular outflow tract (LVOT), with continuous wave spectral Doppler recording demonstrating a peak velocity during late systole
B. The continuous wave Doppler spectrum of the descending thoracic aorta demonstrating persistent turbulent jet throughout diastole
C. Severe eccentric MR likely directed anteriorly
D. Systolic flow reversal noted in the hepatic vein
E. Mitral inflow CW Doppler spectral display with a prolonged pressure half time and elevated mean gradient

9. A 29-year-old female with no significant past medical history initially presented to her primary care physician with complaints of palpitations and decreased exercise tolerance. She was referred for cardiac MRI after the transthoracic echocardiogram demonstrated a mildly dilated right ventricle. The cardiac images are shown in FIGURE 57.9. Which of the following findings can definitively establish the condition?

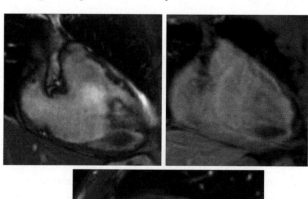

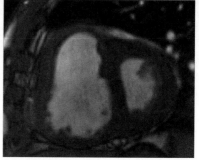

FIGURE 57.9

A. Right ventricular mid–free wall akinesis with normal motion of the apex

B. Mild tricuspid regurgitation

C. Right ventricular pressure overload

D. RV acceleration time of ≤60 ms in the presence of tricuspid insufficiency pressure gradient ≤ 60 mm Hg

E. None of the options

10. A 60-year-old with a history of hypertension was referred to a cardiologist based on complaints of dyspnea and near syncope. His transthoracic echocardiogram demonstrated a right atrial mass. He was subsequently referred for cardiac MRI (FIG. 57.10). The most likely echocardiographic finding in this patient would be

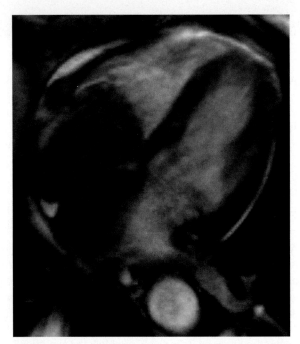

FIGURE 57.10

A. Mitral regurgitation with vena contracta of 0.75 cm

B. Peak tricuspid inflow velocity of 2.1 m/s

C. Inferior vena cava measuring 1.3 cm with normal respiratory collapse

D. Color Doppler indicating flow across the interatrial septum from the right to the left

11. A 41-year-old male with no significant past medical history presented with several-week history of low-grade fever, anorexia, and malaise. His blood cultures grew *Streptococcus solitarius*. His transthoracic echocardiogram showed a left-to-right shunt. He was referred for coronary CT angiography prior to surgery (FIG. 57.11). Where would the defect be expected to be located on the parasternal short-axis view at the level of the aortic valve?

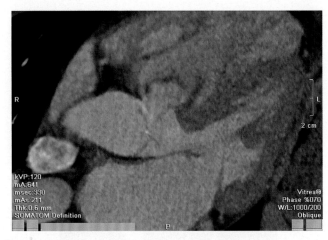

FIGURE 57.11

A. Midportion of the interatrial septum

B. 2 o' clock position with respect to the aortic valve

C. 10 o' clock position with respect to the aortic valve

D. 6 o' clock position with respect to the aortic valve

12. A 59-year-old male with a history of hypertension, dyslipidemia, and atrial fibrillation refractory to medical therapy was referred for cardiac CT prior to ablation. The images are shown in FIGURE 57.12. Based on these images, the patient will likely have which of the following on transesophageal echocardiogram?

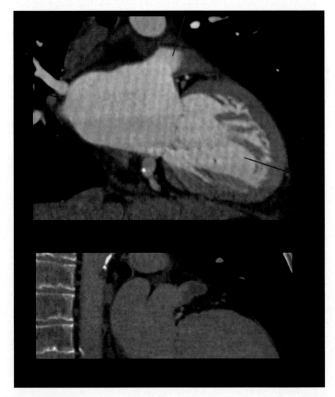

FIGURE 57.12

A. Increased flow velocity in the left upper pulmonary vein
B. A left atrial appendage pulsed-wave Doppler maximal emptying flow velocity likely <20 cm/s
C. Greater than 80% flow duration into the left atrial appendage within a cardiac cycle
D. Systolic flow reversal into the left upper pulmonary vein

13. A 55-year-old male presented with acute anterior wall ST elevation myocardial infarction and underwent urgent percutaneous coronary intervention. He underwent a cardiac MRI 10 days following the event, and the image is shown in FIGURE 57.13. What would be the echocardiographic finding that is equivalent to the finding demonstrated in the image?

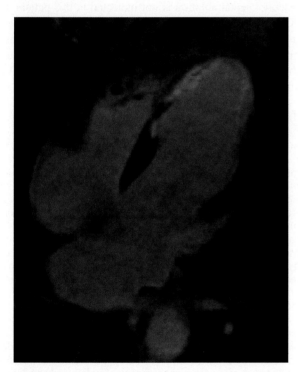

FIGURE 57.13

A. Presence of mural thrombus by contrast echocardiography
B. Mitral regurgitation with color flow filling >40% of the left atrial area
C. End-diastolic wall thickness <0.6 cm
D. Biphasic response to dobutamine infusion

14. A 51-year-old male with a history of hypertension was referred for cardiac MRI based on complaints of dyspnea and lower extremity edema. The short-axis real-time cine images during expiration and inspiration are shown. In addition, tagged MRI cine images during systole are also shown (FIG. 57.14). The most likely echocardiographic findings would be

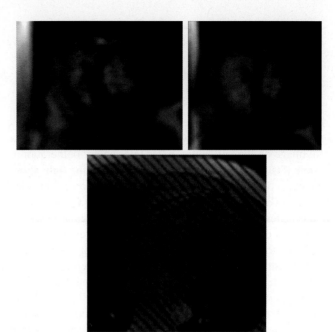

FIGURE 57.14

A. Significantly elevated e′-to-E ratio
B. Markedly diminished e′
C. Lateral e′ > septal e′
D. Septal e′ > lateral e′

15. A 53-year-old woman with a history of hypertension and hyperlipidemia was referred for ^{99m}Tc-sestamibi imaging for evaluation of atypical chest pain. Stress (top row) and rest images (bottom row) are shown in FIGURE 57.15. The most likely echocardiographic finding in this patient would be

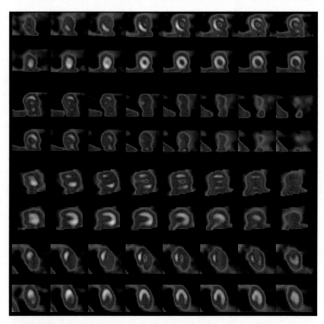

FIGURE 57.15

A. End-diastolic wall thickness <0.6 cm
B. Multiple wall motion abnormality and/or cavity dilation during peak stress
C. Tricuspid velocity of 4 m/s
D. Inferior wall akinesis at rest

Answer 1: A. The images are consistent with apical hypertrophic cardiomyopathy (AHCM) with extensive scarring at the apex. The image on the left demonstrates midcavitary obliteration in systole (FIG. 57.16, small arrow). The image on the right shows significant delayed enhancement at the apex as well as an apical thrombus (FIG. 57.16, large arrow). The coronary CT angiogram in this patient showed only minimal luminal irregularities.

AHCM can be divided into two groups, pure apical hypertrophy or those with coexistent hypertrophy of the interventricular septum (mixed) (1). The diagnostic criteria for AHCM includes demonstration of asymmetric left ventricular (LV) hypertrophy, confined predominantly to the LV apex, with an apical wall thickness ≥15 mm and a ratio of maximal apical to posterior wall thickness ≥1.5 mm, based on an echocardiogram or magnetic resonance imaging (MRI) (1).

The mean age of presentation of AHCM is 41.4 ± 14.5 years and is most commonly seen in males (1). About half the patients are symptomatic, and the most common symptoms are chest pain, followed by palpitations, dyspnea, and syncope (1). The most frequent ECG abnormality is negative T wave in the precordial leads (found in 93% of patients) (1). Transthoracic echocardiogram is usually the initial diagnostic tool for AHCM; however, in cases of suboptimal images, a contrast echocardiogram might be useful for establishing the diagnosis (2), demonstrating the "spade-like" configuration (1). Cardiac MRI (CMR) is also a valuable tool for diagnosing patients with inconclusive echocardiography, with LV apex along with the basal anterolateral free wall being two regions where CMR may provide advantage over echocardiography for identification of hypertrophy (3,4). The majority of the patients with AHCM who suffer myocardial infarction have an apical infarct, some of whom are asymptomatic (1). The patients might have wall motion abnormalities from apical hypokinesis to aneurysm (1).

Unlike other variants of HCM, the prognosis of AHCM is relatively benign; however, ICD has been previously used in AHCM patients with cardiac arrest and nonsustained ventricular tachycardia (5).

Since the MRI shows evidence of apical thrombus, there is an indication for anticoagulation, making answer A correct.

The ACEI and beta-blockers would not lead to regression of LVH in patients with HCM; therefore, answer B is incorrect. Beta-blocking drugs are recommended for the treatment of symptoms (angina or dyspnea) in adult patients with obstructive or nonobstructive HCM but should be used with caution in patients with sinus bradycardia or severe conduction disease (6). The use of ACEI in patients with HCM and preserved LV function is not well established and should be used cautiously in patients with resting or provocable LVOT obstruction due to worsening LVOT obstruction related to fall in peripheral resistance (6). ACEI can be used in HCM patients with low EF (6).

Our patient has no high-risk features; thus, there are no indications for ICD placement. Therefore, answer C is incorrect. Furthermore, there are no indications for long-term antiarrhythmic therapy at this time. In addition, this patient has no indication for cardiac biopsy; hence, answer D is incorrect.

Alcohol septal ablation is not indicated in this patient with AHCM due to lack of LVOT obstruction; therefore, answer E is incorrect. Alcohol septal ablation may be considered as an alternative to surgical myectomy for eligible adult patients with HCM with severe drug-refractory symptoms and LVOT obstruction (based on patient preference [class 2B]) (6).

References

1. Eriksson MJ, Sonnenberg B, Woo A, et al. Long-term outcome in patients with apical hypertrophic cardiomyopathy. *J Am Coll Cardiol* 2002;39(4):638–645.
2. Patel J, Michaels J, Mieres J, et al. Echocardiographic diagnosis of apical hypertrophic cardiomyopathy with optison contrast. *Echocardiography* 2002;19(6):521–524.
3. Rickers C, Wilke NM, Jerosch-Herold M, et al. Utility of cardiac magnetic resonance imaging in the diagnosis of hypertrophic cardiomyopathy. *Circulation* 2005;112(6):855–861.
4. Moon JCC, Fisher NG, McKenna WJ, et al. Detection of apical hypertrophic cardiomyopathy by cardiovascular magnetic resonance in patients with non-diagnostic echocardiography. *Heart* 2004;90(6):645–649.
5. Ridjab D, Koch M, Zabel M, et al. Cardiac arrest and ventricular tachycardia in Japanese-type apical hypertrophic cardiomyopathy. *Cardiology* 2007;107(2):81–86.
6. Gersh BJ, Maron BJ, Bonow RO, et al. 2011 ACCF/AHA guideline for the diagnosis and treatment of hypertrophic cardiomyopathy: a report of the American College of Cardiology Foundation/American Heart Association Task Force on Practice Guidelines. *J Thorac Cardiovasc Surg* 2011;142(6):e153–e203.

Answer 2: B. The MRI image on the left of FIGURE 57.17 demonstrates a defect in the interatrial septum consistent with sinus venosus ASD, while the MRA image on the right demonstrates

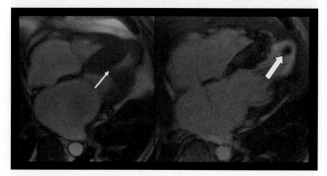

FIGURE 57.16

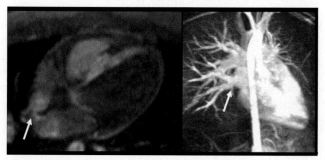

FIGURE 57.17

partial anomalous pulmonary vein return (PAPVR) draining into the right atrium. Patients with sinus venosus ASD often have PAPVR (95% in one study) (1).

The PAPVR defects are often right sided in the majority of cases (1), with bilateral being the least common. The Qp/Qs ratio can reliably be calculated using phase-contrast imaging by MRI, and these values correlate closely to those by invasive oximetry (2). Although 2D TTE has excellent sensitivity for the diagnosis of secundum-type defects (88% to 99%), its sensitivity is significantly less for more uncommon causes of shunting (3). The sinus venosus defect, in contrast to the other types of ASD, is best imaged with the longitudinal plane or the transgastric view to adequately define the overriding relationship of the superior vena cava and identify the pulmonary venous return. The four-chamber image clearly shows defect in the interatrial septum consistent with ASD; therefore, answer A is incorrect.

Ebstein anomaly is a rare congenital heart disease occurring in 1/200,000 live births and accounting for <1% of all cases of congenital heart disease (4). Ebstein anomaly is a malformation of the tricuspid valve and right ventricle characterized by adherence of the septal and posterior leaflets to the underlying myocardium; apical displacement of the functional annulus (septal > posterior > anterior); dilation of the "atrialized" portion of the right ventricle; redundancy, fenestrations, and tethering of the anterior leaflet; and dilation of the right atrioventricular junction (4). The four-chamber image demonstrates normal position of the tricuspid valve; therefore, answer C is incorrect.

Congenitally corrected transposition of the great arteries is a rare congenital abnormality accounting for <1% of cardiac anomalies and is defined as ventriculoarterial and atrioventricular (AV) discordance. The double discordant connection allows for survival with the right ventricle performing as the systemic ventricle and the left ventricle as the pulmonary ventricle. The MRA images demonstrate the aorta arising from the left ventricle; therefore, answer D is incorrect.

References

1. Kafka H, Mohiaddin RH. Cardiac MRI and pulmonary MR angiography of sinus venosus defect and partial anomalous pulmonary venous connection in cause of right undiagnosed ventricular enlargement. *Am J Roentgenol* 2009;192(1):259–266.
2. Debl K, Djavidani B, Buchner S, et al. Quantification of left-to-right shunting in adult congenital heart disease: phase-contrast cine MRI compared with invasive oximetry. *Br J Radiol* 2009;82(977):386–391.
3. Pascoe RD, Oh JK, Warnes CA, et al. Diagnosis of sinus venosus atrial septal defect with transesophageal echocardiography. *Circulation* 1996;94(5):1049–1055.
4. Attenhofer Jost CH, Connolly HM, Dearani JA, et al. Ebstein's anomaly. *Circulation* 2007;115(2):277–285.

Suggested Reading

Stern DR, Steiner C, Bello RA, et al. Congenitally corrected transposition of the great arteries and concomitant coronary artery and valvular disease in the adult patient. *Congenit Heart Dis* 2010;5(6):629–634.

Answer 3: *C.* The CT image demonstrates a thin membrane in the LVOT (Fig. 57.18, arrow) consistent with discrete subaortic stenosis. The color Doppler would demonstrate aliasing in the

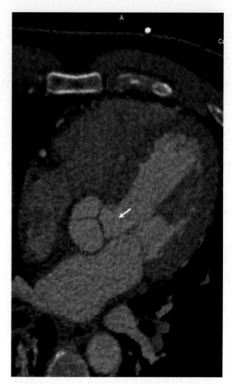

Figure 57.18

LVOT consistent with elevated velocity, and CW velocity demonstrates peak velocity during midsystole.

Subaortic stenosis accounts for approximately 8% to 20% of LVOT obstructions (1,2). Continuous wave Doppler recording from the apical view often demonstrates increased aortic jet velocity during midsystole consistent with a "fixed stenosis." Furthermore, the outflow area had a mosaic pattern indicative of turbulent and high subaortic flow velocities (3). A late-peaking LVOT is usually seen in HOCM/SAM consistent with a "dynamic obstruction." A persistent flow in the descending aorta during diastole is consistent with aortic coarctation, while systolic flow reversal in hepatic veins is seen in severe tricuspid regurgitation.

The current AHA/ACC guidelines for surgical intervention for patients with discrete subaortic stenosis are as follows (4):

CLASS I

1. Surgical intervention is recommended for patients with subaortic stenosis and a peak instantaneous gradient of 50 mm Hg or a mean gradient of 30 mm Hg on echocardiography–Doppler (*Level of Evidence: C*).
2. Surgical intervention is recommended for subaortic stenosis with less than a 50-mm Hg peak or less than a 30-mm Hg mean gradient and progressive AR and an LV dimension at end-systolic diameter of 50 mm or more or LV ejection fraction <55% (*Level of Evidence: C*).

CLASS IIb

1. Surgical resection may be considered in patients with a mean gradient of 30 mm Hg, but careful follow-up is required to detect progression of stenosis or AR (*Level of Evidence: C*).
2. Surgical resection may be considered for patients with less than a 50-mm Hg peak gradient or less than a 30-mm Hg mean gradient in the following situations:
   a. When LV hypertrophy is present (*Level of Evidence: C*)
   b. When pregnancy is being planned (*Level of Evidence: C*)
   c. When the patient plans to engage in strenuous/competitive sports (*Level of Evidence: C*)

CLASS III

1. Surgical intervention is not recommended to prevent AR for patients with subaortic stenosis if the patient has trivial LVOT obstruction or trivial to mild AR (*Level of Evidence: C*).

Elevated velocity at the level of LVOT, with CW recording demonstrating a peak velocity during late systole, would be expected in dynamic obstruction (systolic anterior motion of mitral valve/hypertrophic cardiomyopathy) as opposed to fixed obstruction present in our patient; therefore, answer A is incorrect. In addition, the CW Doppler in LVOT that includes the IVCT and IVRT periods, as well as the systolic ejection period, would be expected in patients with aortic stenosis; therefore, answer E is incorrect.

The CW Doppler of the descending aorta demonstrating persistent turbulent jet throughout diastole is seen in patients with severe aortic regurgitation. Although, subaortic stenosis is associated with aortic regurgitation, additional information would be required; therefore, answer B is incorrect. Finally, systolic flow reversal noted in the hepatic vein is seen in patients with severe tricuspid regurgitation; therefore, answer E is incorrect.

References

1. Leichter DA, Sullivan I, Gersony WM. "Acquired" discrete subvalvular aortic stenosis: natural history and hemodynamics. *J Am Coll Cardiol* 1989;14(6):1539–1544.
2. Sung CS, Price EC, Cooley DA. Discrete subaortic stenosis in adults. *Am J Cardiol* 1978;42(2):283–290.
3. Maréchaux S, Juthier F, Banfi C, et al. Illustration of the echocardiographic diagnosis of subaortic membrane stenosis in adults: surgical and live three-dimensional transesophageal findings. *Eur J Echocardiogr* 2011;12(1):E2.
4. Warnes CA, Williams RG, Bashore TM, et al. ACC/AHA 2008 guidelines for the management of adults with congenital heart disease: a report of the American College of Cardiology/American Heart Association Task Force on Practice Guidelines (Writing Committee to Develop Guidelines on the Management of Adults With Congenital Heart Disease). Developed in Collaboration With the American Society of Echocardiography, Heart Rhythm Society, International Society for Adult Congenital Heart Disease, Society for Cardiovascular Angiography and Interventions, and Society of Thoracic Surgeons. *J Am Coll Cardiol* 2008;52(23):e143–e263.

Answer 4: D. The images demonstrate high-grade ostial left main stenosis with moderate lesions in the left anterior and right coronary arteries. Subsequently, the patient underwent coronary angiography, confirming the presence of ostial left main lesion.

Prior studies have demonstrated that the strongest independent variables for predicting the presence of multivessel CAD during DSE were systolic wall thickening index (WMSI) at peak stress ($P < 0.0001$) and the presence of wall thickening abnormalities in multiple vascular territories ($P = 0.001$) (1).

The American Society of Echocardiography recommends dividing the left ventricle into a 16-segment model (2), and during stress echocardiography, a score is assigned to each segment at baseline, with each stage of stress, and during recovery. Each segment is scored as follows: 1 = normal; 2 = mild to moderate hypokinesis; 3 = severe hypokinesis; 4 = akinesia (no wall thickening and excursion); and 5 = dyskinesia

(paradoxical wall motion away from the center of the LV during systole) (3). A normal response to stress is defined as normal wall motion at rest, with an increase in wall thickening and excursion during stress. The peak WMSI following stress is derived from the cumulative sum score of 16 LV wall segments divided by the number of visualized segments.

Multiple wall motion abnormalities and cavity dilation are seen in patients with multivessel CAD and significant ischemia during stress. In addition, a peak WMSI > 1.7 has been shown to be an independent marker of patients at high risk of an adverse clinical outcome (4).

References

1. Senior R, Khattar R, Lahiri A. Value of dobutamine stress echocardiography for the detection of multivessel coronary artery disease. *Am J Cardiol* 1998;81(3):298–301.
2. Shiller NB, Shah PM, Crawford M, et al. Recommendations for quantitation of the left ventricle by two-dimensional echocardiography. American Society of Echocardiography Committee on Standards, Subcommittee on Quantitation of Two-Dimensional Echocardiograms. *J Am Soc Echocardiogr* 1989;2:358–367.
3. Chaudhry FA, Tauke JT, Alessandrini RS, et al. Prognostic implications of myocardial contractile reserve in patients with coronary artery disease and left ventricular dysfunction. *J Am Coll Cardiol* 1999;34(3):730–738.
4. Yao SS, Qureshi E, Sherrid MV, et al. Practical applications in stress echocardiography: risk stratification and prognosis in patients with known or suspected ischemic heart disease. *J Am Coll Cardiol* 2003;42(6):1084–1090.

Answer 5: E. The images are consistent with noncompaction of the ventricular myocardium. There are currently two sets of diagnostic criteria used for the diagnosis of noncompaction:

1. The Chin criteria require parasternal long-axis, subxiphoid, and apical views, with the absence of any other coexisting cardiac structural abnormality, presence of numerous and excessively prominent trabeculations, and deep intertrabecular recesses. These criteria focus on the depth of the recesses measured in end diastole, and the diagnosis is based on the ratio of the distance from the epicardial surface to the trough of the trabecular recesses and distance from the epicardial surface to peak of the trabeculation ≤ 0.5 (1).

2. The Jenni criteria require parasternal short-axis and apical views. It requires absence of any other coexisting cardiac structural abnormality and presence of numerous and excessively prominent trabeculations and deep intertrabecular recesses. These criteria focus on a two-layer structure measured in end systole, and the diagnosis is made if the ratio of the thick noncompacted layer to thin compacted layer is ≥2 with perfused intertrabecular recesses supplied by intraventricular blood on color Doppler analysis (2).

Although 2D echocardiogram is the most common diagnostic utility, the diagnosis could be missed in half the cases due to poor visualization of the entire myocardium and endocardium as well as misinterpretation of prominent trabeculations as false tendons (3).

The diagnosis of noncompaction could be established by left ventriculography (4), three-dimensional echocardiography

(5), contrast echocardiography (6,7), computed tomography (4), and cardiac MRI (8).

Answer E is not a diagnostic tool that would likely help derive this pathology. The agitated saline bubble study is used to evaluate for shunt physiology and is not a very good agent to define morphology. However, during transition of the microbubbles through the RV, morphology is improved due to superior endocardial definition on the right side, so noncompaction of this ventricle may be noted.

References

1. Chin TK, Perloff JK, Williams RG, et al. Isolated noncompaction of left ventricular myocardium. A study of eight cases. *Circulation* 1990;82(2):507–513.
2. Jenni R, Oechslin E, Schneider J, et al. Echocardiographic and pathoanatomical characteristics of isolated left ventricular noncompaction: a step towards classification as a distinct cardiomyopathy. *Heart* 2001;86(6):666–671.
3. Ichida F, Hamamichi Y, Miyawaki T, et al. Clinical features of isolated noncompaction of the ventricular myocardium: long-term clinical course, hemodynamic properties, and genetic background. *J Am Coll Cardiol* 1999;34(1):233–240.
4. Conces DJ Jr, Ryan T, Tarver RD. Noncompaction of ventricular myocardium: CT appearance. *AJR Am J Roentgenol* 1991;156(4):717–718.
5. Baker GH, Pereira NL, Hlavacek AM, et al. Transthoracic real-time three-dimensional echocardiography in the diagnosis and description of noncompaction of ventricular myocardium. *Echocardiography* 2006;23(6):490–494.
6. Koo BK, Choi D, Ha J-W, et al. Isolated noncompaction of the ventricular myocardium: contrast echocardiographic findings and review of the literature. *Echocardiography* 2002;19(2):153–156.
7. Mulvagh SL, DeMaria AN, Feinstein SB, et al. Contrast echocardiography: current and future applications. *J Am Soc Echocardiogr* 2000;13(4):331–342.
8. Soler R, Rodríguez E, Monserrat L, et al. MRI of subendocardial perfusion deficits in isolated left ventricular noncompaction. *J Comput Assist Tomogr* 2002;26(3):373–375.

Answer 6: D. The image is consistent with coarctation of the aorta. Direct interrogation of the site would demonstrate high systolic velocity, which continues throughout the cardiac cycle (1) (FIG. 57.19A); however, distal to the site one would expect to find parvus tardus waveform with the characteristic prolonged acceleration and deceleration times (2) (FIG. 57.19B).

Diastolic flow reversal in the descending aorta is often seen in patients with severe aortic regurgitation (see FIG. 57.19C).

The current ACC/AHA guidelines for clinical evaluation and follow-up are listed below (3).

Class I

Every patient with systemic arterial hypertension should have the brachial and femoral pulses palpated simultaneously to assess timing and amplitude evaluation to search for the "brachial-femoral delay" of significant aortic coarctation. Supine bilateral arm (brachial artery) blood pressures and prone right or left supine leg (popliteal artery) blood pressures should be measured to search for differential pressure (*Level of Evidence: C*).

- Initial imaging and hemodynamic evaluation by TTE, including suprasternal notch acoustic windows, are useful in suspected aortic coarctation (*Level of Evidence: B*).

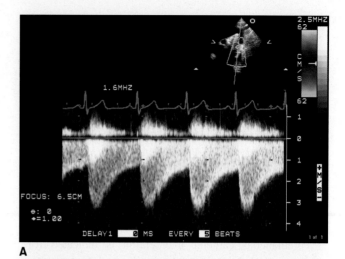

A

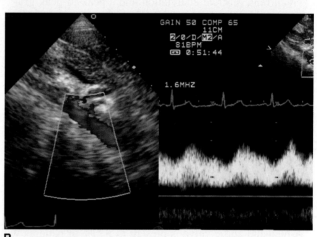

B

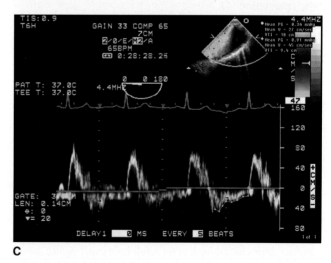

C

FIGURE 57.19 **A:** Suprasternal notch—descending aortic Doppler at the site of coarctation demonstrating high systolic velocity, which continues throughout the cardiac cycle. **B:** Doppler of the descending aorta demonstrating parvus tardus.

- *Every patient with coarctation (repaired or not) should have at least 1 cardiovascular MRI or CT scan for complete evaluation of the thoracic aorta and intracranial vessels (Level of Evidence: B).*

Furthermore, the current ACC/AHA guidelines for intervention/surgery are listed below (3).

Class I

- Intervention for coarctation is recommended in the following circumstances:
- Peak-to-peak coarctation gradient ≥20 mm Hg *(Level of Evidence: C)*.
- Peak-to-peak coarctation gradient <20 mm Hg in the presence of anatomic imaging evidence of significant coarctation with radiologic evidence of significant collateral flow *(Level of Evidence: C)*.
- Choice of percutaneous catheter intervention versus surgical repair of native discrete coarctation should be determined by consultation with a team of ACHD cardiologists, interventionalists, and surgeons at an ACHD center *(Level of Evidence: C)*.
- Percutaneous catheter intervention is indicated for recurrent, discrete coarctation and a peak-to-peak gradient of at least 20 mm Hg *(Level of Evidence: B)*.
- Surgeons with training and expertise in CHD should perform operations for previously repaired coarctation and the following indications:
- Long recoarctation segment *(Level of Evidence: B)*.
- Concomitant hypoplasia of the aortic arch *(Level of Evidence: B)*.

Class IIb

- Stent placement for long-segment coarctation may be considered, but the usefulness is not well established, and the long-term efficacy and safety are unknown *(Level of Evidence: C)*.

A bicuspid aortic valve is present in >50% of patients with aortic coarctation (4).

References

1. Carvalho JS, Redington AN, Shinebourne EA, et al. Continuous wave Doppler echocardiography and coarctation of the aorta: gradients and flow patterns in the assessment of severity. *Br Heart J* 1990;64(2):133–137.
2. Tan J-L, Babu-Narayan SV, Henein MY, et al. Doppler echocardiographic profile and indexes in the evaluation of aortic coarctation in patients before and after stenting. *J Am Coll Cardiol* 2005;46(6):1045–1053.
3. Warnes CA, Williams RG, Bashore TM, et al. ACC/AHA 2008 guidelines for the management of adults with congenital heart disease: a report of the American College of Cardiology/American Heart Association Task Force on Practice Guidelines (Writing Committee to Develop Guidelines on the Management of Adults With Congenital Heart Disease). Developed in Collaboration With the American Society of Echocardiography, Heart Rhythm Society, International Society for Adult Congenital Heart Disease, Society for Cardiovascular Angiography and Interventions, and Society of Thoracic Surgeons. *J Am Coll Cardiol* 2008;52(23):e143–e263.
4. Roos-Hesselink JW, Scholzel BE, Heijdra RJ, et al. Aortic valve and aortic arch pathology after coarctation repair. *Heart* 2003;89:1074–1077.

Answer 7: *D.* The images show a dilated coronary sinus (Fig. 57.20, small arrow) and the superior vena cava (SVC) draining into the coronary sinus (Fig. 57.20, large arrow), consistent with a persistent left SVC. Injection of agitated saline

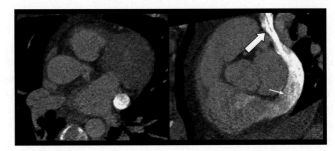

Figure 57.20

via a left antecubital vein will result in opacification of the dilated coronary sinus prior to the right atrium and right ventricle establishing the diagnosis of persistent left SVC.

The injection of saline and evaluation of interatrial septum would be useful for the evaluation of an intracardiac shunt, but this image does not indicate an intracardiac shunt, making answer A incorrect. Mitral valve inflow would be useful for evaluation of diastolic function, while evaluation of tricuspid valve velocity will be useful for the estimation of pulmonary artery systolic pressure. Hence, answers B and C are incorrect.

Persistent left SVC is a congenital anomaly of the thoracic venous system, which occurs due to failure of the left superior cardinal vein to regress to form the ligament of Marshall, and is found in approximately 0.4% of the general population (1). In 90% of the cases, bilateral SVCs are present (2). The drainage of persistent left SVC into the coronary sinus and right atrium has no significant hemodynamic consequences (2).

Agitated saline is used for evaluation of intracardiac shunt; therefore, answer A is incorrect. The mitral valve inflow Doppler is used for assessment of diastolic function; therefore, answer B is incorrect. The assessment of maximal velocity across the tricuspid valve using CW is used to assess right ventricular systolic pressure and, in the absence of pulmonic stenosis, pulmonary artery pressure; therefore, answer C is incorrect.

References

1. Albert M, Geissler W. Persistent left superior vena cava and mitral stenosis. *Z Gesamte Inn Med* 1956;11(19):865–874.
2. Xiong W, Shi C. Concomitant persistent left superior vena cava and agenesis of right superior vena cava a rare congenital anomaly. *Circulation* 2010;121(21):2329–2330.

Answer 8: *A.* The images demonstrate five-chamber cardiac MRI images during systole and diastole. In addition, the patient is noted to have asymmetrical septal hypertrophy (small arrow) and anterior motion of the mitral valve leaflet during systole (Fig. 57.21, large arrow).

The images are consistent with dynamic left ventricular outflow (LVOT) obstruction and systolic anterior motion (SAM) of the mitral valve. SAM is caused by the action of left ventricular flow on mitral valve apparatus. The anterior mitral valve leaflet is displaced by a drag that is directly proportional to the velocity in the LVOT and the angle between the anterior mitral valve leaflet and the direction of flow in the LVOT.

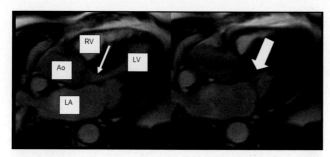

FIGURE 57.21

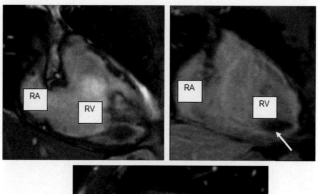

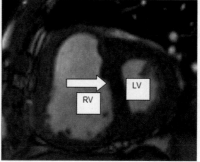

FIGURE 57.22

Furthermore, as the leaflet approaches the septum, a gradient is created that acts as a hydraulic force causing further excursion of the leaflet (1). In addition, the anterior displacement of the leaflet leads to malcoaptation of valvular leaflets during systole, resulting in mitral regurgitation, which is usually laterally or posteriorly directed (2).

The time of onset and the duration of mitral leaflet–septal approach determine the magnitude of the pressure gradient in the left ventricular outflow tract and are used to grade SAM (3,4).

A maximal spectral Doppler velocity in the LVOT that occurs in mid-systole is expected in a fixed obstruction (e.g., aortic stenosis or subaortic membrane). When the maximal velocity occurs in late systole, this suggests a functional obstruction (e.g., systolic anterior motion of the MV in HCM). Answer A is most correct. Answer C is found in aortic coarctation, answer D is found in severe tricuspid regurgitation, and answer E is found in mitral stenosis.

References

1. Sherrid MV, Gunsburg DZ, Moldenhauer S, et al. Systolic anterior motion begins at low left ventricular outflow tract velocity in obstructive hypertrophic cardiomyopathy. *J Am Coll Cardiol* 2000;36(4):1344–1354.
2. Levine RA, Vlahakes GJ, Lefebvre X, et al. Papillary muscle displacement causes systolic anterior motion of the mitral valve. Experimental validation and insights into the mechanism of subaortic obstruction. *Circulation* 1995;91(4):1189–1195.
3. Pollick C, Morgan CD, Gilbert BW, et al. Muscular subaortic stenosis: the temporal relationship between systolic anterior motion of the anterior mitral leaflet and the pressure gradient. *Circulation* 1982;66(5):1087–1094.
4. Nagueh SF, Bierig SM, Budoff MJ, et al. American Society of Echocardiography clinical recommendations for multimodality cardiovascular imaging of patients with hypertrophic cardiomyopathy: endorsed by the American Society of Nuclear Cardiology, Society for Cardiovascular Magnetic Resonance, and Society of Cardiovascular Computed Tomography. *J Am Soc Echocardiogr* 2011;24(5):473–498.

Answer 9: *E.* The images demonstrate right ventricular thrombus (Fig. 57.22, small arrow) along with a D-shaped septum (Fig. 57.22, large arrow) consistent with right ventricular pressure overload. The patient was noted to have massive bilateral pulmonary emboli (PE) in bilateral main pulmonary arteries (not shown).

Right ventricular (RV) mid–free wall akinesis with normal motion of apex, also known as McConnell sign (1), has previously been noted to have very high specificity for acute pulmonary emboli (1,2). In addition, this sign is absent in chronic pulmonary hypertension. However, recent studies have demonstrated that an abnormal pattern of regional RV contractility does not allow one to differentiate between acute PE and RV infarct.

Mild tricuspid regurgitation (TR) is noted in a variety of clinical settings and does not establish the diagnosis. Furthermore, signs of RV overload are also seen in other conditions including chronic pulmonary hypertension. Finally, the so-called 60/60 sign (RV acceleration time of ≤60 ms and TR pressure gradient ≤ 60 mm Hg) reflects increased arterial input impedance and therefore will be abnormal in both acute pulmonary emboli and chronic pulmonary hypertension (3).

Therefore, although both McConnell sign and the 60/60 rule have high specificity for acute PE (2), for bedside evaluation, none of the findings definitively establish the diagnosis.

References

1. McConnell MV, Solomon SD, Rayan ME, et al. Regional right ventricular dysfunction detected by echocardiography in acute pulmonary embolism. *Am J Cardiol* 1996;78(4):469–473.
2. Kurzyna M, Torbicki A, Pruszczyk P, et al. Disturbed right ventricular ejection pattern as a new Doppler echocardiographic sign of acute pulmonary embolism. *Am J Cardiol* 2002;90(5):507–511.
3. Torbicki A, Kurzyna M, Ciurzynski M, et al. Proximal pulmonary emboli modify right ventricular ejection pattern. *Eur Respir J* 1999;13(3):616–621.

Answer 10: *B.* The four-chamber cardiac MRI cine image demonstrates a large right atrial mass protruding through the tricuspid valve (Fig. 57.23, large arrow). In addition, a smaller mass (Fig. 57.23, small arrow) is noted in the left atrium. The patient was also noted to have significant lymphadenopathy on the MRI (not shown). Biopsy confirmed the diagnosis of non-Hodgkin lymphoma.

The mass would result in obstruction of flow from the right atrium into the right ventricle, resulting in an elevated mean gradient between the right atrium and right ventricle. As the normal peak inflow gradient of the tricuspid valve is <1 m/s, the given peak velocity listed is significantly elevated and is consistent

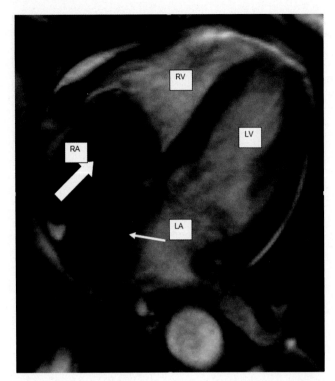

FIGURE 57.23

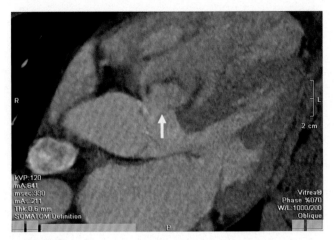

FIGURE 57.24

with stenosis secondary to obstruction from the mass. Hence, answer B is correct. The subsequent right atrial pressure elevation would lead to dilation of IVC. The given IVC diameter of 1.3 cm with respiratory collapse estimates the RA pressure at 3 mm Hg, making answer C incorrect (1). The images are not consistent with severe mitral regurgitation (vena contracta > 0.7 cm) or right-to-left shunt at the interatrial level, as the left atrial volume was normal. Hence, answers A and D are incorrect. An MRI obtained 5 months after showed complete response to chemotherapy with complete resolution of the mass.

Reference

1. Rudski LG, Lai WW, Afilalo J, et al. Guidelines for the echo-cardiographic assessment of the right heart in adults: a report from the American Society of Echocardiography endorsed by the European Association of Echocardiography, a registered branch of the European Society of Cardiology, and the Canadian Society of Echocardiography. *J Am Soc Echocardiogr* 2010;23(7):685–713; quiz 786–788.

Answer 11: C. The five-chamber CT image shows a defect between LVOT and right ventricle (Fig. 57.24, arrow), consistent with membranous ventricular septal defect (VSD).

The patient was noted to have a large vegetation attached to the right ventricular side of the VSD (not seen on image). Parasternal short-axis view of the aortic valve would allow differentiation of membranous (10′) versus supracristal (2′) VSD (1). A defect in the interatrial septum would be expected in patients with atrial septal defect.

Reference

1. Miller LR, Nemeth M, Flamm SD, et al. Supracristal ventricular septal defect. *Tex Heart Inst J* 2006;33(1):96–97.

Answer 12: B. The images demonstrate a filling defect in the left atrial appendage (LAA) (Fig. 57.25, arrow) noted during initial contrast infusion as well as delayed imaging (2 minutes later), confirming the presence of left atrial appendage thrombus.

Patients with left atrial thrombus are noted to have severely reduced emptying and filling velocities within the LAA appendage (<20 versus 50 cm/s in normal patients). Also a reduced flow duration within the LAA is noted with thrombi in LAA (1). Hence, answer C is incorrect as it indicates longer flow duration. Increased flow velocity in the pulmonary vein is seen in pulmonary vein stenosis, which could be a complication of pulmonary vein ablation for atrial fibrillation, and

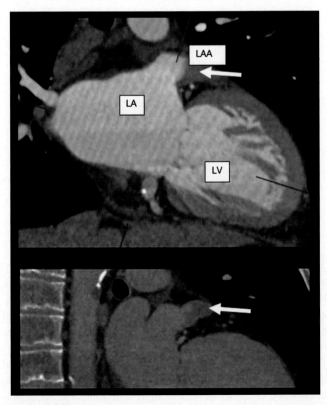

FIGURE 57.25

there is no evidence of this on the images provided. Systolic flow reversal in the pulmonary veins is seen in severe eccentric mitral regurgitation, which is also not depicted in these images.

Systolic flow reversal into the pulmonary veins is associated with severe mitral regurgitation (2), increased flow velocity is seen in patients with pulmonary vein stenosis, and >80% flow duration into LAA during the cardiac cycle is considered normal and not associated with LAA thrombus, making answers A, C, and D incorrect.

References

1. Alessandri N, Mariani S, Ciccaglioni A, et al. Thrombus formation in the left atrial appendage in the course of atrial fibrillation. *Eur Rev Med Pharmacol Sci* 2003;7(3):65–73.
2. Pu M, Griffin BP, Vandervoort PM, et al. The value of assessing pulmonary venous flow velocity for predicting severity of mitral regurgitation: a quantitative assessment integrating left ventricular function. *J Am Soc Echocardiogr* 1999;12(9):736–743.

Answer 13: C. The four-chamber cardiac MRI images demonstrate a large area of delayed enhancement involving the left ventricular apex (Fig. 57.26, arrows) consistent with a large transmural infarct involving the apex.

The degree of delayed enhancement has been shown to be a great predictor of future recovery, with patients with transmural extent of 75% or greater having <10% likelihood of recovery (1). End-diastolic wall thickness of <0.6 cm has been associated with low likelihood of recovery (2).

There is no evidence of mural thrombus on this scan, which would appear as black in this sequence; therefore, answer A is incorrect. Mitral regurgitation with color flow filling >40% of

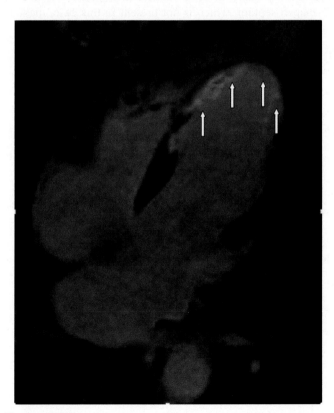

FIGURE 57.26

the left atrial area is associated with severe mitral regurgitation, which is not demonstrated in this image (3). A biphasic cardiac response demonstrates contractile improvement at low-dose dobutamine dose with worsening contractile function at peak dobutamine dose consistent with a viable but ischemic myocardium (4). A biphasic response has been shown to predict recovery following revascularization (4). The images are consistent with transmural MI; therefore, a biphasic response would not be expected in this patient.

References

1. Van Hoe L, Vanderheyden M. Ischemic cardiomyopathy: value of different MRI techniques for prediction of functional recovery after revascularization. *AJR Am J Roentgenol* 2004;182(1):95–100.
2. Cwajg JM, Cwajg E, Nagueh SF, et al. End-diastolic wall thickness as a predictor of recovery of function in myocardial hibernation: relation to rest-redistribution T1-201 tomography and dobutamine stress echocardiography. *J Am Coll Cardiol* 2000;35(5):1152–1161.
3. Zoghbi WA, Enriquez-Sarano M, Foster E, et al. American Society of Echocardiography: recommendations for evaluation of the severity of native valvular regurgitation with two-dimensional and Doppler echocardiography. A report from the American Society of Echocardiography's Nomenclature and Standards Committee and The Task Force on Valvular Regurgitation, developed in conjunction with the American College of Cardiology Echocardiography Committee, The Cardiac Imaging Committee, Council on Clinical Cardiology, The American Heart Association, and the European Society of Cardiology Working Group on Echocardiography, represented by. *Eur J Echocardiogr* 2003;4(4):237–261.
4. Cornel JH, Bax JJ, Elhendy A, et al. Biphasic response to dobutamine predicts improvement of global left ventricular function after surgical revascularization in patients with stable coronary artery disease: implications of time course of recovery on diagnostic accuracy. *J Am Coll Cardiol* 1998;31(5):1002–1010.

Answer 14: D. The free-breathing short-axis real-time MR cine images are shown (in Fig. 57.27, expiration on left, inspiration on right), which demonstrate significant septal bounce and flattening (Fig. 57.27, arrow). In addition, tagged MRI cine images during systole demonstrate no slippage.

These images are consistent with constrictive pericarditis. In constrictive pericarditis, the entire cardiac volume is constrained by the pericardium, leading to significant interventricular dependence. During inspiration, there is increased flow to the right side; however, due to the abovementioned interventricular dependence, the septum shifts to the left (septal bounce, arrow) (1). The septal shift during short-axis real-time cine on MRI has previously been used for the diagnosis of constrictive pericarditis. Furthermore, lack of slippage on tagged MRI imaging has also been used for the diagnosis of constrictive pericarditis (2). Patients with constrictive pericarditis have normal e′ with septal e′ > lateral, the so-called mitral annulus reversus (3). Normally, the lateral e′ is greater than septal e′.

Significantly elevated E/e′ ratio is noted in individuals with elevated LVEDP; therefore, answer A is incorrect. Markedly diminished e′ is seen in individuals with restrictive cardiomyopathy, not constrictive pericarditis.

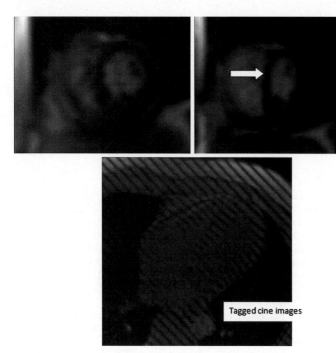

Tagged cine images

FIGURE 57.27

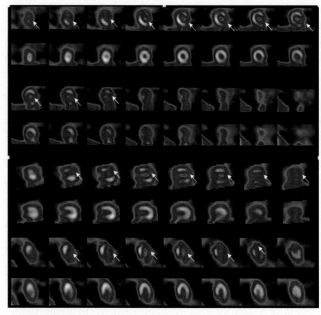

FIGURE 57.28

References

1. Sengupta PP, Eleid MF, Khandheria BK. Constrictive pericarditis. *Circ J* 2008;72(10):1555–1562.
2. Kojima S, Yamada N, Goto Y. Diagnosis of constrictive pericarditis by tagged cine magnetic resonance imaging. *N Engl J Med* 1999;341(5):373–374.
3. Reuss CS, Wilansky SM, Lester SJ, et al. Using mitral "annulus reversus" to diagnose constrictive pericarditis. *Eur J Echocardiogr* 2009;10(3):372–375.

***Answer 15:** B.* The images demonstrate homogenous perfusion at rest. However, during stress, large perfusion defect is noted in the inferolateral and apex (Fig. 57.28, arrows). In addition, significant transient ischemic dilation (TID) during stress is consistent with severe stress-induced ischemia. Cardiac catheterization confirmed significant three-vessel CAD. Based on these images, the best answer is B. The most likely finding on stress echocardiogram would be multiple wall motion abnormalities and/or cavity dilation.

Prior studies have demonstrated that the strongest independent variables for predicting the presence of multivessel CAD during DSE were systolic wall thickening index (WMSI) at peak stress ($P < 0.0001$) and the presence of wall thickening abnormalities in multiple vascular territories ($P = 0.001$) (1).

End-diastolic wall thickness <0.6 cm is seen in patients with prior myocardial infarction and is a poor predictor of recovery following revascularization (2). Based on normal perfusion at rest, answers A and D are less likely, therefore incorrect. Tricuspid regurgitation of 4 m/s would be expected in patients with severe pulmonary hypertension. Patients with severe pulmonary hypertension often have significant right ventricular uptake (secondary to right ventricular hypertrophy) and/or D-shaped septum, which is not present in this case, making answer C incorrect.

References

1. Senior R, Khattar R, Lahiri A. Value of dobutamine stress echocardiography for the detection of multivessel coronary artery disease. *Am J Cardiol* 1998;81(3):298–301.
2. Cwajg JM, Cwajg E, Nagueh SF, et al. End-diastolic wall thickness as a predictor of recovery of function in myocardial hibernation: relation to rest-redistribution T1-201 tomography and dobutamine stress echocardiography. *J Am Coll Cardiol* 2000;35(5):1152–1161.

Suggested Reading

Mazraeshahi RM, Striet J, Oeltgen RC, et al. Myocardial SPECT images for diagnosis of pulmonary hypertension and right ventricular hypertrophy. *J Nucl Med Technol* 2010;38(4):175–180.

Chapter 58

Practice Exam

Vincent L. Sorrell and Niti Aggarwal

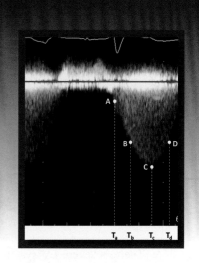

1. Which of the following echo findings in a 50-year-old male evaluated for liver transplant is most suggestive that their cause of dyspnea is related to an elevated LA pressure?

A. Pulmonary vein AR duration greater than mitral inflow A-wave duration
B. Tissue Doppler e' velocity = 6.0 cm/s
C. E/A decrease by <0.5 with Valsalva maneuver
D. Right ventricular systolic pressure > 45 mm Hg
E. Left atrial volume index > 40 mL/m^2

2. Which of the following parameters have outcome-based partition values for mild, moderate, or severe?

A. LVEF
B. LA diameter
C. LV mass
D. LV diameter
E. None of the above

3. A 39-year-old male with a history of intravenous drug abuse presents with high fever and shortness of breath. See VIDEO 58.1 and FIGURES 58.1 TO 58.3.

Based upon these images, which of the following is the most accurate interpretation?

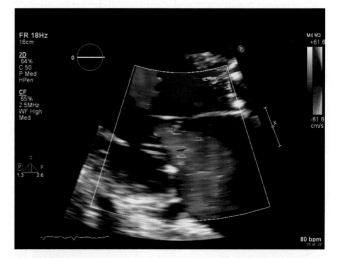

FIGURE 58.1

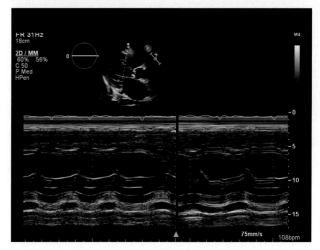

FIGURE 58.2

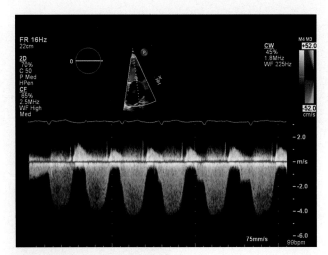

FIGURE 58.3

A. There is severe LV systolic dysfunction with reduced mitral valve opening and a B-bump.
B. There is mitral valve endocarditis with MS and MR.
C. There is aortic valve endocarditis with hemodynamically severe AR.
D. There is a rheumatic mitral valve.
E. There is an acute myocardial infarction.

4. A 19-year-old male with exertional syncope was seen in clinic. A loud systolic murmur was noted on exam. An echocardiogram was obtained and the sonographer asked for your interpretation of the pulsed wave Doppler spectral display shown in Figure 58.4.

What do you tell the sonographer?

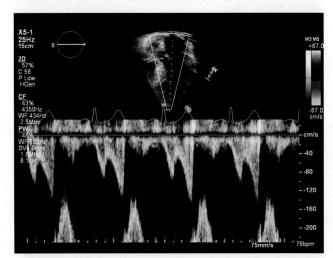

FIGURE 58.4

A. The image is incorrect and inverted.
B. This is due to high pulse repetition frequency.
C. There is severe MR creating a flow alias.
D. This is due to grade I diastolic dysfunction.
E. There is a mid-systolic drop in LV ejection velocity.

5. The M-mode shown in Figure 58.5 was obtained a 31-year-old male with dyspnea. Which of the following is best demonstrated?

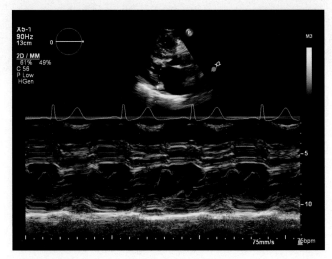

FIGURE 58.5

A. Hypertrophic cardiomyopathy
B. Amyloidosis
C. Hypertensive heart disease
D. Mitral valve prolapse
E. Rheumatic mitral stenosis

6. A 50-year-old male with a known hypertrophic cardiomyopathy on medical therapy underwent a serial 2D and Doppler echocardiogram. Which of the following echo findings would be most consistent with this diagnosis?

A. Figure 58.6
B. Figure 58.7
C. See Video 58.2
D. Figure 58.8

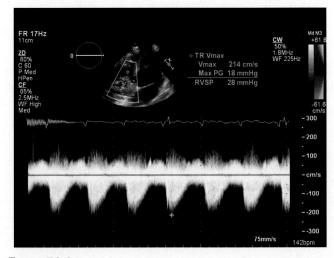

FIGURE 58.6

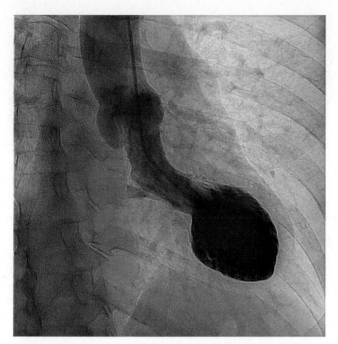

Figure 58.7

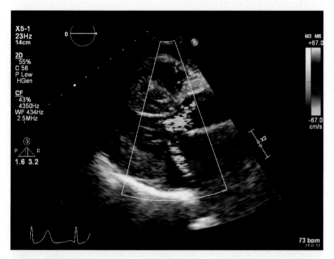

Figure 58.8

7. You are consulted on an obese 84-year-old male who presents to the emergency room after a motor vehicle accident in which he was restrained. There was no loss of consciousness. He has no serious traumatic injuries. His sternum is bruised, but not fractured. His ECG demonstrates sinus tachycardia with diffuse, but nonspecific, ST segment changes. His troponin is mildly increased. He is complaining of mild anterior wall chest pain. His past medical history is only significant for hypertension. He takes carvedilol 25 mg twice daily. You perform a limited point of care echocardiogram in the ER (see Videos 58.3 and 58.4).

Which of the following is the most important next step in the management of this patient?

A. Perform an urgent CT scan of the chest
B. Admit for close observation
C. Repeat echo with a manufactured ultrasound contrast agent
D. Recommend urgent CT surgery consultation
E. Perform coronary angiography

8. A 46-year-old active male presented with acute visual changes and suspected TIA. He admits to mild atypical chest pain and dyspnea. He takes no medications and has no past cardiovascular history. An echocardiogram was obtained and selected images are shown from the apical and subcostal windows (Videos 58.5 and 58.6).

Which of the following is the most appropriate next step in management?

A. Cardiothoracic surgery consultation
B. Administer fibrinolytic therapy
C. Perform coronary angiography
D. Recommend percutaneous thrombectomy
E. Recommend placement of a septal closure device

9. A 39-year-old male presents for ambulatory consultation for increasing dyspnea and cardiomyopathy. He has no relevant past history, but denies close medical attention. On exam, his pulse is notably bouncy and wide and his PMI is displaced laterally. An echocardiogram from his referring physician reports a dilated LA and LV; LVEF = 35%; normal right heart with RV to RA gradient 35 mm Hg. O_2 saturations on room air = 96%. BP 130/50 mm Hg. HR 90 regular. There is a loud systolic and diastolic murmur. A selected parasternal image is shown in the videos (Videos 58.7 and 58.8).

Which of the following would be the most appropriate next step in management?

A. Perform TEE
B. Perform percutaneous closure device
C. Recommend cardiothoracic surgery
D. Initiate low dose ACEi and beta-blocker
E. Initiate nifedipine 30 mg daily

10. A 45-year-old female presents to the emergency department with abrupt chest pain and dyspnea. She denies any emotional triggers or recent illness. ECG demonstrates diffuse T-wave inversions and no STEMI. Initial cardiac biomarkers are above the upper limit of normal. Echocardiography and coronary angiography are shown (Videos 58.9 to 58.12).

Which of the following statements is most accurate when comparing this syndrome to an acute STE myocardial infarction from total coronary artery obstruction?

A. This is a relatively uncommon cause of ACS presentation (<5% in women).
B. There is no reported clustering of events with natural disasters.
C. The troponin elevation is not in a typical "rise and fall" temporal pattern.
D. The initial presentation LVEF is usually lower.
E. Acute myocardial perfusion imaging is normal.
F. Morbidity and mortality is rare (<0.1%).

11. The spectral Doppler pattern shown in FIGURE 58.9 was obtained at baseline and the pattern shown in FIGURE 58.6 (question 8) was immediately following a procedure.

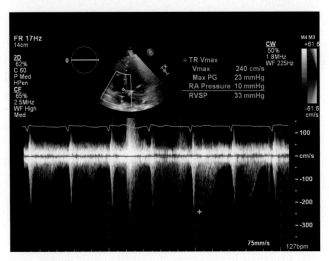

FIGURE 58.9

A. Pulmonary balloon valvuloplasty
B. TAVR
C. Mitral clip procedure
D. Alcohol septal ablation
E. RV biopsy
F. Pulmonary vasodilator test

12. Which of the following is considered to be an "appropriate" indication for the initial use of transesophageal echocardiography over transthoracic echocardiography?

A. A 50-year-old female previously healthy female who presents with difficulty of speaking since this morning
B. A 75-year-old male with a history of moderate COPD and obesity, now presenting with chest pain
C. Intraprocedural guidance of a left main percutaneous coronary intervention in a 52-year-old male
D. An 85-year-old male presenting with fever and blood cultures positive for *Candida albicans*
E. A 48-year-old male with paroxysmal atrial fibrillation anticoagulated with Coumadin and a history of congestive heart failure presenting with urinary tract infection with an INR of 1.4

13. Which of the following risk profiles would have an "appropriate" indication to perform a stress echocardiogram in an asymptomatic patient?

A. A 35-year-old male with no cardiac risk factors or family history of coronary artery disease and a normal electrocardiogram
B. A 45-year-old male with diabetes and hypertension and a normal electrocardiogram
C. A 45-year-old African-American male with longstanding hypertension and electrocardiogram with left ventricular hypertrophy and strain
D. A 65-year-old Caucasian male with diabetes mellitus, hypertension dyslipidemia, and current smoking history and a normal electrocardiogram
E. A 58-year-old male with a CT Agatston coronary artery calcium score of 482

14. A 35-year-old woman with dilated cardiomyopathy undergoes an echocardiogram. She has a dilated left ventricle with an ejection fraction of 35% (by biplane method of discs). Her cardiac index is 5 L/min/m^2. Based on the above information, this patient most likely has which of the following?

A. Severe mitral regurgitation
B. Severe tricuspid regurgitation
C. Severe aortic regurgitation
D. Ventricular septal defect
E. None the above

15. A 42-year-old female, who is new to your clinic, presents with progressive dyspnea on exertion. An echocardiogram performed reveals the following image (below FIG. 58.10). What auscultatory finding is expected in this patient?

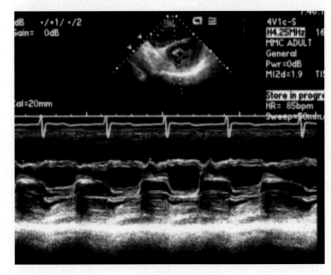

FIGURE 58.10

A. Opening snap
B. Tumor plop
C. Knock
D. Third heart sound

16. In a 45-year-old male with history of hypertension and diabetes, presents with pedal edema and dyspnea on exertion. On exam, BP is 145/75 mm Hg, with heart rate of 65 bpm. The following image (Figure. 58.11) is obtained on M-mode echocardiography. Which of the following is the most likely cause for his clinical symptoms?

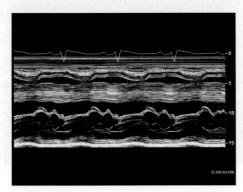

Figure 58.11

A. Mitral stenosis
B. Elevated left ventricular filling pressures
C. Systolic anterior motion of the mitral valve leaflet
D. Atrial flutter
E. Pulmonary hypertension

17. Which of the following statements regarding conditions of increased left ventricular (LV) wall thickness is true?

A. It is common for increased LV wall thickness due to athlete's heart to have an increased wall thickness of >13 mm.
B. In patients with increased LV wall thickness due to cardiac amyloidosis, the basal wall function is better preserved than apical wall function (as assessed by strain imaging).
C. In patients with increased LV wall thickness due to cardiac amyloidosis, basal longitudinal LV strain predicts mortality.
D. It is common for increased LV wall thickness due to athlete's heart to also have severe left atrial enlargement.
E. It is common for increased LV wall thickness due to athlete's heart to also have relatively small LV cavity size.

18. Which of the following is the correct order of the velocity of sound within the medium, from fastest to slowest tissue?

A. Blood, bone, and air
B. Air, bone, and blood
C. Air, blood, and bone
D. Bone, blood, and air
E. Bone, air, and blood

19. Based upon the 2D short axis images shown in Figure 58.12, which of the following statements is most accurate?

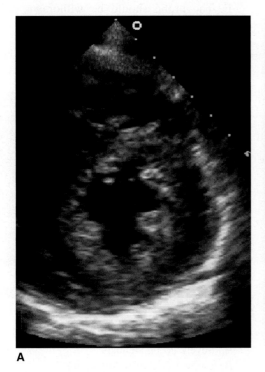

A

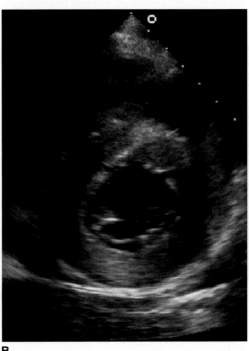

B

Figure 58.12 From Armstrong, WF, Ryan T. Feigenbaum's Echocardiography. 7th ed. Philadelphia, PA: Lippincott Williams & Wilkins, 2010.

A. The image on the left was obtained using much higher gain than the image on the right.

B. The image on the right has the focus much closer to the near field than the image on the left.

C. The image on the left was obtained with fundamental frequency, and the image on the right was obtained using a harmonic multiband imaging probe.

D. The image on the left used a lower-frequency imaging probe compared with the image on the right.

E. The image on the left has higher spatial resolution than the image on the right.

20. Reliable techniques in the diagnosis of ischemic mitral regurgitation (MR) include both 2D and 3D echo. Which of the following statements regarding the diagnosis of ischemic MR is most accurate?

A. There is shortening of the mitral valve apparatus, resulting in failure of the leaflets to close completely and a resultant eccentric MR jet away from the diseased leaflet.

B. By 3D, the pattern of mitral valve deformation is asymmetric in ischemic MR and symmetric in functional MR.

C. By 3D, the LV chamber and mitral annulus are more enlarged in ischemic MR than in functional MR.

D. Exercise Doppler echocardiography may show a marked decrease in MR grade.

E. An ERO ≥ 0.4 cm^2 defines severe ischemic MR.

21. A 76-year-old patient who has a history of coronary artery disease presents for a transesophageal echocardiogram. A regional wall motion abnormality is noted in the segments marked in red (Fig. 58.13). Disease in which coronary artery is *most* commonly responsible for this?

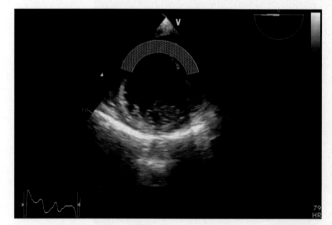

FIGURE 58.13

A. Left anterior descending artery
B. Left circumflex artery
C. Right coronary artery
D. Left main artery
E. Ramus intermedius

22. Choose the best statement that applies to the image (Fig. 58.14, VIDEO 58.13):

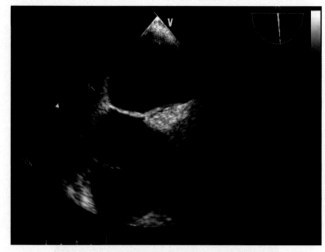

FIGURE 58.14

A. To obtain this view from the short axis view of the aortic valve, the probe should be rotated in a counterclockwise direction.

B. Advancing the probe would better visualize the superior vena cava.

C. Advancing the probe will better visualize the origin of the structure marked with an **asterisk**.

D. Clockwise rotation of the probe from this position will better evaluate the left atrium.

E. The probe should be withdrawn to visualize the coronary sinus.

23. What is the most likely diagnosis of the patient with the M-mode displayed in FIGURE 58.15?

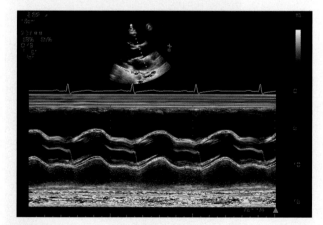

FIGURE 58.15

A. Severe aortic stenosis
B. Large aortic valve vegetation
C. Bicuspid aortic valve
D. Severe LV systolic dysfunction
E. Severe mitral stenosis

24. A patient with asymptomatic severe aortic regurgitation has an echocardiogram to reassess left ventricular size and function. On the 2D echo evaluation, the left ventricular ejection fraction is 45% using a biplane Simpson method. What do you recommend?

A. Continuation of medical therapy
B. Surgical replacement
C. Cardiac rehabilitation
D. Transcutaneous aortic valve replacement (TAVR)
E. None of the above

25. A 44-year-old male with no significant past medical history comes with progressive fatigue over the last 4 months. He denies any chest pain, palpitations, or syncope. His current exercise tolerance is about four blocks on a level ground. He has a strong family history of coronary artery disease with his father undergoing coronary artery grafting at the age of 48 years. Transthoracic echocardiogram shows a dilated left ventricle with global hypokinesis and ejection fraction of 30%. Electrocardiogram shows normal sinus rhythm with 1-mm lateral ST segment depression and T-wave inversion. Which of the following is the best next step in managing this patient?

A. Treadmill exercise echocardiography using Bruce protocol
B. Treadmill exercise EKG using Bruce protocol
C. Dobutamine echocardiography using 2.5 to 40 μg/kg/min
D. Dobutamine echocardiography using 10 to 40 μg/kg/min
E. Dipyridamole echocardiography using 0.84 mg/kg

26. Which aortic valve coronary cusp is starred in Figure 58.16?

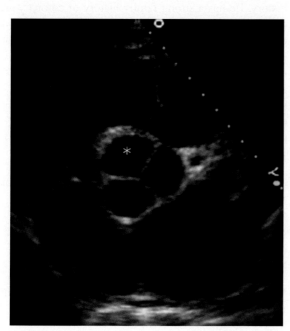

FIGURE 58.16

A. Septal
B. Right
C. Left
D. Noncoronary
E. Anterior

27. Which leaflets are seen in this view (Fig. 58.17)?

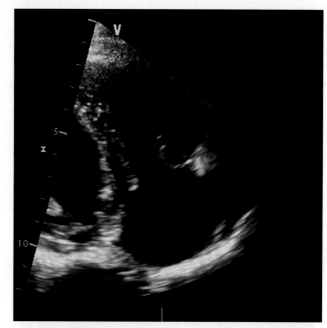

FIGURE 58.17

A. Anterior and posterior
B. Anterior and septal
C. Posterior and septal
D. Anterior and right
E. Posterior and right

28. Which vessel is starred in this view (Fig. 58.18)?

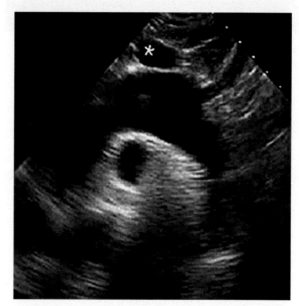

FIGURE 58.18

A. Left atrium
B. Right brachiocephalic vein
C. Right pulmonary artery
D. Left pulmonary artery
E. Left brachiocephalic vein

29. Which of the following statements is correct regarding the relationship between the Doppler frequency shift and the velocity of the object?

    A. Velocity is directly proportional to the angle between the Doppler ultrasound interrogating beam and the direction of the blood flow being interrogated.
    B. The change of speed of sound within the medium is an important factor contributing significantly to the measured Doppler velocity.
    C. The small difference in the transmitted and received frequencies is assumed to be twice the actual transducer frequency.
    D. A decrease in the Doppler frequency shift will decrease the recorded velocity.
    E. Velocity is equal to the frequency shift divided by a speed of sound constant times the cosine of the interrogating beam angle.

30. What should be adjusted to improve the Doppler spectral signal (Fig. 58.19)?

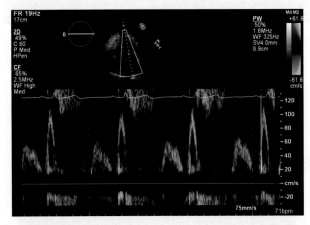

FIGURE 58.19

    A. Increase the wall filter
    B. Reduce the wall filter
    C. Increase the gain
    D. Reduce the gain
    E. Increase the frequency

31. A high-resistance spectral Doppler flow pattern is identified in the:

    A. Left common carotid artery
    B. Right internal carotid artery
    C. Left subclavian artery
    D. Left vertebral artery

32. During transesophageal echo examination, the true left ventricular apex is best visualized in the:

A. Four-chamber view
B. Two-chamber view
C. Transgastric short axis view
D. Deep transgastric (reverse four-chamber view)

33. Which of the following changes will increase the radius of the proximal isovelocity surface area (PISA) when this method is used in estimating the mitral valve area in the apical four-chamber view on a transthoracic echocardiogram?

    A. Shifting the baseline of the velocity scale toward the LV apex.
    B. Shifting the baseline of the velocity scale in the direction of mitral regurgitant flow.
    C. Increasing the Nyquist limit.
    D. Radius of PISA is determined by the transvalvular gradients and cannot be changed.

34. Mitral inflow velocities demonstrate grade I diastolic dysfunction. If you calculate the mitral valve area using the P t½ method in this patient:

    A. The mitral valve area will be underestimated.
    B. The mitral valve stenosis will be severely underestimated.
    C. The pressure half-time will be short relative to other grades of diastolic dysfunction.
    D. The mitral valve area calculation will not change.

35. A 62-year-old male with hypertension and hyperlipidemia complains of exertional chest discomfort. He describes the discomfort as tightness around his chest that is somewhat similar to asthma symptoms that he experiences occasionally. He is an ex-smoker with a 20-pack-year smoking history. He has a strong family history of coronary artery disease. His electrocardiogram shows normal sinus rhythm and nonspecific T-wave changes. He is scheduled for an exercise echocardiogram. Which of the following would decrease the specificity of the test result in this patient?

    A. Hypertensive response to exercise
    B. Left circumflex artery disease
    C. Mitral regurgitation
    D. Suboptimal effort
    E. Use of a beta-blocker prior to exercise

36. One way to reduce the appearance of a grainy 2D image is to:

    A. Turn persistence off
    B. Lower fundamental frequency
    C. Increase compress and/or dynamic range
    D. Foreshorten imaging plane

37. Which of the following is the primary determinant of mitral inflow E-wave and A-wave velocities?

    A. LA compliance
    B. LV compliance
    C. Transmitral pressure gradient
    D. Mitral valve area
    E. LV relaxation

38. Which of the following M-mode and Doppler profiles would NOT be indicative of hemodynamic compromise related to the pericardial effusion?

A. FIGURE 58.20
B. FIGURE 58.21
C. FIGURE 58.22
D. FIGURE 58.23
E. FIGURE 58.24

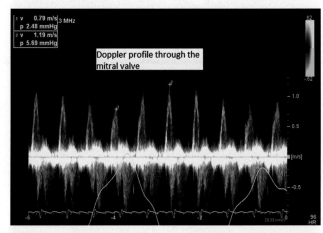

FIGURE **58.20**

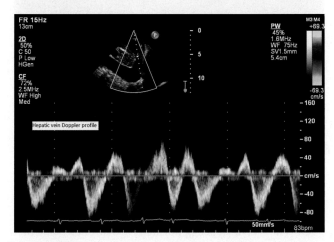

FIGURE **58.21**

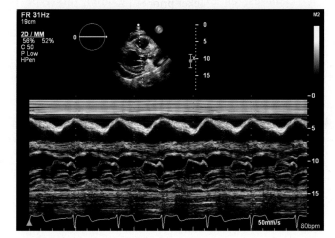

FIGURE **58.22**

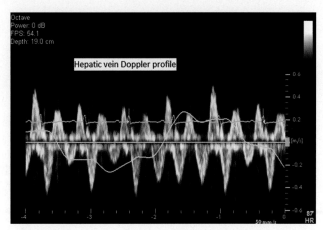

FIGURE **58.23**

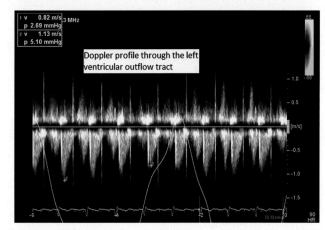

FIGURE **58.24**

39. A 46-year-old male had a #29 bioprosthetic valve replacement 11 years prior to this examination. He remains largely asymptomatic except for shortness of breath with heavy exertion or prolonged walking upstairs. Data from his continuous-wave Doppler exam across the valve are (FIG. 58.25):

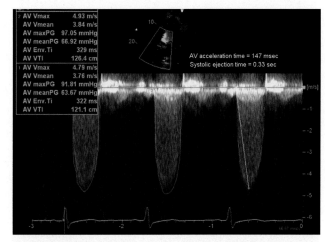

FIGURE **58.25**

Peak gradient 94 mm Hg

Mean gradient 65 mm Hg

Valvular velocity time integral 124 cm

Acceleration time 147 ms

Systolic ejection time 330 ms

Of the following choices, which additional 2D or Doppler echo findings would most likely be found?

A. Significant deterioration of the bioprosthetic leaflets with associated severe aortic valve regurgitation, a high flow state across the valve, and thus a high gradient across the valve

B. Heavy calcific and fibrotic changes on the leaflets, severely limiting leaflet motion, causing severe primary bioprosthetic valve stenosis

C. A significantly abnormal Doppler velocity index >0.35

D. Normal leaflets but evidence of severe patient–prosthetic valve mismatch with an indexed effective valve orifice area >0.85 cm²/m²

40. A 56-year-old male is 2 years status postplacement of a #25 Medtronic-Hall valve for aortic stenosis caused by a bicuspid valve. His aorta was left intact. Since the surgery, he has had no history of complications of either emboli or bleeding. He recently moved and now presents to the emergency department with complaints of occasional fever and night sweats but otherwise normal functional capacity. Laboratory exam is positive for an erythrocyte sedimentation rate of 44, a white blood count of 12,500, and an INR of 2.6. Blood cultures are pending. A transthoracic echocardiogram is ordered and shows normal left ventricular function with normal flow characteristics across the Medtronic-Hall valve, with the expected central jet of aortic regurgitation. No evidence of a perivalvular regurgitation jet is identified. The patient underwent a transesophageal echocardiogram and selected images from that study are shown in FIGURE 58.26 and VIDEO 58.14. Regarding the images shown, what is the most likely diagnosis?

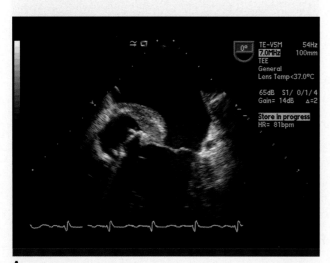

A

FIGURE 58.26

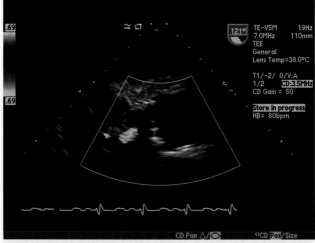

B

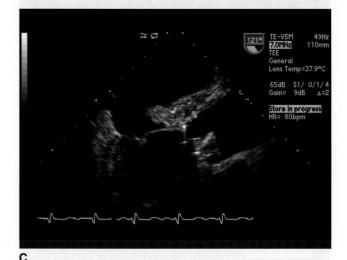

C

FIGURE 58.26 (*Continued*)

A. The Medtronic-Hall valve is normally positioned and normally functioning, with only a small, expected central jet of aortic regurgitation.

B. The valve appears normally positioned, and there is persistent postoperative thickening in the aortic annulus, an expected finding after this type of surgery.

C. The patient has developed an abscess of the native mitral valve, starting at the base of the anterior leaflet.

D. The patient has developed a periprosthetic aortic valve abscess even though there is no evidence of a perivalvular leak or vegetations.

41. The axial resolution at the focus of a single-element ultrasound transducer depends the **least** on which of the following variables?

A. Center frequency of the ultrasound transducer

B. Diameter of the ultrasound transducer

C. Backing material of the ultrasound transducer

D. Speed of sound of the medium

42. Which of the following comorbid conditions will **least** impact the simplified Bernoulli equation ($p = 4v^2$) to measure transaortic valve gradients?

  A. Severe aortic regurgitation
  B. Severe anemia
  C. Thyrotoxicosis
  D. AV fistula
  E. Severe mitral stenosis

43. True or False. Lateral resolution can be improved by reducing the spatial pulse length and increased damping.

  A. True
  B. False

44. Which of the following statements is most appropriate regarding aortic valve gradients?

  A. Aortic valve peak gradients by echo are instantaneous and overestimate the true gradient.
  B. Catheter-based aortic valve peak-to-peak gradients are generally lower than echo-based peak gradients.
  C. Increased cardiac output is more likely to affect measurement of catheter-based gradients rather than echo-based gradients.
  D. Catheter-based aortic valve mean gradients are generally higher than echo-based mean gradients.

45. Which of the following statements regarding etiology of aortic stenosis is most accurate?

  A. Calcific degenerative stenosis of a trileaflet valve is a more common indication for aortic valve replacement than bicuspid aortic valve disease with supraimposed calcification.
  B. Radiation damage typically involves severe aortic valve thickening without calcification.
  C. Commissural fusion is suggestive of an autoimmune etiology.
  D. A preserved second heart sound and a normal pulse typically do not exclude hemodynamically significant calcific degenerative aortic stenosis.

46. Which of the following is the correct slope to measure mitral deceleration time (Fig. 58.27)?

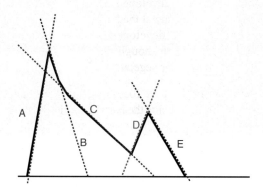

FIGURE 58.27

  A. A
  B. B
  C. C
  D. D
  E. E

47. Which of the following is true regarding the condition present in FIGURE 58.28 and VIDEO 58.15?

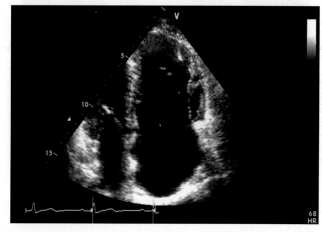

FIGURE 58.28

  A. Findings are limited to the tricuspid valve only.
  B. More than 50% of patients have a shunt at the atrial level with either a patent foramen ovale or secundum ASD, which results in varying degrees of cyanosis.
  C. The posterior leaflet of the tricuspid valve is usually sail-like and larger than normal.
  D. The most reliable echocardiographic indicator is reduced apical displacement of the septal insertion of the tricuspid valve.
  E. A displacement index of 8 mm is invariably associated with this abnormality.

48. What are the wall motion abnormalities in this patient who suffered a myocardial infarction (VIDEO 58.16)?

  A. Right ventricular free wall hypokinesis
  B. Anterior and anteroseptal akinesis
  C. Lateral and inferolateral wall akinesis
  D. Apical akinesis
  E. None of the options

49. Which of the following is a typical finding associated with the image in FIGURE 58.29?

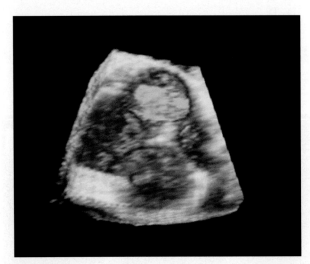

FIGURE **58.29**

A. Absence of associated hemodynamic abnormalities in over half of the cases
B. Aortic stenosis more commonly than aortic regurgitation
C. Concomitant congenital cardiac defects
D. Four equal cusps

50. Match the following imaging artifacts (FIGS. 58.30 through 58.34) with the best description.

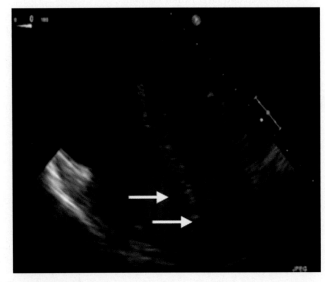

FIGURE **58.30**

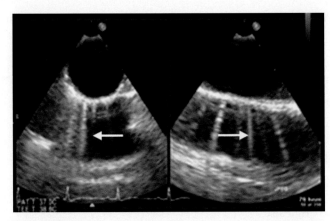

FIGURE **58.31**

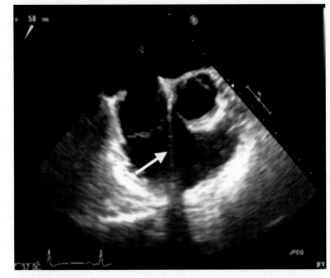

FIGURE **58.32**

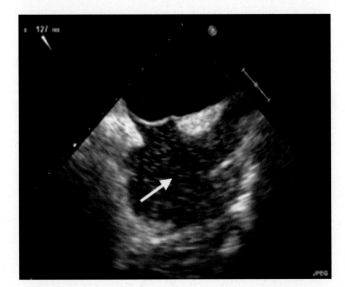

FIGURE **58.33**

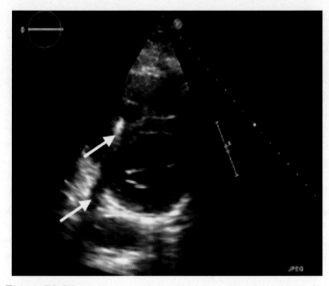

FIGURE 58.34

A. Comet tail (reverberation)
B. Mirror (duplication) artifact and scatter
C. Reverberation and ring down
D. Reverberation artifact and attenuation artifact
E. Lateral resolution artifact

51. A 55-year-old obese female presents with shortness of breath after undergoing right knee replacement. Transthoracic echocardiogram revealed normal left ventricular systolic function, no significant valvular disease, and the right heart findings depicted in FIGURE 58.35.

The left panel represents tissue Doppler recordings of the tricuspid annulus. The right panel shows M-mode recording of the tricuspid annulus. In addition, spectral Doppler of the tricuspid inflow was obtained (not shown); it revealed a peak E-wave velocity of 45 cm/s, a peak A-wave velocity of 28 cm/s, and a deceleration time (DT) of the tricuspid E wave 145 ms.

Which of the following is a correct statement?

A. The findings confirm the diagnosis of massive pulmonary embolism.
B. Tricuspid filling pattern demonstrates abnormal relaxation.
C. There is normal longitudinal RV systolic function.
D. Tricuspid annular tissue peak velocity of S wave is diminished.
E. Tricuspid E-wave DT is abnormally short.

52. Which of the following is true regarding biologic effects of ultrasound?

A. The two primary mechanisms of biologic effects of ultrasound are sound and thermal effect.
B. Stable cavitation is potentially more harmful than transient cavitation.
C. An unfocused beam carries more potential harm than a focused beam.
D. The risk of cavitation is not related to the mechanical index.
E. The most effective method during scanning to reduce biologic effect is to increase scan time.

53. Which of the following causes of tricuspid stenosis is demonstrated in VIDEO 58.17 and FIGURE 58.36?

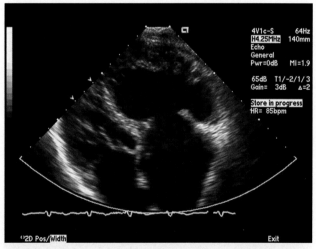

FIGURE 58.36

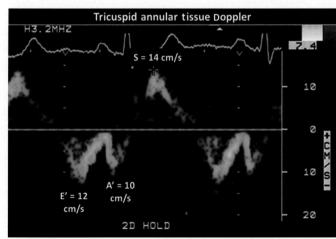

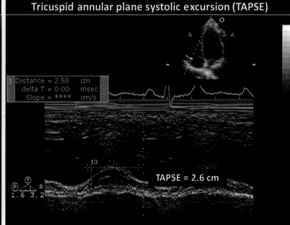

FIGURE 58.35

A. Rheumatic heart disease
B. Carcinoid syndrome
C. Ebstein abnormality
D. Lupus valvulitis
E. Pacemaker-induced adhesions

54. The correct formula to calculate Qp:Qs in a patient with an isolated patent ductus arteriosus (PDA) defect is:

A. RVOT flow/LVOT flow
B. LVOT flow/RVOT flow
C. Right pulmonary artery flow/LVOT flow
D. Tricuspid flow/mitral flow

55. A 45-year-old female is being evaluated for progressive shortness of breath over the past 6 weeks. Transthoracic echocardiography (TTE) was performed, and the following continuous-wave spectral Doppler tracing of the mitral regurgitant (MR) jet was obtained from the apical four-chamber view (FIG. 58.37).

Letters A through D represent Doppler velocities; corresponding time points are labeled Ta through Td.

Which is the correct formula for calculating left ventricular dP/dT, a measure of systolic function?

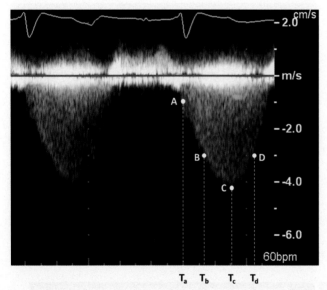

FIGURE 58.37

A. (4C2 to 4A2)/(Tc to Ta)
B. (4B2 to 4A2)/(Tb to Ta)
C. (4D2 to 4C2)/(Td to Tc)
D. (4D2 to 4B2)/(Td to Tb)
E. (4D2 to 4A2)/(Td to Ta)

Answers

Answer 1: D. There is a direct correlation between the PASP and the LAP (with this relationship adjusted by the cardiac output; e.g., the lower the CO, the higher the PCWP/PASP).

The expected LAP for a PASP of 45 mm Hg is approximately 20 mm Hg (for CO ~3.0 L/m) and approximately 40 mm Hg (for CO ~6.0 L/m).

Answer 2: A. The chamber quantification document has an excellent description on the controversial use of partition values for all echo parameters. In the end, due to lack of scientific evidence and limited data, only LVEF and LAVI have outcome-based partitions (e.g., moderate abnormality has a worse outcome than mild; severe is worse than moderate).

Answer 3: C. The video shows a vegetative mass with a possible flail AV leaflet, dilated and reduced LV systolic function, and reduced mitral valve opening due to the severe AR. The color flow Doppler is a diastolic phase and demonstrates low velocity, laminar MR (timed with end of AR). The M-mode confirms that the longer R-R intervals (patient is in AFib) are associated with early MV closure. The CW Doppler MR spectrum demonstrates a late diastolic MR component (again, only seen in the longer R-R intervals when the AR regurgitant volume raises the LVEDP greater than LAP).

Answer 4: E. This is a typical pattern in the LVOT in patients with true obstruction to flow as in hypertrophic "obstructive" cardiomyopathy and may be referred to as the "Lobster Claw Doppler pattern." See *J Am Soc Echocardiogr* 1997;10:707–712 for additional details.

Answer 5: A. There is systolic anterior motion (SAM) with prolonged septal contact (which is only noted in patients with severe LVOT obstruction). Although other causes of LV wall thickening may be seen with SAM, they rarely remain in contact with the septum that long to cause that degree of LVOT obstruction (90 mm Hg in this patient).

Answer 6: D. This still frame systolic color flow Doppler figure demonstrates turbulent flow in the LVOT and a typical eccentric MR jet timed with the increased outflow velocity and directed opposite (posterior) to this LVOT (anterior) jet (relating to the underlying etiology from systolic anterior motion of the MV). A is severe TR; B is takotsubo; C is an acute posterior wall infarct.

Answer 7: E. Although limited, this echocardiogram clearly demonstrates a large wall motion abnormality in the lateral, and inferolateral myocardial wall segments. Given his elevated cardiac biomarker and continued chest pain, urgent coronary revascularization for an acute coronary syndrome should be recommended. If there were additional features on the echocardiogram to suggest an aortic dissection (as a potential cause for the coronary infarction) such as an intimal dissection flap, acute aortic regurgitation, etc., then option A may have been reasonable. Option B would be reasonable if a diagnosis of ACS was not likely (or a cardiac contusion was being considered). Option C is not needed at this point but should be considered on his next echo exam. There is no reason for Option D at this time (see VIDEO 58.18).

Answer 8: A. This patient has a large left atrial mass arising from the atrial septum demonstrated on the apical four-chamber view. The most common cause for this, although relatively rare, is an atrial myxoma. The subcostal view confirms an additional large, frond-like, mobile mass arising from the atrial septum raising the possibility for biatrial myxoma (or possibly a thrombus-in-transit through a PFO). This latter diagnosis would be uncommon without risk factors or diagnosis of DVT and/or pulmonary emboli. Further, the 2D appearance is more random in shape ("myxoma like") rather than cavity-forming shape ("thrombus like").

See: http://dx.doi.org/10.1016/S0003-4975(98)00206-9 for additional reading.

Answer 9: B. The images demonstrate a moderate-sized patent arterial duct from the aorta to the pulmonary artery. There is left heart volume overload that should resolve with closure of this shunt. Without closure, this will evolve to Eisenmenger physiology ("large" PDA). Once visualized on transthoracic echo, there is no need for TEE (which may be more difficult than TTE). Surgery is rarely required except in failed attempt of closure in the cath lab. Therapy for either heart failure or aortic regurgitation (sometimes misdiagnosed on exam) is not adequate.

Answer 10: D. This patient has a typical takotsubo (apical ballooning syndrome) stress cardiomyopathy (SC) without a trigger (10% of presentations have no triggers). The initial LVEF has been demonstrated to be lower and this may represent the multivessel distribution less common in STEMI. Since both STEMI and SC may occur with stress, both are increased in natural disasters. Both have typical rise and fall biomarkers, but SC values are lower. It is now recognized that serious M&M is not uncommon and occurs at a 2% to 4% event rate in various registries. MPI may be abnormal initially, but normalizes quickly after presentation.

Additional reading: https://www.jstage.jst.go.jp/article/circj/78/9/78_CJ-14-0770/_pdf

Answer 11: E. This patient has mild TR at baseline and severe, free TR after the procedure. The only procedure that could do this from the list above is an RV biopsy with iatrogenic flail TV leaflets from torn major chordae.

Answer 12: D. According to the 2011 AUC guidelines, transesophageal echocardiography is rarely the first imaging test recommended. However, diagnosis of infective endocarditis with a moderate to high pretest probability with Staph bacteremia, fungemia prosthetic heart valve are intracardiac devise is deemed an appropriate indication.

Hence, the patient with *Candida albicans* bacteremia could directly proceed for transesophageal echocardiography.

Answer 13: E. There are no indications for asymptomatic patients listed in the 2011 AUC for echocardiography that are deemed "appropriate" for stress echocardiography for the purpose of coronary artery disease detection/cardiovascular risk assessment except an Agatston calcium score of > 400. Agatston scores > 400 are considered "appropriate" indications for stress echocardiography; scores < 100 are considered rarely appropriate; scores of 100 to 400 are of uncertain appropriateness.

Answer 14: C. In a patient with an elevated cardiac index (and hence stroke volume), but low ejection fraction, the LVEDD volume must be elevated. These parameters are consistent with aortic regurgitation. Both mitral regurgitation and ventricular septal defects result in increased stroke volumes and falsely increase the ejection fraction. Hence, these choices are incorrect. Tricuspid regurgitation does not directly affect the left ventricular ejection fraction.

Answer 15: A. The image represents an M-mode through the mitral valve demonstrating decrease slope (flattening) of the valve opening, and thickened anterior mitral valve leaflet consistent with mitral stenosis. Clinically, an opening snap would be auscultated. Tumor plop is incorrect and is heard with an atrial myxoma. A pericardial knock is heard with constriction, and third heart sound with restrictive heart disease, and there is no evidence of those on this study.

Answer 16: B. The M-mode image through the mitral valve shows a patient with hypertrophic cardiomyopathy. There is evidence of asymmetric hypertrophy of the septum. However, this is no evidence of systolic anterior motion of the mitral valve leaflet making choice C incorrect. There is an extra bump (B-bump) after the mitral valve opening, consistent with high left ventricular filling pressures. There is no evidence of mitral valve pathology, and based on the ECG, the patient is normal sinus rhythm (choice D is incorrect). There is no evidence of elevated pressures on the right side to suggest pulmonary hypertension, making choice E incorrect as well.

Answer 17: C. Basal LV longitudinal strain predicts mortality in patients with cardiac amyloidosis.

In the study by Koyama et al., basal LV longitudinal strain predicted mortality in patients with cardiac amyloidosis (Fig. 58.38). It is not common for athletes to have increased left ventricular wall thickness >13 mm (Fig. 58.39). The increased wall thickness seen in athletes regresses quickly with deconditioning.

In patients with increased LV wall thickness from cardiac amyloidosis, it is apical wall function that is better preserved than basal wall function (the opposite of what is written in response B). This can often better be demonstrated by strain imaging (Videos 58.19 and 58.20, Figs. 58.40 and 58.41). It is uncommon for athletes to have severe left atrial enlargement and uncommon for athletes to have a relatively small LV cavity size (Fig. 58.42).

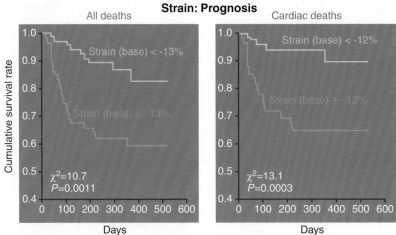

Strain: Prognosis

All deaths

Strain (base) < -13%

Strain (base) ≥ -13%

$\chi^2=10.7$
$P=0.0011$

Cumulative survival rate

Days

Cardiac deaths

Strain (base) < -12%

Strain (base) ≥ -12%

$\chi^2=13.1$
$P=0.0003$

Days

n = 119 patients with biopsy-proven AL amyloidosis
32 deaths (27%) over ~10-month follow-up

FIGURE 58.38

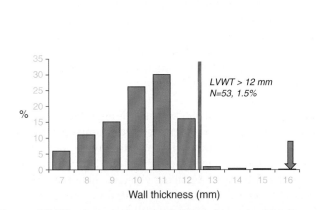

LVWT > 12 mm
N=53, 1.5%

Wall thickness (mm)

FIGURE 58.39

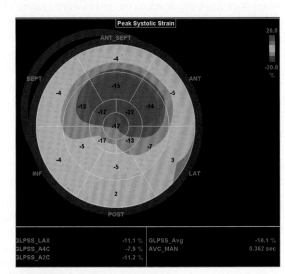

FIGURE 58.40

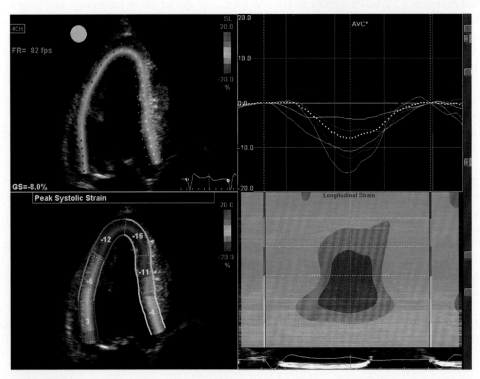

FIGURE 58.41

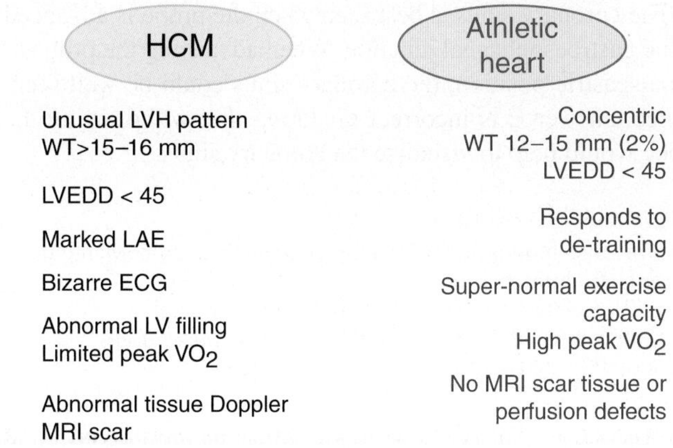

FIGURE 58.42

Suggested Readings

Basavarajaiah S, Wilson M, Whyte G, et al. Prevalence of hypertrophic cardiomyopathy in highly trained athletes: relevance to pre-participation screening. *J Am Coll Cardiol* 2008;51(10):1033–1039.

Koyama J, Falk RH. Prognostic significance of strain Doppler imaging in light-chain amyloidosis. *JACC Cardiovasc Imaging* 2010;3(4):333–342.

Maron BJ. Distinguishing hypertrophic cardiomyopathy from athlete's heart: a clinical problem of increasing magnitude and significance. *Heart* 2005;91(11):1380–1382.

Pelliccia A. Athlete's heart and hypertrophic cardiomyopathy. *Curr Cardiol Rep* 2000;2(2):166–171.

Pelliccia A, Maron BJ, De Luca R, et al. Remodeling of left ventricular hypertrophy in elite athletes after long-term deconditioning. *Circulation* 2002;105(8):944–949.

Pelliccia A, Maron BJ, Di Paolo FM, et al. Prevalence and clinical significance of left atrial remodeling in competitive athletes. *J Am Coll Cardiol* 2005;46(4):690–696.

Pelliccia A, Maron MS, Maron BJ. Assessment of left ventricular hypertrophy in a trained athlete: differential diagnosis of physiologic athlete's heart from pathologic hypertrophy. *Prog Cardiovasc Dis* 2012;54(5):387–396.

Phelan D, Collier P, Thavendiranathan P, et al. Relative apical sparing of longitudinal strain using two-dimensional speckle-tracking echocardiography is both sensitive and specific for the diagnosis of cardiac amyloidosis. *Heart* 2012;98(19):1442–1448.

***Answer 18:** D.* Velocity is fastest in bone (>4,000 m/s) and slowest in air (<350 m/s). Most soft tissue organs and blood are the same, and blood travels at 1,540 m/s (or 1.54 km/s).

The velocity of sound varies depending on the density of tissue as it travels through the medium. Table 58.1 represents the velocity of sound and various tissues.

Table 58.1	Velocity of Sound and Various Tissues
TISSUE TYPE	**VELOCITY (M/S)**
Air	330
Fat	1,450
Soft tissues	1,540
Blood	1,570
Muscle	1,580
Bone	4,080

Suggested Readings

King DL. Cardiac ultrasonography. Cross-sectional ultrasonic imaging of the heart. *Circulation* 1973;47:843–847.

vonRamm OT, Thurstone FL. Cardiac imaging using a phased array ultrasound system. I. System design. *Circulation* 1976;53:258–262.

***Answer 19:** D.* This is an example of the impact transducer frequency changes will have on 2D image quality. The parasternal short axis image on the left was recorded using a 3.0-MHz transducer, while the image on the right, a similar image, was obtained with a 5.0-MHz probe. The higher-frequency image has superior spatial resolution, which is very noticeable within the myocardium, where the lower-frequency image appears more "grainy" and the higher-frequency image is more "smooth." This smooth appearance is due to the ability of the higher spatial resolution to separate "two points very close together" into "two points" as opposed to "one point." The "points" or targets on this image reside within the heterogeneity of the normal LV myocardium.

Options A to C are incorrect since the focal point, the gain, and the probe were unchanged. Option E is incorrect since the LV myocardial image on the *right* has a noticeably higher spatial resolution (thus, confirming that Option D is the only correct answer).

Suggested Reading

Pye SD, Wild SR, McDicken WN. Adaptive time gain compensation for ultrasonic imaging. *Ultrasound Med Biol* 1992;18:205–212.

***Answer 20:** B.* Option A is incorrect since with tethering and shortening, the leaflets will fail to close completely, and the resultant MR jet will be directed toward the diseased leaflet. Option B is correct since the pattern of deformation of the mitral valve is symmetric in functional cardiomyopathy and asymmetric in ischemic MR. Option C is incorrect since the LV chamber and mitral annulus are more enlarged in functional rather than ischemic MR. Exercise Doppler may show a marked increase in MR grade. Option E is incorrect as the ERO of more than 0.2 cm² defines severe ischemic MR.

Suggested Reading

Kwan J, Shiota T, Agler DA, et al. Geometric differences of the mitral apparatus between ischemic and dilated cardiomyopathy with significant mitral regurgitation: real-time three-dimensional echocardiography study. *Circulation* 2003;107(8):1135.

***Answer 21:** C.* The image is a transgastric view. The marked segments are the midinferior and inferior septal segments, which are commonly supplied by the right coronary artery. Rarely, a dominant circumflex artery may also supply these segments. It is important to be cognizant of the fact that the segments will be reversed in the transgastric short axis view in TEE when compared to transthoracic short axis views (Video 58.21).

Suggested Reading

Lang RM, Bierig M, Devereux RB, et al. Recommendations for chamber quantification: a report from the American Society of Echocardiography's Guidelines and Standards Committee and the Chamber Quantification Writing Group, Developed in Conjunction with the European Association of Echocardiography, a Branch of the European Society of Cardiology. *J Am Soc Echocardiogr* 2005;18(12):1440–1463.

Answer 22: *C.* The image is close to a midesophageal bicaval view.

As noted in the image (Fig. 58.43), the left atrium (LA), right atrium (RA), and the interatrial septum (IAS) are visualized in this view. The SVC is to the right of the screen, while the IVC is to the left. In this patient, the structure marked with an asterisk is the eustachian valve, which is an embryologic remnant, attached to the IVC to RA junction. To better visualize this structure, the probe should be advanced toward the IVC. Therefore, answer C is correct.

To obtain this view, from a view of the short axis aortic valve, the probe should be rotated, so the ultrasound beam is directed more to the right of the patient. Clockwise rotation enables structures on the right side to be better visualized. Hence, answer A is incorrect in stating that counterclockwise rotation would obtain this view.

To visualize the SVC, the probe should be withdrawn from this position as the SVC is a superior structure. Further advancing the probe would help to better study the IVC and not the SVC. Hence, answer B is incorrect. In the video accompanying this question, a central catheter is seen in the SVC.

Clockwise rotation of the probe would not help to better evaluate the LA since the ultrasound beam needs to be focused to the left of the patient for this purpose. Hence, counterclockwise rotation would help to better evaluate the LA. Answer D is therefore incorrect.

The coronary sinus is best seen when the probe is advanced to the gastroesophageal junction. When advancing the probe to a transgastric position, the coronary sinus could be well seen. Hence, answer E is incorrect in stating that withdrawing the probe would help to visualize the coronary sinus.

Suggested Readings

http://pie.med.utoronto.ca/TEE/TEE_content/TEE_probeManipulation_intro.html
Peters PJ, Reinhardt S. The echocardiographic evaluation of intracardiac masses: a review. *J Am Soc Echocardiogr* 2006;19(2):230–240.

Answer 23: *C.* This is an M-mode across the aortic valve and aorta. In this image, the coaptation line of the aortic valve in diastole demonstrates significant eccentricity and is closer to the anterior border of the aorta (straight arrow, Fig. 58.44). This is a common characteristic finding in a bicuspid aortic valve. Therefore, answer C is the most correct answer.

A stenotic aortic valve would have reduced valve opening, which is not the case in this patient (blue arrow). Although M-mode is not able to directly correlate with the severity of AS, an opening >1.0 cm is not possible in a patient with an area <1.0 cm^2. Therefore, answer A is incorrect.

Although a small vegetative mass may be missed on M-mode echo, a large mass should be evident. There is no evidence of a high-frequency (independently mobile) echo-dense mass (vegetation) on this M-mode image. Answer B is therefore incorrect.

The motion of the aorta demonstrates a normal anterior–posterior motion, and the aortic valve opening is persistent through the entire systolic ejection. Both findings suggest a normal LV stroke volume. Therefore, answer D is incorrect.

Likewise, a normal-sized LA cavity (slightly >4.0 cm on this M-mode) rules out severe mitral stenosis. Answer E is incorrect.

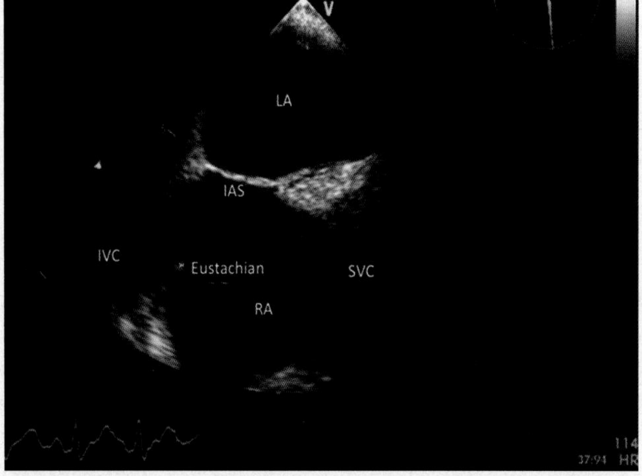

FIGURE 58.43

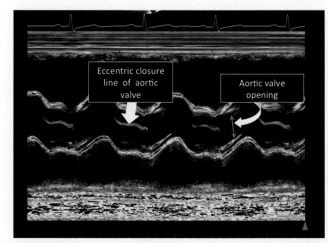

FIGURE 58.44 It is very uncommon for athletes to have significantly increased left ventricular wall thickness (LVWT); *n* = 3,500 elite athletes.

Suggested Readings

Corya BC, Rasmussen S, Phillips JF, et al. Forward stroke calculated from aortic valve echocardiograms in normal subjects and patients with mitral regurgitation secondary to left ventricular dysfunction. *Am J Cardiol* 1981;47:1215.

Nanda MC, Gramiak R, Manning J, et al. Echocardiographic recognition of the congenital bicuspid aortic valve. *Circulation* 1974;49:870–875.

Answer 24: B. Medical therapy with vasodilators has limited indications. It is indicated in patients with symptomatic severe aortic regurgitation or left ventricular dysfunction when valve replacement is not recommended (class I). Aortic valve replacement is indicated for symptomatic severe aortic regurgitation, asymptomatic severe aortic regurgitation, and LV systolic dysfunction (EF < 50%), and in those with severe aortic regurgitation while undergoing CABG or aortic surgery. Therefore, the single best choice to the above question is answer B.

Suggested Readings

Bonow RO, et al.; American College of Cardiology/American Heart Association Task Force on Practice Guidelines. 2008 focused update incorporated into the ACC/AHA 2006 guidelines for the management of patients with valvular heart disease: a report of the American College of Cardiology/American Heart Association Task Force on Practice Guidelines (Writing Committee to revise the 1998 guidelines for the management of patients with valvular heart disease). *J Am Coll Cardiol* 2008;52:e1–e142.

Answer 25: C. In patients with systolic left ventricular dysfunction and significant resting wall motion abnormalities, dobutamine echocardiography allows assessment of both viability and ischemia. Inclusion of low-dose stages (2.5 and 5 µg/kg/min) facilitates identification of viability and ischemia in segments that are abnormal at rest (1–3). Treadmill exercise EKG, treadmill echocardiography, and vasodilator stress echocardiography have poor sensitivity in identifying both viable and ischemic myocardium.

Suggested Readings

Afridi I, Kleiman NS, Raizner AE, et al. Dobutamine echocardiography in myocardial hibernation. Optimal dose and accuracy in predicting recovery of ventricular function after coronary angioplasty. *Circulation* 1995;91:663–670.

Pellikka PA, Nagueh SF, Elhendy AA, et al. American Society of Echocardiography recommendations for performance, interpretation, and application of stress echocardiography. *J Am Soc Echocardiogr* 2007;20:1021–1041.

Chaudhry FA, Iskandrian AE. Assessing myocardial viability in ischemic cardiomyopathy. *Echocardiography* 2005;22:57.

Answer 26: B. The basal short axis view allows for visualization of the aortic annulus. The aortic valve is trileaflet, comprised of the left, right, and noncoronary cusps. The noncoronary cup is easily recognized since it is intersected by the interatrial septum. ED comment: It is important to remember that the interatrial septal cusp is the NCC since this helps to identify anatomic leaflets regardless of view or type of echo (TTE or TEE). The right coronary cusp is the most anterior and adjacent to the right ventricular outflow tract. The left coronary cusp is the only one remaining. Superior angulation occasionally will allow visualization of the left main and right coronary arteries.

Suggested Readings

Netter FH. *Atlas of Human Anatomy*. 2nd ed. Teterboro, NJ: Icon Learning Systems, 2001:200–217.

Otto C. Transthoracic views, normal anatomy and flow patterns. In: *Textbook of Clinical Echocardiography*. 3rd ed. Philadelphia, PA: Elsevier Saunders, 2004:70–95.

Answer 27: B. The right ventricular inflow is obtained by starting in the parasternal long axis view; medial angulation of the probe allows for visualization of the right side of the heart. The scan plane courses through (as in this example) the posterior segment of the interventricular septum. The septal and anterior tricuspid valve leaflets are seen. Further clockwise rotation is necessary to remove the left ventricle (RV inflow is not parallel to LV), leaving only the right atrium and right ventricle. Now, the anterior and posterior TV leaflets will be seen as well as the posterior structures of the right atrium (eustachian valve and IVC) (Fig. 58.45).

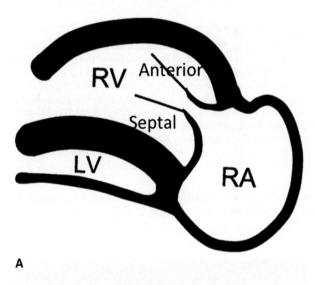

A

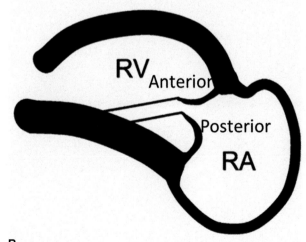

B

Figure 58.45

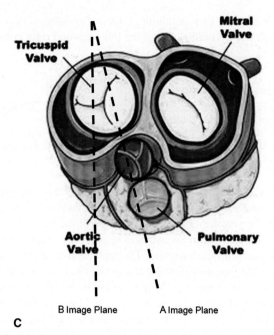

Tricuspid Valve
Mitral Valve

Aortic Valve
Pulmonary Valve

B Image Plane   A Image Plane

C

FIGURE 58.45 (*Continued*)

Suggested Readings

Anwar A, Geleijnse M, Soliman O, et al. Assessment of normal tricuspid valve anatomy in adults by real-time three-dimensional echocardiography. *Int J Cardiovasc Imaging* 2007;23(6):717–724.

Badano L, Agricola E, Perez L, et al. Evaluation of the tricuspid valve morphology and function by transthoracic real-time three-dimensional echocardiography. *Eur J Echocardiogr* 2009;10:477–484.

Feigenbaum H, Armstrong WF, Ryan T. The echocardiographic examination. In: Feigenbaum H, Armstrong WF, Ryan T, eds. *Feigenbaum's Echocardiography*. 7th ed. Philadelphia, PA: Lippincott Williams & Wilkins, 2010:91–122.

Answer 28: *E.* The suprasternal notch view is obtained with the probe pointed at the left shoulder and tilted down to parallel the aortic arch (FIG. 58.46, AA). Structures that can be

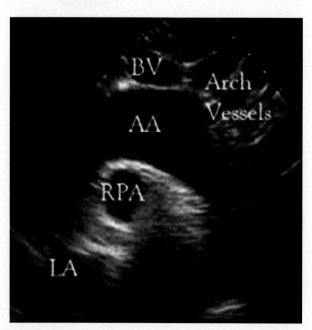

FIGURE 58.46

visualized in this view include the left brachiocephalic vein (BV) emptying into the SVC, right pulmonary artery (RPA) coursing under the arch, left atrium, and arch vessels. The arch vessels are difficult to identify unless all three are seen. The left pulmonary artery and right common carotid artery (branch of innominate artery) are not seen in this view.

Suggested Readings

Feigenbaum H, Armstrong WF, Ryan T. The echocardiographic examination. In: Feigenbaum H, Armstrong WF, Ryan T, eds. *Feigenbaum's Echocardiography*. 7th ed. Philadelphia, PA: Lippincott Williams & Wilkins, 2010:91–122.

Otto C. Transthoracic views, normal anatomy and flow patterns. In: *Textbook of Clinical Echocardiography*. 3rd ed. Philadelphia, PA: Elsevier Saunders, 2004:70–95.

Answer 29: *D.* Velocity of flow as determined by Doppler echocardiography honors the following equation:

$$V = \Delta f \times c / 2f_o \times \cos \theta$$

where V = velocity in m/s; Δf = the difference in the transmitted and received frequencies (shifted frequencies expressed in kHz); c = velocity of sound in the medium (which for blood is assumed to be 1,560 m/s); $2f_o$ = twice the frequency transmitted by the transducer (expressed in kHz); $\cos \theta$ is the cosine formed by the angle between the Doppler ultrasound interrogating beam and the actual true direction of the blood flow being interrogated.

Answer A is incorrect. Velocity is *inversely* proportional to the angle between the Doppler ultrasound interrogating beam and the direction of the blood flow being interrogated.

Answer B is incorrect. The speed of sound within the medium is not an important factor contributing significantly to the measured Doppler velocity, and blood flow is assumed to be 1,560 m/s. Since the actual Doppler frequency shift is very small and this is multiplied to such a proportionally large value, it is the change in frequency shift that primarily determines the velocity.

Answer C is incorrect. The small difference in the transmitted and received frequencies, or the *Doppler frequency shift*, is multiplied by the speed of sound and divided by twice the actual transducer frequency.

Answer D is correct. The measured velocity of blood flow is directly proportional to the Doppler shift, and, therefore, a decrease (or increase) in the Doppler frequency shift will decrease (or increase) the recorded velocity.

Answer E is incorrect. Velocity is equal to the frequency shift *multiplied by*, *not divided by*, a speed of sound constant times the cosine of the interrogating beam angle (and also times $2f_o$).

This formula is important and one of many the readers need to recite. It provides the basic understanding of the relationships between Doppler ultrasound frequency shifts and the subsequently determined blood flow velocity. This velocity is then converted to pressure using the Bernoulli equation, which is essential in nearly every echo examination.

Suggested Readings

Hatle L, Angelsen B. *Doppler Ultrasound in Cardiology: Physical Principles and Clinical Applications.* Philadelphia, PA: Lea & Febiger, 1985:32.

Hoskins PR. A review of the measurement of blood velocity and related quantities using Doppler ultrasound. *Proc Inst Mech Eng H* 1999;213:391–400.

Answer 30: ***B.*** Wall filter or high-pass filter eliminates frequency shifts below the set threshold. This definitely helps in eliminating low-frequency tissue movements from the spectral display but may also eliminate low-frequency shifts from slow flow. Increasing the wall filter threshold decreases the sensitivity to detect slow flow (Fig. 58.47).

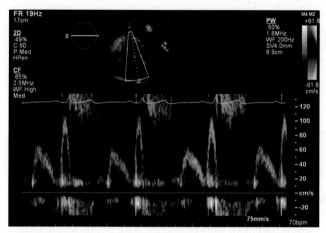

Figure 58.47

Suggested Reading

Armstrong WF. *Feigenbaum's Echocardiography.* 7th ed. Philadelphia, PA: Lippincott Williams & Wilkins, 2009.

Answer 31: ***C.*** The left subclavian artery, which supplies the face and left upper limb, demonstrates high-resistance flow signals with conventional spectral Doppler. This means flow signals are oriented in one direction in systole and in the opposite direction in diastole. The other vessels named supply the brain and characteristically show low-resistance flow; that is, flow signals are oriented in the same direction in both systole and diastole. Both internal and external carotid arteries show low-resistance flow signals. However, the external carotid artery generally shows sharper systolic velocity waveforms and lower velocity diastolic velocities as compared to the internal carotid vessel. Also, the internal carotid artery frequently has a more vertically oriented course compared to the external branch. This facilitates parallel placement of the Doppler beam resulting in accurate recording of velocities and is a potential advantage over the surface approach where it is impossible to align the Doppler beam parallel to flow direction. The external carotid is also differentiated from the internal carotid by the presence of branches. On the other hand, no branches originate from the initial carotid in its extracranial course.

Suggested Readings

Nanda NC, Biederman RW, Thakur AC, et al. Examination of left external and internal carotid arteries during transesophageal echocardiography. *Echocardiography* 1998;15:755–758.

Nanda NC, Thakur AC, Thakur D, et al. Transesophageal echocardiographic examination of left subclavian artery branches. *Echocardiography* 1999;16:217–277.

Answer 32: ***B.*** This view generally provides the maximum length between the mitral annulus and the apex and is the view with the least foreshortening. In general, TEE is inferior to TTE for comprehensive examination of the left ventricular apex. The other views often provide a foreshortened image of the left ventricle, resulting in nonvisualization or partial visualization of the apex.

Suggested Reading

Nanda NC, Domanski M. *Atlas of Transesophageal Echocardiography.* 2nd ed. Baltimore, MD: Lippincott Williams & Wilkins, 2007:304–325.

Answer 33: ***A.*** As the blood from the left atrium converges toward the stenotic mitral valve during diastole, blood velocity gradually increases forming a series of hemispheres. The velocity is equal along the surface of any one hemisphere, hence the name isovelocity.

Color flow imaging can be used to identify the isovelocity hemisphere. The red-blue aliasing interface (blue-red on TEE orientation) identifies one hemisphere. The velocity along this hemisphere is equal to the aliasing velocity. For all hemispheres, the surface velocity multiplied by the surface area is constant, for any valve. When the aliasing velocity is lower, the hemisphere is larger and farther away from the stenotic valve. The aliasing velocity can be altered by shifting the baseline. Generally, the baseline should be shifted in the direction of jet flow. Since diastolic flow is toward the left ventricular cavity or toward the transducer in TTE, the baseline should be shifted in this direction to obtain an optimally visualized and contoured hemispheric PISA. Answer A is therefore correct. If TEE is used, then the baseline will have to be shifted downward ("away" from the transducer, in the direction of blood flow). Note that the reverse is true in mitral regurgitation.

Aliasing velocity should be decreased in order to increase the radius of PISA. Answer (C) is therefore not true. Answer (D) is incorrect since it is possible to change the PISA radius as explained above.

Suggested Reading

Messika-Zeitoun D, Fung Yiu S, Cormier B, et al. Sequential assessment of mitral valve area during diastole using color M-mode flow convergence analysis: new insights into mitral stenosis physiology. *Eur Heart J* 2003;24:1244–1253.

Answer 34: ***A.*** Grade I diastolic dysfunction results in mitral inflow E/A ratio reversal and denotes the presence of mildly impaired left ventricular relaxation. Consequently, more time is required for pressure equalization to take place between the LA and the LV. Both mitral stenosis and mildly impaired LV relaxation prolong THE deceleration time and the pressure half-time. This results in an overestimation of the severity of mitral stenosis and an underestimation of mitral valve area.

The pressure half-time will be prolonged due to combination of delayed relaxation and mitral stenosis.

Suggested Readings

Karp K, Teien D, Bjerle P, et al. Reassessment of valve area determinations in mitral stenosis by the pressure half-time method: impact of left ventricular stiffness and peak diastolic pressure difference. *J Am Coll Cardiol* 1989;13:594–599.

Thomas JD, Wilkins GT, Choong CY, et al. Inaccuracy of mitral pressure half-time immediately after percutaneous mitral valvotomy. Dependence on transmitral gradient and left atrial and ventricular compliance. *Circulation* 1988;78:980–993.

Answer 35: A. The specificity of a test is determined by the false-positivity rate, whereas the sensitivity is determined by the false-negativity rate. Abnormal increase in blood pressure during stress can cause global or regional left ventricular dysfunction in the absence of epicardial coronary disease (1). This is due to increased myocardial oxygen demand exceeding the myocardial perfusion reserve (afterload mismatch). Other answer options list potential causes of a false-negative test (decreased sensitivity). The list of potential reasons for false-positive and false-negative stress echocardiography results is given in Table 58.2 (2).

Suggested Readings

1. Ha JW, Juracan EM, Mahoney DW, et al. Hypertensive response to exercise: a potential cause for new wall motion abnormality in the absence of coronary artery disease. *J Am Coll Cardiol* 2002;39:323–327.
2. Pellikka PA, Nagueh SF, Elhendy AA, et al. American Society of Echocardiography recommendations for performance, interpretation, and application of stress echocardiography. *J Am Soc Echocardiogr* 2007;20:1021–1041.

Answer 36: C.

Table 58.2	**Potential Reasons for False-Positive and False-Negative Stress Echocardiography Results**
FALSE-POSITIVE RESULTS	**FALSE-NEGATIVE RESULTS**
Hypertensive response to stress	Inadequate level of stress
Hypertrophic cardiomyopathy	Delays in image acquisition postexercise
Microvascular disease (syndrome X)	Single vessel disease, especially left circumflex
Nonischemic cardiomyopathy	Concentric left ventricular remodeling
Stress-induced cardiomyopathy	Hyperdynamic state in patients with mitral regurgitation or aortic regurgitation
Coronary spasm	
Abnormal septal motion due to pacing, conduction abnormalities, prior surgery, or right ventricular volume overload	Apical foreshortening

A. False. Persistence refers to temporal averaging and will cause the image to have a smoother or blurry appearance. Turning off the persistence will provide a raw unprocessed image that will appear grainy or nonsmoothed.

B. False. Power is the rate at which energy is transferred and describes the magnitude of the wave, which in turn affects the brightness of the image. The unit value of power is noted in watts; however, on ultrasound systems, power is noted by the mechanical index (MI) or thermal index (TI).

C. True. See discussion below.

D. False. Foreshortening the image plane will have no effect on the grainy appearance of the image but will impact appropriate visualization of the true apex.

Increasing compress and/or dynamic range will add shades of gray to the grayscale map and provide a softer or smoother image appearance. Conversely, lowering the compress and/or dynamic range will enhance the raw or grainy appearance of the image in which the image will appear darker without a wide range of shades of gray.

Suggested Readings

Carlsen EN. Ultrasound physics for the physician. A brief review. *J Clin Ultrasound* 1975;3:69–75.
Edelman SK. *Understanding Ultrasound Physics*. 3rd ed. Canada: KnowledgeMasters, 2004.
Kremkau F. Ultrasound physics. *Ultrasound Med Biol* 1991;17:411.
Kremkau FW. *Sonography Principles and Instruments*. 8th ed. China: Jeanne Olson, 2011.
McCulloch ML, Davis R. Practical scanning tips and considerations: a review of the basics. *Cardiac Ultrasound Today* 2003;9/10(9):171–199.

Answer 37: C. While a number of variables affect mitral E-wave and A-wave velocities (e.g., preload, LV compliance, LV relaxation properties, LA contractile function, mitral inflow obstruction), the primary single determinant of the mitral inflow velocities is the pressure gradient between the left atrium and the left ventricle during diastolic filling.

Suggested Readings

Appleton CP, Hatle LK, Popp RL. Relation of transmitral flow velocity patterns to left ventricular diastolic function: new insights from a combined hemodynamic and Doppler echocardiographic study. *J Am Coll Cardiol* 1988;12:426–440.
Nagueh SF, Smiseth OA, Appleton CP, et al. Recommendations for the evaluation of left ventricular diastolic function by echocardiography: an update from the American Society of Echocardiography and the European Association of Cardiovascular Imaging. *J Am Soc Echocardiogr* 2016;29:277–314.

Answer 38: B. It is very important when assessing pericardial effusion to identify if there is hemodynamic compromise related to the effusion. The diagnosis of tamponade is a clinical one, but two-dimensional and Doppler echocardiography play major roles in identifying the location and characteristics of effusions as well as their hemodynamic significance. Certain echocardiographic findings can be indicative of increased intrapericardial pressure, leading to tamponade physiology. Figure 58.48 shows the mitral inflow Doppler signal. Respirometer tracing is seen on the bottom of the view.

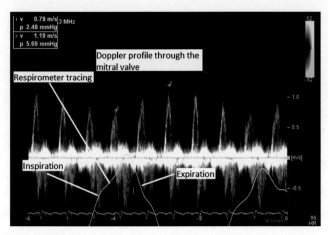

FIGURE 58.48

Mitral inflow E velocity decreases >25% during inspiration (point 1). During inspiration, the flow to the right ventricle increases. In tamponade, this increased RV flow causes a decrease of flow through the left side due to the shift of the ventricular septum leftward (a process called ventricular interdependence). Thus, a decrease in early mitral inflow is seen by a reduction in the E velocity. Accordingly, the flow out of the aortic valve will show a decrease during inspiration as well, which is illustrated in FIGURE 58.49. These changes play a primary role in the finding of pulsus paradoxus seen in clinical tamponade. FIGURE 58.22 reveals an M-mode tracing through the heart from the parasternal long axis view. The still picture shows the pericardial effusion anterior to the right ventricle. The M-mode tracing reveals early right ventricular diastolic collapse (FIG. 58.50 and seen in 2D here in VIDEO 58.22). The hepatic vein Doppler tracing in FIGURE 58.22 shows evidence of end-expiratory diastolic flow reversal (FIG. 58.51). This is seen in constrictive pericarditis as well and reflects the ventricular interdependence and the dissociation between intracardiac and intrathoracic pressures. FIGURE 58.21 is a hepatic vein Doppler tracing in a patient with severe tricuspid regurgitation. Systolic flow reversal within the hepatic vein is seen with each cardiac beat (FIG. 58.52). This pattern is the least likely to be seen in a patient with a hemodynamically significant pericardial effusion.

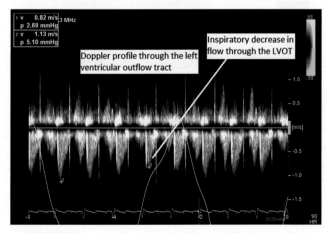

FIGURE 58.49

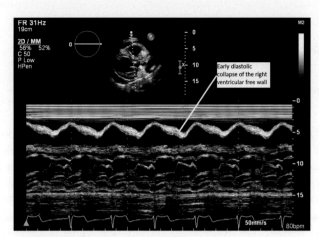

FIGURE 58.50

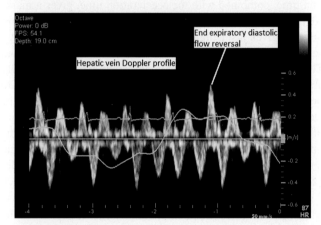

FIGURE 58.51

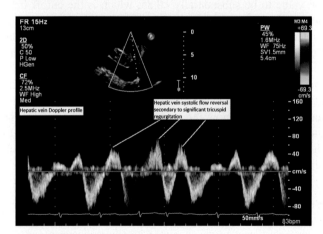

FIGURE 58.52 Proper wall filter setting.

Suggested Readings

Anderson DW, Virmani R, Reilly JM, et al. Prevalent myocarditis at necropsy in the acquired immunodeficiency syndrome. *J Am Coll Cardiol* 1988;11:792.

Cammarosano C, Lewis W. Cardiac lesions in acquired immune deficiency syndrome (AIDS). *J Am Coll Cardiol* 1985;5:703.

De Castro S, Migliau G, Silvestri A, et al. Heart involvement in AIDS: a prospective study during various stages of the disease. *Eur Heart J* 1992;13:1452.

De Castro S, d'Amati G, Gallo P, et al. Frequency of development of acute global left ventricular dysfunction in human immunodeficiency virus infection. *J Am Coll Cardiol* 1994;24:1018.

Eisenberg MJ, Gordon AS, Schiller NB. HIV-associated pericardial effusions. *Chest* 1992;102:956.

Shannon RP, Simon MA, Mathier MA, et al. Dilated cardiomyopathy associated with simian AIDS in nonhuman primates. *Circulation* 2000;101(2):185–193.

Sudano I, Spieker LE, Noll G, et al. Cardiovascular disease in HIV infection. *Am Heart J* 2006;151:1147.

Answer 39: *B.* This patient has severe bioprosthetic valve aortic stenosis. He has gradually developed significant calcific aortic valve disease over the last several years. The flow velocity signal in the figure is consistent with a very high gradient across the valve. In addition, the flow acceleration time is markedly prolonged at 147 ms, highly consistent with aortic stenosis. The shape of the forward flow signal is rounded, peaking in the middle of systole and not early. Systolic ejection time, combined with the acceleration time, gives a markedly abnormal ratio of 0.44. These values would be highly unlikely given just a high flow state across the valve caused by something such as severe anemia or severe aortic regurgitation. Thus, answer A is not correct. One would expect a markedly abnormal Doppler velocity index; however, the index should be markedly reduced and substantially <0.35. Recall that the Doppler velocity index is the ratio of the velocity time integral of the left ventricular outflow tract divided by the velocity time integral of the prosthetic valve. Assuming a relatively typical outflow tract velocity time integral of perhaps 28, the Doppler velocity index would be 0.22. Therefore, option C is incorrect.

Option D is only partially correct. The patient does have severe patient–prosthetic valve mismatch, but the listed value associated with this statement is incorrect. One would expect the value to be substantially <0.85, which is the cutoff for a normal effective orifice area index.

The 2009 American Society of Echocardiography guidelines (see Suggested Reading) suggest the following values for significant prosthetic valve stenosis: peak velocity >4 m/s, mean gradient >35 mm Hg, Doppler velocity index <0.25, effective orifice area <0.8, or an effective orifice area two standard deviations below the reference value for the valve. The guidelines also suggest that the contour of a stenotic valve, as in this case, should be rounded and symmetric and the acceleration time should be >100 ms.

Suggested Reading

Zoghbi WA, Chambers JB, Dumesnil JG, et al. Recommendations for evaluation of prosthetic valves with echocardiography and Doppler ultrasound: a report from the American Society of Echocardiography's Guidelines and Standards Committee and the Task Force on Prosthetic Valves, developed in conjunction with the American College of Cardiology Cardiovascular Imaging Committee, Cardiac Imaging Committee of the American Heart Association, the European Association of Echocardiography, a registered branch of the European Society of Cardiology, the Japanese Society of Echocardiography and the Canadian Society of Echocardiography, endorsed by the American College of Cardiology Foundation, American Heart Association, European Association of Echocardiography, a registered branch of the European Society of Cardiology, the Japanese Society of Echocardiography, and Canadian Society of Echocardiography. *J Am Soc Echocardiogr* 2009;22:975–1014.

Answer 40: *D.*

Editors' Note: *This question is entirely based upon the ability of the test taker to interpret echocardiographic images and provide the most correct option.*

Options A and B are incorrect options given the grossly abnormal appearance of the intervalvular fibrosa between the aorta and mitral valves.

Option C is not the best option since it would be exceedingly rare for a native mitral valve to develop an abscess.

Option D is most correct and importantly emphasizes the need for the echo boards taker to know that this disease process can occur in the absence of a clearly visualized perivalvular regurgitant AR jet or a prosthetic vegetative lesion.

Suggested Readings

Habib G, Badano L, Tribouilloy C, et al. Recommendations for the practice of echocardiography in infective endocarditis. *Eur J Echocardiogr* 2010;11:202–219.

Habib G, Thuny F, Avierinos JF. Prosthetic valve endocarditis: current approach and therapeutic options. *Prog Cardiovasc Dis* 2008;50:274–281.

Piper C, Korfer R, Horstkotte D. Prosthetic valve endocarditis. *Heart* 2001;85:590–593.

Answer 41: *B.*

Option A: True. The axial resolution is inversely proportional to the ultrasound center frequency.

Option B: False. The diameter of the ultrasound transducer does not typically affect axial resolution.

Option C: True. The backing material affects the bandwidth of the transducer, which is inversely proportional to the axial resolution (i.e., larger bandwidth = better resolution).

Option D: True. The speed of sound is proportional to axial resolution.

The *axial resolution* refers to the ability to resolve structures along the axis of ultrasound propagation (Fig. 58.53).

Given depth z, speed of sound c, and propagation time t, the following relations are helpful in understanding spatial resolution along the propagation axis of the ultrasonic wave:

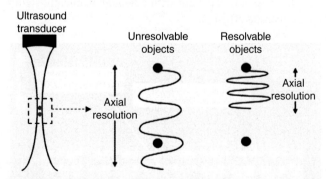

Figure 58.53 Axial resolution depends on the duration of the transmitted pulse. In this example, a single-element focused ultrasound transducer has an ultrasound beam that passes over two objects shown inside the *box* **(left)**. A low ultrasound frequency produces a relatively long transmitted ultrasound pulse, such that the two objects are unresolvable **(middle)**. The shorter pulse with higher ultrasound frequency (and shorter wavelength) is able to resolve the two objects **(right)**.

$z = (c/2)\,(t)$ [**range equation relates z to c and t**]

$\Delta z = (c/2)\,(\Delta t)$ [**axial resolution Δz related to the duration of the transmitted pulse Δt**]

$\Delta z = (\lambda/2)\,(f_0/\Delta f)$ [**relates Δz to wavelength, center frequency f_0, and bandwidth Δf**]

From the last equation, it is clear that the diameter of the ultrasound transducer is not a factor in determining the axial spatial resolution.

Suggested Readings

Hedrick WR, Hykes DL, Starchman DE. *Ultrasound Physics and Instrumentation*. 4th ed. St. Louis, MO: Elsevier/Mosby, 2005.

Szabo TL. *Diagnostic Ultrasound Imaging: Inside Out*. Boston, MA: Boston University Academic Press, 2004: Chapters 6 and 7.

Answer 42: E.

A. False. As in this setting, LVOT velocity is typically not normal.

B. False. As in A.

C. False. As in A.

D. False. As in A.

E. True. See discussion below.

This simplified version of the Bernoulli equation makes several assumptions that need to be considered in certain clinical scenarios. The most clinically relevant assumption is that LVOT velocity is negligible compared to transaortic valve velocity (as is typically the case with severe mitral stenosis). Thus, in conditions where LVOT velocity is increased (>1 m/s) such as in options A to D, a longer version of the formula ($\Delta p = 4(V_{AV}^2 - V_{LVOT}^2)$ should be used. Other assumptions include lack of a significant friction factor (viscosity) and the absence of a significant inertial or convective component to flow across a restrictive orifice.

Suggested Reading

Rijsterborgh H, Roelandt J. Doppler assessment of aortic stenosis: Bernoulli revisited. *Ultrasound Med Biol* 1987;13:241–248.

Answer 43: False. Lateral resolution is dependent on beam width, not on the spatial pulse length. Therefore, the statement is false. Damping (i.e., reducing the number of cycles) will have no effect on lateral resolution. Damping can improve axial resolution.

Suggested Readings

Baun J. *Physical Principles of General and Vascular Sonography*. San Francisco, CA: California Publishing Company, 2004: Chapter 14. ISBN 940471-35-3.

Kremkau FW. *Diagnostic Ultrasound: Physical Principles and Exercises*. New York, NY: Grune & Stratton, 1980. ISBN 0-8089-1233-X.

Answer 44: B.

A. False. Echocardiography by its nature can detect the actual maximal peak gradient at the vena contracta (location of the narrowest orifice, highest velocity, and lowest pressure) "in an instantaneous fashion" with negligible time lag and theoretically characterizes the true degree of stenosis.

B. True. See discussion below.

C. False. Without consideration of the increase in LVOT velocity, echo-based pressure gradients will typically be overestimated in the setting of increased cardiac output. Here, LVOT velocity would likely not be negligible compared to transaortic valve velocity and prohibit the use of the simplified version of the Bernoulli equation.

D. False. Unlike peak gradients, which are measured at one time point only, mean pressure gradients are averaged over systole and tend to be similar by catheterization and echo.

During measurement of peak aortic valve gradients by catheterization, the time lag involved in catheter "pullback" typically results in submaximal values being recorded that are typically lower than those measured by echocardiography. However, it has also been argued that the net pressure drop as obtained by distal pressure measurements including pressure recovery may serve as a better physiologic indicator of the hemodynamic significance of the stenosis.

Suggested Reading

Baumgartner H, Stefenelli T, Niederberger J, et al. "Overestimation" of catheter gradients by Doppler ultrasound in patients with aortic stenosis: a predictable manifestation of pressure recovery. *J Am Coll Cardiol* 1999;33:1655–1661.

Answer 45: C.

A. False. More than 50% of all valve replacements in Europe and the United States relate to bicuspid aortic valve disease although calcification of a trileaflet valve accounts for most of the remainder.

B. False. Radiation is typically associated with severe aortic valve leaflet calcification and also calcification of other structures such as the aorta and the mitral–aortic valve curtain.

C. True. See discussion below.

D. False. The clinical examination remains an important part of the assessment of a patient with suspected aortic stenosis. Signs that may help distinguish aortic sclerosis from hemodynamically significant aortic stenosis include preservation of the second heart sound, a normal pulse, and the absence of a mid to late peak intensity of the murmur.

Rheumatic disease, suggested by commissural fusion and systolic doming, rarely affects the aortic valve in isolation and typically also involves the mitral valve. Radiation-induced aortic stenosis occurs as part of a spectrum of extracardiac and cardiac lesions ("pancarditis") that include radiation-induced atherosclerosis; pericardial, myocardial, and valvular disease; as well as conduction abnormalities. However, concomitant manifestations of atherosclerosis and some degree of mitral regurgitation are commonly seen in patients with degenerative aortic stenosis.

Suggested Reading

Baumgartner H, Hung J, Bermejo J, et al. Echocardiographic assessment of valve stenosis: EAE/ASE recommendations for clinical practice. *Eur J Echocardiogr* 2009;10(1):1–25.

Answer 46: C. The mitral deceleration time is obtained by interrogating mitral inflow by placing a pulsed wave sample at the tips of the mitral leaflets during diastole. The early passive diastolic flow is the E wave, and the late flow, which occurs as a result of atrial contraction, is the A wave.

The deceleration time (DT) is defined as the time taken from the peak E-wave velocity to the baseline obtained by extrapolating along the velocity deceleration slope. Therefore, *answers A, D,* and *E* are all incorrect as they do not measure this slope.

In the event an early short rapid deceleration slope is followed by a slower longer deceleration slope, the time taken from the peak E velocity to the time taken for the slower deceleration slope to intersect the baseline is considered the mitral deceleration time. Therefore, *option B* is incorrect as it extrapolates the initial rapid deceleration slope ("ski slope") and not the slower deceleration slope (Fig. 58.54).

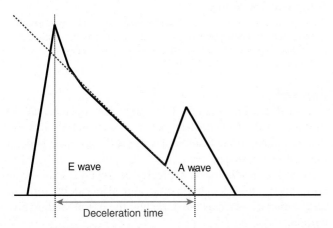

Figure 58.54 Correct slope for measurement of mitral deceleration time.

Suggested Readings

Appleton CP, Hatle LK. The natural history of ventricular filling abnormalities: assessment by two-dimensional and Doppler echocardiography. *Echocardiography* 1992;9:437–457.

Gilman G. Diastolic function: a sonographer's approach to the essential echocardiographic measurements of left ventricular diastolic function. *J Am Soc Echocardiogr* 2007;20(2):199–209.

Nagueh SF. Recommendations for the evaluation of left ventricular diastolic function by echocardiography. *J Am Soc Echocardiogr* 2009;22(2):107–33.

Answer 47: B. More than 50% of patients have a shunt at the atrial level with either a patent foramen ovale or secundum ASD, which results in varying degrees of cyanosis.

The image shows a patient with the typical characteristics of Ebstein anomaly. Although the orientation is not aligned as a standard ASE alignment (and has the RV on the right side of the display), the reader must be able to distinguish echo features to recognize this common variation. Of these features, apical displacement of the tricuspid valve is the most reliable indicator of an anatomic RV. Ebstein anomaly is a malformation of the tricuspid valve and right ventricle characterized by (a) adherence of the septal and posterior tricuspid leaflets to the underlying myocardium (failure of delamination); (b) apical displacement of the functional annulus; (c) dilation of the "atrialized" portion of the right ventricle with various degrees of hypertrophy and thinning of the wall; (d) redundancy, fenestrations, and tethering of the anterior leaflet with sail-like enlargement; and (e) dilation of the right atrioventricular junction. Note that clear diagnostic criteria are commonly tested in exams because they allow for decreased ambiguity of the answers. Answer A is incorrect as the findings are not limited to the tricuspid valve. Answer C is incorrect as the anterior leaflet is usually sail-like and larger. Echocardiography is the diagnostic test of choice for Ebstein anomaly and allows accurate evaluation of the tricuspid valve leaflets and size and function of the cardiac chambers. The principal echocardiographic feature is apical displacement of the septal leaflet of the tricuspid valve from the insertion of the anterior leaflet of the mitral valve by at least 8 mm/m^2 body surface area. Answer D is incorrect, as increased, and not decreased apical displacement is characteristic, and Answer E is incorrect as the tester needs to show awareness of the need to adjust the septal displacement for body surface area. Associated anatomic lesions include a shunt at the atrial level (>50%), ventricular septal defect, varying degrees of anatomic and physiologic RVOT obstruction, mitral valve prolapse, and left ventricular morphologic abnormalities.

Suggested Readings

Attenhofer Jost CH, Connolly HM, Dearani JA, et al. Ebstein's anomaly. *Circulation* 2007;115(2):277–285.

Shiina A, Seward JB, Edwards WD, et al. Two-dimensional echocardiographic spectrum of Ebstein's anomaly. Detailed anatomic assessment. *J Am Coll Cardiol* 1984;3:356–370.

Warnes CA, Williams RG, Bashore TM, et al. ACC/AHA 2008 guidelines for the management of adults with congenital heart disease: executive summary: a report of the American College of Cardiology/American Heart Association Task Force on Practice Guidelines. *Circulation* 2008;118(23):2395–451.

Answer 48: C.

Option A is incorrect since the right ventricle appears normal in size and contracts normally.

Option B is incorrect.

Option C is correct. There is akinesis of the lateral and inferolateral wall when compared to the opposing walls, which appear hyperdynamic.

Option D is incorrect. There are more extensive abnormalities other than just the apex.

Option E is incorrect.

This patient suffered an acute myocardial infarction involving the lateral and inferolateral wall, which in this case was a circumflex obstruction, which was then successfully revascularized.

Suggested Reading

Lang RM, Bierig M, Devereux RB, et al. Recommendations for chamber quantification: a report from the American Society of Echocardiography's Guidelines and Standards Committee and the Chamber Quantification Writing Group, developed in conjunction with the European Association of Echocardiography, a branch of the European Society of Cardiology. *J Am Soc Echocardiogr* 2005;18:1447.

Answer 49: A.

A. True. See discussion below.

B. False.

C. False.

D. False.

The congenital aortic valve demonstrated in the video is a quadricuspid AV. Quadricuspid aortic valve morphology is associated with hemodynamic abnormalities in fewer than half of cases, but when present, aortic regurgitation (44%) is a more common finding than aortic stenosis (VIDEO 58.23A). Quadricuspid aortic valve is not generally associated with other congenital cardiac defects, although concomitant patent ductus arteriosus, subvalvular aortic stenosis, ventricular septal defect, and mitral valve abnormalities have been described. The most common morphology is three equal large cusps and one smaller cusp. It has been suggested that the greater the degree of cusp asymmetry, the higher the risk of complications such as aortic regurgitation or endocarditis due to increased flow disturbance (VIDEO 58.23B).

Suggested Reading

James KB, Centorbi LK, Novoa R. Quadricuspid aortic valve. Case report and review of the literature. *Tex Heart Inst J* 1991;18:141–143.

Answer 50: FIGURE 58.30 = C, FIGURE 58.31 = B, FIGURE 58.32 = A, FIGURE 58.33 = E, FIGURE 58.34 = D.

FIGURE 58.30 depicts the ring-down phenomenon that results from the persistent ringing of the crystal within the transducer, causing the appearance of indiscreet echoes along lines of reverberation near the transducer. FIGURE 58.31 shows duplication of the aorta in orthogonal views. Also shown are bright lines of scatter emanating from the echogenic aortic wall. FIGURE 58.32 demonstrates the typical comet tail reverberation artifact. This artifact results in a diminishing trail of reverberations as the distance from the strongly reflective origin increases. FIGURE 58.33 depicts a splaying pattern of injected microbubbles, causing the bubbles to assume an elongated rather than spherical shape. The artifact results

from the intrinsic limitations of ultrasound lateral resolution. FIGURE 58.34 shows a catheter located within the right ventricle. The catheter is a strongly reflective object and causes the appearance of reverberation artifact seen as the bright, trailing pattern of echoes. It also causes attenuation of the distal soft tissue, specifically the basal inferoseptal LV wall, pericardium, and lung tissue.

Suggested Readings

Baun J. *Physical Principles of General and Vascular Sonography.* San Francisco, CA: California Publishing Company, 2004: Chapter 14. ISBN 940471-35-3.

Hedrick WR, Petersen CL. Image artifacts in real time ultrasound. *J Diagn Med Sonogr* 1995;11:300–308.

Kremkau FW. *Diagnostic Ultrasound: Physical Principles and Exercises.* New York, NY: Grune & Stratton, 1980. ISBN 0-8089-1233-X.

Scanlan KA. Sonographic artifacts and their origins. *Am J Radiol* 1991;156:1267–1272.

Answer 51: C.

Regarding individual answers:

A. Incorrect answer. Although the clinical scenario may suggest the diagnosis of pulmonary embolism, the echocardiographic findings are not confirmatory. Massive pulmonary embolism is typically associated with reduced right ventricular systolic function. This patient has normal TAPSE (≥ 1.6 cm) and peak S-wave velocity (≥ 10 cm/s) values, which argue against right ventricular systolic dysfunction.

B. Incorrect answer. An abnormal relaxation pattern is characterized by a tricuspid E/A ratio of <0.8. In this patient, E/A = 1.6 (normal 0.8 to 2.1). Furthermore, this patient has a normal tricuspid E/E' ratio of 3.8 (normal ≤ 6); this argues against RV diastolic dysfunction.

C. Correct answer. Tricuspid annular plane systolic excursion (TAPSE) is an M-mode technique that measures systolic displacement of the tricuspid annulus. Normal TAPSE values are ≥ 1.6 cm and correspond to normal longitudinal right ventricular systolic function.

D. Incorrect answer. The patient has normal S-wave velocity of 12 cm/s (normal ≥ 10 cm/s). Normal S-wave velocity is indicative of normal RV longitudinal contractility.

E. Incorrect answer. The patient has normal deceleration time (DT) of the tricuspid E wave (145 ms; normal ≥ 120 ms). Values <120 ms indicate restrictive filling pattern when tricuspid E/A >2.1. Note the different cutoff values for mitral versus tricuspid restrictive filling pattern (mitral restrictive pattern has DT <150 ms; tricuspid restrictive pattern has DT <120 ms).

Suggested Reading

Rudski LG, Lai WW, Afilalo J, et al. Guidelines for the echocardiographic assessment of the right heart in adults: a report from the American Society of Echocardiography endorsed by the European Association of Echocardiography, a registered branch of the European Society of Cardiology, and the Canadian Society of Echocardiography. *J Am Soc Echocardiogr* 2010;23(7):685–713.

Answer 52: *C.* The two primary biologic effects of ultrasound are cavitation and thermal effect. Sound, or noise, which is ultrasound produced during diagnostic scanning, is not known to be harmful to humans.

In stable cavitation, resonance of a gas-filled microbubble would expand and contract (compression and rarefaction) with no subsequent rupture of the bubble.

However, in transient cavitation, the gas-filled microbubble ruptures with possible injury to the surrounding tissue. Therefore, transient cavitation is potentially more harmful than stable cavitation.

A focused beam heats a small area of tissue and dissipates rapidly to the surrounding tissue, while an unfocused ultrasound beam heats a larger area with less opportunity for dissipation. Therefore, an unfocused ultrasound beam has a higher potential for biologic effects.

The risk of cavitation is directly related to the mechanical index.

The most effective method during scanning to reduce biologic effect is to decrease scan time.

Suggested Reading

EFSUMB. European Committee of Medical Ultrasound Safety 2006: Clinical Safety Statement for Diagnostic Ultrasound.

Answer 53: *B.* Tricuspid stenosis is the least common of the valvular stenosis lesions in the developed world given the low incidence of rheumatic heart disease. In carcinoid syndrome, the classic appearance of carcinoid involvement of the tricuspid valve involves severe immobility of the leaflets with a thickened, retracted valve and incomplete coaptation, as demonstrated in this clip (option B). Rheumatic tricuspid valve disease echocardiographic features include similar features to mitral valve changes with leaflet thickening, commissural fusion, and variable degrees of calcification. Ebstein anomaly (option C) is associated with tricuspid regurgitation and not stenosis in addition to the following morphologic features: (a) adherence of the septal and posterior tricuspid leaflets to the underlying myocardium (failure of delamination); (b) apical displacement of the functional annulus; (c) dilation of the "atrialized" portion of the right ventricle with various degrees of hypertrophy and thinning of the wall; (d) redundancy, fenestrations, and tethering of the anterior leaflet with sail-like enlargement; and (e) dilation of the right atrioventricular junction. Lupus valvulitis causes endocarditis-like vegetations on the valve and is an exceedingly rare and, hence, an unlikely cause of tricuspid stenosis (option D). No pacemaker lead is present; hence, option E is incorrect.

Suggested Readings

Baumgartner H, Hung J, Bermejo J, et al. Echocardiographic assessment of valve stenosis: EAE/ASE recommendations for clinical practice. *J Am Soc Echocardiogr* 2009;22(1):1–23.
Zoghbi WA, Enriquez-Sarano M, Foster E, et al. Recommendations for evaluation of the severity of native valvular regurgitation with two-dimensional and Doppler echocardiography. *J Am Soc Echocardiogr* 2003;16:777–802.

Answer 54: *B.* In a patient with a PDA, the flow across the pulmonary circulation includes the stroke volume through the pulmonary valve + the flow through the shunt. This cumulative blood volume returns through the pulmonary venous system and left atrium to the left ventricle. Therefore, in the setting of a PDA, the LVOT flow is the pulmonary flow.

The systemic flow comprises of the flow that is the remainder after blood shunts through the PDA from the aorta to the pulmonary artery. This blood volume returns to the heart through the systemic venous circulation and right atrium to the right ventricle. Hence, the RVOT flow is the systemic flow when a PDA is present.

Hence, Qp:Qs in the setting of a PDA is LVOT flow/RVOT flow. Therefore, answer B is correct.

When an atrial septal defect of ventricular septal defect is present, Qp:Qs would be the reverse of this since the shunt is intracardiac. Hence, in this instance, the Qp:Qs would be RVOT flow/LVOT flow.

Formulae in answers C and D are not of any significance.

Suggested Reading

Vargas-Barrón J, Sahn DJ, Valdes Cruz LM, et al. Clinical utility of two-dimensional Doppler echocardiographic techniques for estimating pulmonary to systemic blood flow ratios in children with left to right shunting atrial septal defect, ventricular septal defect or patent ductus arteriosus. *J Am Coll Cardiol* 1984;3:169–178.

Answer 55: *B.*
The rate of left ventricular pressure rise during early systole (dP/dT) is a measure of left ventricular systolic function. dP/dT can be calculated using the continuous-wave Doppler tracing of the MR jet.

dP/dT represents the slope of an MR jet Doppler tracing between two time points in early systole. By convention, the first time point is when the MR jet velocity reaches 1 m/s (point A in Fig. 58.37). The second one when the MR jet velocity reaches 3 m/s (point B in Fig. 58.37).

One can increase accuracy of these measurements by increasing the sweep speed to make the mitral regurgitant jet Doppler envelope as wide as possible and by decreasing the velocity scale to just above 3 m/s.

Using the simplified Bernoulli equation ($dP = 4V^2$), the pressure difference between points A and B can be calculated as follows:

$dP = 4A^2 - 4B^2$

$dP = 4 \times (3 \text{ m/s})^2 - 4 \times (1 \text{ m/s})^2$

$dP = 36 - 4 = 32 \text{ mm Hg}$

Thus, to calculate the left ventricular dP/dT, one only needs to measure the time interval (in seconds) between points A and B.

$dP/dT = 32 \text{ mm Hg}/dT \text{(in seconds)}$

In the patient above, dT = Tb − Ta = 0.12 s.

dP/dT = 32 mm Hg/0.12 s

dP/dT = 267 mm Hg/s

This patient has markedly diminished left ventricular systolic function (flat slope). Normal dP/dT is typically >1,000 mm Hg/s (steep slope).

Suggested Readings

Bargiggia GS, Bertucci C, Recusani F, et al. A new method for estimating left ventricular dP/dt by continuous wave Doppler-echocardiography. Validation studies at cardiac catheterization. *Circulation* 1989;80(5):1287–1292.

Mason DT, Braunwald E, Covell JW, et al. Assessment of cardiac contractility. The relation between the rate of pressure rise and ventricular pressure during isovolumic systole. *Circulation* 1971;44(1):47–58.

Index

Note: Page locators followed by f and t indicates figure and table respectively.

A

AAD (acute aortic dissection) extension, 429, 429f, 432, 433f

AAS. *See* Acute aortic syndromes (AAS)

Abascal score. *See* Wilkins score

Abscess formation, prosthetic valve, 170, 177–178

Acoustic coupling gels, ultrasound, 12, 17

Acquired pulmonary stenosis
  carcinoid disease, 158, 162
  intracardiac tumors, 158, 162

Acute aortic dissection (AAD) extension, 429, 429f, 432, 433f

Acute aortic syndromes (AAS)
  with AAD extension, 429, 429f, 432, 433f
  and acute valvular lesion, 7–8
  aortic root and stenosis, 431, 436–437
  with ascending aortic aneurysm, 432, 437
  asymptomatic patients with, 432, 437
  bicuspid aortic valve, 431, 436–437
  chest pain, 432, 437–438, 438f
  early rupture of aortic aneurysms, 431, 436
  infective endocarditis, 431, 431f, 437
  an intramural hematoma, 430, 430f, 435–436, 435f
  leaflet fusion, 431, 437
  with Marfan syndrome, 432, 437
  medical therapy of, 429–430, 429f–430f, 433, 434f
  patient management of, 429–430, 429f–430f, 433, 434f
  sporadic mutation, 430, 430f, 436
  with thoracic aortic aneurysm, 432, 437
  transcatheter aortic valve replacement, 431, 431f, 437
  transthoracic echocardiogram, 430, 430f, 431, 431f, 437
  Turner syndrome, 436

Adriamycin cardiotoxicity, 277, 284

Agitated saline bubble study, 309, 313
  intracardiac shunt evaluation, 533, 540, 541f
  shunt physiology, 532, 532f, 539

AHCM (apical hypertrophic cardiomyopathy), 531, 536

AIUM. *See* American Institute of Ultrasound Medication (AIUM)

Akinesis, 229, 234

ALARA principle, 72, 73

ALCAPA (anomalous origin of left coronary artery from pulmonary artery), 311, 317, 328, 333

Alcohol septal ablation, 524, 524f, 527

Aliasing velocity
  artifact, pulsed-wave Doppler, 24, 27–28
  mitral valve area calculation, 137, 139
  pulse repetition frequency, 23, 26, 26t

Aliasing velocity. *See also* Nyquist limit

American Institute of Ultrasound Medication (AIUM), 72

American Society of Echocardiography, 532, 538, 554, 568

Amplatz device, 297f–298f, 298, 301

Amplatzer septal occluder device, 231, 231f, 236

Amyloidosis, 276, 276f, 279
  diagnosis of, 289, 289f, 293
  pericardiocentesis, 278, 284
  subtypes, 289, 289f, 293

Aneurysmectomy, 234, 238

Aneurysms, 326, 326f, 329–330

Annular dilation, 148

Anomalous origin of left coronary artery from pulmonary artery (ALCAPA), 311, 317, 328, 333

Anterior mitral valve leaflet, 533, 540

Anterolateral papillary muscle, 229, 234

Anthracycline-related cardiomyopathy, 287, 291–292

Anthracyclines, 262, 266
  cardiotoxicity, 287, 291–292

Antibiotic prophylaxis, 367–368, 378

Anticoagulation, 230, 235

Anticramming, optimal standardized test-taking, 2

Aorta
  diastolic flow, 425, 427f, 428
  embolic events risk of, 423, 425
  FAP study criteria, 423, 426
  innominate artery, 424, 424f, 426
  Loeys-Dietz syndrome, 424, 427
  luminal narrowing, 423, 425
  Marfan syndrome, 425, 427
  midesophageal TEE view, 423, 423f, 426

  peak systolic, 423, 423f, 425
  pericardial cyst, 425, 428, 428f
  plaque, 423, 425
  right common carotid artery, 424, 424f, 426
  sinus of Valsalva aneurysms, 425, 428
  structure identification, 424, 424f, 426
  subcostal views, 424f, 425, 428
  TEE views, 423, 426
  thoracic (*See* Thoracic aorta)
  Turner syndrome, 424, 424f, 426
  valve abnormalities, 423, 423f, 425

Aortic aneurysm repair, 252, 252f

Aortic arch, plane orientation, 94, 97

Aortic dissection
  linear echo with irregular motion, wiggling worm, 103, 104
  pericardial effusions, 399, 403
  Stanford classification, 8

Aortic regurgitant jet, 208, 208f, 214, 214f

Aortic regurgitation (AR), 295, 299, 551, 563
  ascending aorta, dissection flap, 7–8
  assessment parameters, 129, 133
  CW Doppler, 369, 369f, 370, 378, 379
  diastolic flow, 532–533, 533f, 539, 539f
  echocardiographic evaluation indications, 129, 133
  etiology, 129, 134
  holodiastolic flow reversal, 369, 369f, 379
  mild/moderate, M-mode, 128, 132, 132f
  moderate to severe, 128, 133, 133f
  vena contracta, 129, 134

Aortic root dilation and aortic coarctation, 119, 126–127

Aortic root replacement, 447, 464

Aortic stenosis (AS)
  calcification, moderate to severe, 118, 124
  commissural fusion, 118, 125
  continuous-wave Doppler signal, 210, 210f, 215
  continuous-wave spectral Doppler tracings, 115, 115f, 120
  dimensionless index, 117, 122
  echocardiographic assessment, 170, 178

575

Aortic stenosis (AS) (*Continued*)
  fixed subvalvular, 118, 125
  low-output low-gradient severe, 117, 123
  pseudosevere, 117, 122
  pulmonary stenosis, 193, 199
  severity assessment, 116, 116f, 120, 120f–121f
  spectral Doppler signals, 147, 153, 153f
  subclavian artery stenosis, 193, 199
  supravalvular aortic stenosis, 193, 199
  TTE, 189, 189f, 196
  ventricular septal defect, 193, 199
Aortic syndrome, acute, 7–8
Aortic transection, 103, 104
Aortic translocation. *See* Nikaidoh repair
Aortic valve
  balloon dilation, 523, 523f, 526
  continuity equation, 117, 121
  continuous-wave Doppler, 193, 199, 210, 210f, 215
  contrast administration, 193, 199
  coronary cusp, 85, 86f, 89
  Doppler gradient optimization, 193, 199
  echocardiographic assessment, 170, 178
  emergent surgical replacement, 523–524, 523f, 526
  endocarditis, 369, 369f, 370, 379
  M-mode measurements, 204, 207
  papillary fibroelastoma, 367, 374, 376
  parasternal short-axis, 534, 534f, 542, 542f
  patient positioning, 193, 199
  peak and mean gradients, 193, 199
  peak aortic valve gradients, 117, 122
  Pedoff probe, 193, 199
  quadricuspid morphology, 118, 126
  suprasternal notch imaging, 193, 199
  unicuspid morphology, 118, 126
  vegetation, 370, 370f, 380–381
Aortic valve area (AVA), 193, 198
Aortic valve coronary cusp, 551, 551f, 563
Aortic valve gradients, 555, 569–570
Apical ballooning syndrome, 259, 259f, 262
Apical four-chamber view, 87, 87f, 91, 92f
Apical hypertrophic cardiomyopathy (AHCM), 531, 536
Apical thrombus, 531, 536
Apical-variant hypertrophic cardiomyopathy, 289–290, 289f
Appropriate Use Criteria (AUC)
  appropriate imaging test, 75, 77
  for TTE, 156, 160
  valvular heart disease, 75, 78

Area–length method, 224, 227
Arrhythmogenic right ventricular cardiomyopathy/dysplasia (ARVC/ARVD), 262, 265, 266, 286, 286f, 291
Arterial anomalies
  aortic dissection, 327, 330
  arterial hypertension, 326, 326f, 330
  bicuspid aortic valve, 326, 330
  cerebral aneurysms, 326, 326f, 329–330
  complete heart block, 327, 331
  complete transposition of, 326, 329
  coronary artery aneurysm, 328, 331–332
  Mustard/Senning repair, 326, 329
  pulmonary valve stenosis, 327, 330
  renal abnormalities, 327, 330
  rib notching, 326, 330
Arterial hypertension
  ACC/AHA guidelines, 533, 539
  arterial anomalies, 326, 326f, 330
Arterial switch operation (ASO), 340, 439, 450
Artifact, 556–557, 556f, 557f, 571
  aliasing, pulsed-wave Doppler, 24, 27–28
  aorta duplication, 58, 58f, 66
  attenuation, 55, 62, 63f
  comet tail, 58, 58f, 61, 66
  description, ultrasound, 13, 13f–14f, 19–22
  with Doppler echo
    bidirectional flow artifact, 68, 69
    vs. conventional 2D, 69, 70
    ECMO, 68–69, 68f, 70, 70f
    mechanical prosthetic aortic valve, 69, 69f, 70
    shift, 69–71
    transducer frequency, 69, 71
  enhancement, 13, 19, 21, 56, 64–65
  infused microbubbles, 57–58, 57f, 66
  injected microbubbles, 58, 58f, 66
  mirror, 56, 64–65
  mirror-image artifacts, 21, 21f
  misregistration, returning ultrasound, 57, 65, 65f
  real pathology as, 13, 20
  refraction (or lens) artifacts, 21, 22f
  resolution axial, 54, 54f, 59–60
  reverberation, 20, 20f, 21f, 55, 56, 58, 58f, 60–61, 61f, 63f, 64–66
  ring-down, 13, 19–21, 56, 58, 58f, 65, 66
  shadowing, 13, 19, 21, 57, 57f, 66
  side-lobe, 13, 20–21, 21f, 55, 60, 63, 63f

speckle artifact, wave interference, 55, 60
  stitch, 67
ARVC/ARVD (arrhythmogenic right ventricular cardiomyopathy/dysplasia), 262, 265
Ascending aorta, 97, 101
Ascending aortic aneurysm, 97, 101
ASCeXAM, 1, 2
ASO (arterial switch operation), 340, 439, 450
Aspirin, 349, 351
Atelectatic lung segment, 106, 106f, 109
Atria, pathologic masses in, 355–358
Atrial baffle leak, 326
Atrial fibrillation
  clinical setting of, 138, 142, 143f
  echo-relevant guidelines, 446, 463–464
  exercise echocardiography, 250, 255
  hypertrophic cardiomyopathy, 271, 274
  metoprolol, 370, 379
  transesophageal echo study, 356, 356f, 358
  transesophageal echocardiography, 356, 356f, 358
  warfarin, 370, 381
Atrial flutter, 326
  ablation, right ventricle, 225, 229, 229f
Atrial septal defect (ASD), 555, 570
  anatomy, 499, 499f, 508
  echocardiographic signs, 309, 312
  echo-relevant guidelines, 443, 456
  heart rate, 309, 313
  largest-sized defect, 297f–298f, 298, 300
  mitral valve pathology, 499, 499f, 508
  ostium secundum, 297f–298f, 298, 300
  patch surgical closure with, 526, 526f, 529
  pressure gradient, 309, 313
  pulmonary vascular resistance, 309, 313
  rim of tissue size, 299f–300f, 298, 300
  secundum, 309, 312–313
  sinus venosus, 297f–298f, 298, 300, 309, 312, 531, 536, 537
  size, 309, 313
  surgical view, 439, 449
  transcatheter, 297f–298f, 298, 300
Atrioventricular canal defects, 326, 341, 344, 349, 351
Atrioventricular dyssynchrony, 296–297, 297f, 300
Atrioventricular optimization, 303, 307

Atropine, 242, 246, 247
Attenuation coefficient, tissue, 39, 40
Audio signal, Doppler ultrasound, 24, 27, 27f
AVA (aortic valve area), 193, 198
A-wave velocities, 552, 566
Axial resolution, 55, 62, 554, 569

B
Bacterial endocarditis, tricuspid valve resection, 156, 156f, 161
Balloon aortic valvuloplasty, 326, 330
Balloon valvuloplasty, 318–319, 318f, 321, 431, 431f, 437
Basal septal hypertrophy, 445, 460–461
Baseline dyssynchrony, 303, 306, 306f
BAV. *See* Bicuspid aortic valve (BAV)
Benign premature atrial contractions, 349, 351
Benign tumor, 355, 355f, 356
Bernoulli equation, 555, 558, 569, 572–573
    beam angulation, 32, 37, 37f
    transaortic valve gradients measurement, 116, 121
Berry aneurysms, 330
Bicaval technique, 290, 294
Bicuspid aortic valve (BAV), 318, 318f, 319–321, 323–324
    AAS, 431, 436–437
    arterial anomalies, 326
    congenital valve anomaly, M-mode, 128, 132
    echocardiographic finding, 318, 318f, 320–321
Bicuspid valves, 170, 178
Bioprosthetic aortic valve
    aortic paravalvular abscess, 372, 372f, 383
    endocarditis, 373, 383, 387
    fistulous flow, 372, 372f, 383
    stenosis, 553–554, 553f, 568
        calcific and fibrotic change, 164–165, 164f, 173
        continuous-wave Doppler examination, 164–165, 164f, 173
        Doppler velocity index, 164–165, 164f, 173
        patient-prosthetic valve mismatch, 164, 164f, 173
    vegetation, 372, 372f, 383
Bioprosthetic valves, dense structures, 166, 174–175, 174f
Biphasic cardiac response, 535, 535f, 543, 543f
Biphasic pattern, 448, 467

Biplane modified Simpson method, 359, 363
Biplane Simpson method, 181, 186, 233–234, 237
Blood velocity measurement, color Doppler imaging, 39, 41–42, 42f
Brachiocephalic vein, left, 87, 87f, 91
Breast cancer, echo-relevant guidelines, 442, 455

C
CAD. *See* Coronary artery disease (CAD)
Calcification, 370, 381–382
    moderate to severe, aortic stenosis, 118, 124
Cancer therapeutic–related cardiac dysfunction (CTRCD), 442, 455
Candida albicans bacteremia, 559
Carcinoid syndrome, 557–558, 557f, 572
    acquired pulmonary stenosis, 158, 162
    RA pressure, 224, 224f, 227
    tricuspid stenosis, 156, 156f, 160
    tricuspid valve appearance, 155, 158
    valvular involvement, 155, 158
Cardiac amyloidosis, 278, 284, 549, 559, 560f
    diagnosis of, 289, 291f, 293
    echocardiographic diagnosis of, 277f, 278, 284
    left ventricular wall thickness, 261, 266
    strain and strain rate Doppler imaging method, 277f, 278, 284
Cardiac biomarker (troponin)
    elevation, 396, 399–400
    tamponade and myocyte damage, 396, 400
Cardiac chambers, 442, 455, 460
Cardiac devices
    Amplatz device, 297f–299f, 298, 301
    LARIAT, 298, 301
    pericardial effusion, 298, 301
Cardiac magnetic resonance imaging (CMR), 410, 419, 420f, 472, 479
Cardiac malformation, L-transposition of great vessels, 319, 322
Cardiac papilloma, 367, 376
Cardiac resynchronization therapy (CRT), 302, 304
    baseline dyssynchrony, 303, 306, 306f
    clinical benefits, 304, 307
    echo strain, 487, 494
    intra-atrial conduction delay, 303, 303f, 307
    papillary muscle closing forces, 303, 305f, 307

TARGET and STARTER trial, 304, 307
    women with nonischemic cardiomyopathy, 303, 307
    Yu index, 302, 305
Cardiac sarcoidosis. *See* Sarcoidosis
Cardiac shunt lesions
    agitated saline bubble study, 309, 313
    ASD, 309, 313
    desaturation of patient, 311, 314–315
    left-to-right shunting, 311, 315
    muscular VSD, 310, 310f, 314
    pulmonary artery systolic pressure, 311, 311f, 316
    secundum ASD, 309, 312–313
    sinus venosus ASD, 309, 312
    stroke volume measurement, 310, 310f, 313–314
    ventricular septal defect velocity, 310, 310f, 314
Cardiac silhouette, 396, 400
Cardiac surgery, echo-relevant guidelines, 443, 456–457
Cardiac valves, 370, 381, 382
Cardiomyopathy, 362, 367. *See* Anthracycline-related cardiomyopathy; Apical hypertrophic cardiomyopathy (AHCM); Apical-variant hypertrophic cardiomyopathy; Arrhythmogenic right ventricular cardiomyopathy/dysplasia (ARVC/ARVD); Chemotherapy-induced cardiomyopathy; Dilated cardiomyopathy; Eosinophilic cardiomyopathy; Familial dilated cardiomyopathy; Hypertrophic cardiomyopathy (HCM); Hypertrophic obstructive cardiomyopathy; Idiopathic restrictive cardiomyopathy; Infiltrative cardiomyopathy; Ischemic cardiomyopathy; Obstructive hypertrophic cardiomyopathy; Peripartum cardiomyopathy; Restrictive cardiomyopathy; Stress-induced cardiomyopathy
Cardiothoracic surgery consultation, 362–363, 363f, 366, 547, 559
Cardiotoxicity, anthracycline therapy, 287, 291–292
Cardiovascular disease
    complications, 241, 246
    preoperative risk assessment, 242, 246
    transthoracic 2D echo, 242, 246
Cardiovascular implantable electronic device (CIED) infection, 296, 296f, 299–300

Carotid artery flow velocity pattern, 501, 502f, 510
Carotid bulb examination, 94, 98
Carpentier classification, 145, 149, 149f, 149t
CAVC (complete atrioventricular canal defect), 319, 323
Cavitation, 557, 572
Cavity obliteration, 365
Ceftriaxone, 367, 374
CFD (color flow Doppler), 32, 38, 39, 41–42, 72, 74, 295, 299, 302, 305, 305f, 552, 565–566
Chagas disease, 288–289, 288f, 292–293
Chelation therapy, 276, 279–280
Chemotherapy-induced cardiomyopathy, 262, 266, 267f
Chest pain, 547, 559
   etiology of, 107, 107f, 110
   saddle pulmonary embolus, 107, 107f, 110
   thrombolysis, 107, 107f, 110
Chest x-ray, cardiac silhouette, 396, 400
Chiari network, 86, 90, 356, 357
Chondroectodermal dysplasia. *See* Ellis–van Creveld syndrome
Chronic obstructive lung disease (COPD), 211, 217
CIED (cardiovascular implantable electronic device) infection, 296, 296f, 299–300
Circular mitral orifice, 189, 195
CMR (cardiac magnetic resonance imaging), 410, 419, 420f
Coarctation
   aorta, 501, 501f, 510
   M-mode, 128, 132
Cocktail personality, 346
Coefficients of variation, echo-relevant guidelines, 442–443, 456
Color flow Doppler (CFD), 32, 38, 39, 41–42, 72, 74, 295, 299, 302, 305, 305f, 552, 565
Comet tail artifacts, 58, 58f, 61, 66
Commissural fusion, aortic stenosis, 118, 125
Complete atrioventricular canal defect (CAVC), 319, 323
Complete heart block, 327, 331
Congenital aortic valve, 556, 556f, 571
Congenital heart defect
   acute coronary syndrome (*See* Acute coronary syndromes)
   acute valvular lesion, 7–8
   apical ballooning syndrome, 259, 259f, 262
   Dressler syndrome, 391–392, 392f, 394

echo-relevant guidelines, 439, 449
   hypereosinophilic syndrome (HES), 289–290, 289f, 293
   hypoplastic left heart syndrome, 349, 352, 353
   Noonan syndrome (*See* Noonan syndrome)
   right axis deviation, 297f–299f, 298, 300
   scimitar syndrome, 335, 337
   sinus venosus atrial septal defects, 297f–299f, 298, 300
   Uhl anomaly, 319, 322
Congenital syndromes
   DiGeorge syndrome, 342, 342f, 347
   Down syndrome, 341, 341f, 344
   Ellis–van Creveld syndrome, 341, 341f, 344
   Loeys–Dietz syndrome, 344, 431, 436
   Marfan syndrome, 341, 341f, 344
   Noonan syndrome (*See* Noonan syndrome)
   Turner syndrome, 342, 342f, 344, 344f, 345, 346, 348
   Williams syndrome, 342, 342f, 348
Congenital valve lesions
   in adult congenital heart, 319, 320f, 324, 324f
   bicuspid aortic valve (BAV), 319, 323–324
   bicuspid aortic valve and subaortic membrane, 318, 318f, 320
   with fractured arm, 320, 325
   Marfan syndrome, 319, 324
   Noonan syndrome (*See* Noonan syndrome)
   subaortic membrane resection, 319, 321
   trisomy 21, 319, 323
   unrepaired pulmonary atresia, 319, 324–325, 325f
Congestive heart failure
   amplatzer septal occluder device, 231, 231f, 236
   muscular VSD, 231, 231f, 236
   pseudoaneurysm, 230–231, 230f, 235–236
Connective tissue disorders, 137, 138
Consensus committee, 442, 455
Constrictive pericarditis, 210, 212, 216, 218, 277, 281–282, 281f
   annular velocities, 212, 218
   annulus reversus, 212, 218
   cardiac volume, 535, 535f, 543, 543f
   hepatic flow reversal, 212, 218
   respiratory flow variation, 212, 218

vs. restrictive cardiomyopathy, 277, 283
   septal bounce, 212, 218
Continuity equation, aortic valve area, 193, 198
Continuous-wave spectral Doppler tracing, 188, 188f, 194
Contrast echocardiography, 230, 235
COPD (chronic obstructive lung disease), 211, 217
Coronary angiography, 448, 449, 466, 468, 547, 559
Coronary artery aneurysm, 240, 244, 328, 331–332
Coronary artery bypass grafting, 204, 204f, 207, 207f
Coronary artery disease (CAD), 550, 552, 561, 566
   atrial fibrillation, 250, 255
   embolic event, 239, 242–243
   impaired regional myocardial relaxation, 248, 253, 253f
   incidence of LV thrombus, 239, 242–243
   mobility and protrusion of LV thrombus, 239, 242–243
   right ventricular involvement, 239, 243
Coronary artery fistula, 311, 317
Coronary artery involvement, 231, 236
Coronary catheterization
   artery involvement, 231, 236
   cardiovascular surgery consultation, 231, 236
   occlusion, 231, 236
   TEE image, 232, 232f, 236
Coronary ischemia, 440, 450, 451
Coronary sinus (CS)
   dilation, TTE, 85, 85f, 88–89
   superior vena cava, 533, 540, 540f
Coronary syndromes
   acute
      acute myocarditis, 229, 234
      angina, 230, 235
      diastolic LV dysfunction, 230, 235
      ECG changes, 230, 235
      echocardiography, 229, 235
      mitral regurgitation development, 230, 235
      primary/metastatic cardiac tumors, 229, 234
      stress-induced cardiomyopathy, 229, 234
      symptoms, 230, 235
      systolic LV dysfunction, 230, 235
      systolic thickening impairment, 229, 234
      type A aortic dissection, 229, 234

Coumadin ridge (Q tip), 94, 98
CRT. *See* Cardiac resynchronization therapy (CRT)
Cryptogenic stroke, 96–97, 101
CTRCD (cancer therapeutic-related cardiac dysfunction), 442, 455
Cube (cuboid) formula, 187
Cyanosis, tricuspid valve, 155, 155f, 158

D

2D echo investigation secundum atrial septal defect, 309, 312–313
2D echocardiography, 230, 235
2D measurements
    biplane Simpson method, 181, 186
    3D echocardiography, 181, 186
    2D midventricular ratio, 179, 181–182
    3D-based formula, 181, 186
    end diastole and systole, 180, 180f, 184
    fractional shortening, 181, 186
    global and regional LV function, 179, 184
    left ventricular dimensions, 180, 184, 185f
    LV ejection fraction, 179, 183, 184t
    LV global systolic function, 179, 182
    LV volumetric measurements, 181, 186
    M-mode measurements, 181, 186
    modified Simpson method, 182, 187
    TEE, 181, 181t, 186
    visual assessment, 181, 186
    wall motion scoring, 181, 182
2D short axis, 549–550, 549f, 561
3D-based formula, 181, 186
3D echocardiography
    advantageous, 471, 477–478
    aortic valve and root, 474, 482
    vs. cardiac MRI, 472, 479
    clinical setting, 472, 478
    critical anatomic landmarks, 472, 479
    vs. 2D TEE, 472, 480, 481
    3DE imaging, 472, 478
    flail P3 scallop, 473, 481
    incremental diagnostic value, 474, 482
    indications for, 474, 482, 485t, 484, 525, 528, 528t
    left ventricle, 472, 479
    left ventricular ejection fraction, 471, 471f, 472, 474, 475, 479, 482
    mitral valve, 473, 480
    pulmonary stenosis valvuloplasty, 525, 528
    real-time imaging size, 471, 477–478
    right ventricular systolic function assessment, 472, 479

with spatial resolution, 473, 478, 481
    stitch artifact, 472, 472f, 479
    tricuspid valve function, 474, 482
3D transesophageal echocardiography. *See* Transesophageal echocardiography (TEE)
Deceleration time (DT), 555, 555f, 570
Degenerative diseases, 137, 138
Degenerative mitral valve disease, 145, 148
Device embolization, 443, 456
Device erosion, 443, 457
Diabetes, 549, 549f, 559
    type 2, M-mode measurements, 204, 204f, 207, 207f
Diastole, mitral valve leaflet, 533, 538
Diastolic deformation, 290, 294
Diastolic dysfunction
    IVRT, 210, 216
    mitral inflow pattern, 209, 209f, 214–215
Diastolic exercise testing, 441, 453
Diastolic flow
    aortic regurgitation, 533, 539, 539f
    mitral regurgitation causes, 154, 154f
Diastology
    E/A ratio, 213, 220–221
    LVEDP, 208, 208f, 214, 214f
    mitral inflow pattern, 209, 209f, 214–215
    pulmonary artery diastolic pressure, 211, 211f, 217, 217f
    pulmonic regurgitant interval, 208, 214
Diffuse concentric hypertrophy, 268, 272
DiGeorge syndrome, 342, 342f, 347
Dilated cardiomyopathy, 203, 206, 286, 286f, 290, 548, 559
    apical ballooning syndrome, 259, 259f, 262
    HIV/AIDS-related heart disease, 260, 263
    with left bundle branch block, 210, 210f, 216
    LVOT gradient, 259, 259f, 263
    mitral inflow pattern, 209, 209f, 214–215
    pericardial effusion, 259, 260, 263, 264
    with stage D heart failure, 210, 210f, 216
2-Dimensional imaging
    grainy appearance reduction, 29, 33
    nonstandard views, 29, 34
    over gain, 29, 32
    quality, 29, 33
3-Dimensional imaging, planar array, 39, 42, 43f

2-Dimensional scanning (2D), 72, 74
Direct current cardioversion, 57, 65, 65f
Dobutamine echocardiography
    aortic valve replacement, 250, 250t, 256
    biphasic response for regional systolic function, 248, 248f, 253
    nonsustained ventricular tachycardia, 249, 254
    sensitivity, 250, 255
    viability and ischemia assessment, 249, 255
Dobutamine stress echocardiography (DSE)
    atropine, 242, 247
    hibernating myocardium, 241, 246
    LV function, 241, 245
    sensitivity, 241, 246
Doppler, 546, 552, 558, 564–565
    continuous-wave Doppler, 72, 74
        bioprosthetic valve aortic stenosis, 164–165, 164f, 173
        pulmonary stenosis, 155, 159
        signals, hypertrophic cardiomyopathy, 270, 270f, 274
    flow pattern, 94, 98
    frequency shift, 69–71, 552, 564–565
    intracardiac blood flow pathophysiology, 405–406, 406f, 413
    measurements
        aortic stenosis, 193, 198
        Doppler gradient optimization, 193, 199
        Doppler-based strain curve, 191, 191f, 197
        effective systemic cardiac output, 188, 194–195
        Flow propagation velocity (Vp), 190, 190f, 196–197
        left ventricular outflow tract, 188, 188f, 194–195
        left ventricular systolic pressure (LVSP), 191, 191f, 197
        LVEDP estimation, 194, 200
        mean PA pressure estimation, 194, 200
        mitral orifice cross-sectional area, 189, 195
        mitral regurgitant jet, 188, 188f, 194
        myocardial performance index (MPI), 190, 190f, 196
        PA systolic pressure estimation, 194, 200
        PADP estimation, 194, 200
        pulmonary artery wedge pressure, 190, 190f, 196–197

Doppler (*Continued*)
tricuspid annular plane systolic
excursion, 192, 192f, 196
mitral regurgitation, 146, 146f–147f,
153
parameters, 155, 158, 159t
paravalvular leak closure procedure,
502, 510–511
paravalvular leak location, 502, 502f,
503, 504f, 512–514
pattern, 29, 35
principles
aliasing, pulse repetition frequency,
23, 26, 26t
audio signal, 24, 27, 27f
beam alignment, flow direction,
23–24, 24f, 27
deviation velocity, 23, 25, 25t
frequency shift *vs.* velocity, 23, 25
pulse repetition frequency, 23, 26
spectral signal, 24, 27, 27f
transducer, higher-frequency, 24,
27–28
pulsed wave, 29, 35, 72, 74
aliasing artifacts, 41, 42f
left atrial appendage, 355, 355f, 357
spectral signal, 552, 552f, 565
tissue Doppler echocardiography
(TDE), 241, 245
variation
measurement, 396–397, 397f, 400
tamponade, 397, 399–400
velocity index
bioprosthetic valve aortic stenosis,
164–165, 164f, 173
mitral valve, 168–169, 168f,
175–176
Doppler velocity index, 554, 568
Down syndrome (DS)
atrioventricular canal defect, 326, 341,
344
echocardiography, 341, 341f, 344
fetal echocardiography, 349, 351
ventricular septal defect, 343, 345
Dressler syndrome, 391–392, 392f, 394
DSE. *See* Dobutamine stress echocardiography (DSE)
D-shaped septum, cardiac MRI, 533,
533f, 540–541, 541f
DT (deceleration time), 555, 555f, 570
d-Transposition of the great arteries
(d-TGA), 336, 340
Duke criteria, modified
coagulase-negative *Staphylococcus*
bacteremia, 370, 380
Enterococcus, 369, 379
injectable drug abuse, 370, 380

mycotic aneurysm, 370, 380
predisposing heart condition, 370, 380
Staphylococcus aureus, 369, 379
Streptococcus viridans, 369, 379–380
Dynamic obstructive spectral Doppler
pattern, 324, 324f
Dyspnea, 169, 169f, 176–177, 545, 548,
558, 559
echo-relevant guidelines, 440, 452
etiology of, 107, 107f, 110
M-mode measurements, 203, 206
saddle pulmonary embolus, 107, 107f,
110
thrombolysis, 107, 107f, 110
Dyssynchrony
baseline, 303, 306, 306f
interventricular mechanical delay,
302, 304, 305f
intraventricular dyssynchrony, 302,
305, 305f
speckle tracking echocardiography,
303, 306–307
Yu index, 302, 305

E

Ebstein anomaly, 555, 570
echocardiography, 156, 156f, 160
fetal echocardiography, 350, 350f, 353
tricuspid regurgitation, 156, 160
tricuspid valve malformation, 531, 537
Echo contrast agents, 45, 47
Echo Doppler patterns, pulmonary vasodilator test, 548, 548f, 559
Echo strain
aortic stenosis, 486, 494
calculation, 486, 490
cardiology clinical, 487, 497
chemotherapy, 489, 490, 497
clinical variables, 487, 487f, 495
contrast-enhanced MRI, 486, 493
CRT, 487, 494
dobutamine stress, 486, 493
ejection fraction, 491, 497
Fabry disease, 498
HCM, 486, 493
left ventricular global longitudinal
strain, 489, 496
light chain amyloidosis, 486, 493–494
longitudinal strain, 486, 494
LVH, 486, 493
map of, 487, 488f, 495
mitral regurgitation, 486, 494
myocardial contractility, 488, 495
myocardial deformation imaging, 488,
495
myocardial regional mechanics, 486,
491f, 492

prognosis, 486, 493
radial, 488, 495
rate, 486, 493
risk prediction, 486, 494
speckle-tracking echocardiography,
486, 488, 492, 496
STE, 486, 487, 487f, 492–493
subclinical myocardial evidence, 486,
494
TDI, 488, 495
valvular heart disease, 486, 494
Echo-bright myocardium, 363, 366
Echocardiography, 555, 570
Echo-dense mass, 106, 106f, 109
Echo-relevant guidelines
aortic root replacement, 447, 464
ASD, 439, 443, 449, 456
atrial fibrillation, 446, 463–464
basal septal hypertrophy, 445,
460–461
biphasic pattern, 448, 467
breast cancer, 442, 455
cardiac surgery, 443, 456–457
coefficients of variation, 442–443, 456
congenital heart diseases, 439, 440,
449
consensus committee and, 442, 455
coronary angiography, 448, 449, 466,
468
coronary ischemia, 439, 450, 451
CTRCD, 442, 455
diastolic exercise testing, 441, 453
Doppler parameters, 440–441, 452
D-TGA, 440, 450
dyspnea, 440, 445, 452, 460–461
embolic potential risk, 441, 453, 454
endocarditis, 442, 454
exercise, 448, 468
familial cardiomyopathies, 447–448,
466
giant Lambl excrescences, 441, 453
HCM, 449, 468–469
hypertension, 440, 441, 443, 444, 447,
451, 453, 457, 459, 464
Imdur/add beta-blocker, 447, 464
intravenous drug abuse, 441, 453
ischemic *vs.* nonischemic cardiomyopathy, 449, 469
LAA, 446, 464
LAP, 440, 450–451
LVEF, 442, 455
mitral annular calcification, 442, 454
mitral valve replacement, 446, 463
Mustard operation, 439–440, 449–450
myocardial infarction and LVEF, 440,
451–452
non–severe aortic stenosis, 445, 462

obesity and respiratory failure, 444, 459

palpitations and frequent PVCs, 440, 450

peak instantaneous LV outflow gradient, 448, 467

percutaneous closure, limitations to, 443, 456

POCUS, 442, 454

radiation exposure, 444, 464

restrictive filling pattern, 440, 452

17-segment model, 445, 460

SPB response, 448, 468

stage D AS, 445, 462

stress echocardiography, 449, 468

TAVR, 445, 462

transcranial Doppler, 444, 459

valvular heart diseases, 441, 452–453

wall motion assessment, 2D echo for, 444, 460

WMSI, 444, 460

ECMO (extracorporeal membrane oxygenation), 58, 66–69, 68f, 70, 70f, 290, 294

Effective orifice area (EOA), 168–169, 168f, 175–176

Effective regurgitant orifice (ERO), 232–233, 233f, 236

Effective systemic cardiac output, 188, 194–195

Ehlers–Danlos syndrome, 431, 436

Elfin facies, 342, 346

Ellipsoid mitral orifice, 189, 195

Ellipsoid model, 187

Ellis–van Creveld syndrome, 341, 341f, 344

Embolism, 169, 169f, 176–177

Embolization, 230, 235

EMS, 290, 294

Enalapril, 443, 457

Endocardial cushion defects, 349, 349f, 351

Endocarditis

with acute severe aortic regurgitation, 210, 210f, 216

antimicrobial therapy, 380t, 383

complications of, 372, 382

diagnosis of, 367–377, 382

echo-relevant guidelines, 442, 454

embolic risk, 371, 371f, 383

with hypotension, 210, 210f, 216

indications for, 370, 380

intravenous drug use, 373, 373f, 377, 389

left-sided native valve, 370, 380

predictors of, 373, 383, 388

prosthetic valve, 167, 167f, 175

PVE, 373, 373f, 386, 387, 389t

transesophageal echocardiogram, 167, 167f, 175, 367, 374, 374t

treatment of, 367, 374, 374t, 375f

vegetation size, 371, 383, 383f

Endomyocardial fibrosis, 277, 277f, 281, 283

hypereosinophilic syndrome, 277, 283

End-stage renal disease (ESRD)

atropine, 242, 246

benefits of, 242, 246

dobutamine stress echo, 242, 246

ischemic segments percentage, 242, 246

transthoracic 2D echo, 242, 246

troponin, 242, 246

Enhancement artifacts, 13, 19, 21

Enterococcus bacteremia, 369, 379, 387

EOA (effective orifice area), 168–169, 168f, 175–176

Eosinophilic cardiomyopathy. *See* Loeffler endocarditis

Eosinophilic endomyocardial disease. *See* Loeffler endocarditis

Eosinophilic myocarditis, 277, 283

ERO (effective regurgitant orifice), 232–233, 233f, 236

ESE. *See* Exercise stress echocardiogram (ESE)

ESRD. *See* End-stage renal disease (ESRD)

Eustachian valve, 85, 85f, 89

E-wave velocities, 552, 567

Exercise stress echocardiogram (ESE)

Kawasaki diseas, 240, 245

prognostic value, 242, 247

wall motion score index, 8, 9

Exercise testing, 449, 468

Extracardiac Fontan procedure, 319, 321–322

Extracorporeal membrane oxygenation (ECMO), 58, 66–69, 68f, 70, 70f, 290, 294

F

Fabry disease, 262, 268, 273, 277, 280, 280f, 498

Falciform ligament, 106, 106f, 109

False aneurysm, 290, 294

False-negative stress echocardiography, 249, 254, 254t

False-negative test, 552, 566, 566t

False-positive stress echocardiography, 249, 254, 254t

False-positivity test, 552, 566, 566t

Familial dilated cardiomyopathy, 261, 265, 447–448, 466

Familial restrictive cardiomyopathy, 282

Fetal echocardiography

abnormal umbilical arterial Doppler pattern, 350, 350f, 352, 353

Ebstein anomaly of tricuspid valve, 350, 350f, 353

familial indications, 349, 351

gestational diabetes, 349–351

hypoplastic left heart syndrome, 349, 352, 353

maternal indications, 349, 351

pericardial effusions, 350, 352

primary fetal indications, 349, 351

pulmonary stenosis, 350, 353

trisomy 21, 349, 349f, 351

Fetal M-mode tracing, 349, 351

Fetal ventricular tachycardia, 349, 351

Fixed obstructive spectral Doppler pattern, 324, 324f

Flow propagation velocity (Vp), 190, 190f, 196–197

Fluorodeoxyglucose (FDG)-positron emission tomography (PET) sensitivity, 241, 246

Focused ultrasound (FOCUS) mitral regurgitation, 152, 152t

Fontan fenestration, 336, 340

Fractional shortening, 202, 202f, 205, 233–234, 237

Framingham risk score-, 255

Friedreich ataxia, 268, 272–273

Fulminant sepsis, 335

Fundamental B-mode image, 46, 49, 49f

Furosemide, intravenous, 261, 265

G

Gastrointestinal bleeding, 295, 299

Grade I diastolic dysfunction, 138, 144, 552, 566

H

Harmonic B-mode imaging, 46, 49, 49f

Harmonic power Doppler imaging, 46, 50, 50f

Hatle equation, 137, 141

Heart failure

class II, 362, 365–366

congestive

amplatzer septal occluder device, 231, 231f, 236

muscular VSD, 231, 231f, 236

pseudoaneurysm, 230–231, 230f, 235–236

HeartMate, 290, 294

HeartWare, 290, 294

Hematoma, 232, 236

Hemochromatosis, 276, 279–280

Hemorrhagic pericardial effusion, 431, 431f, 437
Hemorrhagic stroke, 295, 299
Heparin, 360, 363
Hepatic vein (HV)
  atrial fibrillation, 409, 419–420, 420f
  Doppler assessment of, 408–409, 408f, 417–418, 417f–419f
  normal flow, 408–409, 408f, 417
  normal sinus rhythm, 408–409, 408f, 418, 419f
  restrictive cardiomyopathy, 409, 418, 419f
  severe flow, 408–409, 408f, 418, 418f
Hepatoma, 110
HES (hypereosinophilic syndrome), 186, 277, 283, 289–290, 289f, 293
Hiatal hernia, 108, 108f, 111
Hodgkin lymphoma, 278, 284
Human immunodeficiency virus infection and acquired immune deficiency syndrome (HIV/AIDS), 553, 553f, 567, 567f
Hydrops fetalis, 350, 352
Hypereosinophilic syndrome (HES), 186, 277, 283, 289–290, 289f, 293
Hyperlipidemia, 552, 566
Hypernephroma, 110
Hypertension, 549, 552, 559, 566
  echo-relevant guidelines, 440, 441, 451, 453
  history of, 429, 432
Hyperthyroidism
  methimazole, 261, 261f, 264
  propranolol, 261, 261f 6
Hypertrophic cardiomyopathy (HCM), 203, 206, 262, 267f, 268, 277, 280, 280f, 486, 493
  alcohol septal ablation procedure, 272, 275
  asymmetric septal hypertrophy, 270, 274
  athlete's heart, 268, 272–273, 288, 292
  atrial fibrillation, 271, 274
  CW Doppler signals, 270, 270f, 274
  diagnosis of, 268, 273
  diastolic and systolic LV heart failure, 271, 274
  diffuse concentric hypertrophy, 268, 272
  echo strain, 486, 493
  echo-relevant guidelines, 449, 468–469
  Fabry disease, 268, 273
  Friedreich ataxia, 268, 273

genotype, 268, 269f, 273
  ischemic heart disease, 268, 273
  with LV outflow tract (OT), 516, 518
  with midcavitary obstruction, 516, 518
  mitral regurgitation, 268, 270, 273, 274
  M-mode, 546, 548f, 549f, 558
  myectomy, 271, 274–275, 516, 518
  Noonan syndrome, 268, 273
  Pompe disease, 268, 272–273
  screening echocardiograms, 271, 275
  sudden cardiac death, 271, 271f–272f, 274, 275
  systolic anterior motion, 146, 151–152, 152f, 268, 273
  takotsubo, 268, 273
  tissue Doppler imaging signal, 268, 269f, 273
  Valsalva maneuver, 270, 274
  VSD, 516, 518
  wall motion abnormalities, 268, 273
  without LVOT obstruction, 516, 518
Hypertrophic obstructive cardiomyopathy, 524, 524f, 527
Hypokinesis, 229, 234
Hypoplastic left heart syndrome, 349, 352, 353
Hypotension, pericardial effusions, 396–397, 400

I
ICE. *See* Intracardiac echocardiography (ICE)
Idiopathic restrictive cardiomyopathy, 277, 282
Image acquisition, 112–113
Impaired regional myocardial relaxation, 248, 253, 253f
Impella device, 295–296, 296f, 299, 502, 506, 510, 513–514
Infective endocarditis
  American Heart Association guidelines, 367, 378
  diagnosis of, 370, 382–384
  modified Duke criteria, 369, 379–381
  and pericardial effusions, 398–399, 402
  possible IE, 372, 372f, 385
  prophylaxis, 367–368, 378
Inferior vena cava
  hepatoma, 110
  hypernephroma, 110
  leiomyosarcoma, 108, 110
  renal cell carcinomas, 108, 110
Infiltrative cardiomyopathy, 276, 278
Infundibular ventricular septal defects, 231, 231f, 236

Inlet ventricular septal defects, 231, 231f, 236
Instrumentation, monitor adjustment, 29, 32
Interatrial septal closure device, 56–57, 66
Interobserver variability (IOV), 442–443, 456
Intersocietal Commission for the Accreditation of Echocardiography Laboratories (ICAEL) standards and guidelines, 76, 80
Interventricular mechanical delay (IVMD), 302, 304, 305f
Intracardiac echocardiography (ICE)
  with LAA, 525, 527–528
  risk of, 523, 526
  vs. TEE, 523, 526
  tissue heating levels, 524, 527
Intravenous dobutamine administration, 250, 250t, 256
Intravenous drug abuse, 545–546, 548f, 558
Intraventricular dyssynchrony
  color-coded tissue Doppler, 302, 305, 305f
  ischemic mitral regurgitation, 240, 243–244
IOV (interobserver variability), 442–443, 456
Ischemia, 248, 253, 253f
  acute myocardial, 230, 235
  coronary, 439, 450, 451
  myocardial
    echocardiography, 229, 235
    systolic thickening impairment, 229, 234
Ischemic cardiomyopathy, 241, 245, 290, 294, 449, 469
Ischemic cascade, 230, 235
  angina, 242, 247
  biochemical changes, 242, 247
  diastolic dysfunction, 242, 247
  electrocardiogram changes, 242, 247
Ischemic mitral regurgitation
  diagnosis of, 240, 245
  increased depth of tenting, 240, 243–244
  intraventricular dyssynchrony, 240, 243–244
  mitral valve deformation, 240, 245
  papillary muscle dislocation, 240, 243–244
  septolateral dilation, 240, 243–244
Ischemic mitral regurgitation, acute, 145, 148

Ischemic stroke, 295, 298

Isovolumic relaxation time (IVRT) measurements, 212–213, 212f–213f, 219–220, 219f–220f

IVMD (interventricular mechanical delay), 302, 304, 305f

IVRT (isovolumic relaxation time) measurements, 212–213, 212f–213f, 219–220, 219f–220f

K

Kawasaki disease (KD), 331, 334
  diagnosis of, 240, 244
  exercise stress test, 240, 245
  patient size, 240, 244
  SE *vs.* SPECT, 240, 245
  stress test, 240, 245

Konno procedure, 319, 322

L

LAA. *See* Left atrial appendage (LAA)

LAD (left anterior descending) artery territory ischemia, 248, 253–254

Lambl excrescences, 370, 374, 381

Large perfusion defect during stress, 535–536, 536f, 544, 544f

LARIAT cardiac device, 298, 301

Lateral resolution, 555, 569

LAVI (left atrial volume index), 182, 186

Leaflet dysfunction, mitral regurgitation, 145, 149, 149t

Left anterior descending (LAD) artery territory ischemia, 248, 253–254

Left atrial appendage (LAA)
  cardiac CT, 534–535, 534f, 542, 542f
  ICE with, 525, 527–528
  occlusion, LARIAT device, 298, 301
  waveform, 355, 355f, 357

Left atrial size and function, 212, 219

Left atrial thrombus, 534–535, 534f, 542, 542f

Left atrial volume index (LAVI), 181, 186

Left brachiocephalic vein, 87, 87f, 91

Left subclavian artery, 552, 565

Left superior vena cava (LSVC)
  left-to-right shunt, 335
  pulmonary hypertension, 335, 338
  Tetralogy of Fallot, 335, 337

Left ventricular aneurysm, 262, 264

Left ventricular apex
  cardiac MRI, 535, 535f, 543, 543f
  transducer, 29, 35

Left ventricular assist device (LVAD), 203, 206, 295, 295f, 298, 299

Left ventricular dimensions, 180, 184, 185f

Left ventricular dysfunction, 202–203, 202f–203f, 206

Left ventricular (LV) dyssynchrony. *See* Dyssynchrony

Left ventricular ejection fraction (LVEF), 179, 183, 183t, 359, 359f, 363
  continuous-wave Doppler tracing, 210, 210f, 216
  3D echocardiography, 471, 471f, 472, 474, 475, 479, 482
  echo-relevant guidelines, 440, 451–452
  endocardium, 153

Left ventricular end diastolic pressure (LVEDP)
  end-diastolic AR jet velocity, 208, 208f, 214, 214f
  estimation, 194, 200

Left ventricular (LV) function
  dobutamine stress echocardiography, 241, 245
  filling pressure estimation, 213, 220
  strain rate imaging, 241, 245
  tissue Doppler echocardiography, 241, 245

Left ventricular hypertrophy (LVH), 486, 493

Left ventricular noncompaction (LVNC), 262, 268, 286, 286f, 290, 362, 365–366

Left ventricular opacification
  faster saline flush, 230, 235
  mechanical index, 230, 235

Left ventricular outflow tract (LVOT)
  cardiac MRI, 533, 533f, 540–541, 541f
  continuous wave Doppler in, 533, 537
  CT images, 534, 534f, 542, 542f
  diameter, 118, 123
  elevated velocity level, 532, 533, 537, 538
  mitral valve area calculation, 137, 139
  parasternal long-axis window, 193, 199
  pulsed-wave Doppler tracing, 188, 188f, 194–195
  subaortic stenosis, 531, 532, 537, 538

Left ventricular remodeling
  end-diastolic dimension and volume, 240, 244
  end-systolic dimension and volume, 240, 244
  mass and ejection fraction, 240, 244
  measurement of, 240, 244
  myocardial strain, 240, 244

Left ventricular stroke volume, 193, 199–200

Left ventricular systolic dysfunction, 550, 550f, 562, 562f, 563

Left ventricular systolic function, 261, 265

Left ventricular thrombus, 239, 242–243

Left ventricular (LV) wall thickness, 261, 266, 549, 559

Left-sided native valve endocarditis. *See* Endocarditis

Leiomyosarcoma, 108, 110

Libman–Sacks endocarditis, 372, 372f, 385

Lipomatous hypertrophy, interatrial septum, 57, 65, 65f

Lisinopril, 146–147, 146f–147f, 153

Lithium, 349, 351, 353

Liver transplant, 545, 558

Lobster Claw Doppler pattern, 546, 558

Loeffler endocarditis, 277, 283

Loeys-Dietz syndrome, 344, 424, 427, 431, 436

LPA stenosis, 312, 317

LSVC. *See* Left superior vena cava (LSVC)

Lupus valvulitis, 156, 160, 557–558, 572

LV function. *See* Left ventricular (LV) function

LV internal diameter at end diastole (LVIDD), 442, 455

LVAD (left ventricular assist device), 203, 206, 295, 295f, 298, 299

LVEDP. *See* Left ventricular end diastolic pressure (LVEDP)

LVEF. *See* Left ventricular ejection fraction (LVEF)

LVH (left ventricular hypertrophy), 486, 493

LVNC (left ventricular noncompaction), 262, 268, 286, 286f, 290, 362, 365–366

LVOT. *See* Left ventricular outflow tract (LVOT)

M

Main pulmonary artery (MPA) flow, 309, 313

Marantic endocarditis, 372, 372f, 385

Marfan syndrome, 319, 324, 341, 341f, 344
  abnormal fibrillin protein, 341, 341f, 344
  aorta, 425, 427

MAs (mycotic aneurysms), 373, 388

MBV (mitral balloon valvuloplasty), 502, 502f, 504, 510–512

McConnell sign, 533, 541, 541f

Mechanical aortic valve prosthesis, 203, 206

Mechanical index (MI), 72, 74, 230, 235

Mechanical prosthetic aortic valve, 69, 69f, 70

Medtronic-Hall valve, 554, 568–569
tilting disc valve, 169–170, 170f, 177

Membranous ventricular septal defects, 231, 231f, 236

Metastatic melanoma, 396–397, 400

Methimazole, 261, 261f, 264

Method of disks (MOD), 179, 183

Microbubbles, 45–53, 45f–46f, 48f–49f
apical four-chamber view
with agent, 45, 45f, 49
without agent, 46, 46f
bioeffect of, 46, 52–53
clinical applications, 45, 48–49
clinical scenarios, 47, 53
contrast administration, 8–9
destruction of, 38
echo contrast agents, 45, 47
indications, 46, 52
interaction of, 45, 48
left ventricular thrombus, 46, 52f
side effect, 46, 51–52
ultrasound, impact of, 45, 47–48

Microcavitation. *See* Free gas microbubbles

Mid-cavitary obliteration, 531, 536, 536f

Midwall fractional shortening (MWFS), 202, 205

Mirror-image artifacts, 21, 21f

Mitral annular calcification, 442, 454

Mitral annulus pulsed wave, 212–213, 212f–213f, 219–220, 219f–220f

Mitral balloon valvuloplasty (MBV), 502, 502f, 504, 510–512

Mitral inflow pattern
abnormal relaxation, 209, 209f, 211, 211f, 214–216, 216f
color M-mode flow propagation rate, 211, 211f, 216–217
Doppler patterns, 405, 411
E/A wave velocities, transmitral pressure gradient, 210, 215
exudative effusive-pericardial constraint, 412, 414f, 419
left atrial volume index, 211, 211f, 216–217
measurements for, 212–213, 212f–213f, 219–220, 219f–220f
pseudonormal pattern, 209, 209f, 215
pulmonary venous flow, 211, 211f, 216–217
restrictive physiology, 209, 209f, 214

Mitral leaflet, aortic valve, 500–501, 501f, 509

Mitral regurgitation (MR), 329, 332
acute severe aortic regurgitation, 147, 147f, 153–154, 154f
anatomical lesions, 145, 145f, 149, 149t
Carpentier classification, 145, 149, 149f, 149t
causes, 145, 148
with color flow, 535, 535f, 543, 534f
continuous-wave Doppler images, 146–147, 146f–147f, 153, 558, 558f, 572–573
coronary revascularization, 146, 152
degenerative mitral valve disease, 145, 148
diagnosis, 208, 208f–209f, 214, 550, 561
diastolic, 154, 154f
Doppler signal, 147, 153, 153f, 208, 208f, 214
echo strain, 486, 494
effective regurgitant orifice calculation, 146, 149–150, 150f, 232–233, 233f, 236
etiology, 145, 145f, 148, 148f, 232, 236
flail posterior leaflet, 232, 236
inferior wall myocardial infarction, 232, 236
leaflet dysfunction, 145, 149, 149t
left atrial volume, 534, 534f, 542, 542f
left ventricular dilation, 230, 235
lisinopril, 146–147, 146f–147f, 153
M-mode images, 148, 148f
moderately dilated LA and LV, 517, 520
myectomy, 146, 152
Nyquist limit, 517, 520
papillary muscle closing forces, 303, 304f, 307
papillary muscle dysfunction, 230, 235
papillary muscle rupture, 146, 152
posteromedial papillary muscle, 146, 153
pressure half-time and ejection fraction, 166, 166f, 175
prolapse of posterior leaflet, 145, 145f, 148, 148f
segmental wall motion abnormalities, 230, 235
stunned myocardium, 145, 145f, 148
surgical indications for, 146, 150–151, 151f

with systolic anterior motion, 146, 151–152, 152f
systolic pressure gradient, 210, 215–216, 215f
3DE assessment, 473, 475f, 480
transesophageal color-flow Doppler after mitral valve surgery, 103, 104
transesophageal echocardiography, 146, 151–152
transmitral Doppler image, 138, 142–143, 143f
transthoracic echocardiography, 146, 149–150, 150f
type IIIb
apical leaflet tethering, 240, 244
features, 240, 244
severe, 130, 273, 341, 344
velocity, 166, 166f, 175
vena contracta width, 517, 520

Mitral scallop, 525, 525f, 529

Mitral stenosis, 506, 507f, 514
associated mitral regurgitation, 138, 142–143, 143f
in atrial fibrillation, 138, 142, 143f
chordal structures, 138, 142
continuity equation, 138, 142
etiology of, 137, 138
hyperdynamic circulation, 138, 143, 143f
indications for, 138, 142
leaflet mobility and thickness, 137, 142
mitral valve leaflets, 138, 143–144
nonrestrictive ventricular septal defect, 138, 142–143
planimetry, 137, 140, 141f
pressure half-time method, 137, 138, 140, 141
reduced EF slope, 13, 13f, 138
thyrotoxicosis, 138, 143
transaortic *vs.* transmitral gradients, 117, 122
transmitral Doppler image, 138, 142–143, 143f
transthoracic echocardiography, 138, 142
Wilkins score, 137, 139, 139t

Mitral valve
annulus, septolateral dilation, 240, 243–244
carpentier functional classification, 517, 520
of chordal preservation, 516, 520
diastolic function evaluation, 533, 538
hypertrophic cardiomyopathy, 203, 206

M-mode images, 368, 368f, 379, 381, 383

pathology, 517, 519, 520f

with pulmonary artery, 516, 519

RV dysfunction, 517, 520

surgical view, 499, 500, 502, 508–511, 509f

TEE, 239–240, 243

3D echocardiography, 472, 473, 480, 525, 525f, 529

Mitral valve area calculation

aliasing velocity, 137, 139–140

Hatle equation, 137, 141

leaflet segments, 138, 141–142

left ventricular outflow tract method, 137, 140

planimetry, 137, 140, 141f

pressure half-time, 137–141, 142f, 144

proximal isovelocity surface area, 137, 138, 140, 144

severe aortic regurgitation, 138, 144

severe tricuspid regurgitation, 137, 139

velocity measurement, 137, 140

Mitral valve clipping procedure, 502, 502f, 504, 505, 511, 513

Mitral valve disease, 166, 174–175, 174f

Mitral valve inflow, 406, 406f, 411

Mitral valve leaflets, 233, 236

M-mode, 128, 132, 132f

Mitral valve prolapse, 341, 341f, 344, 355, 356

Mitral valve repair, 150–151, 150f

Mitral valve replacement, 168–169, 168f, 175–176, 446, 463

Mitral valve stenosis, 168–169, 168f, 175–176

M-mode image, 368, 368f, 379, 381, 383

aortic regurgitation color, 407–408, 415, 416f

bicuspid aortic valve, 128, 132

coarctation, 128, 132

diagnosis of, 550, 550f, 562, 562f

hypertrophic cardiomyopathy, 546, 546f, 547f, 558

mitral valve leaflets, 128, 132, 132f, 148, 148f

parasternal long-axis view, 225, 225f, 228, 228f

pericardial effusion, 391, 393, 394, 394f

pulmonary valve, 406–407, 407f, 414, 415f

PV motion characterization, 406, 406f, 414

regurgitant jet, 145, 145f, 148

rheumatic mitral stenosis, 138, 143–144, 144f

right ventricle, 225, 227–228, 228f

tricuspid annulus, 192, 192f, 196

M-mode measurements

aortic valve, 204, 207

coronary artery bypass grafting, 204, 204f, 207, 207f

diabetes type 2, 204, 204f, 207, 207f

dyspnea, 203, 206

fractional shortening, 202, 202f, 205

hypertension and diabetes, 203–204, 204f, 206f, 207, 207f

LV global systolic function, 202, 205

multiple cardiac surgeries, 203, 206

MOD (method of disks), 179, 183

Moderator band, 88, 88f, 93

Modified Duke criteria. *See* Duke criteria, modified

Modified Simpson method, 182, 187

MPI (myocardial performance index), 190, 190f, 196

MR. *See* Mitral regurgitation (MR)

Multimodal imaging

CCTA, 532, 532f, 538

CT, 531–534, 536, 536f, 537, 537f, 539, 542, 542f

MRA, 531, 536, 536f, 537

MRI, 531–537, 531f–537f, 539

9mTc-sestamibi, 535–536, 536f, 543, 543f

PAPVR defects, 531, 537, 537f

short-axis real-time MR cine, 535, 535f, 543, 545f

stress and rest, 535–536, 535f, 544, 544f

tagged MRI cine, 535, 535f, 543, 544f

Multiple myeloma, 277, 277f, 284

Multiple wall motion abnormalities, 532, 535–536, 538, 544

Mural thrombus, 535, 535f, 543, 543f

Muscular ventricular septal defects, 231, 231f, 236

Mustard operation, 326, 329, 439–440, 449–450

MWFS (midwall fractional shortening), 202, 205

Mycotic aneurysms (MAs), 373, 388

Myectomy

hypertrophic cardiomyopathy, 271, 274–275

mitral regurgitation, 146, 152

Myocardial contractility, 488, 495

Myocardial contrast echocardiography, 272, 275

Myocardial infarction

acute, 231, 236

echo-relevant guidelines, 440, 451–452

transesophageal echocardiography, 229, 235

ventricular septal defect, 229, 235

wall motion abnormalities, 233, 236–237

Myocardial ischemia

acute, 230, 235

echocardiography, 229, 235

systolic thickening impairment, 229, 234

Myocardial performance index (MPI), 190, 190f, 196

Myocardial perfusion imaging, 242, 247

Myocardial rupture

pericardial effusion, 232, 236

wall motion abnormalities, 232, 236

Myocardial segment viability

contrast echocardiography, 230, 235

regional functions, 230, 235

resting two-dimensional echocardiography, 230, 235

stunned myocardium, 230, 235

Myocardial stunning, 145, 145f, 148

Myocarditis, 229, 234

Myxomas, 355, 355f, 357

Myxomatous degeneration, 370, 370f, 382

N

NCFs. *See* Noncardiac findings (NCFs)

Nikaidoh repair, 320, 325

Nonbacterial thrombotic endocarditis (NBTE). *See* Marantic endocarditis

Noncardiac findings (NCFs)

atelectatic lung segment, 106, 106f, 109

falciform ligament, 106, 106f, 109

hiatal hernia, 108, 108f, 111

inferior vena cava, 107, 107f, 108, 110

oblique sinus, 9, 108, 108f

prevalence of, 106, 109

thoracic descending aorta, 107–108, 108f, 110

transthoracic echocardiograms, 106, 109

venous thrombosis, 107, 109

Nonischemic cardiomyopathy, 449, 469

Non–severe aortic stenosis, 445, 462

Non-ST elevation myocardial infarction (NSTEMI), 229, 234–235

Nonstenotic intercostal artery, 94, 98

Nonsustained ventricular tachycardia, 249, 254

Noonan syndrome, 349, 349f, 351
  diagnosis, 343, 346
  echocardiography, 343, 343f, 346
  hypertrophic cardiomyopathy, 268, 273
  pulmonary artery stenosis, 155, 159–160
  pulmonary valve stenosis, 327, 331
Norepinephrine therapy, 295–296, 296f, 299
NSTEMI (non-ST elevation myocardial infarction), 229, 234–235
Nuclear SPECT, 241, 246
Nyquist limit, 32, 37–38, 157, 157f, 161

O
Obesity, 444, 459
Oblique sinus, 9, 108, 108f
Obstructive hypertrophic cardiomyopathy. See Hypertrophic cardiomyopathy (HCM)
Optimal standardized test-taking
  anticramming, 2
  cued guessing, 1
  informed guessing, 1
  random guessing, 1
  stress and anxiety handling, 4–6
  study tips, 6
  tricks, 3–4
Ostium secundum atrial septal defect (OS-ASD), 298, 300
Outcome-based partition values, 545, 558

P
Pacemaker, 356, 358
PADP (pulmonary artery diastolic pressure), 194, 200
Papillary endocardial tumors. See Papillary fibroelastoma (PFE)
Papillary fibroelastoma (PFE), 367, 374, 376
Papillary fibroma, 367, 376
Papillary muscle dysfunction, 230, 235
Papilloma. See Papillary fibroelastoma (PFE)
PAPVR (partial anomalous pulmonary venous return), 335, 336
Parasternal long-axis, Chin criteria, 532, 538
Parasternal short-axis
  aortic valve, 534, 534f, 542, 542f
  Jenni criteria, 532, 538
Parietal pericardium, 397, 401
Partial anomalous pulmonary venous return (PAPVR), 335, 336, 531, 537, 537f

Patent ductus arteriosus (PDA), 311, 312, 317, 327, 331, 558, 572
Patent foramen ovale (PFO), 8, 9, 444, 459, 460
  defect, 505, 505f, 509, 513
  TEE bubble study, severe mitral regurgitation, 103, 104
Patient-prosthetic mismatch (PPM)
  bioprosthetic valve aortic stenosis, 164, 164f, 173
  effective orifice area, 163, 171
  prosthetic valve, 163, 170–171
  severity determination, 163, 171, 171t
PAWP (pulmonary artery wedge pressure), 190, 190f, 196–197
PDA (patent ductus arteriosus), 311, 317
Peak aortic valve gradients, 117, 122
Pedoff probe, 193, 199
Percutaneous closure
  device, 547, 559
  limitations to, 443, 456
Pericardial constraint
  with chronic constrictive physiology, 406–407, 406f–407f, 414, 414f
  classic Doppler, 405–406, 405f–406f, 413
  constrictive and restrictive physiology, 411, 421, 421t
  Doppler patterns, 405, 406f, 411
  exudative effusive, 412, 412f, 419
  mitral valve E-wave deceleration time, 411, 420–421, 421t
  M-mode display, 407–408, 408f, 414–416, 415f, 416f
  M-mode echocardiogram, 406–407, 407f, 414, 415f
  right heart catheterization and vasodilator challenge, 410, 421
  survival rate, 405, 411
Pericardial cyst
  aorta, 425, 428, 428f
  pericardium, 393, 393f, 395
Pericardial effusions, 298, 301, 553, 553f, 567, 567f
  aortic dissection, 399, 403
  AV groove, 398, 398f, 402
  cardiac silhouette, 396, 400
  chest pain and hypotension, 396, 400
  chronic venous thromboembolism, 399, 403
  classic clinical signs, 398, 402
  conventional epilepsy therapy, 396, 400
  dilated cardiomyopathy, 259, 260, 263, 264
  Doppler, 396–398, 398f, 400–402
  end atrial diastole, 399, 403
  fetal echocardiography, 350, 352

fibrinous adhesions, 398, 398f, 402
fibrinous strands, 398, 398f, 401
hemodynamic condition, 398, 402
hypotension and tachycardia, 396–397, 400
infective endocarditis and, 398–399, 402
intravenous drug use, 398–399, 399f, 402
LV dysfunction, 397, 400
measurement, 397, 397f, 400
metastatic melanoma, 396–397, 400
metastatic tumors, 398, 398f, 402
NSAIDs, 399, 403
parasternal long-axis view, 397–398, 398f, 401–402
parietal, 397–398, 398f, 401
pregnancy, 397, 397f, 400
respiratory variation, 398, 404
sarcoidosis, 396, 400
tamponade, 397, 397f, 398, 399, 401–403
with 2D echocardiographic features, 397, 397f, 400–401
visceral, 398, 398f, 401
Pericardial space evaluation, 9
Pericardial tamponade, 211, 211f, 217
Pericardiocentesis, 295, 299
  circumferential pericardial effusion, 525–526, 526f, 529
  needle location, 523, 523f, 526
Pericardium
  cardiac MRI axial image, 392, 395, 395f
  congenital absence of, 392, 394, 395, 395f
  constriction, 399, 403
  constrictive and restrictive physiology, 411, 421, 421t
  diagnosis, 392, 394
  Doppler patterns, 405, 406f, 411
  echocardiographic evaluation of, 392, 394
  epicardial fat, 392, 394
  evaluation of, 391, 393
  M-mode display, 391, 393, 394, 394f, 407–408, 408f, 414–416, 415f, 416f
  M-mode echocardiogram, 406–407, 407f, 414, 415f
  pericardial cyst, 393, 393f, 395
  reflective structure, 391–392, 391f, 394
  right heart catheterization and vasodilator challenge, 410, 421
Peripartum cardiomyopathy, 261, 261f, 265, 288, 292

Periprosthetic aortic valve abscess, 169–170, 170f, 177

Perivalvular aortic valve regurgitation
  Doppler features, 165f, 173–174
  severity evaluation, 165f, 173–174

Perivalvular regurgitant, 169–170, 170f, 177

PFO (patent foramen ovale), 8, 9, 444, 459, 460
  defect, 505, 505f, 509, 513
  TEE bubble study, severe mitral regurgitation, 103, 104

Phlebotomy, 276, 279–280

Physical principles of ultrasound
  artifacts, 54–67, 54f–59f, 61f–65f
  2D ultrasound, 11–22, 12f–14f, 20f–22f
  Doppler, 23–28, 23f–27f
  knobology, 29–38, 30f–34f, 36f–37f
  spatial and temporal resolution, 39–44, 39f–44f

Physics
  alias artifacts, 24, 27–28, 41, 42f
  attenuation artifacts, 55, 62, 63f
  bidirectional flow artifact, 68, 69
  comet tail artifacts, 58, 58f, 61, 66
  duplication artifacts, 58, 58f, 66
  equations
    Bernoulli, 32, 37, 37f, 116, 121
    continuity, 117, 121, 138, 142, 193, 198
    Hatle, 137, 141
    PISA, 232–233, 233f, 236
  mirror artifacts, 56, 64–65
  misregistration artifacts, 57, 65, 65f
  Nyquist limit, 32, 37–38, 157, 157f, 161
  principles, Doppler
    aliasing, pulse repetition frequency, 23, 26, 26t
    audio signal, 24, 27, 27f
    beam alignment, flow direction, 23–24, 24f, 27
    deviation velocity, 23, 25, 25t
    frequency shift *vs.* velocity, 23, 25
    pulse repetition frequency, 23, 26
    spectral signal, 24, 27, 27f
    transducer, higher-frequency, 24, 27–28, 69, 71
  refraction (or lens) artifacts, 21, 22f
  reverberation artifacts, 20, 20f, 21f, 55, 56, 58, 58f, 60–61, 61f, 63f, 64–66
  ring-down artifacts, 13, 19–21, 56, 58, 58f, 65, 66
  shadowing artifacts, 13, 19, 21, 57, 57f, 66

side-lobe artifacts, 13, 20–21, 21f, 55, 60, 63, 63f

spatial and temporal resolution, 39–44, 39f–44f

speckle artifacts, 55, 60

stitch artifacts, 67

2D and Doppler ultrasound principles, 11–22, 12f–14f, 20f–22f, 69, 70

Planar array, 3D imaging, 39, 42, 43f

Planimetry method, 137, 140, 141f

Polysplenia syndrome, 338

Pompe disease, 268, 272–273

Posteromedial papillary muscle, 88, 88f, 92, 92f, 146, 153

Post-myocardial infarction
  echocardiogram, left ventricular aneurysm, 262, 268
  ventricular septal defect occurrence, 241, 245

Power pulse inversion imaging, 46, 49, 50

PPM. *See* Patient-prosthetic mismatch (PPM)

Pressure half-time (P t½) method, 135
  mitral valve area calculation, 137–141, 142f, 144
  velocity measurement, 137, 140

Pressure recovery, 118, 124, 164, 164f, 172

PRF. *See* Pulse repetition frequency (PRF)

Primary cardiac lymphoma, 356, 356f, 357

Primum atrial septal defect, 341, 345

Prophylaxis, infective endocarditis, 367–368, 378

Propranolol, 261, 261f, 264

Prosthetic mitral valve disease, 166, 174–175, 174f

Prosthetic valve(s)
  abscess formation, 170, 177–178
  bileaflet mechanical valve, 163–164, 164f, 172
  echocardiography, 164, 172
  endocarditis, 167, 167f, 175
  evaluation of, 164, 172
  follow-up of, 164, 172
  outflow tract velocity, 163, 171
  patient-prosthetic mismatch, 163, 171, 171t
  peak gradient calculation, 163, 171
  physiologic regurgitation, 163–164, 164f, 172
  pressure recovery, 164, 164f, 172
  size, 163–164, 171
  sutures of, 370, 370f, 382
  thrombus, 169, 169f, 176–177

transesophageal echocardiography, 163–164, 164f, 172
  valve number, 163, 170–171
  vegetations, 167, 167f, 175

Prosthetic valve endocarditis (PVE), 373, 373f, 386, 387, 387t

Prosthetic vegetative lesion, 169–170, 170f, 177

Proximal isovelocity surface area (PISA) method, 552, 565
  aliasing velocity alteration, 137, 139–140
  effective regurgitant orifice, 146, 149–150, 150f
  mitral valve area calculation, 137, 138, 140, 144
  overestimation of flow rate, 138, 144
  radius measurement, 150, 150f

Pseudoaneurysm (PA), 230–231, 230f, 235–236, 290, 294

Pseudonormal pattern, 209, 209f, 214–215

Pseudosevere aortic stenosis, 117, 122

Pulmonary artery(ies), 88, 88f, 92

Pulmonary artery diastolic pressure (PADP), 194, 200, 211, 211f, 217, 217f

Pulmonary artery stenosis, 351

Pulmonary artery systolic pressure
  cardiac shunt lesions, 311, 311f, 316
  RA pressure, 224, 224f, 227

Pulmonary artery wedge pressure (PAWP), 190, 190f, 196–197

Pulmonary atresia, 319, 324–325, 325f

Pulmonary emboli (PE), 533–534, 534f, 541

Pulmonary hypertension, 335, 337, 338

Pulmonary insufficiency end-diastolic (PIED) velocity of, 311, 316–317, 316f

Pulmonary regurgitation
  Doppler envelope, 194, 200, 200f
  flow signal evaluation, 156, 160
  post-tetralogy of Fallot repair, 157, 157f, 161
  pulmonary vascular resistance, 156, 160
  severity evaluation, 157, 157f, 161

Pulmonary stenosis, 350, 353
  congenital heart defect (*See* Congenital heart defect)
  congenital syndromes (*See* Congenital syndromes)
  congenital valve lesions (*See* Congenital valve lesions)
  continuous-wave spectral Doppler measurement, 155, 159

Pulmonary stenosis (*Continued*)
  Noonan syndrome (*See* Noonan syndrome)
  post-tetralogy of Fallot repair, 157, 157f, 161
  pulmonary artery stenosis, 155, 159
  pulmonary valve stenosis
    balloon valvuloplasty, 318–319, 318f, 321
    echocardiography, 318–319, 321
    Noonan syndrome (*See* Noonan syndrome)
    Williams syndrome (*See* Williams syndrome)
  RVOT, 157, 161
Pulmonary valve regurgitation, 319, 321
Pulmonary valve stenosis, 327, 330
Pulmonary vasodilator test, 548, 548f, 559
Pulmonary veins, systolic flow reversal, 534–535, 535f, 543
Pulmonary venous flow, 31, 31f–32f, 36, 36f
  D wave velocity, 212, 218–219
  measurements for, 212–213, 212f–213f, 219–220, 219f–220f
  mitral stenosis, 212, 218–219
  S1 flow, 212, 218
Pulmonary venous return, 327, 329
Pulmonic regurgitant (PR) interval, 208, 214
Pulmonic valve (PV)
  characterization of, 406–407, 407f, 414
  leaflets, 85, 89
  pulmonary branch artery stenosis, 155, 159–160
  valvular involvement, 155, 158
Pulse repetition frequency (PRF)
  aliasing, 23, 26, 26t
  color Doppler flow acquisition, 24, 27
  systolic Doppler signal, 23, 26
Pulsed-wave Doppler, 29, 35, 72, 74
  aliasing artifacts, 41, 42f
  left atrial appendage, 355, 355f, 357
Pulsed-wave spectral Doppler display, 157, 157f, 161
PVE (prosthetic valve endocarditis), 373, 373f, 386, 387, 387t

Q

22q11 deletion syndrome, 343, 346, 347
Quadricuspid aortic valve morphology, 118, 126

R

Radiation, 555, 570
Radiation exposure, echo-relevant guide-lines, 444, 464

Radiation-induced aortic stenosis, 555, 570
Rastelli procedure, 319, 320, 323, 325
Refraction (or lens) artifacts, 21, 22f
Regurgitant jet, 145, 145f, 148
Relative wall thickness (RWT), 181, 181t, 186
Renal abnormalities, 327, 330
Renal cell carcinomas, 108, 110
Resolution
  axial, 39, 40f, 54, 54f, 59–60
  lateral, 39, 40, 56, 63–64
  spatial and temporal, 39–44, 39f–44f
Respiratory failure, echo-relevant guide-lines, 444, 459
Respiratory flow variation, 211, 217
Restrictive cardiomyopathy
  atria enlargement, 276, 279
  vs. constrictive pericarditis, 277, 281–282, 281f
  definition and classification, 276, 278–279
  endomyocardial fibrosis, 277, 277f, 281, 283
  hemochromatosis, 276, 279–280
  idiopathic restrictive cardiomyopathy, 277, 282
  radiation cardiotoxicity, 277, 281–282, 281f
Resynchronization therapy. *See* Cardiac resynchronization therapy (CRT)
Retroactive inhibition, ASCeXAM, 1
REV repair, 320, 325
Reverberation, 20, 20f, 21f, 55, 56, 58, 58f, 60–61, 61f, 63f, 64–66
Rhabdomyomas, 356, 356f, 357
Rheumatic disease, 555, 570
Rheumatic fever, 137, 138
Rheumatic mitral stenosis, 138, 143–144, 144f
Rheumatic tricuspid valve disease, 156, 160
Rib notching, 326, 330
Right atrial (RA) pressure
  carcinoid heart disease, 224, 224f, 227
  echocardiographic evaluation, 222, 226
  estimation of, 222–223, 222f, 226
  hepatic vein flow pattern, 222–223, 222f, 226
  IVC diameter measurement, 222, 222f, 226
  pulmonary artery systolic pressure, 224, 224f, 227
Right ventricle
  atrial flutter ablation, 225, 229, 229f
  constrictive physiology, 225, 227–228, 228f

dyssynchrony, 296–297, 297f, 300
echocardiography *vs.* MRI, 224, 227
infarction
  hemodynamical significance, 229, 235
  hypotension, 229, 235
  with inferior wall myocardial infarction, 229, 235
  with myocardial infarction, 211, 216
  nitroglycerin administration, 229, 235
  right-to-left shunt, 229, 235
inflow image, 223, 223f, 226
linear measurements, 225, 227
M-mode, 225, 227–228, 228f
normal grade of diastolic function, 223, 223f, 226–227
RA pressure (*See* Right atrial (RA) pressure)
TAPSE value, 223, 223f, 225–227
thrombus, 535, 541, 542, 542f
tissue Doppler S' wave, 225, 227
tricuspid valve leaflets, 223, 223f, 226
Right ventricular inflow, 551, 563, 563f-564f
Ring-down, reverberation artifacts, 13, 19–21, 56, 58, 58f, 65, 66
Ross procedure, 319, 320, 322, 325
RWT (relative wall thickness), 181, 181t, 186

S

Saddle pulmonary embolus, 107, 107f, 110
Saline contrast injection, 444, 459, 460
SAM. *See* Systolic anterior motion (SAM)
Sarcoidosis, 277, 278, 282–283, 282f, 284–285
  clinical manifestations of, 261, 261f, 264–265
  pericardial effusions, 396, 400
  wall motion abnormalities, 289, 293
Scimitar syndrome, 335, 337
Secundum atrial septal defect, 309, 312–313
Secundum-type defects, 531, 537
17-segment model, 242, 247, 445, 460
Senile calcific aortic stenosis, 501, 501f, 509
Senning repair, 326, 329
Septic emboli, 168–169, 168f, 175–176
Serum ferritin test, 276, 280
Shadowing artifacts, 13, 19, 21
Short-axis real-time MR cine, 535, 535f, 543, 544f

Side-lobe artifacts, 13, 20–21, 21f, 55, 60, 63, 63f
Simpson rule, 179, 183
Single-element ultrasound transducer, 554, 568–569
Sinus node dysfunction, Mustard/Senning repair, 326, 329
Sinus of Valsalva aneurysms, 425, 428
Sinus tachycardia, 349, 349f, 352, 547, 558
Sinus venosus atrial septal defects, 297f–298f, 298, 300, 309, 312
Spade-like systolic pattern, 361, 365
Speckle artifact, 55, 60
Speckle tracking echocardiography, 233–234, 237, 303, 306–307
Speckle tracking radial strain method, 303, 306–307, 306f
Spectral Doppler flow pattern, 552, 565
Spectral Doppler modalities, 29, 35
Specular reflector tissues, 12, 17
Splitability index. *See* Wilkins score
Spongy myocardium, 262, 268
Stanford classification, 8
Staphylococcus aureus bacteremia, 367, 369, 374, 442, 454
Stenotic aortic valve, 550, 550f, 562, 562f
STICH trial, 238
Stitch artifact, 472, 472f, 479
Strain rate imaging (SRI), 241, 245
Streptococcus bovis bacteremia, 367, 374
Streptococcus pneumoniae, 335, 338
Streptococcus viridans bacteremia, 367, 369, 374
Stress echocardiography, 449, 468
   absence of hyperkinesia, 242, 247
   appropriate indication, 548, 559
   coronary angiography, 241, 246
   coronary artery anatomy, 250, 251f, 256–257, 256f–257f
   exercise-induced ischemia, 241, 246
   exertional dyspnea, 250, 255
   hypertensive response to exercise, 249, 254, 254t
   impaired regional myocardial relaxation, 248, 253, 253f
   inappropriate of exercise, 250, 255
   left anterior descending territory ischemia, 248, 253–254
   LV wall motion abnormalities, 241, 246
   multivessel disease with transient ischemic dilation, 248, 253–254
   myocardial infarction/cardiac death probability, 248, 254

reassurance and routine care, 249, 255
   right ventricular wall motion abnormalities, 249, 255
   sensitivity of, 242, 247
   specificity of, 249, 254, 254t
   transaortic and left ventricular outflow tract velocities, 250, 255
Stress test
   exercise capacity and duration, 241, 246
   Kawasaki disease, 240, 245
   LV end-systolic volume, 241, 246
   postexercise LVEF, 241, 246
   postexercise WMSI, 241, 246
Stress-induced cardiomyopathy, 229, 234, 239, 243, 287, 287f, 291
Stroke
   atria masses, 355, 355f, 357
   right atrium, 355, 355f, 357
Subaortic membrane, 203, 206
Subaortic stenosis, 531, 537, 538
Subclavian artery stenosis, 193, 199
Subendocardial myocardial infarctions, 229, 234–235
Superior vena cava (SVC), 86–87, 87f, 91
   coronary sinus, 533, 540, 540f
   TEE, 517, 522
Suprasternal notch acoustic windows, 532–533, 539
Suprasternal notch imaging, aortic valve, 193, 199
Supravalvular aortic stenosis, 342, 346, 348
   aortic stenosis, 193, 198
Supraventricular tachycardia, 349, 349f, 351
S-wave velocity, 557, 557f, 571
Syncope, 546, 558
Syndromes
   acute aortic syndromes (*See* Acute aortic syndromes (AAS))
   acute valvular lesion and acute aortic syndrome, 7–8
   apical ballooning syndrome, 259, 259f, 262
   carcinoid, 557–558, 557f, 572
   congenital syndromes (*See* Congenital syndromes)
   DiGeorge syndrome, 342, 342f, 347
   Down syndrome (*See* Down syndrome (DS))
   Ehlers–Danlos syndrome, 431, 436
   Ellis–van Creveld syndrome, 341, 341f, 344
   hypereosinophilic syndrome, 277, 283, 289–290, 289f, 293

hypoplastic left heart syndrome, 349, 352, 353
   Loeys–Dietz syndrome, 344, 431, 436
   Marfan syndrome, 341, 341f, 344
   Noonan syndrome (*See* Noonan syndrome)
   22q11 deletion syndrome, 343, 346, 347
   Scimitar, 335, 337
   Takotsubo syndrome, 287, 287f, 291
   Turner syndrome, 344, 344f, 346, 348
   velocardiofacial syndrome, 343, 347
   Williams syndrome, 342, 342f, 348
   Wolff–Parkinson–White syndrome, 349, 349f, 351
Systemic venous return, 329, 331
Systemic ventricular failure, 326, 329
Systolic anterior motion (SAM), 546, 558
   causes, 533, 535f, 540, 543f
   color M-mode images, 268, 270f, 274
   hypertrophic cardiomyopathy, 146, 151–152, 152f, 268, 273
   mitral regurgitation, 146, 151–152, 152f, 268, 270, 273, 274
Systolic flow reversal, 534–535, 535f, 543

T

Tachycardia, pericardial effusions, 396–397, 400
Takotsubo syndrome, 287, 287f, 291
TandemHeart, 290, 294
TAPSE (tricuspid annular plane systolic excursion), 192, 192f, 196
TAPVR (total anomalous pulmonary venous return), 336, 339
TAVR (transcatheter aortic valve replacement), 431, 431f, 437
TEE. *See* Transesophageal echocardiography (TEE)
Tei index. *See* Myocardial performance index (MPI)
Tetralogy of Fallot (TOF)
   atrial septal defect, 335, 337
   left SVC, 335, 336
   right ventricular enlargement, 318, 321
Thermal index (TI), 73
Thoracic aorta, 94, 98
   descending, 107–108, 108f, 110
Thrombi valves, 370, 370f, 382
Thrombolysis, 107, 107f, 110
Thrombosis, 505–506, 513
Thrombus
   risk of, 355–357
   transesophageal echocardiography, 169, 169f, 176–177
   waveform velocity, 355, 355f, 357

TID (transient ischemic dilation), 535–536, 535f, 544, 546f

Tissue Doppler imaging (TDI), 486, 488, 490, 490f, 492, 492f, 495
  Eustachian valve, 85, 85f, 89
  medial annulus measurements, 212–213, 212f–213f, 219–220, 219f–220f

Tissue Doppler S' wave, 225, 227

Tissue harmonic imaging, 39, 43, 43f–44f

TOF (Tetralogy of Fallot)
  atrial septal defect, 335, 337
  left SVC, 335, 336
  right ventricular enlargement, 318, 321

Total anomalous pulmonary venous return (TAPVR), 336, 339

Transcatheter aortic valve replacement (TAVR), 431, 431f, 437, 445, 462

Transcatheter atrial septal defect, 299f–300f, 298, 300

Transcranial Doppler (TCD), echo-relevant guidelines, 444, 459

Transducer
  attenuation coefficient, tissue, 39, 40
  axial resolution, 39, 40f
  lateral resolution, 39, 40
  left ventricular apex, 29, 35

Transesophageal color-flow Doppler, 103, 104

Transesophageal echo examination, 552, 565

Transesophageal echocardiography (TEE)
  abscess formation, 170, 177–178
  alcohol septal ablation, 516, 519
  amyl nitrite, 516, 519
  anticoagulation, indication, 518, 522
  aorta, 423, 426
  aortic atheroma, 518, 521
  aortic dissection, 232, 232f, 236
  aortic incompetence, 517, 521
  aortic valve leaflets, 516, 521
  appropriate indication, 548, 559
  asymptomatic, 518, 522
  atrial fibrillation, 356, 356f, 358
  bacterial vegetation, 367, 374–375, 374t, 375f
  bileaflet mechanical valve, 163–164, 164f, 172
  cardioplegia, 517, 521
  carney complex, 516, 521
  central line, 95, 99
  complexity of, 517, 521
  coronary artery disease, 96, 100
  coronary artery involvement, 231, 236

coronary sinus, 518, 522
deep transgastric position, 518, 522
emergent pericardiocentesis, 524–525, 525f, 527
endarterectomy, 518, 521
endocarditis, 167, 167f, 175
guidance, 523, 526
heart block rate of, 516, 519
vs. ICE, 523, 526
infective endocarditis, 517, 521
intraoperative, heating in US system, 13, 19
laminated thrombus, 233, 233f, 237
left atrial appendage structure, 500, 500f, 509–512
left atrial mass, 516, 520–521
left innominate vein, 94, 98
lipomatous hypertrophy, interatrial septum, 57, 65, 65f
meta-analysis stroke, 518, 522
midesophageal view, 423, 423f, 426
mitral valve evaluation, 239–240, 243, 472, 481, 481f
moderate MR, 518, 522
myocardial infarction, 229, 235
myxoma, 517, 521
paravalvular abscess, 7, 8
paravalvular leak closure procedure, 502, 510–511
patent foramen ovale, 8, 9
pectinate muscles *vs.* thrombi, 94, 98
pericardial thickness evaluation, 392, 393
perindopril, 516, 519
periprosthetic aortic valve abscess, 169–170, 170f, 177
phenylephrine, 516, 519
propranolol, 516, 519
protamine, 517, 521
quality, 94, 98
RCT, 516, 519
retrograde cardioplegia, 518, 522
SAM and LVOT obstruction, 516, 519
scallops structure, 500–501, 501f
sensitivity and specificity, 367, 377, 379t
severe mitral regurgitation, 96, 100
severe MR postrepair, 518, 522
Shone syndrome, 517, 520–521
sinus rhythm, 516, 521
SVCs, 518, 522
Swan–Ganz catheter, 518, 522
thrombus, 169, 169f, 176–177
transgastric, RV inflow view, 95, 99
2D measurements, 181, 181t, 186
ventricular apex view, 94, 98–99

Transferrin saturation test, 276, 280
Transient apical ballooning. *See* Stress-induced cardiomyopathy
Transient ischemic dilation (TID), 535–536, 535f, 544, 546f
Transmitral continuous-wave Doppler image, 143f
Transmitral Doppler image
  mitral regurgitation, 138, 142–143, 143f
  mitral stenosis, 138, 142–143, 143f
Transposition of the great arteries (TGA), echo-relevant guidelines, 440, 450
Transseptal puncture procedure, 504, 504f, 512
Transthoracic bubble study, 103, 104
Transthoracic echocardiography (TTE), 440, 450, 551, 563
  AAS, 430, 430f, 431, 431f, 437–438
  alcohol septal ablation, 524, 527
  aortic stenosis, 189, 189f, 196
  apical hypertrophic cardiomyopathy, 531, 536
  2011 AUC, echocardiography, 75–79, 156, 160
  cardiovascular disease, 242, 246
  coronary sinus dilation, 85, 85f, 88–89
  Eustachian valve, 85, 85f, 89
  falciform ligament, 106, 106f, 109
  hematoma, 232, 236
  hiatal hernia, 108, 108f, 111
  left-sided and right-sided intracardiac filling pressures, 290, 294
  mitral regurgitant, 188, 188f, 194
  mitral regurgitation, 146, 149–150, 150f
  mitral stenosis, 138, 142
  muscular VSD, 231, 231f, 236
  noncardiac findings, 106, 109
  Noonan syndrome, 341, 342, 344
  oblique sinus, 9, 108, 108f
  PLSVC, 85, 89
  sensitivity, 7, 7t, 8
  vs. transesophageal echocardiogram accuracy, 7, 7t, 8
  ventricles, masses and tumors, 360, 360f, 364
Transvalvular and central venous flow velocities, 406–407, 406f–407f, 413–414, 413f
Transvenous pacemaker, 296, 296f, 299–300
Trastuzumab, 262, 266
Traumatic injuries, 547, 558
Tricuspid annular plane systolic excursion (TAPSE), 192, 192f, 196

Tricuspid inflow, 398, 401, 402
Tricuspid regurgitation (TR), 290, 294
    atrial and ventricular size, 155, 158
    atrioventricular dyssynchrony, 296–297, 297f, 300
    AUC guidelines, 156, 160
    biopsy-induced, post-cardiac transplant, 157, 157f, 161
    clinical settings, 533–534, 534f, 541, 543f
    Doppler features, 156, 156f, 161
    Ebstein anomaly, 156, 160
    echocardiographic and Doppler parameters, 155, 158, 159t
    etiology, 157, 157f, 161
    flow signal evaluation, 156, 160
    hepatic vein flow, 157, 157f, 161
    interfering with closure of leaflet mechanism, 296–297, 297f, 300
    Nyquist limit, 157, 157f, 161
    pulmonary vascular resistance, 156, 160
    pulsed-wave spectral Doppler display, 157, 157f, 161
    right ventricular dyssynchrony, 296–297, 297f, 300
    right ventricular infarction, 229, 235
    with severe pulmonary hypertension, 535–536, 535f, 544, 544f
    severity evaluation, 155, 158, 159t
    spearing of leaflet, 296–297, 297f, 300
Tricuspid stenosis, 557–558, 557f, 572
    with atrial fibrillation, 156, 160
    carcinoid syndrome, 156, 156f, 160
    causes of, 156, 156f, 160
    Doppler signal, 193, 199
    heart rate measurement, 156, 160
    inflow velocity measurements, 156, 160
    sweep speed measurements, 156, 160
Tricuspid valve, 350, 352, 353, 373, 389
    bacterial endocarditis, 156, 156f, 161
    cyanosis, 155, 155f, 159
    Ebstein anomaly, 156, 156f, 160
    isolated pulmonary carcinoid, 155, 158
    peak inflow gradient, 534, 534f, 541
    redundancy of, 361, 364–365
    valvular involvement, 155, 158
Tricuspid valve inflow, 406, 406f, 412, 412f, 419
Tricuspid valve malformation, 531, 537
Trisomy 21, 319, 323, 341, 342, 345
Troponin
    end-stage renal disease, 242, 246
    test, 239, 243
Truncus arteriosus, 319, 322

Trypanosoma cruzi, 288, 288f, 292
TTE. *See* Transthoracic echocardiography (TTE)
Turbulent color Doppler flow, 107, 110
Turner syndrome, 342, 342f, 345, 349, 349f, 351, 436
    aorta, 424, 424f, 426
    echocardiography, 342, 342f, 345
Type A dissection, 431, 431f, 432, 435, 437

U
UCA (ultrasound contrast agent), 361–362, 365
Uhl anomaly, 319, 322
Ultrasound
    absorption, defined, 11, 16, 16t
    acoustic coupling gels, 12, 17
    acoustic impedance, defined, 11, 16, 16t
    artifact description, 13, 13f–14f, 19–22
    attenuation, defined, 11, 16, 16t
    axial resolution, 55, 62
    backscatter, 47, 53
    beam biologic effects, 72, 73
    beam intensity, AIUM, 72
    characteristics, 11, 15
    disadvantages, 11, 15
    fundamental B-mode image, 46, 49, 49f
    gain, defined, 11, 16, 16t
    gel use, 12, 17
    harmonic B-mode imaging, 46, 49, 49f
    harmonic power Doppler imaging, 46, 50, 50f
    imaging probe comparison, 12, 12f, 17–18
    intensity, defined, 11, 16, 16t
    interaction of, 45, 48
    line density, 13, 19
    mechanical index, 45, 47–48, 48f
    physical principles of
        artifacts, 54–67, 54f–59f, 61f–65f
        2D ultrasound, 11–22, 12f–14f, 20f–22f
        Doppler, 23–28, 23f–27f
        knobology, 29–38, 30f–34f, 36f–37f
        spatial and temporal resolution, 39–44, 39f–44f
    power pulse inversion imaging, 46, 49, 50
    pulse repetition rates, 12, 18
    thermal bioeffects, 72, 74
    vs. tissue interaction, attenuation, 11, 16–17
    velocity of sound, tissue, 11, 15, 15t

Ultrasound contrast agent (UCA), 361–362, 365
Unicuspid aortic valve morphology, 118, 126

V
Valve masses
    bacterial vegetation, 367, 374–375, 374t, 375f
    papillary fibroelastoma, 367, 374, 376
Valvular heart diseases, 486, 494
    echo-relevant guidelines, 441, 452–453
Valvular lesion, acute, 7–8
Vegetations, 370, 370f, 382
    aortic valve, 370, 370f, 380–381
    bioprosthetic aortic valve placement, 372, 372f, 385
    definition of, 367, 374–375, 374t, 375f
    echocardiography, 367, 374, 377, 377t
    transesophageal echocardiography, 367, 374, 377, 377t
Velocardiofacial syndrome (VCFS), 343, 347
Velocity, 552, 564–565
Velocity of sound, 549, 561, 561t
Velocity time integral (VTI), 188
Venous malformations
    left SVC, 335, 336
    LSVC, 335–337
    PAPVR, 335, 336
    polysplenia syndrome, 338
    Scimitar syndrome, 335, 337
    TAPVR, 336, 339
    tetralogy of Fallot, 335, 337
    TGA, 336, 340
Venous thrombosis, 107, 109
Ventricles, masses and tumors of
    CAD, 360, 363
    cardiothoracic surgery consultation, 362–363, 363f, 366
    echo-bright myocardium, 363, 366
    heparin, 360, 363
    nonpathologic finding, 359, 363
    pacemaker/defibrillator, 360, 360f, 364
    right ventricular volume overload, 361, 365
    tricuspid valve, redundancy of, 361, 364–365
    ultrasound contrast agent, 361–362, 365
Ventricular myocardium, 532, 538–539
Ventricular septal defect (VSD), 231, 231f, 236, 534, 534f, 542, 542f
    aortic stenosis, 193, 199

Ventricular septal defect (VSD)
(*Continued*)
    closure procedure, 503, 503f, 510–511
    diagnoses, 311, 311f, 315–316,
        315f–316f
    Down syndrome, 341, 345, 346
    HCM, 516, 518
    leak, 367–368, 378
    muscular VSD, 310, 310f, 314
    myocardial infarction, 229, 235
    unrepaired pulmonary atresia, 319,
        324–325, 325f
    velocity measurement, 310, 310f, 314
    velocity pattern, 501–502, 502f, 510,
        511
Ventriculoarterial concordance, 326, 329
Verrucous endocarditis, 372, 372f, 385

VSD (ventricular septal defect), 231,
    231f, 236
VTI (velocity time integral), 188

W
Wall akinesis, lateral and inferolateral,
    555, 571
Wall motion score index (WMSI), 8, 9,
    230, 235
    semi-quantitative evaluation, 242, 247
    stress test, 241, 246
Wall motion scoring, 2D measures, 181,
    185
Warfarin, 230, 235
Wave interference, speckle artifact,
    55, 60
Wilkins score, 137, 139, 139t

Williams syndrome, 97, 101
    pulmonary artery stenosis, 155,
        159–160
Williams–Beuren/simply Williams syn-
    drome, 349, 349f, 351
WMSI (wall motion score index), 8, 9,
    230, 235
    semi-quantitative evaluation, 242, 247
    stress test, 241, 246
Wolff–Parkinson–White (WPW) syn-
    drome, 349, 349f, 351

Y
Yu index, 302, 305

Z
Z-scores, 240, 244